The Sociology of Health and Illness

10th Edition

The Sociology of Health and Illness

Critical Perspectives

10th Edition

Editors

Peter Conrad
Brandeis University

Valerie Leiter
Simmons College

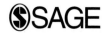

Los Angeles | London | New Delhi
Singapore | Washington DC | Melbourne

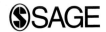

FOR INFORMATION:

SAGE Publications, Inc.
2455 Teller Road
Thousand Oaks, California 91320
E-mail: order@sagepub.com

SAGE Publications Ltd.
1 Oliver's Yard
55 City Road
London, EC1Y 1SP
United Kingdom

SAGE Publications India Pvt. Ltd.
B 1/I 1 Mohan Cooperative Industrial Area
Mathura Road, New Delhi 110 044
India

SAGE Publications Asia-Pacific Pte. Ltd.
3 Church Street
#10-04 Samsung Hub
Singapore 049483

Acquisitions Editor: Jeff Lasser
Editorial Assistant: Tiara Beatty
Production Editor: Jane Haenel
Copy Editor: Diane Wainwright
Typesetter: Hurix Digital
Proofreader: Tricia Curry-Knight
Indexer: Nancy Fulton
Cover Designer: Candice Harman
Marketing Manager: Kara Kindstrom

Printed in the United States of America

Library of Congress Cataloging-in-Publication Data

Names: Conrad, Peter, 1945– editor. | Leiter, Valerie, 1965– editor.

Title: The sociology of health and illness : critical perspectives / [edited by] Peter Conrad, Brandeis University, Valerie Leiter, Simmons College.

Description: Thousand Oaks, California : SAGE, [2019] | Includes bibliographical references and index.

Identifiers: LCCN 2018008053 | ISBN 9781544326245 (pbk. : alk. paper)

Subjects: LCSH: Social medicine.

Classification: LCC RA418 .S6739 2019 | DDC 362.1—dc23

LC record available at https://lccn.loc.gov/2018008053

This book is printed on acid-free paper.

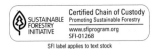

18 19 20 21 22 10 9 8 7 6 5 4 3 2 1

CONTENTS

PART III • CONTEMPORARY CRITICAL DEBATES

PREFACE

In the past five decades, medical sociology has grown from a small subspecialty to a major area of scholarly and student interest. Thirty-five years ago, there were few good teaching resources, and none from a critical perspective. The first edition of *The Sociology of Health and Illness: Critical Perspectives* was published in 1981 and has been revised numerous times, culminating with this tenth edition. From the beginning, there has been a strong commitment to drawing on diverse sources: Articles are primarily by sociologists but also by public health specialists, health activists, feminists, and social critics. Selections must be interesting, readable, and make important sociological and conceptual points about health and health care. For each section, we provide substantive introductions that contextualize the issues at hand and highlight each selection's main points.

There are few areas of society changing as rapidly as the health care system. Health care costs have risen more rapidly than virtually any other part of society, new treatments and technologies continually become available, health insurance politics remain contentious, professional power has declined while corporate power has increased, and pressures remain on the health care system to change in ways that are not always in patients' interest. Although health and medical care do not stand still for our sociological study, it is possible to examine the health care system as it is being transformed.

The tenth edition of this book reflects the continuities and changes in the sociology of health and illness. Only seven articles remain from the original edition; the other 39 were added in subsequent editions as older selections were dropped. In the first edition, issues like environmental disease, HIV/AIDS, sexual dysfunction, rationing, genetics, managed care, and alternative medicine had not yet moved to the fore, but they are all central to this edition.

While we maintain the overall framework that has characterized the book since its inception, changes in health and medicine are reflected in this new edition. For this edition, we have added a new section on global issues, reflecting the growing importance of globalization in health. We have also added new selections on fundamental causes of health inequalities, racism and health, cancer and end-of-life care, health policy, medical technologies, and cesarean sections. Altogether, there are 17 new selections and one updated selection. Throughout the volume, we continue to believe that a critical and conceptual sociological orientation is necessary to understand the problems with our health care system. The book's purpose continues to be to help students better understand issues underlying our health care dilemmas and to promote an informed discussion on the potential changes in health and health care.

ACKNOWLEDGMENTS

As you may notice from the cover, we have a new publisher and are now working with SAGE Publishing on this tenth edition of the volume. We thank Jeff Lasser, our editor at SAGE, for his patient encouragement, and Adeline Wilson, Diane Wainwright, and Tiara Beatty for their assistance with the entire process of producing the volume. We also wish to thank Sarah Berger, our previous editor at Macmillan, for helping with this transition. We are grateful to many colleagues and adopters who were kind enough to share their reactions to previous editions and whose comments helped strengthen this edition. We want to especially acknowledge those adopters who reviewed the previous edition and suggested new additions and revisions. While we couldn't follow all of the suggestions, these comments helped us rethink some sections and selections for the tenth edition. Peter wants to thank Libby Bradshaw, a physician committed to examining the social context of medical care (and also his wife and partner), for more than forty years of dialogue about critical perspectives on health and illness. Val thanks John Gilbert (her spouse) for absorbing discussions about medical devices and methodology, and Wally Gilbert (her father-in-law) for his enthusiastic support. We also thank our editorial assistant, Meagan Wilber, for helping us organize the materials for this edition.

INTRODUCTION

Three major themes underlie the organization of this book: that the conception of medical sociology must be broadened to encompass a sociology of health and illness; that medical care in the United States is presently in crisis; and that the solution of that crisis requires that our health care and medical systems be reexamined from a critical perspective.[1]

TOWARD A SOCIOLOGY OF HEALTH AND ILLNESS

Today, medical sociology is one of the three largest sections of the American Sociological Association (out of more than 30). However, this was not always so. In the 1950s, medical sociology was an esoteric subspecialty taught in a few graduate departments. But in less than two decades it became a central concern of sociologists and sociology students (Bloom 2002), and continues to be today. The causes of this growth are too many and too complex to be within the scope of this book. However, a few of the major factors underlying this development are noted next.

The rise of chronic illness as a central medical and social problem has led physicians, health planners, and public health officials to look to sociology for help in understanding and dealing with this major health concern. In addition, increased government involvement in medical care has created research opportunities and funding for sociologists to study the organization and delivery of medical care. Sociologists have also become increasingly involved in medical education, as evidenced by the large number of sociologists currently on medical school faculties. Furthermore, since the 1960s, the social and political struggles over health and medical care have become major social issues, as evidenced

in most presidential campaigns since, thus drawing additional researchers and students to the field. Indeed, some sociologists have come to see the organization of medicine and the way medical services are delivered as social problems in themselves.

Traditionally, the sociological study of illness and medicine has been called, simply, *medical sociology*. Straus (1957) differentiated between sociology "of" medicine and sociology "in" medicine. Sociology *of* medicine focuses on the study of medicine to illuminate some *sociological issue* (e.g., patient–practitioner relationships, the role of professions in society). Sociology *in* medicine, on the other hand, focuses primarily on *medical concerns* (e.g., the sociological causes of disease and illness, reasons for delay in seeking medical aid, patient compliance or noncompliance with medical regimens). As one might expect, the dichotomy between these two approaches is more distinct conceptually than in actual sociological practice.

A recent overview of the status of medical sociology (Rosich and Hankin 2010) organized key findings of the discipline under two major categories: (1) persistence of health inequalities among social groups and (2) challenges in the contemporary health care system in the United States. The findings reported under each category are as follows.

Persistence of Health Inequalities in the United States

1. Health inequalities are deeply rooted in society.

2. Stressors substantially damage health.

3. Social relationships are linked to health behaviors and outcomes.

4. Race is linked to the very large disparities in health in the United States.

Challenges in the Contemporary Health Care System in the United States

1. Disease and illness are social constructs as well as medical constructs.

2. How the public accesses and uses health care has changed dramatically.

3. The authority of the medical profession has been eroded.

4. Health care is costly and of inconsistent quality.

5. Advances in health and health care technology have transformed health care.

6. Ethical challenges and controversies have emerged with advances in medical science.

7. The challenges of comprehensive health care reform in the United States are complex.

The authors conclude that sociological research is key to reducing disparities and inequities in health, and sociology suggests what is needed to achieve comprehensive health reform (Rosich and Hankin 2010, S7–S8).

Most of the selections in this book reflect one or more of these concerns. In this volume, rather than focusing on physicians and the physician's work, we emphasize a more general concern with how health and illness are dealt with in our society. This broadened conceptualization of the relationship between sociology and medicine encourages us to examine problems such as the social causation of illness, the economic basis of medical services, and the influence of medical industries. It also allows us to direct our primary attention to the social production of disease and illness, as well as the social organization of the medical care system.

Both disease and medical care are related to the structure of society. The social organization of society influences, to a significant degree, the type and distribution of disease (Kawachi et al. 2008). It also shapes the organized response to disease and illness—the

medical care system. To analyze either disease or medical care without investigating its connection with social structure and social interaction is to miss what is unique about the sociology of health and illness. To make the connection between social structure and health, we must investigate how social factors such as the political economy, the corporate structure, the distribution of resources, and the uses of political, economic, and social power influence health and illness, and society's response to health and illness. To make the connection between social interaction and health, we need to examine people's experiences, face-to-face relationships, cultural variations within society, and how society constructs "reality" in general. Social structure and interaction are, of course, interrelated, and making this linkage clear is a central task of sociology. Both health and the medical system should be analyzed as integral parts of society. In short, instead of a "medical sociology," in this book we posit and profess a *sociology of health and illness.*

THE CRISIS IN U.S. HEALTH CARE

It should be noted at the outset that, by any standard, the U.S. medical system and the U.S. medical profession are among the best in the world. Our society invests a great amount of its social and economic resources in medical care; has some of the world's finest physicians, hospitals, and medical schools; is no longer plagued by most deadly infectious diseases that still exist in developing countries (e.g., cholera, dysentery, malaria); and is in the forefront in developing medical and technological advances for the treatment of disease and illness.

However, it must also be noted that U.S. health care is in a state of crisis. At least that is the judgment not of a small group of social and political critics but of concerned social scientists, thoughtful political leaders, leaders of labor and industry, and members of the medical profession itself. But although there is general agreement that a health care crisis exists, there is, as one would expect, considerable disagreement as to what caused this crisis and how to deal with it. For example, some see the latest health reform—the 2010 Patient Protection and Affordable Care Act (ACA)—as a major and essential step toward the solution to some of our health care problems, while others call it "Obamacare" and see it as a "government takeover" of health care, creating a new health care crisis. While we clearly support the current health reform efforts, we also know that they are only a beginning of the needed reform in the United States. The ACA attempts to mediate and even eliminate some aspects of our persistent health care crisis.

What major elements and manifestations of this crisis are reflected in the concerns expressed by the contributors to this volume?

Medical costs have risen exponentially; in five decades, the amount people in the United States spent annually on medical care increased from 4 percent to 17.8 percent of the nation's gross national product. In 2016, the total cost was $3.3 trillion (Centers for Medicare & Medicaid Services 2017a). Medical problems contribute to almost half of all U.S. bankruptcies (Himmelstein et al. 2009).

Access to medical care remains a serious problem. Prior to the ACA, there were over 48 million people without health insurance (National Center for Health Statistics 2016), and perhaps an equal number were underinsured and thus without adequate financial access to health care when they needed it. While the ACA reduced the number of uninsured people substantially—to 24.5 million (National Center for Health Statistics 2017)—disparities in access remain. U.S. health care suffers from "the inverse coverage law": the more people need insurance coverage, the less likely they are to get it (Light 1992; Watt 2002). That is, the poorest and sickest individuals often have less health insurance coverage than those who are wealthier and well.

Increasing specialization of doctors has made *primary care* medicine scarcer. Just one-third of physicians are in primary care with no subspecialty (Bureau of Labor Statistics 2011). In many rural and inner-city areas, the only primary care available is in hospital emergency departments where waits are long, treatment is often impersonal, continuity of care is minimal, and the cost of service delivery is

very high. Nurse practitioners and physician assistants are now filling some of these gaps in primary care, taking the place of primary care physicians.

Although the quality of health and medical care is difficult to measure, a few standard measures are helpful. *Life expectancy,* the number of years a person can be expected to live, is at least a crude measure of a nation's health. According to World Health Organization data (2017), the United States ranks thirty-first overall among nations in life expectancy, at 79.3 years, with life expectancy at birth declining by .1 years in 2015 (Centers for Disease Control 2016), the first decline in twenty years. *Infant mortality,* infant death in the first year, is one of our best indicators of health and medical care, particularly prenatal care. The United States ranked twelfth in 1963, falling to twenty-third in 1990 and twenty-sixth in 2016 (World Bank 2018). It currently falls at the bottom of the Organisation for Economic Co-operation and Development countries, which include countries in Europe, plus Israel, Japan, and Korea (Centers for Disease Control 2014). Large racial disparities persist in the United States. Infant mortality is lowest for Asian or Pacific Islander infants (4.0 per 1,000 live births), compared with 5.0 among White and Latinx infants, 7.9 among American Indian or Alaska Native infants, and 11.1 among Black or African American infants (Centers for Disease Control 2014).

Our medical system is organized to deliver "medical care" (actually, "sick care") rather than "health care." Medical care is that part of the system "which deals with individuals who are sick or who think they may be sick." Health care is that part of the system "which deals with the promotion and protection of health, including environmental protection, the protection of the individual in the workplace, the prevention of accidents, [and] the provision of pure food and water" (Sidel and Sidel 1983, xxi–xxii).

Very few of our resources are invested in "health care"—that is, in *prevention* of disease and illness. Yet with the decrease in infectious disease and the subsequent increase in chronic disease (especially cancer and heart disease), prevention is becoming ever more important to our nation's overall health and would probably prove more cost-effective than "medical care" (healthypeople.gov/2020).

There is little public accountability in medicine. Innovations such as Health Systems Agencies, regional organizations designed to coordinate medical services (now defunct), and Peer Review Organizations, boards mandated to review the quality of (mostly) hospital care, had limited success in their efforts to control the quality and cost of medical care. These efforts at accountability, either through public or government regulations, were abandoned or revised due to opposition or lack of efficacy. (The incredible rise in the number of malpractice suits may be seen as an indication not of increasing poor medical practice but of the fact that such suits are about the only form of medical accountability presently available to the consumer.) Numerous other attempts to control medical costs—in the form of health maintenance organizations, diagnostic-related groups, evidence-based medicine, and "managed care"—have also largely failed. The most significant attempt, managed care, is changing how medicine is delivered. But it has not yet controlled costs, and it is most unlikely to increase public accountability. Most recently, the ACA attempted to create Accountable Care Organizations, groups of providers who organized voluntarily to create coordinated care for patients and would share in any savings that they created for the Medicare program (Centers for Medicare & Medicaid Services 2017b).

Another element of our crisis in health care is the "medicalization" of society. Many, perhaps far too many, of our social problems (e.g., alcoholism, drug addiction, and child abuse) and of life's normal, natural, and generally nonpathological events (e.g., birth, death, and sexuality) have come to be seen as "medical problems." It is by no means clear that such matters constitute appropriate medical problems per se. Indeed, there is evidence that the medicalization of social problems and life's natural events has itself become a social problem (Zola 1972; Conrad 2007).

Many other important elements and manifestations of our current health care situation are described in the works contained in this volume, including the uneven distribution of disease and health care, the role of the physical environment in disease and illness, the monopolistic history of the medical profession, the role of government in financing health care, inequalities in medical care, the growth of the pharmaceutical industry, the role of the Internet, and global issues in health. The particularities of the U.S. health crisis aside, most contributions to this volume reflect the growing conviction that the social organization of medicine in the United States has been central to perpetuating that crisis.

CRITICAL PERSPECTIVES ON HEALTH AND ILLNESS

The third major theme of this book is the need to examine the relationship between our society's organizations and institutions and its medical care system from a "critical perspective." What do we mean by a critical perspective?

A critical perspective is one that does not consider the present fundamental organization of medicine as sacred and inviolable. Nor does it assume that some other particular organization would necessarily be a panacea for all our health care problems. A critical perspective accepts no "truth" or "fact" merely because it has hitherto been accepted as such. It examines what is, not as something given or static, but as something out of which change and growth can emerge. In contrast, any theoretical framework that claims to have all the answers to understanding health and illness is not a critical perspective. The social aspects of health and illness are too complex for a monolithic approach.

Furthermore, a critical perspective assumes that a sociology of health and illness entails societal and personal values, and that these values must be considered and made explicit if illness and health care problems are to be dealt with satisfactorily. Since any critical perspective is informed by values and assumptions, we would like to make ours explicit: (1) The problems and inequalities of health and medical care are connected to the particular historically located social arrangements and the cultural values of any society. (2) Health care should be oriented toward the prevention of disease and illness. (3) The priorities of any medical system should be based on the needs of the consumers and not the providers. A direct corollary of this is that the socially based inequalities of health and medical care must be eliminated. (4) Ultimately, society itself must change for health and medical care to improve.

Although economic concerns have dominated the health policy debate since the 1980s, the development of critical perspectives on health and illness are central to the reform of health care in the twenty-first century (Mechanic and McAlpine 2010). In 2010, President Obama did what seemed impossible 10 years ago: he succeeded in getting the ACA passed through Congress and signed it into law. Yet the future of that law is very uncertain as the current Congress and administration attempt to dismantle it.

Bringing such critical perspectives to bear on the sociology of health and illness has thus informed the selection of readings contained in this volume. It has also informed the editorial comments that introduce and bind together the book's various parts and subparts. Explicitly and implicitly, the goal of this work is to generate awareness that informed social change is a prerequisite for the elimination of socially based inequalities in health and medical care.

Note

1. Inasmuch as we define the sociology of health and illness in such a broad manner, it is not possible to cover adequately all the topics it encompasses in one volume. Although we attempt to touch on the most important sociological aspects of health and illness, space limitations preclude presenting all potential topics. For instance, we do not include sections on professional socialization, the social organization of hospitals, and the use of health care services. Discussions of these are easily available in standard medical sociology textbooks. We have made a specific decision not to include material on mental health and illness. Although mental and physical health are not as separate as was once thought, the sociology of mental health comprises a separate literature and raises some different issues from the ones developed here.

References

Bloom, Samuel W. 2002. *The Word as Scalpel*. New York: Oxford University Press.

Bureau of Labor Statistics, U.S. Department of Labor. 2011. *Occupational Outlook Handbook, 2010–11 Edition: Physicians and Surgeons*. Accessed July 25, 2011. http://www.bls.gov/oco/ocos074.htm#emply.

Centers for Disease Control. 2014. *International Comparisons of Infant Mortality and Related Factors: United States and Europe, 2010*. Accessed January 15, 2018. https://www.cdc.gov/nchs/data/nvsr/nvsr63/nvsr63_05.pdf.

Centers for Disease Control. 2016. *Health, United States, 2016*. Accessed January 15, 2018. https://www.cdc.gov/nchs/data/hus/hus16.pdf#015.

Centers for Medicare & Medicaid Services. 2017a. *National Health Expenditures 2015*

Highlights. Accessed November 10, 2017. https://www.cms.gov/Research-Statistics-Data-and-Systems/Statistics-Trends-and-Reports/NationalHealthExpendData/downloads/highlights.pdf.

Centers for Medicare & Medicaid Services. 2017b. *Accountable Care Organizations (ACO).* Accessed January 15, 2018. https://www.cms.gov/Medicare/Medicare-Fee-for-Service-Payment/ACO/.

Conrad, Peter. 2007. *The Medicalization of Society: On the Transformation of Human Conditions Into Treatable Disorders.* Baltimore: Johns Hopkins University Press.

Himmelstein, David U., Deborah Thorne, Elizabeth Warren, and Steffie Woolhandler. 2009. "Medical Bankruptcy in the United States, 2007: Results of a National Study." *American Journal of Medicine* 122: 741–46.

Kawachi, Ichiro, S.V. Subramian, and D. Kim. 2008. *Social Capital and Health.* New York: Springer.

Light, Donald W. 1992. "The Practice and Ethics of Risk-Rated Health Insurance." *Journal of the American Medical Association* 267: 2503–08.

Mechanic, David, and Donna D. McAlpine. 2010. "Sociology of Health Care Reform: Building on Research and Analysis to Improve Health Care." *Journal of Health and Social Behavior* 51 (extra issue): S147–59.

National Center for Health Statistics. 2016. *Health Insurance Coverage: Early Release of the Estimates From the National Health Interview Survey, January–June 2016.* Accessed March 2, 2018. https://www.cdc.gov/nchs/data/nhis/earlyrelease/insur201611.pdf.

National Center for Health Statistics. 2017. *Early Release of Selected Estimates Based on Data From the 2016 National Health Interview Survey.* Accessed November 10, 2017. https://www.cdc.gov/nchs/data/nhis/earlyrelease/earlyrelease201705.pdf.

Rosich, Katherine J., and Janet R. Hankin. 2010. "Executive Summary: What Do We Know? Key Findings From 50 Years of Medical Sociology." *Journal of Health and Social Behavior* 51 (extra issue): S1–29.

Sidel, Victor W., and Ruth Sidel. 1983. *A Healthy State,* rev. ed. New York: Pantheon Books.

Straus, Robert. 1957. "The Nature and Status of Medical Sociology." *American Sociological Review* 22 (April): 200–204.

Watt, G. 2002. "The Inverse Care Law Today." *The Lancet* 360: 252–54.

World Bank. 2018. *Mortality Rate, Infant (per 1,000 Live Births).* Accessed March 2, 2018. https://data.worldbank.org/indicator/SP.DYN.IMRT.IN?order.

World Health Organization. 2017. *Life Expectancy at Birth: 2000–2015.* Accessed January 15, 2018. http://gamapserver.who.int/gho/interactive_charts/mbd/life_expectancy/atlas.html.

Zola, Irving Kenneth. 1972. "Medicine as an Institution of Social Control." *Sociological Review* 20: 487–504.

THE SOCIAL PRODUCTION OF DISEASE AND MEANINGS OF ILLNESS

Part I of this book is divided into five sections. While the overriding theme is "the social production of disease and meanings of illness," each section develops a particular aspect of the sociology of disease production. For the purposes of this book, we define *disease* as the bio-physiological phenomena that manifest themselves as changes in and malfunctions of the human body. *Illness,* on the other hand, is the experience of being sick or diseased. Accordingly, we can see disease as a physiological state and illness as a social psychological state presumably caused by the disease. Thus, pathologists and public health doctors deal with disease, patients experience illness, and, ideally, clinical physicians treat both. Furthermore, such a distinction is useful for dealing with the possibility of people feeling ill in the absence of disease, or being "diseased" without experiencing illness. Obviously, disease and illness are related, but separating them as concepts allows us to explore the objective level of disease and the subjective level of illness. The first three sections of Part I focus primarily on disease; the last two focus on illness.

All the selections in Part I consider how disease and illness are socially produced. The so-called *medical model* focuses on organic pathology in individual patients, rarely taking societal factors into account. In the face of increased concern about chronic disease and its prevention, the selections suggest that a shift in focus from the internal environment of individuals to the interaction between external environments in which people live and the internal environment of the human body will yield new insights into disease causation and prevention. Clinical medicine locates disease as a problem in the individual body, but although this is clearly important and useful, it provides an incomplete and sometimes distorted picture. A *social model* of health must complement that clinical perspective if we are to reduce health disparities.

THE SOCIAL NATURE OF DISEASE

When we look historically at the extent and patterns of disease in Western society, we see enormous changes. In the early nineteenth century, the infant mortality rate was very high, life expectancy was short (approximately 40 years), and life-threatening epidemics were common. Infectious diseases, especially those of childhood, were often fatal. Even at the beginning of the twentieth century the U.S. annual death rate was 28 per 1,000 population, compared with 8 per 1,000 today, and the cause of death was usually pneumonia, influenza, tuberculosis, typhoid fever, or one of the various forms of dysentery (Miniño et al. 2007). But patterns of *morbidity* (disease rate) and *mortality* (death rate) have changed. Today we have "conquered" most infectious diseases; they are no longer feared, and few people die from them. Chronic diseases such as heart disease, cancer, and stroke are now the major causes of death in the United States (see Figure 1.3 in Chapter 1).

Medicine usually receives credit for the great victory over infectious diseases. After all, certain scientific discoveries (e.g., germ theory) and medical interventions (e.g., vaccinations and drugs) developed and used to combat infectious diseases must have been responsible for reducing deaths from those diseases, or so the logic goes. While this view may seem reasonable from a not too careful reading of medical history, it is contradicted by some important social scientific work.

René Dubos (1959) was one of the first to argue that social changes in the environment rather than medical interventions led to the reduction of mortality by infectious diseases. He viewed the nineteenth-century sanitary movement's campaign for clean water, air, and proper sewage disposal as a particularly significant public health measure. Thomas McKeown (1971) showed that biomedical interventions were not the cause of the decline in mortality in England and Wales in the nineteenth century. This viewpoint, or the "limitations of modern medicine" argument (Powles 1973), is now well known in public health circles. The argument is essentially a simple one: discoveries and interventions by *clinical medicine* were not the cause of the decline of mortality for various populations. Rather, it seems that social and environmental factors such as sanitation, improved housing and nutrition, and a general rise in the standard of living were the most significant contributors. This does not mean that clinical medicine did not reduce some people's suffering or prevent or cure diseases in others; we know it did. But social factors appear much more important than medical interventions in the conquest of infectious disease. There are current concerns that life expectancies in the United States may begin to decline in the future as a result of higher rates of obesity (Olshansky et al. 2005).

In the keynote selection in this book, John B. McKinlay and Sonja M. McKinlay assess "Medical Measures and the Decline of Mortality." They offer empirical evidence to support the limitations of medicine argument and point to the social nature of disease. We must note that mortality rates, the data on which they base their analysis, only crudely measure "cure" and don't measure "care" at all. But it is important to understand that much of what is attributed to "medical intervention" seems not to be the result of clinical medicine per se (cf. Levine, Feldman, and Elinson 1983). The limitations of medicine argument underlines the need for a broader, more comprehensive perspective on understanding disease and its treatment (see also Tesh 1988), a perspective that focuses on the significance of social structure and change in disease causation and prevention. (See also Link and Phelan 2002.) The second chapter in this section, "Social Conditions as Fundamental Causes of Health Inequalities: Theory, Evidence, and Practice" by Jo C. Phelan, Bruce G. Link, and Parisa Tehranifar, explains why the strong connection between socioeconomic status (SES) and mortality has persisted. They examine the range of resources that accompany SES and protect health, such as wealth, income, status, and power. While they acknowledge the role of medicine, they stress the need for policies that weaken the link between socioeconomic resources and health.

References

Dubos, René. 1959. *Mirage of Health.* New York: Harper & Row.

Levine, Sol, Jacob J. Feldman, and Jack Elinson. 1983. "Does Medical Care Do Any Good?" In *Handbook of Health, Health Care, and the Health Professions*, edited by David Mechanic, 394–404. New York: Free Press.

Link, Bruce, and J. Phelan. 2002. "McKeown and the Idea That Social Conditions Are Fundamental Causes of Disease." *American Journal of Public Health* 92: 730–32.

McKeown, Thomas. 1971. "A Historical Appraisal of the Medical Task." In *Medical History and Medical Care: A Symposium of Perspectives*, edited by G. McLachlan and T. McKeown, 29–55. New York: Oxford University Press.

Miniño, Arialdi M., Melonie P. Heron, Sherry L. Murphy, and Kenneth D. Kochanek. 2007.

"Deaths: Final Data for 2004." *National Vital Statistics Reports.* Accessed February 18, 2008. http://www.cdc.nchs/data/nvsr/nvsr55/nvsr55_19/pdf.

Olshansky, S. Jay, Douglas J. Passaro, Ronald C. Hershow, Jennifer Layden, Bruce A. Carnes, Jacob Brody, Leonard Hayflick, Robert N. Butler, David B. Allison, and David S. Ludwig. 2005. "A Potential Decline in Life Expectancy in the United States in the 21st Century." *New England Journal of Medicine* 352: 1138–45.

Powles, John. 1973. "On the Limitations of Modern Medicine." *Science, Medicine and Man* 1: 1–30.

Tesh, Sylvia Noble. 1988. *Hidden Arguments: Political Ideology and Disease Prevention.* New Brunswick, NJ: Rutgers University Press.

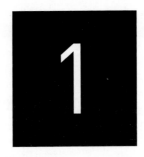

MEDICAL MEASURES AND THE DECLINE OF MORTALITY

John B. McKinlay and Sonja M. McKinlay

By the time laboratory medicine came effectively into the picture the job had been carried far toward completion by the humanitarians and social reformers of the nineteenth century. Their doctrine that nature is holy and healthful was scientifically naive but proved highly effective in dealing with the most important health problems of their age. When the tide is receding from the beach it is easy to have the illusion that one can empty the ocean by removing water with a pail.

—R. Dubos, *Mirage of Health* (New York: Perennial Library, 1959), p. 23

INTRODUCING A MEDICAL HERESY

The modern "heresy" that medical care (as it is traditionally conceived) is generally unrelated to improvements in the health of populations (as distinct from individuals) is still dismissed as unthinkable in much the same way as the so-called heresies of former times. And this is despite a long history of support in popular and scientific writings as well as from able minds in a variety of disciplines. History is replete

This article originally appeared in *Milbank Memorial Fund Quarterly/Health and Sociology* under the title "The Questionable Contribution of Medical Measures to the Decline of Mortality in the United States in the Twentieth Century," John B. McKinlay and Sonja M. McKinlay, Summer 1977, pp. 405–428. Reprinted by permission of John Wiley & Sons.

This paper reports part of a larger research project supported by a grant from the Milbank Memorial Fund (to Boston University) and the Carnegie Foundation (to the Radcliffe Institute). The authors would like to thank John Stoeckle, M.D. (Massachusetts General Hospital) and Louis Weinstein, M.D. (Peter Bent Brigham Hospital) for helpful discussions during earlier stages of the research.

with examples of how, understandably enough, self-interested individuals and groups denounced popular customs and beliefs which appeared to threaten their own domains of practice, thereby rendering them heresies (for example, physicians' denunciation of midwives as witches, during the Middle Ages). We also know that vast institutional resources have often been deployed to neutralize challenges to the assumptions upon which everyday organizational activities were founded and legitimated (for example, the Spanish Inquisition). And since it is usually difficult for organizations themselves to directly combat threatening "heresies," we often find otherwise credible practitioners, perhaps unwittingly, serving the interests of organizations in this capacity. These historical responses may find a modern parallel in the way everyday practitioners of medicine, on their own altruistic or "scientific" grounds and still perhaps unwittingly, serve present-day institutions (hospital complexes, university medical centers, pharmaceutical houses, and insurance companies) by spearheading an assault on a most fundamental challenging heresy of our time: *that the introduction of specific medical measures and/or the expansion of medical services are generally not responsible for most of the modern decline in mortality.*

In different historical epochs and cultures, there appear to be characteristic ways of explaining the arrival and departure of natural vicissitudes. For salvation from some plague, it may be that the gods were appeased, good works rewarded, or some imbalance in nature corrected. And there always seems to be some person or group (witch doctors, priests, medicine men) able to persuade others, sometimes on the basis of acceptable evidence for most people at that time, that they have *the* explanation for the phenomenon in question and may even claim responsibility for it. They also seem to benefit most from common acceptance of the explanations they offer. It is not uncommon today for biotechnological knowledge and specific medical interventions to be invoked as *the major reason* for most of the modern (twentieth century) decline in mortality.[1] Responsibility for this decline is often claimed by, or ascribed to, the present-day major beneficiaries of this prevailing explanation. But both in terms of the history of knowledge and on the basis of data

presented in this paper, one can reasonably wonder whether the supposedly more sophisticated explanations proffered in our own time (while seemingly distinguishable from those accepted in the past) are really all that different from those of other cultures and earlier times, or any more reliable. Is medicine, the physician, or the medical profession any more entitled to claim responsibility for the decline in mortality that obviously has occurred in this century than, say, some folk hero or aristocracy of priests sometime in the past?

AIMS

Our general intention in this paper is to sustain the ongoing debate on the questionable contribution of specific medical measures and/or the expansion of medical services to the observable decline in mortality in the twentieth century. More specifically, the following three tasks are addressed: (a) selected studies are reviewed which illustrate that, far from being idiosyncratic and/or heretical, the issue addressed in this paper has a long history, is the subject of considerable attention elsewhere, attracts able minds from a variety of disciplines, and remains a timely issue for concern and research; (b) age- and sex-adjusted mortality rates (standardized to the population of 1900) for the United States, 1900–1973, are presented and then considered in relation to a number of specific and supposedly effective medical interventions (both chemotherapeutic and prophylactic). So far as we know, this is the first time such data have been employed for this particular purpose in the United States, although reference will be made to a similar study for England and Wales; and (c) some policy implications are outlined.

BACKGROUND TO THE ISSUE

The beginning of the serious debate on the questionable contribution of medical measures is commonly associated with the appearance, in Britain, of Talbot Griffith's (1967) *Population Problems in the Age of Malthus.* After examining certain medical activities associated with the eighteenth century—particularly the growth of hospital, dispensary, and midwifery services, additions to knowledge of physiology and anatomy, and the introduction of smallpox inoculation—Griffith concluded that they made important contributions to the observable decline in mortality at that time. Since then, in Britain and more recently in the United States, this debate has continued, regularly engaging scholars from economic history, demography, epidemiology, statistics, and other disciplines. Habakkuk (1953), an economic historian, was probably the first to seriously challenge the prevailing view that the modern increase in population was due to a fall in the death rate attributable to medical interventions. His view was that this rise in population resulted from an increase in the birth rate, which, in turn, was associated with social, economic, and industrial changes in the eighteenth century.

McKeown, without doubt, has pursued the argument more consistently and with greater effect than any other researcher, and the reader is referred to his recent work for more detailed background information. Employing the data and techniques of historical demography, McKeown (a physician by training) has provided a detailed and convincing analysis of the major reasons for the decline of mortality in England and Wales during the eighteenth, nineteenth, and twentieth centuries (McKeown et al., 1955, 1962, 1975). For the eighteenth century, he concludes that the decline was largely attributable to improvements in the environment. His findings for the nineteenth century are summarized as follows:

> [T]he decline of mortality in the second half of the nineteenth century was due wholly to a reduction of deaths from infectious diseases; there was no evidence of a decline in other causes of death. Examination of the diseases which contributed to the decline suggested that the main influences were: (a) rising standards of living, of which the most significant feature was a better diet; (b) improvements in hygiene; and (c) a favorable trend in the relationship between some micro-organisms

and the human host. *Therapy made no contributions, and the effect of immunization was restricted to smallpox which accounted for only about one-twentieth of the reduction of the death rate.* (Emphasis added, McKeown et al., 1975, p. 391)

While McKeown's interpretation is based on the experience of England and Wales, he has examined its credibility in the light of the very different circumstances which existed in four other European countries: Sweden, France, Ireland, and Hungary (McKeown et al., 1972). His interpretation appears to withstand this cross-examination. As for the twentieth century (1901–1971 is the period actually considered), McKeown argues that about three-quarters of the decline was associated with control of infectious diseases and the remainder with conditions not attributable to microorganisms. He distinguishes the infections according to their modes of transmission (air-, water- or food-borne) and isolates three types of influences which figure during the period considered: medical measures (specific therapies and immunization), reduced exposure to infection, and improved nutrition. His conclusion is that:

> The main influences on the decline in mortality were improved nutrition on airborne infections, reduced exposure (from better hygiene) on water- and food-borne diseases and, less certainly, immunization and therapy on the large number of conditions included in the miscellaneous group. Since these three classes were responsible respectively for nearly half, one-sixth, and one-tenth of the fall in the death rate, it is probable that the advancement in nutrition was the major influence. (McKeown et al., 1975, p. 422)

More than twenty years of research by McKeown and his colleagues recently culminated in two books—*The Modern Rise of Population* (1976a) and *The Role of Medicine: Dream, Mirage or Nemesis* (1976b)—in which he draws together his many excellent contributions. That the thesis he advances remains highly newsworthy is evidenced by recent editorial reaction in *The Times* of London (1977).

No one in the United States has pursued this thesis with the rigor and consistency which characterize the work by McKeown and his colleagues in Britain. Around 1930, there were several limited discussions of the questionable effect of medical measures on selected infectious diseases like diphtheria (Lee, 1931; Wilson & Miles, 1946; Bolduan, 1930) and pneumonia (Pfizer and Co., 1953). In a presidential address to the American Association of Immunologists in 1954 (frequently referred to by McKeown), Magill (1955) marshalled an assortment of data then available—some from England and Wales— to cast doubt on the plausibility of existing accounts of the decline in mortality for several conditions. Probably the most influential work in the United States is that of Dubos who, principally in *Mirage of Health* (1959), *Man Adapting* (1965), and *Man, Medicine and Environment* (1968), focused on the nonmedical reasons for changes in the health of overall populations. In another presidential address, this time to the Infectious Diseases Society of America, Kass (1971), again employing data from England and Wales, argued that most of the decline in mortality for most infectious conditions occurred prior to the discovery of either "the cause" of the disease or some purported "treatment" for it. Before the same society and largely on the basis of clinical experience with infectious diseases and data from a single state (Massachusetts), Weinstein (1974), while conceding there are some effective treatments which seem to yield a favorable outcome (e.g., for poliomyelitis, tuberculosis, and possibly smallpox), argued that despite the presence of supposedly effective treatments some conditions may have increased (e.g., subacute bacterial endocarditis, streptococcal pharyngitis, pneumococcal pneumonia, gonorrhea, and syphilis) and also that mortality for yet other conditions shows improvement in the absence of any treatment (e.g., chickenpox). With the appearance of his book, *Who Shall Live?* (1974), Fuchs, a health economist, contributed to the resurgence of interest in the relative contribution of medical care to the modern decline in mortality in the United States. He believes there has been an unprecedented improvement in health in the United States since about the middle of the eighteenth century, associated primarily with a rise in real income. While agreeing with much of Fuchs' thesis, we will present evidence which seriously questions his belief that "beginning in the mid '30s, major therapeutic discoveries made significant contributions independently of the rise in real income."

Although neither representative nor exhaustive, this brief and selective background should serve to introduce the analysis which follows. Our intention is to highlight the following: (a) the debate over the questionable contribution of medical measures to the modern decline of mortality has a long history and remains topical; (b) although sometimes popularly associated with dilettantes such as Ivan Illich (1976), the debate continues to preoccupy able scholars from a variety of disciplines and remains a matter of concern to the most learned societies; (c) although of emerging interest in the United States, the issue is already a matter of concern and considerable research elsewhere; (d) to the extent that the subject has been pursued in the United States, there has been a restrictive tendency to focus on a few selected diseases, or to employ only statewide data, or to apply evidence from England and Wales directly to the United States situation.

HOW RELIABLE ARE MORTALITY STATISTICS?

We have argued elsewhere that mortality statistics are inadequate and can be misleading as indicators of a nation's overall health status (McKinlay and McKinlay). Unfortunately, these are the only types of data which are readily accessible for the examination of time trends, simply because comparable morbidity and disability data have not been available. Apart from this overriding problem, several additional caveats in the use of mortality statistics are: (a) difficulties introduced by changes in the registration area in the United States in the early twentieth century; (b) that often no single disease, but a complex of conditions, may be responsible for death (Krueger, 1966); (c) that studies reveal considerable inaccuracies in recording the cause of death (Moriyama et al., 1958); (d) that there are changes over time in what it is fashionable to diagnose (for example, ischaemic heart disease and cerebrovascular disease); (e) that changes in disease classifications (Dunn and Shackley, 1945) make it difficult to compare some conditions over time and between countries (Reid and Rose, 1964); (f) that some conditions result in immediate death while others have an extended period of latency; and (g) that many conditions are severely debilitating and consume vast medical resources but are now generally nonfatal (e.g., arthritis and diabetes). Other obvious limitations could be added to this list.

However, it would be foolhardy indeed to dismiss all studies based on mortality measures simply because they are possibly beset *with known limitations*. Such data are preferable to those the limitations of which are either unknown or, if known, cannot be estimated. Because of an over-awareness of potential inaccuracies, there is a timorous tendency to disregard or devalue studies based on mortality evidence, even though there are innumerable examples of their fruitful use as a basis for planning and informed social action (Alderson, 1976). Sir Austin Bradford Hill (1955) considers one of the most important features of Snow's work on cholera to be his adept use of mortality statistics. A more recent notable example is the study by Inman and Adelstein (1969) of the circumstantial link between the excessive absorption of bronchodilators from pressurized aerosols and the epidemic rise in asthma mortality in children aged ten to fourteen years. Moreover, there is evidence that some of the known inaccuracies of mortality data tend to cancel each other out.[2] Consequently, while mortality statistics may be unreliable for use in individual cases, when pooled for a country and employed in population studies, they can reveal important trends and generate fruitful hypotheses. They have already resulted in informed social action (for example, the use of geographical distributions of mortality in the field of environmental pollution).

Whatever limitations and risks may be associated with the use of mortality statistics, they obviously apply equally to all studies which employ them—both those which attribute the decline in mortality to medical measures and those which argue the converse, or something else entirely. And, if such data constitute acceptable evidence in support of the presence of medicine, then it is not unreasonable, or illogical, to employ them in support of some opposing position. One difficulty is that, depending on the nature of the results, double standards of rigor seem to operate in the evaluation of different studies. Not surprisingly, those which challenge prevailing myths or beliefs are subject to the most stringent methodological and statistical scrutiny, while supportive studies, which frequently employ the flimsiest impressionistic data and inappropriate techniques of analysis, receive general and uncritical acceptance. Even if all possible "ideal" data were available (which they never will be) and if, after appropriate analysis, they happened to support the viewpoint of this paper, we are doubtful that medicine's protagonists would find our thesis any more acceptable.

THE MODERN DECLINE IN MORTALITY

Despite the fact that mortality rates for certain conditions, for selected age and sex categories, continue to fluctuate, or even increase (U.S. Dept. HEW, 1964; Moriyama and Gustavus, 1972; Lilienfeld, 1976), there can be little doubt that a marked decline in overall mortality for the United States has occurred since about 1900 (the earliest point for which reliable national data are available).

Just how dramatic this decline has been in the United States is illustrated in Fig. 1.1 which shows age-adjusted mortality rates for males and females separately.[3] Both sexes experienced a marked decline in mortality since 1900. The female decline began to level off by about 1950, while 1960 witnessed the beginning of a slight increase for males. Figure 1.1 also reveals a slight but increasing divergence between male and female mortality since about 1920.

Figure 1.2 depicts the decline in the overall age- and sex-adjusted rate since the beginning of this century. Between 1900 and 1973, there was a 69.2 percent decrease in overall mortality. The average annual rate of decline from 1900 until 1950 was .22

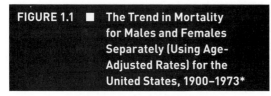

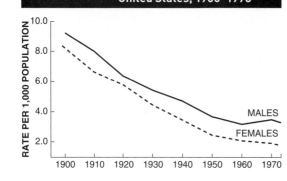

FIGURE 1.1 ■ The Trend in Mortality for Males and Females Separately (Using Age-Adjusted Rates) for the United States, 1900–1973*

*For these and all other age- and sex-adjusted rates in this paper, the standard population is that of 1900.

per 1,000, after which it became an almost negligible decline of .04 per 1,000 annually. Of the total fall in the standardized death rate between 1900 and 1973, 92.3 percent occurred prior to 1950. Figure 1.2 also plots the decline in the standardized death rate *after* the total number of deaths in each age and sex category has been reduced by the number of deaths attributed to the eleven major infectious conditions (typhoid, smallpox, scarlet fever, measles, whooping cough, diphtheria, influenza, tuberculosis, pneumonia, diseases of the digestive system, and poliomyelitis). It should be noted that, although this latter rate also shows a decline (at least until 1960), its slope is much more shallow than that for the overall standardized death rate. A major part of the decline in deaths from these causes since about 1900 may be attributed to the virtual disappearance of these infectious diseases.

An absurdity is reflected in the third broken line in Fig. 1.2 which also plots the increase in the proportion of Gross National Product expended annually for medical care. *It is evident that the beginning of the precipitate and still unrestrained rise in medical care expenditures began when nearly all (92 percent) of the modern decline in mortality this century had already occurred.*[4]

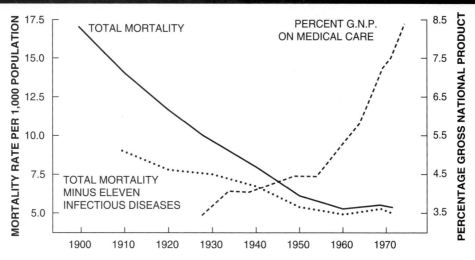

FIGURE 1.2 ■ Age- and Sex-Adjusted Mortality Rates for the United States, 1900–1973, Including and Excluding Eleven Major Infectious Diseases, Contrasted with the Proportion of the Gross National Product Expended on Medical Care

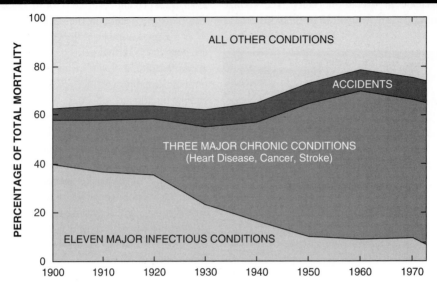

FIGURE 1.3 ■ **Pictorial Representation of the Changing Contribution of Chronic and Infectious Conditions to Total Mortality (Age- and Sex-Adjusted) in the United States, 1900–1973**

Figure 1.3 illustrates how the proportion of deaths contributed by the infectious and chronic conditions has changed in the United States since the beginning of the twentieth century. In 1900, about 40 percent of all deaths were accounted for by eleven major infectious diseases, 16 percent by three chronic conditions 4 percent by accidents, and the remainder (37 percent) by all other causes. By 1973, only 6 percent of all deaths were due to these eleven infectious diseases, 58 percent to the same three chronic conditions, 9 percent to accidents, and 27 percent were contributed by other causes.[5]

Now to what phenomenon, or combination of events, can we attribute this modern decline in overall mortality? Who (if anyone), or what group, can claim to have been instrumental in effecting this reduction? Can anything be gleaned from an analysis of mortality experience to date that will inform health care policy for the future?

It should be reiterated that a major concern of this paper is to determine the effect, if any, of specific medical measures (both chemotherapeutic and prophylactic) on the decline of mortality. It is clear from Figs. 1.2 and 1.3 that most of the observable decline is due to the rapid disappearance of some of the major infectious diseases. Since this is where most of the decline has occurred, it is logical to focus a study of the effect of medical measures on this category of conditions. Moreover, for these eleven conditions, there exist clearly identifiable medical interventions to which the decline in mortality has been popularly ascribed. No analogous interventions exist for the major chronic diseases such as heart disease, cancer, and stroke. Therefore, even where a decline in mortality from these chronic conditions may have occurred, this cannot be ascribed to any specific measure.

THE EFFECT OF MEDICAL MEASURES ON TEN INFECTIOUS DISEASES WHICH HAVE DECLINED

Table 1.1 summarizes data on the effect of major medical interventions (both chemotherapeutic and prophylactic) on the decline in the age- and sex-adjusted death rates in the United States, 1900–1973, for ten of the eleven major infectious diseases listed previously. Together, these diseases accounted for approximately 30 percent of all deaths at the turn of the century and nearly 40 percent of the total decline in the mortality rate since then. The ten diseases were selected on the following criteria: (a) some decline in the death rate had occurred in the period 1900–1973; (b) significant decline in the death rate is commonly attributed to some specific medical measure for the disease; and (c) adequate data for the disease over the period 1900–1973 are available. The diseases of the digestive system were omitted primarily because of lack of clarity in diagnosis of specific diseases such as gastritis and enteritis.

Some additional points of explanation should be noted in relation to Table 1.1. First, the year of medical intervention coincides (as nearly as can be determined) with the first year of widespread or commercial use of the appropriate drug or vaccine.[6] This date does *not* necessarily coincide with the date the measure was either first discovered, or subject to clinical trial. Second, the decline in the death rate for smallpox was calculated using the death rate for 1902 as being the earliest year for which this statistic is readily available (U.S. Bureau of the Census, 1906). For the same reasons, the decline in the death rate from poliomyelitis was calculated from 1910. Third, the table shows the contribution of the decline in each disease to the total decline in mortality over the period 1900–1973 (column b). The overall decline during this period was 12.14 per 1,000 population (17.54 in 1900 to 5.39 in 1973). Fourth, in order to place the experience for each disease in some perspective, Table 1.1 also shows the contribution of the relative fall in mortality after the intervention to the overall fall in mortality since 1900 (column e). In other words, the figures in this last column represent the percentage of the total fall in mortality contributed by each disease after the date of medical intervention.

It is clear from column b that only reductions in mortality from tuberculosis and pneumonia contributed substantially to the decline in total mortality between 1900 and 1973 (16.5 and 11.7

percent, respectively). The remaining eight conditions *together* accounted for less than 12 percent of the total decline over this period. Disregarding smallpox (for which the only effective measure had been introduced about 1800), only influenza, whooping cough, and poliomyelitis show what could be considered substantial declines of 25 percent or more after the date of medical intervention. However, even under the somewhat unrealistic assumption of a constant (linear) rate of decline in the mortality rates, only whooping cough and poliomyelitis even approach the percentage which would have been expected. The remaining six conditions (tuberculosis, scarlet fever, pneumonia, diphtheria, measles, and typhoid) showed negligible declines in their mortality rates subsequent to the date of medical intervention. The seemingly quite large percentages for pneumonia and diphtheria (17.2 and 13.5, respectively) must of course be viewed in the context of relatively early interventions—1935 and 1930.

In order to examine more closely the relation of mortality trends for these diseases to the medical interventions, graphs are presented for each disease in Fig. 1.4. Clearly, for tuberculosis, typhoid, measles, and scarlet fever, the medical measures considered were introduced at the point when the death rate for each of these diseases was already negligible. Any change in the rates of decline which may have occurred subsequent to the interventions could only be minute. Of the remaining five diseases (excluding smallpox with its negligible contribution), it is only for poliomyelitis that the medical measure appears to have produced any noticeable change in the trends. Given peaks in the death rate for 1930, 1950 (and possibly for 1910), a comparable peak could have been expected in 1970. Instead, the death rate dropped to the point of disappearance after 1950 and has remained negligible. The four other diseases (pneumonia, influenza, whooping cough, and diphtheria) exhibit relatively smooth mortality trends which are unaffected by the medical measures, even though these were introduced relatively early, when the death rates were still notable.

It may be useful at this point to briefly consider the common and dubious practice of projecting estimated mortality trends (Witte and Axnick, 1975).

TABLE 1.1 ■ The Contribution of Medical Measures (Both Chemotherapeutic and Prophylactic) to the Fall in the Age- and Sex-Adjusted Death Rates (S.D.R.) of Ten Common Infectious Diseases and to the Overall Decline in the S.D.R., for the United States, 1900–1973

Disease	Fall in S.D.R. per 1,000 Population, 1900–1973 (a)	Fall in S.D.R. as % of the Total Fall in S.D.R. $(b) = \dfrac{(a)}{12.14} \times 100\%$	Year of Medical Intervention (Either Chemotherapy or Prophylaxis)	Fall in S.D.R. per 1,000 Population After Year of Intervention (c)	Fall in S.D.R. After Intervention as % of Total Fall for the Disease $(d) = \dfrac{(c)}{(a)}$	Fall in S.D.R. After Intervention as % of Total Fall in S.D.R. for All Causes $(e) = \dfrac{(b)(c)\%}{(a)}$
Tuberculosis	2.00	16.48	Isoniazid/Streptomycin, 1950	0.17	8.36	1.38
Scarlet Fever	0.10	0.84	Penicillin, 1946	0.00	1.75	0.01
Influenza	0.22	1.78	Vaccine, 1943	0.05	25.33	0.45
Pneumonia	1.42	11.74	Sulphonamide, 1935	0.24	17.19	2.02
Diphtheria	0.43	3.57	Toxoid, 1930	0.06	13.49	0.48
Whooping Cough	0.12	1.00	Vaccine, 1930	0.06	51.00	0.51
Measles	0.12	1.04	Vaccine, 1963	0.00	1.38	0.01
Smallpox	0.02	0.16	Vaccine, 1800	0.02	100.00	0.16
Typhoid	0.36	2.95	Chloramphenicol, 1948	0.00	0.29	0.01
Poliomyelitis	0.03	0.23	Vaccine, Salic/Sabin, 1955	0.01	25.87	0.06

In order to show the beneficial (or even detrimental) effect of some medical measure, a line, estimated on a set of points observed prior to the introduction of the measure, is projected over the period subsequent to the point of intervention. Any resulting discrepancy between the projected line and the observed trend is then used as some kind of "evidence" of an effective or beneficial intervention. According to statistical theory on least squares estimation, an estimated line can serve as a useful predictor, but the prediction is only valid, and its error calculable, within the range of the points used to estimate the line. Moreover, those predicted values which lie at the extremes of the range are subject to much larger errors than those nearer the center. It is, therefore, probable that, even if the projected line was a reasonable estimate of the trend after the intervention (which, of course, it is not), the divergent observed

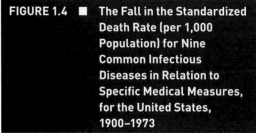

FIGURE 1.4 ■ **The Fall in the Standardized Death Rate (per 1,000 Population) for Nine Common Infectious Diseases in Relation to Specific Medical Measures, for the United States, 1900–1973**

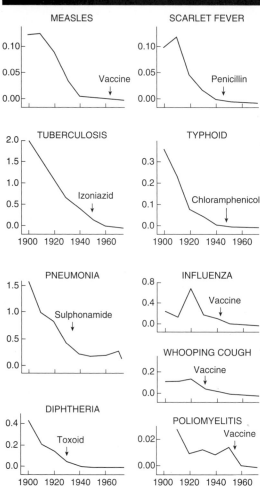

and a relatively large prediction error cannot be estimated, which is required in order to objectively judge the extent of divergence of an observed trend.

With regard to the ten infectious diseases considered in this paper, when lines were fitted to the nine or ten points available over the entire period (1900–1973), four exhibited a reasonably good fit to a straight line (scarlet fever, measles, whooping cough, and poliomyelitis), while another four (typhoid, diphtheria, tuberculosis, and pneumonia) showed a very good quadratic fit (to a curved line). Of the remaining two diseases, smallpox showed a negligible decline, as it was already a minor cause of death in 1900 (only 0.1 percent), and influenza showed a poor fit because of the extremely high death rate in 1920. From Fig. 1.4 it is clear, however, that the rate of decline slowed in more recent years for most of the diseases considered—a trend which could be anticipated as rates approach zero.[7]

Now it is possible to argue that, given the few data points available, the fit is somewhat crude and may be insensitive to any changes subsequent to a point of intervention. However, this can be countered with the observation that, given the relatively low death rates for these diseases, any change would have to be extremely marked in order to be detected in the overall mortality experience. Certainly, from the evidence considered here, only poliomyelitis appears to have had a noticeably changed death rate subsequent to intervention. Even if it were assumed that this change was entirely due to the vaccines, then only about one percent of the decline following interventions for the diseases considered here (column d of Table 1.1) could be attributed to medical measures. Rather more conservatively, if we attribute some of the subsequent fall in the death rates for pneumonia, influenza, whooping cough, and diphtheria to medical measures, then perhaps 3.5 percent of the fall in the overall death rate can be explained through medical intervention in the major infectious diseases considered here. Indeed, given that it is precisely for these diseases that medicine claims most success in lowering mortality, 3.5 percent probably represents a reasonable upper-limit estimate of the total contribution of medical measures to the decline in mortality in the United States since 1900.

trend is probably well within reasonable error limits of the estimated line (assuming the error could be calculated), as the error will be relatively large. In other words, this technique is of dubious value as no valid conclusions are possible from its application,

TABLE 1.2 ■ Pair-Wise Correlation Matrix for 44 Countries, Between Four Measures of Health Status and Three Measures of Medical Case Input

Variable		Matrix of Coefficients							
1.	Infant Mortality Rate (1972)								
2.	Crude Mortality Rate (1970–1972)	−0.14							
3. (a)	Life Expectancy (Males) at 25 years	−0.14	−0.12						
3. (b)	Life Expectancy (Females) at 25 years	−0.12	0.04	0.75					
4. (a)	Life Expectancy (Males) at 55 years	−0.01	0.10	0.74	0.93				
4. (b)	Life Expectancy (Females) at 55 years	−0.13	0.01	0.75	0.98	0.95			
5.	Population per Hospital Bed (1971–1973)	0.64	−0.30	0.05	−0.02	0.17	0.0		
6.	Population per Physician (1971–1973)	0.36	−0.30	0.11	0.04	0.16	0.07	0.70	
7.	Per Capita Gross National Product: In $U.S. Equivalent (1972)	−0.66	0.26	0.16	0.18	0.07	0.22	−0.56	−0.46
	Variable (by number)	1	2	3a	3b	4a	4b	5	6

Sources: 1. *United Nations Demographic Yearbook: 1974,* New York, United Nations Publications, 1975. (For the Crude and Infant Mortality Rates). 2. *World Health Statistics Annual: 1972,* Vol. 1, Geneva, World Health Organization, 1975, pp. 780–783. (For the Life Expectancy Figures). 3. *United Nations Statistical Yearbook, 1973 and 1975,* New York, United Nations Publications, 25th and 27th issues, 1974 and 1976. (For the Population Bed/Physician Ratios). 4. *The World Bank Atlas,* Washington, D.C., World Bank, 1975. (For the Per Capita Gross National Product).

CONCLUSIONS

Without claiming they are definitive findings, and eschewing pretentions to an analysis as sophisticated as McKeown's for England and Wales, one can reasonably draw the following conclusions from the analysis presented in this paper:

In general, medical measures (both chemotherapeutic and prophylactic) appear to have contributed little to the overall decline in mortality in the United States since about 1900—having in many instances been introduced several decades after a marked decline had already set in and having no detectable influence in most instances. More specifically, with reference to those five conditions (influenza, pneumonia, diphtheria, whooping cough, and poliomyelitis) for which the decline in mortality appears substantial after the point of intervention—and on the unlikely assumption that all of this decline is attributable to the intervention—it is estimated that at most 3.5 percent of the total decline in mortality since 1900 could be ascribed to medical measures introduced for the diseases considered here.

These conclusions, in support of the thesis introduced earlier, suggest issues of the most strategic significance for researchers and health care legislators. Profound policy implications follow from either a confirmation or a rejection of the thesis. If one subscribes to the view that we are slowly but surely eliminating one disease after another because of medical interventions, then there may be little commitment to social change and even resistance to some reordering of priorities in medical expenditures. If a disease X is disappearing primarily because of the presence of a particular intervention or service *Y,* then clearly *Y* should be left intact, or, more preferably, be expanded. Its demonstrable contribution justifies its presence. But, if it can be shown convincingly, and on commonly accepted grounds, that the major part of the decline in mortality is unrelated to medical care activities, then some commitment to social change and a reordering of priorities may ensue. For, if the disappearance of *X* is largely unrelated to the presence of *Y,* or even occurs in the absence of *Y,* then clearly the expansion and even the continuance of *Y* can be reasonably questioned. Its demonstrable ineffectiveness justifies some reappraisal of its significance and the wisdom of expanding it in its existing form.

In this paper we have attempted to dispel the myth that medical measures and the presence of medical services were primarily responsible for the modern decline of mortality. The question now remains: if they were not primarily responsible for it, then how is it to be explained? An adequate answer to this further question would require a more substantial research effort than that reported here, but is likely to be along the lines suggested by McKeown which were referred to early in this paper. Hopefully, this paper will serve as a catalyst for such research, incorporating adequate data and appropriate methods of analysis, in an effort to arrive at a more viable alternative explanation.

Notes

1. It is obviously important to distinguish between (a) advances in knowledge of the cause and natural course of some condition and (b) improvements in our ability to effectively treat some condition (that is, to alter its natural course). In many instances these two areas are disjoint and appear at different stages of development. There are, on the one hand, disease processes about which considerable knowledge has been accrued, yet this has not resulted (nor necessarily will) in the development of effective treatments. On the other hand, there are conditions for which demonstrably effective treatments have been devised in the absence of knowledge of the disease process and/or its causes.

2. Barker and Rose cite one study which compared the ante-mortem and autopsy diagnoses in 9,501 deaths which occurred in 75 different hospitals. Despite lack of a concurrence on *individual* cases, the *overall* frequency was very similar in diagnoses obtained on either an ante-mortem or post-mortem basis. As an example they note that clinical diagnoses of carcinoma of the rectum were confirmed at autopsy in only 67 percent of cases, but the incorrect clinical diagnoses were balanced by an almost identical number of lesions diagnosed for the first time at autopsy (Barker and Rose, 1976).

3. All age and sex adjustments were made by the "direct" method using the population of 1900 as the standard. For further information on this method of adjustment, see Hill (1971) and Shryock et al. (1971).

4. Rutstein (1967), although fervently espousing the traditional view that medical advances have been largely responsible for the decline in mortality, discussed this disjunction and termed it "The Paradox of Modern Medicine." More recently, and from a perspective that is generally consistent with that advanced here, Powles (1973) noted the same phenomenon in England and Wales.

5. Deaths in the category of chronic respiratory diseases (chronic bronchitis, asthma, emphysema, and other chronic obstructive lung diseases) could not be included in the group of chronic conditions because of

insurmountable difficulties inherent in the many changes in disease classification and in the tabulation of statistics.

6. In determining the dates of intervention we relied upon: (a) standard epidemiology and public health texts; (b) the recollections of authorities in the field of infectious diseases; and (c) recent publications on the same subject.

7. For this reason, a negative exponential model is sometimes used to fit a curved line to such data. This was not presented here as the number of points available was small and the difference between a simple quadratic and negative exponential fit was not, upon investigation, able to be detected.

References

Alderson, M. 1976. *An Introduction to Epidemiology*. London: Macmillan Press, pp. 7–27.

Barker, D.J.P., and Rose, G. 1976. *Epidemiology in Medical Practice*. London: Churchill Livingstone, p. 6.

Bolduan, C.F. 1930. *How to Protect Children From Diphtheria*. New York: N.Y.C. Health Department.

Dubos, R. 1959. *Mirage of Health*. New York: Harper and Row.

Dubos, R. 1965. *Man Adapting*. New Haven, Connecticut: Yale University Press.

Dubos, R. 1968. *Man, Medicine and Environment*. London: Pall Mall Press.

Dunn, H.L., and Shackley, W. 1945. *Comparison of cause of death assignments by the 1929 and 1938 revisions of the International List: Deaths in the United States, 1940 Vital Statistics—Special Reports* 19:153–277, 1944, Washington, D.C.: U.S. Department of Commerce, Bureau of the Census.

Fuchs, V.R. 1974. *Who Shall Live?* New York: Basic Books, p. 54.

Griffith, T. 1967. *Population Problems in the Age of Malthus*. 2nd ed. London: Frank Cass.

Habakkuk, H.J. 1953. English Population in the Eighteenth Century. *Economic History Review*, 6.

Hill, A.B. 1971. *Principles of Medical Statistics*. 9th ed. London: Oxford University Press.

Hill, A.B. 1955. Snow—An Appreciation. *Proceedings of the Royal Society of Medicine* 48:1008–1012. Illich, I. 1976. *Medical Nemesis*. New York: Pantheon Books.

Inman, W.H.W., and Adelstein, A.M. 1969. Rise and fall of asthma mortality in England and Wales, in relation to use of pressurized aerosols. *Lancet* 2:278–285.

Kass, E.H. 1971. Infectious diseases and social change. *The Journal of Infectious Diseases*, 123(1):110–114.

Krueger, D.E. 1966. New enumerators for old denominators—multiple causes of death. In *Epidemiological Approaches to the Study of Cancer and Other Chronic Diseases*, edited by W. Haenszel. National Cancer Printing Office, pp. 431–443.

Lee, W.W. 1931. Diphtheria immunization in Philadelphia and New York City. *Journal of Preventive Medicine* (Baltimore) 5:211–220.

Lilienfeld, A.M. 1976. *Foundations of Epidemiology*. New York: Oxford University Press, pp. 51–111.

McKeown, T. 1976a. *The Modern Rise of Population*. London: Edward Arnold.

McKeown, T. 1976b. *The Role of Medicine: Dream, Mirage or Nemesis.* London: Nuffield Provincial Hospitals Trust.

McKeown, T.; Brown, R.G.; and Record, R.G. 1972. An interpretation of the modern rise of population in Europe. *Population Studies* 26: 345–382.

McKeown, T., and Record, R.G. 1955. Medical evidence related to English population changes in the eighteenth century. *Population Studies* 9:119–141.

McKeown, T., and Record, R.G. 1962. Reasons for the decline in mortality in England and Wales during the nineteenth century. *Population Studies* 16:94–122.

McKeown, T.; Record, R.G.; and Turner, R.D. 1975. An interpretation of the decline of mortality in England and Wales during the twentieth century. *Population Studies* 29:391–422.

McKinlay, J.B., and McKinlay, S.M. *A refutation of the thesis that the health of the nation is improving.*

Magill, T.P. 1955. The immunologist and the evil spirits. *Journal of Immunology* 74:1–8.

Moriyama, I.M.; Baum, W.S.; Haenszel, W.M.; and Mattison, B.F. 1958. Inquiry into diagnostic evidence supporting medical certifications of death. *American Journal of Public Health* 48:1376–1387.

Moriyama, I.M., and Gustavus, S.O. 1972. *Cohort Mortality and Survivorship: United States Death—Registration States, 1900–1968.* National Center for Health Statistics, Series 3, No. 16. Washington, D.C.: U.S. Government Printing Office.

Pfizer, C., and Company. 1953. *The Pneumonias, Management with Antibiotic Therapy.* Brooklyn.

Powles, J. 1973. On the limitations of modern medicine. *Science, Medicine and Man.* 1:2–3.

Reid, O.D., and Rose, G.A. 1964. Assessing the comparability of mortality statistics. *British Medical Journal* 2:1437–1439.

Rutstein, D. 1967. *The Coming Revolution in Medicine.* Cambridge, Massachusetts: MIT Press.

Shryock, H., et al. 1971. *The Methods and Materials of Demography.* Washington, D.C.: U.S. Government Printing Office.

The Times (London). 1977. The Doctors Dilemma: How to Cure Society of a Life Style That Makes People Sick. Friday, January 21.

U.S. Bureau of the Census. 1906. *Mortality Statistics 1900–1904.* Washington, D.C.: Government Printing Office.

U.S. Department of Health, Education and Welfare. 1964. *The Change in Mortality Trend in the United States.* National Center for Health Statistics, Series 3, No. 1. Washington, D.C.: U.S. Government Printing Office.

Weinstein, L. 1974. Infectious Disease: Retrospect and Reminiscence. *The Journal of Infectious Diseases.* 129 (4):480–492.

Wilson, G.S., and Miles, A.A. 1946. In Topley and Wilson's *Principles of Bacteriology and Immunity.* Baltimore: Williams and Wilkins.

Witte, J.J., and Axnick, N.W. 1975. The benefits from ten years of measles immunization in the United States. *Public Health Reports* 90 (3):205–207.

SOCIAL CONDITIONS AS FUNDAMENTAL CAUSES OF HEALTH INEQUALITIES

Theory, Evidence, and Practice

Jo C. Phelan, Bruce G. Link, and Parisa Tehranifar

As we mark the fiftieth anniversary of the Medical Sociology Section of the American Sociological Association, one of the most basic and critical problems addressed by medical sociologists is a very old one: the fact that society's poorer and less privileged members live in worse health and die much younger than the rich and more privileged ones. Socioeconomic inequalities in health and mortality are very large, very robust, and very well documented. Typically, age-adjusted risk of death for those in the lowest socioeconomic level is double to triple that for the highest level (Antonovsky 1967; Sorlie, Backlund, and Keller 1995; Kunst, Feikje, and Mackenbach 1998). To illustrate, in 2005,

all-cause, age-adjusted death rates for individuals between the ages of 25 and 64 were strongly related to education level for both men (at < 12 years, 821 per 100,000; at 12 years, 605; and at > 12 years, 249) and women (at < 12 years, 472; at 12 years, 352; and at > 12 years, 165) (National Center for Health Statistics 2008). Similar levels of inequality are observed between income groups.

These inequalities in overall health and mortality are not only very common in modern times, but they have persisted at similar levels at least since the early nineteenth century (Antonovsky 1967). This persistence is puzzling because major diseases and risk factors that appeared to account for the inequalities seen in earlier periods (i.e., deadly infectious diseases such as diphtheria, measles, typhoid fever, and tuberculosis fueled by overcrowding and poor sanitation in low socioeconomic status homes and communities) have been virtually eradicated in the developed world. Rather than disappearing, socioeconomic status (SES) inequalities in mortality have persisted and now reflect new major causes of death including cancers and cardiovascular illness, fueled by risk factors such as poor diet, inadequate exercise, and smoking that are more common in lower SES groups. Socioeconomic inequalities in health and mortality have even survived concerted efforts to eliminate them, such as institution of the United Kingdom's National Health Service, their vast publicly-funded health care system (Black et al. 1982).

It is this persistence across time that Link and Phelan (1995) aimed to explain with their theory of fundamental causes. They reasoned that we cannot claim to understand why health inequalities exist if we cannot explain why they persist under conditions that should eliminate or reduce them, and if we can understand why they persist, this may provide clues to the more general problem of the causes of health inequalities. That is, the remarkable persistence of inequalities may provide a lever for understanding the more general fact of their existence.

In this article, we will explicate the theory as it has developed over the past 15 years, review key empirical findings, develop some refinements of the theory, address potential limits of the theory, and discuss implications for health policies that might reduce health inequalities.

THE THEORY

The theory of fundamental causes is rooted in Lieberson's (1985) concept of basic causes, which was first applied to the association between SES and mortality by House and colleagues (House et al. 1990, 1994). The theory has been developed primarily by Link and Phelan (Link and Phelan 1995; Phelan et al. 2004; Link

and Phelan, forthcoming), with significant elaboration and extension by Lutfey and Freese (2005).

The primary statement of the theory appeared in 1995 in a previous special issue of the *Journal of Health and Social Behavior*. According to Link and Phelan (1995), a fundamental social cause of health inequalities has four essential features. First, it influences multiple disease outcomes, meaning that it is not limited to only one or a few diseases or health problems. Second, it affects these disease outcomes through multiple risk factors. Third, it involves access to resources that can be used to avoid risks or to minimize the consequences of disease once it occurs. Finally, the association between a fundamental cause and health is reproduced over time via the replacement of intervening mechanisms (Link and Phelan 1995). It is the persistent association of SES with overall health in the face of dramatic changes in mechanisms linking SES and health that led Link and Phelan to call SES a "fundamental" cause of health inequalities.

The Central Role of Flexible Resources for SES Inequalities in Health

According to the theory of fundamental causes, an important reason that SES is related to multiple disease outcomes through multiple pathways that change over time is that individuals and groups deploy resources to avoid risks and adopt protective strategies. Key resources such as knowledge, money, power, prestige, and beneficial social connections can be used no matter what the risk and protective factors are in a given circumstance. Consequently, fundamental causes affect health even when the profile of risk and protective factors and diseases changes radically. If the problem is cholera, for example, a person with greater resources is better able to avoid areas where the disease is rampant, and highly resourced communities are better able to prohibit entry of infected persons. If the problem is heart disease, a person with greater resources is better able to maintain a heart-healthy lifestyle and get the best medical treatment available. Because these resources can be used in different ways in different situations, we call them flexible resources.

It is their capacity to be used flexibly by individuals and groups that places resources of knowledge, money, power, prestige, and beneficial social connections at the center of fundamental cause theory. Their flexible use tells us why SES gradients tend to reproduce themselves over time. This focus on resources and their deployment does not deny the importance of antecedent causes of the resources themselves that lie in the social, economic, and political structures of society. In fact, fundamental cause theory is deeply connected to the sociological study of stratification in this way—the resources highlighted in fundamental cause theory must come from somewhere, and theories of the origins of inequalities are the best source for understanding these processes. To understand how flexible resources might facilitate the creation of new mechanisms linking SES and health, consider the following example. Screening for several cancers has become possible over the past few decades, making it feasible to detect cancer or its precursors earlier, thereby helping to prevent mortality from these cancers. Since the screening procedures represent relatively recent technological advances, one can imagine a time before the procedures existed, when resources had no bearing on access to cancer screening because the procedures did not exist. There was no mechanism linking SES to screening access to health. But after the screening procedures were developed, people with more resources could use those resources to gain access to the life-saving screens. Link et al. (1998) presented evidence from the Behavioral Risk Factor Survey showing that screening rates for cervical and breast cancer are indeed associated with education and income.[1] A new mechanism had emerged to link social conditions to health outcomes. The idea is that this process extends beyond this example to many, many others.

The flexible resources that are central to fundamental cause theory operate at both individual and contextual levels. At the individual level, flexible resources can be conceptualized as the "cause of causes" or "risk of risks" that shape individual health behaviors by influencing whether people know about, have access to, can afford, and receive social support for their efforts to engage in health-enhancing or health-protective behaviors. In addition, resources shape access to broad contexts

that vary dramatically in associated risk profiles and protective factors. For example, a person with many resources can afford to live in a high SES neighborhood where neighbors are also of high status and where, collectively, enormous clout is exerted to ensure that crime, noise, violence, pollution, traffic, and vermin are minimized, and that the best health-care facilities, parks, playgrounds, and food stores are located nearby. Once a person has used SES-related resources to locate in an advantaged neighborhood, a host of health-enhancing circumstances comes along as a package deal. Similarly, a person who uses educational credentials to procure a high-status occupation inherits a package deal that is more likely to include excellent health benefits and less likely to involve dangerous conditions and toxic exposures. In these circumstances, the person benefits in numerous ways that do not depend on his or her own initiative or ability to personally construct a healthy situation; it is an "add on" benefit operative at the contextual level. These contexts may be meso (families) or macro levels (a congressional block that opposes changes in health care policy that would shift the distribution of health care away from high SES groups to the uninsured), formal (employer or trade union), or informal (social networks). The clearest example of fundamental cause theory occurs when groups explicitly push for better health conditions for their members. But the health-enhancing use of group resources can operate at a less explicit level. Consider Cockerham's (2005) ideas about the influence of status groups on health lifestyles. According to Cockerham, social norms and other social supports, such as the health-product industry, reinforce distinctive health lifestyles in different status groups, and the lifestyles of high SES groups are particularly healthy ones. In these instances, status groups do not explicitly advocate for health-enhancing conditions, but rather members form cultural practices around food, exercise, and other health-related circumstances that influence the behavior of status-group members. These lifestyles are shaped by the extant stock of health knowledge and pecuniary resources generally available in particular status groups—a circumstance that generally leads to healthier lifestyles in higher status groups. For example, it is almost unheard of for snacks offered at meetings held at the Mailman School of Public Health at Columbia University to not include multiple varieties of fruits; Dunkin Donuts, in contrast, are rare indeed. It is not as if the people who order these snacks explicitly consider the health impact of their choices each time a decision is made. Instead, cultural practices shaped over time lead them to order the conventional, and the conventional in this context is generally healthy fare.

KEY EMPIRICAL FINDINGS

Empirical tests of the theory are not obvious or straightforward. A demonstration of socioeconomic inequalities in health or mortality, even ones that persist over time, does not in itself constitute support for the theory. It is precisely the nearly ubiquitous inverse association between SES and mortality that the theory attempts to explain. Demonstrating this association in any particular circumstances cannot adjudicate between fundamental causes and other possible explanations of those facts.

Empirical support for the theory relies on evaluating the four essential features of a fundamental cause of health inequalities (Link and Phelan 1995). In the following sections, we present key findings bearing on each of these components: (1) evidence that SES influences multiple disease outcomes; (2) evidence that SES is related to multiple risk factors for disease and death; (3) evidence that the deployment of resources plays a critical role in the association between SES and health/mortality; and (4) evidence that the association between SES and health/mortality is reproduced over time via the replacement of intervening mechanisms.

Evidence That SES Is Related to Multiple Disease Outcomes via Multiple Risk Factors

The first two propositions are strongly supported by empirical data. Low SES is related to a multiplicity of diseases and other causes of death. The broad generality of this association can be summarized with two sets of facts: (1) Low SES is related to mortality from each of the broad categories of chronic diseases, communicable diseases, and injuries (Pamuk et al. 1998; National Center for Health Statistics 2008), and (2) low SES is related to mortality from each of the 14 major causes of death in the International Classification of Diseases (Illsley and Mullen 1985).

There is also clear evidence that SES is associated with numerous risk and protective factors for disease and other causes of death, both currently and in the past. These include smoking, sedentariness, and being overweight (Lantz et al. 1998; Link 2008); stressful life conditions (Turner, Wheaton, and Lloyd 1995; House and Williams 2000); social isolation (House and Williams 2000; Ruberman et al. 1984); preventive health care (Dutton 1978; Link et al. 1998); and crowded and unsanitary living conditions, unsanitary water supplies, and malnutrition (Rosen 1979).

Lutfey and Freese (2005) describe this component of the theory as involving a "massive multiplicity of mechanisms." They suggest that, because fundamental cause processes are "holographic," such a multiplicity of mechanisms should be found in all or most particular instances in which SES and health outcomes are connected. Using an ethnographic analysis, they use the example of routine diabetes care in two socioeconomically contrasting clinics to articulate several concrete ways in which differential health outcomes emerge in the two clinics. For example, the clinic serving higher SES patients provided better continuity of care, and the higher SES patients encountered fewer costs of complying with treatment regimens and had more knowledge about diabetes. Similar analyses conducted in a variety of contexts relating to treatment or prevention of a variety of diseases would enrich our understanding of the pathways through which SES influences health and longevity.

Evidence That the Deployment of Resources Plays a Critical Role in the Association Between SES and Health

Central to fundamental cause theory is the idea that resources of money, knowledge, power, prestige, and beneficial social connections are critical to maintaining a health advantage. Empirically testing the importance of resources per se is difficult, because it requires the identification of situations in which the ability to use socioeconomic resources can be analytically separated from SES itself (e.g., situations in which high SES persons are prevented from using their resources to gain a health advantage). If the utilization of resources is critical in maintaining health or prolonging life, then in situations in which the resources associated with higher status are of no use, high SES should confer no advantage, and the usually robust association between SES and health or mortality should be greatly reduced.

One such situation occurs when the causes and cures of fatal diseases are unknown. In these circumstances, socioeconomic resources cannot be used to avoid death due to these diseases, because it is not known how the resources should be deployed. Thus, to the extent that the ability to use socioeconomic resources is critical in maintaining SES inequalities in mortality, there should be strong SES gradients in mortality for causes of death that are highly preventable—for which we have good knowledge and effective measures for prevention or treatment. However, for causes of death about which we know little regarding prevention or treatment, SES gradients in mortality should be much weaker. Consistent with this prediction, Phelan et al. (2004) found that socioeconomic inequalities in mortality were significantly more pronounced for causes of death that were reliably rated by two physician-epidemiologists as being highly preventable (such as lung cancer and ischemic heart disease), and thus more amenable to the application of flexible resources than for causes that were rated as not very preventable (such as brain cancer and arrhythmias). Although they do not address or explicitly test fundamental cause theory, three other studies that reported evidence on this issue also found that the SES-mortality association was stronger for preventable causes of death (Dahl,

Hofoss, and Elstad 2007; Marshall et al. 1993; Song and Byeon 2000).

Evidence for the validity and generality of these findings is strengthened by another study that employed a similar research strategy but (1) examined a different set of causes of death, (2) confined attention to treatment rather than including prevention, (3) used a different and more objective measure of amenability to treatment, and (4) examined racial and ethnic differences as opposed to socioeconomic ones.[2] Tehranifar et al. (2009) identified, prior to hypothesis testing, cancers that are more or less amenable to treatment and examined whether racial-ethnic differences in disease-specific mortality varied according to the degree to which that disease is amenable to available medical intervention. This study used five-year survival rates for 53 different cancer sites as a measure of effectiveness of treatment and/or early detection methods. Consistent with fundamental cause theory, survival disparities comparing disadvantaged minority groups (African Americans, American Indians, and Hispanics) to whites were substantially greater for cancers that were more amenable to treatment (e.g., cancers with five-year relative survival rates ≥ 70%, such as bladder, breast, and prostate cancers) than they were for cancers that were less so (e.g., cancers with five-year relative survival rates < 40%, such as liver, pancreatic, and esophageal cancers).

These studies show that, somewhat ironically, one way in which fundamental cause theory can be tested is by looking for exceptions to the strong SES gradient in health or mortality that is almost always observed—exceptions in which the ability to use resources to gain a health advantage is blocked. In these examples, the use of socioeconomic resources to improve health is blocked because risk factors are unknown and treatments do not exist (Phelan et al. 2004; Tehranifar et al. 2009). Other situations in which resources may be unhelpful or even harmful may be exploitable for testing of the theory. Examples are situations in which prevailing medical recommendations are subsequently discovered to be harmful (Carpiano and Kelly 2007) and the case of old age, when the growing frailty of the body may place limits on the effectiveness of interventions (Phelan et al. 2004).

Evidence That the Association Between SES and Health/Mortality Is Reproduced Over Time via the Replacement of Intervening Mechanisms

The fourth essential feature of SES as a fundamental cause of health inequalities is that the association between SES and health/mortality is reproduced over time via the replacement of intervening mechanisms. This key element of the theory arose from two sets of observations: (1) The SES-mortality association persisted over time despite the decline of mechanisms (e.g., poor sanitation and widespread death from infectious disease) that formerly provided important links between SES and mortality; and (2) new, previously weak or absent mechanisms currently link SES and mortality (e.g., smoking, exercise, diet, and cardiovascular disease). These observations are consistent with the idea that socioeconomic inequalities in health are reproduced via the replacement of intervening mechanisms. To more fully evaluate this component of the theory, however, more direct evidence was needed showing the emergence of new mechanisms. In particular, the theory predicts that new mechanisms arise following the development of new knowledge or medical intervention related to some disease, because higher SES individuals and groups are better equipped to take advantage of the new knowledge. Therefore, a key empirical question is whether the SES-health gradient shifts in favor of high SES individuals following the development of new knowledge. This evidence is particularly persuasive if the health outcome for which a shifted gradient is observed is directly related to the emergent knowledge, for example, if an advance in heart disease treatment furthers the advantage of high SES individuals in terms of heart disease mortality. Just as important is evidence that, in the absence of advances in knowledge, the SES gradient in relevant health outcomes remains fairly steady.

Several such analyses have now been conducted. Phelan and Link (2005) examined selected causes of death for which great strides in prevention or treatment were made over the last half of the twentieth century (heart disease, lung cancer, and colon cancer), and for which much less progress had been made over the same period (brain cancer, ovarian cancer, and pancreatic cancer). Looking at age-adjusted death rates by race and by county-level SES, they reported that, for the causes of death where little had been learned about treatment or prevention, mortality rates stayed fairly steady, and the degree of inequality based on race and SES stayed fairly steady as well. By contrast, for the causes of death where gains in treatment and prevention had been significant, overall mortality rates declined while race and SES gradients shifted in the direction of relatively higher mortality for the less advantaged group.

Subsequent studies have gone much further in drawing specific connections between gains in knowledge and subsequent changes in relevant disease outcomes. Carpiano and Kelly (2007) analyzed changes in breast cancer incidence following the widely publicized findings from the Women's Health Initiative (WHI) that linked hormone replacement therapy to increased breast cancer risk (Haas et al. 2004). In the following two years, consistent with the racial pattern in the use of hormone replacement therapy (Haas et al. 2004; Hulley et al. 1998), breast cancer incidence among white women age 50 and older, the age group most likely to have been using hormone therapy before the WHI study results were publicized, dropped precipitously, while incidence among black women in that age group stayed fairly steady (Carpiano and Kelly 2007). These findings were confirmed by another study that also considered county-level median household income and breast tumor estrogen (ER) receptor status (Krieger, Chen, and Waterman 2010). That study found the decline in breast cancer incidence after the WHI study publication to be limited to white women, aged 50 and older, who were residents of high income counties and had estrogen-positive breast tumors (the type of tumor most likely to be affected by hormone replacement).

Chang and Lauderdale (2009) studied the impact of statins (an effective and expensive medication to lower cholesterol) on socioeconomic gradients in cholesterol levels. Using nationally representative data from 1976 to 2004, they found that those with higher income initially had higher cholesterol levels, but that the SES-cholesterol association then reversed and became negative in the era of widespread statin use.

Link (2008) traced changes in knowledge, beliefs, and behavior that followed the discovery of a causal link between cigarette smoking and lung cancer, and that eventually led to strong socioeconomic gradients in smoking. Scientific evidence strongly linking smoking to lung cancer emerged in the early 1950s. To assess changes that may have occurred in the decades following the production of this new knowledge, Link (2008) analyzed multiple public opinion polls assessing smoking beliefs and behaviors. Evidence from the first surveys conducted just as the scientific evidence was emerging in 1954 showed that, while most people had heard about the findings, only a minority believed that smoking was a cause of lung cancer, and no educational gradient in this belief was evident. Nor was smoking behavior strongly linked to educational attainment in 1954. Over the subsequent 45 years, as people began to adopt the belief that smoking is a cause of lung cancer, sharp educational gradients opened up in this belief. Additionally, people of higher education were less likely to start smoking and more likely to quit, thereby generating a strong SES gradient in smoking behavior (Link 2008). A new and powerful mechanism linking SES to an important health behavior had emerged.

The studies just described are particularly valuable for their ability to pinpoint temporal connections between particular developments in knowledge and technology surrounding specific diseases, on the one hand, and changes in SES-related health gradients predicted by the theory, on the other. Moreover, these studies address major diseases that are important causes of death. However, there is always the possibility that these cases are not representative of the situation that holds more generally when new health knowledge or technology develops. For this reason, the more systematic and comprehensive analysis of Glied and Lleras-Muney (2008) is particularly valuable. This study provides evidence that the results of the case studies reported previously are indeed generalizable. Like Phelan

et al. (2004) and Tehranifar et al. (2009), Glied and Lleras-Muney conducted a systematic test based on a comprehensive set of diseases. In fact, Glied and Lleras-Muney repeated their analysis with two separate data sets: the Mortality Detail Files from the National Center for Health Statistics, and the Surveillance Epidemiology and End Results cancer registry. They operationalized the development of life-saving knowledge and technology, or "innovation," in two ways. In the first, they used the rate of change in mortality over time to indicate progress in addressing mortality due to particular diseases, the assumption being that the greater the decline in mortality, the greater the progress that has been made. In the second, they used the number of active drugs approved to treat particular diseases, with the assumption that more progress has been made where more new drugs have been developed to treat disease. They found, consistent with the theory of fundamental causes, that educational gradients became larger for diseases where greater innovation had occurred.

In summary, evidence has accumulated that is consistent with each of the four components of fundamental cause theory. Empirical testing of the theory is accelerating, and studies are now being conducted by researchers other than the theory's originators. This is a desirable development, as it raises confidence that the theory is being subjected to scientific scrutiny.

RETURNING TO THE THEORY: REFINEMENTS AND LIMITATIONS

Refinements to Fundamental Cause Theory

The theory has two sets of implications for continuity and change in health inequalities over time. The theory's basic principle—that a superior collection of flexible resources held by higher SES individuals and the collectivities to which they belong allow those of higher SES to avoid disease and death in widely divergent circumstances— leads to the prediction that, at any given time, greater resources will produce better health, and consequently, inequalities in health and mortality will persist as long as resource inequalities do.

At the same time, this long-term stability in the association between SES and health/mortality results from the amalgamation of effects across many specific processes and conditions. New knowledge and technology relating to innumerable diseases emerges constantly. The nature of the new knowledge varies, and the social conditions in which this knowledge emerges also vary. As a result, while in general new knowledge and medical development about a disease will lead to a shift in the disease gradient in favor of higher SES individuals and groups, they will not all have an identical impact on this gradient. Another reason for the long-term stability in the SES-mortality association is that old mechanisms wane to be replaced by new ones. Again, the demise of mechanisms is not a uniform process: Some mechanisms have long lives, others short ones. In this section, we take steps toward understanding some of the conditions that lead to variations in the processes of mechanism generation and demise. Our aim is not only to strengthen the theory but to understand how it may be possible to weaken new mechanisms connecting SES and disease/mortality, and how old ones may be undermined.

Specifying Conditions That Modify the Impact of New Knowledge on Health Inequalities

The situation that most clearly exemplifies fundamental cause processes is one in which we initially know nothing about how to prevent or cure a disease, and there is no association between SES and morbidity or mortality due to that disease. Then, upon discovery of modifiable risk or protective factors, an inverse association between SES and the disease in question emerges. But other situations that differ from this prototype are not only possible but to be expected.

One factor that should modify the impact of emergent knowledge is the pre-existing SES distribution of the disease at the time of a new advance in prevention or treatment.[3] The pre-existing association between the disease and SES is unlikely to be null for two reasons. First, when new knowledge and technology emerge, it is often the case that prior knowledge and technology have already shaped the association between SES and disease; the new knowledge will further shape this association. Second, even in the absence of previous knowledge about its risk and protective factors, a disease may be influenced by factors that are associated with SES, either directly or inversely. Second, even in the absence of previous knowledge about its risk and protective factors, a disease may be influenced by unknown factors that are associated with SES, either directly or inversely. For example, before cholesterol was identified as a risk factor for cardiovascular disease, its levels were likely higher in higher SES populations because such populations had greater access to relatively expensive fatty foods.

The reason that prior associations between risk factors or diseases and SES are important for fundamental cause theory is that the new knowledge has greater utility for those who have the disease or risk factor. Notably, if the initial association between SES and the disease is *inverse* such that people of lower SES are at greater risk, an effective intervention can reduce inequalities in that disease. This is because more people of low SES are likely to benefit from the intervention, because more of them have the disease initially. This can be true even if persons of higher SES who have the disease are more likely to gain access to and benefit from the intervention than lower SES persons who have the disease. We call this a "give back effect" (Link and Phelan, forthcoming), because the initial inverse SES-to-disease association provides a starting point that allows the new knowledge about the disease to "give back" some equality, even though it may also exemplify a fundamental cause process in which the knowledge is not distributed equally across socioeconomic groups. For example, smoking is a risk factor that has been influenced by knowledge of its harmful effects such that what was once a direct SES-to-smoking association has become a sharply graded inverse association, and one reason that SES is related to smoking-related diseases.

In this context a "give back" effect would arise if a new intervention blocked the effect of smoking on heart disease or lung cancer mortality. Even if this new intervention was itself maldistributed by SES, a "give back" effect might arise because smoking is so much more common in low SES populations; in other words, there are more people at the low end who can benefit from the new intervention. Importantly, from a fundamental cause perspective, if the intervention had been discovered earlier, before an SES-to-disease association in smoking emerged, and if the intervention had been maldistributed by SES at that time, the intervention would have created an inverse association between SES and lung cancer or heart disease.

Mechanism Demise and Death

Whereas it is understandable that empirical tests have focused on the creation of mechanisms that produce health inequalities, fundamental cause theory is predicated on the idea that mechanisms are *replaced*. Replacement requires that old mechanisms wane in importance over time. In fact, the theory emerged in part *because* prominent risk-factor mechanisms associated with vicious infectious diseases declined in significance as germ theory, improved sanitation, and vaccination came into existence. Thus, understanding the demise and death of mechanisms linking flexible resources to disease is an important area that needs more development and testing. We offer two examples that may help others develop this area of inquiry more fully.

Salk's discovery of the polio vaccine is an example of a mechanism that was very short-lived. Before his discovery, people of all resource levels could be afflicted, including, for example, President Franklin Roosevelt. After the discovery, resource-rich individuals were more likely to receive the vaccine and be protected. A mechanism linking resources to health existed, but only for a short time. The vaccine was quickly approved for widespread distribution to the U.S. population, and polio was virtually eradicated here. Other mechanisms

remain potent for a very long time. For example, the discovery of the pap test for the early detection and prevention of cervical cancer has existed since the 1940s. Early on, access to the test was shaped by flexible resources creating an inequality in the use of this life-saving screen that remains prominent today. As these examples suggest, some mechanisms become long-lasting while others have short lives. If we can understand what leads to the demise of mechanisms, and especially how that decline is related to flexible resources, we may open avenues to speed such a demise and reduce health inequalities. Indeed, much of the public health significance of fundamental cause theory may reside in understanding how the link between flexible resources and health-relevant risk and protective factors has been broken.

Limits on Fundamental Cause Theory: Countervailing Mechanisms

Whereas the previous sections elaborated fundamental cause theory, here we consider conditions that place limits on the theory.

We believe readers will agree that health and longevity are desirable, but they are not all that a person may want. Other things being equal, those with more resources can be expected to deploy those resources to increase health. But there are undoubtedly situations in which the goals of health and long life compete with and may cede dominance to other important life goals. Perhaps desiderata such as power, manliness, or beauty are sometimes more powerful motivators than health, and are pursued to the detriment of health. Lutfey and Freese (2005) refer to these competing goals as "countervailing mechanisms." The potential for countervailing mechanisms does not threaten the truth-value of fundamental cause theory, because "fundamental relationships do not require that all of the pathways between X and Y support the relationship. The only requirement is that the effects of [countervailing] mechanisms are cumulatively smaller than the effects of mechanisms producing the fundamental relationship" (Lutfey and Freese 2005: 1365). However, to the extent that countervailing mechanisms are called upon *post hoc* to explain results that do not support the theory, countervailing mechanisms pose a challenge to the falsifiability of the theory. For this reason, as well as for the fuller understanding of health inequalities, it is desirable to attend to countervailing mechanisms systematically, as Lutfey and Freese argue, and attempt to move the consideration of countervailing mechanisms from *post hoc* to *a priori*.

We first note that the connection between SES and health is an extremely powerful one and that goals that successfully compete with those of health and long life must surely be quite potent. For example, the goal of health attainment has been powerful enough to override or socially reconstruct many aspects of pleasure and pain—which would seem to be basic and powerful forces in their own right—among the socioeconomically privileged. Erstwhile pleasures such as well-marbled steaks are eschewed by higher SES groups in favor of sushi-grade tuna. Similarly, in the past, exhausting physical activity was considered something that high SES people were fortunate enough to be able to avoid. Now, "no pain, no gain" prevails in the most expensive health clubs. Cigarette smoking, although highly addictive, as well as sexual practices that increase the risk of HIV/AIDS, have also been significantly altered by high SES groups in the name of health attainment. We also note that the goals of health and longevity are strongly supported by social norms and other forms of social support among high status groups as part of the beneficial health lifestyle associated with high SES (Cockerham 2005). We suggest that the power of health attainment to shape the behavior of high SES individuals is largely due to these social forces, and we propose that successful countervailing mechanisms are also likely to be embedded in strong social norms and support.

One such motivation that may meet these conditions is status attainment. In Lutfey and Freese's (2005) ethnographic analysis of diabetes treatment, the pursuit of status, for example, occupational success or staying thin, sometimes led higher SES diabetic patients to behave in ways detrimental to the management of their disease. Similarly, Courtenay (2000) suggests that signifiers of masculinity such as the denial of weakness and engagement in risky or aggressive behavior often undermine men's health. Thus, the pursuit of masculine status may help explain the fact that women, who are generally lower resourced than men, live longer than men, a fact that would not be predicted by fundamental cause theory.[4] It seems, then, that status pursuit is one potential countervailing mechanism to the SES-health association. In the context of particular empirical studies, researchers may be able to consider *a priori* whether the situation under study is one in which the goals of health and social status are likely to collide. Additional motivations that might potentially be powerful enough to operate as countervailing mechanisms to SES include power, affiliation, self-esteem, identity, freedom, creation, and leisure (Maslow 1943; Max-Neef, Elizalde, and Hopenhayn 1989).

Note that, in most circumstances, we would expect the goal of good health to be compatible with goals of power, self-esteem, and so on, and we would expect higher SES individuals to use their resources to achieve more of all these desiderata than lower SES persons would be able to. Still, the example of status pursuit as a countervailing mechanism suggests that there will be instances when other powerful motivations that are more readily attained by high SES persons work to the detriment of health. In those situations, the usual association between resources and health should be attenuated. Also note that these countervailing mechanisms may create conditions when SES will not operate as a fundamental cause of health and mortality, but they do not negate the power of SES as a fundamental cause of unequal life chances more generally.

IMPLICATIONS FOR HEALTH POLICY

The fundamental cause approach leads to very different policies for addressing health inequalities than does an individually oriented risk-factor approach. The latter asks us to locate modifiable risk factors that lie between distal cause (such as SES) and disease, and to intervene in those risk factors. By addressing intervening factors, the logic goes, we will eliminate health disparities.

Our approach points to the pitfalls of this logic and suggests that developing new interventions, even when beneficial to health, is very likely to increase social inequalities in health outcomes. The idea that medical progress often leads to increased health inequality leads to an obvious conundrum: Must we choose between improving overall levels of health and reducing inequalities in health? Some argue that continued inequalities in health outcomes are acceptable as long as overall health improves or that some improvement is achieved for most social groups. We, on the other hand, are committed to reducing health inequalities, but it seems wrong-headed to oppose advances in health knowledge and technology because those may increase inequalities. We see no reason not to make both outcomes important goals, simultaneously pursuing better overall health and reduced inequalities.

We suggest some general strategies that we believe will lead to improved overall population health without further widening social inequalities in health. Our approach points to policies that encourage advances while breaking or weakening the link between these advances and socioeconomic resources, either by reducing disparities in socio-economic resources themselves, or by developing interventions that, by their nature, are more equally distributed across SES groups.

Reduce Resource Inequalities

The first recommendation falls outside the explicit domain of health policy, but according to fundamental cause theory is intimately tied to it. The theory stipulates that people and collectivities use their knowledge, money, power, prestige, and social connections to gain a health advantage, and thereby reproduce the SES gradient in health. The most direct policy implication of the theory is that, if we redistribute resources in the population so as to reduce the degree of resource inequality, inequalities in health should also decrease. Policies relevant to fundamental causes of disease form a major part of

the national agenda, whether this involves the minimum wage, housing for homeless and low-income people, capital-gains and estate taxes, parenting leave, social security, head-start programs and college-admission policies, regulation of lending practices, or other initiatives of this type. We argue that all these policies are health-relevant policies and that understanding how they are relevant should be claimed as an essential part of the domain of medical sociology.

Contextualize Risk Factors

Potential interventions that seek to change individual risk profiles should first identify factors that put people at risk of risks, for example, power disadvantages that prevent some people from adopting safe sex strategies or neighborhood environments that make healthful foods unavailable. This will avoid the enactment of interventions aimed at changing behaviors that are powerfully influenced by factors left untouched by the intervention.

Prioritize the Development of Interventions That Do Not Entail the Use of Resources or That Minimize the Relevance of Resources

As we seek to create interventions to improve health, we need to ask if an intervention is something that anyone can potentially adopt, or whether the benefit will only be available to people with the necessary resources. Fundamental cause theory suggests that health inequalities based on SES can be reduced by instituting health interventions that automatically benefit individuals irrespective of their own resources or behaviors. Examples are the manufacture of automobiles with air bags as opposed to relying on the use of seatbelts; providing health screenings in schools, workplaces, and other community settings rather than only through private physicians; providing health care to all citizens rather than only to those with the requisite resources; requiring window guards in all high-rise apartments rather than advising parents to watch their children carefully; thoroughly inspecting meat rather than advising consumers to wash cutting boards and cook meat thoroughly; adding folic acid to grains rather than recommending that supplements be taken by pregnant women to prevent neural tube defects in developing embryos; requiring landlords to keep homes free of lead paint hazards rather than warning parents to protect their toddlers from chipped paint. In some cases, such as this last example, existing risks will be greater in low-income neighborhoods and contexts, and special enforcement of these policies may be required in those contexts. In each example, the former solution does not give an advantage to those with greater resources, because individual resources are unrelated and irrelevant to benefiting from the intervention.

However, even if we become far more creative in developing contextually based interventions that blanket an entire population with health benefits, addressing many health problems will still require individual resources and action. In these cases, resource-rich persons are likely to fare better. Even in these cases, however, we can influence the trajectory of inequalities by attending to the type of interventions we adopt. When we create interventions that are expensive, complicated and time-consuming to carry out, and difficult to distribute broadly, we are likely to create health disparities (Chang and Lauderdale 2009). Conversely, to the extent that we develop interventions that are relatively affordable and easy to disseminate and use, we should be able to reduce the degree to which new interventions give advantage to high SES persons. Goldman and Lakdawalla (2005) analyzed two case studies supporting the idea that the introduction of difficult-to-implement treatments (in their analysis, HAART treatment for HIV/AIDS) lead to increased SES inequalities in health outcomes, whereas treatments that are simpler and require less effort (in their analysis, beta-blockers to reduce hypertension) reduce such inequalities. As Chang and Lauderdale (2009) suggest, this principle should also apply to cost: New interventions that are less expensive should result in smaller SES-based health inequalities than those that are more expensive. Chang and Lauderdale also point out,

importantly, that "technologies that have the potential to contract disparities will not do so unless they also diffuse broadly" (Chang and Lauderdale 2009:257). We add that a necessary ingredient of successful diffusion will be broadly disseminated and clearly stated information about how an intervention can help one's health, where that intervention is available, whether and how much of it is covered by health insurance plans, and, if not, how much it will cost individuals.

CONCLUSION

The theory of fundamental causes attempts to explain why the association of SES to health and mortality has persisted despite the demise of risk factors and diseases that appeared to explain the association. Mounting evidence in support of the theory of fundamental causes begins to suggest that the theory is not just an interesting idea but very possibly a valid explanation of persistent SES inequalities in health and mortality. We believe this empirical support warrants the investment of medical sociologists in (1) further empirical analyses using a variety of methodologies to give greater weight to the body of research, to specify and elaborate the processes at work, and to find conditions that may block these processes; and (2) developing elaborations, extensions, and modifications of the theory itself. We also believe the accumulated evidence warrants serious attention to the implications of the theory for health policy. Those implications are that, to achieve greater equality in matters of life, death, and health, the connection between socioeconomic resources and health-beneficial preventive measures and treatments must be broken or diminished, by reducing the magnitude of inequalities in socioeconomic resources themselves and/or by minimizing the extent to which socioeconomic resources buy a health advantage. By attending to these principles, we believe we can move toward the important dual goals of continuing to improve overall population health while distributing that health more equally.

Notes

1. We acknowledge recent debate and changes in guidelines with regard to screening interval and age at initiation of screening mammography and pap tests. However, convincing evidence supports the effectiveness of these screens in reducing cancer mortality and morbidity (U.S. Preventive Services Task Force 2009; ACOG Committee on Practice Bulletins— Gynecology 2009).

2. Fundamental cause theory was developed to explain the enduring effects of SES on health and mortality. It is possible that other social statuses, such as race, ethnicity, or gender, also have enduring associations with resources of money, knowledge, power, prestige, and beneficial social connections, and with health and mortality, and that they may also operate as fundamental causes. Even if not, however, race and ethnicity are currently strongly related to resources and consequently would be expected to behave similarly to SES in analyses such as Tehranifar's (Tehranifar et al. 2009), which focus on the current health context.

3. We thank David Mechanic for this insight.

4. Recent research suggests that when health behaviors of women come to resemble those of men more closely, the female mortality advantage declines (Preston and Wang 2006).

References

ACOG Committee on Practice Bulletins— Gynecology. 2009. "ACOG Practice Bulletin No. 109: Cervical Cytology Screening." *Obstetrics and Gynecology* 114: 1409–20.

Antonovsky, A. 1967. "Social Class, Life Expectancy, and Overall Mortality." *Milbank Memorial Quarterly* 45:31–73.

Black, Douglas, J. N. Morris, Cyril Smith, and Peter Townsend. 1982. *Inequalities in Health: The Black Report*. Middlesex, England: Penguin.

Carpiano, Richard M. and Brian C. Kelly. 2007. "Scientific Knowledge as Resource and Risk: What Does Hormone Replacement Tell Us About Health Disparities." Presented at the annual meeting of the American Sociological Association, August 2007, New York.

Chang, Virginia W. and Diane S. Lauderdale. 2009. "Fundamental Cause Theory, Technological Innovation, and Health Disparities: The Case of Cholesterol in the Era of Statins." *Journal of Health and Social Behavior* 50:245–60.

Cockerham, William. 2005. "Health Lifestyle Theory and the Convergence of Agency and Structure." *Journal of Health and Social Behavior* 46:51–67.

Courtenay, Will H. 2000. "Constructions of Masculinity and Their Influence on Men's Well-Being: A Theory of Gender and Health." *Social Science and Medicine* 50:1385–1401.

Dahl, Espen, Dag Hofoss, and Jon I. Elstad. 2007. "Educational Inequalities in Avoidable Deaths in Norway: A Population Based Study." *Health Sociology Review* 16:146–59.

Dutton, Diana H. 1978. "Explaining the Low Use of Health Services by the Poor: Costs, Attitude, or Delivery Systems." *American Sociological Review* 43:348–68.

Glied, Sherry and Adriana Lleras-Muney. 2008. "Technological Innovation and Inequality in Health." *Demography* 45:741–61.

Goldman, D. P. and D. N. Lakdawalla. 2005. "A Theory of Health Disparities and Medical

Technology." *Contributions to Economic Analysis and Policy* 4:1–30.

Haas, J. S., C. P. Kaplan, E. P. Gerstenberger, and K. Kerlikowske. 2004. "Changes in the Use of Postmenopausal Hormone Therapy after the Publication of Clinical Trial Results." *Annals of Internal Medicine* 140:184–88.

House, James S., Ronald C. Kessler, A. R. Herzog, R. P. Mero, A. M. Kinney, and M. J. Breslow. 1990. "Age, Socioeconomic Status, and Health." *The Milbank Quarterly* 68:383–411.

House, James S., James M. Lepkowski, Ann M. Kinney, Richard P. Mero, Ronald C. Kessler, and A. Regula Herzog. 1994. "The Social Stratification of Aging and Health." *Journal of Health and Social Behavior* 35:213–34.

House, James S. and David R. Williams. 2000. "Understanding and Reducing Socioeconomic and Racial/Ethnic Disparities in Health." Pp. 81–124 in *Promoting Health: Intervention Strategies from Social and Behavioral Research*, edited by B. D. Smedley and S.L. Syme. Washington, DC: National Academy Press.

Hulley, S., D. Grady, T. Bush, C. Furberg, D. Herrington, B. Riggs, and E. Vittinghoff. 1998. "Randomized Trial of Estrogen Plus Progestin for Secondary Prevention of Coronary Heart Disease in Postmenopausal Women: Heart and Estrogen/Progestin Replacement Study (HERS) Research Group." *Journal of the American Medical Association* 280:605–13.

Illsley, Raymond and Ken Mullen. 1985. "The Health Needs of Disadvantaged Client Groups." Pp. 389–402 in *Oxford Textbook of Public Health*, edited by W. W. Holland, R. Detels, and G. Know. Oxford, England: Oxford University Press.

Krieger, N., J.T. Chen, P.D. Waterman. 2010. "Decline in U.S. Breast Cancer Rates after the Women's Health Initiative: Socioeconomic and Racial/Ethnic Differentials." *American Journal of Public Health* 100: S132–S139.

Kunst, A. E., G. Feikje, and J. P. Mackenbach [EU Working Group on Socioeconomic Inequalities

in Health]. 1998. "Occupational Class and Cause Specific Mortality in Middle Aged Men in 11 European Countries: Comparison of Population Based Studies." *British Medical Journal* 316:1636–42.

Lantz, P. M., J. S. House, J. M. Lepkowski, D. R. Williams, R. P. Mero, and J. Chen. 1998. "Results from a Nationally Representative Prospective Study of U.S. Adults." *Journal of the American Medical Association* 279: 1703–08.

Lieberson, Stanley. 1985. *Making It Count: The Improvement of Social Research and Theory.* Berkeley: University of California Press.

Link, Bruce G. 2008. "Epidemiological Sociology and the Social Shaping of Population Health." *Journal of Health and Social Behavior* 49:367–84.

Link, Bruce G, M. Northridge, J. Phelan, and M. Ganz. 1998. "Social Epidemiology and the Fundamental Cause Concept: On the Structuring of Effective Cancer Screens by Socioeconomic Status." *The Milbank Quarterly* 76:375–402.

Link, Bruce G. and Jo C. Phelan. 1995. "Social Conditions as Fundamental Causes of Disease." *Journal of Health and Social Behavior* 35(Extra Issue):80–94.

———. Forthcoming. "Social Conditions as Fundamental Causes of Health Inequalities." In *Handbook of Medical Sociology*, 6th ed., edited by C. Bird, P. Conrad, and A. Fremont. Nashville, TN: Vanderbilt University Press.

Lutfey, Karen, and Jeremy Freese. 2005. "Toward Some Fundamentals of Fundamental Causality: Socioeconomic Status and Health in the Routine Clinic Visit for Diabetes." *American Journal of Sociology* 110: 1326–72.

Marshall, Stephen W., Ichiro Kawachi, Neil Pearce, and Barry Borman. 1993. "Social Class Differences in Mortality from Diseases Amenable to Medical Intervention in New Zealand." *International Journal of Epidemiology* 22: 255–61.

Maslow, A. H. 1943. "A Theory of Human Motivation." *Psychological Review* 50: 370–96.

Max-Neef, Manfred, Antonio Elizalde, and Martín Hopenhayn. 1989. "Human Scale Development: An Option for the Future." *Development Dialogue: A Journal of International Development Cooperation* 1: 7–80.

National Center for Health Statistics. 2008. *Health United States 2008: With Chartbook on Trends in the Health of Americans.* Hyattsville, MD.

Pamuk, E. R., D. Makuc, K. Heck, C. Reuben, and K. Lochner. 1998. *Socioeconomic Status and Health Chartbook: Health, United States, 1998.* Hyattsville, MD: National Center for Health Statistics.

Phelan, Jo C., and Bruce G. Link. 2005. "Controlling Disease and Creating Disparities: A Fundamental Cause Perspective." *The Journals of Gerontology* 60B (special issue II): 27–33.

Phelan, Jo C., Bruce G. Link, Ana Diez-Roux, Ichiro Kawachi, and Bruce Levin. 2004. "Fundamental Causes of Social Inequalities in Mortality: A Test of the Theory." *Journal of Health and Social Behavior* 45: 265–85.

Preston, S. H., and H. Wang. 2006. "Sex Mortality Differences in the United States: The Role of Cohort Smoking Patterns." *Demography* 43: 631–46.

Rosen, G. 1979. "The Evolution of Social Medicine." In *The Handbook of Medical Sociology,* 3rd ed., edited by H. Freeman, S. Levine, and L. Reeder, 23–50. Englewood Cliffs, NJ: Prentice Hall.

Ruberman, William, Eve Weinblatt, Judith D. Goldberg, and Banvir S. Chaudhary. 1984. "Psychological Influences on Mortality after Myocardial Infarction." *New England Journal of Medicine* 311: 552–59.

Song, Yun-Mi, and Jai Jun Byeon. 2000. "Excess Mortality from Avoidable and Non-Avoidable Causes in Men of Low Socioeconomic Status: A Prospective Study in Korea." *Journal of Epidemiology and Community Health* 54: 166–72.

Sorlie, P., M. Backlund, and J. Keller. 1995. "U.S. Mortality by Economic, Demographic, and Social Characteristics: The National Longitudinal Mortality Study." *American Journal of Public Health* 85: 949–56.

Tehranifar, P., A. I. Neugut, J. C. Phelan, B. G. Link, Y. Liao, M. Desai, and M. B. Terry. 2009. "Medical Advances and Racial/Ethnic Disparities in Cancer Survival." *Cancer Epidemiology, Biomarkers and Prevention* 18: 2701–08.

Turner, R. Jay, Blair Wheaton, and Donald A. Lloyd. 1995. "The Epidemiology of Social Stress." *American Sociological Review* 60: 104–25.

U.S. Preventive Services Task Force. 2009. "Screening for Breast Cancer: U.S. Preventive Services Task Force Recommendation Statement." *Annals of Internal Medicine* 151: 716–26.

WHO GETS SICK? THE UNEQUAL SOCIAL DISTRIBUTION OF DISEASE

Disease is not distributed evenly throughout populations. Certain groups of people get sick more often, and some populations are more likely than others to die prematurely. The study of which groups of people get sick with what diseases is called *epidemiology* and has been defined by one expert as "the study of the distributions and determinants of states of health in human populations" (Susser 1973, 1). By studying populations rather than individuals, epidemiologists seek to identify characteristics of groups of people or their environments that make them more or less vulnerable to disease (morbidity) or death (mortality).

A growing body of research has found significant associations between a range of social and cultural factors, and the risk for disease and death. The term *social epidemiology* has been adopted by some researchers to emphasize the importance of social variables in the patterning of disease (Berkman and Kawachi 2000). Social epidemiologists ask "Why is this society unhealthy?" (Kawachi 2002, 1,739). By focusing on the social factors that affect the social production of disease, social epidemiology provides the social scientist with an important opportunity to understand more fully the relationship between society and the individual. Among the historical predecessors of today's social epidemiology was the emergence in the nineteenth century of "social medicine" with a number of important studies in Western Europe. In England, Edwin Chadwick studied the death rates of populations and identified relationships between disease and social problems—most notably poverty—thus laying an important foundation for the developing public health movement, a nineteenth-century movement to prevent infectious disease, particularly through sanitation reforms (Chadwick 1842). Another early investigator in social medicine was Rudolf Virchow (1958), who was asked by the Prussian government to study the causes of a terrible typhus epidemic. His pioneering research identified connections between disease and a number of social factors, including the economy, conditions of work, and the organization of agriculture (Virchow 1868, 1879, in Waitzkin 1978). The readings in this section examine contemporary social factors that affect the distribution of disease, including social class, race, and gender. These studies highlight the relevance of a social epidemiological perspective and point to several promising directions for future research.

Across nations and across history, one of the most striking and consistent patterns in the distribution of disease is its relationship to poverty. By and large, death and disease rates vary inversely with social class; that is, the poorer the population, the higher the risk for sickness and death (Wagstaff 2002). While it has been known for well over a century that poor people suffer from more disease than others, just how poverty influences health is not yet well understood. There is also some evidence of the reverse relationship as well, that poor health may predict poorer economic outcomes (Subramanian, Belli, and Kawachi 2002).

Despite an overall decline in death rates in the United States, the poor are still dying at higher rates than those with higher incomes; in fact, the disparity between socioeconomic groups has actually increased (Pappas et al. 1993). Where once researchers thought that it was only poverty that created poor health outcomes, now there is evidence that there is a continuous impact of social class on health (Adler et al. 1994). That is, the health effects of socioeconomic status extend to all classes along a gradient from the lower to higher classes, although with more negative impacts in the lower classes. And now, some suggest that inequality is bad for society, including negative impacts on health (Wilkinson and Pickett 2010). While research on the links between social stratification and health is becoming more sophisticated and subtle, the evidence of the impact of social class on health remains stronger than ever (Robert and House 2000). In "Social

Class, Susceptibility, and Sickness," S. Leonard Syme and Lisa F. Berkman explore the relationship between social class and sickness, examining the influence of stress, living conditions, nutrition, and medical services on the patterns of death and disease among the poor. They focus on how the living conditions of the lower class may compromise the body's "disease defense systems" and engender greater vulnerability to disease.

In U.S. society, race and class are highly associated in that a disproportionate number of African Americans and other people of color are living in poverty. In general, African Americans have higher morbidity and mortality rates than do whites, and a shorter life expectancy (women 81.3 to 78.5, men 76.6 to 72.2 in 2015; National Center for Health Statistics 2016). Although the infant mortality (death before the age of one) rate in the United States has declined dramatically in this century, it remains over twice as high among African Americans compared to whites: 10.7 versus 4.9 per 1,000 live births (National Center for Health Statistics 2016). Between 1983 and 2003 the black–white life expectancy gap increased sharply and then declined. The decline resulted from mortality improvements in homicide, HIV, and unintentional injuries (Harper et al. 2007). Segregation plays an important part in shaping black–white health outcomes, and exposure to discrimination affects both physical and mental health (Williams and Sternthal 2010).

David R. Williams and Selina A. Mohammed review recent empirical research about how racism affects the health of people of color in "Racism and Health: Pathways and Scientific Evidence." They examine how institutional racism resulted in policies and procedures that reduced access to valuable resources in U.S. society, including housing, education, and neighborhood quality. At the cultural level, they demonstrate how hostile policy environments, negative stereotypes, and discrimination can result in health-damaging individual responses such as internalized racism. There is also increasing evidence that racial discrimination results in psychosocial stress, behavioral patterns, and adverse changes in health status. These efforts to explain the pathways between race and health have important implications for reducing racial and ethnic health disparities.

Gender is another powerful social determinant of health and illness. In the United States and other Western societies, women have higher illness rates than men, while men have higher death rates. There is a great deal of disagreement about the explanation for these patterns, including debates over whether women actually do get sick more often than men or whether they are more likely to report symptoms or seek medical care (e.g., Muller 1991; Waldron 2000; Gove and Hughes 1979). Growing feminist scholarship on women's health and more recent epidemiological interest in studying patterns of physical disease in female populations have begun to clarify the debate. It now appears that women *do* in fact have higher rates of sickness than men *and* that they are more likely than men to report symptoms and use medical services. Rachel C. Snow broadens this inquiry into the connections between gender and health in "Sex, Gender, and Vulnerability." Snow uses international data to compare health outcomes for males and females, disentangling the ways in which biological and social factors may make individuals vulnerable to chronic illness and disability. She is heartened that many of the differences between males and females can be attributed to gender rather than biology, because that makes them more amenable to social intervention. For example, it is well known that men's greater propensity to risky behaviors (e.g., smoking, drinking, occupational hazards) affects male longevity; it is also true that changing women's and men's behaviors narrowed the gap of life expectancy in developed countries (cf. Trovato and Lalu 2001). The question of longevity posed here is not only how long people live but how healthy their life expectancies will be (Crimmins and Saito 2001). While it is important to acknowledge *intergender* differences (that is, differences between male and female populations), we must be careful not to ignore *intragender* patterns (that is, patterns among men or among women). The distribution of disease and death within male and female populations is patterned by other social factors, including social class, race, age, marital status, presence and number of children in the home, employment outside the home, and other social roles (e.g., Rieker, Bird, and Lang 2010; Waldron 2000).

In medical sociology and social epidemiology, we have amassed tremendous evidence regarding the social determinants of health. Now that we documented extensively the ways in which social factors shape health outcomes, there are increasing attempts to make this knowledge relevant to health care providers. In "Structural Violence and Clinical Medicine," Paul Farmer and his colleagues point out the urgent need for biosocial understandings of health phenomena, bringing the analysis of social determinants of health into clinical medicine. In doing so, they rely on the concept of "structural violence," the ways in which social structures can inflict harm upon individuals, such as unequal access to education, political power, and health care. They argue that clinicians are not trained to understand these forces, nor to alter them, and go on to describe the social and political context behind the HIV/AIDS epidemics in the United States, Rwanda, and Haiti. Their call for "resocializing" our understandings of disease is an attempt to apply our knowledge about social epidemiology.

Clearly, there is a need for a new and broader conceptualization of disease production than the traditional medical model can provide. Attention must shift from the individual to the social and physical environments in which people live and work. The development of an adequate model of disease production must draw on the conceptual and research contributions of multiple disciplines not only to identify the social production of diseases, but to elaborate this process and provide important information on which to base effective primary intervention and prevention strategies.

The final selection in this section, John B. McKinlay's "A Case for Refocusing Upstream: The Political Economy of Illness," is a classic medical sociology article that frames prevention in structural terms. McKinlay argues that we need to change the way we think about prevention and start to "refocus upstream," beyond lifestyle and healthy habits to the structure of society. He suggests that we concentrate on and investigate political–economic aspects of disease, paying particular attention to what he calls "the manufacturers of illness." In this article, he singles out the food industry as a major manufacturer of illness; one could examine the tobacco (McKinlay and Marceau 2000) or the alcohol industries in this manner as well. McKinlay's major contribution in this selection is to go beyond the conventional view of prevention as a biomedical or lifestyle problem to conceptualize prevention as a socioeconomic issue.

References

Adler, Nancy E., Thomas Boyce, Margaret A. Chesney, Sheldon Cohen, Susan Folkman, Robert L. Kahn, and Leonard Syme. 1994. "Socioeconomic Status and Health: The Challenge of the Gradient." *American Psychologist* 49: 15–24.

Berkman, Lisa F., and Ichiro Kawachi. 2000. *Social Epidemiology.* New York: Oxford University Press.

Chadwick, Edwin. 1842. *Report on the Sanitary Condition of the Labouring Population of Great Britain.* Reprinted 1965. Edinburgh: Edinburgh University Press.

Crimmins, Eileen M., and Yasuhiko Saito. 2001. "Trends in Healthy Life Expectancy in the United States, 1970–1990: Gender, Racial and Educational Differences." *Social Science and Medicine* 52: 1629–41.

Gove, Walter, and Michael Hughes. 1979. "Possible Causes of the Apparent Sex Differences in Physical Health: An Empirical Investigation." *American Sociological Review* 44: 126–46.

Harper, Sam, John Lynch, Scott Burris, and Georg Davey Smith. 2007. "Trends in the Black-White Life Expectancy Gap in the United States:

1983–2003." *Journal of the American Medical Association* 297: 1224–32.

Kawachi, Ichiro. 2002. "What Is Social Epidemiology?" *Social Science & Medicine* 54:1739–41.

McKinlay, John B., and Lisa D. Marceau. 2000. "Upstream Healthy Public Policy: Lessons from the Battle of Tobacco." *International Journal of Health Services* 30: 49–69.

Muller, Charlotte. 1991. *Health Care and Gender.* New York: Russell Sage.

National Center for Health Statistics. 2016. *Health, United States, 2016: With Special Chartbook on Long-Term Trends in Health.* Hyattsville, MD. Accessed November 10, 2017. https://www.cdc.gov/nchs/data/hus/hus16.pdf#015.

Pappas, Gregory, Susan Queen, Wilbur Hadden, and Gail Fisher. 1993. "The Increasing Disparity in Mortality Between Socioeconomic Groups in the United States, 1960 and 1986." *New England Journal of Medicine* 329: 103–9.

Rieker, Patricia P., Chloe E. Bird, and Martha E. Lang. 2010. "Understanding Gender and Health: Old Patterns, New Trends, and Future Directions." In *Handbook of Medical Sociology,* 6th edition, edited by Chloe E. Bird, Peter Conrad, Allen M. Fremont, and Stefan Timmermans, 52–74. Upper Saddle River, NJ: Prentice Hall.

Robert, Stephanie A., and James S. House. 2000. "Socioeconomic Inequalities in Health: An Enduring Sociological Problem." In *Handbook of Medical Sociology,* 5th edition, edited by Chloe E. Bird, Peter Conrad, and Allen M. Fremont, 79–97. Upper Saddle River, NJ: Prentice Hall.

Subramanian, S.V., P. Belli, and I. Kawachi. 2002. "The Macroeconomic Determinants of Health. *Annual Review of Public Health* 23: 287–302.

Susser, Mervyn. 1973. *Causal Thinking in the Health Sciences: Concepts and Strategies in Epidemiology.* New York: Oxford University Press.

Trovato, Frank, and N. M. Lalu. 2001. "Narrowing Sex Differences in Life Expectancy: Regional Variations, 1971–1991." *Canadian Studies in Population* 28: 89–110.

Virchow, Rudolf. 1958. *Disease, Life and Man.* Translated by Lelland J. Rather. Stanford: Stanford University Press.

Wagstaff, Adam. 2002. "Poverty and Health Sector Inequalities." *Bulletin of the World Health Organization* 80: 97–105.

Waitzkin, Howard. 1978. "A Marxist View of Medical Care." *Annals of Internal Medicine* 89: 264–278.

Waldron, Ingrid. 2000. "Trends in Gender Differences in Mortality: Relationships to Changing Gender Differences in Behavior and Other Causal Factors." In *Gender Inequalities in Health,* edited by E. Annandale and K. Hunt. Buckingham: Open University Press.

Wilkinson, Richard G., and Kate Pickett. 2010. *The Spirit Level: Why Equality is Better for Everyone.* London: Penguin.

Williams, David R., and Michelle Sternthal. 2010. "Understanding Racial-Ethnic Disparities in Health: Sociological Contributions. *Journal of Health and Social Behavior* 51: S15-S27.

SOCIAL CLASS, SUSCEPTIBILITY, AND SICKNESS

S. Leonard Syme and Lisa F. Berkman

Social class gradients of mortality and life expectancy have been observed for centuries, and a vast body of evidence has shown consistently that those in the lower classes have higher mortality, morbidity, and disability rates. While these patterns have been observed repeatedly, the explanations offered to account for them show no such consistency. The most frequent explanations have included poor housing, crowding, racial factors, low income, poor education and unemployment, all of which have been said to result in such outcomes as poor nutrition, poor medical care (either through non-availability or non-utilization of resources), strenuous conditions of employment in non-hygienic settings, and increased exposure to noxious agents. While these explanations account for some of the observed relationships, we have found them inadequate to explain the very large number of diseases associated with socioeconomic status. It seemed useful, therefore, to reexamine these associations in search of a more satisfactory hypothesis.

Obviously, this is an important issue. It is clear that new approaches must be explored emphasizing the primary prevention of disease in addition to those approaches that merely focus on treatment of the sick (1). It is clear also that such preventive approaches must involve community and environmental interventions rather than one-to-one preventive encounters (2). Therefore, we must understand more precisely those features of the environment that are etiologically related to disease so that interventions at this level can be more intelligently planned.

Of all the disease outcomes considered, it is evident that low socioeconomic status is most strikingly associated with high rates of infectious and parasitic diseases (3–7) as well as with higher infant mortality rates (8, 9). However, in our review we found higher rates among lower class groups of a very much wider range of diseases and conditions for which obvious explanations were not as easily forthcoming. In a comprehensive review of over 30

Social Class, Susceptibility, and Sickness, S. Leonard Syme and Lisa F. Berkman in *The American Journal of Epidemiology,* Vol. 104, No. 1, pp. 1–8, July 1976. With permission from Oxford University Press.

studies, Antonovsky (10) concluded that those in the lower classes invariably have lower life expectancy and higher death rates from all causes of death, and that this higher rate has been observed since the 12th century when data on this question were first organized. While differences in infectious disease and infant mortality rates probably accounted for much of this difference between the classes in earlier years, current differences must primarily be attributable to mortality from noninfectious disease.

Kitagawa and Hauser (11) recently completed a massive nationwide study of mortality in the United States. Among men and women in the 25–64-year age group, mortality rates varied dramatically by level of education, income, and occupation, considered together or separately:

> For example, ... white males at low education levels had age-adjusted mortality rates 64 per cent higher than men in higher education categories. For white women, those in lower education groups had an age-adjusted mortality rate 105 per cent higher. For nonwhite males, the differential was 31 per cent and, for non-white females, it was 70 per cent. These mortality differentials also were reflected in substantial differences in life expectancy, and ... for most specific causes of death. ... White males in the lowest education groups have higher age-adjusted mortality rates for every cause of death for which data are available. For white females, those in the lowest education group have an excess mortality rate for all causes except cancer of the breast and motor vehicle accidents.

These gradients of mortality among the social classes have been observed over the world by many investigators (12–18) and have not changed materially since 1900 (except that non-whites, especially higher status non-whites, have experienced a relatively more favorable improvement). This consistent finding in time and space is all the more remarkable since the concept of "social class" has been defined and measured in so many different ways by these investigators.

That the same findings have been obtained in spite of such methodological differences lends strength to the validity of the observations; it suggests also that the concept is an imprecise term encompassing diverse elements of varying etiologic significance.

In addition to data on mortality, higher rates of morbidity also have been observed for a vast array of conditions among those in lower class groups (19–28). This is an important observation since it indicates that excess mortality rates among lower status groups are not merely attributable to a higher case fatality death rate in those groups but are accompanied also by a higher prevalence of morbidity. Of special interest in this regard are data on the various mental illnesses, a major cause of morbidity. As shown by many investigators (29–35), those in lower as compared to higher socioeconomic groups have higher rates of schizophrenia, are more depressed, more unhappy, more worried, more anxious, and are less hopeful about the future.

In summary, persons in lower class groups have higher morbidity and mortality rates of almost every disease or illness, and these differentials have not diminished over time. While particular hypotheses may be offered to explain the gradient for one or another of these specific diseases, the fact that so many diseases exhibit the same gradient leads to speculation that a more general explanation may be more appropriate than a series of disease-specific explanations.

In a study reported elsewhere (36), it was noted that although blacks had higher rates of hypertension than whites, blacks in the lower classes had higher rates of hypertension than blacks in the upper classes. An identical social class gradient for hypertension was noted among whites in the sample. In that report, it was concluded that hypertension was associated more with social class than with racial factors, and it was suggested that the greater prevalence of obesity in the lower class might be a possible explanation. The present review makes that earlier suggestion far less attractive since so many diseases and conditions appear to be of higher prevalence in the lower class groups. It seems clear that we must frame hypotheses of sufficient generality to account for this phenomenon.

One hypothesis that has been suggested is that persons in the lower classes either have less access to medical care resources or, if care is available, that they do not benefit from that availability. This possibility should be explored in more detail, but current evidence available does not suggest that differences in medical care resources will entirely explain social class gradients in disease. The hypertension project summarized previously was conducted at the Kaiser Permanente facility in Oakland, California, which is a prepaid health plan with medical facilities freely available to all study subjects. The data in this study showed that persons in lower status groups had utilized medical resources more frequently than those in higher status categories (37). To study the influence of medical care in explaining these differences in blood pressure levels, all persons in the Kaiser study who had ever been clinically diagnosed as hypertensive, or who had ever taken medicine for high blood pressure, were removed from consideration. Differences in blood pressure level between those in the highest and lowest social classes were diminished when hypertensives were removed from analysis, but those in the lowest class still had higher (normal) pressures. Thus, while differences in medical care may have accounted for some of the variation observed among the social class groups, substantial differences in blood pressures among these groups nevertheless remained. Similar findings have been reported from studies at the Health Insurance Plan of New York (38).

Lipworth and colleagues (39) also examined this issue in a study of cancer survival rates among various income groups in Boston. In that study, low-income persons had substantially less favorable one and three-year survival rates following treatment at identical tumor clinics and hospitals; these differences were not accounted for by differences in stage of cancer at diagnosis, by the age of patients, or by the specific kind of treatment patients received. It was concluded that patients from lower income areas simply did not fare as well following treatment for cancer. While it is still possible that lower class patients received less adequate medical care, the differences observed in survival rates did not seem attributable to the more obvious variations in quality of treatment. Other studies support this general conclusion but not enough data are available to assess clearly the role of medical care in explaining social class gradients in morbidity and mortality; it would seem, however, that the medical care hypothesis does not account for a major portion of these gradients.

Another possible explanation offered to explain these consistent differences is that persons in lower socioeconomic groups live in a more toxic, hazardous and non-hygienic environment resulting in a broad array of disease consequences. That these environments exert an influence on disease outcome is supported by research on crowding and rheumatic fever (5), poverty areas and health (40), and on air pollution and respiratory illnesses (41). While lower class groups certainly are exposed to a more physically noxious environment, physical factors alone are frequently unable to explain observed relationships between socioeconomic status and disease outcome. One example of this is provided by the report of Guerrin and Borgatta (16) showing that the proportion of people who are illiterate in a census tract is a more important indicator of tuberculosis occurrence than are either economic or racial variables. Similarly, the work of Booth (42) suggests that perceived crowding which is not highly correlated with objective measures of crowding may have adverse effects on individuals.

There can be little doubt that the highest morbidity and mortality rates observed in the lower social classes are in part due to inadequate medical care services as well as to the impact of a toxic and hazardous physical environment. There can be little doubt, also, that these factors do not entirely explain the discrepancy in rates between the classes. Thus, while enormous improvements have been made in environmental quality and in medical care, the mortality rate gap between the classes has not diminished. It is true that mortality rates have been declining over the years, and it is probably true also that this benefit is attributable in large part to the enormous improvements that have been made in food and water purity, in sanitary engineering, in literacy and health education, and in medical and surgical knowledge. It is important to recognize, however, that these reductions in mortality rates have not eliminated the gap between the highest and the lowest social class groups; this gap remains very substantial and has apparently stabilized during the last 40 years. Thus, while improvements in the environment and in medical care clearly have been of value, other factors must be identified to account for this continuing differential in mortality rate and life expectancy.

The identification of these new factors might profitably be guided by the repeated observation of social class gradients in a wide range of disease distributions. That so many different kinds of diseases are more frequent in lower class groupings directs attention to generalized susceptibility to disease and to generalized compromises of disease defense systems. Thus, if something about life in the lower social classes increases vulnerability to illness in general, it would not be surprising to observe an increased prevalence of many different types of diseases and conditions among people in the lower classes.

While laboratory experiments on both humans and animals have established that certain "stressful events" have physiologic consequences, very little is known about the nature of these "stressful events" in non-laboratory settings. Thus, while we may conclude that "something" about the lower class environment is stressful, we know much less about what specifically constitutes that stress. Rather than attempting to identify *specific* risk factors for *specific* diseases in investigating this question, it may be more meaningful to identify those factors that affect *general* susceptibility to disease. The specification of such factors should rest on the identification of variables having a wide range of disease outcomes. One such risk factor may be life change associated with social and cultural mobility. Those experiencing this type of mobility have been observed to have higher rates of diseases and conditions such as coronary heart disease (43–46), lung cancer (47), difficulties of pregnancy (48, 49), sarcoidosis (50), and depression (30). Another risk factor may be certain life events; those experiencing what are commonly called stressful life events have been shown to have higher rates of a wide variety of diseases and conditions (51–57).

Generalized susceptibility to disease may be influenced not only by the impact of various forms of life change and life stress, but also by differences in the way people cope with such stress. Coping, in this sense, refers not to specific types of psychological responses but to the more generalized ways in which people deal with problems in their everyday life. It is evident that such coping styles are likely to be products of environmental situations and not independent of such factors. Several coping responses that have a wide range of disease outcomes have been described. Cigarette smoking is one such coping response that has been associated with virtually all causes of morbidity and mortality (58); obesity may be another coping style associated with a higher rate of many diseases and conditions (59, 60); pattern A behavior is an example of a third coping response that has been shown to have relatively broad disease consequences (61). There is some evidence that persons in the lower classes experience more life changes (62) and that they tend to be more obese and to smoke more cigarettes (63, 64).

To explain the differential in morbidity and mortality rates among the social classes, it is important to identify additional factors that affect susceptibility and have diverse disease consequences; it is also important to determine which of these factors are more prevalent in the lower classes. Thus, our understanding would be enhanced if it could be shown not only that those in the lower classes live in a more toxic physical environment with inadequate medical care, but also that they live in a social and psychological environment that increases their vulnerability to a whole series of diseases and conditions.

In this paper, we have emphasized the variegated disease consequences of low socioeconomic status. Any proposed explanations of this phenomenon should be capable of accounting for this general outcome. The proposal offered here is that those in the lower classes consistently have higher rates of disease in part due to compromised disease defenses and increased general susceptibility. To explore this proposal further, systematic research is needed on four major problems:

1. The more precise identification and description of subgroups within the lower socioeconomic classes that have either markedly higher or lower rates of disease:

Included in what is commonly called the "lower class" are semiskilled working men with stable work and family situations, unemployed men with and without families, the rural and urban poor, hard core unemployed persons, and so on. The different disease experiences of these heterogeneous subgroups would permit a more precise understanding of the processes involved in disease etiology and would permit a more precise definition of social class groupings.

2. The disentanglement of socio-environmental from physical-environmental variables: It is important to know whether high rates of illness and discontent in a poverty area, for example, are due to the poor physical circumstances of life in such an area, to the social consequences of life in such an area, or to the personal characteristics of individuals who come to live in the area.

3. The clarification of "causes" and "effects": The implication in this paper has been that the lower class environment "leads to" poor health. Certainly, the reverse situation is equally likely. Many measures of social class position may be influenced by the experience of ill health itself. Further research is needed to clarify the relative importance of the "downward drift" hypothesis. One way of approaching such study is to use measures of class position that are relatively unaffected by illness experience. An example of one such measure is "educational achievement" as used by Kitagawa and Hauser (11). In this

study, educational level was assumed to be relatively stable after age 20 and was felt to be a measure relatively unaffected by subsequent illness experience.

4. The more comprehensive description of those psycho-social variables that may compromise bodily defense to disease and increase susceptibility to illness: The possible importance of life events, life changes, and various coping behavior has been suggested but systematic research needs to be done to provide a more complete view of the factors involved in this process. Of particular interest would be research on the ways in which social and familial support networks (48, 55) mediate between the impact of life events and stresses and disease outcomes.

The research that is needed should not be limited to the study of the specific risk factors as these affect specific diseases. Instead, the major focus of this research should be on those general features of lower class living environments that compromise bodily defense and thereby affect health and well-being in general. This research should go beyond the superficial description of demographic variables associated with illness and should attempt the identification of specific etiologic factors capable of accounting for the observed morbidity and mortality differences between the social classes.

The gap in mortality and life expectancy between the social classes has stabilized and may be increasing; the identification of those factors that render people vulnerable to disease will hopefully provide a basis for developing more meaningful prevention programs aimed toward narrowing the gap.

References and Notes

1. Winkelstein W Jr, French FE: The role of ecology in the design of a health care system. Calif Med 113:7–12, 1970.
2. Marmot M, Winkelstein W Jr: Epidemiologic observations on intervention trials for

prevention of coronary heart disease. Am J Epidemiol 101:177–181, 1975.
3. Tuberculosis and Socioeconomic Status. Stat Bull, January 1970.

4. Terris M: Relation of economic status to tuberculosis mortality by age and sex. Am J Public Health 38:1061–1071, 1948.

5. Gordis L, Lilienfeld A, Rodriquez R: Studies in the epidemiology and preventability of rheumatic fever. II. Socioeconomic factors and the incidence of acute attacks. J Chronic Dis 21:655–666, 1969.

6. Influenza and Pneumonia Mortality in the U.S., Canada and Western Europe. Stat Bull, April 1972.

7. Court SDM: Epidemiology and natural history of respiratory infections in children. J Clin Pathol 21:31, 1968.

8. Chase HC (ed): A study of risks, medical care and infant mortality. Am J Public Health 63: supplement, 1973.

9. Lerner M: Social differences in physical health. *In:* Poverty and Health. Edited by J Kozsa, A Antonovsky, IK Zola. Cambridge, Harvard University Press, 1969, pp 69–112.

10. Antonovsky A: Social class, life expectancy and overall mortality. Milbank Mem Fund Q 45: 31–73, 1967.

11. Kitagawa EM, Hauser PM: Differential Mortality in the United States. Cambridge, Harvard University Press, 1973.

12. Nagi MH, Stockwell EG: Socioeconomic differentials in mortality by cause of death. Health Serv Rep 88:449–465, 1973.

13. Ellis JM: Socio-economic differentials in mortality from chronic disease. *In:* Patients, Physicians and Illness. Edited by EG Jaco. Glencoe, Ill, The Free Press, 1958, pp 30–37.

14. Yeracaris J: Differential mortality, general and cause-specific in Buffalo, 1939–1941. J Am Stat Assoc 50:1235–1247, 1955.

15. Brown SM, Selvin S, Winkelstein W Jr: The association of economic status with the occurrence of lung cancer. Cancer 36:1903–1911, 1975.

16. Guerrin RF, Borgatta EF: Socio-economic and demographic correlates of tuberculosis incidence. Milbank Mem Fund Q 43:269–290, 1965.

17. Graham S: Socio-economic status, illness, and the use of medical services. Milbank Mem Fund Q 35:58–66, 1957.

18. Cohart EM: Socioeconomic distribution of stomach cancer in New Haven. Cancer 7:455–461, 1954.

19. Socioeconomic Differentials in Mortality. Stat Bull, June 1972.

20. Hart JT: Too little and too late. Data on occupational mortality, 1959–1963. Lancet 1:192–193, 1972.

21. Wan T: Social differentials in selected work-limiting chronic conditions. J Chronic Dis 25: 365–374, 1972.

22. Hochstim JR, Athanasopoulos DA, Larkins JH: Poverty area under the microscope. Am J Public Health 58:1815–1827, 1968.

23. Burnight RG: Chronic morbidity and socioeconomic characteristics of older urban males. Mil-bank Mem Fund Q 43:311–322, 1965.

24. Elder R, Acheson RM: New Haven survey of joint diseases. XIV. Social class and behavior in response to symptoms of osteoarthritis. Milbank Mem Fund Q 48:499–502, 1970.

25. Cobb S: The epidemiology of rheumatoid disease. *In:* The Frequency of Rheumatoid Disease. Edited by S Cobb. Cambridge, Harvard University Free Press, 1971, pp 42–62.

26. Graham S: Social factors in the relation to chronic illness. *In:* Handbook of Medical Sociology. Edited by HE Freeman, S Levine, LG Reeder. Englewood Cliffs, NJ, Prentice-Hall Inc, 1963, pp 65–98.

27. Wan T: Status stress and morbidity: A sociological investigation of selected categories of working-limiting conditions. J Chronic Dis 24:453–468, 1971.

28. Selected Health Characteristics by Occupation, U.S. July 1961–June 1963.

National Health Center for Health Statistics, Series 10 21:1–16, 1965.

29. Abramson JH: Emotional disorder, status inconsistency and migration. Milbank Mem Fund Q 44:23–48, 1966.

30. Schwab JJ, Holzer CE III, Warheit GJ: Depression scores by race, sex, age, family income, education and socioeconomic status. (Personal communication, 1974).

31. Srole L, Langner T, Michael S, et al: Mental Health in the Metropolis: the Midtown Study. New York, McGraw-Hill, 1962.

32. Jackson EF: Status consistency and symptoms of stress. Am Sociol Rev 27:469–480, 1962.

33. Hollingshead AB, Redlich FC: Social Class and Mental Illness. New York, John Wiley and Sons Inc. 1958.

34. Gurin G, Veroff J, Feld S: Americans View Their Mental Health. New York, Basic Books Inc. 1960.

35. Langner TS: Psychophysiological symptoms and the status of women in two Mexican communities. *In:* Approaches to Cross-cultural Psychiatry. Edited by AH Leighton, JM Murphy. Ithaca, Cornell University Press, 1965. pp 360–392.

36. Syme SL, Oakes T, Friedman G, et al: Social class and racial differences in blood pressure. Am J Public Health 64:619–620, 1974.

37. Oakes TW, Syme SL: Social factors in newly discovered elevated blood pressure. J Health Soc Behav 14:198–204, 1973.

38. Fink R, Shapiro S, Hyman MD, et al: Health status of poverty and non-poverty groups in multiphasic health testing. Presented at the Annual Meeting of the American Public Health Association, November 1972.

39. Lipworth L, Abelin T, Connelly RR: Socioeconomic factors in the prognosis of cancer patients. J Chronic Dis 23:105–116, 1970.

40. Hochstim JR: Health and ways of living. *In:* Social Surveys. The Community as an Epidemiological Laboratory. Edited by I Kessler, M Levine. Baltimore, Johns Hopkins Press, 1970, pp 149–176.

41. Winkelstein W Jr, Kantor S, Davis EW, et al: The relationship of air pollution and economic status to total mortality and selected respiratory system mortality in men. I. Suspended particulates. Arch Environ Health 14:162–171, 1967.

42. Booth A: Preliminary Report: Urban Crowding Project. Canada, Ministry of State for Urban Affairs, August 1974 (mimeographed).

43. Syme SL, Hyman MM, Enterline PE: Some social and cultural factors associated with the occurrence of coronary heart disease. J Chronic Dis 17:277–289, 1964.

44. Tyroler HA, Cassel J: Health consequences of cultural change. II. The effect of urbanization on coronary heart mortality in rural residents. J Chronic Dis 17:167–177, 1964.

45. Nesser WB, Tyroler HA, Cassel JC: Social disorganization and stroke mortality in the black populations of North Carolina. Am J Epidemiol 93: 166–175, 1971.

46. Shekelle RB, Osterfeld AM, Paul O: Social status and incidence of coronary heart disease. J Chronic Dis 22:381–394, 1969.

47. Haenszel W, Loveland DB, Sirken N: Lung-cancer mortality as related to residence and smoking histories. I. White males. J Natl Cancer Inst 28: 947–1001, 1962.

48. Nuckolls KB, Cassel J, Kaplan BH: Psychosocial assets, life crisis, and the prognosis of pregnancy. Am J Epidemiol 95:431–441, 1972.

49. Gorusch RL, Key MK: Abnormalities of pregnancy as a function of anxiety and life stress. Psychosom Med 36:352–362, 1974.

50. Terris M, Chaves AD: An epidemiologic study of sarcoidosis. Am Rev Respir Dis 94:50–55, 1966.

51. Rahe RH, Gunderson EKE, Arthur RJ: Demographic and psychosocial factors in acute illness reporting. J Chronic Dis 23:245–255, 1970.

52. Wyler AR, Masuda M, Holmes TH: Magnitude of life events and seriousness of illness. Psychosom Med 33:115–122, 1971.

53. Rahe RH, Rubin RT, Gunderson EKE, et al: Psychological correlates of serum cholesterol in man: A longitudinal study. Psychosom Med 33: 399– 410, 1971.

54. Spilken AZ, Jacobs MA: Prediction of illness behavior from measures of life crisis, manifest distress and maladaptive coping. Psychosom Med 33:251–264, 1971.

55. Jacobs MA, Spilken AZ, Martin MA, et al: Life stress and respiratory illness. Psychosom Med 32: 233–242, 1970.

56. Kasl SV, Cobb S: Blood pressure changes in men undergoing job loss; A preliminary report. Psychosom Med 32:19–38, 1970.

57. Hinkle LE, Wolff HG: Ecological investigations of the relationship between illness, life experiences, and the social environment. Ann Intern Med 49:1373–1388, 1958.

58. US Dept of Health, Education, and Welfare: The Health Consequences of Smoking. National Communicable Disease Center, Publication No 74-8704, 1974.

59. US Public Health Service, Division of Chronic Diseases: Obesity and Health. A Source Book of Current Information for Professional Health Personnel. Publication No 1485. Washington DC, US GPO, 1966.

60. Build and Blood Pressure Study. Chicago, Society of Actuaries, Vol I and II, 1959.

61. Rosenman RH, Brand RH, Jenkins CD, et al: Coronary heart disease in the Western collaborative group study: Final follow-up experience of 81/2 years. (Manuscript).

62. Dohrenwend BS (ed): Stressful Life Events: Their Nature and Effects. New York, Wiley-Interscience, 1974.

63. US Dept of Health, Education, and Welfare: Adult Use of Tobacco 1970, Publication No HSM-738727, 1973.

64. Khosla T, Lowe CR: Obesity and smoking habits by social class. J Prev Soc Med 26:249–256, 1972.

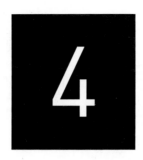

RACISM AND HEALTH

Pathways and Scientific Evidence

David R. Williams and Selina A. Mohammed

In the United States, as in other racialized countries in the world, racially stigmatized and disenfranchised populations have worse health than their more advantaged counterparts (D. Williams, 2012). The poorer health of these racial minority populations is evident in higher rates of mortality, earlier onset of disease, greater severity and progression of disease, and higher levels of comorbidity and impairment. In addition, disadvantaged racial populations tend to have both lower levels of access to medical care and to receive care that is poorer in quality. In U.S. data, these patterns tend to be evident for African Americans (or Blacks), American Indians (or Native Americans), Native Hawaiians and other Pacific Islanders, and economically disadvantaged Hispanic (or Latino) and Asian immigrants with long-term residence in the United States (D. Williams, 2012). These striking disparities are persistent over time and, although reduced, are evident at every level of income and education (Braveman, Cubbin, Egerter, Williams, & Pamuk, 2010; D. Williams, 2012). In recent years, increased attention has been given to the role of racism as a determinant of these patterns of racial inequality in health.

This article describes the complex nature of contemporary racism in the United States. To identify the leverage points for intervention, it outlines the multiple ways in which racism can affect health. First, it provides a brief overview of the empirical evidence that reveals that institutional racism shapes socioeconomic status (SES) and opportunities in a variety of ways. Next, it shows that research reveals that cultural racism, with its associated, negative images, stereotypes, and prejudice, can be damaging to health. Finally, it highlights the research indicating that interpersonal discrimination is a potent psychosocial stressor that has pervasive negative effects on health.

Racism and Health: Pathways and Scientific Evidence, David R. Williams and Selina A. Mohammed in *American Behavioral Scientist* S7(8), 1152–1173. Copyright © 2013 SAGE Publications. Reprinted with permission.

OVERVIEW OF THE NATURE OF RACISM AND ITS PERSISTENCE

Racism is an organized system premised on the categorization and ranking of social groups into races and devalues, disempowers, and differentially allocates desirable societal opportunities and resources to racial groups regarded as inferior (Bonilla-Silva, 1996; D. Williams, 2004). Racism often leads to the development of negative attitudes (prejudice) and beliefs (stereotypes) toward nondominant, stigmatized racial groups and differential treatment (discrimination) of these groups by both individuals and social institutions. These multiple dimensions of racism do not always co-occur. For example, it is possible for racism to exist in institutional structures and policies without the presence of racial prejudice or negative racial stereotypes at the individual level.

Despite progress in the reduction of explicit public support of racism in the United States, there is also strong evidence of its persistence. National data on the racial attitudes of Whites reveal positive changes over time in support of the principle of racial equality (Schuman, Steeh, Bobo, & Krysan, 1997). For example, the percentage of Whites supporting the view that "White people should have the first chance at any kind of job" fell from 55% in 1944 to 3% in 1972. At the same time, support for laws and policies to achieve equality lags behind the support for the principle of equality (Schuman et al., 1997). For example, in spite of increased support for the principle of equality and the advent of laws that prohibit discrimination, Whites' support for the federal government's efforts to ensure that Black people get fair treatment in jobs declined from 38% in 1964 to 28% in 1996.

Several lines of evidence support the notion that racism persists in contemporary society. First, many Americans believe that racism remains a problem in the United States. At the time of President Obama's inauguration in 2009, 85% of Blacks and 71% of Whites saw racism as a somewhat big (41% vs. 49%, respectively) or big problem (44% vs. 22%,

respectively) in the United States (Washington Post Company, 2009). A 2012 national survey found that 67% of Whites and 90% of Blacks agreed that Blacks and Hispanics currently experience discrimination in the United States, and 74% of Blacks and 31% of Whites indicated that they had personally experienced racial discrimination (Schoen, 2012). At the same time, other national data reveal that Whites now believe that they are more likely to be victims of racial discrimination than Blacks (Norton & Sommers, 2011).

Documenting the persistence of racism is a challenge because the nature of racism in contemporary society has also changed in ways that make it not readily recognizable to most adults. Scientific evidence indicates that in addition to conscious, deliberate cognitive processes, humans also engage in implicit (unconscious), effortless, automatic, evaluative processes in which they respond to a stimulus based on images stored in their memory (Dovidio & Gaertner, 2004). For example, Americans manifest high levels of negative feelings and beliefs about Blacks, Latinos, obese people, and homosexuals (Nosek et al., 2007). *Aversive racism* is one of the terms used to characterize contemporary racism (Dovidio & Gaertner, 2004). An aversive racist lacks explicit racial prejudice (that is, has sympathy for those who were victimized by injustice in the past and is committed to principles of racial equality) but has implicit biases that favor Whites over Blacks. Research suggests that almost 70% of Americans have implicit biases that favor Whites over Blacks (Nosek et al., 2007). The pattern is most pronounced among Whites but is also evident for Asians, Hispanics, and American Indians. These high levels of implicit bias suggests that discrimination is likely to be commonplace in American society, with much of it occurring through behaviors that the perpetrator does not experience as intentional (Dovidio & Gaertner, 2004).

Discrimination

Second, racial discrimination persists in contemporary society, with Whites continuing to self-report that they discriminate against minorities (Pager

& Shepherd, 2008). In addition, there is considerable high-quality scientific evidence documenting the persistence of racial discrimination. A recent review of audit studies—those in which researchers carefully select, match, and train individuals to be equally qualified in every respect but to differ only in race—provide striking examples of contemporary racial discrimination (Pager & Shepherd, 2008). For example, audit studies in employment document that a White job applicant with a criminal record is more likely to be offered a job than a Black applicant with an otherwise identical resume whose record was clean. Similarly, job applicants with distinctively Black names (e.g., Aisha, Darnell) are less likely to get callbacks for job interviews than applicants with identical resumes who have distinctively White names (e.g., Alison, Brad). Other audit studies reveal racial discrimination in renting apartments, purchasing homes and cars, obtaining mortgages and medical care, applying for insurance, and hailing taxis. Research has also found that even the price of a fast food meal increases with the percentage Black of a zip code (Pager & Shepherd, 2008). Minority homebuyers and residential areas were also explicitly targeted for subprime and predatory loans (Pager & Shepherd, 2008). Between 1993 and 2000, 78% of the new housing loans in minority neighborhoods and 72% of the increase in refinancing to Blacks were from subprime lenders.

Institutional Racism

Third, racial discrimination also persists in institutional mechanisms and processes. Residential segregation by race is a prime example (Massey & Denton, 1993). *Segregation* refers to the physical separation of the races in racially distinctive neighborhoods and communities that was developed to ensure that Whites were safeguarded from residential closeness to Blacks (Cell, 1982). This enforced residence in separate areas developed in both northern and southern urban areas in the late 19th and early 20th centuries and has remained strikingly stable since then but with small declines in recent years (Glaeser & Vigdor, 2001; Lieberson, 1980; Massey & Denton, 1993). Although segregation has

been illegal since the Fair Housing Act of 1968, it is perpetuated today through an interlocking set of individual actions, institutional practices, and governmental policies. In the 2010 Census, residential segregation was at its lowest level in 100 years, and declines in segregation were evident in all of the nation's largest metropolitan areas (Glaeser & Vigdor, 2012). However, recent declines in segregation in have been driven by a few Blacks moving to formerly all-White census tracts but have had little impact on the very high percentage of Black census tracts, the residential isolation of most African Americans, and the concentration of urban poverty (Glaeser & Vigdor, 2001). The forced removal and relocation of American Indians to reservations is another example of institutionalized isolation of a marginalized racial population.

The high level of incarceration of Blacks and other minorities is another example of institutional racism. The United States imprisons a higher proportion of its population than any other country in the world. Racial disparities in the criminalization and investigation of certain behaviors combined with discrimination in prosecution and sentencing have led to the inordinately high levels of incarceration of minorities in the United States (Alexander, 2010). Immigration policy in the United States, historically and currently, has been another form of institutional racism (Gee & Ford, 2011). These policies have ranked racial groups; excluded, segregated, and incarcerated some racial populations; and limited the rights and privileges of those deemed dangerous or undesirable.

Cultural Racism

The persistence of institutional and interpersonal discrimination is driven by the racism that remains deeply ingrained in American culture. Ideas of Black inferiority and White superiority have historically been embedded in multiple aspects of American culture, and many images and ideas in contemporary popular culture continue to devalue, marginalize, and subordinate non-White racial populations (Dirks & Mueller, 2007). Moreover, anti-Black ideology and representation is distinctive because it is typically the benchmark to which other groups are compared. Findings from surveys and studies employing experimental or quasi-experimental design have found that greater exposure to TV programs that describe Blacks negatively was associated with higher levels of racial prejudice toward Blacks (Mutz & Goldman, 2010). Although Blacks and other minorities appear more frequently on TV than in the past, a recent study that examined characters in 11 popular TV programs found that more negative nonverbal behavior (facial expressions and body language) is directed toward Black characters than toward status-matched White characters and that exposure to nonverbal bias increased viewers' bias—even though viewers were not consciously aware of patterns of nonverbal behavior (Weisbuch, Pauker, & Ambady, 2009). Another study documented that a dehumanizing bias that associates Blacks with apes persists and that this dehumanization matters (Goff, Eberhardt, Williams, & Jackson, 2008). The study found that newspaper stories of defendants convicted of capital crime over a 20-year period were more likely to describe Black convicts than White ones with *ape*-like words (e.g., *beast, brute, monster, prowl*). Importantly, adjusting for defendant SES, victim SES, crime severity, aggravating circumstances, and mitigating circumstances, researchers found that Blacks implicitly portrayed as more ape-like were more likely to be executed than those whose lives were spared (Goff et al., 2008). A similar trend was evident for Whites.

Blacks and other minorities are also negatively stereotyped in the United States. The 1990 General Social Survey (GSS) found that 29% of Whites viewed Blacks as unintelligent, 45% saw them as lazy, 57% believed that Blacks prefer to live off welfare, and 51% believed that Blacks are prone to violence (Davis & Smith, 1990). Questions were asked on a 7-point scale from a positive to a negative stereotype, with 4 on the scale representing agreeing with neither side. Strikingly, one in five Whites or fewer saw Blacks as intelligent (21%), hardworking (17%), preferring to be self-supporting (13%), and not prone to violence (14%). Across the various stereotypes, Whites viewed Blacks, Hispanics, and Asians more negatively than themselves, with Blacks viewed the most negatively and Hispanics twice as negatively as Asians.

Data available in the GSS for two of the stereotypes since 1990 show very limited change over time (Smith, Marsden, & Hout, 2011). In 2010, 32% of Whites agreed that Blacks were lazy, down from 45% in 1990. However, the percentage of Whites endorsing the view that Blacks were hardworking changed from 17% in 1990 to 16% in 2010, with a higher proportion of Whites endorsing the *neither* category (49% vs. 34%). Some progress was evident on the intelligence stereotype, with the rate of Whites who viewed Blacks as unintelligent declining from 29% in 1990 to 13% in 2010 and that of Whites agreeing that Blacks were intelligent increasing from 21% in 1990 to 27% in 2010. The percentage of Whites endorsing the neutral response increased from 44% to 56%.

A recent study documents that negative stereotypes of Blacks are commonplace in American culture. The BEAGLE (Bound Encoding of the Aggregate Language Environment) Project constructed a database of about 10 million words from a sample of books, newspapers, and other materials that is a good representation of American culture and equivalent to what the average college-level student would read in his or her lifetime (Verhaeghen, Aikman, & Van Gulick, 2011). Statistical analysis of the associative strength between pairs of words revealed the following order of the frequency of the pairing of the word *Black* with these 10 words in American culture: *poor, violent, religious, lazy, cheerful, dangerous, charming, merry, ignorant,* and *musical.* Thus, the negative stereotypes of Blacks in the GSS (violent, lazy, dangerous, and unintelligent) probably reflects how often Americans have seen or heard these words paired with *Black* in their lifetime.

MECHANISMS BY WHICH RACISM CAN AFFECT HEALTH AND EVIDENCE OF HEALTH EFFECTS

Figure 4.1 outlines the multiple pathways by which racism can affect health. It indicates that racism is one of several fundamental or basic determinants

FIGURE 4.1 ■ A Framework for the Study of Racism and Health

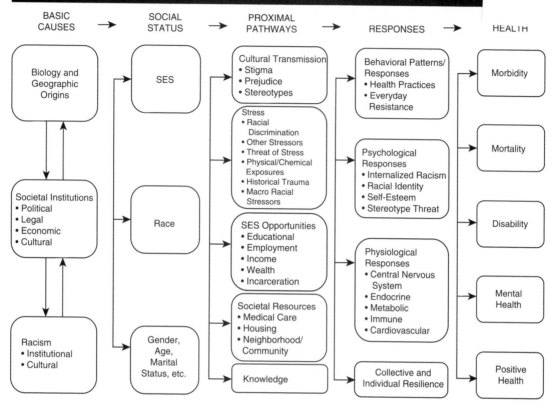

of health, and it gives emphasis to institutional and cultural racism (D. Williams, 1997). The model emphasizes the importance of distinguishing basic causes from surface or intervening causes (proximal pathways). Whereas changes in fundamental causes lead to changes in outcomes, interventions in the intermediate or proximal pathways, without corresponding changes in fundamental causes, are unlikely to produce long-term improvements in population health. The model argues that race and other social status categories, such as SES, gender, age, and marital status, are created by the larger macro forces in society and are linked to health through several intervening mechanisms. Racism and other fundamental causes operate through multiple mechanisms to affect health, and the pathways through which distal causes affect health can change over time. Institutional and cultural racism can adversely affect health through stigma, stereotypes, prejudice,

and racial discrimination. These aspects of racism can lead to differential access to SES and to a broad range of societal resources and opportunities. Racism is not the only determinant of intervening mechanisms, but its presence as a fundamental cause in a society can alter and transform other social factors and can exacerbate the negative effects of other risk factors for health. For example, stress is posited as one of the intervening pathways. Racism creates some types of stressors, such as discrimination and historical trauma, but it can also affect the levels, clustering, and impact of stressors, such as unemployment, neighborhood violence, or physical and chemical exposures in residential and occupational environments.

The model acknowledges that social inequalities in knowledge and communication play an insufficiently recognized role in contributing to and exacerbating social inequalities in health

(Viswanath, 2006). Much of the contemporary disease burden is linked to behaviors that are potentially modifiable with the appropriate opportunities and access to preventive care and health information. Communication factors that shape health knowledge, attitudes, and behavior, such as access to and the use of various media sources, attention to health information, trust in the sources of information, and the processing of information, all vary by race-ethnicity and SES. Moreover, members of stigmatized racial groups are less able to act on and benefit from relevant health knowledge because they often lack the necessary resources to do so.

Much research on the determinants of health focuses on the responses (behavioral, psychological, physiological) to the proximal pathways. Figure 4.1 reminds us that these responses can be optimally understood and contextualized in the light of the upstream factors that initiate and sustain the conditions that population groups are responsive to. It also indicates that attention should be given to both individual and collective resistance and resilience. For example, some recent research suggests that some unhealthy behaviors of minority populations may reflect everyday resistance—an effort to express opposition to the larger society, assert independence, and reject the dominant society's norms (Factor, Kawachi, & Williams, 2013).

Institutional Racism and Health

Residential segregation is a potent institutional legacy of racism that is a driver of the persistence of racial economic inequality and thus racial inequities in health (D. Williams & Collins, 2001). Segregation was one of the most successful domestic policies of the 20th century in the United States (Cell, 1982), and it can affect health through multiple pathways (D. Williams & Collins, 2001). First, it restricts socioeconomic mobility by limiting access to quality elementary and high school education, preparation for higher education, and employment opportunities. For example, segregated schools are unequal on multiple dimensions, including teacher quality, educational resources, per-student spending, and neighborhood violence, crime, and poverty (Orfield, Frankenberg, & Garces, 2008). Segregation also

reduces access to employment opportunities. It has facilitated the exodus of low-skill, high-pay jobs from areas of minority concentration, and it has facilitated discrimination based on place of residence (Pager & Shepherd, 2008; Wilson, 1987). One study found that the elimination of segregation would erase Black-White differences in earnings, high school graduation rate, and unemployment, and reduce racial differences in single motherhood by two thirds (Cutler & Glaeser, 1997).

Segregation is also associated with residence in poorer-quality housing and in neighborhood environments that are deficient in a broad range of resources that enhance health and well-being, including medical care. The concentration of poverty in segregated environments can lead to exposure to elevated levels of chronic and acute stressors. A recent study documented, for example, that compared to Whites, Blacks and U.S.-born Latinos had higher exposure to a broad range of psychosocial stressors and greater clustering of multiple stressors (Sternthal, Slopen, & Williams, 2011). This stress exposure accounted for some of the residual effect of race on health after income and education were controlled. In addition, segregation leads minorities to have higher risk of exposure to toxic chemicals at the individual, household, and neighborhood level (Morello-Frosch & Jesdale, 2006). Research also reveals that segregation directly and indirectly contributes to lower access and poorer quality of health care across the entire continuum of care from prevention services through end-of-life care (White, Haas, & Williams, 2012). The poor health of minorities is further exacerbated by these racial differences in access and quality of care.

Segregation in the United States is also a fundamental cause of the high rates of violent crime and homicide for African Americans. Differences at the neighborhood level, driven by segregation, in the availability of jobs (especially for males), opportunities for marriage, concentrated poverty, family structure, and the supervision of adolescent males are the key determinants of elevated risk of violent crime and homicide (Sampson, 1987). These factors lead to the concentration of urban violence in a few "hot spots." Research in Boston documented that

3% of street segments and intersections accounted for more than 50% of all gun violence incidents (Braga, Papachristos, & Hureau, 2010). A study in Seattle found that most crime was concentrated in a few street segments, and 84% of these segments had stable concentrations of crime over a 14-year period, with increases in crime in a very few street segments accounting for overall city trends in crime (Weisburd, Bushway, Lum, & Yang, 2004).

Incarceration has a range of adverse impacts on the health of incarcerated people and of the communities to which they return after their release (Dumont, Brockmann, Dickman, Alexander, & Rich, 2012). When incarcerated individuals return to their communities, their access to public and private housing, employment opportunities, voting rights, welfare- and food-assistance programs, health services, and financial aid for higher education is limited (N. Williams, 2006). Most incarcerated adults are parents of children younger than 18 years of age, and these children are at increased risk for social and emotional difficulties and for engaging in criminal behavior in the future (Travis & Waul, 2003). When a parent is imprisoned, families often suffer from financial instability and social stigma, and are deprived of social and caregiving support of the incarcerated parent (Travis & Waul, 2003). High rates of incarceration also adversely affect communities by reducing the availability of male partners for marriage.

Although institutional racism is arguably the most important mechanism by which racism adversely affects health, it is challenging to capture in traditional epidemiological research, and we have not fully quantified the impact of institutional racism on health. Some studies have found a positive association between area-level measures of residential segregation and infant and adult mortality rates, and other health outcomes, after adjusting for demographic and socioeconomic variables (Kramer & Hogue, 2009). A recent analysis estimated that segregation is responsible for 176,000 deaths annually (Galea, Tracy, Hoggatt, DiMaggio, & Karpati, 2011). Efforts have also been made, with limited success, to operationalize other aspects of institutional racism in epidemiological studies (e.g., Gee,

2002; Mendez, Hogan, & Culhane, 2012; Wallace, 2011). Recent reviews have provided a roadmap for the needed research to better conceptualize and measure the complex ways in which segregation can affect health and health care (Kramer, Cooper, Drews-Botsch, Waller, & Hogue, 2010; Osypuk & Acevedo-Garcia, 2010; White et al., 2012; White & Borrell, 2011). Implementing these recommendations is an important priority. Similar research attention needs to be given to other aspects of institutional racism.

Cultural Racism and Health

Research is needed to fully understand the multiple ways in which representations of race in popular culture affect persons who are exposed to them, but there is growing evidence that these effects can be decisive for the thoughts, feelings, and behavior of both dominant and subordinate groups. Cultural racism is likely to be a major contributor to negative racial stereotypes and the absence of positive emotion for stigmatized racial groups that can shape the policy preferences of the larger society and contribute to the lack of political will to address racial inequalities in society, including those in health. The absence of positive emotions has been identified as an important component of subtle prejudice (Pettigrew & Meertens, 1995). Research indicates that emotions have a large impact on decision making in general and on race-related attitudes and policy in particular. A recent meta-analysis found that emotional prejudice was twice as strongly predictive of discriminatory behavior as racial beliefs and stereotypes (Talaska, Fiske, & Chaiken, 2008). A study in Germany, the Netherlands, France, and the United Kingdom found that the absence of positive emotions (measured by two items that captured the absence of feelings of sympathy and admiration toward the out-group) was a strong predictor of opposition to policies regarding immigrant outgroups (Pettigrew & Meertens, 1995). Similarly, a study of Detroit-area Whites found that a two-item measure that assessed the lack of sympathy and admiration for Blacks was the strongest predictor of opposition to affirmative action in employment and to an active role of government in reducing racial inequalities (D. Williams et al., 1999). Moreover, recent research reveals that racial prejudice is a driver of opposition to President Obama's health care reform legislation, with the racial divide in attitudes toward health care being 20 percentage points larger now than it was for President Clinton's plan back in the early 1990s (Tesler, 2012).

One response of stigmatized racial populations to the pervasive negative racial stereotypes in the culture is to accept as true the dominant society's beliefs about their biological and/or cultural inferiority. This internalized racism or self-stereotyping is one mechanism by which negative stereotypes about race in the larger society can adversely affect health. By fostering the endorsement of beliefs about the innate deficiencies of one's self and one's group, internalized racism can lead to lower self-esteem and psychological well-being, which in turn could adversely affect health and health behavior in multiple ways (Kwate & Meyer, 2011). A recent review of existing research found that internalized racism was positively associated with alcohol consumption, psychological distress, being overweight, abdominal obesity, blood pressure, and fasting glucose (D. Williams & Mohammed, 2009). It has also been suggested that internalized stereotypes could also indirectly affect health by decreasing motivation for socioeconomic attainment (Kwate & Meyer, 2011).

However, the health consequences of internalized racism have received very limited research attention, and there are many unanswered questions. We currently have limited understanding of which groups are most vulnerable, the range of outcomes most affected, and how internalized racism combines with other aspects of racism to affect health. Some limited research has found that internalized racism is adversely related to cardiovascular risk factors for females but not males, and we do not have a clear understanding of the determinants of these gender differences (Chambers et al., 2004; Tull, Cort, Gwebu, & Gwebu, 2007). A recent study found a positive association between internalized racism and violence and delinquent behavior among adolescents (Bryant, 2011), suggesting that it may be a risk factor for a broad range of outcomes. Another recent study found that internalized racism interacted with

perceived discrimination to affect cardiovascular disease risk (Chae, Lincoln, Adler, & Syme, 2010).

The term *stereotype threat* refers to the activation of negative stereotypes among stigmatized groups that creates expectations, anxieties, and reactions that can adversely affect social and psychological functioning (Fischer et al., 1996; Steele, 1997). U.S. research indicates that when a stigma of inferiority is activated for African Americans in experimental conditions, performance on an examination is adversely affected (Steele, 1997). Similarly, women who were told that they perform more poorly than men, and White men who were told that they do worse than Asians, had lower scores on an examination than control groups (Fischer et al., 1996; Steele, 1997). Research indicates that stereotype threat occurs only when a group is stereotype vulnerable. The activation of negative stereotypes about Blacks enhances academic performance for Black Caribbean immigrants who were not socialized in America's racism-filled culture, but it reduces it for the children of Caribbean Black immigrants (Deaux et al., 2007). Similarly, for Asian American women, making gender salient reduces academic performance, but making their race salient enhances it (Shih, Pittinsky, & Ambady, 1999).

There has been little systematic attention to the direct effects of stereotype threat on health. However, existing research suggests the plausibility of two pathways. First, the psychological stress created by stereotype threat could lead to physiological arousal. One experimental study found that the activation of the stigma of inferiority led to increases in blood pressure for African American but not White students (Blascovitch, Spencer, Quinn, & Steele, 2001). Other limited evidence indicates that stereotype threat can increase anxiety, reduce self-regulation, and impair decision-making processes in ways that can increase aggressive behavior and overeating (Inzlicht & Kang, 2010). Second, stereotype threat can adversely affect the patient-provider relationship. In clinical encounters, stereotype threat can impair patients' communication abilities, leading to discounting of information from the provider, delays, or failure to obtain needed medical care and lower levels of adherence (Aronson, Burgess, Phelan, &

Juarez, 2013; Burgess, Warren, Phelan, Dovidio, & van Ryn, 2010).

Cultural racism can trigger unconscious bias that can lead to unequal access to health-enhancing economic opportunities and resources. Many Whites have automatic, rapid, and unconscious emotional and neural reactions to Blacks, noticing an individual's race and whether he or she is trustworthy in less than 100 ms (Fiske, Bergsieker, Russell, & Williams, 2009). Research indicates that when one holds a negative stereotype about a group and meets someone who fits the stereotype, he or she will discriminate against that individual (van Ryn et al., 2011). This stereotype-linked unconscious or unthinking bias can occur among persons who are not prejudiced and is activated automatically (without intent) with individuals being unaware of its activation and the impact on their behavior (van Ryn et al., 2011). Cultural racism also undergirds the findings from the audit studies reviewed earlier that documented the pervasive societal presence of discrimination that lead to reduced opportunities for socioeconomic advancement, higher costs of goods and services, and poorer quality of life. For example, the discrimination in mortgage lending noted earlier that led to a high level of subprime loans for minorities has contributed to the marked losses in home equity for these populations during the recent housing crisis. Between 2005 and 2009, the median wealth of White households declined by 16% compared to 53% for Black and 66% for Hispanic households (Pew Research Center, 2011). The median wealth of Whites is now 20 times that of Blacks and 18 times that of Hispanics. Wealth is a critical component of SES that has been shown to affect health over and above income and education (Pollack et al., 2007). Thus, the declining wealth of racial minorities is likely to have had adverse health consequences.

Unconscious (as well as conscious) bias can also lead to unequal access to high-quality medical care. A 2003 report from the Institute of Medicine concluded that across virtually every therapeutic intervention, ranging from high-technology procedures to the most basic forms of diagnostic and treatment interventions, Blacks and other minorities receive fewer procedures and poorer-quality medical care than Whites (Smedley, Stith, & Nelson, 2003). Strikingly, these differences persist even after statistical adjustment for variations in health insurance, SES, stage and severity of disease, co-occurring illness, and the type of health care facility are taken into account. Analyses of data from a large, volunteer, and nonrepresentative sample of persons who took the Implicit Association Test (IAT) reveal that physicians have an implicit preference for Whites over Blacks, similar to the pattern observed for other professionals (lawyers and others with PhDs) and the general population (Sabin, Nosek, Greenwald, & Rivara, 2009). Research reveals that higher implicit bias scores among physicians is associated with biased treatment recommendations in the care of Black patients (van Ryn et al., 2011), although the pattern is not uniform (Haider et al., 2011). This highlights the importance of research to better understand the conditions under which these biases are likely to occur. In addition, provider implicit bias is also associated with poorer quality of patient provider communication and lower patient evaluation of the quality of the medical encounter, including provider nonverbal behavior (Cooper et al., 2012; van Ryn et al., 2011). Research is needed to identify optimal strategies of raising health providers' awareness of subtle, unconscious discrimination and providing them with strategies to minimize its occurrence.

Experiences of Discrimination

Individuals are aware of at least some of the experiences of discrimination created by institutional and cultural racism. Research reveals that these subjective experiences of discrimination are psychosocial stressors that adversely affect a very broad range of health outcomes and health risk behaviors (Pascoe & Richman, 2009; D. Williams & Mohammed, 2009). For example, Tené Lewis and colleagues have shown that chronic everyday discrimination is positively associated with coronary artery calcification (Lewis et al., 2006), C-reactive protein (Lewis, Aiello, Leurgans, Kelly, & Barnes, 2010), blood pressure (Lewis et al., 2009), giving birth to lower-birth-weight infants (Earnshaw et al., 2013), cognitive impairment (Barnes et al., 2012), subjective and objective indicators of poor sleep (Lewis et al., 2012), visceral fat (Lewis, Kravitz, Janssen, & Powell, 2011), and mortality (Barnes et al., 2008).

Research on discrimination has also shed light on some puzzles in the literature. For example, prior research reveals that African Americans are more likely than Whites to manifest no blood pressure decline or a blunted blood pressure decline during sleep, a pattern that has been associated with increased risk for mortality and cardiovascular outcomes (Profant & Dimsdale, 1999). Recent studies reveal that exposure to discrimination contributes to the elevated levels of nocturnal blood pressure among Blacks (Brondolo et al., 2008; Tomfohr, Cooper, Mills, Nelesen, & Dimsdale, 2010). Decreases in blood pressure dipping during sleep have also been associated with low SES and other psychosocial stressors (Tomfohr et al., 2010). Prior research has also found lower levels of health care seeking and adherence behaviors among racial minorities, and research on discrimination now documents that racial bias is a contributor to these patterns. Moreover, research in the United States, South Africa, Australia, and New Zealand reveals that discrimination makes an incremental contribution over SES in accounting for racial disparities in health (D. Williams et al., 2008; D. Williams & Mohammed, 2009).

Many questions remain unanswered. Research suggests that across multiple societal contexts, perceptions of unfair treatment, regardless of whether they are attributed to race or other social reasons, are adversely related to health for both racial minorities and Whites (D. Williams & Mohammed, 2009). However, it is unclear whether the occasional experiences of discrimination by Whites are truly equivalent with the insidious and systematic experiences reported by stigmatized minority populations. Moreover, some studies find a more adverse impact of discrimination on mental health for Whites compared to Blacks (Kessler, Mickelson, & Williams, 1999; D. Williams, Yu, Jackson, & Anderson, 1997). One recent study found that discrimination was associated with a flatter (less healthy) diurnal slope of cortisol for Whites than for Blacks, with the healthier cortisol profile being more evident for low-SES Blacks than for their higher-SES counterparts

(Fuller-Rowell, Doan, & Eccles, 2012). This highlights the importance of understanding the conditions under which specific aspects of discrimination are pathogenic for particular social groups as well as the extent to which socialization experiences, resilience resources, coping strategies, and co-occurring exposures may modify the relationship between exposure to discrimination and health.

There are several critical measurement issues with regard to discrimination that need to be addressed in future research. First, fully capturing the impact of discrimination will require greater attention to developing measures that capture not only actual exposure but the threat of exposure (D. Williams & Mohammed, 2009). The threat of discrimination is an understudied aspect of discriminatory stress. Recent research reveals that anticipating being a target of discrimination can produce heightened vigilance that can lead to the activation of negative emotional states, increases in blood pressure, and sympathetic nervous system activation (Sawyer, Major, Casad, Townsend, & Mendes, 2012). Second, exposure to race-related stressors should be captured comprehensively. The stress literature has identified macro stressors—large-scale societal events, such as natural disasters, that can be stressful for individuals. Major negative race-related events can also be macro stressors that lead to adverse changes in health status. For example, in 2006, a Black woman accused White male members of the Duke University lacrosse team of racial derogation, rape, and violence. There was considerable racially divisive media coverage and rhetoric about the incident. Duke's Black students were stressed and had concerns about their safety. An experimental study at Duke found that after the media attention to the incident, Black students, especially females, had higher levels of cortisol and were unresponsive to an experimental task compared to students who participated in the experiment before the lacrosse team incident (Richman & Jonassaint, 2008). Research has also found that historical trauma experienced by Native American communities in the past can reach across generations and adversely affect the physical and mental health of contemporary Native Americans (Walters et al., 2011).

The backdrop of cultural racism can also racialize presumably nonracial societal events so that they have negative health consequences. A study of birth outcomes in California found that infants born to Arab American women 6 months after September 11, 2001 (a period of increased discrimination of Arab Americans), had an increased risk of low birth weight and preterm birth compared to those born in the 6 months before (Lauderdale, 2006). Women of other racial and ethnic groups in California had no change in birth outcome risk, pre- and post-September 11. Personal experiences of abuse and discrimination linked to September 11 were also positively associated with psychological distress and poor health status and inversely associated with happiness among Arab Americans (Padela & Heisler, 2010). Some evidence also suggests that immigration policies hostile to immigrant groups can adversely affect their quality of life (Garcia & Keyes, 2012). Analyses of data collected in California in 2001 (a time of multiple anti-immigrant legislative proposals) found that inconsistent with prior research, Latino and some other immigrant groups reported higher psychological distress than native-born respondents (D. Williams & Mohammed, 2008). Research is needed to systematically assess the health consequences, if any, of the negative climate and hostile policies toward immigrants.

Third, efforts to comprehensively measure discrimination should also seek to assess exposure to racial bias over the life course. A large study of fifth graders found that 7% of Whites, 15% of Hispanics, and 20% of Blacks reported experiences of racial discrimination and that racial bias was associated with increased risk of mental disorder (Coker et al., 2009). Similarly, research on adolescents find high exposure to racial discrimination in online contents and that these experiences were positively associated with symptoms of depression and anxiety (Tynes, Giang, Williams, & Thompson, 2008). At the present time, we do not clearly understand how the age of onset of experiences of discrimination and the accumulation of such experiences over the life course affect the onset and course of illness. Gee, Walsemann, and Brondolo (2012) have recently outlined a comprehensive agenda for empirically assessing how racism

can affect health using a life course lens. They highlight the importance of attending to sensitive periods, the interdependence in exposures among persons, latency periods, stress proliferation processes, and historical period and birth cohort.

Fourth, to the extent feasible, we need to develop measures to assess exposure to discrimination independent of self-report. A significant new development in the assessment of discrimination is the attempt to capture implicit measures of discrimination. A novel application of the IAT is its use to capture the extent to which individuals see themselves and their racial-ethnic group as a perpetrator versus a target of discrimination (Krieger et al., 2011). This measure seeks to minimize the limitations of self-reported data by capturing experiences of racial bias that respondents are unwilling or unable to report. So far, implicit measures of discrimination show weak or modest associations with health outcomes (Krieger et al., 2010, 2011). Nevertheless, the IAT promises a glimpse of the health effects of racial bias that might otherwise be hidden. However, important issues need to be resolved. In contrast to correlations of about .25 between implicit and explicit measures of racial prejudice (Hofmann, Gawronski, Gschwendner, Le, & Schmitt, 2005; Nosek et al., 2007), most of the correlations between the implicit measures attempting to capture racial discrimination and validated explicit measures of discrimination are .10 or less (Krieger et al., 2011). While we know that the IAT measures unconscious processes related to race, these very low correlations raise the question of whether these implicit measures are capturing actual past exposure to racial discrimination, the perceived threat of discrimination, vigilance regarding discrimination, the burden of prior experiences of discrimination, the severity of prior exposure, or some other processes related to race. In addition, much of the literature on discrimination assumes that it operates through processes triggered by the psychological appraisal of an environmental stressor, but we do not know if unconscious processes linked to race generate similar stress responses. More research is needed to provide a deeper understanding of exactly what the IAT is capturing and how we should optimally combine it with explicit measures of discrimination.

CONCLUSION

A major research challenge is the need for the conceptual and analytic models used to study racism and other determinants of disparities in health to reflect the actual clustering of diseases and their determinants. The co-occurrence of multiple diseases is commonplace, increase with age, and is evident at younger ages among low-SES and minority populations (Barnett et al., 2012). Moreover, advantage and disadvantage, resources and risks, tend to co-occur with each other and to cumulate within the same individuals and social spaces over time. Failure to model this accumulation of adversity may fail to capture, and effectively address, the full burden of social exposure. Unhealthy behaviors, such as poor nutrition, physical inactivity, cigarette smoking, and excessive alcohol intake, are clustered in individuals with and without chronic diseases (Héroux et al., 2012). Similarly, discrimination and other psychosocial stressors are clustered with each other and co-occur more frequently in disadvantaged racial populations (Sternthal et al., 2011). Inadequate research attention has been given to the ways in which multiple aspects of racism relate to each other and combine, additively and interactively, with other psychosocial risks and resources to affect health. New analytic models that reflect the complexity of the determinants of health and the clustering and accumulation of risk factors and health outcomes are urgently needed (Adler, Bush, & Pantell, 2012). The model in Figure 4.1 suggests that there are likely to be multiple causal pathways by which a given distal upstream factor, such as racism, can affect health status. Thus, the configuration of intervening mechanisms may vary over time, in different contexts, and for different outcomes.

Historically, racial variations in health were often viewed as genetic or biological, and some current observers view them as intractable and deeply embedded in cultural values and behaviors. The research reviewed here indicates that racism in its institutional and cultural forms have been and continue to be major contributors to initiating and sustaining racial inequalities in a broad range of societal outcomes that combine to create inequalities in health. We need a deeper understanding of how cultural norms and institutional policies and procedures with regard to race shape interpersonal relations and the quality of living conditions in ways that affect health. It follows that we are unlikely to make significant progress in reducing the well-documented large racial disparities in health without intensive, comprehensive, and sustained initiatives to eliminate racial inequalities in a broad range of social, political, and economic indicators. We therefore need more concerted efforts to develop the science base that would enable us to effectively intervene to reduce and ultimately eliminate the pathogenic effects of racism and health. We consider the evidence and research opportunities for effective intervention in a companion article (D. Williams & Mohammed, in press).

References

Adler, N., Bush, N. R., & Pantell, M. S. (2012). Rigor, vigor, and the study of health disparities. *Proceedings of the National Academy of Sciences, 109*(Suppl. 2), 17154–17159.

Alexander, M. (2010). *The new Jim Crow: Mass incarceration in the age of colorblindness.* New York, NY: New Press.

Aronson, J., Burgess, D., Phelan, S. M., & Juarez, L. (2013). Unhealthy interactions: The role of stereotype threat in health disparities. *American Journal of Public Health, 103*(1), 50–56.

Barnes, L. L., de Leon, C. F. M., Lewis, T. T., Bienias, J. L., Wilson, R. S., & Evans, D. A. (2008). Perceived discrimination and mortality in a population-based study of older adults. *American Journal of Public Health, 98*(7), 1241–1247.

Barnes, L. L., Lewis, T. T., Begeny, C. T., Yu, L., Bennett, D. A., & Wilson, R. S. (2012). Perceived discrimination and cognition in older African Americans. *Journal of the International Neuropsychological Society, 18*(5), 856–865.

Barnett, K., Mercer, S. W., Norbury, M., Watt, G., Wyke, S., & Guthrie, B. (2012). Epidemiology of multimorbidity and implications for health care, research, and medical education: A cross-sectional study. *The Lancet, 380*(9836), 37–43.

Blascovitch, J., Spencer, S. J., Quinn, D., & Steele, C. (2001). African Americans and high blood pressure: The role of stereotype threat. *Pschological Science, 12*(3), 225–229.

Bonilla-Silva, E. (1996). Rethinking racism: Toward a structural interpretation. *American Sociological Review, 62*(3), 465–480.

Braga, A. A., Papachristos, A., & Hureau, D. (2010). The concentration and stability of gun violence at micro places in Boston, 1980–2008. *Journal of Quantitative Criminology, 26*(1), 33–53.

Braveman, P. A., Cubbin, C., Egerter, S., Williams, D. R., & Pamuk, E. (2010). Socioeconomic disparities in health in the United States: What the patterns tell us. *American Journal of Public Health, 100*, S186–196.

Brondolo, E., Libby, D. J., Denton, E.-G., Thompson, S., Beatty, D. L., Schwartz, J., & Gerin, W. (2008). Racism and ambulatory blood pressure in a community sample. *Psychosomatic Medicine, 70*(1), 49–56.

Bryant, W. W. (2011). Internalized racism's association with African American male youth's propensity for violence. *Journal of Black Studies, 42*(4), 690–707.

Burgess, D., Warren, J., Phelan, S., Dovidio, J., & van Ryn, M. (2010). Stereotype threat and health disparities: What medical educators and future physicians need to know. *Journal of General Internal Medicine, 25*(Suppl. 2), S169–177.

Cell, J. W. (1982). *The highest stage of White supremacy: The origin of segregation in South Africa and the American South.* New York, NY: Cambridge University Press.

Chae, D. H., Lincoln, K. D., Adler, N. E., & Syme, S. L. (2010). Do experiences of racial discrimination predict cardiovascular disease among African American men? The moderating role of internalized negative racial group attitudes. *Social Science and Medicine, 71*(6), 1182–1188.

Chambers, E. C., Tull, E. S., Fraser, H. S., Mutunhu, N. R., Sobers, N., & Niles, E. (2004). The relationship of internalized racism to body fat distribution and insulin resistance among African adolescent youth. *Journal of the National Medical Association, 96*(12), 1594–1598.

Coker, T. R., Elliott, M. N., Kanouse, D. E., Grunbaum, J. A., Schwebel, D. C., Gilliland, M. J., & Schuster, M. A. (2009). Perceived racial/ethnic discrimination among fifth-grade students and its association with mental health. *American Journal of Public Health, 99*(5), 878–884.

Cooper, L. A., Roter, D. L., Carson, K. A., Beach, M. C., Sabin, J. A., Greenwald, A. G., & Inui, T. S. (2012). The associations of clinicians' implicit attitudes about race with medical visit communication and patient ratings of interpersonal care. *American Journal of Public Health, 102*(5), 979–987.

Cutler, D. M., & Glaeser, E. L. (1997). Are ghettos good or bad? *Quarterly Journal of Economics, 112*, 827–872.

Davis, J. A., & Smith, T. W. (1990). *General social surveys, 1972–1990 NORC ed.* Chicago, IL: National Opinion Research Center.

Deaux, K., Bikmen, N., Gilkes, A., Ventuneac, A., Joseph, Y., Payne, Y. A., & Steele, C. M. (2007). Becoming American: Stereotype threat effects in Afro-Caribbean immigrant groups. *Social Psychology Quarterly, 70*(4), 384–404.

Dirks, D., & Mueller, J. C. (2007). Racism and popular culture. In J. Feagin & H. Vera (Eds.), *Handbook of racial and ethnic relations* (pp. 115–129). New York, NY: Springer.

Dovidio, J. F., & Gaertner, S. L. (2004). Aversive racism. In M. Zanna (Ed.), *Advances in experimental social psychology* (Vol. 36, pp. 1–51). San Diego, CA: Academic Press.

Dumont, D. M., Brockmann, B., Dickman, S., Alexander, N., & Rich, J. D. (2012). Public health and the epidemic of incarceration. *Annual Review of Public Health, 33*(1), 325–339.

Earnshaw, V., Rosenthal, L., Lewis, J., Stasko, E., Tobin, J., Lewis, T., & Ickovics, J. (2013). Maternal experiences with everyday discrimination and infant birth weight: A test of mediators and moderators among young, urban women of color. *Annals of Behavioral Medicine, 45*(1), 13–23.

Factor, R., Kawachi, I., & Williams, D. R. (2013). The social resistance framework for understanding high-risk behavior among non-dominant minorities: Preliminary evidence. *American Journal of Public Health*, e1-e7.

Fischer, C. S., Hout, M., Jankowski, M. S., Lucas, S. R., Swidler, A., & Voss, K. (1996). Race, ethnicity and intelligence. In *Inequality by design: Cracking the bell curve myth*. Princeton, NJ: Princeton University Press.

Fiske, S. T., Bergsieker, H. B., Russell, A. M., & Williams, L. (2009). Images of Black Americans. *Du Bois Review: Social Science Research on Race, 6*(1), 83–101.

Fuller-Rowell, T. E., Doan, S. N., & Eccles, J. S. (2012). Differential effects of perceived discrimination on the diurnal cortisol rhythm of African Americans and Whites. *Psychoneuroendocrinology, 37*(1), 107–118.

Galea, S., Tracy, M., Hoggatt, K. J., DiMaggio, C., & Karpati, A. (2011). Estimated deaths attributable to social factors in the United States. *American Journal of Public Health, 101*(8), 1456–1465.

Garcia, A. S., & Keyes, D. G. (2012). *Life as an undocumented immigrant: How restrictive local immigration policies affect daily life*. Washington, DC: Center for American Progress. Retrieved from http://www.americanprogress.org/issues/2012/03/pdf/life_as_undocumented.pdf

Gee, G. C. (2002). A multilevel analysis of the relationship between institutional and individual racial discrimination and health status. *American Journal of Public Health, 92*(4), 615–623.

Gee, G. C., & Ford, C. L. (2011). Structural racism and health inequities. *Du Bois Review: Social Science Research on Race, 8*(1), 115–132.

Gee, G. C., Walsemann, K. M., & Brondolo, E. (2012). A life course perspective on how racism may be related to health inequities. *American Journal of Public Health, 102*(5), 967–974.

Glaeser, E. L., & Vigdor, J. L. (2001). *Racial segregation in the 2000 Census: Promising news*. Washington, DC: Brookings Institution.

Glaeser, E. L., & Vigdor, J. (2012). The end of the segregated century: Racial separation in America's neighborhoods, 1890–2010. *Civic Report, 66*. Retrieved from http://www.manhattan-institute.org/html/cr_66.htm

Goff, P. A., Eberhardt, J. L., Williams, M. J., & Jackson, M. C. (2008). Not yet human: Implicit knowledge, historical dehumanization, and contemporary consequences. *Journal of Personality and Social Psychology, 94*(2), 292–306.

Haider, A. H., Janel, S. N. S., Cooper, L. A., Efron, D. T., Swoboda, S., & Cornwell, E. E., III. (2011). Association of unconscious race and social class bias with vignette-based clinical assessments by medical students. *JAMA: The Journal of the American Medical Association, 306*(9), 942–951.

Héroux, M., Janssen, I., Lee, D.-C., Sui, X., Hebert, J. R., & Blair, S. N. (2012). Clustering of unhealthy behaviors in the Aerobics Center Longitudinal Study. *Prevention Science*, 13(2), 183–195.

Hofmann, W., Gawronski, B., Gschwendner, T., Le, H., & Schmitt, M. (2005). A meta-analysis on the correlation between the implicit association test and explicit self-report measures. *Personality and Social Psychology Bulletin*, 31(10), 1369–1385.

Inzlicht, M., & Kang, S. K. (2010). Stereotype threat spillover: How coping with threats to social identity affects aggression, eating, decision making, and attention. *Journal of Personality and Social Psychology*, 99(3), 467–481.

Kessler, R. C., Mickelson, K. D., & Williams, D. R. (1999). The prevalence, distribution, and mental health correlates of perceived discrimination in the United States. *Journal of Health and Social Behavior*, 40(3), 208–230.

Kramer, M. R., Cooper, H. L., Drews-Botsch, C. D., Waller, L. A., & Hogue, C. R. (2010). Do measures matter? Comparing surface-density-derived and census-tract-derived measures of racial residential segregation. *International Journal of Health Geographics*, 9(29), 1–15.

Kramer, M. R., & Hogue, C. R. (2009). Is segregation bad for your health? *Epidemiologic Reviews*, 31(1), 178–194.

Krieger, N., Carney, D., Lancaster, K., Waterman, P. D., Kosheleva, A., & Banaji, M. (2010). Combining explicit and implicit measures of racial discrimination in health research. *American Journal of Public Health*, 100(8), 1485–1492.

Krieger, N., Waterman, P. D., Kosheleva, A., Chen, J. T., Carney, D. R., Smith, K. W., & Samuel, L. (2011). Exposing racial discrimination: Implicit and explicit measures. The My Body, My Story Study of 1005 US-born Black and White community health center members. *PLoS ONE*, 6(11), e27636.

Kwate, N. O. A., & Meyer, I. H. (2011). On sticks and stones and broken bones: Stereotypes and

African American health. *Du Bois Review: Social Science Research on Race*, 8(1), 191–198.

Lauderdale, D. S. (2006). Birth outcomes for Arabic-named women in California before and after September 11. *Demography*, 43(1), 185–201.

Lewis, T. T., Aiello, A. E., Leurgans, S., Kelly, J., & Barnes, L. L. (2010). Self-reported experiences of everyday discrimination are associated with elevated C-reactive protein levels in older African-American adults. *Brain, Behavior, and Immunity*, 24(3), 438–443.

Lewis, T. T., Barnes, L. L., Bienias, J. L., Lackland, D. T., Evans, D. A., & Mendes de Leon, C. F. (2009). Perceived discrimination and blood pressure in older African American and White adults. *Journals of Gerontology Series A: Biological Sciences and Medical Sciences*, 64A(9), 1002–1008.

Lewis, T., T. Everson-Rose, S., Powell, L. H., Matthews, K. A., Brown, C., Karavolos, K., & Wesley, D. (2006). Chronic exposure to everyday discrimination and coronary artery calcification in African-American women: The SWAN Heart Study. *Psychosomatic Medicine*, 68, 362–368.

Lewis, T. T., Kravitz, H. M., Janssen, I., & Powell, L. H. (2011). Self-reported experiences of discrimination and visceral fat in middle-aged African-American and Caucasian women. *American Journal of Epidemiology*, 173(11), 1223–1231.

Lewis, T. T., Troxel, W. M., Kravitz, H. M., Bromberger, J. T., Matthews, K. A., & Hall, M. H. (2012). Chronic exposure to everyday discrimination and sleep in a multiethnic sample of middle-aged women. *Health Psychology*. Advance online publication.

Lieberson, S. (1980). *A piece of the pie: Black and White immigrants since 1880*. Berkeley: University of California Press.

Massey, D. S., & Denton, N. A. (1993). *American apartheid: Segregation and the making of the underclass*. Cambridge, MA: Harvard University Press.

Mendez, D. D., Hogan, V. K., & Culhane, J. F. (2012). Stress during pregnancy: The role of institutional racism. *Stress and Health*. Advance online publication.

Morello-Frosch, R., & Jesdale, B. M. (2006). Separate and unequal: Residential segregation and estimated cancer risks associated with ambient air toxics in US metropolitan areas. *Environmental Health Perspectives, 114*(3), 386–393.

Mutz, D. C., & Goldman, S. K. (2010). Mass media. In J. F. Dovidio, M. Hewstone, P. Glick, & V. M. Esses (Eds.), *The Sage handbook of prejudice, stereotyping and discrimination* (pp. 241–257). Thousand Oaks, CA: Sage.

Norton, M. I., & Sommers, S. R. (2011). Whites see racism as a zero-sum game that they are now losing. *Perspectives on Psychological Science, 6*(3), 215–218.

Nosek, B. A., Smyth, F. L., Hansen, J. J., Devos, T., Lindner, N. M., Ranganath, K. A., & Banaji, M. R. (2007). Pervasiveness and correlates of implicit attitudes and stereotypes. *European Review of Social Psychology, 18*, 36–88.

Orfield, G., Frankenberg, E., & Garces, L. M. (2008). Statement of American social scientists of research on school desegregation to the U.S. Supreme Court in *Parents v. Seattle School District* and *Meredith v. Jefferson County. Urban Review, 40*(1), 96–136.

Osypuk, T. L., & Acevedo-Garcia, D. (2010). Beyond individual neighborhoods: A geography of opportunity perspective for understanding racial/ethnic health disparities. *Health Place, 16*(6), 1113–1123.

Padela, A. I., & Heisler, M. (2010). The association of perceived abuse and discrimination after September 11, 2001, with psychological distress, level of happiness, and health status among Arab Americans. *American Journal of Public Health, 100*(2), 284–291.

Pager, D., & Shepherd, H. (2008). The sociology of discrimination: Racial discrimination in employment, housing, credit, and consumer markets. *Annual Review of Sociology, 34*, 181–209.

Pascoe, E. A., & Richman, L. S. (2009). Perceived discrimination and health: A meta-analytic review. *Psychological Bulletin, 135*(4), 531–554.

Pettigrew, T. F., & Meertens, R. W. (1995). Subtle and blatant prejudice in western Europe. *European Journal of Social Psychology, 25*, 57–75.

Pew Research Center. (2011). *Wealth gaps rise to record highs between Whites, Blacks and Hispanics*. Washington, DC: Author.

Pollack, C. E., Chideya, S., Cubbin, C., Williams, B., Dekker, M., & Braveman, P. (2007). Should health studies measure wealth? A systematic review. *American Journal of Preventive Medicine, 33*(3), 250–264.

Profant, J., & Dimsdale, J. E. (1999). Race and diurnal blood pressure patterns: A review and meta-analysis. *Hypertension, 33*(5), 1099–1104.

Richman, L. S., & Jonassaint, C. (2008). The effects of race-related stress on cortisol reactivity in the laboratory: Implications of the Duke lacrosse scandal. *Annals of Behavioral Medicine, 35*(1), 105–110.

Sabin, J. A., Nosek, B. A., Greenwald, A. G., & Rivara, F. P. (2009). Physicians' implicit and explicit attitudes about race by MD race, ethnicity, and gender. *Journal of Health Care for the Poor and Underserved, 20*(3), 896–913.

Sampson, R. J. (1987). Urban Black violence: The effect of male joblessness and family disruption. *American Journal of Sociology, 93*(2), 348–382.

Sawyer, P. J., Major, B., Casad, B. J., Townsend, S. S. M., & Mendes, W. B. (2012). Discrimination and the stress response: Psychological and physiological consequences of anticipating prejudice in interethnic interactions. *American Journal of Public Health, 102*(5), 1020–1026.

Schoen, D. E. (2012). *Race in America*. Retrieved from http://www.thedailybeast.com/content/dam/

dailybeast/2012/04/06/Newsweek_DailyBeast_Race_In_America_Survey.pdf

Schuman, H., Steeh, C., Bobo, L., & Krysan, M. (1997). *Racial attitudes in America: Trends and interpretations* (Rev. ed.). Cambridge, MA: Harvard University Press.

Shih, M., Pittinsky, T. L., & Ambady, N. (1999). Stereotype susceptibility: Identity salience and shifts in quantitative performance. *Psychological Science, 10*(1), 80–83.

Smedley, B. D., Stith, A. Y., & Nelson, A. R. (2003). *Unequal treatment: Confronting racial and ethnic disparities in health care*. Washington, DC: National Academy Press.

Smith, T. W., Marsden, P. V., & Hout, M. (2011). *General Social Survey, 1972–2010*. Retrieved from Inter-university Consortium for Political and Social Research http://www.icpsr.umich.edu/icpsrweb/ICPSR/studies/31521

Steele, C. M. (1997). A threat in the air: How stereotypes shape intellectual identity and performance. *American Psychologist, 52*(6), 613–629.

Sternthal, M. J., Slopen, N., & Williams, D. R. (2011). Racial disparities in health: How much does stress really matter? *Du Bois Review, 8*(1), 95–113.

Talaska, C., Fiske, S., & Chaiken, S. (2008). Legitimating racial discrimination: Emotions, not beliefs, best predict discrimination in a meta-analysis. *Social Justice Research, 21*(3), 263–296.

Tesler, M. (2012). The spillover of racialization into health care: How President Obama polarized public opinion by racial attitudes and race. *American Journal of Political Science, 56*(3), 690–704.

Tomfohr, L., Cooper, D. C., Mills, P. J., Nelesen, R. A., & Dimsdale, J. E. (2010). Everyday discrimination and nocturnal blood pressure dipping in Black and White Americans. *Psychosomatic Medicine, 72*(3), 266–272.

Travis, J., & Waul, M. (2003). Prisoners once removed: The children and families of prisoners. In J. Travis & M. Waul (Eds.), *Prisoners once removed: The impact of incarceration and reentry on children, families and communities* (pp. 1–32). Wahington, DC: Urban Institute Press.

Tull, E. S., Cort, M. A., Gwebu, E. T., & Gwebu, K. (2007). Internalized racism is associated with elevated fasting glucose in a sample of adult women but not men in Zimbabwe. *Ethnicity and Disease, 17*(4), 731–735.

Tynes, B. M., Giang, M. T., Williams, D. R., & Thompson, G. N. (2008). Online racial discrimination and psychological adjustment among adolescents. *Journal of Adolescent Health, 43*(6), 565–569.

van Ryn, M., Burgess, D. J., Dovidio, J. F., Phelan, S. M., Saha, S., Malat, J., & Perry, S. (2011). The impact of racism on clinician cognition, behavior, and clinical decision making. *Du Bois Review, 8*(1), 199–218.

Verhaeghen, P., Aikman, S. N., & Van Gulick, A. E. (2011). Prime and prejudice: Co-occurrence in the culture as a source of automatic stereotype priming. *British Journal of Social Psychology, 50*(3), 501–518.

Viswanath, K. (2006). Public communications and its role in reducing and eliminationg health disparities. In G. E. Thomson, F. Mitchell, & M. B. Williams (Eds.), *Examining the health disparities research plan of the National Institutes of Health: Unfinished business* (pp. 215–253). Washington, DC: Institute of Medicine.

Wallace, D. (2011). Discriminatory mass dehousing and low-weight births: Scales of geography, time, and level. *Journal of Urban Health, 88*(3), 454–468.

Walters, K. L., Mohammed, S. A., Evans-Campbell, T., Beltrán, R. E., Chae, D. H., & Duran, B. (2011). Bodies don't just tell stories, they tell histories: Embodiment of historical trauma among American Indians and

Alaska Natives. *Du Bois Review: Social Science Research on Race*, *8*(1), 179–189.

Washington Post Company. (2009). Washington Post–ABC News poll: Race relations. Retrieved from http://www.washingtonpost.com/wp-srv/politics/polls/postpoll_042609.html

Weisbuch, M., Pauker, K., & Ambady, N. (2009). The subtle transmission of race bias via televised nonverbal behavior. *Science*, *326*(5960), 1711–1714.

Weisburd, D., Bushway, S., Lum, C., & Yang, S.-M. (2004). Trajectories of crime at places: A longitudinal study of street segments in the City of Seattle. *Criminology*, *42*(2), 283–321.

White, K., & Borrell, L. N. (2011). Racial/ethnic residential segregation: Framing the context of health risk and health disparities. *Health and Place*, *17*(2), 438–448.

White, K., Haas, J. S., & Williams, D. R. (2012). Elucidating the role of place in health care disparities: The example of racial/ethnic residential segregation. *Health Services Research*, *47*(3, Part 2), 1278–1299.

Williams, D. R. (1997). Race and health: Basic questions, emerging directions. *Annals of Epidemiology*, *7*(5), 322–333.

Williams, D. R. (2004). Racism and health. In K. E. Whitfield (Ed.), *Closing the gap: Improving the health of minority elders in the new millennium* (pp. 69–80). Washington, DC: Gerontological Society of America.

Williams, D. R. (2012). Miles to go before we sleep: Racial inequities in health. *Journal of Health and Social Behavior*, *53*(3), 279–295.

Williams, D. R., & Collins, C. (2001). Racial residential segregation: A fundamental cause of racial disparities in health. *Public Health Reports*, *116*(5), 404–416.

Williams, D. R., Gonzalez, H. M., Williams, S., Mohammed, S. A., Moomal, H., & Stein, D. J. (2008). Perceived discrimination, race and health in South Africa: Findings from the South Africa Stress and Health Study. *Social Science and Medicine*, *67*(3), 441–452.

Williams, D. R., Jackson, J. S., Brown, T. N., Torres, M., Forman, T. A., & Brown, K. (1999). Traditional and contemporary prejudice and urban Whites' support for affirmative action and government help. *Social Problems*, *46*(4), 503–527.

Williams, D. R., & Mohammed, S. A. (2008). Poverty, migration, and health. In A. C. Lin & D. R. Harris (Eds.), *The colors of poverty* (pp. 135–169). New York, NY: Russell Sage Foundation.

Williams, D. R., & Mohammed, S. A. (2009). Discrimination and racial disparities in health: Evidence and needed research. *Journal of Behavioral Medicine*, *32*(1), 20–47.

Williams, D. R., & Mohammed, S. A. (in press). Racism and health II: A needed research agenda for effective interventions. *American Behavioral Scientist*.

Williams, D. R., Yu, Y., Jackson, J., & Anderson, N. (1997). Racial differences in physical and mental health: Socioeconomic status, stress, and discrimination. *Journal of Health Psychology*, *2*(3), 335–351.

Williams, N. (2006). Where are the men? The impact of incarceration and reentry of African-American men and their children and families. *Community Voices: Healthcare for the Underserved*. Retrieved from http://www.communityvoices.org/uploads/wherearethemen2_00108_00144.pdf

Wilson, W. J. (1987). *The truly disadvantaged*. Chicago, IL: University of Chicago Press.

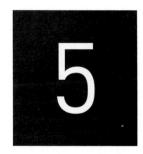

SEX, GENDER, AND VULNERABILITY

Rachel C. Snow

INTRODUCTION

Gender is a particularly complex social determinant of health because it interacts, and is closely identified, with biologic dimensions of vulnerability. Research efforts to understand 'what gender does' to health are particularly challenging for several reasons. Principal among these is that sex and gender are frequently conflated in the epidemiologic and medical literature. While a growing number of health studies claim to include an analysis of gender, they use the terms sex and gender interchangeably, and go no further than including sex/gender as one bivariate category in their analysis. By using the terms gender and sex interchangeably, the public health literature implicitly endorses the notion that gender is an extension of sex. Recent studies offer us disaggregated data by sex, but such data alone do little to further our understanding of whether observed sex differentials are attributable to

underlying chromosomal sex differences, to gender experience, or a combination of factors.

Why would this matter? Because our approach to interventions could be different depending on the answer; sex-linked vulnerabilities, attributable to *gendered experience*, may open debate about prevailing gender norms, and whether gendered expectations may be leading to more harm than good. An acknowledgment that certain aspects of gendered behavioural expectations are harmful to health, or even potentially fatal, begs a discussion on whether re-visioning gender may be warranted for public health purposes.

It is the intention of this paper to compare the 2002 global Disability-Adjusted Life Years (DALYs) for males and females, and to discuss how biologic differences in sex chromosomes contribute to a subset of these differentials through intrinsic vulnerabilities (e.g. birth asphyxia among males, glaucoma among females). A further subset of health conditions, with

Sex, Gender, and Vulnerability, Rachel C. Snow in *Global Public Health*, Vol. 3, Issue Sup. 1, pp. 58–74, January 1, 2008. With permission from Taylor & Francis.

large differentials by sex, are more directly attributable to gendered patterns of work and social experience (e.g. road traffic accidents among males, trachoma among females), while another subset of health conditions illustrates how sex and gender vulnerabilities may be overlaid on one another in ways that can exacerbate sex differences in outcome, or mitigate risks (e.g. the female excess in blindness). A residual group of health outcomes that disproportionately affect one sex remain mystifying (e.g. the high burden of gout among males, the high burden of depression among females), because our current understanding of causality is incomplete.

In the second part of the paper, it is argued that gender effects on health are characterized by a capacity for adaptation over time and space, in response to fashion, media, or public policy. As such, they invite the possibility for interventions that directly target health risks due to gendered behaviours. Yet, even when the impact of gender on health is substantial, and appears amenable to intervention, there have been limited such efforts to intervene. This hesitation to intervene, when gendered socialization and gender discrimination harms, is not only costly to human health, but suggests an abiding unwillingness to design policies or programmes that might instrumentally challenge gendered identities. A more open reflection on gender interventions is called for in the interest of health.

DEFINITIONS

Before proceeding, let me affirm the definitions used in this paper. The term *biologic sex* refers to the developmental differentiations in anatomy and physiology that are a direct consequence of the inherited composition of sex chromosomes (46, XX versus 46, XY karyotypes). It is this difference in sex chromosomes that leads to differentiation of the gonads, steroid production, and, eventually, secondary sex characteristics. The cascade of differentiating events is well underway in the unborn foetus at 20 weeks, and accelerates once again at puberty. Both before birth and after puberty it is the dramatic quantitative differences in the production of hormones (i.e.

androgens and estrogens) that serve as the intermediaries between the sex genotype (i.e. the inherited sex chromosomes) and the manifestation of physical characteristics observed in post-pubertal males and females (Federman 2006). It is the phenotype of sex[1], or whether an individual is judged to look male or female by others, that evokes a constellation of gendered social expectations, responsibilities, and obstacles; such a gendered experience incurs health risks unrelated to chromosomal sex itself.

SEX DIFFERENCES IN DISEASES

To conduct a review of sex, gender, and vulnerability, one must have sex-disaggregated data. Such data are increasingly available in the health field, but not in all countries or international databases. The aggregate data, used for this analysis, are taken from the World Health Organization's (WHO) Global Burden of Disease (2004) estimates of disability adjusted life years (DALYs), by age, sex, and cause, *without age-weighting or discounting* (DALYs [0,0]). DALYs provide an aggregate measure of healthy years of life lost due to premature death or disability. These estimates are extremely rough, as they reflect the many extant gaps in regional, and, thereby global, epidemiologic data. Epidemiologic data may be subject to systematic biases, including intrinsic sex and gender biases (Sundby 1998, Hanson 2002). For example, select conditions are known to be under-reported, by one sex or another, due to gender-based fears of stigma and discrimination (e.g. infertility or domestic violence among females, sexual dysfunction among males). In select regions of northwest India, China, and South Korea, child health data may be more accurate for male children, given the persistent evidence of son preference (Das Gupta et al. 2003), and the discrimination against health-seeking for girl children (Chen et al. 1981, Das Gupta 1987, Das Gupta et al. 2003).

Furthermore, the estimation of DALYs requires the generation of disability weights, i.e. subjective estimations of how 'burdensome' a given illness is for a human life. These estimations have been found to vary substantially, depending on the local culture and professional status of those undertaking the estimations (Sadana 1998, Jelsma et al. 2000). In Zimbabwe and Cambodia, for example, non-professionals weighted infertility as substantially more burdensome than did the Burden of Disease experts. Other conditions affecting marriage prospects for women, such as vitiligo, were also ranked higher by local evaluators in Cambodia, leading to criticism that disability weights reflect the gender biases of elite male health professionals[2].

Substantial criticism has also been raised over the use of age-weighting and discounting in the DALY, but use of these adjustments is optional, and the present analysis makes use of DALYs *without* weighting or discounting (DALYs [0,0]). While a full account of the arguments against age-weighting and discounting are beyond the scope of this paper, the rationale for age-weighting, i.e. an a priori assumption that a given year of life at different ages has greater or lesser value to society, is persuasively rejected by Anand and Hanson (1997, 1998). With regard to discounting, it is sufficient to quote Beermann (1999): 'Ethical criteria become relevant to this question, because, health (or life-years) is a basic aspect of life, so that correspondingly there exists a basic right to health. The *specific* ethical problem in this context is the problem of justice between generations and the general answer to the problem is that current and future generations must be treated equally'.

Acknowledging the underlying weaknesses in epidemiologic coverage of the DALY, and possibilities for systematic underreporting for the poor, and for women's conditions, these estimates still remain the best available source on the relative global status of health outcomes, especially if used without age-weighting or discounting, as provided here. Based on the 2002 global data for all ages combined, the 10 leading causes of lost DALYs, among females and males, are listed in Table 5.1. The first three leading causes are similar for males and females, at least when viewed in large aggregate ICD-10[3] categories: lower respiratory conditions, HIV, and diarrhoeal disease, top the list for both sexes. Thereafter, sex

differences of relative magnitude emerge, with ischemic heart disease, low birth weight, malaria, cerebrovascular disease, and birth trauma, on both lists, but with differences in absolute numbers of DALYs, as well as relative rank order. The overall greater DALY burden, among males worldwide, is evident in the absolute numbers of DALYs lost in the top 10 conditions (e.g. the tenth ranked condition for males is still accounting for 44 million DALYs worldwide); females, on the other hand, have two conditions on their list that contribute less than 35 million DALYs.

The top 10 lists are also distinct in tell-tale ways, i.e. in the appearance of two injury-related categories on the male list (unintentional injury and road traffic accidents), and the appearance of unipolar depressive disorders on the female list. The relative and absolute importance, of accident and injury to men's health, emerges under many separate conditions in the Global Burden of Disease (GBD) statistics. Alcohol contributes to road traffic accidents, especially fatal accidents. A cluster of health outcomes, that include substance abuse (alcohol or drug), and their direct or indirect consequences (such as traffic accidents), are consistently in excess among males (see next section for further discussion).

Women's vulnerability to unipolar depression, in the top 10 list, is echoed by excess female DALYs for a range of other psychiatric conditions, including panic disorder, post-traumatic stress disorder, and obsessive compulsive disorder (see Table 5.2b); the excess female DALYs for these outcomes is found in many national and cross-national studies (Hallstrom 2001, Angst et al. 2002, Hopcraft and Bradley 2007). Several authors have highlighted possible gender biases, in current diagnostic instruments, that would lead to under-diagnosis of male depression (Rutz 1999, Bech 2001, Moeller Leimkuehler et al. 2007). The feminist community, in fact, has questioned, for some time, assumptions that women are inherently vulnerable to mental illness (Chessler 1972). Ironically, the diagnosis and gendered causes of depression may receive more concerted attention, given the growing interest in male depression (van Grootheest et al. 1999, Han et al. 2006, Moeller Leimkuehler et al. 2007). A more

	Males (all ages)		**Females (all ages)**	
	TABLE 5.1 ■ Top 10 Causes of Disease or Disability for Males and Females, Based on the Number of Total Global DALYS Lost at All Ages; Data Based on DALYS [0,0] Published in 2002			
	Cause	DALYs	Cause	DALYs
1	Lower respiratory infections	99,057,981	Lower respiratory infections	97,801,108
2	HIV	78,020,596	HIV	73,516,955
3	Diarrhoeal diseases	71,883,930	Diarrhoeal diseases	67,296,145
4	Ischaemic heart disease	64,504,498	Malaria	52,646,469
5	Low birth weight	58,925,647	Low birth weight	51,321,438
6	Other unintentional injuries	49,236,025	Ischaemic heart disease	50,082,860
7	Malaria	47,184,421	Cerebrovascular disease	47,623,180
8	Cerebrovascular disease	46,437,060	Other infectious diseases	45,068,486
9	Road traffic accidents	45,112,383	Birth asphyxia and birth trauma	34,940,346
10	Birth asphyxia and birth trauma	44,068,687	Unipolar depressive disorders	32,507,673

compelling perspective, on male/female sex differences, is provided by looking at conditions for which there are large disparities in DALYs by sex. Tables 5.2a and 5.2b include all conditions for which the male/female discrepancy in total DALYs is more than 25% of the lesser value; they list conditions for which males or females, respectively, have a 25%, or greater, excess in overall DALYs.

ATTRIBUTING HEALTH OUTCOMES TO SEX OR GENDER

As shown among the conditions listed in Tables 5.2a and 5.2b, one can start to parse out a subset of outcomes that are intrinsically linked to an XX or XY genotype and sex-linked differences in function (and vulnerability). For others, vulnerabilities are clearly associated with specific types of jobs and social exposures that are socially divided between

the sexes. A further group of conditions are impossible to classify as attributable to sex or gender, either because both dimensions are involved in complex ways, or because the level of fundamental research is inadequate.

Differences in health outcomes, that are linked to an XX or XY karyotype (see Table 5.3a), include the risk of haemophilia among XY karyotypes, and the vulnerability to testicular and prostate cancers made possible by the karyotypes encoding the growth and development of a prostate and testes; likewise, corresponding XX karyotypes allow the development of a cervix and ovaries. Male foetal lung development is also distinct from that of females in utero, such that male pulmonary function matures more slowly, contributing to more respiratory distress syndromes and lung-related injuries among male newborns. The male excess of 35–50%, for a wide range of respiratory-related causes of death in the newborn, including infant respiratory distress syndrome (IRDS), sudden infant death syndrome (SIDS), upper respiratory infections, and asphyxia

(Stevenson et al. 2000), are increasingly theorized to reflect an X-linked recessive allele, i.e. a sex-linked chromosomal vulnerability (Mage and Donner 2004), contributing to the 'newborn male disadvantage' in low birth weight as well[4]. Conversely, differences in the biology of male and female lungs also suggest that an equivalent exposure to tobacco smoke leads to a greater risk of molecular aberrations (i.e. mutations) in female lungs (Patel et al. 2004). While the sex genotype does not cause these outcomes, it is a necessary pre-condition to the outcome, distinguishing a sex-linked vulnerability, i.e. a vulnerability not experienced by members of the opposite sex. Health outcomes, such as testicular cancer or low birth weight, for example, may also

be caused by environmental risks or poverty, respectively, but they also reflect sex-specific vulnerabilities.

Gendered expectations, imposed on members of each sex, impact health in a variety of ways. Divisions of labour between the sexes underlie some of the most obviously gendered differences in health outcomes, such as the greater risk of drowning among males worldwide, because of their roles as fishermen and boatmen, and, by contrast, the greater number of burnings among women, due to their responsibility for cooking and fire-tending (see Table 5.3b).

Gendered differences in occupational health risk are, however, only the tip of the iceberg. Gendered leisure activities and ways of coping with life stress,

TABLE 5.2A ■ **Select Health Conditions for Which DALYS Lost to Males Are at Least 25% Above Those Lost to Females**

Condition	Male DALYs	Female DALYs	Male DALYS/ Female DALYS
War	9,306,296	1,131,676	8.223
Gout	4,246,359	572,741	7.414
Alcohol use disorders	14,810,111	2,662,637	5.562
Road and traffic accidents	45,112,383	9,532,961	4.732
Violence	27,470,156	6,810,306	4.034
Other intentional injuries	496,974	126,953	3.915
Drug use disorders	6,006,662	1,616,742	3.715
Lymphatic filariasis	6,248,138	2,056,275	3.039
Mouth and propharynx cancers	4,751,823	1,991,476	2.386
Lung cancer (trachea & bronchus)	15,232,399	6,687,840	2.278
Liver cancer	9,409,480	4,208,880	2.236
Drowning	13,983,352	6,795,333	2.058
Bladder cancer	1,913,556	964,949	1.983
Anorectal atresia	49,504	25,843	1.916
Hepatitis B	2,645,774	1,408,635	1.878

(Continued)

TABLE 5.2A ■ **(Continued)**

Condition	Male DALYs	Female DALYs	Male DALYS/ Female DALYS
Poisoning	8,927,574	5,011,169	1.782
Oesophagus cancer	5,266,748	3,049,496	1.727
Trypanosomiasis	1,741,306	1,043,857	1.668
TB	37,298,748	22,944,907	1.626
Peptic ulcer disease	4,574,045	2,939,246	1.556
Stomach cancer	9,576,685	6,171,105	1.552
Schistosomiasis	1,025,505	666,404	1.539
Other unintentional injuries	49,236,025	32,020,194	1.538
Falls	14,429,845	9,532,961	1.514
Cirrhosis of the liver	14,613,849	9,734,719	1.501
Renal agenesis	104,192	69,973	1.489
Self-inflicted injuries	21,665,217	15,201,138	1.425
Leprosy	198,328	142,864	1.388
Leishmaniasis	1,970,613	1,462,594	1.347
Onchocerciasis	355,411	264,327	1.345
Other malignant neoplasm's	9,324,018	6,993,333	1.333
Inflammatory heart disease	5,650,277	4,387,989	1.288
Appendicitis	359,687	281,805	1.276
Benign prosthetic hypertrophy	3,747,386		
Prostate cancers	3,254,128		

shaped by social messaging about what leisure activities a male or female should undertake, result in differential rates of cigarette smoking, alcohol, and drug use, and a cascade of associated health risks. Cigarette smoking continues to be more common among men in much of the world, contributing not only to lung, mouth, and bladder cancer (Meisel 2002), but also to an estimated one-third of the male excess in reported tuberculosis (TB) cases

(Watkins and Plant 2006). Differential gendered obligations to children, the sick, and the community affect exposure to infections (e.g. trachoma, influenza), and the structure and responsiveness of the health system itself biases care. For example, there is evidence of more renal transplantation for males than females, controlling for medical need and patient interest (Alexander and Sehgal 1998), and fewer referrals for women than men for angiography,

TABLE 5.2B ■ Select Health Conditions for Which DALYS Lost to Females Are at Least 25% Above Those Lost to Males			
Condition	Female DALYs	Male DALYs	Female DALYs/ Male DALYs
Breast cancer	11,733,351	44,483	263.772
Gonorrhoea	2,888,421	264,196	10.933
Chlamydia	2,888,421	264,196	10.933
Trachoma	2,475,721	811,980	3.049
Migraine	8,802,838	3,146,812	2.797
Post-traumatic stress disorder	1,883,391	720,628	2.614
Rheumatoid arthritis	4,259,468	1,672,682	2.546
Panic disorder	3,594,381	1,844,713	1.948
Alzheimer and other dementias	12,818,790	7,213,869	1.777
Osteoarthritis	15,629,274	9,149,400	1.708
Other musculoskeletal disorders	3,518,880	2,093,852	1.681
Fires	12,768,433	8,223,566	1.553
Unipolar depressive disorders	32,507,673	21,133,650	1.538
Iron-deficiency anaemia	9,025,199	6,077,808	1.485
Other oral diseases	95,088	65,503	1.452
Insomnia (primary)	1,894,676	1,362,610	1.390
Multiple sclerosis	1,000,898	722,796	1.385
OCD	2,330,821	1,705,743	1.366
Other intestinal diseases	88,928	65,128	1.365
Cataracts	21,454,199	15,729,865	1.364
Rheumatic heart disease	6,184,772	4,548,016	1.360
Vision disorders, age-related	12,714,330	9,413,331	1.351
Glaucoma	3,304,452	2,464,786	1.341
Other genitourinary systems diseases	3,668,296	2,842,889	1.290
Japanese encephalitis	658,357	522,117	1.261
Other maternal conditions	15,062,497		

(Continued)

TABLE 5.2B   ■   (Continued)

Condition	Female DALYs	Male DALYs	Female DALYs/ Male DALYs
Maternal sepsis	8,688,660		
Maternal haemorrhage	7,602,986		
Cervix uteri cancer	6,322,294		
Abortion	5,967,628		
Obstructed labour	4,851,864		
Hypertensive disorders	3,889,105		
Ovary cancer	3,174,156		
Corpus uteri cancer	2,075,423		

TABLE 5.3A   ■   Sex-Specific Vulnerabilities

XY Vulnerabilities	XX Vulnerabilities
Haemophilia	Breast cancer
Prostate cancer	Ovarian cancer
Testicular cancer	All maternal causes
Birth asphyxia and trauma	Chlamydia
Low birth weight	Rheumatoid arthritis
Acute starvation	Osteoarthritis
Renal agenesis	Glaucoma Cataracts (in part)

TABLE 5.3B   ■   Gendered Vulnerabilities

Male Gender Vulnerabilities	Female Gender Vulnerabilities
Falls Drowning Road traffic accidents Self-inflicted injuries Lung cancer Drug use disorders	Fires Trachoma Cataracts (in part) • Panic disorders • Depressive disorders • Post-traumatic stress disorders • Insomnia • Migraine
Alcohol use disorders Cirrhosis of the liver Bladder cancer (in part) TB (in part)	

despite identical clinical characteristics (Schulman et al. 1999). The literature provides substantial documentation of gendered divisions in health care experience (see Doyal 1995, Annendale and Hunt 2000, Östlin et al. 2001, Sen et al. 2002, among others).

One of the challenges in studying how gender affects health, is the near-ubiquitous assumption that sex-linked genetic differences in biologic capabilities (e.g. women's ability to give birth and breastfeed, men's upper body strength), justify professional and social exclusions that, in turn, come with certain health risks. It is tempting to treat sex and gender as if the latter is a natural extension of the former, especially for health conditions that result from women's roles in homemaking (e.g. fires) and childrearing (e.g. trachoma), or men's work in heavy labour (e.g. falls, drowning). This extends to subtle but widespread assumptions about the inevitability of interpersonal violence, i.e. that males are naturally inclined to violence, and even genetically motivated to control the women in their lives, at times by force. Use of the terms 'gender' and 'sex' interchangeably endorses such a perspective, implying that gendered behaviours and vulnerabilities are an organic consequence of genetic sex; there is much support for such an approach among social conservatives, rationalized as a division of labour rooted in nature, or divine intent.

The excess incidence of depressive and other mental health difficulties among females, begs research on the relative contributions of sex chromosome-linked vulnerabilities versus gendered experience, or the possibility that the relevant diagnostic criteria are, themselves, gender-biased, leading to over-diagnosis of women, or under-diagnosis of men (Moeller Leimkuehler et al. 2007). Astbury comments, 'notions of women's biologically based vulnerability or proneness to [mental] disorder have proved rather resistant to change', while not subjected to empirical investigation (Astbury 2002: 147). Rising interest in men and depression will certainly heighten the attention to possible gender biases in diagnoses, but more analysis is warranted on at least two other questions: whether there are social advantages (for men) in constructing women as vulnerable to mental illness and whether the world is organized in ways that so limit women's options, and so heighten their fears that depression (and panic-disorder) are understandable.

Men's greater vulnerability to alcohol-related disorders has been commented on by Astbury (2002, citing Allen et al. 1994) as possibly exaggerated by reporting bias, i.e. if women selectively avoid reporting alcohol problems. While this may be the case, the DALYs for alcohol-related outcomes, including cirrhosis, gout, and road traffic accidents, are each consistently and strongly in excess for males, supporting the likelihood of greater alcohol-related disorders among males, even in the event of under-reporting by females.

Traffic accidents are not only one of the 10 highest causes of global DALYs for males, but they offer a potent area for gendered analysis of cause and debates over policy. The following case draws on a paper by this author, prepared for the WHO in 2002 (Snow 2002). Globally, males sustain approximately 70% of all traffic accident deaths, and over 70% of all traffic-related DALYs per year. Much of the male excess in traffic accidents can be attributed to men's greater access to vehicles, and their roles as drivers. In general, males have more experience than females in driving all types of vehicles, and socialization of males emphasizes mastery over motorized transport of all kinds. So, does the excess male involvement in traffic accidents simply reflect more (gendered) driving time? US data allow an analysis of crashes, adjusted for total vehicle miles travelled: when controlling for males' excess exposure, the sex difference in crash involvement disappears. However, the same adjustment fails to account for excess male involvement in fatal crashes. The excess risk for fatal crashes among males is especially dramatic among the youngest drivers, and largely attributable to speed and alcohol (Maio et al. 1997, Odero 1998). Males are not only more likely than females to drive after they have been drinking but, when simulated driving was evaluated among 18-year-olds who had their blood alcohol raised experimentally, girls were found to drive more cautiously as they got drunker, while boys became more reckless (Oei Tian and Kerschbaumer 1990).

To what extent is such risk-taking encouraged as part of masculine identity, i.e. a way of 'doing' male gender, or a sex-linked predisposition of the genotype? Investigations of the biologic basis of male risk-taking have been largely inconclusive. Complex studies of twins find more sensation-seeking behaviour among those with greater in utero exposure to androgens (Daitzman et al. 1978, Resnick et al. 1993), but the magnitude of the effects are small, and variations in childrearing cannot be excluded. Even in the event of a sex-linked genetic predisposition to risk-taking among males, we also have powerful social and media messages that promote risk-taking as a signature means of demonstrating masculinity. Courtenay (2000) argues that dismissing risks, in general, is a crucial means by which males construct their gender. Recognizing that some degree of risk-taking has positive value in modern life, the outstanding question may be whether, and how, risk-taking tendencies might be shaped or regulated to avoid endangering males and, more generally, society (Snow 2002).

For a range of health outcomes, with large differences between the sexes, sex and gender vulnerabilities may both be, in effect, compounding or mitigating one another. The challenge here is to undertake a careful desegregation of measured affects that may be caused by sex or gender, often in the midst of other independent causes. Blindness offers a compelling example of a health outcome, attributable to a combination of sex and gendered causes that heightens female risk, resulting in almost 150 blind women for every 100 blind men in the world. This example draws on the research of Courtright, Lewallen, and colleagues who have undertaken a model effort to disentangle sex and gendered causes of blindness (see Abou-Gareeb et al. 2001, Courtright and Lewallen 2002, Lewallen and Courtright 2002).

Women bear approximately two-thirds of the global burden of blindness; results of a metaanalysis suggest a pooled age-adjusted odds ratio of 1.43 (95% CI 1.33-1.53) (Abou-Gareeb et al. 2001). This reflects several dimensions of heightened risk for women: a 10–15% greater incidence of cataracts, the leading cause of global blindness which, Courtright and Lewallen (2002) propose, is due to sex-linked inherent risks for women. To this is added a 2.5–3 times greater risk of trachoma-related blindness among adult women than men. As the proportion of active infections is similar among boys and girls, the greater number of active infections among adult women is attributed to their greater contact with infected children. These disparities in vulnerability are compounded by men's greater access to cataract surgery in many parts of the developing world. Hence, the global excess of female blindness is attributed to an (hypothesized) sex-linked vulnerability to cataract, a gendered risk of trachoma, and a gendered distribution of eye care services. This analysis is particularly helpful in that the authors have identified gendered dimensions which, by definition, are amenable to intervention, such as delivering more cataract surgical services to women.

IMPLICATIONS FOR RESEARCH AND POLICY

The causal factors responsible for many of the sex differences in health, listed in Tables 5.2a and 5.2b, remain poorly understood, including those causing TB, depression, osteoarthritis, Alzheimer's and dementia, migraine, and gout. TB and depression deserve special concern, due to the magnitude of global DALYs lost to these two conditions. The higher proportion of male cases of reported TB may reflect underlying sex-based genetic vulnerabilities, or cultural and service barriers that limit case-reporting among women, or some combination of both (Thorson et al. 2004, Weiss et al. 2006). Given the high global burden of TB for both sexes, there should be sustained efforts to explore all social vulnerabilities, including those attributable to gender. Better understanding of systematic biases in diagnosis, willingness to screen, or access to care would shed light on male and female vulnerabilities alike, furthering TB control for all patients. Recent data, from Malawi, Bangladesh, India, and Colombia, found that women were more likely than men to drop out of care during TB diagnosis, while men were less likely than women to complete treatment once diagnosed (Weiss et al. 2006). The way that gender interacts with stigma, to affect compliance with care, can differ significantly by locale, depending on local confidence about TB treatment, and gendered aspects of the marriage and job markets (Thorson et al. 2004, Weiss et al. 2006). A cautionary lesson from the emerging data on gender and TB is the apparent local mutability of how gender affects health seeking. In the case of TB, generalizations seem difficult. Variations don't preclude national or even regional interventions, but they do call for robust specification of *how* gender impacts health seeking in a given setting.

With regard to depression, substantial gender biases in diagnosis cannot be excluded. Some diagnostic scales include questions about frequent crying or irritability, behaviours that are already laden with gender implications. It is tempting to parallel the female DALYs lost to depression, and other mental health conditions, with the excess of male DALYs lost to negative coping behaviours, such as alcohol or drug use, violence, and risk-taking. The possibility has been raised by several authors (Rutz 1999, Bech 2001, Moeller Leimkuehler et al. 2007), that depression in women, and alcohol use and risk-taking in men, are gendered manifestations for similar underlying distress. Pollack (1998) argues that current cultural standards, in the west, trap boys into a 'boy code' of macho, self-negating behaviours, that emphasize bravado, extreme daring, and attraction to violence, and it remains an active social norm to shame boys who fail to comply with such behaviours. Pollack states that such codes lead to loneliness and distress for a large proportion of boys, putting them at social risks throughout life. Such theories are supported by evidence that males progress to depression after periods of aggression and alcohol abuse that are not observed in females (Bech 2001), and by evidence that depressed men are more likely than women to cope by increasing their sports activity and alcohol consumption (Angst et al. 2002). The social or genetic determinants of these differences warrant much closer scrutiny. In the event that gender socialization itself contributes substantially to depression or negative coping, public information (at the least), and possibly regulation, warrant consideration[5].

THE MUTABILITY OF GENDER

If one agrees that gendered behaviours are subject to socialization then, at least theoretically, the DALYs attributable to gendered behaviours that endanger people should be responsive to intervention. Recent history suggests that gendered health behaviours can change in response to marketing, fashion, or public legislation. In the case of smoking, both the percentage of smokers and the incidence of lung cancer in many high-income countries, such as the USA, have shifted towards equity, even as overall rates of smoking have declined. In the USA, for example, the proportion of adult males who smoke has dropped

by 55% in the past 40 years, from just over half of all adult males in 1965 to fewer than a quarter in 2004 (American Lung Association 2006). Impressively, a large proportion of US males dropped smoking as a requisite accessory of masculinity; over the same period, however, women's relation to smoking has been less clear-cut. Women have always smoked less than males; in fact, smoking was a means of doing 'maleness' precisely because it was something most women did not do. Therefore, smoking has been associated with rebellion from restrictive gender norms, and effectively marketed by the cigarette companies as a symbol of liberation[6] (Brown 2000). The decline in female smokers since 1965 has been less than among males (about 45%), leaving the percentage of adult male and female smokers in the USA closer to equity than ever before (e.g. 23.4% of males and 18.5% of females currently smoke) (American Lung Association 2006).

In middle- and low-income countries, there is typically a much larger sex gap in smoking; the percentage of male and female smokers, respectively, is 51% and 18% in Mexico, 40% and 7% in Zambia, 22% and 2% in Iran, and 29% and 2% in India (Pampel 2006). In many countries, female smoking continues to be regarded as immodest and unfeminine, and is strongly discouraged in all but quite elderly women. Given that similar social constraints on western women's smoking gradually lifted as women moved into public and professional roles, there is concern that women's emerging autonomy in poorer countries will also lead to increased smoking (Patel et al. 2004, Pampel 2006), aided by cigarette companies' efforts to sell smoking as an attractive attribute of a modern woman.

While cigarette companies readily promote change in gender norms to sell smoking, public health advocacy has made only a few concerted attempts to explicitly address gendered imagery to promote health. One such programme, that targeted female smoking, was undertaken by the Irish National Health Promotion Strategy 2000–2005, with a campaign that concentrated on the unattractiveness of smoking, to challenge media images of female smoking as fashionable. Following the campaign, the percentage of young women, aged

18–35, who smoked, dropped by an average of 4%, with proponents encouraged that the gender-targeted approach was a contributing factor.

A much more expanded and long-term effort was initiated in Sweden two decades ago, to promote healthy gender norms. The Swedish Government initiated educational policies in the 1980s that explicitly sought to end stereotyped gender patterns in society. Curricula are required to challenge traditional gender messages. These policies were extended to Swedish pre-schools in 1998 (Lpfo 1998), and both Sweden and France now claim that their pre-schools avoid war toys and fashion dolls. The long-term impact of these efforts deserves scrutiny, not the least for how they impact health behaviours and outcomes.

In the African context, anti-HIV campaigns explicitly challenge aspects of gender identity that endanger young people. The loveLife billboards in South Africa, question gendered assumptions about male control in sexual and romantic relationships, and provide young people (and all viewers) with an alternative gender vision of equitable, negotiated partnerships. However, loveLife is not alone, though perhaps more innovative in their messaging than others. Social marketing firms, such as New Start, promote condom use, HIV testing, and family planning, with ads that incorporate images of a new responsible male. The longer-term impact of such messages is largely untested and warrants evaluation, and it would be particularly worthwhile to examine how such expanded messaging efforts may evoke behaviour change in non-reproductive and non-sexual domains. What, for example, might be the impact on female depression, or men's negative coping behaviours? The health and social costs of gender stereotyping warrant more systematic enquiry, and more quantitative evaluation.

In the West, most restrictions on men's or women's behaviours (e.g. employment or mobility) have now been disallowed in the interest of gender equity, with the exception of restricting pregnant women's exposure to occupational hazards. Yet, the magnitude of the global DALYs lost to road traffic accidents among males (and the acknowledged impact of restrictive licensing) might

warrant another exception. Current legislated and non-binding health policies for traffic accidents and alcohol consumption are sex-neutral. Licensing and alcohol restrictions when driving are the same for both sexes in all countries, with the important exception of several states in the Middle East. Automobile insurance companies have long differentiated between males and females, compensating for the excess male risk of traffic accidents through sex disaggregated premium scales, and close scrutiny of risky behaviour among young males. An intervention looking for high impact on sex-specific DALYs would entertain sex-specific applications of graduated licensing, a higher age for licensing males, a higher age for legal consumption of alcohol by males, or a policy of zero-tolerance for male drinking and driving.

Gender equality legislation in the USA currently disallows such sex-specific discriminations unless sex-specific risk behaviours are proven to be genetically or biologically based (Kommers and Finn 1998); occupational restrictions of pregnant women are allowed under this exception, i.e. because only females become pregnant. This is a somewhat ironic exception in the case of dangerous masculine behaviours, such as drinking and driving, because the logical extension of the restriction is that those arguing that male risk-taking is programmed 'in their genes', are, in fact, offering a rationale for sex-specific restrictions. Arguments that such behaviours are socialized negate any legal chance at regulation (at least in the USA), but place the DALYs due to men's risk taking (or violence, or negative coping) on our doorstep, as a public pathology that we have created, and that we are responsible for changing. Trials that examine efforts to reduce gender stereotyping of males as risk-takers, and promote 'doing gender' in less dangerous ways, are plausible at a significant scale.

A parallel argument might apply to female depression, panic disorder, or OCD. Again, if it's 'all in her genes', then special protections may need to be retrieved from the dustbin of recent history. Conversely, if these excess female DALYs are judged to be a consequence of gendered experience, then public health considerations alone might prompt a re-examination of the health and social costs of gendered expectations and discriminations.

In many respects, the loveLife campaign already offers a radical challenge to female vulnerability, identifying female stereotypes of positive subservience to be deadly, and encouraging self-regard. It is notable that the loveLife campaigns have been particularly controversial, with accusations of using 'overly intellectual' and 'obscure' messages. Gender stereotyping in literature, television, and curricula are increasingly under fire, but much of modern media continues to re-enforce gender messages that can only exacerbate the health patterns observed in the global DALYs. Despite the eloquent reasoning of legal theorists, such as MacKinnon (1987), who have challenged the free-speech defence of sexist media on the principle that such 'speech' endangers women, even violently sexist images remain protected. Such arguments may be more persuasive if they gave greater emphasis to the extent that gender stereotyping endangers the healthy lives of both women and men.

little attention given to the potential impact of interventions that offer alternative gender images for both males and females, and evaluate their public health impact. The global changes underway in smoking offer evidence that gendered health behaviours change with social messaging, marketing, and fashion; such mutability challenges suggestions that gender is simply an organic extension of sex.

To the extent that chromosomal sex dictates human capability, it would appear to provide an impressive array of options for 'doing gender', suggesting that the species, at the least, is highly adaptive and amenable to experimentation and adoption of new habits. Given the extent of psychiatric conditions leading to lost DALYs among females, and the extent of male DALYs lost to negative coping, one has to wonder at the paucity of larger-scale efforts to examine how these health costs might be mitigated by a concerted effort at alternative social messaging about gender. Interventions that would explore and promote affirming ways of 'doing gender' may ultimately constitute 'best buys' for health and society.

CONCLUSION

While a longstanding academic and activist discourse has emphasized that gender stereotypes and discrimination are harmful to women's health, the global DALYs underscore negative health effects of gender for both males and females. In the various treatments of gender and health to date, there has been far too

ACKNOWLEDGMENTS

I thank Piroska Ostlin, Gita Sen, and members of the Women & Gender Equity Network for encouraging this paper, and for their many helpful comments on an earlier draft. I also thank the anonymous reviewers of the Network, and of this journal, for editorial suggestions that significantly improved the paper.

Notes

1. Phenotype is the observable physical characteristics of an organism, or the appearance of an organism resulting from the interaction of genotype and the environment. At birth, infants are typically identified as being male or female, based on the appearance (i.e. phenotype) of their external genitalia; a minority of infants have 'ambiguous' genitalia, and require genotyping to identify their chromosomal sex as male or female.

2. Others have criticized the very notion of characterizing an 'every-person's' response to any given illness, because the true human burden of disability is so affected by social context (Sundby 1998).

3. ICD-10, i.e. the International Statistical Classification of Diseases and Related Health Problems, 10th Revision.

4. Which includes, in this coding, an unspecified proportion of premature births in which the maturation of the lungs informs survival.

5. One can anticipate that legislation to restrict gender imagery in the media would spark debate along lines already drawn over the regulation of pornography and other violence.

6. For example, the Virginia Slims ad copy that read . . . *You've come a long way baby!*

References

Abou-Gareeb, I., Lewallen, S., Bassett, K. and Courtright, P. (2001) Blindness and Gender: A Meta-Analysis of Published Surveys. *Ophthalmic Epidemiology*, 8, 39–56.

Alexander, G.C. and Sehgal, A.R. (1998) Barriers to Cadaveric Renal Transplantation among Blacks, Women and the Poor. *Journal of the American Medical Association*, 280, 1148–1152.

American Lung Association (2006) *Trends in Tobacco Use*. American Lung Association Epidemiology and Statistic Unit, Research and Program Services.

Anand, S. and Hanson, K. (1997) Disability-Adjusted Life Years: A Critical Review. *Journal of Health Economics*, 16, 685–702.

Anand, S. and Hanson, K. (1998) DALYs: Efficiency Versus Equity. *World Development*, 26, 307–310.

Angst, J., Gamma, A., Gastpar, M., Lepine, J.P., Mendlewicz, J. and Tylee, A. (2002) Gender Differences in Depression. *European Archives of Psychiatry and Clinical Neuroscience*, 252, 201–209.

Annendale, E. and Hunt, K. (eds) (2000) *Gender Inequalities in Health* (Buckingham: Open University Press).

Astbury, J. (2002) Mental health: Gender bias, social position and depression. In G. Sen, George, A. and Ostlin, P. (eds) *Engendering International Health: The Challenge of Equity* (Cambridge: MIT Press, 143–166).

Bech, P. (2001) Male depression: stress and aggression as pathways to major depression. In A. Dawson and Tylee, A. (eds) *Depression— Social and Economic Timebomb* (London: British Medical Journal Books, 63–66).

Beermann, W. (1999) Discounting in health economics: An ethical approach. Paper presented at the Workshop of Measuring Health and Disability, University of Heidelberg (July).

Brown, C. (2000) 'Judge me all you want': Cigarette smoking and the stigmatization of smoking. Paper presented at the Society for the Study of Social Problems, Santa Cruz.

Chen, L., Huq, E. and D'Souza, S. (1981) Sex Bias in the Family Allocation of Food and Health Care in Rural Bangladesh. *Population and Development Review*, 7, 55–70.

Chessler, P. (1972) *Women and Madness* (New York: Four Walls Eight Windows).

Courtenay, W. (2000) Constructions of Masculinity and their Influence on Men's Well-Being: A Theory of Gender and Health. *Social Science & Medicine*, 50, 1385.

Courtright, P. and Lewallen, S. (2002) Sex, gender and blindness, eye disease and use of eye care services. Paper presented at a World Health Organization conference, Geneva.

Daitzman, R., Zuckerman, M., Sammelwitz, O. and Ganjam, V. (1978) Sensation-Seeking and Gonadal Hormones. *Journal of Biosocial Science*, 10, 401–408.

Das Gupta, M. (1987) Selective Discrimination against Female Children in Rural Punjab, India. *Population and Development Review*, 13, 77–100.

Das Gupta, M., Zhenghua, J., Bohua, L., Zhenming, X., Chung, W. and Hwa-Ok, B. (2003) Why is Son Preference so Persistent in East and South Asia? A Cross-Country Study of China, India and the Republic of Korea. *Journal of Development Studies*, 40, 153–187.

Doyal, L. (1995) *What Makes Women Sick: Gender and the Political Economy of Health* (New Brunswick: Rutgers University Press).

Federman, D.D. (2006). The Biology of Human Sex Differences. *New England Journal of Medicine*, 354, 1507.

Hallstrom, T. (2001) Gender differences in mental health. In P. Östlin, Danielsson, M., Diderichsen, F., Härenstam, A. and Lindberg, G. (eds) *Gender Inequalities in Health* (Boston: Harvard School of Public Health, 117–135).

Han, H.-R., Kim, M.T., Rose, L., Dennison, C., Bone, L. and Hill, M. (2006) Effects of Stressful Life Events in Young Black Men with High Blood Pressure. *Ethnicity & Disease*, 16, 64–70.

Hanson, K. (2002). Measuring up: gender, burden of disease, and priority setting. In G. Sen, George, A. and Östlin, P. (eds) *Engendering International Health: The Challenge of Equity* (Cambridge: MIT Press, 313–345).

Hopcraft, R.L. and Bradley, D.B. (2007) The Sex Difference in Depression across 29 Countries. *Social Forces*, 85, 1483–1507.

Jelsma, J., Chivaura, V., Mhundwa, K., De Weerdt, W. and de Cock, P. (2000) The Global Burden of Disease Disability Weights. *The Lancet*, 355, 2079–2080.

Kommers, D.P. and Finn, J.E. (1998) *American Constitutional Law* (Belmont: Wadsworth Publishing).

Lewallen, S. and Courtright, P. (2002) Gender and Use of Cataract Surgical Services in Developing Countries. *Bulletin of the World Health Organization*, 80, 300–303.

Lpfo (1998) Curriculum for the pre-school Lpfo 98. National Agency for Education (SKOLFS 2006:22), Fritzes kundservice, Stockholm.

MacKinnon, C.A. (1987) *Feminism Unmodified: Discourses on Life and Law* (Cambridge: Harvard University Press).

Mage, D.T. and Donner, E.M. (2004) The Fifty Percent Male Excess of Infant Respiratory Mortality. *Acta Pediatrica*, 93, 1210–1215.

Maio, R., Waller, F., Blow, F., Hill, E. and Singer, K. (1997) Alcohol Abuse/Dependence in Motor Vehicle Crash Victims Presenting to the Emergency Department. *Academic Emergency Medicine*, 4, 256–262.

Meisel, P. (2002) Letter to the Editor: Cancer, Genes and Gender. *Carcinogenesis*, 23, 1087–1088.

Moeller Leimkuehler, A.M., Heller, J. and Paulus, N. (2007) Subjective Well-Being and 'Male Depression' in Male Adolescents. *Journal of Affective Disorders*, 98, 65–72.

Odero, W. (1998) Alcohol-Related Road Traffic Injuries in Eldoret, Kenya. *East African Medical Journal*, 75, 708–711.

Oei Tian, P.S. and Kerschbaumer, D.M. (1990) Peer Attitudes, Sex, and the Effects of Alcohol on Simulated Driving Performance. *American Journal of Drug and Alcohol Abuse*, 16, 135–146.

Östlin, P., Danielsson, M., Diderichsen, F., Härenstam, A. and Lindberg, G. (eds) (2001) *Gender Inequalities in Health: A Swedish Perspective* (Boston: Harvard School of Public Health).

Pampel, F.C. (2006) Global Patterns and Determinants of Sex Differences in Smoking. *International Journal of Comparative Sociology*, 47, 466–487.

Patel, J.D., Bach, P.B. and Kris, M.G. (2004) Lung Cancer in US Women. *Journal of the American Medical Association*, 291, 1763–1768.

Pollack, W. (1998) *Real Boys: Rescuing our Sons from the Myths of Boyhood* (New York: Random House).

Resnick, S., Gottesmann, I. and McGue, M. (1993) Sensation Seeking in Opposite-Sex Twins: An Effect of Prenatal Hormones? *Behavioral Genetics*, 23, 323–329.

Rutz, W. (1999) Improvement of Care for People Suffering from Depression: The Need for Comprehensive Education. *International Clinical Psychopharmacology*, 14, 27–33.

Sadana, R. (1998) A closer look at the WHO/ World Bank Global Burden of Disease Study's methodologies: How do poor women's values in a developing country compare with international public health experts? Conference presentation at the Public Health Forum, *Reforming Health Sectors*, London School of Hygiene and Tropical Medicine.

Schulman, K.A., Berlin, J.A., Harless, W., Kerner, J.F., Sistrunk, S. and Gersh, B.J. (1999) The Effect of Race and Sex on Physicians Recommendations for Cardiac Catheterization. *New England Journal of Medicine*, 340, 618–626.

Sen, G., Östlin, P. and George, A. (eds) (2002) *Engendering International Health: The Challenge of Equity* (Cambridge: MIT Press).

Snow, R.C. (2002) Sex, gender and traffic accidents: addressing male risk behaviour. Paper presented at a conference for the World Health Organization, Geneva.

Stevenson, D.K., Verter, J., Fanaroff, A.A., Oh, W., Ehrenkranz, R.A., Shankaran, S., et al. (2000) Sex Differences in Outcomes of Very Low Birth-weight Infants: The Newborn Male Disadvantage. Archives of Disease in Childhood. *Fetal and Neonatal Edition*, 83, 182–185.

Sundby, J. (1998) A gender perspective on disability adjusted life years and the global burden of disease. Paper presented at a conference for the World Health Organization, Geneva.

Thorson, A., Hoa, N.P., Long, N.H., Allebeck, P. and Diwan, V.K. (2004) Do Women with Tuberculosis have a Lower Likelihood of Getting Diagnosed? Prevalence and Case Detection of Sputum Smear Positive Pulmonary TB, A Population Based Study from Vietnam. *Journal of Clinical Epidemiology*, 57, 398–402.

van Grootheest, D.S., Beekman, A.T.F., Broese van Groenou, M.I. and Deeg, D.J.H. (1999) Sex Differences in Depression after Widowhood. Do Men Suffer More? *Social Psychiatry and Psychiatric Epidemiology*, 34, 391–398.

Watkins, R.E. and Plant, A.J. (2006) Does Smoking Explain Sex Differences in the Global Tuberculosis Epidemic? *Epidemiology and Infection*, 134, 333–339.

Weiss, M.G., Auer, C., Somma D. and Abouihia, A. (2006) Gender and Tuberculosis: Cross-Site Analysis of a Multi-Country Study in Bangladesh, India, Malawi and Columbia. World Health Organization. *TDR/SDR/SEB/RP/06.1*.

World Health Organization Department of Measurement and Health Information, December 2004. Global Burden of Disease 2004 Update, http://www.who.int/healthinfo/statistics (accessed 2006).

STRUCTURAL VIOLENCE AND CLINICAL MEDICINE

Paul E. Farmer, Bruce Nizeye, Sara Stulac, and Salmaan Keshavjee

Because of contact with patients, physicians readily appreciate that large-scale social forces—racism, gender inequality, poverty, political violence and war, and sometimes the very policies that address them—often determine who falls ill and who has access to care. For practitioners of public health, the social determinants of disease are even harder to disregard.

Unfortunately, this awareness is seldom translated into formal frameworks that link social analysis to everyday clinical practice. One reason for this gap is that the holy grail of modern medicine remains the search for the molecular basis of disease. While the practical yield of such circumscribed inquiry has been enormous, exclusive focus on molecular-level phenomena has contributed to the increasing "desocialization" of scientific inquiry: a tendency to ask only biological questions about what are in fact *biosocial* phenomena [1].

Biosocial understandings of medical phenomena are urgently needed. All those involved in public health sense this, especially when they serve populations living in poverty. Social analysis, however rudimentary, occurs at the bedside, in the clinic, in field sites, and in the margins of the biomedical literature. It is to be found, for example, in any significant survey of adherence to therapy for chronic diseases [2, 3] and in studies of what were once termed "social diseases" such as venereal disease and tuberculosis (TB) [4–8]. The emerging phenomenon of acquired resistance to antibiotics—including antibacterial, antiviral, and antiparasitic agents—is perforce a biosocial process, one which began less than a century ago as novel treatments

Structural Violence and Clinical Medicine, Paul F. Farmer, Bruce Nizeye, Sara Stulac, and Salmaan Keshavjee in *PLoS Med 3*(10): e449. October 24, 2006. Copyright © 2006 Farmer et al.

were introduced [9]. Social analysis is heard in discussions about illnesses for which significant environmental components are believed to exist, such as asthma and lead poisoning [10–15]. Can we speak of the "natural history" of any of these diseases without addressing social forces, including racism, pollution, poor housing, and poverty, that shape their course in both individuals and populations? Does our clinical practice acknowledge what we already know—namely, that social and environmental forces will limit the effectiveness of our treatments? Asking these questions needs to be the beginning of a conversation within medicine and public health, rather than the end of one.

DEFINING STRUCTURAL VIOLENCE

The term "structural violence" is one way of describing social arrangements that put individuals and populations in harm's way (see Box 1) [16]. The arrangements are *structural* because they are embedded in the political and economic organization of our social world; they are *violent* because they cause injury to people (typically, not those responsible for perpetuating such inequalities). With

few exceptions, clinicians are not trained to understand such social forces, nor are we trained to alter them. Yet it has long been clear that many medical and public health interventions will fail if we are unable to understand the social determinants of disease [17, 18].

The good news is that such biosocial understandings are far more "actionable" than is widely recognized. There is already a vast and growing array of diagnostic and therapeutic tools born of scientific research; it is possible to use these tools in a manner informed by an understanding of structural violence and its impact on disease distribution and on every step of the process leading from diagnosis to effective care. This means working at multiple levels, from "distal" interventions—performed late in the process, when patients are already sick—to "proximal" interventions—trying to prevent illness through efforts such as vaccination or improved water and housing quality.

As with many other concepts, structural violence has its limitations [19]. Nevertheless, we seek to apply the concept to what remain the primary tasks of clinical medicine: preventing premature death and disability and improving the lives of those we care for. Using the concept of structural violence, we intend to begin, or revive, discussions about social forces beyond the control of our patients.

BOX 1. WHAT IS STRUCTURAL VIOLENCE?

Structural violence, a term coined by Johan Galtung and by liberation theologians during the 1960s, describes social structures—economic, political, legal, religious, and cultural—that stop individuals, groups, and societies from reaching their full potential [57]. In its general usage, the word *violence* often conveys a physical image; however, according to Galtung, it is the "avoidable impairment of fundamental human needs or . . . the impairment of human life, which lowers the actual degree to which someone is able to meet their needs below that which would otherwise be possible" [58]. Structural violence is often embedded in longstanding "ubiquitous social structures, normalized by stable institutions and regular experience" [59]. Because they seem so ordinary in our ways of understanding the world, they appear almost invisible. Disparate access to resources, political power, education, health care, and legal standing are just a few examples. The idea of *structural violence* is linked very closely to *social injustice* and the social machinery of oppression [16].

22. Oppenheimer G (1998) In the eye of the storm: The epidemiological construction of AIDS. In: Fee E, Fox DM, editors. AIDS: The burdens of history. Berkeley: University of California Press. pp. 267–300.

23. Oppenheimer G (1992) Causes, cases, and cohorts: The role of epidemiology in the historical construction of AIDS. In: Fee E, Fox DM, editors. AIDS: The making of a chronic disease. Berkeley: University of California Press. pp. 49–83.

24. Farmer PE (2006) AIDS and accusation: Haiti and the geography of blame. 2nd edition. Berkeley: University of California Press. 338 p.

25. Farmer P, Connors M, Simmons J, editors (1996) Women, poverty, and AIDS: Sex, drugs, and structural violence. Monroe (ME): Common Courage Press. 473 p.

26. Stryker J, Jonsen AR, editors (1993) The social impact of AIDS in the United States. Washington, DC: National Academies Press. 336 p.

27. Toltzis P, Stephens RC, Adkins I, Lombardi E, Swami S, et al. (1999) Human immunodeficiency virus (HIV)-related risk-taking behaviors in women attending inner-city prenatal clinics in the mid-west. J Perinatol 19: 483–487.

28. Gottlieb SL, Douglas JM Jr, Schmid DS, Bolan G, Iatesta M, et al. (2002) Seroprevalence and correlates of herpes simplex virus type 2 infection in five sexually transmitted-disease clinics. J Infect Dis 186:1381–1389.

29. National Center for Health Statistics (1994) Annual summary of births, marriages, divorces, and deaths: United States, 1993. Hyattsville (MD): US Department of Health and Human Services, Public Health Service, CDC. pp. 18–20.

30. Wiktor SZ, Sassan-Morokro M, Grant AD, Abouya L, Karon JM, et al. (1999) Efficacy of trimethoprim-sulphamethoxazole prophylaxis to decrease morbidity and mortality in HIV-1-infected patients with tuberculosis in Abidjan, Côte d'Ivoire: A randomised controlled trial. Lancet 353: 1469–1475.

31. Moore RD, Stanton D, Gopalan R, Chaisson RE (1994) Racial differences in the use of drug therapy for HIV disease in an urban community. N Engl J Med 330: 763–768.

32. Lucas SB, Hounnou A, Peacock C, Beaumel A, Djomand G, et al. (1993) The mortality and pathology of HIV infection in a west African city. AIDS 7: 1569–1579.

33. Scheper-Hughes N, Lock M (1987) The mindful body: A prolegomenon to future work in medical anthropology. Med Anthropol Q 1: 6–41.

34. French L (1994) The political economy of injury and compassion: amputees on the Thai-Cambodian border. In: Csordas TJ, editor. Embodiment and experience: The existential ground of culture and self. Cambridge: Cambridge University Press. pp. 69–99.

35. Chaisson RE, Keruly JC, Moore RD (1995) Race, sex, drug use, and progression of human immunodeficiency virus disease. N Engl J Med 333: 751–756.

36. Bangsberg D, Tulsky JP, Hecht FM, Moss AR (1997) Protease inhibitors in the homeless. JAMA 278: 63–65.

37. Behforouz HL, Farmer PE, Mukherjee JS (2004) From directly observed therapy to accompagnateurs: Enhancing AIDS treatment outcomes in Haiti and in Boston. Clin Infect Dis 38: S429–S436.

38. Mitty JA, Macalino GE, Bazerman LB, Loewenthal HG, Hogan JW, et al. (2005) The use of community-based modified directly observed therapy for the treatment of HIV-infected persons. J Acquir Immune Defic Syndr 39: 545–550.

39. Little SJ, Holte S, Routy JP, Daar ES, Markowitz M, et al. (2002) Antiretroviral-drug

resistance among patients recently infected with HIV. N Engl J Med 347: 385–394.

40. Neu C (1992) The crisis in antibiotic resistance. Science 257:1064–1073.

41. del Rio C, Green S, Abrams C, Lennox J (2001) From diagnosis to undetectable: The reality of HIV/ AIDS care in the inner city [abstract]. 8th Annual Conference on Retroviruses and Opportunistic Infections; 2001 4–8 February; Chicago, Illinois, United States of America. Available: http://gateway. nlm.nih.gov/ MeetingAbstracts/102244586.html. Accessed 20 September 2006.

42. Walton DA, Farmer PE, Dillingham R (2005) Social and cultural factors in tropical medicine: Reframing our understanding of disease. In: Guerrant RL, Walker DH, Weller PF, editors. Tropical infectious diseases: Principles, pathogens, and practice. 2nd edition. New York: Elsevier. pp. 26–35.

43. Farmer P, Léandre F, Mukherjee JS, Claude MS, Nevil P, et al. (2001) Community-based approaches to HIV treatment in resource-poor settings. Lancet 358: 404–409.

44. Walton DA, Farmer PE, Lambert W, Léandre F, Koenig SP, et al. (2004) Integrated HIV prevention and care strengthens primary health care: Lessons from rural Haiti. J Public Health Policy 25: 137–158.

45. Mitnick C, Bayona J, Palacios E, Shin S, Furin J, et al. (2003) Community-based therapy for multidrug-resistant tuberculosis in Lima, Peru. N Engl J Med 348:119–128.

46. Shin S, Furin J, Bayona J, Mate K, Kim JY, et al. (2004) Community-based treatment of multidrugresistant tuberculosis in Lima, Peru: Seven years of experience. Soc Sci Med 59: 1529–1539.

47. Wilson DP, Kahn J, Blower SM (2006) Predicting the epidemiological impact of antiretroviral allocation strategies in KwaZulu-Natal: The effect of the urban-rural divide. Proc Nat Acad Sci 103:14228–14233.

48. Raymonville M, Léandre F, Saintard R, Colas M, Louissaint M, et al. (2004) Prevention of mother to-child transmission of HIV in rural Haiti: The Partners In Health experience [poster]. A Multicultural Caribbean United Against HIV/AIDS; 2004 5–7 March; Santo Domingo, Dominican Republic.

49. Farmer P (2001) The major infectious diseases in the world—to treat or not to treat? N Engl J Med 345: 208–210.

50. Farmer PE (2005) Pathologies of power: Health, human rights, and the new war on the poor. 2nd edition. Berkeley: University of California Press. 402 p.

51. Shkilnyk A (1985) A poison stronger than love: The destruction of an Ojibwa community. New Haven (CT): Yale University Press. 276 p.

52. Chien A, Connors M, Fox K (2000) The drug war in perspective. In: Kim JY, Millen JV, Gershman J, Irwin A, editors. Dying for growth: Global inequalities and the health of the poor. Monroe (ME): Common Courage Press. pp. 293–327.

53. Lacey M (2005 February 26) Women's voices rise as Rwanda reinvents itself. The New York Times; Sect A: 1 (col 3). Available: http://www. peacewomen.org/news/Rwanda/Feb05/voicesrise.html. Accessed 20 September 2006.

54. Kim JY, Gilks C (2005) Scaling up treatment—why we can't wait. N Engl J Med 353: 2392–2394.

55. McKeown T (1980) The role of medicine: Dream, mirage, or nemesis? Princeton (NJ): Princeton University Press. 224 p.

56. Porter D (2006) How did social medicine evolve, and where is it heading? PLoS Med 3: e399. DOI: 10.1371/journal.pmed.0030399

57. Galtung J (1969) Violence, peace and peace research. J Peace Res 6:167–191.

58. Galtung J (1993) Kultuerlle Gewalt. Der Burger im Staat 43: 106.

59. Gilligan J (1997) Violence: Reflections on a national epidemic. New York: Vintage Books. 306 p.

A CASE FOR REFOCUSING UPSTREAM

The Political Economy of Illness

John B. McKinlay

My friend, Irving Zola, relates the story of a physician trying to explain the dilemmas of the modern practice of medicine:

"You know," he said, "sometimes it feels like this. There I am standing by the shore of a swiftly flowing river and I hear the cry of a drowning man. So I jump into the river, put my arms around him, pull him to shore and apply artificial respiration. Just when he begins to breathe, there is another cry for help. So I jump into the river, reach him, pull him to shore, apply artificial respiration, and then just as he begins to breathe, another cry for help. So back in the river again, reaching, pulling, applying, breathing and then another yell. Again and again, without end, goes the sequence. You know, I am so busy jumping in, pulling them to shore, applying artificial respiration, that I have *no* time to see who the hell is upstream pushing them all in."[1]

I believe this simple story illustrates two important points. *First,* it highlights the fact that a clear majority of our resources and activities in the health field are devoted to what I term "downstream endeavors" in the form of superficial, categorical tinkering in response to almost perennial shifts from one health issue to the next, without really solving anything. I am, of course, not suggesting that such efforts are entirely futile, or that a considerable amount of short-term good is not being accomplished. Clearly, people and groups have

A Case for Refocusing Upstream: The Political Economy of Illness, John B. McKinlay in *Patients, Physicians and Illness: A Sourcebook in Behavioral Science and Health,* ed. E. Gartley Jaco (New York: The Free Press, 1979), 9–25. Reprinted with permission from the author.

important immediate needs which must be recognized and attended to. Nevertheless, one must be wary of the *short-term nature* and *ultimate futility* of such downstream endeavors.

Second, the story indicates that we should somehow cease our preoccupation with this short-term, problem-specific tinkering and begin focussing our attention upstream, where the real problems lie. Such a reorientation would minimally involve an analysis of the means by which various individuals, interest groups, and large-scale, profit-oriented corporations are "pushing people in," and how they subsequently erect, at some point downstream, a health care structure to service the needs which they have had a hand in creating, and for which moral responsibility ought to be assumed.

In this paper two related themes will be developed. *First,* I wish to highlight the activities of the "manufacturers of illness"—those individuals, interest groups, and organizations which, in addition to producing material goods and services, also produce, as an inevitable by-product, widespread morbidity and mortality. Arising out of this, and *second,* I will develop a case for refocussing our attention away from those individuals and groups who are mistakenly held to be responsible for their condition, toward a range of broader upstream political and economic forces.

The task assigned to me for this conference was to review some of the broad social structural factors influencing the onset of heart disease and/or at-risk behavior. Since the issues covered by this request are so varied, I have, of necessity, had to make some decisions concerning both emphasis and scope. These decisions and the reasoning behind them should perhaps be explained at this point. With regard to what can be covered by the term "social structure," it is possible to isolate at least three separate levels of abstraction. One could, for example, focus on such subsystems as the family, and its associated social networks, and how these may be importantly linked to different levels of health status and the utilization of services.[2] On a second level, one could consider how particular organizations and broader social institutions, such as neighborhood and community structures, also affect the social distribution of pathology and at-risk behavior.[3] Third, attention could

center on the broader political-economic spectrum, and how these admittedly more remote forces may be etiologically involved in the onset of disease. . . .

. . . [In this paper] I will argue, for example, that the frequent failure of many health intervention programs can be largely attributed to the inadequate recognition we give to aspects of social context. . . . The most important factor in deciding on the subject area of this paper, however, is the fact that, while there appears to be a newly emerging interest in the political economy of health care, social scientists have, as yet, paid little attention to the *political economy of illness.*[4] It is my intention in this paper to begin to develop a case for the serious consideration of this particular area.

A political-economic analysis of health care suggests that the entire structure of institutions in the United States is such as to preclude the adequate provision of services.[5] Increasingly, it seems, the provision of care is being tied to the priorities of profit-making institutions. For a long time, criticism of U.S. health care focussed on the activities of the American Medical Association and the fee for service system of physician payment.[6] Lately, however, attention appears to be refocussing on the relationship between health care arrangements and the structure of big business.[7] It has, for example, been suggested that:

> . . . with the new and apparently permanent involvement of major corporations in health, it is becoming increasingly improbable that the United States can redirect its health priorities without, at the same time, changing the ways in which American industry is organized and the ways in which monopoly capitalism works.[8]

It is my impression that many of the political-economic arguments concerning developments in the organization of health care also have considerable relevance for a holistic understanding of the etiology and distribution of morbidity, mortality, and at-risk behavior. In the following sections I will present some important aspects of these arguments in the hope of contributing to a better understanding of aspects of the political economy of illness.

AN UNEQUAL BATTLE

The downstream efforts of health researchers and practitioners against the upstream efforts of the manufacturers of illness have the appearance of an unequal war, *with a resounding victory assured for those on the side of illness* and the creation of disease-inducing behaviors. The battle between health workers and the manufacturers of illness is unequal on at least two grounds. In the *first* place, we always seem to arrive on the scene and begin to work after the real damage has already been done. By the time health workers intervene, people have already filled the artificial needs created for them by the manufacturers of illness and are habituated to various at-risk behaviors. In the area of smoking behavior, for example, we have an illustration not only of the lateness of health workers' arrival on the scene, and the enormity of the task confronting them, but also, judging by recent evidence, of the resounding defeat being sustained in this area.[9] To push the river analogy even further, the task becomes one of furiously swimming against the flow and finally being swept away when exhausted by the effort or through disillusionment with a lack of progress. So long as we continue to fight the battle downstream, and in such an ineffective manner, we are doomed to frustration, repeated failure, and perhaps ultimately to a sicker society.

Second, the promoters of disease-inducing behavior are manifestly more effective in their use of behavioral science knowledge than are those of us who are concerned with the eradication of such behavior. Indeed, it is somewhat paradoxical that we should be meeting here to consider how behavioral science knowledge and techniques can be effectively employed to reduce or prevent at-risk behavior, when that same body of knowledge *has already* been used to create the at-risk behavior we seek to eliminate. How embarrassingly ineffective are our mass media efforts in the health field (e.g., alcoholism, obesity, drug abuse, safe driving, pollution, etc.) when compared with many of the tax exempt promotional efforts on behalf of the illness generating activities of large-scale corporations.[10] It is a fact that we are demonstrably more effective in persuading people to purchase items they never dreamt they would need, or to pursue at-risk courses of action, than we are in preventing or halting such behavior. Many advertisements are so ingenious in their appeal that they have entertainment value in their own right and become embodied in our national folk humor. By way of contrast, many health advertisements lack any comparable widespread appeal, often appear boring, avuncular, and largely misdirected.

I would argue that one major problem lies in the fact that we are overly concerned with the war itself, and with how we can more effectively participate in it. In the health field we have unquestioningly accepted the assumptions presented by the manufacturers of illness and, as a consequence, have confined our efforts to only downstream offensives. A little reflection would, I believe, convince anyone that those on the side of health are in fact losing. . . . But rather than merely trying to win the war, we need to step back and question the premises, legitimacy and utility of the war itself.

THE BINDING OF AT-RISKNESS TO CULTURE

It seems that the appeals to at-risk behavior that are engineered by the manufacturers of illness are particularly successful because they are constructed in such a way as to be inextricably bound with essential elements of our existing dominant culture. This is accomplished in a number of ways: (a) Exhortations to at-risk behavior are often piggybacked on those legitimized values, beliefs, and norms which are widely recognized and adhered to in the dominant culture. The idea here is that if a person *would only do X,* then they would also be doing Y and Z. (b) Appeals are also advanced which claim or imply that certain courses of at-risk action are subscribed to or endorsed by most of the culture heroes in society (e.g., people in the entertainment industry), or by those with technical competence in that particular field (e.g., "doctors" recommend it). The idea here is that if a person *would only do X,* then he/she would be doing pretty much the same as is done or recommended by such prestigious people as A and B. (c) Artificial needs are manufactured, the fulfilling of which becomes absolutely essential if one is to be a meaningful and useful member of society. The idea here is that if a person *does not do X, or will not do X,* then they are either deficient in some important respect, or they are some kind of liability for the social system.

Variations on these and other kinds of appeal strategies have, of course, been employed for a long time now by the promoters of at-risk behavior. The manufacturers of illness are, for example, fostering the belief that if you want to be an attractive, masculine man, or a "cool," "natural" woman, you will smoke cigarettes; that you can only be a "good parent" if you habituate your children to candy, cookies, etc.; and that if you are a truly loving wife, you will feed your husband foods that are high in cholesterol. All of these appeals have isolated some basic goals to which most people subscribe (e.g., people want to be masculine or feminine, good parents, loving spouses, etc.) and make claim, or imply, that their realization is only possible through the exclusive use of their product or the regular display of a specific type of at-risk behavior. Indeed, one can argue that certain at-risk behaviors have become so inextricably intertwined with our dominant cultural system (perhaps even symbolic of it) that the routine public display of such behavior almost signifies membership in this society.

Such tactics for the habituation of people to at-risk behavior are, perhaps paradoxically, also employed to elicit what I term *"quasi-health behavior."* Here again, an artificially constructed conception of a person in some fanciful state of physiological and emotional equilibrium is presented as the ideal state to strive for, if one is to meaningfully participate in the wider social system. To assist in the attainment of such a state, we are advised to consume a range of quite worthless vitamin pills, mineral supplements, mouthwashes, hair shampoos, laxatives, pain killers, etc. Clearly, one cannot exude radiance and success if one is not taking this vitamin, or that mineral. The achievement of daily regularity is a prerequisite for an effective social existence. One can only compete and win after a good night's sleep, and this can only be ensured by taking such and such. An entrepreneurial pharmaceutical industry appears devoted to the task of making people overly conscious of these quasi-health concerns, and to engendering a dependency

on products which have been repeatedly found to be ineffective, and even potentially harmful.[11]

There are no clear signs that such activity is being or will be regulated in any effective way, and the promoters of this quasi-health behavior appear free to range over the entire body in their never-ending search for new areas and issues to be linked to the fanciful equilibrium that they have already engineered in the mind of the consumer. By binding the display of at-risk and quasi-health behavior so inextricably to elements of our dominant culture, a situation is even created whereby to request people to change or alter these behaviors is more or less to request abandonment of dominant culture.

The term "culture" is employed here to denote that integrated system of values, norms, beliefs and patterns of behavior which, for groups and social categories in specific situations, facilitate the solution of social structural problems.[12] This definition lays stress on two features commonly associated with the concept of culture. The *first* is the interrelatedness and interdependence of the various elements (values, norms, beliefs, overt life-styles) that apparently comprise culture. The *second* is the view that a cultural system is, in some part, a response to social structural problems, and that it can be regarded as some kind of resolution of them. Of course, these social structural problems, in partial response to which a cultural pattern emerges, may themselves have been engineered in the interests of creating certain beliefs, norms, life styles, etc. If one assumes that culture can be regarded as some kind of reaction formation, then one must be mindful of the unanticipated social consequences of inviting some alteration in behavior which is a part of a dominant cultural pattern. The request from health workers for alterations in certain at-risk behaviors may result in either awkward dislocations of the interrelated elements of the cultural pattern, or the destruction of a system of values and norms, etc., which have emerged over time in response to situational problems. From this perspective, and with regard to the utilization of medical care, I have already argued elsewhere that, for certain groups of the population, underutilization may be "healthy" behavior, and the advocacy of increased utilization an "unhealthy" request for the abandonment of essential features of culture.[13]

THE CASE OF FOOD

Perhaps it would be useful at this point to illustrate in some detail, from one pertinent area, the style and magnitude of operation engaged in by the manufacturers of illness. Illustrations are, of course, readily available from a variety of different areas, such as: the requirements of existing occupational structure, emerging leisure patterns, smoking and drinking behavior, and automobile usage.[14] Because of current interest, I have decided to consider only one area which is importantly related to a range of large chronic diseases—namely, the 161 billion dollar industry involved in the production and distribution of food and beverages.[15] The present situation, with regard to food, was recently described as follows:

> The sad history of our food supply resembles the energy crisis, and not just because food nourishes our bodies while petroleum fuels the society. We long ago surrendered control of food, a vital resource, to private corporations, just as we surrendered control of energy. The food corporations have shaped the kinds of food we eat for their greater profits, just as the energy companies have dictated the kinds of fuel we use.[16]

From all the independent evidence available, and despite claims to the contrary by the food industry, a widespread decline has occurred during the past three decades in American dietary standards. Some forty percent of U.S. adults are overweight or downright fat.[17] The prevalence of excess weight in the American population as a whole is high—so high, in fact, that in some segments it has reached epidemic proportions.[18] There is evidence that the food industry is manipulating our image of "food" away from basic staples toward synthetic and highly processed items. It has been estimated that we eat between 21 and 25 percent fewer dairy products, vegetables, and fruits than we did twenty years ago, and from 70 to 80 percent

more sugary snacks and soft drinks. Apparently, most people now eat more processed and synthetic foods than the real thing. There are even suggestions that a federal, nationwide survey would have revealed how serious our dietary situation really is, if the Nixon Administration had not cancelled it after reviewing some embarrassing preliminary results.[19] The survey apparently confirmed the trend toward deteriorating diets first detected in an earlier household food consumption survey in the years 1955–1965, undertaken by the Department of Agriculture.[20]

Of course, for the food industry, this trend toward deficient synthetics and highly processed items makes good economic sense. Generally speaking, it is much cheaper to make things look and taste like the real thing, than to actually provide the real thing. But the kind of foods that result from the predominance of economic interests clearly do not contain adequate nutrition. It is common knowledge that food manufacturers destroy important nutrients which foods naturally contain, when they transform them into "convenience" high profit items. To give one simple example: a wheat grain's outer layers are apparently very nutritious, but they are also an obstacle to making tasteless, bleached, white flour. Consequently, baking corporations "refine" fourteen nutrients out of the natural flour and then, when it is financially convenient, replace some of them with a synthetic substitute. In the jargon of the food industry, this flour is now "enriched." Clearly, the food industry employs this term in much the same way that coal corporations ravage mountainsides into mud flats, replant them with some soil and seedlings, and then proclaim their moral accomplishment in "rehabilitating" the land. While certain types of food processing may make good economic sense, it may also result in a deficient end product, and perhaps even promote certain diseases. The bleaching and refining of wheat products, for example, largely eliminates fiber or roughage from our diets, and some authorities have suggested that fiber-poor diets can be blamed for some of our major intestinal diseases.[21]

A vast chemical additive technology has enabled manufacturers to acquire enormous control over the food and beverage market and to foster phenomenal profitability. It is estimated that drug companies alone make something like $500 million a year through chemical additives for food. I have already suggested that what is done to food, in the way of processing and artificial additives, may actually be injurious to health. Yet, it is clear that, despite such well-known risks, profitability makes such activity well worthwhile. For example, additives, like preservatives, enable food that might perish in a short period of time to endure unchanged for months or even years. Food manufacturers and distributors can saturate supermarket shelves across the country with their products because there is little chance that they will spoil. Moreover, manufacturers can purchase vast quantities of raw ingredients when they are cheap, produce and stockpile the processed result, and then withhold the product from the market for long periods, hoping for the inevitable rise in prices and the consequent windfall.

The most widely used food additive (although it is seldom described as an additive) is "refined" sugar. Food manufacturers saturate our diets with the substance from the day we are born until the day we die. Children are fed breakfast cereals which consist of 50 percent sugar.[22] The average American adult consumes 126 pounds of sugar each year—and children, of course, eat much more. For the candy industry alone, this amounts to around $3 billion each year. The American sugar mania, which appears to have been deliberately engineered, is a major contributor to such "diseases of civilization" as diabetes, coronary heart disease, gall bladder illness, and cancer—all the insidious, degenerative conditions which most often afflict people in advanced capitalist societies, but which "underdeveloped," nonsugar eaters never get. One witness at a recent meeting of a U.S. Senate Committee, said that if the food industry were proposing sugar today as a new food additive, its "metabolic behavior would undoubtedly lead to its being banned."[23]

In sum, therefore, it seems that the American food industry is mobilizing phenomenal resources to advance and bind us to its own conception of food. We are bombarded from childhood with $2 billion worth of deliberately manipulative advertisements each year, most of them urging us to consume, among other things, as much sugar as possible. To highlight the magnitude of the resources involved,

one can point to the activity of one well-known beverage company, Coca-Cola, which alone spent $71 million in 1971 to advertise its artificially flavored, sugar-saturated product. Fully recognizing the enormity of the problem regarding food in the United States, Zwerdling offers the following advice:

> Breaking through the food industry will require government action—banning or sharply limiting use of dangerous additives like artificial colors and flavors, and sugar, and requiring wheat products to contain fiber-rich wheat germ, to give just two examples. Food, if it is to become safe, will have to become part of politics.[24]

THE ASCRIPTION OF RESPONSIBILITY AND MORAL ENTREPRENEURSHIP

So far, I have considered, in some detail, the ways in which industry, through its manufacture and distribution of a variety of products, generates at-risk behavior and disease. Let us now focus on the activities of health workers further down the river and consider their efforts in a social context, which has already been largely shaped by the manufacturers upstream.

Not only should we be mindful of the culturally disruptive and largely unanticipated consequences of health intervention efforts mentioned earlier, but also of the underlying ideology on which so much of this activity rests. Such intervention appears based on an assumption of the *culpability of individuals* or groups who either manifest illness, or display various at-risk behaviors.

From the assumption that individuals and groups with certain illnesses or displaying at-risk behavior are responsible for their state, it is a relatively easy step to advocating some changes in behavior on the part of those involved. By ascribing culpability to some group or social category (usually ethnic minorities and those in lower socio-economic categories) and having this ascription legitimated by health professionals and accepted by other segments of society, it is possible to mobilize resources to change the offending behavior. Certain people are responsible for not approximating, through their activities, some conception of what *ought* to be appropriate behavior on their part. When measured against the artificial conception of what ought to be, certain individuals and groups are found to be deficient in several important respects. They are *either* doing something that they ought not to be doing, *or* they are not doing something that they ought to be doing. If only they would recognize their individual culpability and alter their behavior in some appropriate fashion, they would improve their health status or the likelihood of not developing certain pathologies. On the basis of this line of reasoning, resources are being mobilized to bring those who depart from the desired conception into conformity with what is thought to be appropriate behavior. To use the upstream-downstream analogy, one could argue that people are blamed (and, in a sense, even punished) for not being able to swim after they, perhaps even against their own volition, have been pushed into the river by the manufacturers of illness.

Clearly, this ascription of culpability is not limited only to the area of health. According to popular conception, people in poverty are largely to blame for their social situation, although recent evidence suggests that a social welfare system which prevents them from avoiding this state is at least partly responsible.[25] Again, in the field of education, we often hold "dropouts" responsible for their behavior, when evidence suggests that the school system itself is rigged for failure.[26] Similar examples are readily available from the fields of penology, psychiatry, and race relations.[27]

Perhaps it would be useful to briefly outline, at this point, what I regard as a bizarre relationship between the activities of the manufacturers of illness, the ascription of culpability, and health intervention endeavors. *First,* important segments of our social system appear to be controlled and operated in such a way that people must inevitably fail. The fact is that there is often no choice over whether one can find employment, whether or not to drop out of college, involve oneself in untoward behavior, or become sick. *Second,* even though individuals and groups lack such choice, they are still blamed for not approximating the artificially contrived norm and are treated as if responsibility for their state lay entirely with them. For example, some illness conditions may be the result of particular behavior and/or involvement in certain occupational role relationships over which those affected have little or no control.[28] *Third,* after recognizing that certain individuals and groups have "failed," we establish, at a point downstream, a substructure of services which are regarded as evidence of progressive beneficence on the part of the system. Yet, it is this very system which had a primary role in manufacturing the problems and need for these services in the first place.

It is around certain aspects of life style that most health intervention endeavors appear to revolve and this probably results from the observability of most at-risk behavior. The modification of at-risk behavior can take several different forms, and the intervention appeals that are employed probably vary as a function of which type of change is desired. People can *either* be encouraged to stop doing what they are doing which appears to be endangering their survival (e.g., smoking, drinking, eating certain types of food, working in particular ways); *or* they can be encouraged to adopt certain new patterns of behavior which seemingly enhance their health status (e.g., diet, exercise, rest, eat certain foods, etc.). I have already discussed how the presence or absence of certain life styles in some groups may be a part of some wider cultural pattern which emerges as a response to social structural problems. I have also noted the potentially disruptive consequences to these cultural patterns of intervention programs. Underlying all these aspects is the issue of behavior control and the attempt to enforce a particular type of behavioral conformity. It is more than coincidental that the at-risk life styles, which we are all admonished to avoid, are frequently the type of behaviors which depart from and, in a sense, jeopardize the prevailing puritanical, middle-class ethic of what ought to be. According to this ethic, activities as pleasurable as drinking, smoking, overeating, and sexual intercourse must be harmful and ought to be eradicated.

The important point here is which segments of society and whose interests are health workers serving, and what are the ideological consequences of their actions.[29] Are we advocating the modification of behavior for the *exclusive* purpose of improving health status, or are we using the question of health as a means of obtaining some kind of moral uniformity through the abolition of disapproved behaviors? To what extent, if at all, are health workers actively involved in some wider pattern of social regulation?[30]

Such questions also arise in relation to the burgeoning literature that links more covert personality characteristics to certain illnesses and at-risk behaviors. Capturing a great deal of attention in this regard are the recent studies which associate heart disease with what is termed a Type A personality. The Type A personality consists of a complex of traits which produces: excessive competitive drive, aggressiveness, impatience, and a harrying sense of time urgency. Individuals displaying this pattern seem to be engaged in a chronic, ceaseless and often fruitless struggle with themselves, with others, with circumstances, with time, sometimes with life itself. They also frequently exhibit a free-floating, but well-rationalized form of hostility, and almost always a deep-seated insecurity.[31]

Efforts to change Type A traits appear to be based on some ideal conception of a relaxed, non-competitive, phlegmatic individual to which people are encouraged to conform.[32] Again, one can question how realistic such a conception is in a system which daily rewards behavior resulting from Type A traits. One can clearly question the ascription of near exclusive culpability to those displaying Type A behavior when the context within which such behavior is manifest is structured in such a way as to guarantee its production. From a cursory reading of job advertisements in any newspaper, we can see that employers actively seek to recruit individuals manifesting Type A characteristics, extolling them as positive virtues.[33]

My earlier point concerning the potentially disruptive consequences of requiring alterations in life style applies equally well in this area of personality and disease. If health workers manage to effect some changes away from Type A behavior in a system which requires and rewards it, then we must be aware of the possible consequences of such change in terms of future failure. Even though the evidence linking Type A traits to heart disease appears quite conclusive, how can health workers ever hope to combat and alter it when such characteristics are so positively and regularly reinforced in this society?

The various points raised in this section have some important moral and practical implications for those involved in health related endeavors. *First,* I have argued that our prevailing ideology involves the ascription of culpability to particular individuals and groups for the manifestation of either disease or at-risk behavior. *Second,* it can be argued that so-called "health professionals" have acquired a mandate to determine the morality of different types of behavior and have access to a body of knowledge and resources which they can "legitimately" deploy for its removal or alteration. (A detailed discussion of the means by which this mandate has been acquired is expanded in a separate paper.) *Third,* [it] is possible to argue that a great deal of health intervention is, perhaps unwittingly, part of a wide pattern of social regulation. We must be clear both as to whose interests we are serving, and the wider implications and consequences of the activities we support through the application of our expertise. *Finally,* it is evident from arguments I have presented that much of our health intervention fails to take adequate account of the social contexts which foster and reinforce the behaviors we seek to alter. The literature of preventive medicine is replete with illustrations of the failure of context-less health intervention programs.

THE NOTION OF A NEED HIERARCHY

At this point in the discussion I shall digress slightly to consider the relationship between the utilization of preventive health services and the concept of need as manifest in this society. We know from available evidence that upper socioeconomic groups are generally more responsive to health intervention activities than are those of lower socio-economic status. To partially account for this phenomenon, I have found it useful to introduce the notion of a *need hierarchy*. By this I refer to the fact that some needs (e.g., food, clothing, shelter) are probably universally recognized as related to sheer survival and take precedence, while other needs, for particular social groups, may be perceived as less immediately important (e.g., dental care, exercise, balanced diet). In other words, I conceive of a *hierarchy of needs,* ranging from what could be termed "primary needs" (which relate more or less to the universally recognized immediate needs for survival) through to "secondary needs" (which are not always recognized as important and which may be artificially engineered by the manufacturers of illness). Somewhere between the high priority, primary needs and the less important, secondary needs are likely to fall the kinds of need invoked by preventive health workers. Where one is located at any point in time on the need hierarchy (i.e., which particular needs are engaging one's attention and resources) is largely a function of the shape of the existing social structure and aspects of socio-economic status.

This notion of a hierarchy of needs enables us to distinguish between the health and illness behavior of the affluent and the poor. Much of the social life of the wealthy clearly concerns secondary needs, which are generally perceived as lower than most health related needs on the need hierarchy. If some pathology presents itself, or some at-risk behavior is recognized, then they naturally assume a priority position, which eclipses most other needs for action. In contrast, much of the social life of the poor centers on needs which are understandably regarded as being of greater priority than most health concerns on the need hierarchy (e.g., homelessness, unemployment). Should some illness event present itself, or should health workers alert people and groups in poverty to possible further health needs, then these needs inevitably assume a position of relative low priority and are eclipsed, perhaps indefinitely, by more pressing primary needs for sheer existence.

From such a perspective, I think it is possible to understand why so much of our health intervention fails in those very groups, at highest risk to morbidity, whom we hope to reach and influence. The appeals that we make in alerting them to possible future needs simply miss the mark by giving inadequate recognition to those primary needs which daily preoccupy their attention. Not only does the notion of a need hierarchy emphasize the difficulty of contextless intervention programs, but it also enables us to view the rejection as a non-compliance with health programs, as, in a sense, rational behavior.

HOW PREVENTIVE IS PREVENTION?

With regard to some of the arguments I have presented, concerning the ultimate futility of downstream endeavors, one may respond that effective preventive medicine does, in fact, take account of this problem. Indeed, many preventive health workers are openly skeptical of a predominantly curative perspective in health care. I have argued, however, that even our best preventive endeavors are misplaced in their almost total ascription of responsibility for illness to the afflicted individuals and groups, and through the types of programs which result. While useful in a limited way, the preventive orientation is itself largely a downstream endeavor through its preoccupation with the avoidance of at-risk behavior in the individual and with its general neglect of the activities of the manufacturers of illness which foster such behavior.

Figure 7.1 is a crude diagrammatic representation of an overall process starting with (1) the activities of the manufacturers of illness, which (2) foster and habituate people to certain at-risk behaviors, which (3) ultimately result in the onset of certain types of morbidity and mortality.[34] The predominant curative orientation in modern medicine deals almost exclusively with the observable patterns of morbidity and mortality, which are the *end-points* in the process. The much heralded preventive orientation focuses

FIGURE 7.1 ■

1	2	3
The activities of the manufacturers of illness	Various at-risk behaviors	Observable morbidity and mortality

Intervention with a political economic focus → Intervention with a preventive focus → Intervention with a curative focus

on those behaviors which are known to be associated with particular illnesses and which can be viewed as the *midpoint* in the overall process. Still left largely untouched are the entrepreneurial activities of the manufacturers of illness, who, through largely unregulated activities, foster the at-risk behavior we aim to prevent. This *beginning point* in the process remains unaffected by most preventive endeavors, even though it is at this point that the greatest potential for change, and perhaps even ultimate victory, lies.

It is clear that this paper raises many questions and issues at a general level—more in fact than it is possible to resolve. Since most of the discussion has been at such an abstract level and concerned with broad political and economic forces, any ensuing recommendations for change must be broad enough to cover the various topics discussed. Hopefully, the preceding argument will also stimulate discussion toward additional recommendations and possible solutions. Given the scope and direction of this paper and the analogy I have employed to convey its content, the task becomes of the order of constructing fences upstream *and* restraining those who, in the interest of corporate profitability, continue to push people in. In this concluding section I will confine my remarks to three selected areas of recommendations.

RECOMMENDED ACTION

a. Legislative Intervention

It is probably true that one stroke of effective health legislation is equal to many separate health intervention endeavors and the cumulative efforts of innumerable health workers over long periods of time. In terms of winning the war which was described earlier, greater changes will result from the continued politicization of illness than from the modification of specific individual behaviors. There are many opportunities for a legislative reduction of at-riskness, and we ought to seize them. Let me give one suggestion which relates to earlier points in this paper. Widespread public advertising is importantly related to the growth and survival of large corporations. If it were not so demonstrably effective, then such vast sums of money and resources would not be devoted to this activity. Moreover, as things stand at present, a great deal of advertising is encouraged through granting it tax exempt status on some vague grounds of public education.[35] To place more stringent, enforceable restrictions on advertising would be to severely curtail the morally abhorrent pushing in activities of the manufacturers of illness. It is true that large corporations are ingenious in their efforts to avoid the consequences of most of the current legislative restrictions on advertising which only prohibit certain kinds of appeals.

As a possible solution to this and in recognition of the moral culpability of those who are actively manufacturing disease, I conceive of a ratio of advertising to health tax or a ratio of risk to benefit tax (RRBT). The idea here is to, in some way, match advertising expenditures to health expenditures. The precise weighting of the ratio could be determined by independently ascertaining the severity of the health effects produced by the manufacture and distribution of the product by the corporation. For example, it is clear that smoking is injurious to health and has no redeeming benefit. Therefore, for this product, the ratio could be determined as say, 3 to 1, where, for example, a company which spends a non-tax deductible $1 million to advertise its cigarettes would be required to devote a non-tax deductible $3 million to the area of health. In the area of quasi-health activities, where the product, although largely useless, may not be so injurious (e.g., nasal sprays, pain killers, mineral supplements, etc.), the ratio could be on, say, a 1 to 1 basis.

Of course, the manufacturers of illness, at the present time, do "donate" large sums of money for the purpose of research, with an obvious understanding that their gift should be reciprocated. In a recent article, Nuehring and Markle touch on the nature of this reciprocity:

> One of the most ironic pro-cigarette forces has been the American Medical Association. This powerful health organization took a position in 1965 clearly favorable to the tobacco interests. . . . In addition, the A.M.A. was, until 1971, conspicuously absent from the membership of the National Interagency Council on Smoking and Health, a coalition of government agencies and virtually all the national health organizations, formed in 1964. The A.M.A.'s largely pro-tobacco behavior has been linked with the acceptance of large research subsidies from the tobacco industry—amounting, according to the industry, to some 18 million dollars.[36]

Given such reciprocity, it would be necessary for this health money from the RRBT to be handled by a supposedly independent government agency, like the FDA or the FTC, for distribution to regular research institutions as well as to consumer organizations in the health field, which are currently so unequally pitted against the upstream manufacturers of illness. Such legislation would, I believe, severely curtail corporate "pushing in" activity and publicly demonstrate our commitment to effectively regulating the source of many health problems.

b. The Question of Lobbying

Unfortunately, due to present arrangements, it is difficult to discern the nature and scope of health lobbying activities. If only we could locate (a) who is lobbying for what, (b) who they are lobbying with, (c) what tactics are being employed, and (d) with what consequences for health legislation. Because these activities are likely to jeopardize the myths that have been so carefully engineered and fed to a gullible public by both the manufacturers of illness *and* various health organizations, they are clothed

in secrecy.[37] Judging from recent newspaper reports, concerning multimillion dollar gift-giving by the pharmaceutical industry to physicians, the occasional revelation of lobbying and political exchange remains largely unknown and highly newsworthy. It is frequently argued that lobbying on behalf of specific legislation is an essential avenue for public input in the process of enacting laws. Nevertheless, the evidence suggests that it is often, by being closely linked to the distribution of wealth, a very one-sided process. As it presently occurs, many legitimate interests on a range of health related issues do not have lobbying input in proportion to their numerical strength and may actually be structurally precluded from effective participation. While recognizing the importance of lobbying activity and yet feeling that for certain interests its scope ought to be severely curtailed (perhaps in the same way as the proposed regulation and publication of political campaign contributions), I am, to be honest, at a loss as to what should be specifically recommended. . . . The question is: quite apart from the specific issue of changing individual behavior, *in what ways could we possibly regulate the disproportionately influential lobbying activities of certain interest groups in the health field?*

c. Public Education

In the past, it has been common to advocate the education of the public as a means of achieving an alteration in the behavior of groups at risk to illness. Such downstream educational efforts rest on "blaming the victim" assumptions and seek to *either* stop people doing what we feel they "ought not" to be doing, *or* encourage them to do things they "ought" to be doing, but are not. Seldom do we educate people (especially schoolchildren) about the activities of the manufacturers of illness and about how they are involved in many activities unrelated to their professed area of concern. How many of us know, for example, that for any "average" Thanksgiving dinner, the turkey may be produced by the Greyhound Corporation, the Smithfield Ham by ITT, the lettuce by Dow Chemical, the potatoes by Boeing, the fruits and vegetables by Tenneco or the Bank of America?[38] I would reiterate that I am not opposed to the education of people who are at risk to illness, with a view to altering their behavior to enhance life chances (if this can be done successfully). However, I would add the proviso that if we remain committed to the education of people, we must ensure that they are being told the whole story. And, in my view, immediate priority ought to be given to the sensitization of vast numbers of people to the

upstream activities of the manufacturers of illness, some of which have been outlined in this paper. Such a program, actively supported by the federal government (perhaps through revenue derived from the RRBT), may foster a groundswell of consumer interest which, in turn, may go some way toward checking the disproportionately influential lobbying of the large corporations and interest groups.

References and Notes

1. I.K. Zola, "Helping Does It Matter: The Problems and Prospects of Mutual Aid Groups." Addressed to the United Ostomy Association, 1970.

2. See, for example, M.W. Susser and W. Watson, *Sociology in Medicine,* New York: Oxford University Press, 1971. Edith Chen, et al., "Family Structure in Relation to Health and Disease." *Journal of Chronic Diseases,* Vol. 12 (1960), p. 554–567; and R. Keelner, *Family III Health: An Investigation in General Practice,* Charles C. Thomas, 1963. There is, of course, voluminous literature which relates family structure to mental illness. Few studies move to the level of considering the broader social forces which promote the family structures which are conducive to the onset of particular illnesses. With regard to utilization behavior, see J.B. McKinlay, "Social Networks, Lay Consultation and Help-Seeking Behavior," *Social Forces,* Vol. 51, No. 3 (March, 1973), pp. 275–292.

3. A rich source for a variety of materials included in this second level is H.E. Freeman, S. Levine, and L.G. Reeder (Eds.), *Handbook of Medical Sociology,* New Jersey: Prentice-Hall, 1972. I would also include here studies of the health implications of different housing patterns. Recent evidence suggests that housing—even when highly dense—may not be directly related to illness.

4. There have, of course, been many studies, mainly by epidemiologists, relating disease patterns to certain occupations and industries. Seldom, however, have social scientists pursued the consequences of these findings in terms of a broader political economy of illness. One exception to this statement can be found in studies and writings on the social causes and consequences of environmental pollution. For a recent elementary treatment of some important issues in this general area, see H. Waitzkin and B. Waterman, *The Exploitation of Illness in Capitalist Society,* New York: Bobbs-Merrill Co., 1974.

5. Some useful introductory readings appear in D.M. Gordon (Ed.), *Problems in Political Economy: An Urban Perspective,* Lexington: D.C. Heath & Co., 1971, and R. C. Edwards, M. Reich and T. E. Weisskopf (Eds.), *The Capitalist System,* New Jersey: Prentice-Hall, 1972. Also, T. Christoffel, D. Finkelhor and D. Gilbarg (Eds.), *Up Against the American Myth,* New York: Holt, Rinehart and Winston, 1970. M. Mankoff (Ed.), *The Poverty of Progress: The Political Economy of American Social Problems,* New York: Holt, Rinehart and Winston, 1972. For more sophisticated treatment see the collection edited by D. Mermelstein, *Economics: Mainstream Readings and Radical*

Critiques, New York: Random House, 1970. Additionally useful papers appear in J. B. McKinlay (Ed.), *Politics and Law in Health Care Policy.* New York: Prodist, 1973, and J. B. McKinlay (Ed.), *Economic Aspects of Health Care,* New York: Prodist, 1973. For a highly readable and influential treatment of what is termed "the medical industrial complex," see B. and J. Ehrenreich, *The American Health Empire: Power, Profits and Politics,* New York: Vintage Books, 1971. Also relevant are T. R. Marmor, *The Politics of Medicare,* Chicago: Aldine Publishing Co., 1973, and R. Alford, "The Political Economy of Health Care: Dynamics Without Change," *Politics and Society,* 2 (1972), pp. 127–164.

6. E. Cray, *In Failing Health: The Medical Crisis and the AMA,* Indianapolis: Bobbs-Merrill, 1970. J.S. Burrow, *AMA—Voice of American Medicine,* Baltimore: Johns Hopkins Press, 1963. R. Harris, *A Sacred Trust,* New York: New American Library, 1966. R. Carter, *The Doctor Business,* Garden City, New York: Dolphin Books, 1961. "The American Medical Association: Power, Purpose and Politics in Organized Medicine," *Yale Law Journal,* Vol. 63, No. 7 (May, 1954), pp. 938–1021.

7. See references under footnote 5, especially B. and J. Ehrenreich's *The American Health Empire,* Chapter VII, pp. 95–123.

8. D.M. Gordon (Ed.), *Problems in Political Economy: An Urban Perspective,* Lexington: D.C. Heath & Co., 1971, p. 318.

9. See, for example, D. A. Bernstein, "The Modification of Smoking Behavior: An Evaluative Review," *Psychological Bulletin,* Vol. 71 (June, 1969), pp. 418–440; S. Ford and F. Ederer, "Breaking the Cigarette Habit," *Journal of American Medical Association,* 194 (October, 1965), pp. 139–142; C. S. Keutzer, et al., "Modification of Smoking Behavior: A Review," *Psychological Bulletin,* Vol. 70 (December, 1968), pp. 520–533. Mettlin considers evidence concerning the following techniques for modifying smoking behavior: (1) behavioral conditioning, (2) group discussion, (3) counselling, (4) hypnosis, (5) interpersonal communication, (6) self-analysis. He concludes that: Each of these approaches suggests that smoking behavior is the result of some finite set of social and psychological variables, yet none has either demonstrated any significant powers in predicting the smoking behaviors of an individual or led to techniques of smoking control that considered alone, have significant long-term effects. In C. Mettlin, "Smoking as Behavior: Applying a Social Psychological Theory," *Journal of Health and Social Behavior,* 14 (June, 1973), p. 144.

10. It appears that a considerable proportion of advertising by large corporations is tax exempt through being granted the status of "public education." In particular, the enormous media campaign, which was recently waged by major oil companies in an attempt to preserve the public myths they had so carefully constructed concerning their activities, was almost entirely non-taxable.

11. Reports of the harmfulness and ineffectiveness of certain products appear almost weekly in the press. As I have been writing this paper, I have come across reports of the low quality of milk, the uselessness of cold remedies, the health dangers in frankfurters, the linking of the use of the aerosol propellant, vinyl chloride, to liver cancer. That the Food and Drug Administration (F.D.A.) is unable to effectively regulate the manufacturers of illness is evident and illustrated in their inept handling of the withdrawal of the drug, betahistine hydrochloride, which supposedly offered symptomatic relief of Meniere's Syndrome

(an affliction of the inner ear). There is every reason to think that this case is not atypical. For additionally disquieting evidence of how the Cigarette Labeling and Advertising Act of 1965 actually curtailed the power of the F.T.C. and other federal agencies from regulating cigarette advertising and nullified all such state and local regulatory efforts, see L. Fritschier, *Smoking and Politics: Policymaking and the Federal Bureaucracy*, New York: Meredith, 1969, and T. Whiteside, *Selling Death: Cigarette Advertising and Public Health*, New York: Liveright, 1970. Also relevant are Congressional Quarterly, 27 (1969) 666, 1026; and U.S. Department of Agriculture, Economic Research Service, *Tobacco Situation*, Washington: Government Printing Office, 1969.

12. The term "culture" is used to refer to a number of other characteristics as well. However, these two appear to be commonly associated with the concept. See J. B. McKinlay, "Some Observations on the Concept of a Subculture." (1970).

13. This has been argued in J. B. McKinlay, "Some Approaches and Problems in the Study of the Use of Services," *Journal of Health and Social Behavior*, Vol. 13 (July, 1972), pp. 115–152; and J. B. McKinlay and D. Dutton, "Social Psychological Factors Affecting Health Service Utilization," chapter in *Consumer Incentives for Health Care*, New York: Prodist Press, 1974.

14. Reliable sources covering these areas are available in many professional journals in the fields of epidemiology, medical sociology, preventive medicine, industrial and occupational medicine and public health. Useful references covering these and related areas appear in J. N. Morris, *Uses of Epidemiology*, London: E. and S. Livingstone Ltd., 1967; and M. W. Susser and W. Watson, *Sociology in Medicine*, New York: Oxford University Press, 1971.

15. D. Zwerling, "Death for Dinner," *The New York Review of Books*, Vol. 21, No. 2 (February 21, 1974), p. 22.

16. D. Zwerling, "Death for Dinner." See footnote 15 above.

17. This figure was quoted by several witnesses at the *Hearings Before the Select Committee on Nutrition and Human Needs*, U.S. Government Printing Office, 1973.

18. The magnitude of this problem is discussed in P. Wyden, *The Overweight: Causes, Costs and Control*, Englewood Cliffs: Prentice-Hall, 1968; National Center for Health Statistics, *Weight by Age and Height of Adults:* 1960–62. Washington: *Vital and Health Statistics*, Public Health Service Publication #1000, Series 11, #14, Government Printing Office, 1966; U.S. Public Health Service, Center for Chronic Disease Control, *Obesity and Health*, Washington: Government Printing Office, 1966.

19. This aborted study is discussed in M. Jacobson, *Nutrition Scoreboard: Your Guide to Better Eating*, Center for Science in the Public Interest.

20. M.S. Hathaway and E. D. Foard, *Heights and Weights for Adults in the United States*, Washington: Home Economics Research Report 10, Agricultural Research Service, U.S. Department of Agriculture, Government Printing Office, 1960.

21. This is discussed by D. Zwerling. See footnote 16.

22. See *Hearings Before the Select Committee on Nutrition and Human Needs*, Parts 3 and 4, "T.V. Advertising of Food to Children," March 5, 1973 and March 6, 1973.

23. Dr. John Udkin, Department of Nutrition, Queen Elizabeth College, London University. See p. 225, *Senate Hearings*, footnote 22 above.

24. D. Zwerling, "Death for Dinner." See footnote 16 above, page 24.

25. This is well argued in F. Piven and R. A. Cloward, *Regulating the Poor: The Functions of Social Welfare,* New York: Vintage, 1971; L. Goodwin, *Do the Poor Want to Work?,* Washington: Brookings, 1972; H. J. Gans, "The Positive Functions of Poverty," *American Journal of Sociology,* Vol. 78, No. 2 (September, 1972), pp. 275–289; R. P. Roby (Ed.), *The Poverty Establishment,* New Jersey: Prentice-Hall, 1974.

26. See, for example, Jules Henry, "American Schoolrooms: Learning the Nightmare," *Columbia University Forum,* (Spring, 1963), pp. 24–30. See also the paper by F. Howe and P. Lanter, "How the School System is Rigged for Failure," *New York Review of Books,* (June 18, 1970).

27. With regard to penology, for example, see the critical work of R. Quinney in *Criminal Justice in America,* Boston: Little Brown, 1974, and *Critique of Legal Order,* Boston: Little Brown, 1974.

28. See, for example, S. M. Sales, "Organizational Role as a Risk Factor in Coronary Disease," *Administrative Science Quarterly,* Vol. 14, No. 3 (September, 1969), pp. 325–336. The literature in this particular area is enormous. For several good reviews, see L.E. Hinkle, "Some Social and Biological Correlates of Coronary Heart Disease," *Social Science and Medicine,* Vol. 1 (1967), pp. 129–139; F. H. Epstein, "The Epidemiology of Coronary Heart Disease: A Review," *Journal of Chronic Diseases,* 18 (August, 1965), pp. 735–774.

29. Some interesting ideas in this regard are in E. Nuehring and G. E. Markle, "Nicotine and Norms: The Reemergence of a Deviant Behavior" *Social Problems,* Vol. 21, No. 4 (April, 1974), pp. 513–526. Also, J.R. Gusfield, *Symbolic Crusade: Status Politics and the American Temperance Movement,* Urbana, Illinois: University of Illinois Press, 1963.

30. For a study of the ways in which physicians, clergymen, the police, welfare officers, psychiatrists and social workers act as agents of social control, see E. Cumming, *Systems of Social Regulation,* New York: Atherton Press, 1968.

31. R. H. Rosenman and M. Friedman, "The Role of a Specific Overt Behavior Pattern in the Occurrence of Ischemic Heart Disease," *Cardiologia Practica,* 13 (1962), pp. 42–53; M. Friedman and R. H. Rosenman, *Type A Behavior and Your Heart,* Knopf, 1973. Also, S. J. Zyzanski and C. D. Jenkins, "Basic Dimensions Within the Coronary-Prone Behavior Pattern," *Journal of Chronic Diseases,* 22 (1970), pp. 781–795. There are, of course, many other illnesses which have also been related in one way or another to certain personality characteristics. Having found this new turf, behavioral scientists will most likely continue to play it for everything it is worth and then, in the interests of their own survival, will "discover" that something else indeed accounts for what they were trying to explain and will eventually move off there to find renewed fame and fortune. Furthermore, serious methodological doubts have been raised concerning the studies of the relationship between personality and at-risk behavior. See, in this regard, G. M. Hochbaum, "A Critique of Psychological Research on Smoking," paper presented to the American Psychological Association, Los Angeles, 1964. Also B. Lebovits and A. Ostfeld, "Smoking and Personality: A Methodologic Analysis," *Journal of Chronic Diseases* (1971).

32. M. Friedman and R.H. Rosenman. See footnote 31.

33. In the *New York Times* of Sunday, May 26, 1974, there were job advertisements seeking "aggressive self-starters," "people who stand real challenges," "those who like to compete," "career oriented specialists," "those with a spark of determination to someday run their own show," "people with the success drive," and "take charge individuals."

34. Aspects of this process are discussed in J. B. McKinlay, "On the Professional Regulation of Change," in *The Professions and Social Change,* P. Halmos (Ed.), Keele: Sociological Review Monograph, No. 20, 1973, and in "Clients and Organizations," chapter in J.B. McKinlay (Ed.), *Processing People— Studies in Organizational Behavior,* London: Holt, Rinehart, and Winston, 1974.

35. There have been a number of reports recently concerning this activity. Questions have arisen about the conduct of major oil corporations during the so-called "energy crisis." See footnote 10. Equally questionable may be the public spirited advertisements sponsored by various professional organizations which, while claiming to be solely in the interests of the public, actually serve to enhance business in various ways. Furthermore, by granting special status to activities of professional groups, government agencies and large corporations may effectively gag them through some expectation of reciprocity. For example, most health groups, notably the American Cancer Society, did not support the F.C.C.'s action against smoking commercials because they were fearful of alienating the networks from whom they receive free announcements for their fund drives. Both the American Cancer Society and the American Heart Association have been criticized for their reluctance to engage in direct organizational conflict with pro-cigarette forces, particularly before the alliance between the television broadcasters and the tobacco industry broke down. Rather, they have directed their efforts to the downstream reform of the smoker. See E. Nuehring and G. E. Markle, cited in footnote 29.

36. E. Nuehring and G. E. Markle, cited in footnote 29.

37. The ways in which large-scale organizations engineer and disseminate these myths concerning their manifest activities, while avoiding any mention of their underlying latent activities, are discussed in more detail in the two references cited in footnote 34 above.

38. For a popularly written and effective treatment of the relationship between giant corporations and food production and consumption, see W. Robbins, *The American Food Scandal,* New York: William Morrow and Co., 1974.

OUR SICKENING SOCIAL AND PHYSICAL ENVIRONMENTS

In the previous section, we explored the relationship between society and the distribution of disease and death. We saw that in U.S. society, diseases are patterned by sociocultural factors, including social class, gender, and race. Here, we continue to search for an understanding of the interface between diseases and society by examining the sociological contexts of having asthma and of mortality.

Social scientists have little difficulty analyzing the social nature of problems such as homicide, suicide, and automobile accidents. Less often, however, have they applied sociological perspectives to understanding the causes and prevention of diseases such as cancer or diabetes. The selections in this section share the theme that at least some of these chronic diseases have developed as a result of modern industrialization, and so are deeply connected to the organization and characteristics of social life.

Chronic health conditions—heart disease, cancer, and chronic lower respiratory diseases—are the top three causes of death in the United States (Xu et al. 2016). One in ten people have fair to poor health in the United States, and 29% report at least one limitation in doing basic actions or completing everyday activities (National Center for Health Statistics 2016). These data give us a general picture of the significant impact of chronic disease on our population's health. Chronic diseases generally develop and persist over a long period of time. Their signs often go unnoticed or unidentified until they cause serious damage to the victim's body, and they usually have complex rather than simple or single causes. Medical treatment generally aims to alleviate symptoms, prevent or slow down further organic damage, or minimize physical discomfort, primarily through treatments with medications or surgery. Treatment rather than prevention is the dominant medical approach to these diseases.

Although *prevention* of chronic diseases seems to be the most logical, safe, and perhaps the most moral approach, few financial resources have been devoted in the United States to the elimination of the physical and social causes of chronic health disorders. The growing recognition of the environmental component in many chronic diseases has led some critics to question the priorities of our current medical care system, as well as the limits of its approach to the treatment, let alone prevention, of these conditions.

For example, Samuel Epstein has argued that the "epidemic" of cancer in the United States is both a medical and social issue, involving as it does a range of political and economic factors including the use of chemicals in manufacturing to increase profits, economic and political pressures on industry scientists, and the relatively low priority given to cancer prevention research (Epstein 1979; Patterson 1989). If many cancers are environmentally produced, and the federal government has estimated that as many as 90 percent may be so, why has medical research and treatment focused on cure rather than prevention (Muir and Sasco 1991; McCormick 2009)? We need to look "upstream" to learn more about how environments cause disease rather than focusing most of our efforts "downstream," on treating people after they become sick.

In recent years, evidence has accumulated that the social environment may produce ill health. For example, studies have shown that the social organization of the work environment (House and Cottington 1984), social stress (Kasl 1984), and social support (Cohen and Syme 1985) can affect health status and outcomes. Among the most intriguing work in this area are the studies that show the importance of social relationships to health. There is continuing evidence that individuals with few social relationships are at increased risk for disease (morbidity) and death (mortality). In "Social Relationships and Health," James S. House, Karl R. Landis, and Debra Umberson review the existing research and conclude that a significant causal relationship exists between social relationships and health. They contend the evidence is as strong as that for cigarette smoking and health in 1964, when the surgeon general issued the first report on the dangers of smoking, although the specificity of the associations is not yet as well known. For example, social support may have a moderating effect on individuals who experience stress, helping them weather it with fewer ill effects (Thoits 2010). While we don't really know how social relationships affect health, it is increasingly clear that these factors need to be considered seriously in terms of etiology and prevention. This awareness is especially important because evidence exists that the quantity and quality of social relationships in our society may be declining. One in every seven adults in the United States lives alone, and there are more single-person households than there are nuclear families (Klinenberg 2013).

Public health analysts have long known that the physical environment can produce disease. Asthma is a disease that is often triggered by environmental factors, both indoor and outdoor. In the second selection in this section, "The Health Politics of Asthma: Environmental Justice and Collective Illness Experience in the United States," Phil Brown and his colleagues examine the health politics of asthma, focusing on two environmental justice

organizations' attempts to combat community-level pollution. These groups arose in poor communities of color in response to "transit racism"—air pollution that was created in those neighborhoods by public policies. Through this work, the groups attempted to shift perceptions of asthma within their communities, using education to empower community members to take action to eliminate local sources of air pollution.

In the third selection, "Dying Alone: The Social Production of Urban Isolation," Eric Klinenberg presents a dramatic and tragic illustration of the impact of an extreme lack of social relationships. In this article, he searches for the root causes of the deaths of over 700 Chicago residents during a devastating heat wave in 1995. He conducts what he calls a "social autopsy" to examine the underlying factors of why these residents died, beyond the immediate medical causes that would be listed on the death certificates. Klinenberg found that urban isolation combined with a culture of fear and political neglect created a chronic situation that made poor, elderly people particularly vulnerable to death in this disaster (see also Klinenberg 2002). With a greater number of people living alone, many of them poor and elderly, this type of social susceptibility to disease and death may become a greater problem despite advances in medical care.

References

Cohen, Sheldon, and S. Leonard Syme. 1985. *Social Support and Health*. New York: Academic Press.

Epstein, Samuel. 1979. *The Politics of Cancer*. New York: Anchor/Doubleday.

House, James S., and Eric M. Cottington. 1984. "Health and the Workplace." In *Applications of Social Science to Clinical Medicine and Health Policy*, edited by David Mechanic and Linda H. Aiken. New Brunswick, NJ: Rutgers University Press.

Kasl, Stanislav. 1984. "Stress and Health." *Annual Review of Public Health* 5: 319–41.

Klinenberg, Eric. 2002. *Heat Wave: A Social Autopsy of Disaster in Chicago*. Chicago: University of Chicago Press.

Klinenberg, Eric. 2013. *Going Solo: The Extraordinary Rise and Surprising Appeal of Living Alone*. New York: Penguin Books.

McCormick, Sabrina. 2009. *No Family History: The Environmental Links to Breast Cancer*. Lanham, MD: Rowman and Littlefield.

Muir, C. S., and A. J. Sasco. 1991. "Prospects for Cancer Control in the 1990s." *Annual Review of Public Health* 11: 143–64.

National Center for Health Statistics. 2016. *Health, United States, 2016: With Special Chartbook on Long-Term Trends in Health.* Hyattsville, MD. Accessed November 10, 2017. https://www.cdc.gov/nchs/data/hus/hus16.pdf#015.

Patterson, James. 1989. *The Dread Disease: Cancer and American Culture.* Cambridge: Harvard University Press.

Thoits, Peggy. 2010. "Stress and Health: Major Findings and Policy Implications." *Journal of Health and Social Behavior* 51: S41–53.

Xu, Jiaquan, Sherry L. Murphy, Kenneth D. Kochanek, and Elizabeth Areas. 2016. *Mortality in the United States, 2015.* NCHS Data Brief No. 267. Accessed November 10, 2017. https://www.cdc.gov/nchs/data/databriefs/db267.pdf.

SOCIAL RELATIONSHIPS
AND HEALTH

James S. House, Karl R. Landis, and Debra Umberson

[M]y father told me of a careful observer, who certainly had heart-disease and died from it, and who positively stated that his pulse was habitually irregular to an extreme degree; yet to his great disappointment it invariably became regular as soon as my father entered the room.

—Charles Darwin (1)

Scientists have long noted an association between social relationships and health. More socially isolated or less socially integrated individuals are less healthy, psychologically and physically, and more likely to die. The first major work of empirical sociology found that less socially integrated people were more likely to commit suicide than the most integrated (2). In subsequent epidemiologic research age-adjusted mortality rates from all causes of death are consistently higher among the unmarried than the married (3–5). Unmarried and more socially isolated people have also manifested higher rates of tuberculosis (6), accidents (7), and psychiatric disorders such as schizophrenia (8, 9). And as the previous quote from Darwin suggests, clinicians have also observed potentially health-enhancing qualities of social relationships and contacts.

The causal interpretation and explanation of these associations has, however, been less clear. Does a lack of social relationships cause people to

Social Relationships and Health, James S. House, Karl R. Landis, and Debra Umberson in *Science,* Vol. 241, Issue 4865, pp. 540–545. July 29, 1988. With permission from the American Association for the Advancement of Science.

become ill or die? Or are unhealthy people less likely to establish and maintain social relationships? Or is there some other factor, such as a misanthropic personality, which predisposes people both to have a lower quantity or quality of social relationships and to become ill or die?

Such questions have been largely unanswerable before the last decade for two reasons. First, there was little theoretical basis for causal explanation. Durkheim (2) proposed a theory of how social relationships affected suicide, but this theory did not generalize to morbidity and mortality from other causes. Second, evidence of the association between social relationships and health, especially in general human populations, was almost entirely retrospective or cross-sectional before the late 1970s. Retrospective studies from death certificates or hospital records ascertained the nature of people's social relationships after they had become ill or died, and cross-sectional surveys of general populations determined whether people who reported ill health also reported a lower quality or quantity of relationships. Such studies used statistical control of potential confounding variables to rule out third factors that might produce the association between social relationships and health, but could do this only partially. They could not determine whether poor social relationships preceded or followed ill health.

In this article, we review recent developments that have altered this state of affairs dramatically: (i) emergence of theoretical models for a causal effect of social relationships on health in humans and animals; (ii) cumulation of empirical evidence that social relationships are a consequential predictor of mortality in human populations; and (iii) increasing evidence for the causal impact of social relationships on psychological and physiological functioning in quasi-experimental and experimental studies of humans and animals. These developments suggest that social relationships, or the relative lack thereof, constitute a major risk factor for health—rivaling the effects of well-established health risk factors such as cigarette smoking, blood pressure, blood lipids, obesity, and physical activity. Indeed, the theory and evidence on social relationships and health increasingly approximate that available at the time of the U.S. Surgeon General's 1964 report on smoking and health (10), with similar implications for future research and public policy.

THE EMERGENCE OF "SOCIAL SUPPORT" THEORY AND RESEARCH

The study of social relationships and health was revitalized in the middle 1970s by the emergence of a seemingly new field of scientific research on "social support." This concept was first used in the mental health literature (11, 12), and was linked to physical health in separate seminal articles by physician-epidemiologists Cassel (13) and Cobb (14). These articles grew out of a rapidly developing literature on stress and psychosocial factors in the etiology of health and illness (15). Chronic diseases have increasingly replaced acute infectious diseases as the major causes of disability and death, at least in industrialized countries. Consequently, theories of disease etiology have shifted from ones in which a single factor (usually a microbe) caused a single disease, to ones in which multiple behavioral and environmental as well as biologic and genetic factors combine, often over extended periods, to produce any single disease, with a given factor often playing an etiologic role in multiple diseases.

Cassel (13) and Cobb (14) reviewed more than 30 human and animal studies that found social relationships protective of health. Recognizing that any one study was open to alternative interpretations, they argued that the variety of study designs (ranging from retrospective to experimental), of life stages studied (from birth to death), and of health outcomes involved (including low birth weight, complications of pregnancy, self-reported symptoms, blood pressure, arthritis, tuberculosis, depression, alcoholism, and mortality) suggested a robust, putatively causal, association. Cassel and Cobb indicated that social relationships might promote health in several ways, but emphasized the role of social relationships in moderating or buffering potentially deleterious health effects of psychosocial stress or other health hazards. This idea of "social support," or something that maintains or sustains the organism by promoting adaptive behavior or neuroendocrine responses in the face of stress or other health hazards, provided a general, albeit simple, theory of how and why social relationships should causally affect health (*16*).

Publications on "social support" increased almost geometrically from 1976 to 1981. By the late 1970s, however, serious questions emerged about the empirical evidence cited by Cassel and Cobb and the evidence generated in subsequent research. Concerns were expressed about causal priorities between social support and health (since the great majority of studies remained cross-sectional or retrospective and based on self-reported data), about whether social relationships and supports buffered the impact of stress on health or had more direct effects, and about how consequential the effects of social relationships on health really were (*17–19*). These concerns have been addressed by a continuing cumulation of two types of empirical data: (i) a new series of prospective mortality studies in human populations and (ii) a broadening base of laboratory and field experimental studies of animals and humans.

PROSPECTIVE MORTALITY STUDIES OF HUMAN POPULATIONS

Just as concerns began to surface about the nature and strength of the impact of social relationships on health, data from long-term, prospective studies of community populations provided compelling evidence that lack of social relationships constitutes a major risk factor for mortality. Berkman and Syme (*20*) analyzed a probability sample of 4775 adults in Alameda County, California, who were between 30 and 69 in 1965 when they completed a survey that assessed the presence or extent of four types of social ties—marriage, contacts with extended family and friends, church membership, and other formal and informal group affiliations. Each type of social relationship predicted mortality through the succeeding 9 years. A combined "social network" index remained a significant predictor of mortality

(with a relative risk ratio for mortality of about 2.0, indicating that persons low on the index were twice as likely to die as persons high on the index) in multivariate analyses that controlled for self-reports in 1965 of physical health, socioeconomic status, smoking, alcohol consumption, physical activity, obesity, race, life satisfaction, and use of preventive health services. Such adjustment or control for baseline health and other risk factors provides a conservative estimate of the predictive power of social relationships, since some of their impact may be mediated through effects on these risk factors.

The major limitation of the Berkman and Syme study was the lack of other than self-reported data on health at baseline. Thus, House *et al.* (*21*) sought to replicate and extend the Alameda County results in a study of 2754 adults between 35 and 69 at their initial interview and physical examinations in 1967 through 1969 by the Tecumseh (Michigan) Community Health Study. Composite indices of social relationships and activities (as well as a number of the individual components) were inversely associated with mortality during the succeeding 10- to 12-year follow-up period, with relative risks of 2.0 to 3.0 for men and 1.5 to 2.0 for women, after adjustment for the effects of age and a wide range of biomedically assessed (blood pressure, cholesterol, respiratory function, and electrocardiograms) as well as self-reported risk factors of mortality. Analyzing data on 2059 adults in the Evans County (Georgia) Cardiovascular Epidemiologic Study, Schoenback *et al.* (*22*) also found that a social network index similar to that of Berkman and Syme (*20*) predicted mortality for an 11- to 13-year follow-up period, after adjustment for age and baseline measures of biomedical as well as self-reported risk factors of mortality. The Evans County associations were somewhat weaker than those in Tecumseh and Alameda County, and as in Tecumseh were stronger for males than females.

Studies in Sweden and Finland have described similar results. Tibblin, Welin, and associates (*23, 24*) studied two cohorts of men born in 1913 and 1923, respectively, and living in 1973 in Gothenberg, Sweden's second largest city. After adjustments for age, baseline levels of systolic blood pressure, serum cholesterol, smoking habits, and perceived health status, mortality in both cohorts through 1982 was inversely related to the number of persons in the household and the men's level of social and outside home activities in 1973. Orth-Gomer *et al.* (*25*) analyzed the mortality experience through 1981 of a random sample of 17,433 Swedish adults aged 29 to 74 at the time of their 1976 or 1977 baseline interviews. Frequency of contact with family, friends, neighbors, and coworkers in 1976–77 was predictive of mortality through 1981, after adjustment for age, sex, education, employment status, immigrant status, physical exercise, and self-reports of chronic conditions. The effects were stronger among males than among females, and were somewhat nonlinear, with the greatest increase in mortality risk occurring in the most socially isolated third of the sample. In a prospective study of 13,301 adults in predominantly rural eastern Finland, Kaplan *et al.* (*26*) found a measure of "social connections" similar to those used in Alameda County, Tecumseh, and Evans County to be a significant predictor of male mortality from all causes during 5 years, again after adjustments for other biomedical and self-reported risk factors. Female mortality showed similar, but weaker and statistically nonsignificant, effects.

These studies manifest a consistent pattern of results, as shown in Figs. 8.1 and 8.2, which show age-adjusted mortality rates plotted for the five prospective studies from which we could extract parallel data. The report of the sixth study (*25*) is consistent with these trends. The relative risks (*RR*) in Figs. 8.1 and 8.2 are higher than those reported previously because they are only adjusted for age. The levels of mortality in Figs. 8.1 and 8.2 vary greatly across studies depending on the follow-up period and composition of the population by age, race, and ethnicity, and geographic locale, but the patterns of prospective association between social integration (that is, the number and frequency of social relationships and contacts) and mortality are remarkably similar, with some variations by race, sex, and geographic locale.

Only the Evans County study reported data for blacks. The predictive association of social integration with mortality among Evans County black males is weaker than among white males in Evans

County or elsewhere (Fig. 8.1), and the relative risk ratio for black females in Evans County, although greater than for Evans County white females, is smaller than the risk ratios for white females in all other studies (Fig. 8.2). More research on blacks and other minority populations is necessary to determine whether these differences are more generally characteristic of blacks compared to whites.

Modest differences emerge by sex and rural as opposed to urban locale. Results for men and women are strong, linear, and similar in the urban populations of Alameda County (that is, Oakland and environs) and Gothenberg, Sweden (only men were studied in Gothenberg). In the predominantly small-town and rural populations of Tecumseh, Evans County, and eastern Finland, however, two notable deviations from the urban results appear: (i) female risk ratios are consistently weaker than those for men in the same rural populations (Figs. 8.1 and 8.2), and (ii) the results for men in more rural populations, although rivaling those in urban populations in terms of risk ratios, assume a distinctly nonlinear, or threshold, form. That is, in Tecumseh, Evans County, and eastern Finland, mortality is clearly elevated among the most socially isolated, but declines only modestly, if at all, between moderate and high levels of social integration.

Explanation of these sex and urban-rural variations awaits research on broader regional or national populations in which the same measures are applied to males and females across the full rural-urban continuum. The current results may have both substantive and methodological explanations. Most of the studies reviewed here, as well as others (*27–29*), suggest that being married is more beneficial to health, and becoming widowed more detrimental, for men than for women. Women, however, seem to benefit as much or more than men from relationships with friends and relatives, which tend to run along same-sex lines (*20, 30*). On balance, men may benefit more from social relationships than women, especially in cross-gender relationships. Small communities may also provide a broader context of social integration and support that benefits most people, except for a relatively small group of socially isolated males.

These results may, however, have methodological rather than substantive explanations. Measures of

FIGURE 8.1 ■ Level of Social Integration and Age-Adjusted Mortality for Males in Five Prospective Studies

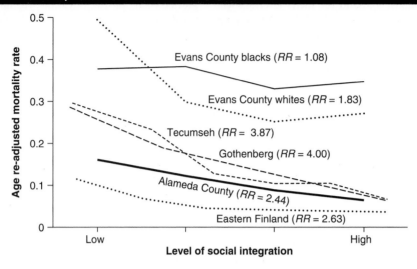

Note: RR, the relative risk ratio of mortality at the lowest versus highest level of social integration.

FIGURE 8.2 ■ Level of Social Integration and Age-Adjusted Mortality for Females in Five Prospective Studies

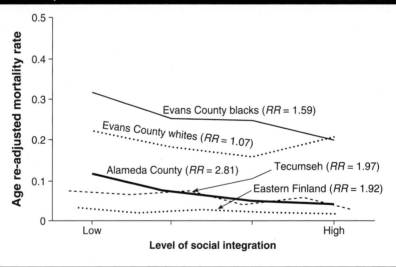

Note: RR, the relative risk ratio of mortality at the lowest versus highest level of social integration.

social relationships or integration used in the existing prospective studies may be less valid or have less variance in rural and small town environments, and for women, thus muting their relationship with mortality. For example, the data for women in Fig. 8.2 are similar to the data on men if we assume that women have higher quality relationships and hence that their true level of social integration is moderate even at low levels of quantity. The social context of small communities may similarly provide a moderate level of social integration for everyone except quite isolated males. Thus measures of frequency of social contact may be poorer indices of social integration for women and more rural populations than for men and urban dwellers.

Variations in the results in Figs. 8.1 and 8.2 should not, however, detract from the remarkable consistency of the overall finding that social relationships do predict mortality for men and women in a wide range of populations, even after adjustment for biomedical risk factors for mortality. Additional prospective studies have shown that social relationships are similarly predictive of all-cause and cardiovascular mortality in studies of people who are elderly (*31–33*) or have serious illnesses (*34, 35*).

EXPERIMENTAL AND QUASI-EXPERIMENTAL RESEARCH

The prospective mortality data are made more compelling by their congruence with growing evidence from experimental and clinical research on animals and humans that variations in exposure to social contacts produce psychological or physiological effects that could, if prolonged, produce serious morbidity and even mortality. Cassel (*13*) reviewed evidence that the presence of a familiar member of the same species could buffer the impact of experimentally induced stress on ulcers, hypertension, and neurosis in rats, mice, and goats, respectively; and the presence of familiar others has also been shown to reduce anxiety and physiological arousal (specifically secretion of free fatty acids) in humans in potentially stressful laboratory situations (*36, 37*). Clinical and laboratory data indicate that the presence of or physical contact with another person can modulate human cardiovascular activity and reactivity in general, and in stressful contexts such as intensive care units (*38*, pp. 122–141). Research also points to the operation of such processes across

species. Affectionate petting by humans, or even their mere presence, can reduce the cardiovascular sequelae of stressful situations among dogs, cats, horses, and rabbits (*38*, pp. 163–180). Nerem *et al.* (*39*) found that human handling also reduced the arteriosclerotic impact of a high fat diet in rabbits. Recent interest in the potential health benefits of pets for humans, especially the isolated aged, is based on similar notions, although the evidence for such efforts is only suggestive (*40*).

Bovard (*41*) has proposed a psychophysiologic theory to explain how social relationships and contacts can promote health and protect against disease. He reviews a wide range of human and animal studies suggesting that social relationships and contacts, mediated through the amygdala, activate the anterior hypothalamic zone (stimulating release of human growth hormone) and inhibit the posterior hypothalamic zone (and hence secretion of adrenocorticotropic hormone, cortisol, catecholamines, and associated sympathetic autonomic activity). These mechanisms are consistent with the impact of social relationships on mortality from a wide range of causes and with studies of the adverse effects of lack of adequate social relationships on the development of human and animal infants (*42*). This theory is also consistent with sociobiological processes which, due to the survival benefit of social relationships and collective activity, would promote genetic selection of organisms who find social contact and relatedness rewarding and the lack of such contact and relatedness aversive (*43*).

The epidemiologic evidence linking social relationships and supports to morbidity in humans is limited and not fully consistent. For example, although laboratory studies show short-term effects of social relationships on cardiovascular functioning that would, over time, produce cardiovascular disease, and prospective studies show impacts of social relationships on mortality from cardiovascular disease, the link between social relationships and the incidence of cardiovascular morbidity has yet to be firmly demonstrated (*19, 44*). Overall, however, the theory and evidence for the impact of social relationships on health are building steadily (*45, 46*).

SOCIAL RELATIONSHIPS AS A RISK FACTOR FOR HEALTH: RESEARCH AND POLICY ISSUES

The theory and data reviewed previously meet reasonable criteria for considering social relationships a cause or risk factor of mortality, and probably morbidity, from a wide range of diseases (*10; 46; 47*, pp. 289–321). These criteria include strength and consistency of statistical associations across a wide range of studies, temporal ordering of prediction from cause to effect, a gradient of response (which may in this case be nonlinear), experimental data on animals and humans consistent with non-experimental human data, and a plausible theory (*41*) of biopsychosocial mechanisms explaining the observed associations.

The evidence on social relationships is probably stronger, especially in terms of prospective studies, than the evidence which led to the certification of the Type A behavior pattern as a risk factor for coronary heart disease (*48*). The evidence regarding social relationships and health increasingly approximates the evidence in the 1964 Surgeon General's report (*10*) that established cigarette smoking as a cause or risk factor for mortality and morbidity from a range of diseases. The age-adjusted relative risk ratios shown in Figs. 8.1 and 8.2 are stronger than the relative risks for all cause mortality reported for cigarette smoking (*10*). There is, however, less specificity in the associations of social relationships with mortality than has been observed for smoking, which is strongly linked to cancers of the lung and respiratory tract (with age-adjusted risk ratios between 3.0 and 11.0). Better theory and data are needed on the links between social relationships and major specific causes of morbidity and mortality.

Although a lack of social relationships has been established as a risk factor for mortality, and probably morbidity, three areas need further investigation: (i) mechanisms and processes linking social relationships to health, (ii) determinants of levels of "exposure" to social relationships, and (iii) the means to lower the prevalence of relative social isolation in the population or to lessen its deleterious effects on health.

MECHANISMS AND PROCESSES LINKING SOCIAL RELATIONSHIPS TO HEALTH

Although grounded in the literature on social relationships and health, investigators on social support in the last decade leaped almost immediately to the interpretation that what was consequential for health about social relationships was their supportive quality, especially their capacity to buffer or moderate the deleterious effects of stress or other health hazards (*13, 14*). Many recent studies have reported either a general positive association between social support and health or a buffering effect in the presence of stress (*49*), but these studies are problematic because the designs are largely cross-sectional or retrospective and the data usually self-reported. The most compelling evidence of the causal significance of social relationships on health has come from the experimental studies of animals and humans in the prospective mortality studies reviewed previously—studies in which the measures of social relationships are merely the presence or absence of familiar other organisms, or relative frequency of contact with them, and which often do not distinguish between buffering and main effects. Thus, social relationships appear to have generally beneficial effects on health, not solely or even primarily attributable to their buffering effects, and there may be aspects of social relationships other than their supportive quality that account for these effects.

We now need a broader theory of the biopsychosocial mechanisms and processes linking social relationships to health than can be provided by extant concepts or theories of social support. That broader theory must do several things. First, it must clearly distinguish between (i) the existence or quantity of social relationships, (ii) their formal structure (such as their density or reciprocity), and (iii) the actual content of these relationships such as social support. Only by testing the effects on health of these different aspects of social relationships in the same study can we understand what it is about social relationships that is consequential for health.

Second, we need better understanding of the social, psychological, and biological processes that link the existence, quantity, structure, or content of social relationships to health. Social support—whether in the form of practical help, emotional sustenance, or provision of information— is only one of the social processes involved here. Not only may social relationships affect health because they are or are not supportive, they may also regulate or control human thought, feeling and behavior in ways that promote health, as in Durkheim's (2) theory relating social integration to suicide. Current views based on this perspective suggest that social relationships affect health either by fostering a sense of meaning or coherence that promotes health (50) or by facilitating health-promoting behaviors such as proper sleep, diet, or exercise, appropriate use of alcohol, cigarettes, and drugs, adherence to medical regimens, or seeking appropriate medical care (51). The negative or conflictive aspects of social relationships need also to be considered, since they may be detrimental to the maintenance of health and of social relationship (52).

We must further understand the psychological and biological processes or mechanisms linking social relationships to health, either as extensions of the social processes just discussed [for example, processes of cognitive appraisal and coping (53)] or as independent mechanisms. In the latter regard, psychological and sociobiological theories suggest that the mere presence of, or sense of relatedness with, another organism may have relatively direct motivational, emotional, or neuroendocrinal effects that promote health either directly or in the face of stress or other health hazards but that operate independently of cognitive appraisal or behavioral coping and adaptation (38, pp. 87–180; 42, 43, 54).

DETERMINANTS OF SOCIAL RELATIONSHIPS: SCIENTIFIC AND POLICY ISSUES

Although social relationships have been extensively studied during the past decade as independent, intervening, and moderating variables affecting stress or health or the relations between them, almost no attention has been paid to social relationships as dependent variables. The determinants of social relationships, as well as their consequences, are crucial to the theoretical and causal status of social relationships in relation to health. If exogenous biological, psychological, or social variables determine both health and the nature of social relationships, then the observed association of social relationships to health may be totally or partially spurious. More practically, Cassel (13), Cobb (14), and others became interested in social support as a means of improving health. This, in turn, requires understanding of the broader social, as well as psychological or biological, structures and processes that determine the quantity and quality of social relationships and support in society.

It is clear that biology and personality must and do affect both people's health and the quantity and quality of their social relationships. Research has established that such factors do not, however, explain away the experimental, cross-sectional, and prospective evidence linking social relationships to health (55). In none of the prospective studies have controls for biological or health variables been able to explain away the predictive association between social relationships and mortality. Efforts to explain away the association of social relationships and supports with health by controls for personality variables have similarly failed (56, 57). Social relationships have a predictive, arguably causal, association with health in their own right.

The extent and quality of social relationships experienced by individuals is also a function of broader social forces. Whether people are employed, married, attend church, belong to organizations, or have frequent contact with friends and relatives, and the nature and quality of those relationships, are all determined in part by their positions in a larger social structure that is stratified by age, race, sex, and socioeconomic status and is organized in terms of residential communities, work organizations, and larger political and economic structures. Older people, blacks, and the poor are generally less socially integrated (*58*), and differences in social relationships by sex and place of residence have been discussed in relation to Figs. 8.1 and 8.2. Changing patterns of fertility, mortality, and migration in society affect opportunities for work, marriage, living and working in different settings, and having relationships with friends and relatives, and can even affect the nature and quality of these relations (*59*). These demographic patterns are themselves subject to influence by both planned and unplanned economic and political change, which can also affect individuals' social relationships more directly—witness the massive increase in divorce during the last few decades in response to the women's movement, growth in women's labor force participation, and changing divorce law (*60, 61*).

In contrast with the 1950s, adults in the United States in the 1970s were less likely to be married, more likely to be living alone, less likely to belong to voluntary organizations, and less likely to visit informally with others (*62*). Changes in marital and childbearing patterns and in the age structure of our society will produce in the 21st century a steady increase of the number of older people who lack spouses or children—the people to whom older people most often turn for relatedness and support (*59*). Thus, just as we discover the importance of social relationships for health, and see an increasing need for them, their prevalence and availability may be declining. Changes in other risk factors (for example, the decline of smoking) and improvements in medical technology are still producing overall improvements on health and longevity, but the improvements might be even greater if the quantity and quality of social relationships were also improving.

References and Notes

1. C. Darwin, *Expression of the Emotions in Man and Animals* (Univ. of Chicago Press, Chicago, 1965 [1872]).
2. E. Durkheim, *Suicide* (Free Press, New York, 1951 [1897]).
3. A. S. Kraus and A. N. Lilienfeld, *J. Chronic Dis.* 10, 207 (1959).
4. H. Carter and P. C. Glick, *Marriage and Divorce: A Social and Economic Study* (Harvard Univ. Press, Cambridge, MA, 1970).
5. E. M. Kitigawa and P. M. Hauser, Differential Mortality in the United States: A Study in Socio-Economic Epidemiology (Harvard Univ. Press, Cambridge, MA, 1973).
6. T. H. Holmes, in *Personality, Stress and Tuberculosis*, P. J. Sparer, Ed. (International Univ. Press, New York, 1956).
7. W. A. Tillman and G. E. Hobbs, *Am. J. Psychiatr.* 106, 321 (1949).
8. R. E. L. Faris, *Am. J. Sociol.* 39, 155 (1934).
9. M. L. Kohn and J. A. Clausen, *Am. Sociol. Rev.* 20, 268 (1955).
10. U.S. Surgeon General's Advisory Committee on Smoking and Health, *Smoking and Health* (U.S. Public Health Service, Washington, DC, 1964).
11. G. Caplan, *Support Systems and Community Mental Health* (Behavioral Publications, New York, 1974).
12. President's Commission on Mental Health, *Report to the President* (Government Printing Office, Washington, DC, 1978), vols. 1 to 5.
13. J. Cassel, *Am. J. Epidemiol.* 104, 107 (1976).
14. S. Cobb, *Psychosomatic Med.* 38, 300 (1976).
15. J. Cassel, in *Social Stress*, S. Levine and N. A. Scotch, Eds. (Aldine, Chicago, 1970), pp. 189–209.

16. J. S. House, *Work Stress and Social Support* (Addison-Wesley, Reading, MA, 1981).

17. K. Heller, in *Maximizing Treatment Gains: Transfer Enhancement in Psychotherapy,* A. P. Goldstein and F. H. Kanter, Eds. (Academic Press, New York, 1979), pp. 353–382.

18. P. A. Thoits, *J. Health Soc. Behav.* 23, 145 (1982).

19. D. Reed et al., Am. J. Epidemiol. 117, 384 (1983).

20. L. F. Berkman and S. L. Syme, *ibid.* 109, 186 (1979).

21. J. S. House, C. Robbins, H. M. Metzner, *ibid.* 116, 123 (1982).

22. V. J. Schoenbach *et al., ibid.* 123, 577 (1986).

23. G. Tibblin *et al.,* in *Social Support: Health and Disease,* S. O. Isacsson and L. Janzon, Eds. (Almqvist & Wiksell, Stockholm, 1986), pp. 11–19.

24. L. Welin *et al., Lancet* i, 915 (1985).

25. K. Orth-Gomer and J. Johnson, *J. Chron. Dis.* 40, 949 (1987).

26. G. A. Kaplan *et al., Am. J. Epidemiol.,* 127, 1131– 1142 (1988).

27. M. Stroebe and W. Stroebe, *Psychol. Bull.* 93, 279 (1983).

28. W. R. Gove, *Soc. Forces* 51, 34 (1972).

29. K. J. Helsing and M. Szklo, *Am. J. Epidemiol.* 114, 41 (1981).

30. L. Wheeler, H. Reis, J. Nezlek, *J. Pers. Soc. Psychol.* 45, 943 (1983).

31. D. Blazer, *Am. J. Epidemiol.* 115, 684 (1982).

32. D. M. Zuckerman, S. V. Kasl, A. M. Ostfeld, *ibid.* 119, 410 (1984).

33. T. E. Seeman *et al., ibid.* 126, 714 (1987).

34. W. E. Ruberman *et al., N. Engl. J. Med.* 311, 552 (1984).

35. K. Orth-Gomer *et al., in Social Support: Health and Disease,* S. O. Isacsson and L. Janzon, Eds. (Almqvist & Wiksell, Stockholm, 1986), pp. 21–31.

36. L. S. Wrightsman, Jr., *J. Abnorm. Soc. Psychol.* 61, 216 (1960).

37. K. W. Back and M. D. Bogdonoff, *Behav. Sci.* 12, 384 (1967).

38. J. J. Lynch, *The Broken Heart* (Basic Books, New York, 1979).

39. R. M. Nerem, M. J. Levesque, J. F. Cornhill, *Science* 208, 1475 (1980).

40. J. Goldmeier, *Gerontologist* 26, 203 (1986).

41. E. W. Bovard, in *Perspectives on Behavioral Medicine,* R. B. Williams (Academic Press, New York, 1985), vol. 2.

42. J. Bowlby, in *Loneliness: The Experience of Emotional and Social Isolation,* R. S. Weiss, Ed. (MIT Press, Cambridge, MA, 1973).

43. S. P. Mendoza, in *Social Cohesion: Essays Toward a Sociophysiological Perspective,* P. R. Barchas and S. P. Mendoza, Eds. (Greenwood Press, Westport, CT, 1984).

44. S. Cohen, *Health Psychol.* 7, 269 (1988).

45. L. F. Berkman, in *Social Support and Health,* S. Cohen and S. L. Syme, Eds. (Academic Press, New York, 1985), pp. 241–262.

46. W. E. Broadhead *et al., Am. J. Epidemiol.* 117, 521 (1983).

47. M. Lilienfeld and D. E. Lilienfeld, *Foundations of Epidemiology* (Oxford Univ. Press, New York, 1980).

48. National Heart, Lung and Blood Institute, *Circulations* 63, 1199 (1982).

49. S. Cohen and S. L. Syme, *Social Support and Health* (Academic Press, New York, 1985).

50. A. Antonovsky, *Health, Stress and Coping* (Jossey-Bass, San Francisco, 1979).

51. D. Umberson, *J. Health Soc. Behav.* 28, 306 (1987).

52. K. Rook, *J. Pers. Soc. Psychol.* 46, 1097 (1984).

53. R. S. Lazarus and S. Folkman, *Stress, Appraisal, and Coping* (Springer, New York, 1984).

54. R. B. Zajonc, *Science* 149, 269 (1965).

55. J. S. House, D. Umberson, K. Landis, *Annu. Rev. Sociol.*, 14, 293–318 (1988).

56. S. Cohen, D. R. Sherrod, M. S. Clark, *J. Pers. Soc. Psychol.* 50, 963 (1986).

57. R. Schultz and S. Decker, *ibid.* 48, 1162 (1985).

58. J. S. House, *Socio Forum* 2, 135 (1987).

59. S. C. Watkins, J. A. Menken, J. Bongaarts, *Am. Sociol. Rev.* 52, 346 (1987).

60. A. Cherlin, *Marriage, Divorce, Remarriage* (Harvard Univ. Press, Cambridge, MA, 1981).

61. L. J. Weitzman, *The Divorce Revolution* (Free Press, New York, 1985).

62. J. Veroff, E. Douvan, R. A. Kulka, *The Inner American: A Self-Portrait from 1957 to 1976* (Basic Books, New York, 1981).

63. Supported by a John Simon Guggenheim Memorial Foundation Fellowship and NIA grant 1-PO1AG05561 (to J.S.H.), NIMH training grant 5-T32-MH16806-06 traineeship (to K.R.L.), NIMH training grant 5-T32-MH16806-05 and NIA 1-F32-AG05440-01 postdoctoral fellowships (to D.U.). We are indebted to D. Buss, P. Converse, G. Duncan, R. Kahn, R. Kessler, H. Schuman, L. Syme, and R. Zajonc for comments on previous drafts, to many other colleagues who have contributed to this field, and to M. Klatt for preparing the manuscript.

9

THE HEALTH POLITICS OF ASTHMA

Environmental Justice and Collective Illness Experience in the United States

Phil Brown, Brian Mayer, Stephen Zavestoski, Theo Luebke, Joshua Mandelbaum, and Sabrina McCormick

Asthma rates have risen so much in the US that medical and public health professionals invariably speak of it as a new epidemic. The number of individuals with asthma in the United States grew to 73.9% between 1980 and 1996, with an estimated 14.6 million people reporting suffering from asthma in 1996 (Mannino et al., 2002). This is widely believed to be a real increase, not an artifact of diagnosis (Woolcock & Peat, 1997; Sears, 1997; Goodman, Stukel, & Chang, 1998; Mannino et al., 2002).* In the same period, hospitalizations for asthma rose to 20%, and by 1995 there were 1.8 million emergency room visits a year. The estimated cost to society from asthma is greater than $11 billion a year (Pew Environmental Health Commission, 2000). As the number of cases has increased, medical and public health professionals and institutions have expanded their treatment and prevention efforts, environmental and community activists have made asthma a major part of their agenda, and media coverage has grown.

The Health Politics of Asthma: Environmental Justice and Collective Illness Experience in the United States, Phil Brown, Brian Mayer, Stephen Zavestoski, Theo Luebke, Joshua Mandelbaum, and Sabrina McCormick in *Social Science & Medicine,* August 2003. With permission from Elsevier.

*Since then, prevalence rates have reached a plateau, with roughly 7.7 percent of the United States population (22 million) suffering from asthma (National Center for Health Statistics, 2008).

In the midst of this attention, there is significant disagreement over the role of environmental factors in causing or triggering asthma. The widely accepted belief in psychogenic causes for asthma has shifted in the last two decades to a focus on environmental conditions, including indoor ones such as animal dander, cockroach infestation, tobacco smoke, mold, and other allergens; and outdoor ones, particularly $PM_{2.5}$ (particles under 2.5 mm in diameter, which penetrate deep into the lungs and are linked to asthma and other chronic respiratory symptoms, especially among children and the elderly). Some environmental groups and community activists have made asthma a key focus, and in several areas, have entered into coalitions with academic research centers, health providers, public health professionals, and even local and state governmental public health agencies. Despite grassroots efforts to highlight environmental factors in asthma, this remains a contentious debate; these disputes are important because they substantially influence public health prevention and government regulation.

As we have written elsewhere (Brown, Zavestoski, Mayer, McCormick, Webster, 2002), most public health education and intervention focuses on the indoor factors, since they are amenable to short-term action that can improve the immediate environment of people with asthma, hence reducing the frequency and severity of attacks, and limiting emergency room visits. Public health professionals and organizations have less capacity to act effectively on outdoor air pollution, which involves regulation of emissions and changes in air-quality standards at local, state, and national levels. Still, many public health agencies and programs increasingly understand that indoor environmental conditions are related to social inequalities, and they seek an intersectoral approach to improve living conditions. By intersectoral, we mean the inclusion of non-medical sectors—housing, transportation, economic development—in dealing with health interventions and preventions.

Activist groups do not provide direct medical and public health services, and can therefore place a different emphasis on air pollution. These groups define themselves as environmental justice organizations, and view asthma within the larger context of community well being. Those groups emphasize the unequal distribution of environmental risks and hazards according to race and class, and the reduction of environmental factors that they believe are responsible for increased asthma in their communities. In their approaches to asthma, such groups combine general education about asthma with political actions to alter local pollution sources.

We frame our paper around the notion that asthma has become for many people a "politicized illness experience" whereby community-based environmental justice organizations show people with asthma how to make direct links between their experience of asthma and the social determinants of their health. Medical sociologists study the illness experience in many ways. They have studied the personal experience of illness and symptoms (Conrad, 1987). Others have examined how individuals adapt to their illnesses in order to function in everyday life (Charmaz, 1991). Beyond the experience of symptoms and subsequent adaptation, sociologists have also studied how illness shapes personal identity (Bury, 1982). Finally, sociologists have studied how individuals search for a cause of their illness and subsequently how they attribute responsibility for the illness (Williams, 1984).

In the case of asthma, we are interested in studying not how the illness shapes the individual experience, but rather how the community-based organizations work to create a collective identity around the experience of asthma. Collective identity links social and physical realities and tends to be a function of shared grievances that might result from discrimination, structural dislocation, shared values, or other social constructions. Through the process of collective framing, these organizations transform the personal experience of illness into a collective identity that is focused on discovering and eliminating the social causes of asthma. This collective framing leads to the politicized illness experience. While our concept of the politicized illness experience is new, it fits well with existing studies by medical sociologists and medical anthropologists on community-based approaches to environmental hazards and catastrophes (Erikson, 1976; Balshem, 1993) and to collective approaches to illness experience, as with breast cancer (Kasper & Ferguson, 2000).

All health social movements take up the experience of illness in some way, and since asthma advocacy is tied up with environmental justice activism, this social movement framework is important. Usually, a health social movement needs some degree of a shared illness experience in order to organize in the first place. When people organize to seek recognition of a disease, obtain increased funding and research for a disease, seek alternatives to traditional treatments, or look for the causes of a disease, they are by definition doing something in terms of illness experience. This may mean that they are casting off a passive patient role, countering stigma of their disease, or fighting against treatments that cause pain, disfigurement, or dangerous side effects. Any of these motivations or actions affect the way that people deal with the disease process.

Connecting a disease with a cause is a powerful effort that shapes illness experience. As Williams (1984) shows in his work on narrative reconstruction, people frame their illness experience through diverse interpretations of cause. The etiological narrative is centrally tied to the daily-lived experience of illness and the way that it alters people's sense of self. We cannot separate the experience of illness from the social construction of illness. In changing the perception of asthma by those who suffer from it, a new and more empowered path of response is revealed.

Our approach integrates several important areas of medical and environmental sociology—illness experience, environmental justice, and lay discovery of environmental health effects—in order to explore two community environmental justice organizations working to reframe the etiology of asthma. We begin by pointing out why asthma is significant for health and social policy. Then we examine the social discovery of asthma and its environmental correlates, the political and economic conflicts surrounding asthma research and regulation, and the transformation of the dominant view of the triggers of asthma. Building on those bases, we explore how activist groups have used the issues raised in terms of asthma and the environment to build a collective "politicized illness experience," in which people with asthma make direct links between their experience of asthma and the social determinants of their health.

METHODS AND DATA

We focus on two community environmental justice organizations—Alternatives for Community and

Environment (ACE) in Boston's Roxbury neighborhood and West Harlem Environmental Action (WE ACT) in New York City, both of which organize around environmental factors in asthma and respiratory health as part of a broader program. We chose these two organizations because they are well-known environmental justice groups that have put significant emphasis into asthma education and organizing, and that maintain connections with academic researchers who study air pollution. We also provide data from our interviews with members of academic-community partnerships that are funded by one or more federal agencies).

Our methods include content analysis of government documents and scientific literature in medical, public health, and epidemiological journals; 16 participant observations of ACE and 2 of WE ACT; and 20 interviews with ACE and WE ACT staff, public health practitioners and researchers, and government officials. The ACE observations were mainly conducted at classes taught by ACE in public schools in minority neighborhoods in Boston. These classes provide basic information on the symptoms of asthma, on how to seek help, and on environmental triggers. They also introduce students to concepts of environmental justice, and offer them opportunities to get involved in community activism. A few observations were made of other public presentations by ACE staff to conferences and workshops. Observations of WE ACT included spending a day in their office and another day with them at a New York area environmental justice meeting. Unreferenced quotes come from our interviews and observations.

THE SIGNIFICANCE OF ASTHMA IN HEALTH AND SOCIAL POLICY

Asthma is very significant in the United States for a number of reasons—it has increased dramatically, it has a differential impact by race and class, it challenges individual responsibility and focuses on social structural factors, and it leads to pressure on Congress for nationwide health tracking.

Asthma, like most diseases, strikes lower income and minority populations more than other groups. This difference is very pronounced in the US, though not in the UK. Although asthma also affects people across all classes, and is not restricted to dense urban areas, the bulk of media and research attention has been focused on the poor and minority sufferers because they are disproportionately affected by recent increases. Many minority people now report asthma as one of their chief health problems. From 1980 to 1994, asthma rates among children aged 5–17 increased 74% nationally, a figure that more than doubles to 160% for children under the age of four (Pew Environmental Health Commission, 2000). People with asthma are more likely to be children aged 5–14 years, blacks compared to whites, and females (Mannino et al., 2002). In many low-income urban areas, especially minority communities, rates are significantly higher than the national average. While national prevalence of childhood asthma in 2005 overall was 6.2% for 0- to 4-year-olds and 9.6% in 5- to 17-year-olds, black children in particular were 60% more likely to have asthma (Alahbami, 2006).

Beyond these already telling statistics, we observe a large degree of community concern about asthma. Asthma has become, for many, poor and minority neighborhoods, one of the most visible and pressing problems. Laypeople have become very active in school-based programs, community clinic programs, novel public health initiatives, and—most central to this paper—activist groups that view asthma as related to social inequalities.

Social movement activism has developed in response to the racial disparities in asthma and the attention to air pollution as a trigger. In its focus on environmental and social determinants, asthma activism challenges the individual responsibility approach. Many well-intentioned public health programs understand the importance of outdoor as well as indoor factors. But they usually feel only able to act on indoor factors due to available resources, political constraints, and the fact that indoor solutions appear to provide rapid health effects. Since this involves parents doing a variety of domestic cleanups, people may be left feeling that they are the primary agents responsible for dealing with the problem. Parents can consequently feel responsible for their children's suffering in spite of domestic cleaning regimens. This type of individual-level solution often obscures the role of corporate pollution and government regulation.

Asthma activism advances the environmental justice approach that originally focused largely on demonstrating race and class differences in toxic exposures and proximity to waste sites (Bryant & Mohai, 1992; Bullard, 1993; Brown, 1995). The environmental justice approach has rapidly become central to US environmental policy and includes a Presidential Executive Order to reduce environmental injustice, as well as Environmental Protection Agency (EPA) programs and guidelines to do so. Further, environmental justice efforts take on a strong intersectoral approach, linking health to neighborhood development, economic opportunity, housing policy, planning and zoning activities, transportation accessibility, sanitation, social services, and education. In this sense, environmental health is a model for intersectoral approaches to health, since so much can be done to reduce or prevent asthma through non-medical action. The EPA, National Institute of Environmental Health Sciences (NIEHS), Department of Housing and Urban Development, and Centers for Disease Control have begun intersectoral approaches, including funding community intervention programs that have explicit anti-racist foundations, and that view social inequality as contributing to the asthma epidemic. Asthma has become perhaps the primary disease in which poor and minority people have pointed to social inequality and have engaged in widespread political action. The case of asthma demonstrates how environmental justice approaches place ethics and rights issues in the center of health policy.

Asthma has been an important impetus to health tracking, a growing public health concern in the US, a country that has minimal national data gathering compared to most industrialized nations. This is particularly critical in the case of asthma, because it also provides us with a vehicle to better understand inequalities of place (c.f. Fitzpatrick & LaGory, 2000). Environmental exposure disparities are typically centered in geographic location—poor and minority people live in concentrated areas, and geography frequently tells us what inequalities we may expect. The growth in GIS methodologies, the use of EPA's toxic release inventory (a federally mandated reporting system that shows what firms have emitted toxic substances; it is widely used in environmental hazards research), and other such geographically based approaches, have increased our awareness of place inequality. As this section shows, there are many reasons why asthma is important to health and other social policy. In the rest of the paper, we will see how environmental asthma activists, academic researchers, and government agencies have addressed these reasons.

SCIENTIFIC INVESTIGATION OF ENVIRONMENTAL CORRELATES AND THE POLITICAL RESPONSE

Unlike other diseases, activists do not have to fight the government concerning the impact of environmental factors. There is much congruence between activist, public health, and government actors on the question of particulates. Government efforts to enact strict air pollution standards have been met by opposition from industry interests that challenge the scientific evidence undergirding new air-quality standards specifically, as well as the government's right to regulate air pollution more generally.

Evidence dating back over 50 years suggests a link between asthma and air pollution. This was demonstrated as early as 1948, in the severe air pollution episode in Donora, Pennsylvania, where 88% of asthmatics suffered exacerbation (Amdur, 1996). Later in 1952, the "London Fog" led to thousands of deaths due to respiratory failure when air particulate levels reached 2800 mg/m³. The evidence from these natural disasters led scientists to estimate a health threshold level of 500 mg/m³. However, as more recent research demonstrates, this threshold was much too high. For instance, one study

suggests that the death rate associated with airborne particulate matter more than triples for every 100 mg/m³ increase (Schwartz, 2000). Furthermore, a 1993 study (Dockery et al., 1993) provided powerful evidence associating pulmonary morbidity and mortality with fine particulate matter, which led the EPA in 1997 to set a new standard targeting air particulate matter larger than 2.5 mg/m³.

Some natural experiments strengthen the evidence linking air pollution and asthma. Pope (1989) observed a significant decrease in asthma morbidity during a steel mill strike in Utah; reduced production resulted in a dramatic drop in airborne particulate matter. Another natural experiment showed that a 23% reduction in automobile traffic due to stringent traffic control during the 1996 Olympic Games in Atlanta, led to a 42% reduction in asthma claims reported to the state's Medicaid program (Friedman, Powell, Hutwagner, Graham, & Teague, 2001). Though such powerful evidence linking asthma with air pollution exists, less is known about the biological mechanisms that cause asthma and trigger asthma attacks. Researchers have produced results suggesting that 25 different substances found in air pollution are related to mortality rates. Using heart monitors on subjects, the researchers found heart rate variability was reduced as particulates increased (Schwartz, 2000). Further research has also shown lung inflammation, increased neutrophils in blood, vascular injury, and toxicity to tissue in the heart and lungs (Godleski, 2000). In total, particulates are estimated to account for over 100,000 deaths annually, more than breast cancer, prostate cancer, and AIDS combined (Schwartz, 2000). While some of the previously mentioned research does not apply specifically to asthma, it is worthy of mention for two reasons: (1) research on particulates is collectively driven by both asthma and other diseases, and (2) we should assume that effects on general pulmonary health might logically also harm people with asthma.

The government agency responsible for monitoring air pollution, the EPA, has only been marginally successful in reducing dangerous particulates. In accordance with the Clean Air Act (CAA), the EPA is required to constantly monitor air quality and to periodically evaluate its current air-quality standards. Following the passage of the 1970 CAA, the EPA regulated only large particles, referring to them as "total suspended particulates," In 1987, based upon new air pollution research the EPA revised its standards to address smaller particulate matter, at 10 mg/m^3. In 1994, the American Lung Association filed suit against the EPA for failing to review the air particulate standards every 5 years, as required by the CAA. In response to the pressure from the American Lung Association and the new evidence emerging from major health researchers mentioned earlier, the EPA revised its standards to include particulate matter at the 2.5 mg/m^3 level. Industry representatives who feared high economic costs of reducing the particulate matter in their airborne effluent feared the 1997 revisions. Immediately following the signing of the new law on July 16, 1997, a series of lawsuits against the EPA were filed. On May 14, 1999, in American Trucking Association, Inc., et al. v. US EPA, a federal appellate court concluded that the EPA had made unconstitutional delegations of legislative power. Though the appellate decision was a major blow for environmental regulation, in early 2001 the Supreme Court overturned the earlier decision (Greenhouse, 2001).

Following the 1997 EPA standard, the National Research Council conducted the Research Priorities for Airborne Particulate Matter Study. In response to the claims made in the lawsuits, the study included a comparison of cost estimates with health effects, although the 1970 CAA did not require cost–benefit analyses. According to the EPA, the cost of 15,000 deaths was higher than the challenger's estimates for the costs of compliance with the stricter standards. Critics of the new standards attacked EPA's ability to set the standards once again, this time charging that the EPA utilized "hidden data," forcing the EPA to ask for a reanalysis of the data by the Health Effects Institute. The second study reaffirmed the previous findings, but the EPA was forced to compromise and postponed the adoption of PM2.5 standard until the next 5-year review in 2002. In preparation for the review, the EPA installed thousands of air monitors across the country, strengthening the scientific evidence supporting the PM2.5 standard (Greenbaum,

2000; more extensive discussion of the scientific literature and the conflicts on regulation are found in Brown et al., 2002).

Despite the legitimacy of the scientific evidence of particulate matter health effects, the illness experience has been framed in individual terms. Public health professionals and activists believe that not enough has been done to treat and prevent asthma. We now turn to a discussion of how activists combine a public health and political perspective to deal with asthma as a politicized illness experience.

APPLYING THE ENVIRONMENTAL JUSTICE FRAME, ALTERNATIVES FOR COMMUNITY AND ENVIRONMENT AND WEST HARLEM ENVIRONMENTAL ACTION

ACE began in 1993 as an environmental justice organization based in the Roxbury–Dorchester area of Boston, MA, and has since become nationally recognized for its work. One of its earliest actions was a successful mobilization to prevent an asphalt plant from being permitted in Dorchester. ACE had initially expected to focus on issues such as vacant lots, and did not intend to focus on asthma, but a year of talking with the community showed ACE that residents established asthma as the number one priority. ACE believes that to address asthma requires addressing housing, transportation, community investment patterns, access to health care, pollution sources and sanitation, as well as health education. As one staff member notes, "everything we do is about asthma."

West Harlem Environmental Action was founded in 1988 in response to environmental threats to the community created by the mismanagement of the North River Sewage Treatment

Plant and the construction of the sixth bus depot in Northern Manhattan. WE ACT quickly evolved into an environmental justice organization with the goal of working to improve environmental protection and public health in the predominately African-American and Latino communities of Northern Manhattan. They identified a wide range of environmental threats, including air pollution, lead poisoning, pesticides and unsustainable development. WE ACT has continued to grow and expand, extending its reach beyond West Harlem to other Northern Manhattan communities.

Developing a Social Structural, Environmental Justice Approach

It is not easy to develop an environmental justice approach that emphasizes social structural causes of asthma, and to spread that approach to others. Many urban asthma coalitions have developed in recent years to treat, prevent, and educate around asthma. Some of these asthma programs openly talk about the racial and class inequalities in asthma incidence, pointing to poverty, racism, poor living conditions, inadequate sanitation, and unequal access to health services. They call for housing reform, in order to provide better living arrangements that will keep children safe from dust, roaches, and poor indoor air. Many people involved in these programs frame their concerns in terms of environmental justice. Several programs train community health workers, reminiscent of the 1960s and early 1970s paraprofessionals, where nonprofessional lay-people in the community were taught considerable public health skills in order to have them carry out intervention work in a culturally/racially/ethnically appropriate way (Cohen & Love, 2000).

But despite that broad political understanding, most asthma projects focus on controlling indoor environmental factors. Given the extent of the asthma epidemic, it is understandable that many clinicians, social workers, and community activists want to do front line work to achieve rapid changes in personal behaviors, which are often effective in reducing asthma suffering. But even if these programs reach a significant fraction of inner-city residents, they cannot offer any protection against the outdoor air pollution that will remain as a trigger for everyone—both outdoors, and when it enters the home and becomes part of the indoor air quality.

This is where the environmental justice groups come in. They focus on sources of outdoor pollution, and engage in local-level intersectoral political organizing. This includes reducing or eradicating diesel buses, pressing for stronger air-quality regulations, and curtailing hazardous plant emissions. While some broad national efforts, such as changing air-quality regulations, will take a long time, local changes in public transportation can be relatively rapid, resulting in benefits to the entire population. ACE has been able to obtain changes in transit policy, such as controlling truck idling and reducing future diesel bus use.

Transit Issues

ACE encourages communities to take ownership of the asthma issue and to push for proactive, empowered solutions. Central to this is the role of direct action and education, such as a campaign in which residents identified idling trucks and buses as a major source of particulate irritants. They organized an anti-idling march and began giving informational "parking tickets" to idling buses and trucks that explained the health effects of diesel exhaust.

Since ACE identifies diesel buses as a problem, they also take up transportation issues more broadly than just air pollution. ACE ran a major campaign targeting local and state government over the allocation of transit resources. Charging "transit racism," ACE argued that the estimated 366,000 daily bus riders in Boston were being discriminated against by the over $12 billion of federal and state money being spent on the "Big Dig" highway project, while the Massachusetts Bay Transit Authority (MBTA) refused to spend $105 million to purchase newer, cleaner buses and bus shelters. In tying dirty buses to higher asthma rates, ACE successfully framed an issue of transit spending priorities into one of health, justice, and racism. In 2000, the Transit Riders' Union, largely created by ACE, got the MBTA to allow free transfers between buses, since the many inner-city residents who relied on two buses for transportation had to pay more than others who had free transfers on subways.

Similarly, WE ACT has identified diesel exhaust as a major factor behind the disparate burden of asthma experienced in their community. Using publicity campaigns such as informative advertisements placed in bus shelters, public service announcements on cable television, and a direct mailing, WE ACT has reached a vast number of community residents and public officials and let them know that diesel buses could trigger asthma attacks. Though their efforts increased public awareness of WE ACT and its efforts to reduce asthma, the media campaign did not lead to a shift in New York's Metropolitan Transit Authority's (MTA) policy towards diesel buses. Thus in November 2000, WE ACT filed a lawsuit against the MTA with the Federal Department of Transportation claiming that the MTA advances a racist and discriminatory policy by disproportionally siting diesel bus depots and parking lots in minority neighborhoods.

Community Empowerment Through Asthma and Other Education

A key component of ACE's education and empowerment efforts is reflected in its Roxbury Environmental Empowerment Project (REEP). REEP teaches classes in local schools, hosts environmental justice conferences, and through its intern program trains high-school students to teach environmental health in schools. Classes are designed to educate students about environmental justice, and use asthma as a focal issue. For example, REEP teachers discuss the potential process for siting a hazardous facility in people's neighborhoods, and ask the students why was this was being sited there, and what would they do about the siting decision. Through their "know your neighborhood" strategy, they teach students how to locate on local maps the potentially dangerous locations in their area. ACE has helped some of its high-school interns get into college as a result of the education they received in the REEP program. ACE also participates in job fairs to help students find good employment prospects. On some occasions, ACE has brought Harvard School

of Public Health air-quality researchers along with them, to present findings to school audiences. In this way, ACE demonstrates to children in underfunded and understaffed schools how important they are, by having important scientists share their relevant work with them.

WE ACT's Healthy Home, Healthy Child campaign reflects a similar community empowerment approach. WE ACT works to address a broad range of issues and does not attempt to separate environmental issues from each other or the community context. The Healthy Home, Healthy Child campaign, developed in partnership with the Columbia Center for Children's Environmental Health, works to educate the community on a variety of risk factors including cigarettes, lead poisoning, drugs and alcohol, air pollution, garbage, pesticides and nutrition (Evans et al., 2000). Educational materials, translated both from English into Spanish and from medical terminology into lay language, inform residents about the effects of risk factors and actions they can take to alleviate or minimize those effects. In the case of air pollution, one of the actions that residents can take is to contact WE ACT and become involved in their clean air campaign. WE ACT believes that focusing solely on air pollution can be a disservice to the community and thus it addresses all of the issues raised in the Healthy Home campaign. As with ACE's experience in identifying community issues, WE ACT's Healthy Home, Healthy Child campaign began by focusing on specific asthma triggers, but soon expanded to include residents' key concerns such as drugs, alcohol, and garbage. . . .

Organizing With Environmental Justice Principles

Although their work has national implications, ACE's promotion of a new approach to asthma remains expressly local in focus. Like other environmental justice organizations, ACE believes that if it becomes too nationally focused or too involved in too many governmental and academic meetings, it would forsake the individuals in the neighborhood that have granted ACE the efficacy in the first place.

ACE is aware that even if there is national implementation of safer PM2.5 air-quality standards, local injustices will remain, and hence local action will always be necessary. Local action can have national impact based on the accumulation of action and research by citizen-science alliances involving national-level research universities. In influencing the way this science itself is done, the organizations can shape how the findings are presented, and in some cases, the findings themselves. Additionally, limited national networking encourages groups to use other groups' issues and strategies—ACE borrowed its "transit racism" campaign from the Bus Rider's Union in Los Angeles, while WE ACT's current challenges to the MTA's bus depot sitings mirror ACE's actions in Roxbury. Thus, strategies are shared, even if there is no national organization. The environmental justice approach to structural factors has ramifications for internalized self-perceptions of people with asthma, and hence for their illness experience. Part of the rationale for ACE's and WE ACT's efforts to change social perceptions of asthma causation is to simultaneously transform the self-perception of people with asthma. One of the REEP interns wrote an essay in which he characterizes the kind of transformation that ACE engenders in people:

> There are things in my environment that truly outrage me. The fact that people have to wait hours for dirty diesel MBTA buses on extremely cold or hot days, the fact that someone I know is being evicted from their home because they can't pay their rent, and the fact that a small child I see every day has died of asthma in a community where asthma rates are 6 times the state average. These things should not be happening where I live or where anyone lives. Everyone no matter what community they reside in should have the right to a safe and healthy neighborhood. So what is environmental justice is a hard question but I know what it is to me. It is allowing everyone the right to have the best life has to offer from affordable housing to safe neighborhoods and clean air.

Reframing Asthma and Creating a Collective Illness Experience

As mentioned earlier, we are not examining how asthma shapes individual illness experience, but rather how activist groups create a collective identity around the experience of asthma. These organizations collectively frame asthma as an environmental justice issue, and therefore transform the personal experience of illness into a collective identity aimed at discovering and eliminating the social causes of asthma. When people view asthma as related to both air pollution and to the living conditions of poor neighborhoods, they reconstruct asthma narratives differently than the narrative reconstruction that occurs with other chronic illnesses. Because asthma is increasingly framed in the language of air pollution and environmental justice, the disparities in asthma suffering are translated into the rhetoric of illness experience. Illness experience in the case of asthma is broader than that of the typical illness narrative. Such narratives typically incorporate perceived causes and effects of the disease with personal perception, work, family, relationships, and schooling. But asthma activists also include the political economic framework surrounding the production of asthma and the political perspectives that situate asthma in terms of housing, transportation, neighborhood development, the general economy, and government regulations. This broader focus on the social and economic factors shaping the illness experience of asthma is reflected in the goals of one ACE organizer:

> I think we have to look at how is it that our society has created such disparate environments for people to live in—from the kind of housing you have, to the kind of school you go to, to the kind of vehicle you ride in, to the kind of air that is outside your door. . . . I think that there's huge changes that are way beyond individual lifestyle changes that we need to look at about production of synthetic chemicals that may play a role, or about the way we're designing and building our cities, towns, and whatnot.

This enables people with asthma to place responsibility in part on social structural forces.

The experience of illness plays a major role in the educational programs conducted by ACE and WE ACT. Because ACE, WE ACT, and various academic-community partnerships hold so many educational sessions to make asthma a very public concern, the stigma and denial normally associated with asthma is lessened. The power of destigmatization is central. We are only a couple of decades removed from the psychoanalytic notion that asthma stems from overprotective mothers and that it is essentially a psychogenic response to family dynamics (Williams, 1989). It took better medical knowledge to overcome the psychogenic definition and to situate asthma in terms of environmental triggers such as household mold, animal dander, roaches, or exposure to second-hand tobacco smoke. Though medical research rejected the psychogenic model for causation, the framing of asthma as a weakness rather than a chronic disease created a stigma that remains today. In an op-ed article in the *New York Times*, Olympic track medalist Jackie Joyner-Kersee (2001) addressed her difficulty in overcoming such stigma in order to be open about her asthma. Draw-A-Breath, a Providence, Rhode Island, asthma outreach program largely focused on schools, runs a summer camp for children with asthma. They point to the powerful message children learn—that they can do athletics despite having asthma.

A common theme to emerge from qualitative studies of people with asthma is the feeling of powerlessness. Both among children and adults, people with asthma are without a potential cure for the disease and can rely only on management to prevent attacks. For children, managing asthma requires reliance upon their doctors, parents, and teachers, which reduces their sense of individuality and exploration (Rudestam, 2001). Children learn to associate various places with asthma exacerbation, leading many children and their families to associate local environmental hazards with their asthma. When observing a child's asthma attacks, parents themselves may feel powerless to help their child breathe normally. Limited access to quality health care also leads parents to feel helpless to reduce their child's asthma suffering. Frequent trips

to the emergency room are the norm for impoverished families seeking asthma treatment, resulting in both poor management and the loss of control (Center, 2000). Inequalities in health polarize the experience of asthma in terms of agency. For children and their families who cannot afford quality management of the disease, asthma becomes another problem beyond their control, exacerbating the feeling of powerlessness. Not only do they not have adequate access to health care, but they have little control of either indoor or outdoor sources of asthma triggers.

Community groups like ACE and WE ACT work to reframe the illness in terms of the larger illness experience. They feel that the medical establishment has a limited ability to address many of the important factors in the experience of asthma, and see their role as a bridge. One WE ACT organizer recounted the experience many people with asthma go through in a medical setting:

> I think that doctors think that there is very little that they can do about [the factors of asthma]. They go through this checklist of risk factors at the beginning of a physical, which now includes, "Do you wear seatbelts?" Like different questions assessing individual behavior and risk taking behavior. They focus on things that they feel they can change somehow. So they ask about the indoor environment.

Groups like ACE and WE ACT realize that doctors are often unable to address larger issues than individual behavior:

> Even if a kid has really terrible asthma, they're in the hospital, you know, once every two weeks. Sometimes doctors aren't trained to say, "Do you have mold in your home—where do you live?"

Organizers at ACE and WE ACT also recognize that even if the medical community incorporated questions about the home environment, many other important factors shaping the illness experience would still be neglected:

It feels like [asthma] has been taken out slightly from the context of everything else that is happening to people ... and I don't think that that is the way that community groups really approach asthma. They see it in the way environment justice sees it, defining the environment where people live, work, play, and breathe. And so it's the underlying conditions of poverty and social injustice that are contributing to all these things. And no matter whose fault it is, you can't just get rid of cockroaches and expect asthma to go away. For that matter, you can't just put in better buses and expect asthma to go away. It's all got to be approached in a social justice framework.

In painting this broad picture of the experience of asthma, ACE and WE ACT create the foundation for an environmental justice-based approach to reducing the burden of asthma.

Through the educational programs held by ACE and WE ACT, people with asthma learn to manage their disease while simultaneously beginning to see themselves as part of a collective of people with asthma who understand the importance of external factors beyond their individual homes. By learning that even their indoor exposures through poor housing are a social phenomenon, they see themselves less as individual sick people and more as part of a group that has unfair disadvantages. The environmental justice approach informs these people that they can act to change their social circumstances, and in that sense asthma becomes a stepping point to a politicized view of the world. For example, ACE got state, regional, and federal agencies to place an air monitor in their Roxbury office. They use this monitor for their educational programs in public school and community after-school programs, showing students the relationships between their results on a pulmonary function test and current levels of outdoor air pollution. The ACE interns and many of the children they teach cannot separate out their experience of wheezing from their knowledge of the harmful effects of diesel exhaust from nearby buses. They cannot think about their inhalers without thinking about the excess of bus depots and trash incinerators located in their neighborhoods.

For a growing number of people and organizations, the experience of illness has transformed asthma from an individual disease into a social movement focused on health inequalities. Their role in building and maintaining this social movement is a growing concern for organizers, as noted by this ACE person:

The other part of ACE that's really emerged probably in the past couple of years is our role as movement builders; building an environmental justice movement both locally and nationally. And the leadership development fits under that as well. But it has changed the way we look at our programs. Now we're trying to figure out how we not only take out interns and train them as educators, but train them as organizers.

People with asthma in Boston and New York are incorporating rhetoric from the environmental justice movement to address the social and political forces responsible for the disparate rates of the disease among urban minority communities. ACE and WE ACT look beyond medical solutions to the overburden of asthma in their communities to the social forces shaping the urban environment. As one organizer noted:

I think our approach has been that if people are suffering from asthma that's something we need to deal with now, today. And yes, part of that answer is a medical solution, figuring out how to get people the right treatment. But in the meantime, if there are things we can do to reduce the level of triggers, if we can figure out how to take more a pollution prevention approach to figure out how to keep these things from getting into the environment, then we ought to do that.

Through community education and direct action campaigns, ACE and WE ACT help people with asthma to overcome the stigma that frames asthma both as a weakness and as a result of living in an unclean household. Asthma activists use the destigmatization process to politicize fellow sufferers and gain allies in their effort to produce a healthy environment for their community.

Based on the illness experience we have described earlier, we believe that many people with asthma have developed what we term a "politicized illness experience," in which their personal experience of illness, symptoms, coping, and adaptation has become linked with a broad social critique. This critique involves assessing responsibility for the causes and/or triggers of the disease, as well as responsibility for treating and preventing the disease.

CONCLUSIONS

As we have shown, a considerable amount of attention to the new asthma epidemic comes from laypeople who are concerned with environmental factors as triggers. Their broad intersectoral approach to asthma includes action in diverse social sectors, such as housing, transportation, and economic development, and is framed in environmental justice terms that emphasize race and class inequities. The environmental asthma activists focus their attention on political and economic action. Although they understand the need for household level attention, they reject the primacy of individual responsibility for asthma control.

ACE and WE ACT exemplify this environmental asthma approach, and define themselves as environmental justice organizations for which asthma activism is only one part of a broader approach. Even though they are not primarily health-oriented, they offer a sociologically informed approach to disease. They are a unique type of health social movement organization, precisely because they are not centered on either a particular disease (as with environmental breast cancer movement groups) or on the health status of a social category (as with the women's health movement). This type of wide-reaching approach to social health, rather than just medical health, provides an important insight into new ways that lay-driven efforts can reframe social conceptions of health.

This environmental focus on asthma has achieved legitimacy in part because of its health inequalities

and environmental justice approach. Because of its express social justice ideology that places issues of ethics and rights in the center of health policy discussion, government officials are pressed to pay attention. Activists' legitimacy was enhanced by not having to struggle for recognition of the epidemic—there was ample attention from medical, public health, and educational institutions and professionals, and there was an excellent science base. In addition, although WE ACT and ACE approached science and scientists differently, these groups have found creative ways to work alongside scientists, while not placing primary emphasis on research.

Asthma has become perhaps the primary disease in which poor and minority people have pointed to social inequality, and it is a useful class and race indicator of health inequalities. The wide-ranging, intersectoral perspective we see in environmental asthma activism offers lessons for future contested illnesses. In cases of isolated community contamination, the intersectoral approach is difficult to adopt. But as more diseases come to be understood as widespread phenomena linked to modern industrial practices and consumer lifestyles, illness activists stand to learn from the approaches of asthma activist organizations such as ACE and WE ACT.

Further, the growing perspective on social and environmental determinants of asthma fosters a different approach to personal illness experience, what we term a politicized illness experience. We expect this politicized illness experience, together with support from public health and science allies, to lead to concrete results in health policy, especially in terms of health tracking, academic-community collaboration, and stronger air-quality regulation. The Trust for America's Health (formerly the Pew Environmental Health Commission) has pointed to asthma as one of the central reasons why the United States needs a national health tracking system, and has garnered much scientific and governmental support for this approach, including recent passage of a health tracking bill in Congress. Innovative academic-community collaborations sponsored by federal grants have developed in recent years as well, with asthma a main focus because there are such strong community organizations available to do joint work with researchers. Last, the growing power of the environmental justice activists, combined with much public health sympathy toward the environmental justice perspective and with a solid science base of particulate researchers, holds the potential to support stronger air-quality regulation.

ACKNOWLEDGMENTS

This is a revised version of a paper presented at the 2001 Annual Meeting of the American Sociological Association, August 19, 2001, Anaheim, CA. This research is supported by grants to the first author from the Robert Wood Johnson Foundation's Investigator Awards in Health Policy Research Program (Grant #036273) and the National Science Foundation Program in Social Dimensions of Engineering, Science, and Technology (Grant # SES-9975518). We thank Meadow Linder and Pamela Webster for their involvement in the larger project from which this research arises. We are grateful to the staff of Alternatives for Community and Environment and West Harlem Environmental Action for granting access to their work. We thank Rachel Morello-Frosch and Rebecca Gasior for comments on the manuscript.

Note

1. Some data have been updated from the original article.

References

Alahbami, L. J. (2006). The state of childhood asthma, United States, 1980–2005. *Advance Data from Vital and Health Statistics*, 381.

Amdur, M. (1996). Animal toxicology. In R. Wilson, & J. Spengler (Eds.). *Particles in our air: Concentrations and health effects* (pp. 85–122). Cambridge: Harvard University Press.

Balshem, M. (1993). *Cancer in the community: Class and medical authority*. Washington, DC: Smithsonian Institution Press.

Brown, P. (1995). Race, class, and environmental health: A review and systematization of the literature. *Environmental Research*, 69, 15–30.

Brown, P., Zavestoski, S., Mayer, B., McCormick, S., Webster, P. (2002). Policy issues in Environmental Health Disputes. Annals of the American Academy of Political and Social Science, 584, 175–202.

Bryant, B., & Mohai, P. (Eds.) (1992). *Race and the incidence of environmental hazards*. Boulder, CO: Westview.

Bullard, R. (Ed.) (1993). *Environmental racism: Voices from the grassroots*. Boston: South End Press.

Bury, M. (1982). Chronic illness as biographical disruption. *Sociology of Health and Illness*, 4, 167–182.

Center, R. (2000). *Poverty, ethnicity, and pediatric asthma in Rhode Island*. Senior Honors thesis, Center for Environmental Studies, Brown University.

Charmaz, K. (1991). *Good days, bad days: The self in chronic illness and time*. New Brunswick, NJ: Rutgers University Press.

Cohen, L., & Love, M. B. (2000). Urban asthma and community health workers. *Presentation at annual meeting of American Public Health Association*, Boston, November 14.

Conrad, P. (1987). The experience of illness: Recent and new directions. *Research in the Sociology of Health Care, 6*, 1–31.

Dockery, D., Pope, C., Xu, X., Spengler, J., Ware, J., Ray, M., Ferris, B., & Speitzer, F. (1993). An association between air pollution and mortality in six US cities. *New England Journal of Medicine, 329*, 1753–1759.

Erikson, K. (1976). *Everything in its path: The destruction of community in the Buffalo Creek flood*. New York: Touchstone.

Evans, D., Fullilove, M., Shepard, P., Corbin-Mark, C., Edwards, C., Green, L., & Perera, F. (2000). Healthy Home, Healthy Child Campaign: A community intervention by the Columbia Center for Children's Environmental Health. Presentation at annual meeting of American Public Health Association, Boston, November 15.

Fitzpatrick, K., & LaGory, M. (2000). *Unhealthy places: The ecology of risk in the urban landscape*. New York: Routledge.

Friedman, M. S., Powell, K. E., Hutwagner, L., Graham, L. M., & Teague, W. G. (2001). Impact of changes in transportation and commuting behaviors during the 1996 Summer Olympic Games in Atlanta on air quality and childhood asthma. *Journal of the American Medical Association, 285*, 897–905.

Godleski, J. (2000). Mechanisms of particulate air pollution health effects. Presentation at annual meeting of American Public Health Association, Boston, November 14.

Goodman, D. C., Stukel, T. A., & Chang, C. H. (1998). Trends in pediatric asthma hospitalization rates: Regional and socioeconomic differences. *Pediatrics, 101*, 208–213.

Greenbaum, D. (2000). Interface of science with policy. Presentation at annual meeting of American Public Health Association, Boston, November 14.

Greenhouse, L. (2001). EPA's authority on air rules wins Supreme Court's backing. New York Times, February 28.

Joyner-Kersee, J. (2001). Asthma and the athlete's challenge. *New York Times*, August 13.

Kasper, A., & Ferguson, S. (Eds.). (2000). *Breast cancer: Society shapes an epidemic*. New York: St. Martin's Press.

Mannino, D., Homa, D., Akinbami, L., Moorman, J., Gwynne, C., & Redd, S. (2002). Surveillance for asthma—United States, 1980–1999. Morbidity and mortality weekly report 51(SS-1), (pp. 1–13), March 29.

National Center for Health Statistics. (2008). Summary Health Statistics for U.S. Adults. Interview Survey, CDC.

Pew Environmental Health Commission. (2000). *Attack asthma report*. Pew Environmental Health Commission.

Pope, C. (1989). Respiratory disease associated with community air pollution and a steel mill, Utah valley. *American Journal of Public Health, 79*(5), 623–628.

Rudestam, K. (2001). *The important of place: Asthmatic children's perceptions of inside and outside environments*. Senior honors thesis, Center for Environmental Studies, Brown University.

Schwartz, J. (2000). Fine particulate air pollution: Smoke and mirrors of the '90s or hazard of the new millennium. Presentation at annual meeting of American Public Health Association, Boston, November 14.

Sears, M. R. (1997). Epidemiology of childhood asthma. *Lancet, 350*, 1015–1020.

Williams, G. H. (1984). The genesis of chronic illness: Narrative reconstruction. *Sociology of Health and Illness, 6*, 175–200.

Williams, J. (1989). Chronic respiratory illness and disability: A critical review of the psychosocial literature. *Social Science & Medicine, 28*, 791–903.

Woolcock, A. J., & Peat, J. K. (1997). Evidence for the increase in asthma worldwide. *Ciba Foundation Symposia, 206*, 122–134.

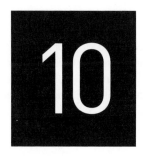

DYING ALONE

The Social Production of Urban Isolation

Eric Klinenberg

There is a file marked "Heat Deaths" in the recesses of the Cook County morgue. The folder holds hundreds of hastily scribbled death reports authored by city police officers in July 1995 as they investigated cases of mortality during the most proportionately deadly heat wave in recorded American history.[1] Over 700 Chicago residents in excess of the norm died during the week of 13th to 20th of July (Whitman et al., 1997),[2] and the following samples of the official reports hint at the conditions in which the police discovered the decedents.

Male, age 65, black, July 16, 1995:

R/Os [responding officers] discovered the door to apt locked from the inside by means of door chain. No response to any knocks or calls. R/Os . . . gained entry by cutting chain.

R/Os discovered victim lying on his back in rear bedroom on the floor. [Neighbor] last spoke with victim on 13 July 95. Residents had not seen victim recently. Victim was in full rigor mortis. R/Os unable to locate the whereabouts of victim's relatives . . .

Female, age 73, white, July 17, 1995:

A recluse for 10 yrs, never left apartment, found today by son, apparently DOA. Conditions in apartment when R/Os arrived thermostat was registering over 90 degrees f. with no air circulation except for windows opened by son [after death]. Possible heat-related death. Had a known heart problem 10 yrs ago but never completed medication or treatment . . .

Dying Alone: The Social Production of Urban Isolation, Eric Klinenberg in *Ethnography*, December 1, 2001. Reprinted with permission from SAGE Publications, Inc.

Male, age 54, white, July 16, 1995:

R/O learned . . . that victim had been dead for quite awhile. . . . Unable to contact any next of kin. Victim's room was uncomfortably warm. Victim was diabetic, doctor unk. Victim has daughter . . . last name unk. Victim hadn't seen her in years. . . . Body removed to C.C.M. [Cook County Morgue].

Male, age 79, black, July 19, 1995:

Victim did not respond to phone calls or knocks on victim's door since Sunday, 16 July 95. Victim was known as quiet, to himself and, at times, not to answer the door. X is landlord to victim and does not have any information to any relatives to victim. . . . Chain was on door. R/O was able to see victim on sofa with flies on victim and a very strong odor decay (decompose). R/O cut chain, per permission of [landlord], called M.E. [medical examiner] who authorized removal. . . . No known relatives at this time.

These accounts rarely say enough about a victim's death to fill a page, yet the words used to describe the deceased—"recluse," "to himself," "no known relatives"—and the conditions in which they were found—"chain was on door," "no air circulation," "flies on victim," "decompose"—are brutally succinct testaments to forms of abandonment, withdrawal, fear, and isolation that proved more extensive than anyone in Chicago had realized, and more dangerous than anyone had imagined. "During the summer heat wave of 1995 in Chicago," the authors of the most thorough epidemiological study of the disaster explained, "anything that facilitated social contact, even membership in a social club or owning a pet was associated with a decreased risk of death" (Semenza et al., 1996: 90). Chicago residents who lacked social ties and did not leave their homes regularly died disproportionately during the catastrophe.

Three questions motivate this article. First, why did so many Chicagoans *die alone* during the heat wave? Second, to expand this question, why do so many Chicagoans, particularly older residents, *live alone*

with limited social contacts and weak support during normal times? What accounts for the social production of isolation? Third, what social and psychological processes organize and animate the experiential make-up of aging alone? How can we understand the lives and deaths of the literally isolated?

DYING ALONE

If "bowling alone," the social trend reported by Robert Putnam and mined for significance by social critics and politicians of all persuasions (Putnam, 1995), is a sign of a weakening American civil society, dying alone—a fate few Americans can confidently elude—carries even more powerful social and symbolic meaning. For while in advanced societies the normative "good death" takes place at home, it is even more crucial that the process of dying is collective, shared by the dying person and his or her community of family and friends.[3] When someone dies alone and at home the death is a powerful symbol of social abandonment and failure. The community to which the deceased belonged, whether familial, friendship-based, or political, is likely to suffer from stigma or shame as a consequence, one which it must overcome with redemptive narratives and rituals that reaffirm the bonds among the living (Seale, 1995).

The issues of aging and dying alone are hardly limited to Chicago. In Milwaukee, where a similar proportion of city residents died during the 1995 heat wave (US Centers for Disease Control and Prevention, 1996), 27 percent of the decedents, roughly 75 percent of whom were over 60, were found alone more than one day after the estimated time of death (Nashold et al., n.d.). Most older people in Western societies, and particularly in the United States, place great value on their independence, a characteristic of sufficient cultural and psychological importance that people for whom independence is objectively dangerous are often willing to risk its consequences in order to remain self-sufficient. The number of older people living alone is rising almost everywhere in the world, making it one of the major demographic trends of the contemporary period. According to the US Census Bureau, the total number of people living alone in the United States rose from 10.9 million

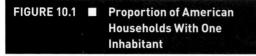

FIGURE 10.1 ■ Proportion of American Households With One Inhabitant

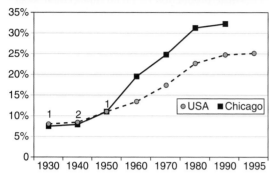

Source: The Statistical Abstract of the United States (1980, 1989, 1999), US Census Bureau.

FIGURE 10.2 ■ Proportion of American Elderly (65+) Living Alone

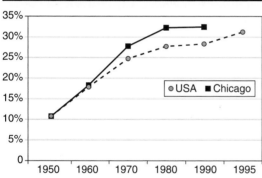

Source: The Statistical Abstract of the United States (1980, 1989, 1999), US Census Bureau.

in 1970 to 23.6 million in 1994 (Wuthnow, 1998); and, as Figures 10.1 and 10.2 show, the proportions of American households inhabited by only one person and of elderly people living alone have soared since the 1950s. Dramatic as these figures are, they are certain to rise even higher in the coming decades as societies everywhere age.

Ethnographers have done little to document the daily routines and practices of people living alone,[4] but a recent study in the *New England Journal of Medicine* (Gurley et al., 1996) suggests that their

solitary condition leaves them vulnerable in emergency situations and times of illness. Researchers in San Francisco, a city about one-quarter the size of Chicago, reported that in a 12 week period emergency medical workers found 367 people who lived alone and were discovered in their apartments either incapacitated or, in a quarter of the cases, dead. The victims, as in the Chicago heat wave, were disproportionately old, white and African American, with older black men most over-represented. Many of them, the researchers reported, suffered tremendously while they waited to be discovered in their homes, suffering that could have been reduced by earlier intervention but was exacerbated by the victims' isolation (Gurley et al., 1996).

In this article I examine the lived experiences of isolated Chicago residents, placing them in the context of the changing demography and ecology of the city and paying special attention to the ways in which migration patterns, increasing life-spans and changes in urban social morphology have altered the structural conditions of social and support networks. I also consider the impact of the spreading *culture of fear* that has transformed the nature of social life and community organization as well as the physical and political structure of cities. To illustrate how city residents experience these conditions and depict how they impact on the social life of the city, I return to the streets and neighborhoods of Chicago, drawing upon ethnographic research to flesh out the haunting spectre of dying alone in the great metropolis. Although we cannot speak with those who perished during the heat wave, we can look closely at the conditions in which they died and then follow up by examining the experiences of people in similar conditions today. Thus my focus moves outward from the heat wave to the years immediately following when I conducted fieldwork alongside seniors living alone in Chicago.

It is important to make distinctions between *living alone, being isolated, being reclusive,* and *being lonely.* I define alone as residing without other people in a household; being isolated as having limited social ties; being reclusive as largely confining oneself to the household; and being lonely as the subjective state of feeling alone.[5] Most people who live alone, seniors included, are neither lonely nor deprived of social contacts.[6] This is significant because seniors who are embedded in active social networks tend to have better health and greater longevity than those who are relatively isolated. Being isolated or reclusive, then, is more consequential than simply living alone. But older people who live alone are more likely than seniors who live with others to be depressed, isolated, impoverished, fearful of crime and removed from proximate sources of support.[7] Moreover, seniors who live alone are especially vulnerable to traumatic outcomes during episodes of acute crisis because there is no one to help recognize emerging problems, provide immediate care or activate support networks.

It is difficult to measure the number of people who are relatively isolated and reclusive because they have few ties to informal or formal support networks or have little exposure to researchers. In surveys and censuses, isolates and recluses are among the social types most likely to be uncounted or undercounted because those with permanent housing often refuse to open their doors to strangers and are unlikely to participate in city or community programs through which they can be tracked. In academic research it is common to underestimate the extent of isolation or reclusion among seniors because most scholars gain access to samples of elderly people who are already relatively connected. One recent book about loneliness in later life, for example, makes generalizations about the prevalence of isolation and loneliness on the basis of a survey of seniors who participate in a university for the aged (Gibson, 2000) and even medical studies of isolation and health are likely to exclude people whom medical doctors and research teams never see or cannot locate. . . .

What social conditions produce isolation? And how can we understand the lived experience of isolation itself? The heat wave mortality patterns pointed to places in the city where isolation proved to be especially dangerous and suggested sites where similarly situated isolates who survived the disaster but remained alone and vulnerable to the problems stemming from reclusiveness were concentrated. In addition, the disaster illuminated a set of demographic, cultural and political conditions that are associated with isolation, forming the broader social context in which social isolation emerges.

There are four key social conditions that contribute to the production of literal and extreme social isolation: first, the aging of the urban population, particularly the increases in the population of African American, Latino and Asian seniors; second, the fear of crime stemming from the violence and perceived violence of everyday life—in extreme forms this fear can result in the retreat from public life altogether and the creation of urban burrows, "safe houses" where the alone and the afraid protect themselves from a social world in which they no longer feel secure; third, the degradation and fortification of public spaces in poor urban areas and specific residential facilities (such as senior public housing units and some single-room-occupancy hotels); fourth, the transformation in the nature of state social services and support systems such as health care, public or subsidized housing and home energy subsidies. The interaction of these conditions with poverty and the daily deprivations it entails renders poor seniors who live alone vulnerable to a variety of dangers whose consequences can be severe.

Our focus on social isolation should not obscure the fact that literal isolation is an uncommon condition. As Claude Fischer has shown, the overwhelming majority of city dwellers are integrated into personal networks that provide them with support during normal times as well as times of crisis (Fischer, 1982, 1984[1976]). There is, by now, compelling evidence that Wirth's general theory of urbanism—the thesis that city living will break down most forms of solidarity, destroying social groups and creating an anomic society and alienated, isolated individuals—is simply not true; nor is there evidence that city residents on the whole are any less socially integrated than residents of rural areas. Whether urbanites remain with their traditional ethnic groups or form new subcultural groups on the basis of shared interests and experiences (Fischer, 1975), decades of research have shown that, despite the common experience of feeling alone in crowded urban areas, in private life most city dwellers have rich and rewarding relationships and social networks (Fischer, 1982). What I want to show here, however, is that literal social isolation arises in certain situations which, although historically unusual, are becoming more common in American cities today.

"THE CLOSEST I'VE COME TO DEATH"

The first of the conditions producing extreme urban isolation and its experiential correlates is the general aging of American society and the willingness of seniors to live alone. For cities there are three specific pre-disposing factors: first, the rise in the number of seniors living alone, often after outliving their social contacts and seeing their children migrate to the suburbs or other regions of the country altering their neighborhood populations so that they feel culturally or linguistically differentiated; second, the rapid increase in the population of "very old" seniors, 85 and above, who are more likely to be both alone and frail, sick, and unable or unwilling to enter into a public world in which they often feel vulnerable and who are, in fact, an historically new group, older than all previous cohorts and subjected to a distinct set of physical constraints; and third, the increase in the population of black and Latino seniors, who are more likely than their white counterparts to live in poverty and be at risk of the related forms of vulnerability, including illness and inadequate access to health care (Ford, et al., 1992; Lawlor et al., 1993). There is a fourth implication for metropolitan areas (as distinct from central cities) which is the growth of the elderly population in the suburban ring which in general lacks the appropriate housing stock and support systems for aged and aging residents.

By 1990, one-third of Chicago's elderly population, roughly 110,000 seniors, lived alone. When a group of researchers from the Heartland Center on Aging, Disability and Long Term Care at Indiana University surveyed Chicago seniors in 1989 and 1990, they found that 48 percent of Chicagoans over 65, and 35 percent of suburbanites over 65, reported having no family members available to assist them (Fleming-Moran et al., 1991).

Pauline Jankowitz is one of the recluses I got to know during my fieldwork in Chicago.[8] Her story helps to illustrate some of the fundamental features of life alone and afraid in the city. I first met Pauline on her 85th birthday, when I was assigned to befriend her for a day by the local office of an international organization that supports seniors living alone by linking them up with volunteers who are willing to become "friends" and inviting them to the organization's center for a birthday party, Christmas and a Thanksgiving dinner every year. A stranger before the day began, I became her closest companion for the milestone occasion when I picked her up at the uptown apartment where she had lived for 30 years.

Pauline and I had spoken on the phone the previous day and she was expecting me when I arrived late in the morning. She lived on a quiet residential street dominated by the small, three and four-flat apartment buildings common in Chicago. The neighborhood, a key site of departure and arrival for suburbanizing and new urban migrants, had changed dramatically in the time she had lived there, and her block had shifted from a predominately white ethnic area in which Pauline was a typical resident to a mixed street with a sizable Asian and increasingly Mexican population. Uptown remained home to her, but she was less comfortable in it because the neighbors, whom she was eager to praise for their responsibility and good character, were no longer familiar to her. "They are good people," she explained, "but I just don't know them." Her situation is similar to that of thousands of Chicago residents and millions of seniors across the country who have *aged in place* while the environment around them changes.

The major sources of her discomfort were her physical infirmities which grew worse as she aged, a bladder problem that left her incontinent and a weak leg that required her to walk with a crutch and drastically reduced her mobility, and her real terror of crime, which she heard about daily on the radio and television shows that she likes. "Chicago is just a shooting gallery," she told me, "and I am a moving target because I walk so slowly." Acutely aware of her vulnerability, Pauline reorganized her life to limit her exposure to the threats outside, bunkering herself in a third-floor apartment (in a building with no elevator) that she had trouble reaching because of the stairs, but which "is much safer than the first floor. . . . If I were on the first floor I'd be even more vulnerable to a break-in." With a home-care support worker, meals-on-wheels and a publicly subsidized helper visiting weekly to do her grocery shopping and help with errands, Pauline has few reasons to leave home. "I go out of my apartment about six times a year," she told me, and three of them are for celebrations sponsored by the support organization.

It is, I would learn, a challenge for service providers and volunteers to help even the seniors with whom they have contact. Pauline and I made it to the birthday celebration after a difficult and painful trip down her stairway, during which we had to turn around and return to the apartment so that she could address "a problem" that she experienced on the stairs. Pauline's grimaces and sighs betrayed the depth of the pain the walk had inflicted, but she was so excited to be going out, and going to her party, that she urged me to get us to the center quickly.

During one visit, Pauline, who knew that I was studying the 1995 heat wave, told me that she wanted to tell me her story. "It was," she said softly, "the closest I've come to death." She has one air conditioner in her apartment which gets especially hot during the summer because it is on the third floor. But the machine "is old and it doesn't work too well," which left her place uncomfortably, if not dangerously warm during the disaster. A friend had told her that it was important for her to go outside if she was too hot indoors, so she woke up very early ("it's safer then") on what would become the hottest day of the heat wave and walked towards the local store to buy cherries ("my favorite fruit, but I rarely get fresh food so they're a real treat for me") and cool down in the air conditioned space. "I was so exhausted by the time I got down the stairs that I wanted to go straight back up again," she recounted, "but instead I walked to the corner and took the bus a few blocks to the store. When I got there I could barely move. I had to lean on the shopping cart to keep myself up." But the cool air revived her and she got a bag of cherries and returned home on the bus.

"Climbing the stairs was almost impossible," she remembers. "I was hot and sweaty and so tired." Pauline called a friend as soon as she made it into her place and as they spoke she began to feel her hands going numb and swelling, a sensation that quickly extended into other parts of her body, alarming her that something was wrong. "I asked my friend to stay on the line but I put the phone down and lied down." Several minutes later, her friend still on the line but the receiver on the floor, Pauline got up, soaked her head in water, directed a fan towards her bed, lay down, and placed a number of wet towels on her body and face. Remembering that she had left her friend waiting, Pauline got up, picked up the phone to report that she was feeling better and to thank her buddy for waiting before she hung up. Finally, she lay down again to cool off and rest in earnest. Before long she had fully recovered.

"Now," she ended her story, "I have a special way to beat the heat. You're going to laugh, but I like to go on a Caribbean cruise," which she does alone and, as she does nearly everything else, without leaving her home.

> I get several wash cloths and dip them in cold water. I then place them over my eyes so that I can't see. I lie down and set the fan directly on me. The wet towels and the wind from the fan give a cool breeze, and I imagine myself on a cruise around the islands. I do this whenever it's hot, and you'd be surprised at how nice it is. My friends know about my cruises too. So when they call me on hot days they all say, "Hi Pauline, how was your trip?" We laugh about it, but it keeps me alive.

Social ecological conditions stemming from migration patterns and the widespread abandonment of urban regions have created new barriers to collective life and social support, particularly for the elderly. In *When Work Disappears* William Julius Wilson noted the significance of depopulation in poor black neighborhoods for both formal and informal social controls (Wilson, 1996: 44–5). Most scholars who have analyzed urban social support systems have focused on provision for children, but the changing demographics of the city suggest that it is increasingly important to consider how these systems work for older neighborhood residents as well. The problems are not exclusive to black and Latino communities. Since the 1950s, many white ethnic groups have experienced a sweeping suburbanization that has undercut the morphological basis for cross-generational support, leaving thousands of white seniors estranged in neighborhoods that their families and friends had left behind, out of reach during times of need but also during everyday life. As the concentration of heat wave deaths among seniors in the traditionally Polish and Slav neighborhoods on the southwest side of Chicago suggests, many of the older Italians, Slavs and Poles whose communities appeared so resilient in the work of Kornblum (1974) and Suttles (1968) have been separated from their children and extended family ties. These patterns are becoming more prevalent in Latino and African American communities as they join the suburban exodus, leaving behind older and poorer people for whom the loss of proximity to family and friends will be compounded by the relatively high rates of poverty and illness in America's so-called minority groups.

In addition to the fraying lines of social support from families experiencing generational rifts due to migration, the changing nature of friendship networks has also undermined the morphological basis of mutual assistance. For decades, community scholars have shown that many communities are no longer place-based, but organized instead around common interests and values. Advanced technology, including the telephone and the internet, ease the process of establishing connections with people in disparate places and therefore increase the probability that new social networks will develop without much regard for spatial proximity. Yet, as much research has established, certain forms of social assistance, particularly emergency care and frequent visitation, are more likely when members of a network are physically close to one another. Indeed, after the heat wave, epidemiologists found that older Chicagoans who had died during the disaster were less likely than those who survived to have had friends in the city (Semenza et al., 1996: 86).

Spatial distance, in other words, imposes real barriers to social support for friends as well as family. Proximity is a life and death matter for some people, particularly for the elderly who suffer from limited mobility.

"I'LL TALK THROUGH THE DOOR"

Although old age, illness and spatial separation from her family and friends established the grounding for Pauline Jankowitz's condition, her isolation became particularly extreme because of her abiding fear of being victimized by crime. Pauline's perception of her own extreme vulnerability heightens her fear, but her concerns are in fact typical of city dwellers throughout the United States at a time when a veritable culture of fear and a powerful cultural industry based on crime have come to influence much of the organizational, institutional and political activity within the country as well as the thought and action of Americans in their everyday lives. By the late 1990s, fear of crime has taken on a paradoxical role in American urban life, on the one hand pushing people to dissociate from their neighbors and extend their social distance from strangers, and on the other hand becoming one of the organizing principles of new collective projects, such as neighborhood watch groups and community policing programs. Regardless of the form it takes, "coping with crime," as Wesley Skogan and Michael Maxfield put it in the title of their book (Skogan and Maxfield, 1981), has become a way of life for Americans in general and for residents of notably violent cities such as Chicago.

Throughout Chicago and especially in the most violent areas, city residents have reorganized their daily routines and behaviors in order to minimize their exposure to crime in an increasingly Hobbesian universe, scheming around the clock to avoid driving, parking or walking on the wrong streets or in the wrong neighborhoods, seeing the wrong people and visiting the wrong establishments and public places. In Chicago, as in most other American cities, "wrong" in this context is associated with blacks in general and young men in particular, especially now that the massive dragnet cast by the drug warrior state has captured so many young blacks and labeled them as permanent public enemies (Wacquant, 2001). Yet doing fieldwork in even the most objectively dangerous streets of Chicago makes it clear that the common depiction of city residents, and particularly those who live in poor and violent areas, as constantly paranoid and so acutely concerned about proximate threats that they can hardly move, is a gross misrepresentation of how fear is managed and experienced. "It's caution, not fear, that guides me," Eugene Richards, a senior citizen living in North Lawndale explained to me during a discussion of managing danger in the area. Eugene will walk a few blocks during the day, but he refuses to go more than four blocks without a car. Alice Nelson, a woman in her 70s who lives in the Little Village, walks during the day and carries small bags of groceries with her. "But I won't go out at night," she told me. "And if someone comes to the door I won't open it. I'll talk through the door because you never know . . ."⁹

Preying on the elderly, who are presumed to be more vulnerable and easier to dupe, is a standard and recurrent practice of neighborhood deviants and legitimate corporations, mail-order businesses and salespersons alike. Several of my informants said that turning strangers away at the door was part of their regular routine, and complained that they felt besieged by the combination of local hoodlums who paid them special attention around the beginning of the month when social security checks were delivered as well as outsiders who tried to visit or call and convince them to spend their scarce dollars. In the United States, where guns are easy to obtain and levels of gun-related violence are among the highest in the world, roughly one-quarter of households are touched by crime each year, and about one-half of the population will be victimized by a violent crime in their life-time (Miethe, 1995). The nature of the association between fear and vulnerability is enigmatic because it is impossible to establish that the lower levels of victimization are not at least partially attributable to fear which causes people to avoid potentially dangerous situations and, in the most extreme cases, pushes people to become recluses, "prisoners of their own fear," as one social worker I shadowed calls them. Nonetheless, many scholars of crime have argued that fear of crime is irrational because of the often-cited finding that the elderly and women, who are the least likely to be victimized, are the most fearful of crime. Yet ethnographic observation and more fine-grained surveys of fear can show what grounds these concerns.

First, community area or neighborhood characteristics influence levels of fear. Just as city residents tend to be more concerned about crime than residents of suburban and rural areas, African Americans and other ethnic groups who live in areas with higher levels of crime are more likely than whites to report fear of crime in surveys (Joseph, 1997; Miethe, 1995). Signs of neighborhood "disorder," such as abandoned buildings, vandalism, litter and graffiti, instill fear in local residents, whereas, as Richard Taub and his colleagues found in Chicago, neighborhood resources, such as stores, safe public spaces, and active collective life provide incentives for city dwellers to overcome their fears and participate in public activities (Joseph, 1997; Miethe, 1995; Skogan, 1990; Taub et al., 1984). Second, as Sally Engle Merry concluded from her study of a high-crime, multi-ethnic urban housing project, once residents of a particular area grow fearful of crime a vicious cycle begins: fear causes people to increase the amount of time they spend at home and reduces their willingness to socialize with their neighbors; reclusiveness increases the social distance between residents and their neighbors creating a community of strangers who grow even more fearful of each other; heightened fear leads to heightened reclusiveness, and so on (Merry, 1981).

In interviews and casual conversations conducted during my fieldwork, Chicago seniors provided their own explanations for the fear that so many criminologists and city officials seem unable to understand. Many of the seniors I got to know said that although they knew that they were unlikely to be robbed or attacked, their heightened concern about victimization stemmed from their knowledge that if they were victimized, the consequences, particularly of violent crime, would be devastating in ways that they would not be for younger people. At the economic level, seniors living on fixed and limited incomes feared that a robbery or burglary could leave them without sufficient resources to pay for such basic needs as food, medication, rent or energy. In Chicago, where hunger, under-medication, homelessness, displacement and energy deprivation are not uncommon among seniors, these are not unfounded concerns. At the physical level, seniors, for whom awareness of bodily frailty is one of the defining conditions of life, are afraid that a violent attack could result in permanent disabilities, crippling and even death. The elderly make it clear that their fears of crime are directly related to their concerns about the difficulty of recovering from crime and that their sensitivities to danger were rational from their points of view.

DEAD SPACE

A cause and consequence of this culture of fear is the degradation and fortification of urban public spaces in which city dwellers circulate. The loss of viable public space is the third condition that gives rise to literal social isolation undermining the social morphological foundations of collective social life and so giving rise to sweeping insecurity in everyday urban life. The real and perceived violence of the city has pushed Chicago residents to remake the sociospatial environment in which they live.[10] In Chicago the degradation of public space has been most rampant in the city's hyperghettos, where the flight of business, the retrenchment of state supports, the out-migration of middle-class residents, the rise of public drug markets, and the concentration of violent crime and victimization have radically reduced the viability of public spaces (Wacquant, 1994). Despite the real decreases in crime that Chicago experienced in the mid-1990s, the overall crime rate in Chicago is falling at a slower pace than in all of the other major American cities. According to the Chicago Community Policing Evaluation Consortium, a major research project directed by Wesley Skogan at Northwestern University, "the largest declines [in

crime] have occurred in the highest-crime parts of the city," and "the greatest decline in gun-related crime has occurred in African-American neighborhoods" (Chicago Community Policing Evaluation Consortium, 1997: 6–8). Nonetheless the levels of violent crime concentrated in poor black areas of the city remain comparatively high, making it difficult for residents to feel safe in the streets. A study by the Epidemiology Program at the Chicago Department of Public Health showed that in 1994 and 1995 the overall violent crime rate as reported to the Chicago Police Department, a likely underestimation of the true victimization levels, was 19 violent crimes for every 100 residents of Fuller Park, the community area that had the highest mortality levels during the heat wave. Other community areas with high heat wave mortalities had similar crime levels: Woodlawn, with the second highest heat mortality rate, reported 13 violent crimes per 100 residents; Greater Grand Crossing reported 11 per 100; Washington Park, Grand Boulevard, and the near south side, all among the most deadly spots during the disaster, listed rates above 15 crimes per 100 residents as well, suggesting, as did the Illinois Department of Public Health, an association between the everyday precariousness of life in these neighborhoods and vulnerability during the heat wave (City of Chicago, 1996). In contrast, Lincoln Park, the prosperous community on the near north side, reported two violent crimes for every 100 residents, and a heat wave mortality rate among the lowest in the city (City of Chicago, 1996).

But the conditions of insecurity are hardly confined to the Chicago ghettos, and constant exposure to images and information about violence in the city has instilled genuine fear in communities throughout the city. Moreover, the depacification of daily life that is concentrated in the city's ghettos has emerged on a smaller scale in other parts of Chicago, affecting a broad set of buildings, blocks, and collective housing facilities as well as neighborhood clusters. Several studies have documented the erosion of the sociospatial infrastructure for public life in low-income barrios and ghettos, therefore I will focus here on showing the ways in which spatial degradation and public crime have fostered reclusiveness in settings, such as senior public housing units, where many of the heat wave deaths occurred.

In the four years leading up to the heat wave conditions in the city's senior public housing facilities bucked all of Chicago's crime trends. Residents of these special units experienced a soaring violent crime rate even as the overall crime levels in the Chicago Housing Authority (CHA) family projects and the rest of the city declined, forcing many residents to give up not only the public parks and streets that once supported their neighborhoods, but the public areas within their own apartment buildings as well. In the 1990s the CHA opened its 58 senior buildings, which house about 100,000 residents and are dispersed throughout the city although generally located in safer areas than the family public housing complexes, to people with disabilities as well as to the elderly. The 1990 Americans with Disabilities Act made people with substance abuse problems eligible for social security insurance and the CHA welcomed them into senior housing units as well. Unfortunately this act of accommodation has proven disastrous for senior residents and the communities they had once established within their buildings: the mix of low-income substance abusers, many of whom continue to engage in crime to finance their habits, and low-income seniors, many of whom keep everything they own, savings included, in their tiny apartments, creates a perfect formula for disaster in the social life of the housing complex.

In March of 1995, just a few months before the heat wave, the Chicago Housing Authority reported that from 1991 to 1994 the number of Part I crimes (in which the US Justice Department includes homicide, criminal sexual assault, serious assault, robbery, burglary, theft and violent theft) committed and reported within CHA housing increased by over 50 percent. "The elderly in public housing," a group of CHA tenants and advisers called the Building Organization and Leadership Development (BOLD) group reported, "are more vulnerable than seniors in assisted or private housing in that they are being victimized in many cases by their neighbors." Moreover, BOLD showed that thefts, forcible entry, armed robbery, "and other crimes of violence are substantially higher in those developments housing a large percentage of non-elderly disabled. . . . The reality appears to be that disabled youth are victimizing seniors" (BOLD, 1995).

Elderly residents of senior buildings throughout the city now voice the same complaint: they feel trapped in their rooms, afraid that if they leave they might be attacked or have their apartment robbed, and the most afraid refuse to use the ground floor common rooms unless security workers are there. The fortification of public space that contributes to isolation all over the city is exacerbated here. Most residents, to be sure, do manage to get out of their units, but they have to limit themselves to secure public areas, elevators and halls. Unable to reduce the structural conditions of insecurity in the buildings, workers at the Chicago Department on Aging recently initiated a program to help residents develop building watch groups in the senior complexes. True to its mission to enable as well as provide, the city has increased the security services in the buildings but has also encouraged the elderly and poor CHA residents to arm themselves with flashlights, cellular phones and badges to patrol their home turf. Yet while one branch of the city government prepares the seniors for a feeble battle against the conditions that another branch of the city has created, the most worried and disaffected residents of the senior buildings respond by sealing off their homes with home-made security systems designed to ward off invaders.

Concern about the proximity of younger residents and their associates who are using or peddling drugs is ubiquitous in Chicago's senior housing complexes. During an interview in her home, one woman, a resident of a CHA building on the near west side, expressed remorse that a formerly pleasant and popular patio on the top floor had been vandalized and looted by younger residents and their friends. The group had first taken the space over and made it their hangout spot, then decided to take some of the furniture and even the fire extinguishers for themselves. Some older residents, she explained to me, did not want to make a big deal out of the problem because they worried that their young neighbors would learn who had informed security and then retaliate. The fear of young people and the demonization of drug users common in contemporary American society rendered the situation more difficult, as many building residents presumed that the younger residents would cause trouble and were scared to approach them. Ultimately, the seniors have been unable to fix up the area or win it back. "Now," she sighed, "no one uses that space. It's just empty, dead."

"I NEVER HAVE ENOUGH TIME TO SEE THEM"

The current array of programs and services is insufficient to provide primary goods such as adequate housing, transportation, energy assistance, reliable health care and medication for the elderly poor, leaving private agencies and numerous charities to address gaps that they have no means to fill. Local welfare state agencies in American cities historically have lacked the resources necessary to meet the needs of impoverished and insecure residents, but in the 1990s the rise of entrepreneurial state programs that required more active shopping services from consumerist citizens created additional difficulties for the most isolated and vulnerable city residents. Studies of Chicago's programs for the poor elderly had warned officials about the dangers of residents falling through gaps in the withering safety net. After conducting a major study of Chicago's support programs and emergency services, social service scholar Sharon Keigher concluded that "city agencies are not equipped to intervene substantially with older persons who do not ask for help, who have no family, or who do not go to senior centers and congregate at meal sites. Yet, increasingly these persons—who tend to be very old, poor and living alone—are in need of multiple services" (Keigher, 1991: 12). Published as both an official city report (in 1987) and a scholarly book (in 1991), Keigher's findings were known to city agencies responsible for serving vulnerable seniors long before the heat wave. But the city government lacked both the resources and the political priorities necessary to respond to them sufficiently, and its agencies were poorly prepared for assisting needy seniors in either the

heat disaster of 1995 or the struggles they take on regularly.

Government policies and procedures that limited the capacity of residents to enter programs and obtain resources they need is the fourth condition that produces literal isolation. These changes have been disproportionately destructive for the city's most impoverished residents, who have had to struggle to secure the basic resources and services necessary for survival that a more generous welfare state would provide. In a political context where private organizations provide most of the human services to elderly city residents, research must shift from state agencies and agents to include the private offices and employees through which local governments reach their constituents. Spending time alongside social workers and home care providers for Chicago seniors, it became clear that the city's incapacity to reach isolated, sick or otherwise vulnerable seniors during the heat wave was by no means an anomaly created by the unusual environmental conditions. Under-service for Chicago's poor elderly is a structural certainty and everyday norm in an era where political pressures for state entrepreneurialism have grown hand-in-hand with social pressures for isolation. Embedded in a competitive market for gaining city contracts which provides perverse incentives for agencies to underestimate the costs of services and overestimate their capacity to provide them, the agencies and private organizations I observed had bargained themselves into responsibilities that they could not possibly meet. "Most entrepreneurial governments promote *competition* between service providers," David Osborne and Ted Gaebler wrote in *Reinventing Government* (Osborne and Gaebler, 1992: 19), but competition undermines the working conditions of human service providers if it fosters efficiency but compromises the time and human resources necessary to provide quality care. "My seniors love to see me," Mandy Evers, an African-American woman in her late 20s who was on her fourth year working as a case manager, told me. "The problem is I never have enough time to get to them."

Stacy Geer, a seasoned advocate of Chicago seniors who spent much of the 1990s helping the elderly secure basic goods such as housing and energy, insists that the political mismatch between more entrepreneurial service systems and isolated seniors contributed to the vulnerability of Chicago seniors during the heat wave. "The capacity of service delivery programs is realized fully only by the seniors who are most active in seeking them out, who are connected to their family, church, neighbors, or someone who helps them get the things they need." In some circumstances, the aging process can hinder seniors who have been healthy and financially secure for most of their lives. Geer continues, "As seniors become more frail their networks break down. As their needs increase, they have less ability to meet them. The people who are hooked into the Department on Aging, the AARP, the senior clubs at the churches, they are part of that word of mouth network and they hear. I know, just from doing organizing in the senior community, that you run into the same people, and the same are active in a number of organizations."[11] Seniors who are marginalized at the first, structural level of social networks and government programs are then doubly excluded at the second, conjunctural level of service delivery because they do not always know of—let alone know how to activate—networks of support. Those who are out of the loop in their daily life are more likely to remain so when there is a crisis. This certainly happened during the heat wave, when relatively active and informed seniors used official cooling centers set up by the city while the more inactive and isolated elderly stayed home.

During the 1990s, however, not even the best-connected city residents knew where to appeal if they needed assistance securing the most basic of primary goods: home, energy and water. In Chicago, the combination of cuts to the budget for the federally-sponsored Low Income Home Energy Assistance Program (LIHEAP) and a market-model managerial strategy for punishing consumers who are delinquent on their bills has placed the poor elderly in a permanent energy crisis. Facing escalating energy costs (even before prices soared in 2000),

declining government subsidies and fixed incomes, seniors throughout the city express great concern about the cost of their utilities bills and take pains to keep their fees down.[12]

Poor seniors I got to know understood that they would face unaffordable utilities costs in the summer if they used air conditioners. Epidemiologists estimate that "more than 50 percent of the deaths related to the heat wave could have been prevented if each home had had a working air conditioner," arguing that surely this would be an effective public health strategy (Semenza et al., 1996: 87). Yet the elderly who regularly struggle to make ends meet explain that they could not use air conditioners even if they owned them because activating the units would push their energy bills to unmanageable levels. But their energy crisis was pressing even during moderate temperatures. The most impoverished seniors I visited kept their lights off during the day, letting the television, their most consistent source of companionship, illuminate their rooms. Fear of losing their energy altogether if they failed to pay the bills has relegated these seniors to regular and fundamental forms of insecurity and duress. Yet their daily crisis goes largely unnoticed.

THE FORMULA FOR DISASTER

The four conditions highlighted here impose serious difficulties for all seniors. But they are particularly devastating for the elderly poor who cannot buy their way out of them by purchasing more secure housing in safer areas, visiting or paying for distant family members to visit, by obtaining private health insurance supplements or by using more expensive and safe transportation such as taxis to get out of the house or the neighborhood. Each one of the key conditions described in this article contributes to the production of the forms of isolation that proved so deadly during the heat wave and that continue to undermine the health and safety of countless older

Chicagoans. But in many cases Chicago residents are subjected to all of the conditions together, and the combination creates a formula for disaster that makes extreme social, physical and psychological suffering a feature of everyday life. If aging alone, the culture of fear, the degradation and fortification of public space and the reduction of redistributive and supportive state programs continue at their current pace, more seniors will retreat to their "safe houses," abandoning a society that has all but abandoned them. Collectively producing the conditions for literal isolation, we have made dying alone a fittingly tragic end.

ACKNOWLEDGMENTS

The National Science Foundation Graduate Research Fellowship, the Jacob Javits Fellowship and a grant from the Berkeley Humanities Division helped to support research for this project. This publication was also supported in part by a grant from the Individual Project Fellowship Program of the Open Society Institute. Thanks go to Loïc Wacquant, Mike Rogin, Jack Katz, Nancy Scheper-Hughes, Kim DaCosta, Dan Dohan, Paul Willis and Caitlin Zaloom for incisive comments on earlier drafts.

Notes

1. For a synthetic sociological account of the conditions that helped produce the historic mortality rates, see Klinenberg (1999); for an epidemiological account, see Semenza et al. (1996).

2. Roughly 70 Chicagoans died on a typical July day during the 1990s. "Excess deaths" measures the variance from the expected death rate. In assessing heat wave mortality, forensic scientists prefer the excess death measure to the heat-related death measure, which is based on the number of deaths examined and recorded by investigators, because many deaths during heat waves go unexamined or are not properly attributed to the heat (Shen et al., 1998).

3. Sherwin Nuland is among the more recent writers to discuss the modern version of the *ars moriendi*. Describing a man dying of AIDS, Nuland writes, "During his terminal weeks in the hospital, Kent was never alone. Whatever help they could or could not provide him at the final hours, there is no question that the constant presence of his friends eased him beyond what might have been achieved by the nursing staff, no matter the attentiveness of their care" (Nuland, 1993: 196).

4. There is, of course, a brighter side to the extension of the life span, which is itself a sign of significant social and scientific progress. Aging alone, as Robert Coles and Arlie Hochschild have argued, can be a rich personal and social experience, albeit one filled with challenges. In *The Unexpected Community*, Hochschild documents the active social lives of a group of Bay Area seniors who, as she emphatically stated, "were not isolated and not lonely" but instead "were part of a community I did not expect to find" (Hochschild, 1973: xiv), one that worked together to solve the problem of loneliness that proves so troublesome for the elderly. There are vital communities of older people and Hochschild's research shows how these groups come into being, portraying them once they are made. But too often readers of Hochschild are so eager to celebrate the community she describes that they forget that she chose to study Merrill Court

precisely because the residents there were an exceptional case. The opening lines of her epilogue explain the goal of her project much better than do many of her interpreters. She wrote, "The most important point I am trying to make in this book concerns the people it does not discuss—the isolated. Merrill Court was an unexpected community, an exception. Living in ordinary apartments and houses, in shabby downtown hotels, sitting in parks and eating in cheap restaurants, are old people in various degrees and sorts of isolation" (Hochschild, 1973: 137). Hochschild leaves it to others to render the social worlds of the isolated as explicit as she makes the world in Merrill Court.

5. This conception of social isolation breaks from both sociological definitions of the term, which generally refer to relations between groups rather than people, and from conventional gerontological definitions of isolation, which define isolation as being single or living alone. There are, however, an increasing number of social network studies and gerontological reports that classify social integration or isolation by relative levels of social contact. Fischer and Phillips, for example, define social isolation as "knowing relatively few people who are probable sources of rewarding exchanges" (Fischer and Phillips, 1982: 22); Rubinstein classifies social integration and activity on a scale ranging from "very low range" to "high range" (Rubinstein, 1986: 172–9); and Gibson lists four types of loneliness: "physical aloneness," "loneliness as a state of mind," "the feeling of isolation due to a personal characteristic," and "solitude" (Gibson, 2004: 4–6).

6. See Gibson (2000) for a review of studies showing that most seniors who live alone are not lonely.

7. Thompson and Krause find that not only do people who live alone report more fear of crime than those who live with others, but also that "the greater sense of security among those who live with others appears to permeate beyond the home because they report less fear of crime than their counterparts" (Thompson and Krause, 1998: 356).

8. All personal names of Chicago residents have been changed.

9. Yet, as Alex Kotlowitz and teenage journalists LeAlan Jones and Lloyd Newman have shown in their accounts of growing up in Chicago's West and South Side housing projects, even young residents of the most violent urban areas are subjected to so much brutality, death and suffering that they have learned from their infancy how to organize their daily routines around the temporal and seasonal variations of the criminal economy (Jones et al., 1997; Kotlowitz, 1991). For Jones and Newman, managing fear and avoiding violence is such a fundamental part of their everyday lives that they decided to introduce and organize their book around it. "They used to shoot a lot in the summertime," Jones begins. Lloyd continues ominously, especially in light of the heat wave, "That's why I stayed in my house most of the time" (Jones et al., 1997: 31).

10. In 1995 Chicago ranked 6th in robbery and 5th in aggravated assaults among all United States cities with a population of over 350,000; in 1998 the city was the national leader in homicide, with the annual figure of 698 exceeding New York City's by about 100 even though Chicago is roughly one-third as populous; and throughout the 1990s its violent crime rate decreased much more slowly than any of the eight largest American cities (New York City, Los Angeles, Chicago,

Houston, Philadelphia, Phoenix, San Diego, Dallas).

11. Internal pressures within state agencies and advocacy organizations push social workers and organizers to reward the most entrepreneurial clients with special attention. Overwhelmed with problem cases and operating in an environment where agencies must show successful outcome measures to garner resources from external funders who expect tangible results, the social

workers I observed engaged in what Lipsky called "creaming," the practice of favoring and working intensively on the cases of people "who seem likely to succeed in terms of bureaucratic success criteria" (Lipsky, 1980: 107).

12. While the average Illinois family spends roughly 6 percent of its income on heat-related utilities during winter months, for low-income families the costs constitute nearly 35 percent (Pearson, 1995).

References

BOLD (1995) "BOLD Group Endorses CHAPS Police Unit," report by the Building Organization and Leadership Development group, Chicago.

Chicago Community Policing Evaluation Consortium (1997) "Community Policing in Chicago, Year Four: An Interim Report," report by the Chicago Community Policing Evaluation Consortium.

City of Chicago (1996) "An Epidemiological Overview of Violent Crimes in Chicago, 1995," report by the Department of Public Health, City of Chicago.

Fischer, Claude (1975) "Toward a Subcultural Theory of Urbanism," *American Journal of Sociology* 80: 1319–41.

Fischer, Claude (1982) *To Dwell among Friends: Personal Networks in Town and City.* Chicago, IL: University of Chicago Press.

Fischer, Claude (1984[1976]) *The Urban Experience.* San Diego: Harcourt, Brace, Jovanovich.

Fischer, Claude and Meredith Phillips (1982) "Who is Alone? Social Characteristics of People with Small Networks," in Leticia Anne

Peplau and Daniel Perlman (eds) *Loneliness: A Sourcebook on Current Theory: Research and Therapy.* New York: Wiley.

Fleming-Moran, Millicent, T. Kenworthy-Bennett and Karen Harlow (1991) "Illinois State Needs Assessment Survey of Elders Aged 55 and Over," report from the Heartland Center on Aging, Disability and Long Term Care, School of Public Health and Environmental Affairs, Indiana University and the National Center for Senior Living, South Bend, IN.

Ford, Amasa, Marie Haug, Paul Jones and Steven Folmar (1992) "New Cohorts of Urban Elders: Are They in Trouble?" *Journal of Gerontology* 47: S297–S303.

Gibson, Hamilton (2000) *Loneliness in Later Life.* New York: Saint Martin's Press.

Gurley, Jan, Nancy Lum, Merle Sande, Bernard Lo and Mitchell Katz (1996) "Persons Found in their Homes Helpless or Dead," *New England Journal of Medicine* 334: 1710–16.

Hochschild, Arlie Russel (1973) *The Unexpected Community: Portrait of an Old-Age Subculture.* Berkeley: University of California Press.

Jones, LeAlan and Lloyd Newman with David Isay (1997) *Our America: Life and Death on the South Side of Chicago*. New York: Washington Square Press.

Joseph, Janice (1997) "Fear of Crime among Black Elderly," *Journal of Black Studies* 27: 698–717.

Keigher, Sharon (1987) "The City's Responsibility for the Homeless Elderly of Chicago," report by the Chicago Department of Aging and Disability.

Klinenberg, Eric (1999) "Denaturalizing Disaster: A Social Autopsy of the 1995 Chicago Heat Wave," *Theory and Society* 28: 239–95.

Kornblum, William (1974) *Blue Collar Community*. Chicago, IL: University of Chicago Press.

Kotlowitz, Alex (1991) *There Are No Children Here: The Story of Two Boys Growing Up in the Other America*. New York: Anchor Books.

Lawlor, Edward, Gunnar Almgren and Mary Gomberg (1993) "Aging in Chicago: Demography," report, Chicago Community Trust.

Lipsky, Michael (1980) *Street-Level Bureaucracy: Dilemmas of the Individual in Public Services*. New York: Russell Sage.

Merry, Sally Engle (1981) *Urban Danger: Life in a Neighborhood of Strangers*. Philadelphia, PA: Temple University Press.

Miethe, Terance (1995) "Fear and Withdrawal," *The Annals of the American Academy* 539: 14–29.

Nashold, Raymond, Jeffrey Jentzen, Patrick Remington and Peggy Peterson (n.d.) "Excessive Heat Deaths, Wisconsin, June 20–August 19, 1995," unpublished manuscript.

Nuland, Sherwin (1993) *How We Die: Reflections on Life's Final Chapter*. New York: Vintage.

Osborne, David and Ted Gaebler (1992) *Reinventing Government: How the Entrepreneurial Spirit is Transforming the Public Sector*. New York: Plume.

Pearson, Rick (1995) "Funding to Help Poor Pay Heating Bills Evaporating," *Chicago Tribune* (20 July): Metro 2.

Perrow, Charles and Mauro Guillen (1990) *The Aids Disaster*. New Haven, CT: Yale University Press.

Putnam, Robert (1995) "Bowling Alone: America's Declining Social Capital," *Democracy* 6: 65–78.

Rubinstein, Robert (1986) *Singular Paths: Old Men Living Alone*. New York: Columbia University Press.

Seale, Clive (1995) "Dying Alone," *Sociology of Health and Illness* 17: 376–92.

Semenza, Jan, Carol Rubin, Kenneth Falter, Joel Selanikio, W. Dana Flanders, Holly Howe and John Wilhelm (1996) "Heat-Related Deaths During the July 1995 Heat Wave in Chicago," *The New England of Medicine* 335: 84–90.

Shen, Tiefu, Holly Howe, Celan Alo and Ronald Moolenaar (1998) "Toward a Broader Definition of Heat-Related Death: Comparison of Mortality Estimates From Medical Examiners" Classification with Those from Total Death Differentials During the July 1995 Chicago Heat Wave', *The American Journal of Forensic Medicine and Pathology* 19: 113–18.

Skogan, Wesley (1990) *Disorder and Decline: Crime and the Spiral of Decay in American Neighborhoods*. Berkeley: University of California Press.

Skogan, Wesley and Michael Maxfield (1981) *Coping with Crime: Individual and Neighborhood Reactions*. Newbury Park, CA: Sage.

Suttles, Gerald (1968) *The Social Order of the Slum: Ethnicity and Territory in the Inner City*. Chicago, IL: University of Chicago Press.

Taub, Richard, D. Garth Taylor and Jan Durham (1984) *Paths of Neighborhood Change: Race and Crime in Urban America*. Chicago, IL: University of Chicago Press.

Thompson, Emily and Neil Krause (1998) "Living Alone and Neighborhood Characteristics as Predictors of Social Support in Later Life," *Journal of Gerontology* 53B(6): S354–S364.

US Centers for Disease Control and Prevention (1996) "Heat-Related Mortality—Milwaukee, Wisconsin, July 1995," *Morbidity and Mortality Weekly Report* 45:505–7.

Wacquant, Loïc (1994) "The New Urban Color Line: The State and Fate of the Ghetto in PostFordist America," in Craig Calhoun (ed.) *Social Theory and the Politics of Identity*. Oxford: Basil Blackwell.

Wacquant, Loïc (2001) "Deadly Symbiosis: When Ghetto and Prison Meet and Mesh," *Punishment and Society* 3(1): 95–134.

Wilson, William Julius (1996) *When Work Disappears: The World of the New Urban Poor*. New York: Alfred Knopf.

Wuthnow, Robert (1998) *Loose Connections: Joining Together in America's Fragmented Communities*. Cambridge, MA: Harvard University Press.

THE SOCIAL AND CULTURAL MEANINGS OF ILLNESS

Medical sociologists draw a distinction between disease and illness. Put simply, *disease* is the biophysiological phenomenon that affects the body, while *illness* is a social phenomenon that accompanies or surrounds the disease. The shape of illness is not necessarily determined by the disease. Illnesses involve the interaction of the disease, sick individuals, and society. To examine illness, we must focus on the subjective worlds of meaning and experience. Here, we investigate the social images and moral meanings that are attributed to illnesses. In this perspective, we view illness as a social construction. While most illnesses are assumed to have a biophysiological basis (i.e., an underlying disease), this is not a necessary condition for something to be defined as an illness. As Joseph Gusfield (1967, 180) notes, "Illness is a social designation, by no means given by the nature of medical fact." Thus, we can conceivably have illnesses without diseases or illnesses whose meaning is completely independent from the actual biomedical entity. For example, illnesses may be contested, in that "sufferers claim to have a specific disease that many physicians do not recognize or acknowledge as distinctly medical" (Conrad and Barker 2010, S67). This group of contested illnesses includes fibromyalgia, chronic fatigue syndrome, irritable bowel syndrome, and multiple chemical sensitivity disorder. In examining the social meaning of illness, we focus on the role of social and cultural values that shape the perception of a disease or malady. Illness can reflect cultural assumptions and biases about a particular group or groups of people, or it can become a cultural metaphor for existing societal problems.

Illnesses may reflect deeply rooted cultural values and assumptions. This is particularly evident in the medical definition and treatment of women and women's maladies. During the nineteenth century, organized medicine achieved a strong dominance over the treatment of women and proceeded to promulgate erroneous and damaging conceptualizations of women as sickly, irrational creatures at the mercy of their reproductive organs (Barker-Benfield 1976; Wertz and Wertz 1989). Throughout history, we can find similar examples of medical and "scientific" explanations of women's health and illnesses that reflect the dominant conceptions of women in society. For example, a century ago common medical knowledge was replete with assumptions about the "fragile" nature of upper-class women, a nature first believed to be dominated by reproductive organs and later by psychological processes innate in women (Ehrenreich and English 1978). Assumptions about women's nature frequently set cultural limits on what women could do. In the late nineteenth century, physicians opposed granting women the right to vote on the grounds that concern about such matters would strain their "fragile" brains and cause their ovaries to shrink! The creation of the "cult of invalidism" among upper-class women in the nineteenth century—at the same time that working-class women were considered capable of working long, hard hours in sweatshops and factories—can be interpreted as physicians acting as agents of social control. Physicians' use of definitions of health and illness kept women of both classes "in their place," both overtly and subtly, through a socialization process in which many women came to accept being sickly as their proper role and in which many unquestioningly accepted the physicians' claim to "expertise" in treating women's health and sexual problems. While physicians did not invent sexism, they reflected common sexist attitudes that they then reinforced in their definition and treatment of women.

While the grossest biases about women and their bodies have diminished, the effects of gender bias on the meanings of illness are now subtler and more complex. Since the 1930s, a significant number of women's problems—childbirth, birth control, abortion, menopause, and premenstrual syndrome—have become "medicalized" (see "The Medicalization of American Society" in Part 3). While the consequences of medicalization are probably mixed (Riessman 1983), various feminist analysts see it as an extension of medicine's control over women (see, for example, Boston Women's Health Book Collective 2011; Riska 2003). Looking at one example, premenstrual syndrome (PMS), we see that medicalization can legitimate the real discomforts of many women who had long been told their premenstrual pain was "all in their head." On the other hand, one consequence of the adoption of PMS as a medical syndrome is the legitimation of the view that all women are potentially physically and emotionally incapacitated each month by menstruation and thus not fully capable of responsibility. Wide adoption of PMS as a syndrome could undercut some important gains of the contemporary women's movement (cf. Figert 1995).

The current treatment of menopause provides another example of the changing medical meanings of women's disorders. Several analysts (Kaufert 1982; McCrea 1983; Bell 1987) have described how menopause, a natural life event for women, became defined as a "deficiency disease" in the 1960s when medical therapy became readily available to treat it. The treatment, estrogen replacement therapy, promised women they could stay "feminine forever" and preserve their "youth and beauty." Feminists argued that menopause is part of the normal aging process and thus not an illness. They also argued that the treatment is usually unnecessary and, since estrogen has been linked to cancer, always dangerous. In recent years, estrogen replacement therapy was found to pose severe risks to women's health, and many women (perhaps half) have discontinued taking it (Houck 2006; Stults and Conrad 2008). Studies have suggested that both the meanings and experience of menopause may be culturally bound. In Japan, for example, cessation of menstruation is not given much importance and is seen as a natural part of aging, not a disease-like condition. Even the experience is different: Japanese women report few hot flashes but rather typically suffer from stiff shoulders (Lock 1993). PMS and menopause

provide contemporary examples of how cultural assumptions of gender can be reflected in the medical definitions of disorder, which affect the medical treatment of women.

The meaning attributed to medical problems often reflects the attitudes of a given culture. Obesity and anorexia have become major health problems in our society. There is strong evidence for a great rise in obesity in the past several decades, so much so it has been considered an epidemic (Caballero 2007). But obesity is inexorably tied in with its social and cultural meanings. In this section's first selection, "Morality and Health: News Media Constructions of Overweight and Eating Disorders," Abigail Saguy and Kjerstin Gruys examine how eating disorders and overweight/obesity are portrayed in the news. Both extreme thinness and extreme fatness are deemed illnesses but are imbued with particular social meanings. In the United States today, thinness is taken as a sign of social virtue, while fatness is seen as a sign of sloth and gluttony. In their research of a decade of news articles, the authors found that anorexia and bulimia are depicted as caused by a complex set of factors beyond an individual's control, while overweight and obesity are typically attributed to bad eating choices, lack of self-control, and blameworthy overeating. Moreover, the typical anorexic is seen as a middle-class white girl, while the obese are seen as poor women of color, extending existing stereotypes of the disorders. This selection illustrates how the meanings of illnesses often reflect societal attitudes toward the social groups who are deemed to have them.

All illnesses are not created and treated equally. Certain illnesses may engender social meanings that affect our perception and treatment of those who suffer from them. One important example of this is "stigmatized illness" (Gussow and Tracy 1968). Certain illnesses, including leprosy, epilepsy, sexually transmitted diseases, and AIDS, have acquired moral meanings that are inherent in the very construction of the illness's image and thus affect our perception of the illness and our reaction to those who have it. These illnesses carry considerable potential to stigmatize individuals, adding social suffering to physical difficulties. Frequently, individuals must invest as much energy in managing the stigma as in managing the disorder itself (e.g., Lee et al. 2002).

The social meaning of an illness can shape the social response to it. Illness can become imbued with a moral opprobrium that makes its sufferers outcasts. For example, Cotton Mather, the celebrated eighteenth-century New England Puritan minister, declared that syphilis was a punishment "which the Just judgment of God has reserved for our later ages" (cited in Sontag 1988, 92). The social definition of epilepsy fostered myths (e.g., epilepsy was inherited or it caused crime) that further stigmatized the disorder (Schneider and Conrad 1983). Finally, the negative image of venereal diseases was a significant factor in the limited funds allocated for dealing with these illnesses (Brandt 1985).

AIDS, perhaps more than any other example in the twentieth century, highlights the significance that social meaning has on the social response to illness. A fear virtually unprecedented in contemporary society led to an overreaction to the disease sometimes bordering on hysteria. When AIDS was first discovered, it was thought to be a "gay disease" and thus was stigmatized and its research underfunded (Perrow and Guillén 1990). Although we have learned a great deal about AIDS in recent years, the image of AIDS remains fundamentally shaped by the stigma attached to it and the fear of contagion (Nelkin et al. 1991; Rushing 1995; Herek 1999; Parker and Aggleton 2003). AIDS-related stigma has been manifested in discrimination, violence, and personal rejection of people with AIDS (PWAs). PWAs, at least in developed countries, are living longer with the disease, and thus the impact of AIDS stigma has a direct effect on individuals' well-being and everyday life (e.g., see Klitzman

1997). Stigma has hindered societies' responses to the AIDS epidemic and continues to impact on the lives of PWAs, their families, and associates, despite the fact that HIV infection has become a disease that when treated properly is largely a chronic illness people can live with for decades.

In the second selection, "Illness Meanings of AIDS Among Women With HIV: Merging Immunology and Life Experience," Alison Scott investigates how women with HIV view AIDS. In an age when HIV has become a disease treatable with highly active antiretroviral therapy (HAART), the negative perception and stigma of AIDS can still be debilitating and counterproductive to proper medication adherence. Thus, as Scott shows, the stigma and moral meanings of AIDS can have a direct effect on treatment and immune system recovery.

The final selection further examines why the social response to diseases differs. In an innovative study, Elizabeth Armstrong and her colleagues, using coverage in the news media as data, asked the question "Whose deaths matter?" They looked at the media attention given to seven diseases over nearly two decades and examined how it related to both the mortality rate of a disease and the organized advocacy activity in response to a disease. They found that both *who* and *how many* suffer from a disease help explain why some diseases get more attention than others. The authors report that diseases that affect blacks more than whites receive less attention in the media, and that AIDS is viewed differently than other diseases.

To understand the effects of disease in society, it is also necessary to understand the impact of illness. For it is in the social world of illness that the sick and the well must face one another and come to terms.

References

Barker-Benfield, G.J. 1976. *The Horrors of the Half-Known Life*. New York: Harper and Row.

Bell, Susan E. 1987. "Premenstrual Syndrome and the Medicalization of Menopause: A Sociological Perspective." In *Premenstrual Syndrome: Ethical and Legal Implications in a Biomedical Perspective*, edited by Benson E. Ginsburg and Bonnie Frank Carter, 151–73. New York: Plenum.

Boston Women's Health Book Collective. 2011. *Our Bodies, Ourselves*. New York: Touchstone.

Brandt, Allen M. 1985. *No Magic Bullet*. New York: Oxford University Press.

Caballero, B. 2007. "The Global Epidemic of Obesity: An Overview." *Epidemiology Review* 29: 1–5.

Conrad, Peter, and Kristin K. Barker. 2010. "The Social Construction of Illness: Key Insights and Policy Implications." *Journal of Health and Social Behavior* 51: S67–79.

Ehrenreich, Barbara, and Deirdre English. 1978. *On Her Own*. New York: Doubleday.

Figert, Ann. 1995. "Three Faces of PMS: The Professional, Gendered and Scientific Structuring of a Psychiatric Disorder." *Social Problems* 42: 56–73.

Gusfield, Joseph R. 1967. "Moral Passage: The Symbolic Process in the Public Designations of Deviance." *Social Problems* 15: 175–88.

Gussow, Zachary, and George Tracy. 1968. "Status, Ideology, and Adaptation to Stigmatized Illness: A Study of Leprosy." *Human Organization* 27: 316–25.

Herek, Gregory. 1999. "AIDS and Stigma." *American Behavioral Scientist* 42: 1106–16.

Houck, Judith A. 2006. *Hot and Bothered: Women, Medicine and Menopause in Modern America*. Cambridge: Harvard University Press.

Kaufert, Patricia A. 1982. "Myth and the Menopause." *Sociology of Health and Illness* 4: 141–66.

Klitzman, Robert. 1997. *Being Positive: Lives of Men and Women with HIV*. Chicago: Ivan R. Dee.

Lee, Rachel S., Arlene Kochman, and Kathleen Sikkema. 2002. "Internalized Stigma Among People Living With HIV-AIDS." *AIDS and Behavior* 6: 309–19.

Lock, Margaret. 1993. *Encounters With Aging: Mythologies of Menopause in Japan and North America*. Berkeley: University of California Press.

McCrea, Frances. 1983. "The Politics of Menopause: The 'Discovery' of a Deficiency Disease." *Social Problems* 31: 111–123.

Nelkin, Dorothy, David P. Willis, and Scott Parris. 1991. *A Disease of Society: Cultural and Social Responses to AIDS*. New York: Cambridge University Press.

Parker, Richard, and Peter Aggleton. 2003. "HIV and AIDS-Related Stigma and Discrimination: A Conceptual Framework and Implications for Action." *Social Science & Medicine* 57: 13–24.

Perrow, Charles, and Mauro F. Guillén. 1990. *The AIDS Disaster*. New Haven: Yale University Press.

Riessman, Catherine K. 1983. "Women and Medicalization." *Social Policy* 14: 3–18.

Riska, Ellaine. 2003. "Gendering the Medicalization Thesis." *Advances in Gender Research* 7: 59–87.

Rushing, William. 1995. *The AIDS Epidemic: Social Dimensions of an Infectious Disease*. Boulder, CO: Westview Press.

Schneider, Joseph W., and Peter Conrad. 1983. *Having Epilepsy: The Experience and Control of Illness*. Philadelphia: Temple University Press.

Sontag, Susan. 1988. *Illness and Its Metaphors*. New York: Farrar, Straus and Giroux.

Stults, Cheryl, and Peter Conrad. 2008. "Medicalization, Pharmaceuticals and Public Risk Scares: The Case of Menopause and HRT." In *The Risks of Prescription Drugs*, edited by Donald Light. New York: Columbia University Press.

Wertz, Richard, and Dorothy Wertz. 1989. *Lying-In: A History of Childbirth in America*. New Haven: Yale University Press.

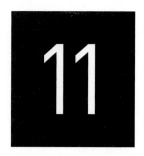

MORALITY AND HEALTH

News Media Constructions of Overweight and Eating Disorders

Abigail C. Saguy and Kjerstin Gruys

In 2005, in the wealthy suburbs of Richmond, Virginia, Emily and Mark Krudys' ten-year-old daughter, Katherine, was diagnosed with anorexia, and her parents were desperate for a cure. "Emily and Mark tried everything. They were firm. Then they begged their daughter to eat. Then they bribed her. We'll buy you a pony, they told her. But nothing worked" (Tyre 2005). Finally, Katherine was admitted for inpatient treatment at a children's hospital in another town. During the two months of her daughter's treatment, Emily stayed nearby so that she could attend family-therapy sessions. After Katherine was released, Emily homeschooled her while Katherine regained strength. Considered a success story, *Newsweek* reported that Katherine entered sixth grade in fall of 2005: "She's got the pony, and she's become an avid horsewoman, sometimes riding five or six times a week . . . But the

anxiety still lingers. When Katherine says she's hungry, Emily has been known to drop everything and whip up a three-course meal" (Tyre 2005).

Only a short drive away, in Washington, DC, Leslie Abbott, a black single mother, was dealing with a very different food battle. She had lost custody of her son Terrell after months of fighting neglect charges related to his body weight. Known to his friends as "Heavy T," Terrell had recently been released from an inpatient weight-loss program, but—once at home—had gained weight. Leslie explained to a reporter why it was unfair for public authorities to blame her for Terrell's backslide: "This boy is 15, going to be 16 years old. I can't watch him 24 hours a day. They want me to hold his hand, take him to the Y, make him eat salad" (Eaton 2007). Leslie said she would have had to quit her minimum-wage job in order to follow

Morality and Health: News Media Constructions of Overweight and Eating Disorders, Abigail C. Saguy and Kjerstin Gruys in *Social Problems*, *57*(2): 231–250, 2010. With permission from Oxford University Press.

the health regimen suggested by Terrell's doctors. But, as noted by the journalist, "How could she afford that? To her thinking, the healthy food Terrell needed meant she needed more money, not less" (Eaton 2007).

These two news articles discuss topics—anorexia and obesity—in which body size (too thin or too heavy) and eating (too little or too much) are treated as medical risks and/or diseases. The American Psychiatric Association (APA) defines anorexia as the refusal to maintain body weight at or above a minimally "normal weight" for age and height, fear of gaining weight or becoming "fat," and denial of the gravity of one's low body weight. The Centers for Disease Control and Prevention (CDC) defines "obesity" among adults as having a body mass index (BMI) (weight in kilograms divided by height in meters squared) equal to or greater than 30, and "overweight" as having a BMI equal or greater than 25 but less than 30.[1] Different measures are used for children and teenagers under 18 years old, which adjust for age.

This research received funding from the Center for the Advanced Study in the Behavioral Sciences at Stanford University, the Center for the Study of Women at UCLA, the Center for American Politics and Public Policy at UCLA, the UCLA Graduate Research Mentorship Program, and the UCLA Senate. This research is part of a larger project funded by a post-doctoral fellowship from the Robert Wood Johnson Foundation Program in Health Policy Research and the Fund for the Advancement of the Discipline (run jointly by the American Sociological Association and the National Science Foundation). Isabelle Huguet Lee, Erika Hernandez, and Roxana Ghashghaei provided invaluable research assistance. Earlier versions of this article were presented at the Van Leer Institute in January 2009 and at the 2008 American Sociological Association annual meeting. The authors wish to thank Rodney Benson, Dana Britton, Paul Campos, Ted Chiricos, Shari Dworkin, Katherine Flegal, Betsy Lucal, Paul McAuley, Joya Misra, Mignon Moore, Stefan Timmermans, and the anonymous *Social Problems* reviewers for comments on previous drafts. The authors take full responsibility for all errors.

While anorexia and overweight/obesity are both medical categories related to body weight and eating, they have strikingly different social and moral connotations. In the contemporary United States, being heavy is seen as the embodiment of gluttony, sloth, and/or stupidity (Crandall and Eshleman 2003; Latner and Stunkard 2003), while slenderness is taken as the embodiment of virtue (Bordo 1993). A deep-seated cultural belief in self-reliance makes body size—like wealth—especially likely to be regarded as being under personal control and as reflecting one's moral fiber (Stearns 1997).

To what extent does the contemporary American social and moral valence of body size shape how the news media report on overweight/obesity and eating disorders as medical issues? Comparing only the two news media articles mentioned previously suggests that the news media treats anorexics as *victims* of a terrible illness beyond their and their parents' control, while obesity is caused by bad individual behavior, including, in the case of children, parental neglect. Second, the difference in class and racial profile of these two families is striking. A young white girl from a well-to-do family provides "the face" of anorexia, while a young boy and his low-earning, black single mother are discussed in an article on obesity. If these reflect typical patterns in reporting, then news reports on eating disorders and obesity may reinforce moral hierarchies based on body size, race, and class. That is, they may reproduce stereotypes of young white female victims and irresponsible, out-of-control lower class minorities. Moreover, articles may represent the issues of eating disorders and overweight differently depending on which demographic groups are the focus of the discussion.

To investigate this issue more systematically, we draw on content analyses of 332 articles published between 1995 and 2005 in *The New York Times* and *Newsweek* on the topic of eating disorders or overweight/obesity. We also draw on qualitative analyses of five additional articles published in these publications in 2006 and 2007 that specifically discuss binge eating disorder and were not included in our larger sample. We examine how news reports on these issues assign blame and responsibility as well as how they discuss gender, race, and class. In so doing, we contribute to sociological understandings of how cultural values shape the construction of social problems and, in turn, reproduce social inequalities.

THEORETICAL PERSPECTIVE

Body weight has long been a marker of social status. However, at most times and in most places, where food is scarce, corpulence signals *high* rather than low status. In these cultures, plumpness in women is especially prized. Among elite Nigerian Arabs, for instance, girls are fattened up in early childhood (Popenoe 2005). A young girl's girth is physical evidence of her father's—and later her husband's—wealth. Being so fat that she is immobile signifies that her labor is not needed, making fat women the ultimate "trophy wives." Similarly, up until the early twentieth century, women in the United States and Europe strived to be fat, not thin. There too, food was scarce and plumpness signaled wealth, while thinness suggested illness (Klein 1996; Stearns 1997). Yet, while thinness was regarded as ungainly in these contexts, especially in women, it did not reflect on one's *moral* character (Stearns 1997), nor have individual women been personally blamed for being too thin (Popenoe 2005).

As the agricultural and industrial revolutions reduced food shortages, fatness was no longer a reliable sign of wealth and, as the poor got fatter, the symbolic meaning of body size flipped. As corpulence increasingly became a marker for *lower* prestige and status, those with greater resources had more ability and motivation to avoid the stigma of fatness (Aronowitz 2008). Moreover, as moral condemnation of consumerism lessened, maintaining a slender body became the new way for Americans to demonstrate their moral virtue. As Historian Peter Stearns (1997) argues, beginning in the late nineteenth and early twentieth century:

People could indulge their taste for fashion and other products with a realization that, if they disciplined their bodies through an

attack on fat, they could preserve or even enhance their health and also establish their moral credentials . . . An appropriately slender figure could denote the kind of firm character, capable of self-control, that one would seek in a good worker in an age of growing indulgence; ready employability and weight management could be conflated (p. 59–60).

This moral association of slenderness with "firm character" and heaviness as the embodiment of gluttony, sloth, and stupidity is still with us today (Bordo 1993; Crandall and Eshleman 2003; Latner and Stunkard 2003). In the United States, where there is a deep-seated cultural belief in self-reliance, body size is especially likely to be regarded as under personal control and reflecting moral fiber (Stearns 1997), despite research suggesting that much of the variation in body size is biologically determined (Kolata 2007). Thinness is a *cultural value* in the contemporary United States—it is a quality that is widely prized by members of this society.

In the contemporary United States, body size intersects with other dimensions of inequality. Stereotypes of fat people as gluttonous and undisciplined echo similar stereotypes of the working classes as "the archetypal 'uncontrolled' body in public health discourse, as lazy, dirty, immoral, incapable of resisting their urges" (Lupton 1995:75). Compared to men, women are held to higher standards of thinness and suffer greater penalties if they fall short, in terms of marriage prospects as well as employment (Conley and Glauber 2007; Puhl, Andreyeva, and Brownell 2008). On average, wealthier white people—especially women—tend to be thinner than poorer people of color (Flegal et al. 1998; Flegal et al. 2002; Sobal and Stunkard 1989). This is, in part, because having a thin and toned body is expensive in contemporary Western contexts, where fresh fruits and vegetables are more expensive than higher calorie processed foods and where physical activity requires leisure time (Drewnowski and Barratt-Fornell 2004). Heavier women are also poorer, however, because of weight-based stigma. For women, higher body mass *predicts* lower personal and spousal earnings (Puhl et al. 2008).

Negative stereotypes of fatness and ethnic minority status often reinforce each other, such that a fat black woman is stigmatized for both her body size and race. However, these stigmas can also be disassociated with various consequences. Thus, a white middle class woman will lose some of her class and racial privilege if she is heavy, while a woman of color can gain status by being thin. Realizing this, some black and Latino families pressure their daughters to be thin as part of a strategy of upward mobility (Thompson 1994).

Yet, white middle class women and girls are more likely than poorer women and girls, women and girls of color, and boys or men to be diagnosed with anorexia or bulimia, also referred to as "thinness-oriented eating disorders" (Bruch 1978; Striegel-Moore et al. 2003).[2] In contrast, rates of binge eating disorder, which are often associated with higher body weight, are similar among black women, white women, and white men (Smith et al. 1998). Indeed, some scholars have found recurrent binge eating to be *more* common among black women than among white women (Striegel-Moore et al. 2000). This makes news media discussions of binge eating disorder important for understanding how discussions of eating and body weight are racialized and gendered.

Anorexia is listed in the *Diagnostic and Statistical Manual of Mental Disorders* (*DSM-IV*) as an eating disorder, along with bulimia, which is defined as recurrent episodes of binge eating (eating extremely large amounts of food in one sitting) followed by "inappropriate compensatory" purging (i.e., by vomiting and/or talking laxatives) and an undue influence of body shape in self-evaluation. Binge eating disorder is categorized in the *DSM-IV* as an "Eating Disorder—Not Otherwise Specified," an umbrella category for various eating disorders that do not meet the precise criteria for either anorexia or bulimia. The APA provides a "provisional diagnosis" of binge eating disorder as bingeing without compensatory purging and/or extreme dietary constraint (APA1994). This provisional diagnosis signals that binge eating disorder is being seriously considered for its own diagnostic category in the *DSM-V* (expected in 2012), while also providing clinical researchers with shared criteria for

studying the disorder. Binge eating is likely to be the object of more public discussions as it gains more attention from clinicians.

The mass media offer important primary sources for cultural and social research. Television, radio, magazines, newspapers, and Internet content provide a sensitive barometer of social process and change. Once created, these texts remain unchanged and available for analysis, making them ideal for the study of attitudes, concerns, ideologies, and power relations, and how they shift over time (Lupton 1994). Aware of these strengths, early feminist work examined the fashion media, demonstrating how fashion magazines and advertisements convey to readers the importance of slenderness and the shame of fatness for women (Bordo 1993). Anthropologist Mimi Nichter (2000) has argued that such images contribute to negative body image and eating problems among young girls; however, she finds that African American girls are buffered from fashion pressures to be thin by a vibrant ethnic culture that values personal style as well as "thicker" body types.

News accounts of health and illness differ from other media texts in that they have the weight of "expert" opinion, making them especially important to study (Lupton 1994; Nelkin 1987). In recent years, a few scholars have begun examining media reporting on the so-called "obesity epidemic" (Boero 2007; Lawrence 2004; Saguy and Almeling 2008). Natalie Boero (2007) finds that news reporting has largely framed obesity as a moral problem of gluttony and sloth. Abigail C. Saguy and Rene Almeling (2008) find that body size is predominantly blamed on individual choices rather than social or biological factors, while Regina Lawrence (2004) shows that there is increasing discussion of social-structural factors over time. Saguy and Almeling (2008) find that news reports on scientific findings are more likely than the original research on which they report to focus on individual blame and to describe obesity as a public health crisis and/or epidemic. They further find that articles discussing the poor, blacks, or Latinos are more likely than articles not discussing these groups to blame body size on individual choices (Saguy and Almeling 2008). Similarly, previous research has shown that news reports are more likely to portray welfare recipients as dependent (and thus unworthy) when they are unmarried or black, compared to when they are widowed or white (Misra, Moller, and Karides 2003). These studies suggest that news reports will blame individuals for overweight and obesity, especially when such individuals are poor and/or from minority ethnic groups, thus reflecting and reinforcing negative stereotypes of fat people, the poor, and ethnic minorities.

While important, extant studies have methodological and conceptual limitations. For instance, Lawrence (2004) does not examine how views about gender, race, or class inform news media reports of obesity, while Boero (2007) draws heavily on qualitative analysis of seven articles published in the fall of 2000 as part of a series on the "Fat Epidemic," thereby limiting the generalizability of her findings. Saguy and Almeling's (2008) analysis of news reporting on two special issues on obesity published in the *Journal of the American Medical Association (JAMA)* in 1999 and 2003 allows for a systematic examination of how scientific research is popularized by the news media, but does not constitute a representative sample of reporting on the topic of overweight/obesity. Moreover, because all of these studies lack a comparative case, it is impossible to know the extent to which these patterns are simply a product of generic news media routines that favor sensationalism and morality tales (Schudson 2003), combined perhaps with health policy tendencies to emphasize individual blame and responsibility (Fitzpatrick 2000; Lupton 1995; Tesh 1988).

Motivated by research on social problem construction (Best 2008; Gusfield 1981; Kitsuse and Spector 1973) and news media framing research (e.g., Benson and Saguy 2005; Entman 1993; Gamson 1992), this article examines how news reports *frame* overweight/obesity and eating disorders in particular ways by drawing attention to some aspects of these issues while obscuring others. It draws on quantitative and qualitative analyses of a random sample of news reports on overweight/obesity or eating disorders published between 1995 and 2005 in *The New York Times* and *Newsweek*. The comparative case study allows us to disentangle general aspects of news reporting from the specific cases at hand. In that anorexics and bulimics are seen as pursuing a culturally valued ideal (slenderness), we expect that the news media will be less likely to blame them—compared to the overweight or obese—for their malady. Rather, we expect anorexics and bulimics to be portrayed as victims of a host of complex factors beyond their control. To the extent that the news media focuses on cases of young, white middle class anorexics and bulimics, they risk reproducing cultural stereotypes of young, white female victims. In contrast, in that the news media frame overweight/obesity as a public health crisis produced by irresponsible individuals, while focusing on cases of overweight among the poor and minorities, they are likely to reinforce negative stereotypes based on body size, ethnicity, and class.

DATA AND METHODS

Our news sample is drawn from *The New York Times* and *Newsweek*. Widely regarded as the newspaper of record, *The New York Times* enjoys among the highest national circulation of any newspaper and is considered authoritative, giving it influence over opinion leaders and policy makers. Reporting in *The New York Times* has also been shown to shape reporting in other news media (Gans 1979). *The New York Times* is known for a relatively high quality of reporting on health issues, biasing our sample towards more sophisticated reporting on these issues. The newsmagazine *Newsweek* has the advantage of publishing longer articles than those a newspaper can usually accommodate. These two publications have the methodological advantage of being available in the Lexis-Nexis database for the entire 1995–2005 time period. This sample does not capture some of the range of the news media, including women's magazines, the ethnic press, or political presses (Rohlinger 2007). Given that the majority of readers of these papers are white and from the middle class, it is possible that these publications are more likely—compared to ethnic presses or presses catering to a more working class audience—to uncritically reproduce negative stereotypes regarding heavier people, the poor, and ethnic minorities. Nonetheless, given their cultural influence, they are critical to study.

We sampled from news articles and opinion pieces published that had the words "anorexia/anorexic/bulimia/bulimic" or "obese/obesity/overweight" in the heading or leading paragraphs. Using these search criteria for the specified time period generated a chronological list of articles by publication and by issue, totaling 1,496 articles. We winnowed down this list using three criteria. First, because there were so many articles published on obesity or overweight in *The New York Times,* we eliminated the first two of every three articles in the chronological *New York Times* list of articles on obesity/overweight, reducing this sample by two thirds. (Cross-publication analyses reveal that the differences between publications on the variables we discuss are minor. Thus, the fact that proportionally more eating disorder articles are from *The New York Times* is unlikely to account for the cross-issue differences we report.) Second, we eliminated articles that were less than 300 words, since it is difficult to develop the themes of interest in such a short article, which reduced the sample further by over one half. Finally, from this list, we eliminated the few articles from the full sample that were completely off topic. This strategy yielded a final sample of 174 articles on obesity and 64 on eating disorders from the *New York Times* and 88 articles on obesity and 6 on eating disorders from *Newsweek,* or a total of 262 articles on overweight/obesity and 70 articles on eating disorders.

This sampling strategy produced seven articles that discussed binge eating disorder—six of which met the sampling criteria for anorexia/bulimia and a seventh that met the criteria for overweight/obesity. An additional search of articles that had "binge eating disorder" anywhere in the full text yielded no new articles. In an effort to expand the number of articles on binge eating disorder, a "newer" eating disorder of growing importance, we further searched for all articles published between January 2006 and November 13, 2007 (the day the search was conducted) that had "binge eating disorder" in the full text. This identified an additional five relevant articles (three from *The New York Times* and

two from *Newsweek*). While these five articles are not included in the core 332 articles that were analyzed quantitatively, they were separately analyzed qualitatively (along with the seven articles from our original sampling technique) to inform the discussion of binge eating disorder below.

We focus on 1995 through 2005, a time frame that includes a long period characterized by a moderate level of press attention to eating disorders and a surge of attention to obesity in the late 1990s and early twenty-first century. It does not include the 1980s, a period when concern over anorexia was arguably at its height among the medical community (Hof and Nicolson 1996) but when news media attention to anorexia/bulimia in *The New York Times* and *Newsweek* was actually lower (see Figure 11.1).

Given that there is considerably more news reporting on overweight/obesity beginning in 2002 (see Figure 11.1), following several high-profile pronouncements from the CDC, the World Health Organization (WHO), and the Surgeon General about the "obesity epidemic" at the end of 2001 (Schlesinger 2005), our overweight sample is weighted towards the latter time period, while our eating disorder sample is spread more evenly across the decade. Comparisons of reporting by time period (1995–2001, 2002–2005) reveal one important change in framing over time: there is more discussion of social-structural causes and policy solutions for overweight in later years (see also Lawrence 2004). Thus, our sample—by virtue of including disproportionately more articles published in later years—may overstate the extent to which, during the entire 1995–2005 time period, the news media emphasized social-structural causes for the "obesity epidemic" and policy solutions.

Coding

A subsample of articles was initially read to develop variables for the content analysis. Knowledge of the obesity and eating disorders literature was also used to develop the variables. Some variables were added or refined during the analyses, requiring additional coding. Coding was done at the article level for over 200 variables for all of

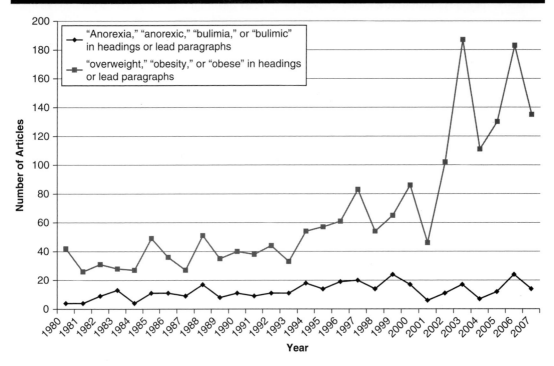

FIGURE 11.1 ■ **News Reporting on Anorexia/Bulimia and Overweight/Obesity, New York Times or Newsweek**

the articles in our sample. In initial "practice" coding, three researchers coded the same articles and discussed differences as a way of arriving at shared agreement. Two coders coded 10 percent of the articles to test for inter-coder reliability, which was very high. The coefficient of reliability (the ratio of coding agreements to the total number of coding decisions) was over .95 (Holsti 1969), and discrepancies were generally due to one person having missed a relevant phrase, rather than to conceptual disagreements about how the variables should be coded. Unless explicitly stated below, variables were dichotomous, coded for whether or not the aspect in question was mentioned at all. Thus all codes are independent of each other. Coders did not determine which themes dominated the article, only if they were present at all. In our discussion, we discuss differences between the overweight/obesity and anorexia/bulimia samples *as differences* only when the chi-square (in cases where cell sizes were 10 or more) or Fisher

exact test (in cases where cell sizes were less than 10) were statistically significant at a level of $p < .05$. We cannot statistically test whether a specific theme is more common than another *within* a given sample, since these observations are not independent of each other, a condition of a chi-square or exact test. Discussions of relative frequency of different themes within each sample should be read with this caveat in mind.

Articles were coded for whether they were standard articles or opinion pieces (i.e., editorials, op-ed, or letters to the editor). Opinion pieces offer a revealing window on issue framing since the editorial page's purpose is to air competing frames (see also Lawrence 2004:60). While journalists themselves do not produce most op-ed pieces and letters to the editor, editors do select who among many contenders will be published. Moreover, their publication in mainstream media gives them cultural authority. We did, nonetheless, replicate our analyses with a sample that excluded the opinion pieces and found consistent results.

To evaluate how news reports assign responsibility for eating disorders and overweight, we coded articles for whether they blamed these things on individual choices or structural factors, such as restaurant portions or messages from the fashion industry. For instance, the following article blames an *individual* for his weight gain, writing "he could look back on decades of binge eating and failed diets" and quoting him as saying "I was killing myself" (Feder 2005). The following would be taken as evidence of blaming *structural* factors: "In many low-income minority neighborhoods, fried carryout is a cinch to find, but affordable fresh produce and nutritious food are not" (*New York Times* 2002). Considered a subset of structural factors, we coded specifically for cultural factors, such as mainstream cultural emphasis on thinness, ethnic culinary practices, or cultural attitudes towards body size, as in the following excerpt: "Being curvy or large was a source of pride within the African American community" (Brodey 2005). We coded for whether articles blamed biological factors, including genetics or prenatal environment, as in the following: "Doctors now compare anorexia to alcoholism and depression, potentially fatal diseases that . . . have their roots in a complex combination of genes and brain chemistry" (Tyre 2005). We coded for whether the article specifically described overweight or eating disorders as a *psychological* problem or labeled either as a (physical or mental) *disease.* Labeling a condition a disease did not necessarily mean that it was ascribed to biological factors. Rather, disease could be attributed to bad lifestyle choices or environmental factors.

By focusing on certain kinds of *solutions,* the news media also convey messages about what sort of problem is being discussed and what should be done about it. If they focus on individual-level solutions, they reinforce the sense that these are problems caused by individuals that individuals need to fix. By discussing policy solutions, they convey that these are collective problems. However, by discussing policy interventions that aim to educate or change bad behaviors of certain groups, they reinforce the sense

that the targeted groups are ignorant. We coded for different types of solutions to weight problems, including behavioral modification (e.g., dieting, increasing exercise), policy changes, inpatient or "intensive outpatient" medical supervision, or prescription drugs and weight-related surgeries. During analyses, we computed a composite variable for any medical intervention, including weight-loss drugs, psychiatric or appetite regulating medications, weight-loss surgery, medical devices such as feeding tubes, or either inpatient or "intensive outpatient" medical supervision.

Finally, to account for how, and to what extent, these issues are associated with different groups, we coded articles for whether they explicitly mentioned specific demographic groups, including men or women; the poor, middle class, or rich; and whites, blacks, Latinos, Asians, and other race. During analyses, we computed composite variables, including "middle class or rich," "nonwhite" and "blacks, Latinos, or the poor."

In addition to the quantitative analysis, we used discourse analysis to get at the subtleties of news reports, including the choice of words and ideologies evident in news reports (Lupton 1994). We created theme sheets that included lengthy quotes that illustrated key themes, such as blame, responsibility, and moral judgment. The quantitative data allows for us to test for statistical significance of differences in reporting across these issues, while the qualitative data permits us to dig deeper into the nuances of reporting.

FINDINGS

Our news sample typically attributes anorexia and bulimia to a host of complex and interrelated factors, thus mitigating individual blame while representing anorexics and bulimics as victims. In contrast, it predominantly blames overweight exclusively on bad individual choices and emphasizes individual-level weight loss solutions. News reports emphasize medical intervention when it comes to anorexia and bulimia *but not* when discussing binge eating disorder, which they tend to deny the status of a real eating disorder and frame instead as *ordinary* overeating caused by lack of self-control and requiring greater personal discipline. After reviewing the quantitative patterns, we examine each case qualitatively.

As shown in Figure 11.2, news reports on both eating disorders and overweight invoke personal choices, with over 40 percent of articles in both categories mentioning personal choices as contributors. However, several factors are described as equally contributing to eating disorders, while individual choice is the *predominant* explanation offered for overweight. Articles about eating disorders discuss structural causes at the same rate as individual choices (47 percent for both), while 19 percent of eating disorder article cite biological causes. In contrast, 41 percent of articles about overweight mention individual choices, with socio-structural and biological causes mentioned in 29 and 16 percent of articles, respectively. Press reports are more likely to describe eating disorders, compared to overweight, as a disease (29 percent versus 4 percent) and/or as a psychological problem (27 percent

versus 3 percent) triggered by cultural messages (30 percent versus 8 percent).

Even more strikingly, as shown in Figure 11.3, the articles were much less likely to hold individuals responsible for curing eating disorders (4 percent of eating disorder sample) than for fixing overweight (56 percent of overweight sample). Articles in the eating disorders sample discuss medical interventions at least *seven times* more frequently than they mention either policy or behavioral solutions (54 percent versus 7 percent and 4 percent, respectively). In contrast, articles on overweight/obesity are over twice as likely to discuss behavioral modification than either medical interventions (24 percent) or policy solutions (21 percent). Forty-six percent of articles on eating disorders, but no articles on overweight, discuss *only* medical solutions.

As is shown in Figure 11.4, 94 percent of eating disorder articles discuss women or girls, compared to 47 percent that mention men or boys. By contrast, articles on overweight mention women/girls and men/boys at similar rates, (47 percent compared to 42 percent). As shown in Figure 11.5, 13 percent

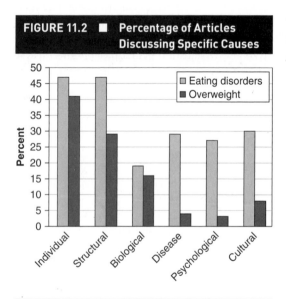

FIGURE 11.2 ■ Percentage of Articles Discussing Specific Causes

Note: With the exception of individual and biological causes, all cross-issue differences are statistically significant (*p* < .05, one-tailed tests).

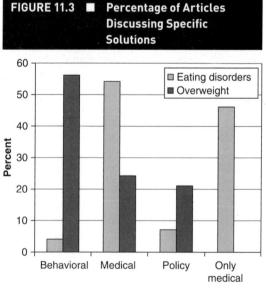

FIGURE 11.3 ■ Percentage of Articles Discussing Specific Solutions

Note: All cross-issue differences are statistically significant (*p* < .05, one-tailed tests).

of articles on eating disorders discuss people from the upper or middle class, compared to the four percent that discuss poor people, and 17 percent

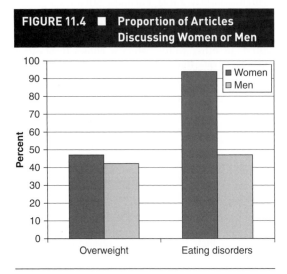

FIGURE 11.4 ■ Proportion of Articles Discussing Women or Men

Note: Frequencies of specific themes *within the same sample* are *not* independent of each other and are therefore unsuitable for a chi-square text of statistical significance.

FIGURE 11.5 ■ Proportion of Articles Discussing Specific Demographic Groups

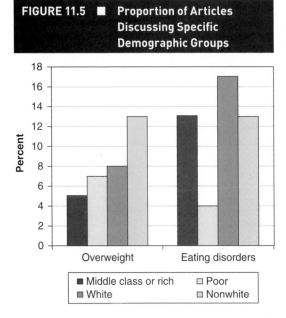

Note: Frequencies of specific themes *within the same sample* are *not* independent of each other and are therefore unsuitable for a chi-square text of statistical significance.

mention whites, compared to 13 percent that discuss minority races, despite the tendency for "white" to function as an unmarked category.[3] In contrast, articles on overweight discuss nonwhites (including blacks, Latino, Asian, and other race) more often than whites (13 percent versus 8 percent) and discuss the poor as frequently as the middle class or rich (7 percent versus 5 percent).

Moreover, as shown in Figure 11.6, we find that news reports mentioning blacks, Latinos, or the poor are more likely to blame social structural factors, but not biological factors, for overweight/obesity. Forty-three percent of articles mentioning these groups, compared to 26 percent of articles that do not mention these groups, cite social structural contributors to obesity, a difference that is statistically significant. Coded as a subset of social-structural factors, cultural causes for overweight/obesity are also significantly more likely to be mentioned when blacks, Latinos, or the poor are cited (17 percent versus 4 percent), often because—as we discuss later—*minority culture* is being blamed. Articles

FIGURE 11.6 ■ Percentage of Overweight Articles Evoking Specific Frames, by Whether or Not They Discuss Blacks, Latinos, or the Poor

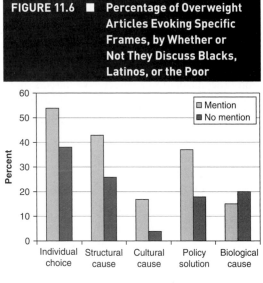

Note: With the exception of biological cause and individual choice, all differences are statistically significant ($p < .05$, one-tailed tests). Thirty-five articles mention blacks, Latinos, or the poor whereas 227 articles do not explicitly mention these groups.

that mention blacks, Latinos, or the poor are also more likely than those that do not mention these groups to discuss obesity policy solutions (37 percent versus 18 percent). As we discuss later, many of these not only address social-structural problems, such as access to affordable fresh fruits and vegetables, but also seek to educate people considered unable to make good food and exercise choices, and to change minority ethnic *cultural attitudes* about food and eating.[4] Fifty-four percent of articles that mention blacks, Latinos, or the poor, compared to 38 percent that do not, discuss how individual choices lead to overweight, but this difference is just shy of statistical significance at $p < .05$ ($p = .055$). Fifteen percent of articles mentioning blacks, Latinos, or the poor discuss biological causes of overweight, compared to 20 percent of articles not mentioning these groups, a difference that is not statistically significant.

Note that the number of articles that *explicitly* mentions blacks, Latinos, or the poor are relatively small, so that most articles that frame obesity as an individual, social-structural, cultural, or biological issue or mention policy solutions do *not* explicitly mention these groups. However, the fact that certain kinds of frames are more or less prevalent depending on the groups being discussed suggests that these news publications may be reproducing common social assumptions about these groups. Next, we flesh out these quantitative patterns with details from the qualitative analyses. We discuss news reporting on (thinness-oriented) eating disorders, overweight, and binge eating disorder, respectively, in three separate sections.

Anorexia and Bulimia: No-One to Blame

A typical article on anorexia evokes "complex webs of cultural factors and psychological processes" (Isherwood 2005), serving to diffuse responsibility amongst several factors. Similarly, a *Newsweek* editorial proclaims: "Good news: scientists are developing a better sense of how genetic and social triggers interact" (Whitaker 2005). In such articles, genetic factors and social constraints are said to work in tandem, jointly diffusing focus away from individual blame.

In contrast to how parents are frequently blamed for their children's (over) weight problems, the article cited in the introduction to this article concludes: "Parents do play a role, but most often it's a genetic one. In the last 10 years, studies of anorexics have shown that the disease often runs in families" (Tyre 2005). In other words, when it comes to anorexia there is, as the title of this article proclaims, "no-one to blame" (Tyre 2005). Contemporary reports on anorexia tend to portray parents as part of the solution, rather than as part of the problem. For instance, an article on anorexia describes how parents of anorexics "are encouraged to think of the disorder as an outside force that has taken over their daughter's life. And they are exhorted to be unwavering in finding ways to feed their child" (Goode 2002).

Even when an eating disorder is described as beginning with a choice (i.e., to start a diet), the choice is depicted as a "normal" response to cultural pressures, rather than as an irresponsible or self-indulgent behavior. For instance, an article titled "When Weight Loss Goes Awry" describes a teenager's anorexia as beginning with an innocent diet: "last summer, as friends started dieting, she decided to lose five to 10 pounds. Within a few months Amelia, now 15, was on the death-march called anorexia nervosa" (Kalb 2000). Of course, in a society where watching one's weight is a moral obligation, it makes sense that Amelia would not be faulted for beginning a diet. Rather, anorexia is viewed as a case in which good intentions go too far. Amelia is described as "a straight-A student and cheerleader" who says "in a weak but determined voice from her bed at the Children's Hospital in Denver" that she "would never want this to happen to anybody else" (Kalb 2000). The article thus describes anorexia as something that "happens to" people, even model teenagers, rather than something people bring upon themselves. The article states, "there's no simple explanation for why intelligent, often highly accomplished kids spiral into such destructive behavior." It considers a host of factors from "obsessive-compulsive disorder, depression, low self-esteem and anxiety" to the "'reduce fat in your diet' drumbeat, which can haunt children who already feel pressure—from gaunt models or each other—to be thin" (Kalb 2000). Similarly, absolving anorexics from blame, the article cited at the start of this article explains that "For some kids, *innocent*-seeming behavior carries enormous risks" (Tyre 2005, emphasis added).

Despite wide acceptance of dieting as normal and desirable, many news articles point the finger at the narrow beauty standards of popular culture. For instance, discussing anorexia and bulimia, one article declares that "the apparent precipitant of these [eating] disorders seems to be an overwhelming desire to be thin, thin enough to walk down a Paris fashion runway, to act in a Hollywood movie, or to dance with a leading ballet company" (Brody 2000). In these discussions, African American subculture, and specifically an alleged preference for larger female bodies among black Americans, is cast in a positive light, as protecting minority girls from internalizing mainstream pressures to be thin. Quoting a medical doctor, one article reads:

Dr. Brooks said experts traditionally had thought that "anorexia and bulimia didn't happen to black, Asian or Hispanic women, that they were somehow immune." . . . "Curvy African-American women were celebrated," Dr. Brooks said. "These girls didn't experience anxiety and shame about their bodies. Being curvy or large was a source of pride within the African-American community" (Brodey 2005).

Those black (and sometimes Latina) girls who do develop eating disorders are often seen as being especially vulnerable to "white" pressures. The article quoted earlier, for instance, describes how one black teenage girl developed bulimia because, as one of nine black students in a high school of 3,000, she was "struggling simply to be accepted. [In her words:] 'When it came to body image, my perception of beauty was based on my white peers and images of white celebrities in the media'" (Brodey 2005). Thus a mainstream diet culture is implicated in (thinness-oriented) eating disorders, while African American culture is praised as offering some cultural buffering.

Yet, even such blaming of mainstream cultural pressures is tempered by arguing that they only result in eating disorders among people with a biological or psychological predisposition. For example, after noting that doctors have observed a "disturbing trend: a growing group of women in their 30s, 40s and 50s who have eating disorders," one article reassures readers that many of these newly diagnosed older women have actually had lifelong psychological problems and that "lots of people in our culture diet, [but] relatively few end up with an eating disorder" (Rothman Morris 2004). Here, not only are individual dieters not blamed for their behavior but the *culture of dieting* is normalized. Another similar article writes that:

While everyone is exposed to similar societal pressures to be thin, only a small percentage develop eating disorders. Those who succumb typically are prompted by extreme career pressures, as often happens to ballerinas, models, actresses, and jockeys, or they have some underlying emotional and/or physical vulnerability" (Brody 2000).

Similarly, the article cited in the introduction to this article compares anorexia to alcoholism and depression, "potentially fatal diseases that may be set off by environmental factors such as stress or trauma, but have their roots in a complex combination of genes and brain chemistry" (Tyre 2005). It continues:

Many kids are affected by pressure-cooker school environments and a culture of thinness promoted by magazines and music videos, but most of them don't secretly scrape their dinner into the garbage. The environment "pulls the trigger," . . . but it's a child's latent vulnerabilities that "load the gun."

By stressing the complex interplay between individual factors, biological predisposition, and macro-level environmental factors, this type of reporting mitigates blame of individual anorexics and their parents.

As victims of a complex illness, sufferers of eating disorders are not expected to "pull themselves up by their bootstraps." Rather, they are depicted as needing medical intervention. For example, one article describes an anorexic 14-year-old who, despite wanting "to improve," had failed to recover when going it alone: "It took a second hospitalization at Schneider, the following spring, before Molly could maintain a healthy weight" (Hochman 1996). The article cited at the start of this article similarly describes how young Katherine was only able to recover after *repeated* hospitalizations, because she frequently relapsed when not under direct medical supervision (Tyre 2005). Such failures are not seen as evidence of weak-will, as failed diet attempts are, nor are they blamed on their parents. Rather, they are used to underscore the seriousness of anorexia as a medical illness that requires medical intervention.

Even when eating disorder articles explicitly state that individuals can cure themselves, it is almost always under the guidance of a doctor. Thus, we read about new therapies for bulimia in which specially trained nurses coach bulimics to help themselves: "Many bulimics do not need traditional psychiatric therapy. Instead, he said, patients will learn to help themselves. 'What we've done is change the treatment into a self-help format,' said Dr. Fairburn" (Liotta 1999). Yet, when "self-help" for eating disorders is enacted under medical supervision, curing disordered individuals is still presented as the responsibility of an expert physician.

Obesity: No-One to Blame but Yourself (and Your Parents)

In contrast to reporting on eating disorders, even when articles mention more than one cause for overweight, individual blame usually predominates. For instance, a *Newsweek* article explains that "you can't pick your parents, but you can pick what you eat and how often you exercise" (Barrett Ozols 2005). Thus, genetics does not provide an excuse for body weight. Rather, the article emphasizes people's ability (and, seemingly, their obligation) to make *choices* regarding diet and exercise. Similarly, another article cites new research on "race and weight," explaining that

"on average, black women burn nearly 100 fewer calories a day than white women do when their bodies are at rest" but cautions that "the new findings do not mean that controlling and losing weight is a hopeless task for people with lower metabolic rates, just that it may require *more attention to diet and exercise*" (Brody 1997, emphasis added). Again, the reader is reminded that managing her weight is her responsibility. In that pursuing health has become a moral obligation (Edgley and Brissett 1990), this responsibility carries moral connotations.

Moreover, while heaping the blame on individuals, news reports also draw upon and reproduce stereotypes of fat people as gluttonous, slothful, and ignorant, and of parents of fat children as neglectful and irresponsible. Thus, such reports reproduce the negative moral valence of fatness. For instance, one *Newsweek* article writes:

> Bruce and Lisa Smith never skimped much on food. Chips, fried chicken, canned fruit, sodas—they ate as much as they wanted, whenever they wanted. Exercise? Pretty much nonexistent, unless you count working the TV remote or the computer mouse. "We were out of control," says Bruce, 42. And so was their son, Jarvae, who is 5 feet 4 and weighs 176 pounds (Springen 2007).

The Smiths' obesity is portrayed as the direct consequence of a lifestyle of sloth and gluttony. Few readers would consider working a TV remote or a computer mouse physical exercise. Rather, sarcasm is employed to convey disdain and contempt for the Smiths, who are portrayed as lazy and irresponsible individuals and parents. This same article is unrepentant in its blaming of parents for an alleged impending crisis of global proportions. It continues: "The problem [of childhood obesity] is so grave that some researchers predict that the life expectancy of today's children could shrink by as much as five years. The key to reversing the trend? Parents" (Kalb and Springen 2005). Thus, individuals and parents are not only blamed for the onset of obesity, they are held responsible for "reversing the trend."

The fix is presented as a matter of common sense: "One simple way to get the entire family fit is to turn off the television and shut down the computer" (Kalb and Springen 2005). By describing solutions as "simple," the authors imply a logic under which those who have fat children must be stupid, ignorant, or willfully disobedient. Indeed, in the context of childhood obesity, parents (and especially mothers, who are mentioned over twice as often as fathers)[5] are sometimes described as legally unfit to care for their offspring. This was the context in which Heavy T, discussed in the introduction, was removed from his mother's custody. This type of reporting reproduces negative stereotypes. Likewise, from another *New York Times* article:

> [It] is the confounding truth that parents—whether distracted, oblivious or both—are ultimately to blame for what their children eat. "Parents were created for that function," said Dan Jaffe, executive vice president for government relations at the Association of National Advertisers, an organization based in Washington whose members include food companies. "I don't know of any little child who jumps in the car and drives to a supermarket and buys their own food" (Buss 2004).

Again, this article portrays obesity as the product of parental neglect, heaping moral blame on the parents of heavy children. Another article portrays a lawsuit against McDonald's as absurd, arguing that it was the plaintiffs own fault for "gorging themselves so wantonly" on fast food, whether ignorant of, or indifferent to, the likely consequences:

> The [two black-girl plaintiffs from the Bronx] in the McDonald's lawsuit use their ignorance as an argument, claiming that if they'd only known about the nutritional shortcomings of fast food, they certainly would not have gorged themselves so wantonly. (If that's really true, they should consider a lawsuit against their parents for endangering the welfare of their children rather than a suit against McDonald's) (Kuntzman 2002).

The word *wanton* is often used to indicate lewd or bawdy behavior and is clearly moralizing. Similarly, to *gorge* is to consume greedily, thus conjuring up gluttony. Thus, these girls are represented as immorally stuffing themselves with food. That they did not know any better is mentioned as grounds for a lawsuit for neglect against their parents. Also evoking parental responsibility, a letter to the editor in *Newsweek* (2000) asks "Are adults who permit their children to eat as they please (meaning anything and everything) supremely ignorant or genuinely abusive?"

In that heavier body weight is negatively associated with socioeconomic status and given that blacks and Latinos tend to have higher body mass than whites, any discourse that blames people for weighing too much risks reinforcing class and racial stigma. This is even more true when news reports focus on cases of overweight among blacks, Latinos, or the poor. Moreover, many news articles *explicitly* blame ethnic communities for contributing to higher rates of obesity amongst their own. For instance, an article reporting on a women's health study states that "more subtle societal influences, like differences in acceptable body images among different ethnic groups, all contributed to greater obesity among women with lower incomes and those in certain ethnic groups" (Santora 2005). Ethnic culinary practices are also blamed for the alleged obesity epidemic. For instance, a 2003 *New York Times* article discusses how Latino culinary preferences contribute to overweight among Latino children: "[Mr. Batista] says some cultural habits are simply getting the best of his people. Latinos eating vegetables? Come on, he says, raising his hands in frustration. 'We don't eat vegetables. It's rice and beans and meat. It's very natural'" (Richardson 2003).

Another article, discussing the higher rate of overweight among minorities in inner cities, quotes a news source who acknowledges that "it is easier and less expensive to eat fast food and very difficult to find, in some of these neighborhoods, appropriate foods, fruits, and vegetables at a reasonable price" (Braiker 2003). But the article then shifts to a focus on ethnic culture:

In the end, she says, "it will take a culture change" to reverse the trend ... "Eating healthy is synonymous with whiteness for some of these kids," [an activist] says. They'll be like, "Salmon? That's white people food." There are ways to make it more accessible; the first part is about education. (Braiker 2003).

Thus, ethnic minorities are depicted as backward or ignorant and needing to be educated in proper food choices and preparation, thus reproducing stereotypes based on race as well as body size.

Consistent with such stereotypes, many of the policy interventions discussed seek to educate people—and especially ethnic minorities—to make better choices. For instance, an article chronicling a public health intervention in a southern black community describes a recipe for "low-fat catfish" developed by nutritionists as "one of a series [of new recipes] showcasing revered family recipes purged of their sins by two Auburn University nutritionists" and notes how a leader of a public health intervention "recited a litany of virtuous eating for her largely female audience" (Markus 1998). The moral associations with food and eating in this article are striking. As with articles on eating disorders, this article identifies mothers as a crucial part of the solution, recounting how these interventions recruit minority mothers as "cheerleaders for good health" (Markus 1998) and target them as the preparers of food for their families: "We're building on community talent with women who are cooking for their children and passing on behavior patterns to their children and their children's children" (Markus 1998).

Binge Eating Disorder: A Need for Self-Control

Articles that discuss binge eating disorder in detail draw upon frames typical of *both* thinness-oriented eating disorders articles and of articles on overweight, underscoring the extent to which this condition straddles the symbolic space between usually polarized conceptions of body size. Ultimately, however, binge eating disorder is

more firmly situated within an "overeating" frame, depicting sufferers as needing "self-control" more than medical assistance. For instance, in an account of her personal struggle with binge eating disorder, reporter Jane Brody (2007) writes: "My despair was profound, and one night in the midst of a binge I became suicidal. I had lost control of my eating; it was controlling me, and I couldn't go on living that way." A psychologist helped Brody resist suicide but "was not able to help me stop binging. That was something I would have to do on my own." As with eating disorder victims in other accounts, this binge eater is presented as needing help from a doctor or therapist, but ultimately, as with overweight, it is suggested that she needs to control overeating on her own.

Two articles that discuss binge eating disorder argue that the most important reason binge eating disorder needs to be taken seriously is because it makes it more difficult to *succeed at weight-loss*. In other words, the concern with achieving a "normal" weight, which also dominates discussions of overweight, seems to trump more general concerns about eating disorders as psychological problems. One article explains: "The importance of binge eating disorder is that people who fit these criteria do worse than others in weight management programs" (Alter Hubel 1997). By focusing on the importance of weight loss, these articles obscure or downplay the psychiatric symptoms experienced by binge eaters, which have been shown to have negative health effects independent of body size (Telch and Agras 1994). Another article draws upon binge eating disorder's relationship to overweight in order to depict it as a *public* health risk: "Because of the disorder's close link with obesity . . . it's a major public-health burden" (Springen 2007), a theme that we *never* encountered in discussions of anorexia or bulimia.

Further, while feminist authors have identified binge eating and compulsive overeating as serious "eating problems," which—like anorexia and bulimia—often "begin as ways women numb pain and cope with violations of their bodies" and are "a logical response to injustices" (Thompson 1994:26), our news sample describes individuals with binge eating disorder as "overeaters" who have an "ordinary, if unfortunate, human behavior" (Bakalar 2007), and a few articles express concern that binge eating disorder has been "invented" by greedy drug companies. For instance, another article quotes an eating disorders researcher who says, "Outside North America, it's basically a laugh . . . No one thinks it's a serious condition . . . These are overeaters" (Goode 2000). In other words, there is resistance to giving binge eating disorder the status of a full-fledged eating disorder like anorexia or bulimia, for which outside forces of biology or culture—rather than individual choices—are to blame.

DISCUSSION AND CONCLUSION

Previous research has shown that the news media frame obesity as a moral problem of gluttony and sloth (Boero 2007) and overwhelmingly blame bad individual choices (Saguy and Almeling 2008), despite increasing discussion of social-structural factors over time (Lawrence 2004). Extant work, however, has been limited either analytically—by, for instance, not examining the role of gender, class, or race (Lawrence 2004)—or methodologically, by relying heavily on a small (Boero 2007) or non-representative sample (Saguy and Almeling 2008). In contrast, the current study draws on a relatively large and representative sample of news reports in the *New York Times* and *Newsweek*, while harnessing the analytical power of both quantitative and qualitative analysis. Moreover, the systematic comparison of reporting of overweight/obesity with reporting on eating disorders—a first on its kind—allows us to tease out the effects of negative attitudes about fatness from generic media routines that favor morality tales and the tendency in the United States to individualize responsibility for health (Fitzpatrick 2000; Lupton 1995; Tesh 1988). We find that, in the contemporary U.S. society where thinness is highly prized, news articles are less likely to blame individuals for being (or trying to be) too thin than they are to blame them for being too fat. This suggests that, more generally, cultural values shape how the news media assign blame and responsibility. In turn, such reporting is likely to reinforce and naturalize such values. This article further suggests that, depending on how they report on the demographics of a given condition, the news media may reinforce group-based stereotypes.

Specifically, the association of heavier bodies with gluttony and sloth and thinner bodies with discipline and responsibility, leads our news sample to frame anorexics as victims of cultural and biological forces beyond their control, while blaming the obese for their weight, which, in turn, reinforces these original associations. Our sample of news articles tends to deny binge eating disorder, in which sufferers eat large quantities of food and tend to be heavier, the status of a "real" eating disorder, reframing it instead as ordinary and blameworthy overeating. Moreover, because anorexia and bulimia are described as more often affecting middle class white girls and women, the analyzed news reports on these disorders reinforce the image of white middle class girls and women as victims. Since overweight/obesity is described as a problem most common among the poor and minorities, such news reporting on obesity reinforces stereotypes of poor minorities as ignorant or willfully defiant of health guidelines. While articles discussing blacks, Latinos, or the poor are more likely to blame weight on social-structural factors, they are also more likely to blame ethnic preferences for larger women or ethnic cuisine.

These findings have important substantive implications. To the extent that reporting on bigger bodies as a health problem reinforces the negative stigma associated with being heavier, women—who suffer more from weight-based discrimination (Puhl et al. 2008)—will bear the brunt of this stigma. Women, the greater consumers of medical weight-loss interventions, including weight-loss diets, drugs, and surgery (Bish et al. 2005; Santry, Gillen, and Lauderdale 2005), are also likely to increase their use of these costly and often risky interventions. As higher body weight is increasingly discussed as a medical and public health crisis, men may increase their consumption of these products as well. Moreover, characterization of obesity as an "epidemic"—warranted or not—creates a sense of urgency and potentially justifies forms of regulatory intervention that would otherwise appear excessive (Lupton 1995). Given the greater vulnerability of the poor and ethnic minorities to surveillance, we can expect regulatory intervention to target these groups.

Demand for increasingly punitive measures may come in response to images of fat populations as "wantonly gorging" themselves and allowing their children to do the same, thereby bringing diabetes and heart disease upon themselves, their families, and their communities. Removing children from their homes, like Heavy T, discussed in the introduction, is the most chilling example of such punitive measures. Anamarie Regino is another such child who was wrested from her parents by state officials, in her case at the age of four years (Belkin 2001). The state of New Mexico justified putting her in foster care on the grounds that her weight was both life

threatening and her parents' fault (Belkin 2001). In Anamarie's case, her family's Latino ethnicity was taken as further evidence of her parents' ignorance and inability to care for her. Despite the fact that Anamarie's mother was born in the United States and spoke fluent English, the social worker's affidavit stated that, "the family does not fully understand the threat to their daughter's safety and welfare due to language or cultural barriers" (Belkin 2001).

As these examples show, the way in which body size and eating are framed in public discourse has far-reaching consequences for individual behavior, public policy, and social control. Because of their visibility and cultural authority, the news media are important sites of meaning making and merit serious attention from sociologists. We hope that others will join us in investigating, not only the content of news reporting on eating and body size, but also its ramifications for individual behavior, interpersonal relations, public policy, and personal freedoms.

Notes

1. The definition of "overweight" and "obesity," and even these terms themselves, are contested. Fat-acceptance activists, who advocate for civil rights on the basis of body size, argue that these terms pathologize normal biological variation and reclaim the word "fat" as a neutral descriptor like "tall" or "short" (Cooper 1998; Wann 1999). Similarly, many feminist scholars have avoided the term "eating disorder" because it situates "disorder" within individuals rather than in complex social structures. We do not use "overweight," "obesity," or "eating disorders" because we endorse a medical or public health framing, but because we seek to establish how *these particular terms* have been constructed in the news media. We note that a search for articles using the term "fat" produced very few relevant articles, which is not surprising given that

    this word is still taboo in most social circles in the contemporary United States. An article search using the term "eating problems" was similarly unproductive. For stylistic reasons we do not place the terms "overweight," "obesity," or "eating disorder" in quotations throughout the article, but we wish to be clear that this is the spirit in which we use them.

2. However, new evidence suggests that bulimia—but not anorexia—may be more prevalent among poor minority, compared to middle class white women and girls (Goeree, Ham, and Iorio 2009).

3. Note, however, that following research trends, there is increased discussion of nonwhites with eating disorders in our sample over time, with 29 percent of the 2002–2005 sample mentioning nonwhites, compared to 8 percent of the 1995–2001 sample.

4. Race and class are often conflated in news media discussions of obesity, by, for instance, discussing "the poor and minorities" as a group or by using examples of poor members

of ethnic minorities to illustrate larger discussions of, say, "black" or "Latino" culture.

5. On mother blame, see the work of McGuffey (2005).

References

Alter Hubel, Joy. 1997. "Studies Under Way in Fight against Binging Disorder." *The New York Times*, August 3, p. LI13.

American Psychiatric Association (APA). 1994. *Diagnostic and Statistical Manual of Mental Disorders (DSM-IV)*. Washington, DC: American Psychiatric Association.

Aronowitz, Robert. 2008. "Framing Disease: An Underappreciated Mechanism for the Social Patterning of Health." *Social Science & Medicine* 67:1–9.

Bakalar, Nicholas. 2007. "Survey Puts New Focus on Binge Eating as a Diagnosis." *The New York Times*, February 13, p. F5.

Barrett Ozols, Jennifer 2005. "Generation XL." *News-week*, January 6. Retrieved February 12, 2010 (www.newsweek.com/id/47977).

Belkin, Lisa. 2001. "Watching Her Weight." *The New York Times*, July 8, p. 630.

Benson, Rodney and Abigail C. Saguy. 2005. "Constructing Social Problems in an Age of Globalization: A French-American Comparison." *American Sociological Review* 70:233–59.

Best, Joel. 2008. *Social Problems*. New York: Norton.

Bish, Connie L., Heidi Michels Blanck, Mary K. Serdula, Michele Marcus, Harold W. Kohl, and Laura Kettel Khan. 2005. "Diet and Physical Activity Behaviors among Americans Trying to Lose Weight: 2000 Behavioral Risk Factor

Surveillance System." *Obesity Research* 13:596–607.

Boero, Natalie. 2007. "All the News That's Fat to Print: The American 'Obesity Epidemic' and the Media." *Qualitative Sociology* 30:41–60.

Bordo, Susan. 1993. *Unbearable Weight: Feminism, Western Culture, and the Body*. Berkeley: University of California Press.

Braiker, Brian 2003. "Beets, Not Burgers." *Newsweek*, June 25, Retrieved February 12, 21010 (www. newsweek.com/id/58541).

Brodey, Denise. 2005. "Blacks Join the Eating-Disorder Mainstream." *The New York Times*, September 20, p. F5.

Brody, Jane E. 1997. "Health Watch." *New York Times*, March 26, p. C8.

_____. 2000. "Exposing the Perils of Eating Disorders." *New York Times*, December 12, p. F8.

_____. 2007. "Out of Control: A True Story of Binge Eating." *New York Times*, p. F7.

Bruch, Hilde. 1978. *The Golden Cage: The Enigma of Anorexia Nervosa*. Cambridge, MA: Harvard University Press.

Buss, Dale. 2004. "Is the Food Industry the Problem or the Solution?" *New York Times*, August 29, p. 35.

Conley, Dalton and Rebecca Glauber. 2007. "Gender, Body Mass, and Economic Status: New Evidence from the PSID." *Advances in*

Health Economics and Health Services Research 17:253–75.

Cooper, Charlotte. 1998. *Fat and Proud: The Politics of Size.* London, UK: Women's Press.

Crandall, Chris S. and Amy Eshleman. 2003. "A Justification-Suppression Model of the Expression and Experience of Prejudice." *Psychological Bulletin* 129:414–46.

Drewnowski, Adam and Anne Barratt-Fornell. 2004. "Do Healthier Diets Cost More?" *Nutrition Today* 39:161–68.

Eaton, Joe 2007. "The Battle over Heavy T." *Washington City Paper,* September 26. Retrieved January 22, 2010 (www.washingtoncitypaper .com/display.php?id=8136).

Edgley, Charles and Dennis Brissett. 1990. "Health Nazis and the Cult of the Perfect Body: Some Polemic Observations." *Symbolic Interaction* 13:257–79.

Entman, Robert M. 1993. "Framing: Toward Clarification of a Fractured Paradigm." *Journal of Communication* 43:51–58.

Feder, Barnaby J. 2005. "One Alternative: A Ring That Squeezes the Stomach." *The New York Times,* May 27, p. C2.

Fitzpatrick, Michael. 2000. *The Tyranny of Health: Doctors and the Regulation of Lifestyle.* New York: Routledge.

Flegal, K. M., M. D. Carroll, R. J. Kuczmarski, and C.L. Johnson. 1998. "Overweight and Obesity in the United States: Prevalence and Trends, 1960–1994." *International Journal of Obesity* 22:39–47.

Flegal, Katherine M., Margaret D. Carroll, Cynthia L. Ogden, and Clifford L. Johnson. 2002. "Prevalence and Trends in Obesity among U.S. Adults, 1999– 2000." *JAMA* 288:1723–27.

Gamson, William. 1992. *Talking Politics.* Cambridge, UK: Cambridge University Press.

Gans, Herbert. 1979. *Deciding What's News.* New York: Patheon.

Goeree, Michele Sovinky, John C. Ham, and Daniela Iorio. 2009. "Caught in the Bulimic Trap? Socioeconomic Status, State Dependence, and Unobserved Heterogeneity." Pp. 1–41 in *Working Paper Series.* Zurich, Switzerland: Institute for Empirical Research in Economics.

Goode, Erica. 2000. "Watching Volunteers, Experts Seek Clues to Eating Disorders." *The New York Times,* October 24, p. F1.

_____. 2002. "Anorexia Strategy: Family as Doctor." *The New York Times,* June 11, p. F1.

Gusfield, Joseph R. 1981. *The Culture of Public Problems: Drinking-Driving and the Symbolic Order.* Chicago: University of Chicago Press.

Hochman, Nancy S. 1996. "Eating Disorders Strike Younger Girls and Men." *The New York Times,* April 28, p. LI1.

Hof, Sonja van't and Malcolm Nicolson. 1996. "The Rise and Fall of a Fact: The Increase in Anorexia Nervosa." *Sociology of Health and Illness* 18:581–608.

Holsti, Ole R. 1969. *Content Analysis for the Social Sciences and Humanities.* Reading, MA: Addison-Wesley Publishing Co.

Isherwood, Charles. 2005. "A Happy Family Is Stalked by Heartbreak as a Daughter Wastes Herself Away." *The New York Times,* November 1, p. E5.

Kalb, Claudia 2000. "When Weight Loss Goes Awry." *Newsweek,* July 3, p. 46.

Kalb, Claudia and Karen Springen. 2005. "Pump up the Family." *Newsweek,* p. 62.

Kitsuse, John L. and Malcolm Spector. 1973. "Toward a Sociology of Social Problems: Social Conditions, Value Judgments, and Social Problems." *Social Problems* 20:407–19.

Klein, Richard. 1996. *Eat Fat.* New York: Pantheon.

Kolata, Gina. 2007. *Rethinking Thin: The New Science of Weight Loss—and the Myths and*

Realities about Dieting. New York: Farrar, Straus and Giroux.

Kuntzman, Gersh 2002. "American Beat: Food Fight." *Newsweek*, December 9. Retrieved February 12, 2010 (www.newsweek.com/id/66569).

Latner, Janet D. and Albert J. Stunkard. 2003. "Getting Worse: The Stigmatization of Obese Children." *Obesity Research* 11:452–56.

Lawrence, Regina G. 2004. "Framing Obesity: The Evolution of News Discourse on a Public Health Issue." *Press/Politics* 9:56–75.

Liotta, Jarret. 1999. "Searching for a New Way to Treat Bulimia." *The New York Times*, June 6, p. CN3.

Lupton, Deborah. 1994. *Moral Threats and Dangerous Desires: AIDS in the News Media*. Taylor and Francis.

_____. 1995. *The Imperative of Health: Public Health and the Regulated Body*. London, UK: Sage Publications.

Markus, Frances Frank. 1998. "Why Baked Catfish Holds Lessons for Their Hearts." *The New York Times*, June 21, p. 1524.

McGuffey, C. Shawn. 2005. "Engendering Trauma: Race, Class, and Gender Reaffirmation after Child Sexual Abuse." *Gender & Society* 19:621–43.

Misra, Joya, Stephanie Moller, and Marina Karides. 2003. "Envisioning Dependency: Changing Media Depictions of Welfare in the 20th Century." *Social Problems* 50:482–504.

Nelkin, Dorothy. 1987. *Selling Science: How the Press Covers Science and Technology*. New York: Freeman.

New York Times. 2002. "America's Epidemic of Youth Obesity." *The New York Times*, November 29, p. A38.

Newsweek 2000. "Mail Call." *Newsweek*, July 24, p. 14.

Nichter, Mimi. 2000. *Fat Talk: What Girls and the Parents Say About Dieting*. Cambridge, MA: Harvard University Press.

Popenoe, Rebecca. 2005. "Ideal." Pp. 9–28 in *Fat: The Anthropology of an Obsession*, edited by D. Kulick and A. Meneley. New York: Tarcher/Penguin.

Puhl, R. M., T. Andreyeva, and K. D. Brownell. 2008. "Perceptions of Weight Discrimination: Prevalence and Comparison to Race and Gender Discrimination in America." *International Journal of Obesity* 32:992–1000.

Richardson, Lynda. 2003. "Telling Children Not to Inhale Junk Food, Either." *The New York Times*, July 24, p. B2.

Rohlinger, Deana A. 2007. "American Media and Deliberative Democratic Processes." *Sociological Theory* 25:122–48.

Rothman Morris, Bonnie. 2004. "Older Women, Too, Struggle with a Dangerous Secret." *The New York Times*, July 6, p. F5.

Saguy, Abigail C. and Rene Almeling. 2008. "Fat in the Fire? Science, the News Media, and the 'Obesity Epidemic.'" *Sociological Forum* 23:53–83.

Santora, Marc. 2005. "Study Finds More Obesity and Less Exercising among New York City's Women Than Its Men." *The New York Times*, March 8, p. B3.

Santry, Heena P., Daniel L. Gillen, and Diane S. Lauderdale. 2005. "Trends in Bariatric Surgical Procedures." *JAMA* 294:1909–17.

Schlesinger, Mark. 2005. "Editor's Note: Weighting for Godot." *Journal of Health Politics, Policy, and Law* 30:785–801.

Schudson, Michael. 2003. *The Sociology of the News*. New York: W. W. Norton & Company.

Smith, Delia E., Marsha D. Marcus, Cora Lewis, Marian Fitzgibbon, and Pamela Schreiner. 1998. "Prevalence of Binge Eating Disorder,

Obesity, and Depression in a Biracial Cohort of Young Adults." *Annals of Behavioral Medicine* 20:227–32.

Sobal, Jeffery and Albert J. Stunkard. 1989. "Socioeconomic Status and Obesity: A Review of the Literature." *Psychological Bulletin* 105:260–75.

Springen, Karen 2007. "Health: Battle of the Binge." *Newsweek*, February 19, p. 62.

Stearns, Peter N. 1997. *Fat History: Bodies and Beauty in the Modern West*. New York and London: New York University Press.

Striegel-Moore, Ruth H., Denise E. Wilfley, Kathleen M. Pike, Faith-Anne Dohm, and Christopher G. Fairburn. 2000. "Recurrent Binge Eating in Black American Women." *Archives of Family Medicine* 9:83–87.

Striegel-Moore, Ruth H., Faith A. Dohm, Helena C. Kraemer, C. Barr Taylor, Stephen Daniels, Patricia B. Crawford, and George B. Schrieber. 2003. "Eating Disorders in White and Black Women." *American Journal of Psychiatry* 160:1326–31.

Telch, Christy F. and W. Stewart Agras. 1994 "Obesity, Binge Eating, and Psychopathology: Are They Related?" *International Journal of Eating Disorders* 15:53–61.

Tesh, Sylvia Noble. 1988. *Hidden Arguments: Political Ideology and Disease Prevention Policy*. New Brunswick, NJ: Rutgers University Press.

Thompson, Becky W. 1994. *A Hunger So Wide and So Deep: A Multiracial View of Women's Eating Problems*. Minneapolis: University of Minnesota Press.

Tyre, Peg 2005. "Fighting Anorexia: No-One to Blame." *Newsweek*, December 5, p. 50.

Wann, Marilyn. 1999. *Fat! So?: Because You Don't Have to Apologize for Your Size*. Berkeley, CA: Ten Speed Press.

Whitaker, Mark 2005. "The Editor's Desk." *News-week*, December 5, p. 4.

12

ILLNESS MEANINGS OF AIDS AMONG WOMEN WITH HIV

Merging Immunology and Life Experience

Alison Scott

What does "AIDS" mean? This question has had four different "correct" answers since the creation of the acronym by the Centers for Disease Control and Prevention (CDC) in 1982. The term "AIDS" has consistently been used as a clinical and epidemiological tool, and a marker of severe, late-stage disease as a result of HIV infection. Early in the HIV epidemic, the median survival time following an AIDS diagnosis hovered between 12 and 19 months (Lundgren et al., 1994; McNaghten, Hansen, Jones, Dworkin, & Ward, 1999; Mocroft et al., 1997; Schwarcz, Hsu, Vittinghoff, & Katz,

2000). This changed in the mid-1990s with the advent of highly active antiretroviral therapy (HAART). With HAART, the immune system can rally, allowing many with HIV or even AIDS to live on for decades. However, an AIDS diagnosis is permanent once affixed in the clinic, even if the immune system regains strength.

For HAART to be effective, adherence is a critical concern. Patient education about HIV disease is utilized as one tool in efforts to increase adherence rates. Patient education includes careful explication of the definitions of AIDS and other HIV-related

Illness Meaning of AIDS Among Women With HIV: Merging Immunology and Life Experience, Alison Scott in *Qualitative Health Research*, *19*(4), 454–465. Copyright © 2009 SAGE Publications. Reprinted with permission.

Author's Note: Thank you to all the women who participated in the study for sharing their experiences. I also thank the staff at the Tulane Medical Center study site, including Leslie Kozina, Trina Jeanjacques, Alyne Baker, and Dr. Sue Ellen Abdalian for their time and insight. I'm grateful to my mentor, Lori Leonard, for her thoughtful guidance on drafts of this article, and to Kimberly Ashburn, for encouraging me to think about different qualitative approaches. Thanks to the Adolescent Trials Network (ATN), Jonathan Ellen, Gretchen Clum, and Lori Perez. Thanks to Ruth Whitworth for help with the figures.

concepts such as CD4 T cell count and viral load. Patient education seeks to provide disease knowledge; it is predicated on the idea that understanding biomedical concepts will enable rational decision making about adherence and other HIV-related behaviors.

Interventions seeking to improve adherence through increasing disease knowledge have had mixed results. An intervention in France found adherence to increase with disease knowledge; however, CD4 counts, viral loads, and quality-of-life measures remained unchanged (Goujard et al., 2003). In the United States, a trial at 25 outpatient clinics compared adherence in those receiving an HIV educational program and counseling to those receiving counseling alone; they found no differences between the two study arms in terms of adherence rates, viral loads, or CD4 counts (Rawlings et al., 2003).

In this account I ask the question, "What does AIDS mean?" beyond the clinical definition, which, as described earlier, is itself increasingly amorphous; AIDS no longer means imminent death in the presence of HAART. However, as is shown here, the term "AIDS" remains fraught with significance beyond the doors of the clinic.

This query rose out of a larger, multicity interview study with young women attending HIV clinics. The study examined the relationships among AIDS diagnosis, adherence, and receipt of support services such as housing, transport, and cash assistance. In some cities AIDS was extremely salient for instrumental support (Scott, Ellen, Clum, & Leonard, 2007). In New Orleans, the site of this account, this was not the case; relative to other cities, few services of any sort were available to the women interviewed. However, as I reviewed early transcripts, it was clear that the idea of AIDS remained a powerful one to the women there, and was extremely salient to their emotional, social, and clinical experiences. I could not identify literature exploring the shifting meaning of this construct from the perspective of those with HIV. From this emerged the research questions addressed here: In the HAART era, what does AIDS mean to young women with HIV, and how are these meanings integrated into their daily experiences of coping with the illness? How are they reflected in adherence to HAART?

To address these issues, I shifted from the lens of disease knowledge to one of illness meaning. Arthur Kleinman (1988) describes disease as "the problem from the practitioner's perspective," or in this case, the perspective of the biomedical community as a whole. The clinical definitions of AIDS and other HIV terminology are born from epidemiology, immunology, and virology, and have objective, concrete answers at any moment in time; these answers might shift as science evolves. In contrast, according to Kleinman, illness meanings reflect people's personal experiences and explanations of their conditions. Illness meanings are dynamic, situated, and contingent (Kleinman, 1988). They are intertwined with the messiness and complexity of life, and are constructed as illnesses are lived. However, little attention has been paid to illness meaning with regard to HIV, especially in the United States and other developed nations. Most of the literature that does exist provides descriptive comparisons of lay and biomedical ideas surrounding HIV causation, symptoms, and treatment (Baer, Weller, Garcia de Alba Garcia, & Salcedo Rocha, 2004; Mill, 2000, 2001), and does not include the perspective of those infected. This literature also lacks a focus on the AIDS construct, and variations in its meaning across time and context.

Living with HIV, as has been noted by many (Brown, Macintyre, & Trujillo, 2003; Castro & Farmer, 2005; Herek & Glunt, 1988; Madru, 2003; Parker & Aggleton, 2003; Taylor, 2001), often involves social suffering and ostracism. Social experience is reflected strongly in illness meanings. As such, stigma provides a potentially important lens for examining illness meanings of AIDS. Erving Goffman describes stigma as a social process marking those deemed physically or morally blemished, differentiating them from "normals" who do not deviate from social expectations (Goffman, 1963). Within this state of disgrace, Goffman differentiates between those who are discredited and those who are discreditable. To be discredited is to be exposed as stigmatized, whereas the discreditable are able to conceal differences, or "pass" (Goffman, 1963).

The findings here show these social distinctions to be woven intricately into the illness meanings of HIV-positive women.

As discussed previously, there is a dearth of attention given to illness meanings in the context of HIV, especially in the developed world. In addition, the vast literature devoted to HAART adherence pays little attention to illness meanings, focusing instead on disease knowledge and behavioral or contextual predictors. By exploring meanings associated with AIDS among HIV-positive women, I show here that illness meanings, alone and in conjunction with disease knowledge, can enhance our understanding of adherence, and enhance individualized patient care.

In an attempt to capture the complexity of illness meanings, I have used a mixture of qualitative approaches, including drawings as a visual method. This is one of few studies to use drawings to elucidate illness experience, and illustrates the value of this approach. The richness of drawings as a method of data collection was discussed at length by Guillemin (2004), who used drawings in conjunction with interviews to explore Australian women's perceptions of heart disease and menopause. A second example is work by Victora and Knauth (2001), who asked study participants in Brazilian shantytowns to draw images of the male and female reproductive systems. In the study presented here, methodological triangulation of women's drawings of HIV in their bodies, free listing, and in-depth interviewing allowed a deeper exploration of illness meaning than could be pursued by interviewing alone.

METHODS

This research was conducted with HIV-positive young women attending an HIV clinic in New Orleans, Louisiana, as part of a substudy examining instrumental support for women with HIV in urban contexts. The substudy was part of a National Institute on Drug Abuse (NIDA)-funded project examining correlates of engagement in HIV care at four clinic sites. The New Orleans clinic is part of the Adolescent Trials Network (ATN), a group of adolescent HIV clinics that collaborates in research

protocols for the advancement of adolescent HIV care. The study was reviewed by the Institutional Review Boards at the Johns Hopkins Bloomberg School of Public Health and Tulane Medical Center.

I conducted two rounds of in-depth interviews, 4 months apart. Participants were HIV-positive women between 18 and 24 years of age. All were African American or mixed race. Half had not finished high school, and none had degrees beyond a high school diploma or GED. The majority had monthly incomes of less than $500, and were mothers. A purposeful sample of interview participants that varied in duration since HIV diagnosis, family and living situation, education, and level of engagement in care was recruited. Clinic nurses assisted in recruiting participants. The nurses had trusting relationships with the women, and identified potential participants, approached them about the study, and introduced them to me. Women who were recently diagnosed, or by the judgment of the nurses were emotionally or physically vulnerable, were not approached. The nurses were present in the next room during the interviews. Most women spoke freely and with ease during the interviews; if a line of discussion was difficult for a participant, I shifted the conversation, and debriefed the nurses afterwards. In one case the nurses decided to check in with a participant following an interview. The woman's brother had died recently, and she was struggling with grief. Participants were given $30 to help offset any expense and inconvenience of participation.

Interviews were conducted in a private room. A total of 18 interviews were conducted with 10 different women, 9 during the first clinic visit and 9 during the second visit 4 months later. One woman participated in the first interview visit only; one woman participated only during the second visit. In the latter case, an extended interview was conducted. In the former case, data collection unique to the second visit (free listing and drawing) was not completed.

Interviews were conducted with the aid of an interview guide. In the first interview, following discussion of the study and written informed consent, participants shared information about their families, schools and work, life situations growing up, and public assistance; questions also focused on their experiences at the clinic, with HAART, and with HIV. These transcripts were analyzed as described later for themes relevant to the goals of the multisite qualitative substudy examining the relationship between AIDS and instrumental support among women. However, an additional theme that emerged from these transcripts was that of AIDS and its meanings to the women. The second interview guide was adapted to explore this further. In the second interview, participants were asked about AIDS and other HIV-related biomedical terms, including what they meant, how people used them in their communities and in the clinic, and how the terms made them feel. To delve more deeply into the meaning of AIDS, two additional methods were employed: free listing and drawings.

For the free-listing exercise, I asked the women to share the words that "popped into their heads" when they heard various terms, including HIV and AIDS. I probed for additional answers until the women said they couldn't think of anything else. For the drawing exercise, I gave the women white paper, markers, and colored pencils. I asked each woman to draw a "picture she had in her mind" of HIV and how it was in her body; then I asked what AIDS would look like, and the difference. As the women drew, I asked questions, encouraging them to narrate.

Interview recordings were transcribed and analyzed via thematic analysis using the "editing" approach described by Crabtree and Miller (1999) in which sections of text with thematic congruence are extracted and studied together to facilitate interpretation. Segments of text using the word "AIDS" were examined as a group to look for common ideas and patterns. In addition to this decontextualizing approach, narrative summaries of interview transcripts were prepared for each participant to tell the basic story of each woman's life as she presented it, facilitating examination of themes contextualized within women's stories, a form of narrative analysis (Lieblich & Tuval-Mashaiach, 1998). This allowed examination of a woman's "AIDS meanings" within her distinct context. The importance of factors such

as HIV or AIDS status, abuse history, HAART status, and broader social and clinical experience are examples of some issues considered.

Free-listing results were transcribed and examined quantitatively and qualitatively. First, a table was constructed listing all responses and the frequency of each response. Also noted was which responses were given first and second by a participant. Qualitatively, the speed and emphatic nature (or lack thereof) of responses was noted from recordings and transcripts, as well as how the responses were framed; some responses were given as lists, whereas in other cases a woman would give an answer and then elaborate conversationally.

Drawings were scanned for storage in digital form, and analyzed using Guillemin's (2004) adaptation of Rose's critical methodology (Rose, 2001). This involved analysis of (a) the image itself, looking at its content, story, how it was conveyed, and the shapes and colors used; (b) the context of the image's production, in this case how the clinic setting and my presence might have shaped what was drawn; and (c) myself as audience, my unique perspective as a qualitative researcher with extensive training in microbiology and immunology, as well as my relative social position as a White, middle-class academic.

Mixing use of interviews, free lists, and drawings allowed triangulation around major themes related to the meaning of AIDS, which increased my confidence in the credibility of my conclusions. Each method also revealed unique nuances and ambiguities, highlighting the ongoing construction of meanings.

FINDINGS

"There's Really No Hope": AIDS as Death

The free-listing exercise evoked sharply divergent responses to the words HIV and AIDS, reflecting their distinctive meanings to the women; the responses are presented in Table 12.1. When conducting the free-listing exercise, most of the women gave few responses, even when probed; answers they did give often were immediate and emphatic, especially with regard to AIDS. Occasionally the women would elaborate conversationally, restoring the former flow of discussion. Most of the time they would become silent, waiting for the next prompt. The women participated in extensive survey research as part of the larger project, and this exercise seemed to reflect their experience with the "respondent" role.

In Table 12.1, numbers in parentheses indicate repeat responses, and asterisks indicate responses given by the women with AIDS diagnoses. For the word HIV, almost half of the women said "virus." Most other responses related to the active work of managing HIV disease, such as "medication," "peer group," and "counseling." Responses to the word AIDS stand in contrast, and depict a state where disease management has failed. "Death" was the most common response, with other responses invoking images of pain, wasting, and fear. Some women

HIV	AIDS
virus (4)*	death (5)
medication (2)	full-blown disease (2)
counseling sessions	there's really no hope
preventable	excruciating pain
treatment	the last stage
peer group	lose weight, be sick a lot
case manager	"That scares me. That makes the hair on the back of my neck stand up."
doctor's appointments	maybe a little more serious than HIV*
AIDS	mild pains*
BET commercials just a word*	just a word*

TABLE 12.1 ■ Free-Listing Responses to the Words "HIV" and "AIDS"

*Responses from participants with AIDS diagnoses.

recounted experiences of seeing people with AIDS, whereas others explained that they heard people talk about it in a derogatory way. A woman who didn't know the clinical definition, and asked me twice to explain it, said the word nonetheless had great meaning to her:

> When I hear the word AIDS it's like—it's totally—that's when it becomes totally different. . . . Your blood is getting short. So you don't have too much time left.

These images are compatible with the experience of the disease prior to HAART. Though the clinical picture has changed, social meanings surrounding AIDS remain powerful outside the clinic. Although the concept of AIDS is a key component of patient education, a nurse at the clinic said she tried to avoid using the term with patients. She had observed the ability of the word to paralyze the women with fear, making them less receptive to information about their care.

A few responses in the free-list exercise for the word AIDS stand out: AIDS is "just a word," "maybe a little more serious than HIV," and involves "mild pain." The two women giving these responses were the only women in the sample to have received AIDS diagnoses. In the following discussion I explore this contrast, showing how the women negotiate meanings of HIV, AIDS, and HAART according to their own diagnosis status and social experiences, in an ongoing effort to construct illness meanings that support themselves in living "normal" lives.

"I Take Care of Myself": Distance From Discredit

The meanings of AIDS held by the women incorporated not only physical collapse, but also moral and social collapse or discredit. Vanessa,[1] an HIV-positive mother of two, associates AIDS with "not taking care of yourself" or "abusing your body" through behaviors such as poor HAART adherence, taking drugs, drinking, "getting stressed," and not eating right. This is in concordance with patient education messages, which stress adherence and healthy lifestyle to prevent progression to AIDS, linking clinically desirable behaviors and qualities of responsibility and self-control. Vanessa says with pride that she takes care of herself. This will protect her from developing AIDS:

> It [AIDS] mostly comes to people [who] like abuse their bodies—drugs, cigarettes, alcohol—things like that. . . . If you take care of yourself, there will be a chance where you won't—you won't even have to develop to AIDS. So—and I think out of all the years I have not needed a drop of medicine . . . never . . . never.

In this way, AIDS might be seen as a punishment for irresponsible behavior. A similar dynamic has been noted with regard to diabetes, where blood sugar monitoring and the moral imperative of self-control merge. Broom describes this as a facet of "contemporary healthism" (Broom & Whittaker, 2004) in which health is conceived as a virtue and a sign of proper conduct (Broom & Whittaker, 2004; Loewe, Schwartzman, Freeman, Quinn, & Zuckerman, 1998).

The women also identified AIDS as a socially stigmatizing state in which friends and family could desert you, though they had stood by you when you "just" had HIV. This differentiation displaces both death and discrediting social stigma to the state of AIDS, away from HIV. With an HIV diagnosis, Vanessa says she is living a "normal everyday life." This dichotomy is illustrated in Vanessa's drawing (see Figure 12.1). She struggled as she drew, trying to reproduce a poster that depicted HIV in a T cell. She had seen the poster at her clinic.

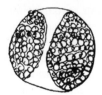

She depicts the virus as attacking the cell's DNA. There are two large cells in her drawing; the one on the left depicts HIV, and the one on the right depicts AIDS. The HIV cell is mostly empty space; the AIDS circle, however, is almost full of large "AIDS viruses." When there's no space left, she explains, you die:

> In the case of AIDS . . . that's supposed to be the AIDS virus with . . . these big ones . . . and why I drew it so big, because . . . it take up most of . . . this is the only thing keeping you from death . . . it's like smaller, like you not far . . . a small space, you know like it's not far. . . . It took over your DNA, and you can't stop it.

What Vanessa expresses both visually and verbally is that with HIV you have "space" between you and death. With AIDS, however, there is little space, and the disappearance of the space is inevitable. By depicting it this way, Vanessa literally gives herself distance, or space, from the ideas of death and stigma, by placing herself in the HIV circle. In this way, her knowledge of HIV disease concepts fuses with her fear of death and perceptions of the rewards of morality, which are both socially and clinically affirmed. Together, they construct a meaning for her illness that fuels her confidence in her own integrity, physical and social.

"This Is What Goes on Inside Me": The Importance of Personal Context

A number of the women with HIV employed the concept of AIDS to portray distance from death and stigma. However, each woman negotiated HIV knowledge in the context of her own personal experience. In this way, life circumstances were mirrored in meanings ascribed to HIV disease concepts, and feelings of confidence, hope, fear, and defeat were expressed through biomedical constructs. Gena has two children, is recently married to a truck driver, and is in school to become a medical assistant. She talks at length about her wedding, decorating her house, bills that eat up their income, and caring for her autistic child. Things are hard, but she has achieved what most of the women only long for: a husband, family, and home. Her health and her counts have been good. She says HIV has not changed her life, either physically or socially:

> Ain't nothing changed. As far as it looks to me everything is still the same. I ain't sick or nothing or anything like that. . . . HIV is like when people look at me . . . you wouldn't know I have it unless I tell you.

She, too, expresses a sense of distance from AIDS through her drawing, which is couched in military language. She depicts AIDS as a lethal general commanding his battalion of HIV warriors in an attack on the innocent T cell (see Figure 12.2). The HIV "troops" come first, but are small and can be repelled; the AIDS "general" will come last and deliver a fatal blow:

> Ok, now. This [pointing to blue circle with frown] is the general, which is the AIDS, and

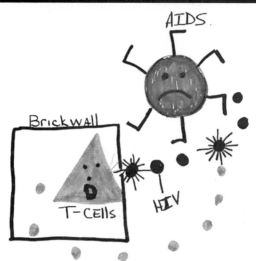

FIGURE 12.2 ■ Gena's Illustration: AIDS as "The General" Attacking Her T Cells With His HIV "Troops"

this is the HIV, which is his troops. That the AIDS is sending his troops to kill off the T cells; the T cells is sending his troops to fight off the HIV and that's like the little HIV exploding . . . dying.

She narrates this drama in the third person, but then makes it personal, emphasizing that the AIDS general has a "long, long, long, long, long way to go" before he reaches her T cell and she dies:

> [B]ut me, this is what goes on inside me, so like he's [the AIDS general] last and he sends all his troops first, which they all dying, because mine is like real real really good, so he's got a long, long, long, long, long way to go.

Gena is keeping the AIDS general at bay in a "fight" that she visualizes going on "around your stomach and intestines and your muscles and your veins." Her optimism and sense of determination are present in her voice, her words, and in her use of the concepts of the T cell, HIV, and AIDS. HAART, if she required it, would add another formidable "brick wall" of protection:

> I will have to put a brick wall and they have to squeeezze through this little bitty tiny tiny tiny tiny tiny tiny hole. That just really hard to get into.

She expresses a sense of insulation from the physical and social ravages of HIV disease, which is supported by the meanings she ascribes to HIV and AIDS. The dichotomy between HIV and AIDS protects her, in this sense, but it also foreshadows a lapse in motivation if she ever does receive an AIDS diagnosis. She reflects that if she had an AIDS diagnosis, she'd be overwhelmed with thoughts of dying, and wouldn't see the sense in trying to work or function:

> Knowing that you about to, you know. . . . I don't think anybody could forget that. You know, I don't think I could keep that off my mind knowing that I'm about to die. . . . I

mean, if they were to tell me that you know, I would be like . . . no sense in doing that. I'm going to die anyway. Ain't no sense in getting a job. I'm going to die anyway.

The emphasis on the distinction between HIV and AIDS possesses both the potential to protect the women before an AIDS diagnosis and to paralyze them after, or to require a fundamental renegotiation of illness meanings. Two women attempting this are discussed later in the paper.

The accounts of others expose the limitations of this metaphor. Casting an HIV diagnosis as a normal precursor to AIDS does not hold up well under the weight of the women's experiences, which include significant physical and social suffering as a result of HIV. Serena was infected when she was 14, after being raped by a man who used drugs with her mother; he has since "died of AIDS." She moved in with her grandmother when she was 16. When her grandmother discovered she had HIV, she made Serena bathe in bleach and forbade her to use household items. She also "told the whole world" Serena had AIDS. She tried living with her cousin, to the same end:

My grandmother when she found out, I couldn't wash my clothes in her washing machine. I had one plate, one fork, one spoon, one knife, one bowl—everything had tape and my name on it and it was mandatory that I didn't wash the things that I eat with—with their things and I had to bleach them and I had to take a bath in bleach. . . . And she just told the whole world. We had this sweet shop downstairs from our house and she went to the sweet shop and she told them don't let me in the sweet shop because I had AIDS. She just told the whole thing. . . . And it was like I went to live with my cousin, Sue, before I went into foster care, and there it was like the same way my grandmother was, so I couldn't take that either.

Serena demonstrates an important disjuncture. On the "street" no distinction is made between HIV

and AIDS. Therefore, to disclose an HIV diagnosis is to risk the same discredited status that the women associate with AIDS. Many of the women had similar stories, being shamed for their disclosure. Goffman (1963) describes this as the tension of the discreditable life; the women must work constantly to manage the selective concealment of their HIV diagnoses, in a quest to find support yet avoid becoming a pariah. As such, the two states of discredited and discreditable intertwine, just as do meanings of AIDS and HIV. Serena also demonstrates that physical suffering is not confined to those with AIDS. She took the antiretroviral drug Sustiva for 2 years, and was plagued by nightmares and night sweats:

It [Sustiva] gives you really horrible nightmares. I had to stop taking it. I took it for like two years and it wouldn't stop. The bad dreams and night sweats and stuff kept coming and the doctor said it was going to be like that for a while and then it was going to stop. But two years. I should have been used to it now. But it wouldn't stop.

As in Gena's case, Serena's drawing of HIV in her body (see Figure 12.3) reflects her life experiences. Only in her case, this includes a sense of powerlessness, contamination, and struggle.

Like Gena, Serena uses military imagery. However, she does not express optimism for her T cell army. She says it's like she's trying to fight a giant, and equates HIV with "gremlins" that keep reproducing in her body:

They're [the yellow dots, T cells] trying to fight with those red dots [HIV], but as you see those red dots are a whole lot bigger than these little bitty light things, so, like, it's me trying to fight a giant. There's no win. [Draws] I don't have armies, like these guys have. [Draws; long pause]. . . . HIV hurts my T cells. Now, we have a lot of HIV, and not that many T cells. Why? Because they're like gremlins. They keep producing.

FIGURE 12.3 ■ Serena's Illustration: HIV as an Army of "Gremlins" Overwhelming Her Body

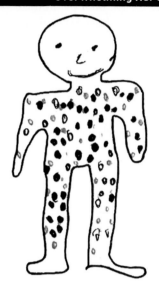

One senses that Serena's "gremlins" function as a metonym for her experiences of social rejection. Other women described this as feeling "germy" or "nasty," or having "germs running all over your body . . . crumbling you up." Serena says that the medications can help her T cells, but HIV keeps reproducing. She ponders the inability of HAART to eliminate the viruses altogether. The medications are helpful, but they can never cleanse her body:

> So if I had 90,000 particles of HIV in my body and then it goes all the way down to und—under 400, where do they go to? . . . How do they get undetectable, because I don't even know how to draw those, because HIV never quite goes away. It don't have nowhere to go. And the meds aren't making them disappear I don't think.

She is happy that her viral load is down, but associates HAART with sufferings of its own, and sees it as an incomplete solution. HIV is always present in her body and in her life. Despite her suffering

with HIV, Serena works to maintain a dichotomy of meaning separating life and death. This is evident when she identifies a challenge to her meaning of AIDS. She describes with horror seeing a woman with AIDS covered in blisters:

> I knew this lady that stayed down the street from me and she used to go to the clinic. Her name was Irene and she had it. I mean she had blisters all on her eyelids, everywhere, all on the back of her neck. I'm like that's going to happen to me? I hope not, because they look really, really scary.

But she also notes there is a woman in her neighborhood who has AIDS yet is big and healthy and has pretty hair:

> There was another lady that used to live in our neighborhood. She had it, but she had AIDS . . . and she was bigger than me and she didn't even—you wouldn't even be able to tell she had it. . . . She's so big now and she's really pretty. She has really pretty hair. You can't even tell.

Serena resolves this discrepancy by a shift in language. She says that what distinguishes the two women is that the healthy woman "takes care of herself," whereas of the woman with the blisters she says, "I don't think she did [take meds]. Uh-uh. She couldn't. I don't think she loved herself too much."

This shifts the focus away from the HIV–AIDS dichotomy, but preserves the notion of taking care of yourself, or self-love, as the key. Moral failing, here, marks the woman with the blisters. She also links self-love seamlessly to taking HAART, showing once again the perceived link between healthy behavior and healthy character.

Vanessa also confronts this dilemma and struggles to resolve it. She has an aunt in Virginia with an AIDS diagnosis. Her aunt still drives a cab and lives an active life, thanks to HAART. Vanessa acknowledges that her aunt looks healthy, but then checks herself and says she looks "different too." She says she can tell her aunt has AIDS, though maybe a stranger couldn't:

> She works every day, so I mean but . . . but at the same time she looks different, too. I can tell—well by me knowing I can look at her and tell, but if a person comes up to me.

In this way she preserves a meaning of AIDS as visible, at least to her, if not quickly fatal. To blur this distinction, as HAART does, has a cost for the HIV-positive women in losing a sense of distance from mortality.

"It's Just a Word": Meanings of AIDS After an AIDS Diagnosis

Another struggle inevitable in this dichotomization is the one reserved for those who receive an AIDS diagnosis. For the women in the study with AIDS diagnoses, the diagnosis was not simply a clinical event. It required a search for a personal illness meaning that could sustain hope in lieu of one that denoted their imminent death.

When Laetitia learned her serostatus, her T cell count was 6 and she was suffering from respiratory and gynecological infections, immediately classifying her as an AIDS patient. She voraciously consumed information about the disease provided her by the clinic and her caseworker. She describes how she collected pamphlets and booklets about HIV and read them in her spare time, storing them in a safe box under her bed:

> They'll have like little pamphlets or little books and stuff and I'll pick up one of them and take them home. . . . I have like a little safe box and all my information—I keep it in a safe box and put it underneath my bed.

She noted that her T cell count had constituted an AIDS diagnosis, though it subsequently rose past 200 with HAART. This frightened her, and she started worrying whether she had AIDS or "just" HIV:

> Well what I read in a book—I'm not sure— depending on how much of the virus was in

the blood was considered AIDS, but I think at one point I was that . . . and so if I'm correct about that—that was considered AIDS, but now it's not. But I was worried; I was like you know do I have AIDS, do I have—is it just HIV?

She doesn't link the word AIDS to herself directly, saying she "was that." She expresses confusion, saying she might have been "that" [AIDS] at one time, but she wasn't anymore, and how can that be? The notion is nonsensical from social meanings ascribed to AIDS. To move past this, she had to reconstruct a meaning of AIDS that gave her a chance to live. She accomplishes this for herself in two ways. First, she resists the distinction between HIV and AIDS. She has something, and it's not going away:

> But you know, after a while it's like you know what? I know I got something, even though it's HIV or whatever, I'm positive, you know, and I just . . . I wasn't really concerned about if I had AIDS, or if I had HIV, or whatever; I just knew I had it, you know, and it's not going away.

She substitutes the word "positive" for HIV and AIDS, acknowledging the presence of the "something" that has changed her life without giving it the implication of her death, and substituting it with, literally, a positive term.

Second, Laetitia copes by backing away from information about the disease. She says she too lives her life as a normal person, trying to stay constantly busy, though acknowledges "it's" still always in the back of her mind:

> It's not like I forgot about it, but if it's not brought up then it's not on my mind . . . so pretty much I live my life, you know, as a normal person would, but it's still in the back of my mind. I know I have it, but I mean I'm kind—I keep myself constantly busy, you know, so it's not on my mind.

Other women also discussed trying not to think about HIV. Backing in and out of engagement with

HIV disease information, which is highly emotionally charged, offered some protection against being overwhelmed.

Laetitia's responses in the word association show well her attempt to rob the word AIDS of its power; she describes AIDS as "maybe a little more serious than HIV." Her drawing also lacks a clear dichotomy between HIV and AIDS (see Figure 12.4). The imagery she uses is that of a battle between good [T cells] and evil [HIV], with HAART as the savior of her T cells. She conveys this through color, language, and shape. HIV is black, which she says is a "bad color" to her, and the T cell is yellow, a bright, good color:

> The HIV virus is black because to me black is like a bad color like a dark color. It doesn't represent anything happy like as far as yellow is bright and colorful and stuff, so that's a good thing. . . . You have the T cell which is good, and you have the virus which is bad.

Other women used similar color schemes. Laetitia's T cells are round, whereas the HIV is drawn as a rectangle, the hard right angles a contrast to the soft circularity. Most striking, the medication is drawn as a series of green hearts, which come in and neutralize the rectangles and support the circles. This

FIGURE 12.4 ■ Laetitia's Illustration: The "Good" T Cells and the "Bad" Virus

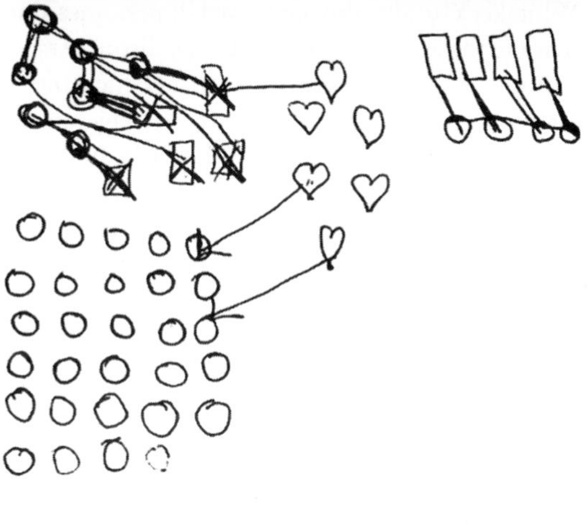

reflects her sense of HAART as a giver of life, having pulled her back from a hard death. By selectively engaging the biomedical concepts that support her and rejecting those that don't, she forges ahead. To her, AIDS means you need HAART. The medicines provide her a sense of strength and comfort. She is devoted to taking them and coming to her clinic appointments to track her T cells as they rise.

This is not always the case; illness meanings might integrate similar disease concepts to different outcomes. Jeanne has an AIDS diagnosis, but finds that taking HAART makes it more, and not less, difficult for her to cope with her diagnosis. She employs a variety of conflicting strategies for negotiating the idea of AIDS. First, in the word association, she takes an approach similar to Laetitia's. She says of both HIV and AIDS that they are "just a word," stripping them of other meaning. In the interview, she simultaneously rejects the notion that AIDS means death, while accepting it and claiming herself exempt because she takes good care of herself. Then in the next breath, she says that some people don't die from AIDS:

> I just know I don't got AIDS yet. . . . It's just I really take care of myself . . . 'cause that— when they say you got AIDS, that's when you pass. Some people don't pass when they have AIDS.

Her sense of conflict is evident, as is her emotional struggle. She, too, says she tries not to think about it. What makes her think about it the most, she says, is taking HAART: "When you take medicine like that you just be thinking—I don't want to think no more."

The medicines remind her that she needs them to live, she says, and of having "a virus." She faces a bind, in that the medicines remind her of the unnamed virus that threatens her life, but in owning that it is threatening her life, she knows she needs to take them. This dilemma is not simply an internal one. She also says that acknowledging she's taking medications for the virus is a "put-down"; she talks of the derogatory talk her family and friends engage in about people with AIDS. She has disclosed to almost no one. She is struggling for more than her physical survival, but to maintain the scant social support that she has, as well as her own sense of integrity. Her attempt at resolving this for herself, so she can go back on HAART, involves resisting not just the words AIDS and HIV, but the whole illness. She's thinking she could go back on HAART and pretend the medication was for another illness, like arthritis, or high blood pressure, or that the pills were vitamins:

> So, I could see it for something else but I do arthritis, you know. I could take it for that or something. . . . I see it as somethin' else or maybe it's these vitamins or something that keeps so, I'll have more like high blood pressure or something. I just think, it'll be crazy stuff but I just keep tryin' to think so I can get that off my mind.

Substituting her illness with one that she doesn't perceive to be fatal or stigmatizing is what she needs to get sufficient distance from her fear and pain. Jeanne's sense of struggle is depicted in her drawing, which is an enlarged view of her stomach (including her navel; see Figure 12.5).

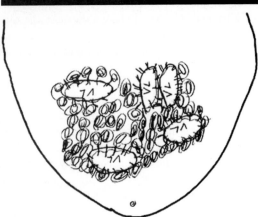

FIGURE 12.5   ■   Jeanne's Illustration: A Fight in Her Stomach Between Her T Cells and Her Viral Load

Inside her stomach, "viral load" cells fight with her T cells. The viral load cells are many times the size of the T cells, and she draws them a dark color with hairy protrusions. The T cells are a cheerful light red. She says they're fighting because she's not taking medications, and it's a bad situation:

> My T cells are fighting my viral load. . . . Because I need to get on my medicine . . . it's bad . . . they fighting right now.

Her depiction of her T cells' struggle against her viral load mirrors her unresolved struggle with the meanings of AIDS and HAART in her life. For her, at this time, this has translated into her living with HIV without the aid of HAART.

DISCUSSION

The findings presented here show women with HIV making a sharp distinction between the meanings of HIV and AIDS, with AIDS being marked as a state of hopelessness and imminent death. These connotations are consistent with images of AIDS before HAART. Though the clinical picture of AIDS has changed, the social meanings of AIDS have not shifted in synchrony. Similar strategies were at play before HAART among a group of HIV-positive Australians described by Whittaker (1992). She describes their inversion of AIDS metaphors to strip HIV-related words of power. Participants in Whitaker's study also employed illness meanings that emphasized HIV and AIDS as distinct stages. Whittaker argues that this allowed participants to regain a sense of control under a "barrage of pro-scriptions and prescriptions" (Whittaker, 1992).

Illness meanings of AIDS incorporate moral components. Irresponsible behavior and lack of self-love are related to getting AIDS, via poor adherence to HAART. Distinctions between HIV and AIDS might serve to distance the women emotionally from a sense of physical, social, and emotional threat.

However, this distinction is limited by the women's very real physical suffering from HAART side effects and other ailments, and the lack of distinction made between HIV and AIDS in their families and communities. In addition, this dichotomy might present real risks to the women if they receive an AIDS diagnosis at some point, and are forced to cross over this "line of meaning." In this case, as is seen with women who have received AIDS diagnoses, meanings must be renegotiated to retain hope and engage in HAART.

Erving Goffman's (1963) ideas of social stigma figure powerfully in the illness meanings described by the women. The HIV-positive women portray an AIDS diagnosis as deeply discrediting; it is held to be a visible state that marks physical failure, moral failure, and social ostracism. Living with only an HIV diagnosis is described as normal. However, it is clear that the women's HIV diagnoses render them discreditable, if not discredited, and make them vulnerable to significant suffering. This suffering includes feelings of contamination, experiences of rejection when they disclose their HIV status, and physical symptoms.

The findings presented here also demonstrate the value of drawings as a visual method in exploring illness meanings. The drawings produced unique insights, enriching the data collected while also adding credibility to themes identified using other methods. Of special interest are the women's depictions of the immune system, and the militaristic language used in descriptions of its function. Both Emily Martin (1994) and Susan Sontag (1988) have written about the pervasive use of war language to describe the immune system, especially in relation to stigmatized illnesses. Both warn against it, as it might lead to conflict between a sense of agency with regard to one's health and a sense of helplessness to control this "invisible inner battle." This is similar to Arthur Frank's concept of "bodyrelatedness" (Frank, 1995; Montez & Karner, 2005), where the body and self are fragmented, leading to a sense of "having a body" rather than "being a body." The women in the study often vacillated back and forth between third- and first-person voice, reflecting this tension. One moment their drawings of bodies and cells depicted "it," and the next moment they depicted "me." However, even in third-person voice, the inner world often reflected elements of the life experienced outside the body.

An exclusive focus on disease knowledge of concepts such as AIDS, T cells, and viruses speaks to the inner mechanics of a body; an exploration of meanings given to these concepts speaks to a life, and the struggle to thrive in the face of a potentially fatal and stigmatizing infection. These results suggest the need to broaden our understanding of how illness meanings function for individual patients, to better support them in adhering to HAART, in engaging in care, and in living fully.

Note

1. All participant names have been changed.

References

Baer, R. D., Weller, S. C., Garcia de Alba Garcia, J., & Salcedo Rocha, A. L. (2004). A comparison of community and physician explanatory models of AIDS in Mexico and the United States. *Medical Anthropology Quarterly, 18*(1), 3–22.

Broom, D., & Whittaker, A. (2004). Controlling diabetes, controlling diabetics: Moral language in the management of diabetes type 2. *Social Science & Medicine, 58*(11), 2371–2382.

Brown, L., Macintyre, K., & Trujillo, L. (2003). Interventions to reduce HIV/AIDS stigma: What have we learned? *AIDS Education and Prevention, 15*(1), 49–69.

Castro, A., & Farmer, P. (2005). Understanding and addressing AIDS-related stigma: From anthropological theory to clinical practice in Haiti. *American Journal of Public Health, 95*(1), 53–59.

Crabtree, B. F., & Miller, W. L. (1999). *Doing qualitative research*. Thousand Oaks, CA: Sage.

Frank, A. (1995). *The wounded storyteller: Body, illness, and ethics*. Chicago: University of Chicago Press.

Goffman, E. (1963). *Stigma: Notes on management of spoiled identity*. New York: Simon & Schuster.

Goujard, C., Bernard, N., Sohier, N., Peyramond, D., Lancon, F., Chwalow, J., et al. (2003). Impact of a patient education program on adherence to HIV medication: A randomized clinical trial. *Journal of Acquired Immune Deficiency Syndrome, 34*(2), 191–194.

Guillemin, M. (2004). Understanding illness: Using drawings as a research method. *Qualitative Health Research, 14*, 272–289.

Herek, G. M., & Glunt, E. K. (1988). An epidemic of stigma. Public reactions to AIDS. *American Psychology, 43*(11), 886–891.

Kleinman, A. (1988). *The illness narratives: Suffering, healing, and the human condition*. New York: Basic Books.

Lieblich, A., & Tuval-Mashaiach, R. (1998). *Narrative: Reading, analysis, and interpretation*. Thousand Oaks, CA: Sage.

Loewe, R., Schwartzman, J., Freeman, J., Quinn, L., & Zuckerman, S. (1998). Doctor talk and diabetes: Towards an analysis of the clinical construction of chronic illness. *Social Science & Medicine, 47*(9), 1267–1276.

Lundgren, J. D., Pedersen, C., Clumeck, N., Gatell, J. M., Johnson, A. M., Ledergerber, B., et al. (1994). Survival differences in European patients with AIDS, 1979–89. *British Medical Journal, 308*, 1068–1073.

Madru, N. (2003). Stigma and HIV: Does the social response affect the natural course of the epidemic? *Journal of the Association of Nurses in AIDS Care, 14*(5), 39–48.

Martin, E. (1994). *Flexible bodies: The role of immunity in American culture from the days of polio to the age of AIDS*. Boston: Beacon Press.

McNaghten, A. D., Hansen, D. L., Jones, J. L., Dworkin, M. S., & Ward, J. W. (1999). Effects of antiretroviral therapy and opportunistic illness primary chemoprophylaxis on survival after AIDS diagnosis. *AIDS, 13*, 1687–1695.

Mill, J. E. (2000). Describing an explanatory model of HIV illness among aboriginal women. *Holistic Nursing Practice, 15*(1), 42–56.

Mill, J. E. (2001). I'm not a "basabasa" woman: An explanatory model of HIV illness in Ghanaian women. *Clinical Nursing Research, 10*(3), 254–274.

Mocroft, A., Youle, M., Morcinek, J., Sabin, C. A., Gazzard, B., Phillips, A. N., et al. (1997). Survival after diagnosis of AIDS: A prospective observational study of 2625 patients. *British Medical Journal, 314*, 409–413.

Montez, J. K., & Karner, T. X. (2005). Understanding the diabetic body-self. *Qualitative Health Research, 15*, 1086–1104.

Parker, R., & Aggleton, P. (2003). HIV and AIDS-related stigma and discrimination: A conceptual framework and implications for action. *Social Science & Medicine, 57*(1), 13–24.

Rawlings, M. K., Thompson, M. A., Farthing, C. F., Brown, L. S., Racine, J., Scott, R. C., et al. (2003). Impact of an educational program on efficacy and adherence with a twice-daily lamivudine/zidovudine/abacavir regimen in underrepresented

HIV-infected patients. *Journal of Acquired Immune Deficiency Syndrome, 34*(2), 174–183.

Rose, G. (2001). *Visual methodologies*. London: Sage.

Schwarcz, S. K., Hsu, L. C., Vittinghoff, E., & Katz, M. H. (2000). Impact of protease inhibitors and other antiretroviral treatments on acquired immunodeficiency syndrome survival in San Francisco, California, 1987–1996. *American Journal of Epidemiology, 152*(2), 178–185.

Scott, A., Ellen, J., Clum, G., & Leonard, L. (2007). HIV and housing assistance in four U.S. cities: Variations in local experience. *AIDS Behavior, 11*(6 Suppl), 140–148.

Sontag, S. (1988). *Illness as metaphor and AIDS and its metaphors*. New York: Picador.

Taylor, B. (2001). HIV, stigma and health: Integration of theoretical concepts and the lived experiences of individuals. *Journal of Advanced Nursing, 35*(5), 792–798.

Victora, C. G., & Knauth, D. R. (2001). Images of the body and the reproductive system among men and women living in Shantytowns in Porto Alegre, Brazil. *Reproductive Health Matters, 9,* 22–33.

Whittaker, A. (1992). Living with HIV: Resistance by positive people. *Medical Anthropology Quarterly, 6*(4), 385–390.

13

WHOSE DEATHS MATTER?

Mortality, Advocacy, and Attention to Disease in the Mass Media*

Elizabeth M. Armstrong, Daniel P. Carpenter, and Marie Hojnacki

Even in today's world of global terrorism, economic crisis and political impasse, the news is often about one of humankind's oldest problems, that of disease. Headlines about disease regularly appear on the front pages of major newspapers. Both newspaper and television news programs rely on reporters who cover "the health beat," and many news venues have dedicated health or science sections that provide regular coverage of diseases. Moreover, organized interest groups, such as ACT UP, the American Lung Association, and the National Breast Cancer Coalition, are ubiquitous in public policy debates. Hollywood celebrities and members of Congress frequently become "sponsors" of various diseases, with their involvement sparking even greater public attention. Indeed, disease captivates the interest of newsmakers, of the public at large, and of policymakers and other political actors.

Most social science research on the process of allocating attention to disease has focused on a single disease at a particular point in time. In this paper, we use a unique dataset that we have collected about print and broadcast media attention to seven diseases across nineteen years in order to address two questions about media attention to disease. First, how (if at all) is the social burden of a disease related to attention? Second, how (if at all) do organized interest groups affect attention? To be sure, many scholars have taken an interest

Whose Deaths Matter? Mortality, Advocacy, and Attention to Disease in the Mass Media, Elizabeth Armstrong, Daniel Carpenter, and Marie Hojnacki in *Journal of Health Politics, Policy and Law, 31*(4), pp. 729–772. Copyright, 2006, Duke University Press. All rights reserved. Republished by permission of the copyright holder, Duke University Press. www.dukepress.edu.

*Some material from this article has been removed. Please consult the original source for full text.

in how the epidemiology and politics of particular diseases—usually examined in case-study form—affect attention from the media. But our project has two unique features. First, the inferences we draw from the impact of social burden and interest groups on media attention to disease are based on a direct comparison of burden, groups, and attention across different diseases. This direct comparison of burden across different "problems" has been difficult for researchers to undertake because most problems lack a common metric for comparison. But we can approximate the social burden of a disease with the number of deaths it causes in order to examine directly the relationship between the social burden a problem inflicts and the attention it receives from the media. Second, given that much research about media attention to disease has been dominated by studies of single, high-profile diseases such as breast cancer or AIDS, we examine whether the process of allocating attention to one of those diseases—HIV/AIDS—is illustrative of the attention-generating process characterizing diseases in general, or whether the attention process to AIDS is distinct from that of the other diseases.

Moreover, studying these seven diseases enables us to escape the constraints of a strict constructionist perspective on the news—that is, that the mass media "create" social problems via their attention to them. Although we are not able to address the content of media attention or the framing of these seven diseases as social problems in this analysis, we are able to examine rigorously and empirically the relationship between "the underlying reality" of a social problem (in this case, a particular disease) and attention to that problem in the public arena. Our analysis suggests that who suffers from a disease as well as how many suffer are critical factors in explaining why some diseases get more attention than others. For example, our data illustrate that both the print and broadcast media tend to be much *less* attentive to diseases that burden blacks more than whites. However, a number of our inferences about media attention are sensitive to the inclusion or exclusion of AIDS observations from the sample, suggesting that scholars should be cautious about generalizing from the AIDS case to the attention process more broadly. We argue that only through a study of why

the media allocates different amounts of attention to different diseases at different points in time is it possible to separate the anomalous aspects of AIDS from those aspects that reflect general tendencies of attention allocation by the media.

VARIATION IN MEDIA ATTENTION TO DISEASE

Public attention to disease in general is expanding over time, yet different diseases capture that attention in varied ways and to varying degrees. Some diseases, such as HIV/AIDS, dominate public discourse, while other diseases, such as pneumonia (which is among the ten leading causes of death in the United States), receive only glancing attention, if any at all. Figure 13.1 demonstrates this variation for the period 1980 through 1998 among the set of seven diseases we study, all of which are leading causes of mortality in the United States: heart disease, lung cancer, cerebrovascular disease (primarily stroke), chronic obstructive pulmonary disease (COPD), diabetes, HIV/AIDS, and Alzheimer's disease. The first row of bars depicts the total number of deaths attributed to each disease over this time period, ranging from 14.2 million for heart disease, to 236,000 for Alzheimer's disease.[1] The second row depicts the total number of stories on each disease appearing in the *New York Times* and the *Washington Post* combined. The third row shows the total number of stories appearing on the major television networks' evening news programs (ABC, CBS, and NBC).

Figure 13.1 illustrates that some diseases get a lot of attention across both print and broadcast venues—most notably, HIV/AIDS, but also heart disease—whereas diabetes, for example, attracts substantial newspaper attention, but almost no attention from the television news. In addition, these data show that at least one measure of social burden—mortality—is not a consistent predictor of media attention to that disease: diseases that cause more deaths do not necessarily get more attention. HIV/AIDS is the clear outlier here, though note as well that while COPD causes almost seven times as

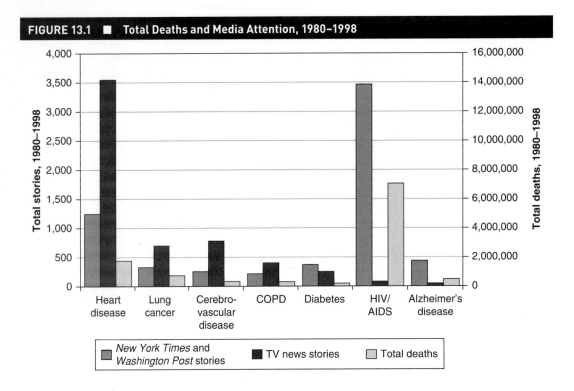

FIGURE 13.1 ■ Total Deaths and Media Attention, 1980–1998

many deaths as Alzheimer's, newspaper stories on Alzheimer's outnumber stories on COPD by about two to one.

Although Figure 13.1 relies on aggregate data for the time period, attention to disease varies over time as well, as shown in Figure 13.2, which depicts the total number of stories devoted to each disease in each year between 1980 and 1998 appearing in the *New York Times* and the *Washington Post*. Again, we can see the unequal levels of attention to these diseases, as well as differences in the extent to which that attention varies over time. In the case of AIDS, Figure 13.2 shows a gradual increase in media attention throughout the early years of the disease, up until attention peaks in the late 1980s. Although media attention to AIDS subsequently begins to decline, the level of attention it commands remains relatively high through the 1990s. The peaks and valleys in attention to the six remaining diseases are much less pronounced. Thus, these diseases are allocated less attention by newspapers than is AIDS, and the annual variation in attention to them is not

nearly as dramatic. Figure 13.2 also illustrates the tremendous growth of annual total stories devoted to disease overall, from fewer than 100 stories in 1980 to about 350 stories in 1998, down from a peak of about 800 stories in 1987 when news writers and producers were giving extensive coverage to the relatively new disease called AIDS.

That disease garners public attention, then, is indisputable. But *how* and *why* do some diseases get more attention from the media than others? Disease itself, as a category of news story, fulfills most of the criteria scholars have associated with newsworthiness. "Newsworthy" problems have been characterized as those that are "new" or current; that affect the general population, or threaten to do so; that are easily described, typically through the use of a "hook" or "human interest" angle; and that can be readily linked to authoritative sources, such as public health officials, scientists or physicians (Gans 1979; Schudson 1978; Tuchman 1978). Diseases typically demonstrate all of these characteristics. Moreover, diseases frequently attract the attention of celebrity advocates, and may be associated with notable people (e.g., sufferers who are known by the general public) and "trigger events" (e.g., a breakthrough in treatment or diagnosis) that researchers have argued are essential for attracting attention to problems (Corbett and Mori 1999; Dearing and Rogers 1996). Yet acknowledging that disease is newsworthy—either inherently or by association with newsworthy individuals or events—does not help us understand the dramatic variation in attention over time, across diseases, and across venues that we observe in Figures 13.1 and 13.2. What propels one newsworthy disease to receive more attention than another newsworthy disease, and what drives these observed shifts in attention levels?[2]

. . . Because most social problems lack a common metric for comparison, researchers have had difficulty sorting out precisely why some problems attract more attention than others. Several studies have described or characterized how variables including interest group involvement, windows of opportunity, shifts in decision-making venues, easily accessible sources of expertise, affected target populations, and definitions or images rooted in

appealing symbols contribute to the ebb and flow in public attention to particular issues and problems (Baumgartner and Jones 1993; Best 1990; Blumer 1971; Cobb and Elder 1983; Cobb and Ross 1997; Cook 1998; Downs 1972; Edelman 1971, 1988; Elder and Cobb 1983; Epstein 1996; Gusfield 1981; Hilgartner and Bosk 1988; Kingdon 1995; Kitsuse and Spector 1973; Schneider and Ingram 1993; Spector and Kitsuse 1973; Terkildsen, Schnell, and Ling 1998). But with no basis for comparing social problems, what we know about the correlates of attention to social issues is drawn from studies that observe attention to individual problems. It is only through implicit comparison that we come to understand why attention is allocated to some social problems more often than others. For example, many researchers claim that empirical indicators of severity are unrelated to the attention a problem receives (Blumer 1971). As evidence for the "relative unimportance" of "real-world indicators," Dearing and Rogers (1996) mention Kerr's (1986) story showing that attention to the war on drugs peaked in response to the death of a young basketball star and Nancy Reagan's "Just Say No" campaign, both

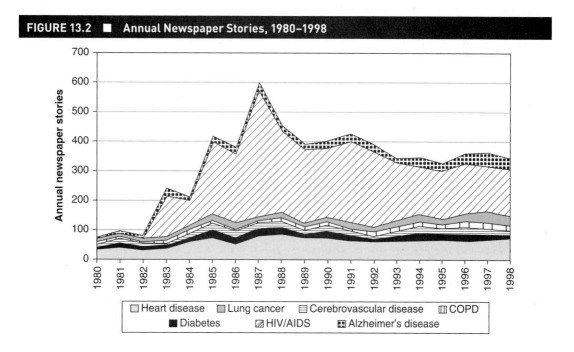

FIGURE 13.2 ■ Annual Newspaper Stories, 1980–1998

of which happened while the number of drug-related deaths declined. Similarly, media attention to environmental issues was shown to increase as pollution decreased (Ader 1993, cited in Dearing and Rogers 1996), lending support to the idea that attention to a problem is uncorrelated or negatively correlated with objective indicators of its severity or that there is a lag between the manifestation of a problem and its recognition in the mass media. But because these studies focus on one social problem at a time, they do not indicate whether variation in the societal burden of drug deaths relative to the societal burden of pollution helps to explain differences in attention to drugs relative to environmental issues; the burden of drug deaths cannot validly be compared with the burden of pollution.

Like these studies, much of what is known about how health problems and diseases capture public attention is drawn from studies of a single disease, particularly AIDS or breast cancer, at a specific point in time (Casamayou 2001; Colby and Cook 1991; Epstein 1996; Lantz and Booth 1998; Lerner 2001). Yet Figures 13.1 and 13.2 suggest that generalizing about how and why diseases capture attention based on any single case—particularly AIDS—could be problematic. AIDS is hardly a "typical" disease. Not only does AIDS command a relatively large amount of public attention and cause far fewer deaths in aggregate than many other diseases, it also is associated with a relatively sizable set of organized groups that advocate on behalf of individuals who suffer from the disease. Moreover, while AIDS mortality may be lower in total than that caused by other diseases, AIDS has powerful cultural associations with death because of its nearly 100 percent case-fatality rate and because it strikes most often in the prime of life. AIDS also enjoys the advantage of a keen news hook via its connection to sex. In addition, as an emerging disease—never seen before—AIDS was both new and "news" in a way that other diseases are not. Yet because scholars have generalized from AIDS, the conventional understanding of how *any disease* gets attention has come to be that the number of deaths associated with it is less important in drawing public attention than is having organized and politically active advocates who work to increase research funding for and public attention to that disease. . . .

DISEASE BURDEN AND MEDIA ATTENTION

From the common cold to AIDS, diseases exact a toll on society as well as on individuals. We believe the burden a disease imposes on the population as a whole, and on specific groups within the population, shapes attention. In other words, diseases garner attention in the public arena precisely because they have *real consequences* for individuals and for society as a whole. However, the burden of a disease is typically distributed unequally across society. This uneven distribution of burden means that diseases have varying degrees of *salience* in the public arena, and this variation in salience may manifest in differential attention from the media.

. . . [There are] at least two fundamental dimensions of burden that we argue may affect the salience of a disease and thus the attention allocation process. First, the nature of the burden itself, whether in the form of morbidity or mortality, impact on quality or length of life, or such direct costs to the health care system as treatment, hospitalization, or pharmaceuticals, may draw the media's attention. Diseases make people sick; morbidity in turn affects the quality of life, labor force productivity, and the care burden that falls on family members or society. Thus, it is important to know how many people suffer from a particular disease, as well as something about the cost of that suffering to them as individuals and to society as a whole; how many and what kinds of societal and health care resources are allocated to the disease? For our purposes, this information is most readily identifiable in data on disease incidence and mortality, hospitalizations, outpatient visits, and drug utilization, though such data do not begin to capture the complete burden of disease. The point is that diseases do exact some burdens that are measurable, even if the true cost of a particular disease to society is itself immeasurable.[3]

Second, we expect the salience of a disease (and subsequent media attention given to a disease) to depend on *who* in society suffers these burdens as described earlier. At the most basic level, the characteristics of the people who suffer or die from a particular disease are important. Are they young or old, male or female, black or white, rich or poor? Few diseases affect all sectors of the population equally. Demographic characteristics of groups on whom the burden of disease falls differentially vary across disease. For example, black mortality from diabetes is significantly higher than white mortality, whereas the reverse is true for mortality from COPD. Men suffer higher death rates from heart disease than women, while women suffer higher death rates from cerebrovascular disease. Thus, the disease burden, reflected in terms of mortality, falls differentially across different population groups, and we believe that not only the numbers of people burdened by a particular disease but also the demographic characteristics of those people (i.e., race, sex, and age) affects the salience of a disease in the public eye.

These two dimensions of burden—its degree and who endures it—map onto distinct ways in which it may affect media attention. First, the overall numbers of those affected (either in terms of deaths, incidence, cost, etc.) by a particular disease may create or shape attention to that disease. Although some research suggests that attention levels do not reflect trends in burden as measured by death (Colby and Cook 1991:222–223), a relatively recent study finds that newspaper coverage of disease *is* responsive to trends in disease mortality (Adelman and Verbrugge 2000). But this study included obituaries and paid death notices in their measure of newspaper coverage, all but ensuring that coverage would map closely with rates of death (indeed, they found that trends in coverage do not correspond to trends in prevalence or incidence of a disease). Thus, the link between attention and burden remains empirically unfounded.

Second, we expect that changes in the burden of a particular disease—either in the form of increases or decreases over time—may affect levels of attention to that disease. This idea is consistent with Adelman and Verbrugge's (2000) suggestion that

the newsworthiness of a decline in cancer deaths may explain why they observe no decrease in news coverage of cancer even as the death rate from cancer decreases, a pattern that is at odds with their central finding that death rates and coverage are linked.

Third, we expect that the groups in society who bear the burden of a disease are likely to have an impact on the amount of attention that is given to a disease. For instance, diseases that affect minority groups may draw less attention than diseases that afflict white males at a greater rate than the general population precisely because "minority" diseases may be regarded as less salient. Diseases affecting minority groups may be perceived as meriting less attention because they pose less of a threat to the general population; less attention to these diseases also may result from the news selection strategies of (predominantly) white broadcast and print media executives who are attentive to problems affecting their own families and friends (Cohen 1999). Editors may also select stories about particular diseases in order to draw readers of a particular social group; diseases that impose a greater burden on women than men may be given more attention as news producers make efforts to attract a female audience. In addition, diseases that are especially burdensome to younger rather than older groups in the population may attract relatively more public attention precisely because the death or illness is premature. Moreover, diseases that affect "sympathetic" social groups such as children, even in a relatively limited way, may garner more attention because of the group affected (Vallabhan 1997). Our analysis, then, examines not only whether death matters in the attention process, but more precisely, *whose* deaths matter.

It is possible that the media respond not to "real" burden but to the perceived burden of a disease. Researchers have demonstrated time and again that the mass media often "get the facts wrong" in portraying social problems (Hubbard et al. 1975) as diverse as child abduction (Best 1990), environmental degradation (Mazur and Lee 1993), and school shootings (Newman 2004). Surely, advocates associated with social problems contribute to these misperceptions. For example, breast cancer is far more likely to strike and kill older women than younger women. But because advocacy groups often emphasize breast cancer deaths among young women, especially young mothers, the public actually misunderstands the epidemiology of the disease (Lantz and Booth 1998). Relatedly, recent public awareness campaigns about heart disease among women have been initiated (at least in part) to clear up the misperception that breast cancer causes more deaths among women than does heart disease. The tendency of politicians and some organizations to link AIDS with children also illustrates how misperceptions can occur. Thus, it is possible that attention is driven not by actual mortality but by a misperception or mischaracterization of that rate. Mistaken portrayals or perceptions of burden could explain why mortality has been observed to be an inconsistent predictor of attention to disease.

ORGANIZED ADVOCACY AND MEDIA ATTENTION

The phenomenon of identifying certain diseases within particular population groups is also reflected in the politics of disease. There has been tremendous attention focused on the politics and politicization of disease, particularly around HIV/AIDS and breast cancer. Researchers and journalists have documented the social movements that emerged to seek more research funding for HIV/AIDS and breast cancer, along with enhanced social service support for those suffering from the diseases, and greater access to drugs and other medical treatments (Epstein 1996; Shilts 1987). Of course, organizations advocating on behalf of victims of disease are not new. Groups such as the March of Dimes, American Lung Association, and American Cancer Society have been around for well over seventy years and have frequently been credited with drawing public and governmental attention to health-related issues (Lerner 2001; Proctor 1995). However, in recent years, organized disease advocates have become a primary focus of those who have sought to understand both the increases in funding for HIV/ AIDS and breast cancer research and the substantial

public attention paid to these diseases. Casamayou (2001), for example, gives nearly sole credit to the National Breast Cancer Coalition, founded in 1991, for increasing federal funding for breast cancer. Epstein (1996) argues that the demographics of those most directly affected by HIV/AIDS (i.e., politically efficacious, white, middle-class men) made possible a movement of "activist experts" rather than of victims. These individuals established themselves as a credible source of knowledge apart from the medical establishment, allowing them to affect policy decisions made about AIDS treatment. More generally, others argue that AIDS advocacy was made relatively easy by the presence of politically active organizations in the gay community that existed prior to the epidemic (Cohen 1999).

Of course, disease sufferers and their advocates are not alone in their interest in drawing public attention to a disease. Physicians, research scientists, fund-raisers, representatives of specialty care centers, and public health officials, among others, have a considerable stake in attracting public attention to particular diseases. Like disease sufferers, specialty associations of physicians and other professionals realize that decisions to allocate resources to a disease may flow from increased public attention. At the same time, reporters and other members of the media most certainly are aware of and attentive to these "authoritative sources" populating many disease communities. Although it is unlikely that these professional associations and institutional interests are distributed evenly across the organizational communities associated with different diseases, they share the incentives of citizen advocates to draw public and governmental attention to health-related issues.[4]

The importance of organized advocates and social movements in drawing public and governmental attention to disease receives support in the broader literature on movements and groups (Best 1990; Cress and Snow 2000; Kitsuse and Spector 1973; Kollman 1998; Wright 1996). Indeed, any social problem that emerges or is recognized as such has associated with it a set of interest groups whose explicit aim it is to draw attention to *their* problem (Best 1990; Kitsuse and Spector 1973). However, the means through which these entities are most successful in drawing attention to their concerns—a strong organization, large numbers, an ability to provide information, protests, headline-grabbing advocacy tactics—is subject to debate (Gamson 1990; Gandy 1982; Montgomery 1989; Piven and Cloward 1977). One way through which organized interests secure attention to particular problems is by acting as noisemakers, communicating to policy makers and members of the media the salience of an issue. Relatively large and proactive organizational communities—like those associated with AIDS and breast cancer—can draw attention to specific issues by communicating, through their claims-making and general advocacy activity, a capacity to stir up public attention and interest, thereby signaling that a problem is salient and of concern to a large (or especially influential) segment of the public (Caldeira and Wright 1988; Kollman 1998; Spector and Kitsuse 1973). Similarly, communities that can give an impression that they will turn out large numbers of voters in response to a particular issue on Election Day are likely to attract attention and agenda space (Donovan 2001; Wright 1996).

Another way in which organized interests can draw attention to problems is by providing information to subsidize the costs of search for those who control access to attention—that is, reporters and government decision makers (Berry 1999; Gandy 1982; Hall 2000). Members of the media operate under tight time schedules. As a result, the expertise, data, and intelligence available from organizations can both fulfill an important need for reporters and make it easier for them to be attentive to groups' concerns. Indeed, just as members of Congress grant access to organized interests who have an information provision advantage relative to their competitors (Hansen 1991), organizations may serve as "authoritative sources" about issues, enhancing the likelihood that "their" problems and concerns become part of the media agenda (Colby and Cook 1991; Cook 1998; Gans 1979). The movement of AIDS activist experts described by Epstein (1996) is especially illustrative of this information subsidy. Politically active groups may be especially valuable information sources since they are able to gather information and convey it to actors in both media outlets and government. Importantly, the ability of different communities of organizations to communicate effectively their concerns will depend on the skills and resources of individual organizations, and whether their message is one that resonates with mainstream public discourse (Barker-Plummer 1995; Gitlin 1980).

DATA

To investigate how disease burden and organized disease advocates affect media attention to disease, we have collected data about seven diseases for each of nineteen years. We have deliberately included diseases that are leading causes of death for the U.S. population as a whole, as well as for different age, gender, and race/ethnicity groups. We examine both chronic and infectious diseases; diseases with low mortality but high morbidity, such as Alzheimer's disease and asthma; diseases that are media-prominent; and diseases that much less often appear in the headlines. Data about media attention to each disease, the organizations with an interest in each disease, and the social burden of each disease have been collected for each year from 1980 to 1998.

Media Attention to Disease

Our analysis rests upon five indicators of the attention allocated to each disease by the broadcast and print media. Broadcast media attention is captured by the number of disease-related stories featured on each of the ABC, CBS, and NBC early evening news broadcasts each week. These data were obtained from the *Vanderbilt Television News Abstracts and Indices* using . . . search terms [that included] words used by laypersons as well as medical professionals . . . [for example, "heart disease" and] "myocardial infarction."

Attention from the print media is measured by the weekly count of disease-related stories appearing in the *New York Times* and in the *Washington Post*.[5] The print data were gathered from Lexis-Nexis using key words. We examined each of the broadcast story abstracts and print stories that were located through our search in order to determine whether the story was actually related to the relevant disease, omitting any stories that were not primarily about the disease in question. For example, our search for HIV/AIDS brought up stories that described efforts to gain support for a housing program that happened to serve individuals with the disease. When those stories focused primarily on the program and only in passing mentioned the clientele served, the stories were not included in our counts. However, if the story dealt with the myriad difficulties faced by HIV/AIDS sufferers, particularly as the disease was emerging, it was included in our counts. In general, when the disease in question was central to the story—either on its own or in conjunction with other topics—only then was that story included in our counts. Although this approach was more time consuming than relying on simple counts of the stories retrieved with each search term, it provides us with a measure that more truly reflects the concept of media attention to a particular disease.

We excluded obituaries and paid death notices from our counts to avoid conflating rising mortality from a particular disease with a genuine increase in attention to that disease outside of the obituaries. Given that we have collected print and broadcast news stories for each week over nineteen years, we have 991 weeks of broadcast abstract counts and print story counts for each disease. Across our seven diseases, then, we have 6,937 weeks of data available for analysis (with each unit representing a broadcast or print story count for a given week of a given year for a given disease).

Disease Burden

In this essay, we focus on mortality as one of the most fundamental measures of the social burden of disease. Death, after all, is the ultimate burden that a disease inflicts on the victim, as well as on the rest of us. We recognize that mortality is *not* the sum-total of social burden. It is not even an appropriate measure for many diseases that cause sickness—the common cold, for example, is estimated to cause 189 million missed school days a year, along with 126 million missed work days and costs the U.S.

economy close to $40 billion annually, a sizable burden that cannot be captured in mortality statistics (Fendrick et al. 2003). However, it is practical to use mortality as our initial measure of the burden of disease because we can very precisely identify deaths from these diseases using national vital statistics. Since deaths are coded by the National Center for Health Statistics using the International Classification of Diseases (ICD-9) codes, we can accurately match deaths to the seven diseases in our sample for the entire time series and for specific population groups.[6] . . .

In addition to measuring the overall mortality rate for a disease, we also expect that the media may be attentive to how death rates change over time and to how different population subgroups bear the burden of disease. Thus, we include in our analysis an indicator of the absolute value of annual changes in the overall mortality rate for each disease, as well as several measures that reflect the differential burden a disease imposed on different subgroups. Specifically, we include an indicator of how each disease affected blacks relative to whites (expressed as the ratio of black mortality to white mortality), and the differential burden each disease imposed on females relative to males (the ratio of female mortality to male mortality). We use ratios rather than including separately the mortality rates for each of these subgroups because we are interested in how attention is affected by the *relative* impact of a disease on particular groups, rather than in how the mortality of individual subgroups affects attention. In other words, in addition to the overall burden inflicted by a disease, we are interested in how attention from the media is shaped by the extent to which a disease affects and comes to be associated with one particular group to the exclusion of other groups.

The seven diseases that we examine exhibit markedly different patterns of mortality change over the time period and across population subgroups. Figure 13.3 shows the mortality rates for each disease across the nineteen years of our series. (Because these death rates are not age-adjusted, changes in the rates may reflect changes in the underlying incidence of the disease, changes in the age structure of the population, or changes in medical treatment.)

Mortality from heart disease and cerebrovascular disease dropped precipitously from 1980 to 1998, while deaths from lung cancer, COPD, diabetes and Alzheimer's disease rose. HIV/AIDS once again exhibits a unique pattern, with mortality rates rising in the first decade and a half of the epidemic and then declining rapidly from 1996 on, due in part to a leveling off in the spread of the disease and in larger part to the success of anti-retroviral treatment at prolonging life. The astronomical rate of increase in Alzheimer's disease is largely an artifact of the growing propensity over time to make this clinical diagnosis, as well as the aging of the population, rather than a true explosion of cases (Ewbank 1999).

Moreover, these diseases exhibit very different demographic patterns. . . . Heart disease affects men more than women (although by 1998 crude death rates are roughly equivalent between men and women) and whites more than blacks. Lung cancer also kills more men than women, though the gap is narrowing over time. Cerebrovascular disease, in contrast, causes higher mortality among women and is also more likely to strike whites than blacks. COPD is initially a "male disease," but by 1998 women caught up and mortality rates are fairly equal by sex. COPD also causes more deaths among whites than blacks. Diabetes shows far greater differences in race than in sex, with blacks much more likely to die of diabetes than whites are. This difference reflects both the higher prevalence of diabetes in the black population, as well as worse care. Alzheimer's disease mortality is higher among women, in part because women are more likely than men to survive to older age. Deaths from Alzheimer's disease are also higher among whites than among blacks. The patterns of HIV/AIDS mortality are much more difficult to summarize. It is well-known that the demography of the AIDS epidemic has shifted dramatically, from a disease of gay, primarily white men, to a disease of minorities that hits women particularly hard.

Communities of Organized Interests

To examine the impact of organized interests on media attention to disease, we identified the organizations that are part of each disease community as well as some of their relevant characteristics by searching the text of national organization entries

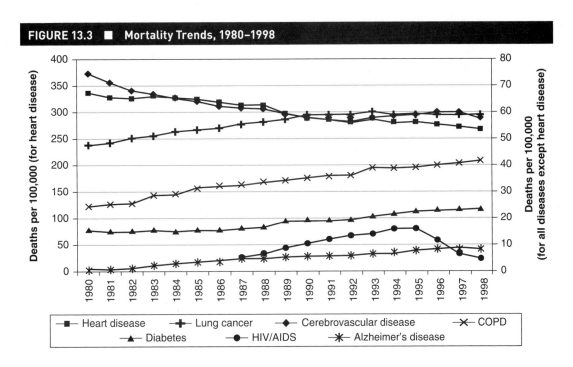

FIGURE 13.3 ■ Mortality Trends, 1980–1998

in the *Associations Unlimited (AU)* database. Relevant organizations could include those that had a direct interest in some aspect of a given disease (e.g., as treatment providers, patient advocates, or seekers of research funding), as well as those with interests that were orthogonal to their primary organizational objectives (e.g., an organization that advocated a particular approach to treating disease that took an interest in cancer patients). The measure we use here focuses solely on the organizations that had a primary interest in a particular disease, a relatively conservative measure of the size of the interested organizational communities. The information about the individual groups was aggregated to obtain counts of the number of organizations expressing some interest in each disease in each year from 1980 to 1998.[7]

Once the relevant organizations associated with each disease community were identified, we also gathered information about some of their characteristics from *Washington Representatives* (2004). For present purposes, we need an indicator of a disease community's capacity for providing expertise and information about a disease to the media or others. Our measure of that capacity is the percentage of groups in each community that registered to lobby Congress as of 2002. Although organized interests may have information to provide to the media even if they do not lobby Congress (Wallack et al. 1993), we believe that politically active organizations are especially likely to work proactively in this way. Because of their political involvement, they would be in a position both to gather information about government activity related to disease, and to obtain information about the priorities and activities of other interested organizations (Heinz et al. 1993). Moreover, because registered groups are engaged in efforts to pursue their policy goals, they would likely be interested in getting attention to their issues on both the political agenda and media agenda.

. . . [Among our seven disease communities, the largest number of groups exist around heart disease and HIV/AIDS.] The growth in groups with a primary interest in AIDS has been most pronounced, increasing from 2 groups in 1982 to more than 40 national organizations in 1998. Although the numbers of organizations with a primary interest in heart disease is large and has grown, this community has not experienced the degree of expansion that occurred among AIDS organizations during the same period. The communities for the remaining five diseases are much smaller, and have experienced little, if any, change over time. However, relative to most other diseases, it appears that many of the groups that take an interest in AIDS are not among the set that register to lobby. . . . As the community of AIDS groups grows, the newer groups tend to be those that do not lobby Congress (e.g., social service providers, various caregivers, foundations). In contrast, the proportion of registered groups is fairly high in the relatively smaller organizational communities associated with the remaining six diseases. This is most obvious in the case of the lung cancer community where one of the two organizations with a primary interest in lung cancer is engaged in legislative advocacy. Thus, lung cancer is a disease with a very small community of interested organizations but it is not an insignificant community from the standpoint of political advocacy given the interests of the American Lung Association.

Control Variables

In addition to the variables that are central to the hypotheses we test, each equation for media attention that we estimate contains some common control variables. To account for secular trends in coverage, we include simple trend variables, namely the year in question and the week of the year. These trend variables are important to include because coverage of health and disease has increased over the time period of our study (see Figure 13.2). We also include dichotomous variables for summer (Memorial Day to Labor Day), and for the first and last weeks of every year (winter vacation) to account for what are commonly considered low periods of readership and viewership. Additional time dependence is taken into account through the inclusion of a lagged dependent variable. The lagged term, which represents the number of stories in the previous week that were broadcast or written by a particular news outlet about a specific disease, allows us to account for patterns of attention continuity over time. In addition, because newspaper reporters and editors as well as television news producers may be responsive to scientific or medical news about disease (Bartlett et al. 2002), we include a measure of the weekly scientific/medical coverage given to each disease, which is simply the average number of articles about each disease that appeared each week in the *New England Journal of Medicine* (*NEJM*), the *Journal of the American Medical Association* (*JAMA*), the *Annals of Internal Medicine* (*AIM*), and *Science* combined. To proxy for technological change, we also include an indicator of the aggregate number of disease-specific drugs that were approved by the FDA in each week of each year in our study. Newspapers and broadcast media alike often carry news of new FDA drug and device approvals. The approvals data allow us to account for the attention to a disease that is given by the media when the government sanctions a new drug treatment.

. . .

The Question of Outliers

Because AIDS is unlike the other six diseases in terms of coverage, organizational community size, and in terms of the rate and change in mortality over the past two decades, we conducted separate analyses upon a full sample of all seven diseases and then replicated the results with the AIDS observations excluded. As will be clear, this often changed our results appreciably.

RESULTS

We have posed two main questions in this paper. We ask, first, how does the social burden of a disease affect attention levels in the mass media; second, how do organized groups affect attention? We summarize our results in Table 13.1. The first set of results, presented in the upper left corner of each cell, is based on a full sample of all seven diseases, including

TABLE 13.1 ■ Summary of Results for All Media	ABC stories	NBC stories	CBS stories	*Washington Post* stories	*New York Times* stories
Total mortality rate	+ −	+ −	+ −	+ −	+ −
Absolute value of annual change in mortality rate		+	+ +		
Black-white mortality ratio	− −	− −	−	−	−
Female-male mortality ratio	− +	− +	 +	 +	+
Number of organizations with primary interest in disease by year	+ +	+	+	+ +	+ +
Percentage of organizations registered to lobby Congress by year	+	+	+ +	+	+ +

Note: The sign of the statistically significant coefficients is reported in each cell of the table. The models with the full sample including AIDS are reported in the upper left section of each cell; the models excluding AIDS are reported in the lower right section. Cells that are shaded indicate changes in direction of effect and/or statistical significance when AIDS is excluded. If the coefficient is not statistically significant, the cell is blank.

AIDS, and the second set of results, presented in the lower right corner of each cell, is based on a restricted sample, excluding AIDS. Cells that are shaded indicate changes in the direction of the effect and/or the statistical significance of the effect when AIDS is excluded. Many of our findings change depending on whether AIDS is included or excluded.

We consider first the effect of social burden, specifically mortality, on attention. When we include AIDS, the total mortality rate has a negative and statistically significant effect on coverage levels in both newspapers and all three television news networks. In other words, the higher the mortality, the less coverage of that disease. Changes in mortality, whether increases or decreases, have no significant effect on attention in the full sample. However, when we exclude AIDS from our estimations, we find very different results: total mortality is again a statistically significant predictor of coverage across all five media outlets, but the sign has shifted from negative to positive, meaning that more deaths generate more attention. In addition, evidence of a positive and significant effect of change in mortality appears for NBC and CBS news stories, but not for the other media outlets. In sum, our results suggest that the relationship between death and news coverage is more complicated than prior research has demonstrated. If AIDS is included in the estimation sample, it is not true that more deaths mean more news; rather, the opposite hypothesis receives support. Yet when AIDS is excluded, we observe a positive relationship between aggregate burden and attention.

In addition to the overall impact of mortality on attention, our results reveal that the relative burden of a disease on different population subgroups also shapes media attention. One of the more consistent findings to emerge from our analyses is that the ratio of black mortality to white mortality tends to be negatively associated with news coverage, a finding that holds true for both the full and the restricted samples. In other words, the greater the burden of disease for blacks relative to whites, the less the attention allocated to that disease. This result is particularly significant in light of how race differentials in media attention have previously been described.

For instance, Cohen (1999) has described how infrequently the nightly news coverage of AIDS through 1993 focused on African-Americans. But our results suggest that this bias in media attention may be even broader: not only are blacks largely absent from the content of coverage of a disease that greatly burdens them, other diseases such as heart disease, stroke, and diabetes that also disproportionately affect blacks are given less attention by television and print news media. The significant race gap in media attention to disease that we observe both reflects and contributes to existing health inequities in the United States.

In contrast to our strong and consistent findings with respect to racial burden and attention, we find considerably more mixed evidence with respect to sex differentials in mortality. In the full samples including AIDS, a greater female burden (as measured by the female/male mortality ratio) is associated with less coverage, but in the restricted sample excluding AIDS, the coefficient for the female/male mortality ratio is positive and statistically significant. The direction of the effect, then, is highly sensitive to the presence of the AIDS data in the models, suggesting that the unique trajectory of AIDS is tilting what otherwise is a positive relationship between female burden and media attention. Coverage of AIDS overall began to decline just as the epidemic was beginning to cause proportionally more female deaths. Thus, the drop-off in attention to AIDS coupled with rising AIDS deaths among women is confounding the relationship between female mortality and attention levels. While this hypothesis clearly deserves investigation in a larger sample, the idea of a positive relationship between relative female burden and media coverage has some plausibility. The cases of breast cancer and hormone replacement therapy, both of which receive extensive media coverage, attest to the power of (certain) women's health issues to command public attention.

To summarize our findings with respect to mortality and attention: the social burden that a disease exacts does affect news coverage. Indeed, it is not enough merely to ask *whether* death matters in the attention process; we must also ask *whose* deaths matter. Most clearly, diseases that claim proportionately more black lives than white lives receive less attention in the mass media. Beyond this observation, our conclusions are complicated by the abundant evidence that the attention process with respect to AIDS differs in significant ways from the attention process with respect to other diseases. Whether AIDS is included in the models or not yields diametrically opposed findings regarding the effect of total mortality on coverage, as well as how gender differentials in burden shape attention.

Our next set of results concerns our second question about the effect of organized interest groups on media attention. We expected to find a positive relationship between the presence of organized interest groups and news coverage of a disease, a hypothesis for which we find mixed support. Here again it is the presence or absence of AIDS in our models that proves crucial to our findings. In the full sample including AIDS, we find that the number of groups with a primary interest in each disease has a very consistent, statistically significant, positive effect on attention. Organized interest groups increase both print and broadcast attention to disease. Yet once we exclude AIDS from the estimation samples, these effects drop to zero for the NBC and CBS equations, but remain positive and statistically significant for the ABC and newspaper equations.

Additional purchase on the nature of the relationship between organizational activity and attention is apparent through our measure of the community's capacity for expertise, the proportion of primary groups registered to lobby by disease-year. Organizational communities in which a greater proportion of groups are registered to lobby tend to attract relatively more attention to "their" diseases than do organizational communities with smaller proportions of politically oriented groups; the effect of this variable is consistently positive in the samples excluding AIDS. When we include AIDS in the model estimation, the impact of the group variables reflects the unique patterns of organizational activity around AIDS. The community of organizations interested in AIDS is the only one in our sample that has increased appreciably over time. Yet, relative to other diseases, far fewer AIDS groups are registered to lobby. This lower proportion reflects the preponderance of AIDS groups devoted to providing direct services to AIDS patients, education about HIV, and fundraising for the disease, among other activities. In sum, the size of the organized interest group community dedicated to a disease appears to increase levels of media coverage of that disease, although the type of organizations in that community may affect the relationship we observe.

Finally, we note the effects of our control variables. When we include AIDS in our estimation of the models, the lagged measure of attention is positive and statistically significant such that stories about a particular disease in one week are likely to continue into the following week. (The extent of continuity is especially strong for stories appearing in the *Post* or the *Times*.) Relative to diseases that are not covered in a given week, those that do receive attention are more likely to be reported on in a subsequent week. All else being equal, the volume of stories will decline over time, but attention to the disease will persist in the relevant media outlet. This pattern of persistence in coverage also is evident when we exclude AIDS from our estimation sample. However, the magnitude of the effect is considerably smaller and evident only for the two newspapers and ABC news.

Scientific attention, in the form of peer-reviewed scientific journal articles, has a positive and statistically significant effect on media coverage. As other researchers before us have demonstrated (Bartlett et al. 2002), the mass media are responsive to scientific/medical attention to a disease. However, FDA attention in the form of new molecular approvals for drugs to treat our sample diseases does not have any effect on media attention.

. . .

CONCLUSION

The mass media play an influential role in the process of agenda setting, by providing one of the primary attention arenas in the public domain, by calling attention to certain problems, and by framing what are seen as the causes of and solutions to those problems. In this paper we have demonstrated that newspapers and the nightly network news programs bring certain diseases into public view, while keeping others out of public sight. Our analysis of the cross-disease and cross-temporal variation in media attention suggests that *who* dies from a disease, as well as *how many* die, are critical factors in explaining why some diseases get more attention than others. Most significantly, our data illustrate that both the print and the broadcast media tend to be much *less* attentive to diseases that burden blacks more than whites, a result that is robust across all of our model specifications. It appears that the news media diminish the agenda space granted to diseases that affect blacks more than whites, thereby curtailing public attention to such diseases. Our data cannot tell us why this pattern of coverage occurs. It may result from the efforts of the predominantly white management of the newspapers and broadcast outlets we study to cater to their predominantly white readers and viewers. But it is also possible that news outlets are reflective of their sources of information. That is, interest organizations and other information providers may not emphasize the diseases and concerns of underrepresented groups.

Our study is unique in that we compare directly the attention allocated to seven diseases across nineteen years as a function of the variation in both the social burden these diseases impose and the interest groups they attract. As a result, we can make inferences about the attention allocation process characterizing diseases in general, as well as to gain leverage on how this process compares to that which characterizes attention to HIV/AIDS.

The results of our investigation underscore the fact that it is problematic to generalize about why disease captures public attention based on any single case, particularly HIV/AIDS. AIDS has a relatively high rate of fatality, there have been dramatic shifts in its incidence and mortality over the past twenty years, and it is a highly stigmatized and moralized disease. Moreover, within our sample, AIDS is the only infectious disease and even more significantly,

it is the only disease to come into existence during the time period we study. The latter fact alone almost guarantees that the attention process to AIDS will be distinct. There is also the tendency of AIDS to kill not only in large numbers, but to kill at young ages. Among the seven diseases that we study here, AIDS is the only one to cause significant levels of premature mortality: over 90 percent of all deaths from AIDS occurred among people under age 55, compared with about 11 percent in the case of diabetes, the next highest. Extreme premature mortality, then, may be one characteristic distinguishing AIDS from other diseases and shaping its distinctive attention process.

Although scholars who focus on AIDS have not explicitly argued that it is representative of other diseases, ideas about why the media pay attention to different diseases often emerge out of studies of AIDS because it has been the focus of so much research. In this regard, the status of AIDS is paradoxical: in terms of the media attention it receives, AIDS is recognized as being distinctly different from other diseases, while at the same time it often serves as a model for understanding the attention allocation process. This dual perception of AIDS has important implications for understanding (and misunderstanding) how and why diseases get attention from the media. . . .

Specifically, an analysis based on the full sample of seven diseases reveals a *negative* relationship between the number of individuals who suffer from a disease and media attention, and diseases that have a greater impact on women relative to men and attention. A *positive* link between the size of the organizational communities that take an interest in the disease and media attention also is apparent but there is also some evidence that the media gives less attention to diseases that are of interest to more politically active organizational communities. When AIDS is excluded from our sample, we observe a *positive* relationship between the number of individuals who die from a disease and media attention, and diseases that have a greater impact on women relative to men and attention, along with the persistent negative relationship between the burden of disease among blacks and attention.

Diseases that are associated with more politically active organizational communities also appear to command more attention; the positive impact of the number of interest organizations on attention observed for the full sample is restricted to attention from the print media when the observations related to AIDS are excluded. The distinct features of AIDS appear to distort the mechanisms that affect the attention process; thus, we argue that our models that exclude AIDS provide a clearer reflection of the mass media attention process to disease.

. . .

In the mass media, the decision of whether to give attention to a particular problem is a key determinant of what makes it onto the public agenda. Attention allocation reflects the distribution of scarce seconds of news coverage or columns of newspaper space to some problem at the expense of others. In this paper, we have demonstrated that certain characteristics associated with problems—namely the segment of society they most burden, and the activity of interested advocacy groups—affect systematically this process of attention allocation, bringing certain diseases into public view, while keeping others out of sight.

Notes

1. This number may in fact be an underestimate of deaths attributable to Alzheimer's disease, which appears to be underreported as a cause of death on death certificates (Ewbank 1999).

2. There are two other elements that are significant in shaping the attention process to any social issue, particularly in the mass media. The first of these are "news shocks"—unanticipated, often calamitous events that dominate the news agenda when they happen, such as Hurricane Katrina in late summer 2005, or the terrorist attacks of September 11, 2001. When such events occur, they crowd other issues off the agenda. The second element is known as "killer issues"—stories that routinely (and somewhat predictably) dominate the news agenda. Examples include both ongoing issues such as the state of the economy, and periodic ones, such as taxation, which routinely overshadows news coverage around April 15 every year. In this paper, we are unable to account for either news shocks or killer issues, though we acknowledge their role in helping to shape the attention cycle to disease.

3. Estimating the burden that any given disease imposes on society and on individuals has long been regarded as a difficult endeavor. There are multiple dimensions of burden— morbidity, mortality, direct costs to the health care system in terms of treatment, indirect costs in terms of lost productivity, quality of life, and so on—and there is no consensus in the literature about how to measure these dimensions of burden. Commonly used multidimensional measures include quality-adjusted life years (QALYs) and disability-adjusted life years (DALYs), both of which attempt to balance morbidity and mortality in the calculus of burden. Although we agree that burden is a complex concept, our point is simply that it is possible to identify, albeit incompletely, some aspect of the social burden of a disease.

4. Readers may wonder whether organization is a simple reflection of burden. Certainly, the burden of a disease and organized interest group attention to that disease *may* be correlated. Diseases that exact large burdens on society may be more likely to have active groups associated with them precisely because of how widespread (or how

deep) that burden is. Cancer is an example of the former, AIDS an example of the latter. Yet there are plenty of counter-examples as well: the common cold costs billions of dollars every year, is experienced by virtually everyone, and yet there are no interest groups for this disease. Breast cancer attracts much more organized interest group attention and activity than does heart disease among women, despite the fact that the latter causes many more deaths than the former. Burden, then, is not the only determinant of interest group presence and activity.

5. We recognize that our measures of media attention are not necessarily representative of the full array of news people read or see. Nightly news viewership has declined over the period of our study. However, for the better part of our time series, we have in effect sampled the entire universe of nightly network news, since we include NBC, ABC, and CBS. Towards the later years in our time period, cable news begins to play a much greater role. In addition, although our indicators of print coverage come from only two sources, these two newspapers have widespread national distribution and are regarded as "papers of record" by many policymakers. In part, the enormous data collection requirements of this project dictated that we confine our initial analysis to these two newspapers, and to network news. We are currently collecting data on a much broader range of newspapers (approximately 12 regional papers and *USA Today*), and on cable news coverage in order to expand our sampling frame.

6. Of course, these national vital statistics are accurate only to the extent that cause of death is correctly reported on death certificates. For a discussion of the accuracy of death certificate reporting, see Smith-Sehdev and Hutchins (2001), Nielsen et al. (1991), and Maudsley and Williams (1996). Although errors certainly do occur on death certificates (as well as arbitrary assignment of cause of death), we believe this misreporting does not affect our results in any particular direction.

7. We recognize that these data about groups from published sources may not provide perfectly accurate information about the composition and character of the organizational communities in each year of our series. For example, when organizations expressed an interest in disease in 2004, we cannot in all cases determine when they first became interested in that disease. For some organizations such as the American Heart Association, it is clear that they have been interested in a disease since their founding. But for organizations such as the ACLU or the National Association of Black County Officials, it is unlikely that formation dates are equivalent to dates of initial interest in a disease. Although this problem exists for a number of organizations in the disease communities we have identified so far, it is especially problematic in the case of HIV/AIDS because many of the organizations that express an interest in AIDS existed long before the virus was identified. Thus, our count of the number of organizations in the AIDS community over time reflects only those organizations that came into being in 1982 or later. Similarly, because we identified disease-related groups in 2004, we cannot account for organizations that existed earlier in our series but have since ceased to exist.

References

Adelman, Richard C., and Lois M. Verbrugge. 2000. "Death Makes News: The Social Impact of Disease on Newspaper Coverage." *Journal of Health and Social Behavior* 41:347–67.

Ader, Christine. 1993. "A Longitudinal Study of Agenda-Setting for the Issue of Environmental Pollution." Presented at the Association for Education in Journalism and Mass Communication, Kansas City.

Associations Unlimited. 2002. Detroit, MI: Gale Research.

Barker-Plummer, Bernadette. 1995. "News as a Political Resource: Media Strategies and Political Identity in the U.S. Women's Movement, 1966–1975." *Critical Studies in Mass Communication* 12:306–324.

Bartlett, Christopher, Jonathan Sterne, and Matthias Egger. 2002. "What is Newsworthy? Longitudinal Study of the Reporting of Medical Research in Two British Newspapers." *British Medical Journal* 325:81–84.

Baumgartner, Frank R., and Bryan D. Jones. 1993. *Agendas and Instability in American Politics*. Chicago: University of Chicago Press.

Berry, Jeffrey M. 1999. *The New Liberalism: The Rising Power of Citizen Groups*. Washington, DC: Brookings.

Best, Joel. 1990. *Threatened Children: Rhetoric and Concern about Child-Victims*. Chicago: The University of Chicago Press.

Blumer, Herbert. 1971. "Social Problems as Collective Behavior." *Social Problems* 18:298–306.

Caldeira, Gregory A., and John R. Wright. 1988. "Organized Interests and Agenda Setting in the U.S. Supreme Court." *American Political Science Review* 82:1109–27.

Casamayou, Maureen Hogan. 2001. *The Politics of Breast Cancer*. Washington, D.C.: Georgetown University Press.

Cobb, Roger W., and Charles D. Elder. 1983. *Participation in American Politics: The Dynamics of Agenda-Building*. 2d ed. Baltimore: Johns Hopkins University Press.

Cobb, Roger W., and Marc Howard Ross. 1997. *Cultural Strategies of Agenda Denial: Avoidance, Attack and Redefinition*. Lawrence: University of Kansas Press.

Cohen, Cathy J. 1999. *The Boundaries of Blackness: AIDS and the Breakdown of Black Politics*. Chicago: University of Chicago Press.

Colby, David C., and Timothy E. Cook. 1991. "Epidemics and Agendas: The Politics of Nightly News Coverage of AIDS." *Journal of Health Politics, Policy, and Law* 16:215–49.

Cook, Timothy E. 1998. *Governing With the News: The News Media as a Political Institution*. Chicago: University of Chicago Press.

Corbett, Julia B., and Motomi Mori. 1999. "Medicine, Media and Celebrities: News Coverage of Breast Cancer, 1960–1995." *Journalism and Mass Communication Quarterly* 76(2) Humanities Module: 229–249.

Cress, Daniel M., and David A. Snow 2000. "The Outcomes of Homeless Mobilization: The Influence of Organization, Disruption, Political Mediation and Framing." *The American Journal of Sociology* 105(4):1063–1104.

Dearing, James W., and Everett M. Rogers. 1996. *Agenda-Setting*. Thousand Oaks, CA: Sage Publications.

Donovan, Mark C. 2001. *Taking Aim: Target Populations and the Wars on AIDS and Drugs*. Washington, DC: Georgetown University Press.

Downs, Anthony. 1972. "Up and Down with Ecology—The 'Issue-Attention Cycle'." *The Public Interest* 28:38–50.

Edelman, Murray. 1971. *Politics as Symbolic Action: Mass Arousal and Quiescence*. Chicago: Markham Publishing Company.

Edelman, Murray. 1988. *Constructing the Political Spectacle*. Chicago: University of Chicago Press.

Elder, Charles D., and Roger W. Cobb. 1983. *The Political Uses of Symbols*. New York: Longman.

Epstein, Steven. 1996. *Impure Science: AIDS, Activism, and the Politics of Knowledge*. Berkeley: University of California Press.

Ewbank, Douglas C. 1999. "Deaths Attributable to Alzheimer's Disease in the United States." *American Journal of Public Health* 89(1):90–91.

Fendrick, A. Mark, Arnold S. Monto, Brian Nightengale, and Matthew Sarnes. 2003. "The Economic Burden of Non-Influenza Related Viral Respiratory Tract Infection in the United States." *Archives of Internal Medicine* 163:487–494.

Gamson, William. 1990. *The Strategy of Social Protest*. 2nd ed. Belmont, CA: Wadsworth Press.

Gandy, Oscar H., Jr. 1982. *Beyond Agenda Setting: Information Subsidies and Public Policy*. Norwood, NJ: Ablex Press.

Gans, Herbert. 1979. *Deciding What's News: A Study of CBS Evening News, NBC Nightly News, News-week and Time*. New York: Vintage.

Gitlin, Todd. 1980. *The Whole World Is Watching: Mass Media in the Making and Unmaking of the New Left*. Berkeley, CA: University of California Press.

Gusfield, Joseph R. 1981. *The Culture of Public Problems: Drinking-Driving and the Symbolic Order*. Chicago: University of Chicago Press.

Hall, Richard L. 2000. *Lobbying as Legislative Subsidy*. Presented at the annual meeting of the American Political Science Association, Washington, DC.

Hansen, John Mark. 1991. *Gaining Access: Congress and the Farm Lobby, 1919–1981*. Chicago: University of Chicago Press.

Heinz, John P., Edward O. Laumann, Robert L. Nelson, and Robert H. Salisbury. 1993. *The Hollow Core: Private Interests in National Policy Making*. Cambridge, MA: Harvard University Press.

Hilgartner, Stephen, and Charles L. Bosk. 1988. "The Rise and Fall of Social Problems: A Public Arenas Model." *American Journal of Sociology* 94:53–78.

Hubbard, Jeffrey C., Melvin L. DeFleur, and Lois B. DeFleur. 1975. "Mass Media Influences on Public Conceptions of Social Problems." *Social Problems* 23(1):22–34.

Kerr, Peter. 1986. "Anatomy of the Drug Issue: How, After Years, It Erupted." *New York Times*, sec. A November 17, 1986.

Kingdon, John W. 1995. *Agendas, Alternatives 2nd and Public Policies*, edition. New York: HarperCollins.

Kitsuse, John I., and Malcolm Spector. 1973. "Toward a Sociology of Social Problems: Social Conditions, Value Judgments, and Social Problems." *Social Problems* 20:407–418.

Kollman, Ken. 1998. *Outside Lobbying: Public Opinion and Interest Group Strategies*. Princeton, NJ: Princeton University Press.

Lantz, Paula M., and Karen M. Booth. 1998. "The Social Construction of the Breast Cancer Epidemic." *Social Science and Medicine* 46:907–918.

Lerner, Barron H. 2001. *The Breast Cancer Wars: Hope, Fear, and the Pursuit of a Cure in Twentieth-Century America*. New York: Oxford University Press.

Maudsley, G., and Williams, E.M. 1996. "Inaccuracy in Death Certification—Where Are We Now?" *Journal of Public Health Medicine* 18(1):59–66.

Mazur, Allan, and Jinling Lee. 1993. "Sounding the Global Alarm: Environmental Issues in the US National News." *Social Studies of Science* 23(4):681–720.

Montgomery, K.C. 1989. *Target: Prime Time.* New York: Oxford University Press.

Newman, Katherine. 2004. *Rampage: The Social Roots of School Shootings.* New York: Basic Books.

Nielsen, G.P., J. Bjornsson, and J.G. Jonasson, 1991. "The accuracy of death certificates: Implications for health statistics." *Virchow Archives* 419(2):143–6.

Piven, Frances Fox, and Richard A. Cloward. 1977. *Poor People's Movements: Why They Succeed, How They Fail.* New York: Pantheon.

Proctor, Robert. 1995. *Cancer Wars: How Politics Shapes What We Know and Don't Know About Cancer.* New York: Basic Books.

Schneider, Anne, and Helen Ingram. 1993. "Social Construction of Target Populations: Implications for Politics and Policy." *American Political Science Review* 87:334–47.

Schudson, Michael. 1978. *Discovering the News: A Social History of American Newspapers.* New York: Basic Books.

Shilts, Randy. 1987. *And the Band Played On: Politics, People and the AIDS Epidemic.* New York: St. Martin's Press.

Smith-Sehdev, A.E., and G.M. Hutchins. 2001. "Problems with Proper Completion and Accuracy of the Cause of Death Statement." *Archives of Internal Medicine* 16(2):277–84.

Spector, Malcolm, and John I. Kitsuse. 1973. "Social problems: A re-formulation." *Social Problems* 21:145–59.

Terkildsen, Nayda, Frauke I. Schnell, and Christina Ling. 1998. "Interest Groups, the Media, and Policy Debate Formation: An Analysis of Message Structure, Rhetoric, and Source Cues." *Political Communication* 15:45–61.

Tuchman, Gaye. 1978. *Making News: A Study in the Construction of Reality.* New York: Free Press.

Vallabhan, Shalini. 1997. *Creating a Crisis: AIDS and Cancer Policymaking in the United States.* Ph.D. dissertation. Texas A&M University.

Wallack, Lawrence, Lori Dorfman, David Jernigan, and Makani Themba. 1993. *Media Advocacy and Public Health: Power for Prevention.* Newbury Park, CA: Sage Publications.

Washington Representatives. 2004. Washington, DC: Columbia Books.

Wright, John R. 1996. Interest Groups and Congress: Lobbying, Contributions, and Influence. Boston: Allyn and Bacon.

THE EXPERIENCE OF ILLNESS

Disease not only involves the body but also affects people's social relationships, self-image, and behavior. The social and psychological aspects of illness are related in part to the biophysiological manifestations of disease but are also independent of them. The very act of defining something as an illness has consequences that are independent of any effects of biophysiology.

When a veterinarian diagnoses a cow's condition as an illness, he does not change the cow's behavior merely by diagnosis; to the cow, illness (disease) remains an experienced biophysiological state and no more. But when a physician diagnoses a human's condition as an illness, he or she changes the person's behavior by diagnosis: a social state is added to a biophysiological state by assigning the meaning of illness to disease (Freidson 1970, 223).

Much of the sociological study of illness has centered on the sick role and illness behavior. Talcott Parsons (1951) argued that to prevent the potentially disruptive consequences of illness on a group or society, there exists a set of shared cultural rules (norms) called the *sick role*. The sick role legitimates the deviations caused by illness and channels the sick into the reintegrating physician–patient relationship. According to Parsons, the sick role has four components: (1) the sick person is exempted from normal social responsibilities, at least to the extent it is necessary to get well; (2) the individual is not held responsible for his or her condition and cannot be expected to recover by an act of will; (3) the person must recognize that being ill is undesirable and must want to recover; and (4) the sick person is obligated to seek and cooperate with "expert" advice, generally that of a physician. Sick people are not blamed for their illness but must work toward recovery. There have been numerous critiques and modifications of the concept of the sick role, such as its inapplicability to chronic illness and disability, but it remains a central sociological way of seeing the illness experience (Williams 2005).

Illness behavior is essentially how people act when they develop symptoms of disease. As one sociologist notes, "Illness behavior refers to the varying ways individuals respond to bodily indications, how they monitor internal states, define and interpret symptoms, make attributions, take remedial actions and utilize various sources of informal and formal care" (Mechanic 1995). Reaction to symptoms, use of social networks in locating help, and compliance with medical advice are some of the activities characterized as illness behavior.

Illness behavior and the sick role, as well as the related concept of *illness career* (the idea that there are different sequential stages to dealing with illness [Suchman 1965]), are all more or less based on a perspective that all (proper) roads lead to medical care. These concepts tend to create a "doctor-centered" picture by making the receipt of medical care the centerpiece of sociological attention. Such concepts are essentially "outsider" perspectives on the experience of illness. Although these viewpoints may be useful in their own right, none of them have as a central concern the actual subjective experience of illness. They don't analyze illness from the sufferer's (or patient's) viewpoint. Over the years, sociologists (e.g., Strauss and Glaser 1975; Schneider and Conrad 1983; Charmaz 1991; Barker 2005) have attempted to develop more subjective "insider" accounts of what it is like to be sick. These accounts focus more on individuals' perceptions of illness, interactions with others, the effects of illness on identity, and people's strategies for managing illness symptoms than do the abstract notions of illness careers or sick roles. Sociologists have produced studies of epilepsy, multiple sclerosis, diabetes, asthma, arthritis, HIV/AIDS, and end-stage renal disease (ESRD) that demonstrate an increasing sociological interest in examining the subjective aspects of illness (see Roth and Conrad 1987; Charmaz 1999; Williams 2000; Pierret 2003; Rier 2010).

The first two selections in this section present different faces of the experience of illness.

Fibromyalgia syndrome (FMS) is a controversial pain disorder. It is a functional pain syndrome or illness for which there is no commonly accepted medical or organic explanation. Since many people suffer from the disorder while physicians tend to be skeptical about its organic origin, sociologists would call it a "contested illness." Yet there are millions of individuals who suffer pain and believe they have the disorder. In the first selection, "Electronic Support Groups, Patient-Consumers, and Medicalization: The Case of Contested Illness," Kristin K. Barker analyzes the role that online electronic support groups (ESGs) play for sufferers of fibromyalgia. She shows how the experiential knowledge of FMS sufferers manifests itself in the interactive posts on the ESG, creating an important lay expertise that challenges dominant medical knowledge. In the context of a contested illness, these ESG participants use their embodied knowledge to empower one another and challenge the ambivalent medical view of FMS, and search for physicians who will accept their views and treat the disorder. This article shows how the experience of illness can differ from medical perspectives and become both a source of collective identity and a challenge to medicine. See the section in Part 4 of this volume titled "Illness, Medicine, and the Internet" for more discussion of how the Internet is changing the experience of health and illness.

The second reading, "The Meaning of Medications: Another Look at Compliance" by Peter Conrad, examines the important issue of how people manage their medication regimens. As part of a study of the experience of epilepsy, Conrad found that a large portion of his respondents did not take their medications as prescribed. From a medical point of view, these patients would be depicted as noncompliant; that is, they do not follow doctors' orders. However, from the perspective of people with epilepsy, the situation looks quite different. Conrad identifies the meanings of medications in people's everyday lives and suggests that from this perspective, it makes more sense to conceptualize these patients' behavior as self-regulation than as noncompliance. By focusing on the experience of illness, we can reframe our understanding of behavior and see what may be deemed a "problem" in a different light.

In the final selection, "Being-in-Dialysis: The Experience of the Machine–Body for Home Dialysis Users," Rhonda Shaw examines home dialysis from the patient's perspective. Dialysis is a lifesaving technology for sufferers of ESRD or failing kidneys. In the United States, most dialysis is done in a special clinic, but there are examples of home dialysis as well. Dialysis is very time consuming and discomforting, and negatively affects patients' quality of life. Patients with home dialysis find greater flexibility, control, and independence. Shaw uses the term *cyborg* to describe the machine–body relationship, though this is not a term patients use. The context of clinic or home dialysis changes the machine–body relationship and patients' experience of illness and treatment.

References

Barker, Kristin. 2005. *The Fibromyalgia Story: Medical Authority and Women's Worlds of Pain.* Philadelphia: Temple University Press.

Charmaz, Kathy. 1991. *Good Days, Bad Days: The Self in Chronic Illness and Time.* New Brunswick, NJ: Rutgers University Press.

Charmaz, Kathy. 1999. "Experiencing Chronic Illness." In *Handbook of Social Studies in Health and Medicine,* edited by Gary L. Albrecht, Ray Fitzpatrick, and Susan C. Scrimshaw, 277–92. Thousand Oaks, CA: Sage.

Freidson, Eliot. 1970. *Profession of Medicine.* New York: Dodd, Mead.

Mechanic, David. 1995. "Sociological Dimensions of Illness Behavior." *Social Science and Medicine* 41: 1207–16.

Parsons, Talcott. 1951. *The Social System*. New York: Free Press.

Pierret, Janine. 2003. "The Experience of Illness: State of Knowledge and Perspectives for Research." *Sociology of Health and Illness* 25: 4–22.

Rier, David A. 2010. "The Patient's Experience of Illness." In *Handbook of Medical Sociology*, 6th edition, edited by Chloe Bird, Peter Conrad, Allen Fremont, and Stefan Timmermans, 163–78. Nashville, TN: Vanderbilt University Press.

Roth, Julius, and Peter Conrad. 1987. *The Experience and Management of Chronic Illness (Research in the Sociology of Health Care*, Volume 6). Greenwich, CT: JAI Press.

Schneider, Joseph W., and Peter Conrad. 1983. *Having Epilepsy: The Experience and Control of Illness*. Philadelphia: Temple University Press.

Strauss, Anselm, and Barney Glaser. 1975. *Chronic Illness and the Quality of Life*. St. Louis: C.V. Mosby.

Suchman, Edward. 1965. "Stages of Illness and Medical Care." *Journal of Health and Social Behavior* 6: 114–28.

Williams, Simon J. 2000. "Chronic Illness as Biographical Disruption or Biographical Disruption as Chronic Illness." *Sociology of Health and Illness* 22: 40–67.

Williams, Simon J. 2005. "Parsons Revisited: From the Sick Role to . . . ?" *Health* 9 (2): 123–44.

ELECTRONIC SUPPORT GROUPS, PATIENT-CONSUMERS, AND MEDICALIZATION

The Case of Contested Illness*

Kristin K. Barker

The Internet is now a principal source of health and medical information. In 2002, for example, approximately 93 million American adults went online to search for information about their health (Fox and Fallows 2003; Wellman and Haythornthwaite 2002). A key component of what is now called "e-health" is electronic support groups (ESGs) for illness sufferers. Accessed as bulletin boards, news-groups, listserves, and chat rooms, ESGs take the form of electronic postings in which individuals—in real or delayed time—write, send, and read textual messages. There are tens of thousands of illness ESGs and many millions of participants (Eysenbach et al. 2004; Fox and Fallows 2003). In effect, nearly any sufferer of nearly any condition can type his or her affliction into a search engine and electronically connect with a group of fellow sufferers.

Even as peer-to-peer ESGs have become a ubiquitous feature of the illness experience, we know remarkably little about them. According to a study published in the *British Medical Journal*, there is a paucity of evidence regarding their therapeutic efficacy and uncertainty about how, or even if, they

Electronic Support Groups, Patient-Consumers, and Medicalization: The Case of Contested Illness, Kristin K. Barker in *Journal of Health and Social Behavior,* 49(1), March 2008, pp. 20–36. Reprinted with permission from The American Sociological Association.

*This study received support from the Center for Humanities and the Faculty Release Grant Program at Oregon State University. For several days of productive collaboration, I extend my gratitude to Pamela Moss, Kathy Teghtsoonian, and other participants in the "Illness at the Contours of Contestation" workshop at the University of Victoria. I also wish to thank Hannah Rosenau for her research assistance, and Peter Conrad, Sally Gallagher, the editor, and three anonymous reviewers for their constructive feedback on earlier drafts of the paper.

can be evaluated in accordance with the clinical standards of evidence-based medicine (Eysenbach et al. 2004). ESGs, after all, are social phenomena, and must be studied, at least in part, using the tools and methods of social science. What is certain is that ESGs provide laypeople with unprecedented opportunities to share information with one another and become experts in their condition (Broom 2005; Fox, Ward, and O'Rourke 2005). As a result, the process of understanding one's embodied distress has been transformed from an essentially private affair between doctor and patient to an increasingly public accomplishment among sufferers in cyberspace.

The spectacular growth of ESGs can be seen as part of a broader contemporary cultural trend; namely, the waxing of lay expertise and the concurrent waning of deference toward expert knowledge systems (Giddens 1991). Laypeople no longer consider expertise to reside exclusively with professionals, including medical experts (Brown 1992; Brown et al. 2004; Collins and Pinch 2005; Kroll-Smith and Floyd 1997). The effects of this trend can only be described as mixed. On the one hand, the democratizing impulse represented by increased access to lay sources of health information is to be applauded; patient self-empowerment and challenges to professional hegemony are rightly seen as positive outcomes (Clarke et al. 2003; Crooks 2006; Hardey 2001; Henwood et al. 2003). The potential for lay ways of knowing to supplement medical knowledge and advance our understanding and management of human suffering is also praiseworthy (Brown 1992; Kroll-Smith and Floyd 1997; Popay and Williams 1996). On the other hand, it is possible that the increased production and exchange of lay information via ESGs and other Internet communities may contribute to "medicalization," or the processes by which an ever wider range of human experiences come to be defined, experienced, and treated as medical conditions. Whereas physicians' professional power and ambition were the principal forces driving medicalization in the twentieth century (Freidson 1972; Illich 1976), Conrad (2005) recently called on sociologists to investigate the role played by consumers, including those who form ESGs, in defining their own problems as medical

and functioning as an important "engine of medicalization" in the twenty-first century.

This article takes up Conrad's charge. More specifically, the following analysis is based on an observational study of a year in the life of an ESG for sufferers of the controversial pain disorder fibromyalgia syndrome (FMS). The data for this study include all the postings to an open bulletin board given the pseudonym *Fibro Spot* from February 2004 to February 2005.[1] *Fibro Spot* is a cyber-community with its own elaborate and distinctive cultural practices, but this investigation expressly addresses the role that these kinds of groups and this new technology play in the process of consumer-driven medicalization.

An ESG run for and by FMS sufferers is an especially instructive case. Fibromyalgia is just one of several increasingly common illnesses characterized by disturbing symptoms for which no specific biomedical mechanism can be found (Barsky and Borus 1999; Manu 2004). As such, these syndromes are medically suspect, even while they are experientially devastating. This case study thus foregrounds a conflict between professional knowledge and lay experience, and how, in the context of such contestation, ESGs can play a crucial role in defining diffuse human suffering in medical terms and engendering patient-consumer demand for medical recognition that physicians are often reluctant to provide. The analysis, therefore, builds on and extends a body of scholarship concerning the growing influence of lay expertise in the context of medical uncertainty (Brown et al. 2000; Brown et al. 2004; Kroll-Smith and Floyd 1997; Zavestoski et al. 2004) by explicitly highlighting its propensity to promote (rather than challenge) medicalization.

BACKGROUND AND CONCEPTUAL FRAMEWORK

Contemporary Medicalization: The Role of Patient-Consumers

Despite a few isolated cases of demedicalization (e.g., masturbation, homosexuality), Western societies have become increasingly medicalized (Clarke et al. 2003; Conrad and Schneider 1992). It is widely recognized, however, that the principal forces behind medicalization in the present era differ from those that expanded medicine's jurisdiction up through the first three quarters of the twentieth century (Clarke et al. 2003; Conrad and Leiter 2004). Dramatic changes in the organization of medicine toward the end of the twentieth century, most notably the rise of corporate managed care and the corresponding decline of physicians' professional power, underlie changing patterns of medicalization. One can summarize (albeit in an overly simplified way) the standard twentieth-century story of medicalization as follows: Physicians carved out a professional niche for themselves by negating lay knowledge and practices and promoting the medical management of natural human experiences, social ills, and personal problems (Conrad and Schneider 1992; Freidson 1972; Illich 1976; Wertz and Wertz 1989). In contrast, when it comes to the forces promoting the expansion of medicine's jurisdiction in the current era, the role of physicians has declined in significance, while that of biotechnology (e.g., pharmaceuticals and genetics) and other corporate health industries (e.g., managed care), in tandem with the markets and consumers they create and serve, have increased in salience (Clarke et al. 2003; Conrad 2005; Conrad and Leiter 2004).

Although there is some disagreement about whether these "shifting engines of medicalization" (Conrad 2005) are the continuation of modernity's march toward rationalization or whether they signify a new, postmodern era of "biomedicalization," there is little disagreement that the transformation of medicine from being primarily professionally directed to being increasingly market-driven places the patient in a new role vis-à-vis medicalization (Ballard and Elston 2005; Clarke et al. 2003; Conrad 2005). Briefly stated, it is increasingly the case that patients contribute to medicalization via their consumer "desire and demand" for medical goods and services (Conrad 2005). Cosmetic surgery, adult attention deficit hyperactive disorder, Gulf War syndrome, multiple chemical sensitivity, and in vitro fertilization are just some of the instances

where patients have played a crucial role in medicalizing their problems and disappointments (Conrad 2005; Conrad and Leiter 2004; Conrad and Potter 2000; Zavestoski et al. 2004). Direct-to-consumer pharmaceutical advertising specifically instructs patients to ask their doctor about particular drugs to treat many previously normal, banal, or benign "symptoms" (e.g., toenail discoloration, heartburn, diminished sexual drive in men) and to consider them as specific medical conditions or diseases (e.g., dermatophytes, acid reflux disease, erectile dysfunction) (Moynihan, Heath, and Henry 2002). The Internet can also fuel consumer demand for medical solutions to a range of human problems (Conrad 2005). When individuals search for online information to help them make sense of common symptoms, troubles, and distresses, an array of commercial and nonprofit Web sites provide them with seemingly endless detail about innumerable medical conditions, diagnoses, and treatments—many of which were previously unknown to the individuals—to discuss with their physicians.

Consequently, physicians increasingly encounter concerned patients who already have information about their problems and how they might be treated. The widespread public availability of such health and medical information alters the traditional doctor–patient relationship and transforms the patient into "a reflexive consumer" who makes "active decisions concerning treatment procedures" (Fox et al. 2005:1300; see also Burrows et al. 2000; Hardey 1999; Hardey 2001; Henwood et al. 2003). More specifically, however, when the informed consumer calls for medical goods and services that fall outside established diagnostic and treatment protocols, there is a risk of medicalizing experiences that would otherwise remain outside of medicine's purview, or intensifying the extent to which already medicalized conditions fall under the medical gaze.

The informed patient-consumer is thus becoming an increasingly potent force in determining what heretofore nonmedical conditions come to be defined and treated in medical terms. What role do ESGs play in this general trend? A small number of studies conclude that the types of information and support individuals receive via ESGs represent challenges to the doctor–patient relationship by subverting the presumed flow of information from doctor to patient and privileging embodied over expert knowledge (Broom 2005; Burrows et al. 2000), but the connection between ESGs and medicalization per se has not yet been explored. As noted, ESGs operated by and for sufferers of contested illnesses, where participants typically struggle to achieve the very medical recognition that physicians often deny them, provide a particularly appropriate context for exploring this connection.

Contested Illness and Lay Expertise: Specifying the Relationship Between ESGs and Medicalization

Recent decades have witnessed a sharp rise in the prevalence of illnesses characterized by a host of disturbing symptoms for which medical experts can find no explanation (Barsky and Borus 1999; Manu 2004). For example, more than ten million Americans are diagnosed with at least one medically unexplained syndrome, including fibromyalgia syndrome, chronic fatigue syndrome, irritable bowel syndrome, chronic pelvic pain, tension headache, multiple chemical sensitivity, Gulf War syndrome, sick building syndrome, chronic Lyme disease, premenstrual dysphoria, and candidiasis sensitivity (Sadovsky 1999; Wesseley 2004). These overlapping disorders are typified by numerous common and diffuse symptoms, ranging from pain and fatigue to cognitive and mood disorders. Because these syndromes are not linked to any known organic abnormality but instead are diagnosed using patients' subjective reports of symptoms, many physicians approach these diagnoses, and those so diagnosed, with considerable skepticism (Asbring and Narvanen 2003; Crofford and Clauw 2002). The fact that patients respond poorly to established treatment protocols further fuels medical suspicions (Goldenberg, Burckhardt, and Crofford 2004). In simple terms, what is at issue in the minds of many physicians is whether these syndromes are "real" (i.e., they have physical origins) or not (i.e., they are psychosomatic).

For these millions of sufferers, living with a medically unexplained syndrome means managing a constellation of chronic and often debilitating symptoms that many physicians consider to be of their own making. As such, these syndromes are important instances of the growing number of cases in which medical expertise and lay experience are profoundly incommensurate (Collins and Pinch 2005; Couch and Kroll-Smith 1997). In an effort to provide answers and solutions to their problems that are consistent with their subjective experiences, laypeople become "citizen scientists" or "patient experts" on their own behalf (Brown 1992; Collins and Pinch 2005; Kroll-Smith and Floyd 1997). This includes drawing on embodied knowledge to challenge medical expertise and producing logical accounts of their own distress (Kroll-Smith and Floyd 1997).

Given the insights of the previously cited research concerning lay expertise and medical uncertainty, it is not surprising that there has been a proliferation of ESGs run for and by sufferers of medically unexplainable syndromes. Anecdotal reports from participants suggest that ESGs provide invaluable information and social support that significantly alleviate distressing symptoms and minimize the self-discrediting impact of living with a contested illness (Barker 2005; WebMD 2005). But what interests us here is the possible relationship between ESGs and the medicalization of common symptoms under the auspices of contested illness classifications.

For a variety of reasons, the scholarship on lay or patient expertise gives little attention to its potential link to medicalization. Medicalization is not its primary substantive concern; rather, the main focus of this literature involves how lay knowledge and expertise are used to make sense of embodied suffering when medical expert systems fail to do so (Brown and Zavestoski 2004; Brown et al. 2000; Kroll-Smith and Floyd 1997; Zavestoski et al. 2004). Medicalization is also underemphasized in this research because its empirical focus is weighted heavily toward illnesses with an environmental component, where patients often attack narrowly biomedical interpretations of their condition in an effort to politicize the environmental causes of their illness. Sufferers of contested environmental illnesses ostensibly resist medicalization (Kroll-Smith and Floyd 1997). In the case of many contested illnesses, however, sufferers are steadfastly committed to framing their problems in strictly conventional biomedical terms. Such is the case for participants at *Fibro Spot*. This study, therefore, builds on and extends our understanding of conflicts between lay and expert knowledge by demonstrating how, in some cases, these conflicts result in patient-consumer initiated medicalization claims.

The analysis that follows highlights how the dominant beliefs and routine practices of *Fibro Spot* simultaneously (and paradoxically) challenge the expertise of physicians and encourage the expansion of medicine's jurisdiction. Drawing on their shared embodied expertise, participants confirm the medical character of their problem and its remedy, and they search, as patient-consumers, for physicians who will recognize and treat their condition accordingly. *Physician compliance*—the expectation that physicians will accept patient expertise—is presented as a useful concept for understanding the link between patient expertise, patient-consumer demand, and contemporary (and future) medicalization trends. The limits of patient expertise and consumer demand are also addressed.

DATA AND METHODS

Lay-run ESGs are organically occurring social phenomena. Hence, there is much to be gained by studying them using methods that capture how they function on a day-to-day basis. This is a task for which field research is particularly well suited. In a published debate concerning the efficacy of ESGs, several leading health researchers suggest that field methods be developed for and applied to the study of these groups (Barak, Grohol, and Pector 2004; Eysenbach 2004). Field research (e.g., ethnography, participant observation, nonparticipant observation) provides a description of a natural social environment based on data that researchers collect by submerging themselves in the very setting being studied. In the case of electronic field research, that social environment is an electronic community, group, or site, such as *Fibro Spot*.

The Setting

Fibro Spot is an open bulletin board system that has been in existence for more than ten years. The Web site's staying power makes clear that it is not one of the many illness ESGs that quickly appear and then disappear into cyberspace. *Fibro Spot* is lay-created and lay-maintained, as is typical of many illness ESGs that have emerged in the last decade (Barak et al. 2004). Without question, lay ESGs are significantly more common than those created and administered by health professionals (Eysenbach et al. 2004). *Fibro Spot* does not display visitor statistics. However, a Google search provides some indication of the group's popularity relative to other fibromyalgia ESGs. *Fibro Spot*'s homepage is among the top fifty highest-ranked pages among 6,710,000 hits for "fibromyalgia" and one of the top five ESGs listed.[2] Although Google's ranking is not a measurement of use per se, it is strongly related to visitor traffic.[3] At the very least, we can say that *Fibro Spot* is among the most electronically visible fibromyalgia ESGs. An additional justification for selecting *Fibro Spot* over other popular groups is found in the emerging ethics guidelines for conducting online research, which I address later.

Nonparticipant Observation

A crucial decision in all fieldwork is whether the researcher will participate in the social setting being studied. Because there are benefits and limitations associated with either approach, the decision to participate (and to what degree) or to be a nonparticipant observer is often determined by particular features of the field or by specific substantive concerns underlying the research (Lofland and Lofland 1995; Marshall and Rossman 1995). When it comes to studying lay-run ESGs, a strong argument can be made for nonparticipation, or what in the online world is called "lurking." The known presence of an online researcher fundamentally changes the peer-to-peer environment of an ESG (Barak et al. 2004; Eysenbach 2004). In a study of an online group for patients with heart defibrillator implants, Dickerson, Flaig, and Kennedy (2001) found that their participation in the ESG significantly altered the character of interactions in terms of both content and structure. In response, the researchers opted not to continue posting to the group but to conduct their research as nonparticipant observers. If we are interested in studying an ESG as a naturally occurring social phenomenon, the direct participation of a researcher is counterproductive. Therefore, this study uses a nonparticipant approach.

Even though there may be a sound substantive reason for conducting a nonparticipant observational study, there are empirical consequences associated with doing so. Insofar as they capture all the public activities of a group, downloaded electronic communications can be thought of as nearly perfect field notes (Stone 1995). Keeping a record of observations is not dependent on the discretions, proclivities, or skills of the researcher. There is effectively a full textual record of what takes place in the public arena of *Fibro Spot*.[4] Nevertheless, under the conditions of nonparticipation, the researcher is unable to follow up on the implied meaning of an author's posting or its implications for readers. This can be particularly problematic when postings are haphazardly and hastily written, as can be the case with computer-mediated communications (Mann and Stewart 2003). Likewise, a nonparticipant researcher cannot ask questions about the nature or significance of private e-mail communications between group members, despite the importance these exchanges may have to online communities. Even as there are widely recognized benefits of unobtrusive measures of social life (Lofland and Lofland 1995), including online social life (Dickerson et al. 2001), simply downloading electronic communications yields data that are stripped of important context. Based as it is on nonparticipant observation, the analysis presented in this article necessarily underappreciates various nuances in the daily life of *Fibro Spot*.

Not interacting with online research subjects also raises a set of ethical concerns. *Fibro Spot* was selected for a number of reasons that exemplify a position in an ongoing debate concerning what obligations researchers have to protect the privacy of ESG participants, given the public nature of the Internet. Using several criteria outlined by Eysenbach and Till (2001), we can say that *Fibro Spot* is significantly more public than private. First, the group is an open bulletin board, which means that it does not require users to register or subscribe. When an ESG requires registration, the group is less public. Second, *Fibro Spot* is a large group. With well over 200 participants, individuals are less likely to think their postings are intimate than would individuals in a group with only a handful of participants. The group also archives its exchanges on its home page. By providing a full electronic history of its postings, *Fibro Spot* intentionally increases its public visibility beyond its current and active participants. Finally, there is nothing posted on *Fibro Spot*'s Web page outlining "netiquette" restrictions concerning who is free to use the materials, who owns or has copyright to the posted materials, and the like. In contrast, *WebMD,* the largest e-health site, operates ESGs that contain the postings of thousands of individuals, but, legally, *WebMD* claims ownership over all the material that appears on their Web site. In sum, the explicit public character of *Fibro Spot* justifies using the group's interactions without their consent (Hewson et al. 2003).

Regardless of how public an ESG is, Eysenbach and Till (2001) maintain that researchers should never lurk and should always seek the informed consent of participants. Unfortunately, this position effectively precludes the study of natural social group dynamics on the Internet. Not only does the known presence of a researcher in a cybercommunity alter routine patterns of interaction, but it would never be possible to gain the consent of all members in a group, especially given the intermittent and infrequent participation patterns of many users. Ultimately, insisting on informed consent in all cases is no less simplistic than its counterpart—namely, that all Internet activity is public and, therefore, ethical guidelines need never be established. It is possible to evaluate where a group falls along a public-private continuum and make nuanced decisions, both about the appropriateness of lurking in specific online contexts and about when informed consent is and is not necessary.

Data and Coding

There are interesting questions about what downloaded electronic communications represent.

In what ways are computer-mediated communications similar to or dissimilar from other types of qualitative data, and how does one go about analyzing them? Electronic support groups exist as texts. Accordingly, electronic field research must rely on textual, discourse, or content analysis (Denzin 1999). Electronic postings, however, are not simply texts. They are also social interactions (Hine 2000; Mann and Stewart 2003). Most postings at *Fibro Spot* are seeking a response or providing one to other participants. A nonobtrusive research method was used in this study precisely to capture the natural interactive character of daily life at *Fibro Spot*. Accordingly, the postings are analyzed in terms of thematic content and in terms of interactive threads that tie individual postings to one another.

All postings to *Fibro Spot* from February 2004 to February 2005 were downloaded and analyzed using NVivo, a computer-assisted qualitative data analysis software program. Two approaches were employed in coding thematic content. First, codes were created for preidentified conceptual concerns, including illness reification, embodied versus professional expertise, and consumer demand for medicalization (Barker 2005; Broom 2005; Clarke et al. 2003; Conrad 2005). I identified postings or sections of postings that addressed the essence of these pre-established codes by closely reading through the entire year of online exchanges. In this process, relevant and pronounced patterns emerged from the data beyond those captured in the pre-established codes. Accordingly, additional codes were created to represent these emerging themes and applied in subsequent readings of the data. For example, the limitations of patient expertise and physician compliance were identified through this strategy. This latter technique more closely approximates an interpretive (Waitzkin, Britt, and Williams 1994) or grounded theoretical approach (Charmaz 2006).

In addition to coding for substantive or thematic content, postings were identified as belonging to particular social threads. A social thread refers to all postings that connect to a particular sequence of social interaction among participants (Denzin 1998). The postings cited in this paper are examples of social threads. The overwhelming majority (more than 90 percent) of messages at *Fibro Spot* are part of at least one social thread; many postings are part of multiple social threads.[5]

Participation at *Fibro Spot*

Between February 2004 and February 2005 there were 249 participants in *Fibro Spot*. Fibromyalgia is highly feminized—approximately 90 percent of those who meet the diagnostic criteria are women (Hawley and Wolfe 2000)—and the participants at *Fibro Spot* reflect this fact. Roughly 92 percent of participants (n = 227) identify themselves as women. Fourteen men participated: Eight were diagnosed with FMS, two were husbands of fibromyalgia sufferers, and four were "third parties" (e.g., individuals posting advertisements for fibromyalgia products or treatments). The gender of eight participants could not be determined either by username or posting content.

Collectively, the 249 participants contributed a total of 1,814 postings. The frequency with which these individuals contributed postings varied considerably (see Table 14.1). One hundred thirteen individuals (45.4 percent) posted only one entry during the entire year; 56 individuals (22.5 percent) posted two or three entries. As measured by actively posting, the overwhelming majority of participants (nearly 70 percent) quickly dropped in and then out of *Fibro Spot*. In contrast, there were some individuals who contributed postings with more regularity, including some who were highly active participants. For example, 16 percent of individuals posted between 4 and 10 entries, slightly more than 8 percent posted between 11 and 20 entries, and slightly less than 8 percent posted more than 20 entries during the course of the year. Only three individuals posted at least one entry a month; the most active participant contributed a total of 145 postings. As seen in Table 14.1, 19 individuals contributed 1,012 of the postings during the year observed, more than 50 percent of all postings. Finally, it is important to acknowledge that, in all likelihood, the most frequent participants of *Fibro Spot* are lurkers—that is, individuals who never

TABLE 14.1 ■ Number of Postings (NOP) to *Fibro Spot*

NOP by Individual	Number of People With This NOP	% of People With This NOP	Cumulative % of People With This NOP	Total NOP	% of Total Postings
1	113	45.4	45.4	113	6.2
2	40	16.1	61.5	80	4.4
3	16	6.4	67.9	48	2.6
4–10	40	16.1	84.0	242	13.3
11–20	21	8.4	92.4	319	17.6
21+	19	7.6	100.0	1,012	56.0
Total	249	100.0	100.0	1,814	100.0

Note: Mean = 7.28; median = 2; mode = 1; maximum = 145.

post a single message but who read the postings of others. In a study that monitored an ESG for smoking cessation, lurkers constituted 95 percent of those who logged onto the group's site (Schneider, Walter, and O'Donnell 1990); other researchers suggest that for every active newsgroup participant there are 20 lurkers (Smith 1999). Even though we can only speak in general terms in the absence of data, it is safe to assume that lurkers are common and frequent visitors at *Fibro Spot*.

FINDINGS

According to Conrad (2005), medicalization happens when some problem gets defined in medical terms, "usually as an illness or disorder, or using a medical intervention to treat it" (p. 3). Electronic support groups provide individuals—active participants and lurkers alike—with the opportunity to come together to make sense of their suffering. By writing and reading about their distress, ESG participants collectively define the nature of their problem and the possible means of its solution. As the following representative exchanges demonstrate, participants at *Fibro Spot* come together to define

their shared suffering and its remedy mainly in ways that encourage medicalization.

Illness Reification

The core symptoms of fibromyalgia (pain, fatigue, headaches, sleep and bowel irregularities, cognitive and mood disorders) are regrettably common in the general (healthy) public and are especially widespread among women (Barsky and Borus 1999; Verbrugge 1990; Waldron 1995). Moreover, the list of additional symptoms said to be associated with fibromyalgia is extensive; one popular self-help book, for instance, proposes nearly 100 common "symptoms" (Starlanyl and Copeland 1996). To say that fibromyalgia symptoms are common and diffuse, however, is not to suggest they are imaginary or inconsequential. There are many within the population who experience such symptoms as both real and troubling, and, when they come together at *Fibro Spot*, they readily forge an alliance. The following exchange is exemplary in this regard:[6]

> Kelly: Hi, all. I'm new here so be gentle with me. I am a 56 year old grandmother of 3, newly diagnosed. I have been suffering for years, but so many different things, all over

the place, that it took a while for my doctor to realize what was happening. I'll give you the short list; sleeplessness, allergies (food, medications, and pets), joint pain, arthritic symptoms, sinus infections, I think that's enough. I was afraid that everyone was starting to see me as a hypocondriac! [. . .] I have been through all the blood tests and x-rays, which of course showed nothing wrong. I hope I hear from others out there. This is good therapy, just putting all this crap in print.

Ruby: Kelly, Hello, Welcome to the group. I am fairly new, and am still amazed to have found that others have the same symptoms. It is such a relief to know that I am not alone. I too suffer from chronic sinus infections, joint pain, sleep troubles, restless legs, and the list goes on. [. . .] I hope this helps you a bit—you aren't alone.

This characteristic exchange both presupposes and corroborates the existence of a *shared* condition, despite the lack of evidence of such a condition in the barrage of medical tests to which most participants, like Kelly, have been subjected. By writing and reading postings at *Fibro Spot*, participants transform a collection of symptoms into a unified entity. At the same time, having described a wide range of possible symptoms, it becomes easy to recognize the overlaps between their own symptoms and those of fellow participants. In this way, routine exchanges at *Fibro Spot* both define what fibromyalgia is and authenticate its existence. From the point of view of participants, shared symptoms, rather than objective medical evidence, substantiate fibromyalgia as an organic disease. This social process is called illness reification.

Reification, or the process by which socially constructed abstractions come to be regarded as actual material things, plays a crucial role in consumer-driven medicalization. Specifically, it is a core feature of lay expertise upon which subsequent consumer demand is based. From the standpoint of clinicians, fibromyalgia is "simply a label"

(Goldenberg 1999) or a "construct" (Bennett 1999). However, it can hardly be experienced as anything less than concrete by *Fibro Spot* participants who come together and endow it with "disease" status. Collective affirmation of the objective, thing-like status of FMS is an essential step in consumer-driven medicalization. In its absence, the certainty that underlies lay expertise and compels consumers to seek medical recognition and treatment would be lacking.

Skeptical Dependency on Medical Expertise

Many physicians will not diagnose patients with fibromyalgia or treat patients who have been so diagnosed (Asbring and Narvanen 2003; Crofford and Clauw 2002). Consequently, like shared symptoms, the shared experience of medical disparagement strengthens participants' sense of illness solidarity. The following exchange reveals this social dynamic:

Sarah: Hello Family! [. . .] my new doctor appointment was today. Was not good!! First of all she is 4 months out of medical school. She looked over my chart and immediately wanted to change all medications that I am taking. . . . I said no, the ones I am taking now are just fine. She wasn't pleased about that. "Now about your fibromyalgia, I will not prescribe pain killers for fibro." I sat there with my mouth open. She went on to tell me the fresh out of med school approach to fibro is excercise, diet. I said what about the pain. She preceeded to tell me the pain was "ALL IN MY HEAD, THERE IS NO PAIN, YOU JUST IMAGINE THERE IS." My first thought was jump up out of this chair and slap the B—!! Instead I said you are an idiot!! Then I walked out. . . . She is a doctor at a large clinic in [city where she lives]. So I called their patient advocacy phone line to report the way I was treated. So if anyone knows a doctor in my town please, please, please e-mail me. I cannot even count the number of doctors I have been to, to just get diagnosed.

Gini: Good Evening FM'ily-Sarah-I am so sorry that you were treated that way. It's scary that some doctor's have so much ego and ignorance about this disease. I hope you have luck finding a new doctor.

Vivian: Sarah—I'm sorry you had to go through that ordeal with your new doctor who truly is ignorant on the subject of fibromyalgia. I hope you find a new one soon who is knowledgeable about fibro instead. I went through the same thing with 2 of my doctors telling me that most doctors did not believe fibromyalgia exists. . . . I really didn't have time to waste with this kind of nonsense. I told one of the docs that he didn't have a clue.

Marilyn: Oh, Sarah, I'm so sorry about your appointment. That has to be one of the worst nightmares of Fibro. It's like having a car that won't start, and standing in front of a mechanic who says, "There's nothing wrong with it." You CAN'T fix it yourself, and now you have to find someone else. [. . .] I think your doc has not seen enough pain in school to be compassionate and willing to deal with pain. You can't truly learn about disease in a book or a school. You should have kicked her in the shins and asked if it felt like it was in her head!

This typical exchange at *Fibro Spot* depicts a number of key dynamics that promote consumer-driven medicalization. For example, the exchange powerfully illustrates participants' insolence when physicians refuse to recognize and treat their suffering as a "real" disease. Vivian recounts telling one doctor that he didn't have a clue, whereas Sarah describes confronting and reporting her doctor before beginning the difficult search for a more knowledgeable replacement. In her retelling of this medical encounter, Sarah reports challenging her doctor's refusal to prescribe pain medications—a perennial complaint of women patients in general and fibromyalgia sufferers in particular (Barker 2005; Calderone 1990). Sarah also rejects her doctor's advice to self-treat fibromyalgia with diet and exercise, and is incensed by the interpretation that her pain is a psychosomatic symptom over which she has control. In other words, Sarah is dismissive of any advice from her doctor that frames her illness as anything other than an organic entity, fully worthy of orthodox medical intervention.

As the exchange unfolds we see participants supporting one another—as "FM'ily"—in the face of medical doubt and derision. Gini, Vivian, and Marilyn appear to be more than casually familiar with "ignorant," "egotistical," and "clueless" doctors. Nearly all fibromyalgia sufferers endure invalidating and discrediting experiences like that described by Sarah (Asbring and Narvanen 2001; Barker 2005; Crooks 2006). The dilemma is straightforward: Patients are certain of their illness but physicians can find nothing wrong. Because medicine doubts the existence of symptoms that cannot be seen or measured, patients' apparent good health is, in Marilyn's words, "one of the worst nightmares of fibromyalgia." Although fibromyalgia eludes medicine's gaze, the experience of fibromyalgia symptoms leaves no room for doubt, a point Marilyn sarcastically drives home by suggesting a kick in the shins for the skeptical doctor. Likewise, Sarah's dismissal of her doctor's "fresh out of medical school" approach, and Marilyn's claim that it isn't possible to learn about "disease" from a book or a school, further accentuate the discrepancy between the foundational basis of lay/experiential and professional/expert knowledge (Brown 1992; Kroll-Smith and Floyd 1997).

Despite participants' criticism of doctors' professional ignorance, this exchange also speaks to their nagging dependency on professionals. After all, they are unable to "fix themselves." Participants' paradoxical stance toward experts—characterized by a combination of distrust and reliance—is identified as a distinguishing feature of the contemporary era (Giddens 1991). Laypeople no longer unquestioningly accept the opinions of experts, yet they face complex problems they are unable to solve on their own. What is insufficiently appreciated, but is exemplified at *Fibro Spot*, is that skeptical dependency can fuel consumer demand for medical solutions to a broad range of individual and social problems. When laypeople seek medical remedies for their hardships, they may be undeterred by medical experts who question the suitability of such a course of action.

Lay/Embodied Versus Professional/Medical Expertise

As foreshadowed in the earlier exchange, another persistent theme found in the postings at *Fibro Spot* is the inherent validity bestowed on embodied expertise. The postings from *Fibro Spot* participants convey, in no uncertain terms, a belief that their shared embodied experience trumps the presumed "expert" knowledge of doctors. The following exchange exemplifies this sentiment:

Angela: One of my doctors warned me about places like this [online groups], telling me I would read what others wrote and then have the same symptoms myself. I can't believe that this is true but while I read some of the old posts, I remember saying to myself, "I have that, or yes that is what I feel."

Yolanda: Don't let doctors treat you like some type of idiot. That's how they deal with not dealing with FMS. It's too big of a pain for some of them to acknowledge they don't know enough about it and can't fix it. What I find in reading others' symptoms, etc. is that i'm not nuts, and this really is happening to me. Find a different doctor.

Susie: Angela, Don't let your doctor tell you that you will "feel" what you read. You will finally find out what you feel is real!! They don't usually like that because then you come back to them saying "HEY! This is wrong and I want us to work on it!" Hang in there dear one. Find a new doctor.

Yolanda and Susie encourage Angela to disregard her doctor's comments about the contaminating influences of ESGs. They explain how, despite expert opinion to the contrary, fibromyalgia is "real" (i.e., not psychosomatic) and reading the posts of others only confirms this reality. If doctors fail to acknowledge this fact, participants are encouraged to find a new doctor. This exchange, therefore, demonstrates the social process of illness reification at work, but it also draws our attention to another paradox: Participants at *Fibro Spot* challenge medical expertise in an effort to have physicians recognize their shared suffering in strictly orthodox medical terms. When Angela raises the possibility that at least some of her fibromyalgia symptoms have a complicated psychosocial origin, the suggestion is quickly and ardently banished by other members of *Fibro Spot*. In effect, the dominant discourse at *Fibro Spot* reproduces the very mind-body dualism through which medicine negates the "reality" of participants' suffering. Rather than critiquing scientific medicine's core assumptions (i.e., "real" illnesses are demarcated by observable pathophysiology), participants simply challenge the competence of particular doctors. In other words, even if physicians have lost a good deal of their cultural omnipotence (McKinlay and Marceau 2002), the strong desire to frame one's suffering within scientific medicine's core assumptions demonstrates that medical discourse still garners significant cultural authority.

There are some important parallels here to the work of Kroll-Smith and Floyd (1997), who explain how persons with multiple chemical sensitivity criticize the medical profession but draw on the "rational, Enlightenment language of biomedicine" (p. 34) in an effort to create a logical account of their somatic suffering. However, unlike those with multiple chemical sensitivity or other contested environmental illnesses, participants at *Fibro Spot* do not resist the depoliticizing and individualizing features of medicalization by drawing attention to the influence of external factors on their well-being (Brown 1992; Brown et al. 2004; Kroll-Smith and Floyd 1997). As seen at *Fibro Spot*, when laypeople "unhinge" (Kroll-Smith and Floyd 1997) or "re-appropriate"

(Giddens 1991) expertise from professional experts, they can also do so in ways that embrace the biological reductionism of medicine and promote rather than deflect medicalization. Fox et al. (2005) came to a similar conclusion in their study of an online support group for individuals taking a weight-loss drug; even though participants were empowered to become expert patients, they paradoxically accepted and perpetrated "a conservative and constraining biomedical perspective" (p. 1305).

Empowerment Without Power

The next exchange further underscores how participants at *Fibro Spot* endorse medicalization by challenging physicians who discredit their embodied experience. At the same time, however, it also demonstrates the limitations on patient empowerment, participants' awareness of those limitations, and the combination of resolve and resignation with which they struggle to make their voices heard.

Becky: I know that several of you have had problems with doctors. I wanted to share my recent experience with a new primary care doctor. . . . She had told me that I could control the pain with my head. She had said to me, "The pain is not killing you. You are not dying from it." She also told me to get a job and that she didn't like couch potatoes. Anyways, I decided to go back to her one last time, but this time was going to be different. This time I was in charge. . . . I explained all about my new diagnosis and my difficulty in showering, dressing, lifting a glass of water, and walking. I explained my done she said, "I don't believe you are disabled." I replied, "Then this conversation is over"!!!. . . . My reason for sharing is that we can not let doctors intim[id]ate us anymore. . . . From now on I will not let this happen. If when I get a new primary he or she isn't listening or treats me in a way that I don't want to be treated then I will tell him or her and I will find a new doctor. I feel that this is important. Instead of letting doctors get us down let

us take control of the situation. After all, we choose them and pay them not the other way around. They are not God and we are not at their mercy.

Gretchen: Thanks Becky for your inspirational words. The hard thing about being sick is that you don't feel good. When you don't feel good it is harder to fight for what you need. It's kind of ironic. The ones that need the most help have the softest voices. God willing, I am going to do something to get FM on the national map. . . . People in chronic pain need chronic pain medicine. . . . Just give us what we need and we'll go away. That is what I would like to say to someone. I don't know who yet. I'll figure it out.

Becky's posting chronicles a single patient's tenacity. She tells the skeptical physician the diagnosis for her condition and her corresponding physical limitations. Becky then encourages others at *Fibro Spot* to follow her lead: Patients must confront doctors who discount their illness. They need to find doctors who are willing to listen to them, believe in what they say, and treat them the way they want to be treated. After all, patients pay doctors; and, as the saying goes, "The customer is always right." At the same time, Becky's frustration and the predicament in which she finds herself illustrate the barriers patients face in the medical marketplace. Patients must negotiate with physicians for access to medical resources, a dependency made all the more palpable in Gretchen's plea for pain medication: "Just give us what we need and we'll go away."

Again the paradoxical nature of *Fibro Spot*'s message is revealed. Participants encourage one another to recognize that they are not at the mercy of doctors, and yet, as their comments plainly reveal, they both recognize and bemoan the power that doctors have over them. *Fibro Spot* participants empower one another to persevere in the face of disparagement, but the only real power they have is the consumer power to search for a less reproachful provider. Even this type of agency can be appreciably restricted by managed care organizations. In sum, participants contribute to the medicalization of their own suffering, but not under conditions of their own choosing.

DISCUSSION

One is necessarily limited to citing only a few examples when presenting qualitative data of this nature. Thus, the previous exchanges represent only a very small fraction of postings to *Fibro Spot* during the course of the year. Although these few exchanges by no means reflect the full breadth of topics and themes discussed by this community, neither is their ethos contradicted elsewhere in the group's routine interactions. These exchanges are highly typical of postings to *Fibro Spot*, even if they are not exhaustive.

These emblematic exchanges reveal mechanisms through which the social life of *Fibro Spot* engenders medicalization. The collective life of *Fibro Spot* contributes to medicalization, not because the symptoms described as fibromyalgia are not real or all in the heads of sufferers. Rather, through routine social interaction on the basis of very real (and yet very common) symptoms, the notion of a disease entity becomes reified, even in the absence of orthodox biomedical evidence. From the perspective of participants, fibromyalgia must be real; otherwise, why would they all experience such similar symptoms? In the process of sharing details about their experiences with common forms of embodied suffering, they define and affirm the existence of fibromyalgia as a medical entity. Stories of medical disparagement, narrated by participant after participant, further solidify a sense of illness camaraderie: Participants become "FM'ily." A host of knowledge claims concerning fibromyalgia circulate and come to be reinforced through routine interactions. For example, participants vigorously defend the physical origins of fibromyalgia and reject contradictory claims. Participants dismiss doctors who claim that fibromyalgia is primarily a mental illness (or even an illness that stands at the mind-body crossroads) or a condition that they can effectively treat themselves

through diet, exercise, or other lifestyle changes. Grounding their claims in their shared embodied expertise, participants challenge the expertise of individual physicians, but they do so in an effort to gain what is frequently denied them: the recognition and treatment of their suffering by members of the medical profession.

These exchanges, therefore, reveal patient-consumers' quest for what I shall call *physician compliance.* Physicians and health researchers have long been interested in improving patient compliance (Gold and McClung 2006). Accordingly, they study ways to increase the likelihood that patients will accept medical expertise and follow doctors' orders. Medical sociologists have criticized much of this research on grounds that it conceptualizes the ideal patient as an "obedient and unquestioning recipient of medical instructions" and attributes noncompliance to patients' lack of knowledge (Stimson 1974:97). In effect, the sociological critique of this research is that the very notion of patient compliance represents a form of social control premised on the unquestioning acceptance of medical authority (Zola 1972).

In the case of fibromyalgia, the tables are turned. *Fibro Spot* participants define the ideal doctor as one who unquestioningly acknowledges patient expertise, and they attribute noncompliance to doctors' lack of knowledge. There is an expectation that doctors will concur with patients' (i.e., consumers') definition of the situation (i.e., they have a discrete physical illness) and the definition of the solution (i.e., they need a fibromyalgia diagnosis and access to the host of medical treatments recommended by fellow sufferers). Discrepancies between their embodied expertise and medical expertise concerning the existence or character of fibromyalgia are swiftly and consistently dismissed.

Of course, it is important not to overstate the power patients have in the context of the health care system or within the doctor–patient relationship. Consumer demand for medical solutions does not go unfettered (Conrad and Leiter 2004); it can be stymied by corporate or public insurance and managed care organizations, as well as by providers within those organizations. As seen in the exchanges at *Fibro Spot*, physicians remain powerful gatekeepers to many medical and social resources upon which patients are dependent. It is precisely this dependency that fuels the existence of groups like *Fibro Spot* and motivates patients in their quest for medical affirmation and treatment. Nevertheless, as seen in these typical exchanges, the search for physician compliance, premised on an unquestioning acceptance of patients' embodied knowledge, represents a significant challenge to the traditional doctor–patient relationship and the epistemological assumptions upon which medical knowledge and practice are based. However circumscribed, patient-consumers seek physician compliance. When such compliance is not forthcoming, many continue to shop for what they really want.

Unfortunately, what they really want offers very little remedy. Even as fibromyalgia sufferers routinely comment on the profound significance of having a name for what is wrong with them (Barker 2005), there is scant evidence that being diagnosed with and treated for fibromyalgia translates into any long-term improvement in health status (Goldenberg et al. 2004; Wolfe et al. 1997). Indeed, many clinicians would argue that the medical diagnosis and treatment of fibromyalgia has little promise of reducing the suffering it represents because fibromyalgia is not, in essence, a discrete medical problem (Bohr 1995; Hadler 1997).

The failure of medical therapeutics to meaningfully lessen the suffering that characterizes fibromyalgia thus points to a well-recognized drawback of medicalization: It can obscure the broader social forces that diminish our health and well-being (Zola 1972). Consistent with this view, I argue elsewhere (Barker 2005) that the fibromyalgia diagnosis medicalizes a vast constellation of common complaints that are associated with social, economic, and personal hardships that characterize the lives of many women. Because *Fibro Spot* participants vigorously defend the conceptualization of fibromyalgia as an organic illness, with origins located in their individual bodies, they effectively preclude any discussion of the social circumstances in which their symptoms emerge. Their strategy makes sense, given that they are commonly disparaged as the likely

culprits of their own predicament. Their strategy is even more understandable given the gender-charged character of the interpretation that their symptoms are "hysterical" or psychosomatic. All the same, by focusing intently on gaining medical legitimatization, *Fibro Spot* participants remain largely silent on the social circumstances in which suffering is grounded and experienced.

Although there is something vaguely political about *Fibro Spot* (i.e., sufferers come together, articulate their collective grievances, and actively seek restitution), it is nevertheless help one another define their collective predicament as located within their individual bodies and encourage one another to seek individual restitution in the form of medical recognition and treatment. *Fibro Spot* participants draw on their embodied expertise to challenge medical expertise, but not in an effort to politicize the causes of their illness or make collective demands, as is the case of sufferers of contested environmental illnesses (Brown et al. 2004; Kroll-Smith and Floyd 1997). Similarly, an enormous gulf separates *Fibro Spot* from the grievances and demands of the women's health movement of the 1970s that explicitly drew attention to the negative impacts of patriarchal society on women's health and called for the demedicalization of women's routine health care (Morgen 2002; Ruzek 1978). In addition to highlighting the dramatic differences between our current neoliberal political climate and the radicalism of the early 1970s, the dissimilarity between the agenda of *Fibro Spot* and the women's health movement brings into focus a central theme of this paper: the increasing role that patient-consumers have come to play in defining their own problems as medical problems in an era characterized by a waning of medical experts' cultural authority.

CONCLUSION

Successful cases of medicalization in the twentieth century required that physicians dismantle lay practices and knowledge in their efforts to promote the medical management of human problems. In contrast, lay practices and knowledge are increasingly crucial factors in advancing consumer demand for the medical management of human problems in the twenty-first century. This article investigated an electronic support group for fibromyalgia sufferers as illustrative of this trend. Several processes have been identified whereby fibromyalgia sufferers utilize ESGs to contribute to the medicalization of their own experiences. These processes include illness reification, patients' skeptical dependency on physicians, and the cultural authority conferred on embodied knowledge. The limitations of patients' empowerment have also been noted. Whether these same processes are also typical of other illness ESGs is a matter for further research.

At a minimum, there are reasons to expect that processes of this sort are also commonplace within ESGs that are managed by and for syndromes. I hypothesize that many new ESGs for sufferers of yet-to-crystallize syndromes will appear in the future, and here, too, we can expect to see similar mechanisms at work. Grounding their claims in embodied expertise, such online communities will demand that new functional somatic syndromes and other contested illness classifications be created and recognized. To give one example, online support groups are now mounting demands for the medical acceptance of Morgellons, a condition that most physicians consider to be delusional. Patients, however, maintain that they suffer from an organic condition characterized by itchy fibers under the skin that often appear blue or red in color but that "fluoresce when viewed under ultraviolet light" (Morgellons Research Foundation 2006). But there will also be less fantastical examples, given our cultural impatience and intolerance for even low-grade pain and suffering, coupled with our strong desire to have these discomforts medically classified and treated (Barsky and Borus 1995; Kleinman 1986). The potential magnitude of this trend is significant. After all, from one-third to half of the physical complaints seen in outpatient clinics are simply medically unexplainable (Kroenke and Rosmalen 2006). As individual sufferers of more and more symptoms (ranging from the mundane to the bizarre) interact with one another in cyberspace, we can anticipate many similar instances of consumer demand for new and controversial medical classifications to capture human suffering.

Some of the social processes by which participants at *Fibro Spot* contribute to medicalization may also be at play in the case of ESGs for accepted illnesses. Consider, for example, ESGs for sufferers of accepted chronic illnesses that lack established and effective treatment protocols. Participants within these ESGs also commiserate, collaborate, and support one another. They share details and information about their symptoms, treatment options, and medical encounters. In the process, they generate and disseminate lay knowledge about the character of their disease and its proper treatment. Because lay knowledge relies on different rules of evidence than does medical and scientific knowledge (Brown 1992; Brown et al. 2004; Kroll-Smith and Floyd 1997; Popay and Williams 1996), ESG participants can easily come to different conclusions about their situation than do their physicians. Because there is no overarching authority to resolve these disputes (Collins and Pinch 2005; Giddens 1991), patient demand for medical goods and services they learn about online but that are not deemed necessary by physicians can broaden and intensify the medical management of already medicalized conditions. Insofar as patients recognize their potential conflict of interest with economizing health care providers and organizations, the managed care environment will increase the likelihood that patient-consumers will persist in realizing their demands; that is, they will seek physician compliance (Barsky and Borus 1995).

The limitations of this study point to a number of important areas for future research. For example, interviewing participants in tandem with observing their online behavior would add depth to our understanding of the influence these groups have on processes of medicalization. What do participants report learning via participation, and how does that knowledge shape their subsequent medical care demands? We also need studies that assess the impacts of ESGs and ESG participation from the point of view of physicians and other health care providers. Are felt pressures for physician compliance experienced as a contributing factor in expanding the jurisdiction of medicine? Finally, studies that directly observe how patient-provider interactions are influenced by ESG participation are needed. To what extent do ESG participants actually challenge their individual doctors by referencing the knowledge claims of their illness communities, and to what effect?

Until there is more systematic research of the sort described earlier, many of the conclusions of this study concerning the current and future role of ESGs in consumer-driven medicalization remain tentative. What is certain is that lay ESGs and other Internet communities will dramatically shape the illness experience and the practice of medicine in the future. Electronic support groups have the potential both to impact the physician-patient relationship and to advance trends toward medicalization. Sociologists must pay attention to these crucial trends as a matter of future research.

Notes

1. *Fibro Spot* and the names of participants used in this paper are pseudonyms. Nevertheless, one can never guarantee the anonymity of research subjects when doing research using public electronic documents, given that online search engines make it possible to trace electronic postings (Walstrom 2004).

2. Specific rankings are not reported to preserve anonymity. This search was conducted in early 2007.

3. Google's listing order is based on a measure of interconnectedness (i.e., how frequently a particular site is linked to other sites, and how well linked those sites are to others). Regarding the relationship between ranking and utilization, the earlier a site appears in a list, the more likely an individual will visit the site. More importantly, the more "in-links" a site has, the more opportunities an individual has to link to that site while visiting other sites to which it is linked.

4. *Fibro Spot* does have a moderator who, according to the group's Web page, can delete messages that violate stated "netiquette." Many posts that clearly violated the group's netiquette standards, however, were not removed. For example, there are several

postings that promote commercial products, as well as several exchanges that capture nasty personal fights. It is impossible to know how many posting violations were removed; clearly, many were not.

5. Less than 10 percent of the postings are not a part of a social thread. These are messages to which no one responded. There are no obvious patterns to these "ignored" messages. Their content ranges from the trivial (e.g., comments about agreeable weather) to the profound (e.g., suicide threats). Likewise, the authors of these ignored messages include regulars as well as first-time posters.

6. The chains of postings presented in this article are not necessarily as they appear on *Fibro Spot*. For example, in some cases there are messages that fall between the postings as presented, but any omitted postings were not a part of that particular social thread. The content of individual postings, however, is presented verbatim. Because *Fibro Spot* participants frequently use ellipses in their postings, I use [. . .] to denote places where I have omitted a section of text from the original posting. Ellipses not in brackets appeared as such in the original posting.

References

Asbring, Pia and Anna-Liisa Narvanen. 2001. "Chronic Illness—A Disruption in Life: Identity-Transformation among Women with Chronic Fatigue Syndrome and Fibromyalgia." *Journal of Advanced Nursing* 34:312–19.

———. 2003. "Ideal versus Reality: Physicians' Perspectives on Patients with Chronic Fatigue Syndrome (CFS) and Fibromyalgia." *Social Science & Medicine* 57:711–20.

Ballard, Karen and Mary Ann Elston. 2005. "Medicalisation: A Multi-dimensional Concept." *Social Theory and Health* 3:228–41.

Barak, Azy, John M. Grohol, and Elizabeth Pector. 2004. "Methodology, Validity, and Applicability: A Critique on Eysenbach et al." *British Medical Journal.* Retrieved May 17, 2005 (http://bmjjournals.com/cgi/eletters/328/7749/1166).

Barker, Kristin. 2005. *The Fibromyalgia Story: Medical Authority and Women's Worlds of Pain.* Philadelphia, PA: Temple University Press.

Barsky, Arthur and Jonathan Borus. 1995. "Somatization and Medicalization in the Era of Managed Care." *Journal of the American Medical Association* 274:1931–34.

———. 1999. "Functional Somatic Syndromes." *Annals of Internal Medicine* 130:910–21.

Bennett, Robert. 1999. "A Contemporary Overview of Fibromyalgia." *National Fibromyalgia Research Foundation.* Retrieved May 1, 2001 (http://www. myalgia.com/NFRA999a.htm).

Bohr, T. 1995. "Fibromyalgia Syndrome and Myofascial Pain Syndrome. Do They Exist?" *Neurologic Clinics* 13:365–84.

Broom, Alex. 2005. "Virtually He@lthy: The Impact of Internet Use on Disease Experience and the Doctor-Patient Relationship." *Qualitative Health Research* 15:325–45.

Brown, Phil. 1992. "Popular Epidemiology and Toxic Waste Contamination: Lay and Professional Ways of Knowing." *Journal of Health and Social Behavior* 33:267–81.

Brown, Phil and Stephen Zavestoski. 2004. "Social Movements in Health: An Introduction." *Sociology of Health and Illness* 26:679–94.

Brown, Phil, Stephen Zavestoski, Sabrina McCormick, Meadow Linder, Joshua Mandelbaum, and Theo Luebke. 2000. "A Gulf of Difference: Disputes over Gulf War-Related Illnesses." *Journal of Health and Social Behavior* 2:235–57.

Brown, Phil, Stephen Zavestoski, Sabrina McCormick, Brian Mayer, Rachel Morello-Frosch, and Rebecca Gesior Altman. 2004. "Embodied Health Movements: New Approaches to Social Movements in Health." *Sociology of Health and Illness* 26:50–80.

Burrows, Roger, Sarah Nettleton, Nicholas Pleace, Brian Loader, and Steven Muncer. 2000. "Virtual Community Care? Social Policy and the Emergence of Computer Mediated Social Support." *Information, Communication and Society* 3:95–121.

Calderone, Karen. 1990. "The Influence of Gender on the Frequency of Pain and Sedative Medication Administered to Postoperative Patients." *Sex Roles* 23:713–25.

Charmaz, Kathy. 2006. *Constructing Grounded Theory: A Practical Guide through Qualitative Analysis.* Thousand Oaks, CA: Sage.

Clarke, Adele, Laura Mamo, Jennifer R. Fishman, Janet K. Shim, and Jennifer Ruth Fosket. 2003. "Biomedicalization: Technoscientific Transformations of Health, Illness, and U.S. Biomedicine." *American Sociological Review* 68:161–94.

Collins, Harry and Trevor Pinch. 2005. *Dr. Golem: How to Think about Medicine.* Chicago, IL: University of Chicago Press.

Conrad, Peter. 2005. "The Shifting Engines of Medicalization." *Journal of Health and Social Behavior* 46:3–14.

Conrad, Peter and Valerie Leiter. 2004. "Medicalization, Markets, and Consumers." *Journal of Health and Social Behavior* 45(extra issue):158–76.

Conrad, Peter and Deborah Potter. 2000. "From Hyperactive Children to ADHD Adults: Observations on the Expansion of Medical Categories." *Social Problems* 47:559–82.

Conrad, Peter and Joseph W. Schneider. 1992. *Deviance and Medicalization: From Badness to Sickness.* Philadelphia, PA: Temple University Press.

Couch, Stephen R. and Steve Kroll-Smith. 1997. "Environmental Movements and Expert Knowledge: Evidence for a New Populism." *International Journal of Contemporary Sociology* 34:185–210.

Crofford, Leslie and Daniel Clauw. 2002. "Fibromyalgia: Where Are We a Decade after the American College of Rheumatology Classification Criteria Were Developed?" *Arthritis and Rheumatism* 46:1136–38.

Crooks, Valorie A. 2006. "'I Go on the Internet; I Always, You Know, Check to See What's New.'" *ACME: An Internet E-Journal for Critical Geographies* 5:50–69.

Denzin, Norman. 1998. "In Search of the Inner Child: Co-Dependency and Gender in a Cyberspace Community." Pp. 97–119 in *Emotions in Social Life,* edited by G. Bendelow and S. Williams. London: Routledge.

———. 1999. "Cybertalk and the Method of Instances." Pp. 107–25 in *Doing Internet Research: Critical Issues and Methods for Examining the Net,* edited by S. Jones. London: Sage.

Dickerson, S. S., D. M. Flaig, and M. C. Kennedy. 2001. "Therapeutic Connection: Help Seeking on the Internet for Persons with Implantable Cardioverter Defibrillators." *Heart Lung* 55:205–17.

Eysenbach, Gunther. 2004." Response to Barak." *British Medical Journal.* Retrieved May 18, 2005 (http://bmjjournals.com/cgi/eletters/328/7449/1166).

Eysenbach, Gunther, John Powell, Marina Englesakis, Carlos Rizo, and Anita Stern. 2004. "Health Related Communities and Electronic Support Groups." *British Medical Journal* 328:1166–70.

Eysenbach, Gunther and J. E. Till. 2001. "Ethical Issues in Qualitative Research on Internet Communities." *British Medical Journal (Clinical Research Edition)* 323:1103–1105.

Fox, N. J., K. J. Ward, and A. J. O'Rourke. 2005. "The 'Expert Patient': Empowerment or Medical Dominance? The Case of Weight Loss, Pharmaceutical Drugs and the Internet." *Social Science & Medicine* 60:1299–1309.

Fox, Susannah and Deborah Fallows. 2003. "Internet Health Resources." *Pew Internet and American Life Project.* Retrieved November 26, 2005 (www. pewinternet.org).

Freidson, Eliot. 1972. *Professional Dominance.* Chicago, IL: Aldine.

Giddens, Anthony. 1991. *Modernity and Self-Identity: Self and Society in the Late Modern Age.* Stanford, CA: Stanford University Press.

Gold, D. T. and B. McClung. 2006. "Approaches to Patient Education: Emphasizing the Long-Term Value of Compliance and Persistence." *American Journal of Medicine* 119:32–37.

Goldenberg, Don. 1999. "Fibromyalgia Syndrome a Decade Later: What Have We Learned?" *Archives of Internal Medicine* 159:777–85.

Goldenberg, Don, Carole Burckhardt, and Leslie Crofford. 2004. "Management of Fibromyalgia Syndrome." *Journal of the American Medical Association* 292:2388–95.

Hadler, N. M. 1997. "La Maladie est Morte, Vive le Malade (The Disease is Dead, Long Live the Disease)." *Journal of Rheumatology* 24:1250–51.

Hardey, Michael. 1999. "Doctor in the House: The Internet as a Source of Lay Health Knowledge and the Challenge to Expertise." *Sociology of Health and Illness* 21:820–35.

_____. 2001. "'E-health': The Internet and the Transformation of Patients into Consumers and Producers of Health Knowledge." *Information, Communication and Society* 4:388–405.

Hawley, Donna and Frederick Wolfe. 2000. "Fibromyalgia." Pp. 1068–83 in *Women and Health,* edited by M. B. Goldman and M. C. Hatch. New York: Academic Press.

Henwood, Flis, Sally Wyatt, Angie Hart, and Julie Smith. 2003. "'Ignorance is Bliss Sometimes': Constraints on the Emergence of the 'Informed Patient' in the Changing Landscapes of Health Information." *Sociology of Health and Illness* 25:589–607.

Hewson, Claire, Peter Yule, Dianna Laurent, and Carl Vogel. 2003. *Internet Research Methods.* Thousand Oaks, CA: Sage.

Hine, Christine. 2000. *Virtual Ethnography.* Thousand Oaks, CA: Sage.

Illich, Ivan. 1976. *Medical Nemesis: The Expropriation of Health.* New York: Pantheon.

Kleinman, Arthur. 1986. *Social Origins of Distress and Disease: Neurasthenia, Depression, and Pain in Modern China.* New Haven, CT: Yale University Press.

Kroenke, K. and J. G. Rosmalen. 2006. "Symptoms, Syndromes, and the Value of Psychiatric Diagnostics in Patients Who Have Functional Somatic Disorders." *Medical Clinics of North America* 90:603–26.

Kroll-Smith, Steve and Hugh H. Floyd. 1997. *Bodies in Protest: Environmental Illness and the Struggle over Medical Knowledge.* New York: New York University Press.

Lofland, John and Lyn Lofland. 1995. *Analyzing Social Settings.* Belmont, CA: Wadsworth.

Mann, Chris and Fiona Stewart. 2003. *Internet Communication and Qualitative Research: A Handbook for Researching Online.* Thousand Oaks, CA: Sage.

Manu, Peter. 2004. *The Psychopathology of Functional Somatic Syndromes.* New York: Haworth Medical Press.

Marshall, Catherine and Gretchen B. Rossman. 1995. *Qualitative Research Design.* Thousand Oaks, CA: Sage.

McKinlay, John B. and L. D. Marceau. 2002. "The End of the Golden Age of Doctoring." *International Journal of Health Services* 32:379–416.

Morgellons Research Foundation. 2006. *Researching an Emerging Infectious Disease.* Retrieved September 15, 2006 (http://www.morgellons.org).

Morgen, Sandra. 2002. *Into Our Own Hands: The Women's Health Movement in the United States, 1969–1990.* New Brunswick, NJ: Rutgers University Press.

Moynihan, Ray, Iona Heath, and David Henry. 2002. "'Selling Sickness': The Pharmaceutical Industry and Disease Mongering." *British Medical Journal* 324:886–91.

Popay, Jennie and Gareth Williams. 1996. "Public Health Research and Lay Knowledge." *Social Science & Medicine* 42:759–68.

Ruzek, Sheryl Burt. 1978. *The Women's Health Movement: Feminist Alternatives to Medical Control.* New York: Praeger.

Sadovsky, Richard. 1999. "An Overall Review of Functional Somatic Syndromes." *American Family Physician* 60:1551.

Schneider, S. J., R. Walter, and R. O'Donnell. 1990. "Computerized Communications as a Medium for Behavioral Smoking Cessation

Treatment: Controlled Evaluation." *Computers in Human Behavior* 6:141–51.

Smith, Mark A. 1999. "Invisible Crowds in Cyberspace: Mapping the Social Structure of the Usenet." Pp. 195–219 in *Communities in Cyberspace,* edited by M. A. Smith and P. Kollock. New York: Routledge.

Starlanyl, Devin J. and Mary Ellen Copeland. 1996. *Fibromyalgia and Chronic Myofascial Pain Syndrome: A Survival Manual.* Oakland, CA: New Harbinger.

Stimson, Gerry V. 1974. "Obeying Doctor's Orders: A View from the Other Side." *Social Science & Medicine* 8:97–104.

Stone, A. R. 1995. "Sex and Death among the Disembodied." Pp. 243–255 in *The Cultures of Computing,* edited by S. L. Star. Oxford, England: Blackwell.

Verbrugge, Lois. 1990. "Pathways of Health and Death." Pp. 41–79 in *Women, Health, and Medicine in America: A Historical Handbook,* edited by R. D. Apple. New York: Garland.

Waitzkin, Howard, Theron Britt, and Constance Williams. 1994. "Narratives of Aging and Social Problems in Medical Encounters with Older Persons." *Journal of Health and Social Behavior* 35:322–48.

Waldron, Ingrid. 1995. "Gender and Health-Related Behavior." Pp. 193–208 in *Health Behavior: Emerging Research Perspectives,* edited by D. S. Gochman. New York: Plenum.

Walstrom, Mary K. 2004. "Ethics and Engagement in Communication Scholarship." Pp. 174–202 in

Readings in Virtual Research Ethics: Issues and Controversies, edited by E. A. Buchanan. Hershey, PA: Information Science Publishing.

WebMD. 2005. "Fibromyalgia Support Group." *WebMD.* Retrieved July 1, 2005 (http://boards . webmd.com/topic.asp? topic_id=13).

Wellman, Barry and Caroline Haythornthwaite. eds. 2002. *The Internet in Everyday Life.* Malden, MA: Blackwell.

Wertz, Richard and Dorothy Wertz. 1989. *Lying In: A History of Childbirth in America.* New Haven, CT: Yale University Press.

Wesseley, Simon and P.D. White. 2004. "There is only one functional somatic syndrome." *British Journal of Psychiatry* 185:95–96.

Wolfe, Frederick, J. Anderson, Daniel Harkness, Robert Bennett, Xavier Caro, Don Goldenberg, I. Jon Russell, and Muhammad Yunus. 1997. "Health Status and Disease Severity in Fibromyalgia: Results of a Six-Center Longitudinal Study." *Arthritis and Rheumatism* 40: 1571–79.

Zavestoski, Stephen, Phil Brown, Sabrina McCormick, Brian Mayer, Maryhelen D'Ottavi, and Jamie C. Lucove. 2004. "Patient Activism and the Struggle for Diagnosis: Gulf War Illnesses and Other Medically Unexplained Physical Symptoms in the US." *Social Science & Medicine* 58:161–75.

Zola, Irving Kenneth. 1972. "Medicine as an Institution of Social Control." *Sociological Review* 20:487–504.

15

THE MEANING OF MEDICATIONS

Another Look at Compliance

Peter Conrad

Compliance with medical regimens, especially drug regimens, has become a topic of central interest for both medical and social scientific research. By compliance we mean "the extent to which a person's behavior (in terms of taking medications, following diets, or executing lifestyle changes) coincides with medical or health advice" [1]. It is noncompliance that has engendered the most concern and attention. Most theories locate the sources of noncompliance in the doctor–patient interaction, patient knowledge or beliefs about treatment and, to a lesser extent, the nature of the regimen or illness.

This paper offers an alternative perspective on noncompliance with drug regimens, one situated in the patient's experience of illness. Most studies of noncompliance assume the centrality of patient–practitioner interaction for compliance. Using data from a study of experience of epilepsy, I argue that from a patient-centered perspective the meanings of medication in people's everyday lives are more salient than doctor-patient interaction for understanding why people alter their prescribed medical regimens. The issue is more one of self-regulation than compliance. After reviewing briefly various perspectives on compliance and presenting a synopsis of our method and sample, I developed the concept of medication practice to aid in understanding patients' experiences with medication regimens. This perspective enables us to analyze "noncompliance" among our sample of people with epilepsy in a different light than the usual medically-centered approach allows.

PERSPECTIVES ON COMPLIANCE

Most studies show that at least one-third of patients are noncompliant with drug regimens; i.e., they do not take medications as prescribed or in their correct

The Meaning of Medications: Another Look at Compliance, Peter Conrad in *Social Science and Medicine,* 20(1), pp. 29–37. Copyright 1985 Elsevier. With permission from Elsevier.

doses or sequences [2–4]. A recent review of methodologically rigorous studies suggests that compliance rates with medications over a large period tend to converge at approximately 50% [5].

Literally hundreds of studies have been conducted on compliance. Extensive summaries and compilations of this burgeoning literature are available [1, 6, 7]. In this section I will note some of the more general findings and briefly summarize the major explanatory perspectives. Studies have found, for example, that noncompliance tends to be higher under certain conditions: when medical regimens are more complex [8]; with asymptomatic or psychiatric disorders [9]; when treatment periods last for longer periods of time [5]; and when there are several troublesome drug side effects [4]. Interestingly, there seems to be little consistent relationship between noncompliance and such factors as social class, age, sex, education and marital status [8].

Two dominant social scientific perspectives have emerged that attempt to explain variations in compliance and noncompliance. One locates the source of the problem in doctor–patient interaction or communication while the other postulates that patients' health beliefs are central to understanding noncompliant behavior. These perspectives each are multicausal and in some ways are compatible.

There have been a series of diverse studies suggesting that noncompliance is a result of some problem in doctor–patient interaction (see [10]). Researchers have found higher compliance rates are associated with physicians giving explicit and appropriate instructions, more and clearer information, and more and better feedback [2, 11]. Other researchers note that noncompliance is higher when patients' expectations are not met or their physicians are not behaving in a friendly manner [12, 13]. Hulka et al. [3], Davis [2] and others suggest that the physician and his or her style of communicating may affect patient compliance. In short, these studies find the source of noncompliance in doctor–patient communication and suggest that compliance rates can be improved by making some changes in clinician–patient interaction.

The importance of patient beliefs for compliant behavior is highlighted by the "health-belief model." The health-belief model is a social psychological perspective first developed to explain preventative health behavior. It has been adapted by Becker [14–16] to explain compliance. This perspective is a "value-expecting model in which behavior is controlled by rational decisions taken in the light of a set of subjective probabilities" [17]. The health-belief model suggests that patients are more likely to comply with doctors' orders when they feel susceptibility to illness, believe the illness to have potential serious consequences for health or daily functioning, and do not anticipate major obstacles, such as side effects or cost. Becker [15] found general support for a relationship between compliance and patients' beliefs about susceptibility, severity, benefits and costs.

Both perspectives have accumulated some supporting evidence, but make certain problematic assumptions about the nature and source of compliant behavior. The whole notion of "compliance" suggests a medically centered orientation; how and why people follow or deviate from doctors' orders. It is a concept developed from the doctor's perspective and conceived to solve the provider defined problem of "noncompliance." The assumption is the doctor gives the orders; patients are expected to comply. It is based on a consensual model of doctor–patient relations, aligning with Parsons' [18] perspective, where noncompliance is deemed a form of deviance in need of explanation. Compliance/noncompliance studies generally assume a moral stance that not following medical regimens is deviant. While this perspective is reasonable from the physicians' viewpoint, when social scientists adopt this perspective they implicitly reinforce the medically centered perspective.

Some assumptions of each perspective are also problematic. The doctor–patient interaction perspective points to flaws in doctor–patient communication as the source of noncompliance. It is assumed that the doctor is very significant for compliance and the research proceeds from there. Although the health belief model takes the patient's perspective into account, it assumes that patients act from a rational calculus based on health-related beliefs. This perspective assumes that health-related beliefs are the most significant aspects of subjective experience and that compliance is a rational decision based on these beliefs. In an attempt to create a succinct and straightforward model, it ignores other aspects of experience that may affect how illness and treatment are managed.

There is an alternative, less-developed perspective that is rarely mentioned in studies of compliance. This patient-centered perspective sees patients as active agents in their treatment rather than as "passive and obedient recipients of medical instructions" [19]. Stimson [19] argues that to understand noncompliance it is important to account for several factors that are often ignored in compliance studies. Patients have their own ideas about taking medication which only in part come from doctors that affect their use of medications. People evaluate both doctors' actions and the prescribed drugs in comparison to what they themselves know about illness and medication. In a study of arthritis patients Arluke [20] found that patients evaluate also the therapeutic efficacy of drugs against the achievement of specific outcomes. Medicines are judged ineffective when a salient outcome is not achieved, usually in terms of the patient's expected time frames. The patient's decision to stop taking medications is a rational-empirical method of testing their views of drug efficacy. Another study found some patients augmented or diminished their treatment regimens as an attempt to assert control on the doctor–patient relationship [21]. Hayes-Bautista [21] notes, "The need to modify treatment arises when it appears the original treatment is somehow not totally appropriate" and contends noncompliance may be a form of patient bargaining with doctors. Others [22] have noted that noncompliance may be the result of particular medical regimens that are not compatible with contexts of people's lives.

These studies suggest that the issue of noncompliance appears very different from a patient-centered perspective than a medically centered one. Most are critical of traditional compliance studies, although still connecting compliance with doctor–patient interactions [19, 21] or with direct evaluation of the drug itself [19, 20]. Most sufferers of illness, especially chronic illness, spend a small fraction of their

lives in the "patient role" so it is by no means certain that the doctor–patient relationship is the only or even most significant factor in their decisions about drug-taking. A broader perspective suggests that sufferers of illness need to manage their daily existence of which medical regimens are only a part (cf. [23]). Such a perspective proposes that we examine the meaning of medications as they are manifested in people's everyday lives.

This paper is an attempt to further develop a patient- or sufferer-centered perspective on adhering to medical regimens. We did not set out to study compliance per se; rather this paper reflects themes that emerged from our larger study of people's experiences of epilepsy [24]. We examine what prescribed medications mean to the people with epilepsy we interviewed; and how these meanings are reflected in their use.

METHOD AND SAMPLE

The larger research project from which these data are drawn endeavors to present and analyze an "insider's" view of what it is like to have epilepsy in our society. To accomplish this we interviewed 80 people about their life experiences with epilepsy. Interviews were conducted over a three-year period and respondents were selected on the basis of availability and willingness to participate. We used a snowball sampling technique, relying on advertisements in local newspapers, invitation letters passed anonymously by common acquaintances, and names obtained from local social agencies, self-help groups and health workers. No pretense to statistical representativeness is intended or sought. Our intention was to develop a sample from which theoretical insight would emerge and a conceptual understanding of epilepsy could be gained (see [25]).

We used an interview guide consisting of 50 open-ended questions and interviewed most of our respondents in their homes. The interviews lasted 1–3 hours and were tape-recorded. The recordings were transcribed and yielded over 2000-single-spaced typed pages of verbatim data.

Our sample ranged in age from 14 to 54 years (average age 28) and included 44 women and 36 men. Most respondents came from a metropolitan area in the Midwest; a small number from a major city on the east coast. Our sample could be described as largely lower-middle class in terms of education and income. None of our respondents were or had been institutionalized for epilepsy; none were interviewed in hospitals, clinics or physicians' offices. In short, our sample and study were independent of medical and institutionalized settings. More detail about the method and sample is available elsewhere [24].

EPILEPSY, MEDICATION AND SELF-REGULATION

The common medical response to a diagnosis of epilepsy is to prescribe various medications to control seizures. Given the range of types of epilepsy and the variety of physiological reactions to these medications, patients often see doctors as having a difficult time getting their medication "right." There are starts and stops and changes, depending on the degree of seizure control and the drug's side effects. More often than not, patients are stabilized on a medication or combination at a given dosage or regimen. Continuing or altering medications is the primary if not sole medical management strategy for epilepsy.

Medications are important to people with epilepsy. They "control" seizures. Most take this medication several times daily. It becomes a routine part of their everyday lives. Although all of our respondents were taking or had taken these drugs, their responses to them varied. The effectiveness of these drugs in controlling seizures is a matter of degree. For some, seizures are stopped completely; they take pills regularly and have no seizures. For most, seizure frequency and duration are decreased significantly, although not reduced to zero. For a very few of our respondents, medications seem to have little impact; seizures continue unabated.

Nearly all our respondents said medications have helped them control seizures at one time or another.

At the same time, however, many people changed their dose and regimen from those medically prescribed. Some stopped altogether. If medications were seen as so helpful, why were nearly half of our respondents "noncompliant" with their doctors' orders?

Most people with illnesses, even chronic illnesses such as epilepsy, spend only a tiny fraction of their lives in the "patient role." Compliance assumes that the doctor–patient relationship is pivotal for subsequent action, which may be the case. Consistent with our perspective, we conceptualize the issue as one of developing a *medication practice*. Medication practice offers a patient-centered perspective of how people manage their medications, focusing on the meaning and use of medications. In this light we can see the doctor's medication orders as the "prescribed medication practice" (e.g., take a 20 mg pill four times a day). Patients interpret the doctor's prescribed regimen and create a medication practice that may vary decidedly from the prescribed practice. Rather than assume the patient will follow prescribed medical rules, this perspective allows us to explore the kinds of practices patients create.[1] Put another way, it sees patients as active agents rather than passive recipients of doctors' orders.

Although many people failed to conform to their prescribed medication regimen, they did not define this conduct primarily as noncompliance with doctors' orders. The more we examined the data, the clearer it was that from the patient's perspective, doctors had very little impact on people's decisions to alter their medications. It was, rather, much more a question of regulation of control. To examine this more closely we developed criteria for what we could call self-regulation. Many of our respondents occasionally missed taking their medicine, but otherwise were regular in their medication practice. One had to do more than "miss" medications now and again (even a few times a week) to be deemed self-regulating. A person had to (1) reduce or raise the daily dose of prescribed drugs for several weeks or more or (2) skip or take extra doses regularly under specific circumstances (e.g., when drinking, staying up late or under "stress") or (3) stop taking the drugs completely for three consecutive days or longer. These criteria are arbitrary, but they allow us to estimate the extent of self-regulation. Using this definition, 34 of our 80 respondents (42%) self-regulated their medication.[2]

To understand the meaning and management of medications we need to look at those who follow a prescribed medications practice as well as those who create their own variations. While we note that 42% of our respondents are at variance with medical expectations, this number is more suggestive than definitive. Self-regulators are not a discrete and separate group. About half the self-regulators could be defined as regular in their practice, whatever it might be. They may have stopped for a week once or twice, or take extra medication only under "stressful" circumstances; otherwise, they are regular in their practice. On the other hand, perhaps a quarter of those following the prescribed medical practice say they have seriously considered changing or stopping their medications. It is likely there is an overlap between self-regulating and medical-regulating groups. While one needs to appreciate and examine the whole range of medication practice, the self-regulators provide a unique resource for analysis. They articulate views that are probably shared in varying degree by all people with epilepsy and provide an unusual insight into the meaning of medication and medication practice. We first describe how people account for following a prescribed medication practice; we then examine explanations offered for altering prescribed regimens and establishing their own practices. A final section outlines how the meaning of medications constructs and reflects the experience of epilepsy.

A TICKET TO NORMALITY

The availability of effective seizure control medications early in this century is a milestone in the treatment of epilepsy (Phenobarbital was introduced in 1912; Dilantin in 1938). These drugs also literally changed the experience of having epilepsy. To the extent the medications controlled seizures, people with epilepsy suffered fewer convulsive disruptions in their lives and were more able to achieve

conventional social roles. To the extent doctors believed medications effective, they developed greater optimism about their ability to treat epileptic patients. To the degree the public recognized epilepsy as a "treatable" disorder, epileptics were no longer segregated in colonies and less subject to restrictive laws regarding marriage, procreation and work [24]. It is not surprising that people with epilepsy regard medications as a "ticket" to normality. The drugs did not, speaking strictly, affect anything but seizures. It was the social response to medications that brought about these changes. As one woman said: "I'm glad we've got [the medications] . . . you know, in the past people didn't and they were looked upon as lepers."

For most people with epilepsy, taking medicine becomes one of those routines of everyday life we engage in to avoid unwanted circumstances or improve our health. Respondents compared it to taking vitamins, birth control pills or teeth brushing. It becomes almost habitual, something done regularly with little reflection. One young working man said: "Well, at first I didn't like it, [but] it doesn't bother me anymore. Just like getting up in the morning and brushing your teeth. It's just something you do."

But seizure control medications differ from "normal pills" like vitamins or contraceptives. They are prescribed for a medical disorder and are seen both by the individual and others, as indicators or evidence of having epilepsy. One young man as a child did not know he had epilepsy "short of taking [his] medication." He said of this connection between epilepsy and medication: "I do, so therefore I have." Medications represent epilepsy: Dilantin or Phenobarbital are quickly recognized by medical people and often by others as epilepsy medications.

Medications can also indicate the degree of one's disorder. Most of our respondents do not know any others with epilepsy; thus they examine changes in their own epilepsy biographies as grounds for conclusions about their condition. Seizure activity is one such sign; the amount of medications "necessary" is another. A decrease or increase in seizures is taken to mean that epilepsy is getting better or worse. So it is with medications. While the two may be related—especially because the common medical response to more seizures is increased medication—they may also operate independently. If the doctor reduces the dose or strength of medication, or vice versa, the patient may interpret this as a sign of improvement or worsening. Similarly, if a person reduces his or her own dose, being able to "get along" on this lowered amount of medication is taken as evidence of "getting better." Since for a large portion of people with epilepsy seizures are considered to be well-controlled, medications become the only readily available measure of the "progress" of the disorder.

TAKING MEDICATIONS

We tried to suspend the medical assumption that people take medications simply because they are prescribed, or because they are supposed to control seizures, to examine our respondents' accounts of what they did and why.

The reason people gave most often for taking medication is *instrumental*: to control seizures, or more generally, to reduce the likelihood of body malfunction. Our respondents often drew a parallel to the reason people with diabetes take insulin. As one woman said, "If it does the trick, I'd rather take them [medications] than not." Or, as a man who would "absolutely not" miss his medications explained, "I don't want to have seizures" (although he continued to have 3 or 4 a month). Those who deal with their medication on instrumental grounds see it simply as a fact of life, as something to be done to avoid body malfunction and social and personal disruption.

While controlling body malfunction is always an underlying reason for taking medications, psychological grounds may be equally compelling. Many people said that medication *reduces worry*, independent of its actually decreasing seizures. These drugs can make people feel secure, so they don't have to think about the probability of seizures. A 20-year-old woman remarked: "My pills keep me from getting hysterical." A woman who has taken seizure control medication for 15 years describes this "psychological" function of medication: "I don't

know what it does, but I suppose I'm psychologically dependent on it. In other words, if I take my medication, I feel better." Some people actually report "feeling better"—clearer, more alert and energetic—when they do not take these drugs, but because they begin to worry if they miss, they take them regularly anyhow.

The most important reason for taking medication, however, is to ensure "normality." People said specifically that they take medications to be more "normal": The meaning here is normal in the sense of "leading a normal life." In the words of a middle-aged public relations executive who said he does not restrict his life because of epilepsy: "Except I always take my medication. I don't know why. I figure if I took them, then I could do anything I wanted to do." People believed taking medicine reduces the risk of having a seizure in the presence of others, which might be embarrassing or frightening. As a young woman explained:

> I feel if it's going to help, that's what I want because you know you feel uncomfortable enough anyway that you don't want anything like [a seizure] to happen around other people; so if it's going to help, I'll take it.

This is not to say people with epilepsy like to take medications. Quite the contrary. Many respondents who follow their medically prescribed medication practice openly say they "hate" taking medications and hope someday to be "off" the drugs. Part of this distaste is related to the dependence people come to feel. Some used the metaphor of being an addict: "I'm a real drug addict"; "I was an addict before it was fashionable"; "I'm like an alcoholic without a drink; I *have* to have them [pills]"; and "I really don't want to be hooked for the rest of my life." Even while loathing the pills or the "addiction" people may be quite disciplined about taking these drugs.

The drugs used to control seizures are not, of course, foolproof. Some people continue to have seizures quite regularly while others suffer only occasional episodes. Such limited effectiveness does not necessarily lead these people to reject medication as a strategy. They continue, with frustration, to express "hope" that "they [doctors] will get it [the medication] right." For some, then, medications are but a limited ticket to normality.

SELF-REGULATION: GROUNDS FOR CHANGING MEDICATION PRACTICE

For most people there is not a one-to-one correspondence between taking or missing medications and seizure activity. People who take medications regularly may still have seizures, and some people who discontinue their medications may be seizure-free for months or longer. Medical experts say a patient may well miss a whole day's medication yet still have enough of the drug in the bloodstream to prevent a seizure for this period.

In this section we focus on those who deviate from the prescribed medication practice and variously regulate their own medication. On the whole, members of this subgroup are slightly younger than the rest of the sample (average age 25 vs 32) and somewhat more likely to be female (59–43%), but otherwise are not remarkably different from our respondents who follow the prescribed medication practice. Self-regulation for most of our respondents consists of reducing the dose, stopping for a time, or regularly skipping or taking extra doses of medication depending on various circumstances.

Reducing the dose (including total termination) is the most common form of self-regulation. In this context, two points are worth restating. First, doctors typically alter doses of medication in times of increased seizure activity or troublesome drug "side effects." It is difficult to strike the optimum level of medication. To people with epilepsy, it seems that doctors engage in a certain amount of trial and error behavior. Second, and more important, medications are defined, both by doctors and patients, as an indicator of the degree of disorder. If seizure activity is not "controlled" or increases, patients see that doctors respond by raising (or changing) medications. The

more medicine prescribed means epilepsy is getting worse; the less means it is getting better. What doctors do does not necessarily explain what patients do, but it may well be an example our respondents use in their own management strategies. The most common rationales for altering a medication practice are drug related: the medication is perceived as ineffective or the so-called side effects become too troublesome.

The efficacy of a drug is a complex issue. Here our concern is merely with perceived efficacy. When a medication is no longer seen as efficacious it is likely to be stopped. Many people continue to have seizures even when they follow the prescribed medication practice. If medication seemed to make no difference, our respondents were more likely to consider changing their medication practice. One woman who stopped taking medications for a couple of months said, "It seemed like [I had] the same number of seizures without it." Most people who stop taking their medicine altogether eventually resume a medication practice of some sort. A woman college instructor said, "When I was taking Dilantin, I stopped a number of times because it never seemed to *do* anything."

The most common drug-related rationale for reducing dose is troublesome "side effects." People with epilepsy attribute a variety of side effects to seizure control medications. One category of effects includes swollen and bleeding gums, oily or yellow skin, pimples, sore throat and a rash. Another category includes slowed mental functioning, drowsiness, slurred speech, dullness, impaired memory, loss of balance and partial impotence.[3] The first category, which we can call body side effects, were virtually never given as an account for self-regulation. Only those side effects that impaired social skills, those in the second category, were given as reasons for altering doctors' medication orders.

Social side effects impinge on social interaction. People believed they felt and acted differently. A self-regulating woman described how she feels when she takes her medication:

> I can feel that I become much more even. I feel like I flatten out a little bit. I don't like

that feeling. . . . It's just a feeling of dull-ness, which I don't like, almost a feeling that you're on the edge of laziness.

If people saw their medication practice as hindering the ability to participate in routine social affairs, they were likely to change it. Our respondents gave many examples such as a college student who claimed the medication slowed him down and wondered if it was affecting his memory, a young newspaper reporter who reduced his medication because it was putting him to sleep at work; or the social worker who felt she "sounds smarter" and more articulate when "off medications."

Drug side effects, even those that impair social skills, are not sufficient in themselves to explain the level of self-regulation we found. Self-regulation was considerably more than a reaction to annoying and uncomfortable side effects. It was an active and intentional endeavor.

SOCIAL MEANINGS OF REGULATING MEDICATION PRACTICE

Variations in medication practice by and large seem to depend on what medication and self-regulation mean to our respondents. Troublesome relation-ships with physicians, including the perception that they have provided inadequate medical informa-tion [14], may be a foundation on which alternative strategies and practices are built. Our respondents, however, did not cite such grounds for altering their doctors' orders. People vary their medication practice on grounds connected to managing their everyday lives. If we examine the social meanings of medications from our respondents' perspective, self-regulation turns on four grounds: testing; con-trol of dependence; destigmatization; and practical practice. While individual respondents may cite one or more of these as grounds for altering medication practice, they are probably best understood as strate-gies common among those who self-regulate.

Testing

Once people with epilepsy begin taking sei-zure-control medications, given there are no special problems and no seizures, doctors were reported to seldom change the medical regimen. People are likely to stay on medications indefinitely. But how can one know that a period without seizures is a result of medication or spontaneous remission of the disorder? How long can one go without medication? How "bad" is this case of epilepsy? How can one know if epilepsy is "getting better" while still taking medication? Usually after a period without or with only a few seizures, many reduced or stopped their medicine altogether to test for themselves whether or not epilepsy was "still there."

People can take themselves off medications as an experiment, to see "if anything will happen." One woman recalled:

> I was having one to two seizures a year on phenobarb . . . so I decided not to take it and to see what would happen . . . so I stopped it and I watched and it seemed that I had the same amount of seizures with it as without it . . . for three years.

She told her physician, who was skeptical but "allowed" her this control of her medication prac-tice. A man who had taken medication three times a day for 16 years felt intuitively that he could stop his medications:

> Something kept telling me I didn't have to take [medication] anymore, a feeling or somethin'. It took me quite a while to work up the nerve to stop takin' the pills. And one day I said, "One way to find out . . ."

After suffering what he called drug withdrawal effects, he had no seizures for 6 years. Others tested to see how long they can go without medication and seizures.

Testing does not always turn out successfully. A public service agency executive tried twice to stop taking medications when he thought he had "kicked" epilepsy. After two failures, he concluded that stopping medications "just doesn't work." But others continue to test, hoping for some change in their condition. One middle-aged housewife said:

> When I was young I would try not to take it . . . I'd take 'em for a while and think, "Well, I don't need it anymore," and I would not take it for, deliberately, just to see if I could do without. And then [in a few days] I'd start takin' it again because I'd start passin' out . . . I will still try that now, when my husband is out of town . . . I just think, maybe I'm still gonna grow out of it or something.

Testing by reducing or stopping medication is only one way to evaluate how one's disorder is progressing. Even respondents who follow the prescribed medication regimen often wonder "just what would happen" if they stopped.

Controlling Dependence

People with epilepsy struggle continually against becoming too dependent on family, friends, doctors or medications. They do, of course, depend on medications for control of seizures. The medications do not necessarily eliminate seizures and many of our respondents resented their dependence on them. Another paradox is that although medications can increase self-reliance by reducing seizures, taking medications can be *experienced* as a threat to self-reliance. Medications seem almost to become symbolic of the dependence created by having epilepsy.

There is a widespread belief in our society that drugs create dependence and that being on chemical substances is not a good thing. Somehow, whatever the goal is, it is thought to be better if we can get there without drugs. Our respondents reflected these ideas in their comments.

A college junior explained: "I don't like it at all. I don't like chemicals in my body. It's sort of like a dependency only that I have to take it because my body forced me to . . ." A political organizer who says medications reduce his seizures commented:

"I've never enjoyed having to depend on anything . . . drugs in particular." A nurse summed up the situation: "The *drugs* were really a kind of dependence." Having to take medication relinquished some degree of control of one's life. A woman said:

> I don't like to have to *take* anything. It was, like, at one time birth control pills, but I don't like to take anything *everyday*. It's just like, y'know, controlling me, or something.

The feeling of being controlled need not be substantiated in fact for people to act upon it. If people *feel* dependent on and controlled by medication, it is not surprising that they seek to avoid these drugs. A high school junior, who once took medicine because he feared having a seizure in the street, commented:

> And I'd always heard medicine helps and I just kept taking it and finally I just got so I didn't depend on the medicine no more, I could just fight it off myself and I just stopped taking it in.

After stopping for a month he forgot about his medications completely.

Feelings of dependence are one reason people gave for regulating medicine. For a year, one young social worker took medication when she felt it was necessary; otherwise, she tried not to use it. When we asked her why, she responded, "I regulate my own drug . . . mostly because it's really important for me not to be dependent." She occasionally had seizures and continued to alter her medication to try to "get it right":

> I started having [seizures] every once in a while. And I thought wow, the bad thing is that I just haven't regulated it right and I just need to up it a little bit and then, you know, if I do it just right, I won't have epilepsy anymore.

This woman and others saw medications as a powerful resource in their struggle to gain control over epilepsy. Although she no longer thinks she can rid herself of epilepsy, this woman still regulates her medication.

In this context, people with epilepsy manipulate their sense of dependence on medications by changing medication practice. But there is a more subtle level of dependence that encourages such changes. Some reported they regulated their medication intake in direct response to interventions of others, especially family members. It was as if others *wanted* them to be more dependent by coaxing or reminding them to take their medications regularly. Many responded to this encouraged greater dependence by creating their own medication practice.

A housewife who said she continues regularly to have petit mal seizures and tremors along with an occasional grand mal seizure, remarked:

> Oh, like most things, when someone tells me I have to do something, I basically resent it. . . . If it's my option and I choose to do it, I'll probably do it more often than not. But if you tell me I have to, I'll bend it around and do it my own way, which is basically what I have done.

Regardless of whether one feels dependent on the drug or dependent because of others' interventions around drug taking, changing a prescribed medication practice as well as continuing self-regulation serve as a form of *taking control* of one's epilepsy.

Destigmatization

Epilepsy is a stigmatized illness. Sufferers attempt to control information about the disorder to manage this threat [38]. There are no visible stigmata that make a person with epilepsy obviously different from other people, but a number of aspects of having epilepsy can compromise attempts at information control. The four signs that our respondents most frequently mentioned as threatening information control were seizures in the presence of others, job or insurance applications, lack of a driver's license and taking medications. People may try to avoid seizures in public, lie or hedge on their applications, develop accounts for not having a driver's license, or

take their medicine in private in order to minimize the stigma potential of epilepsy.

Medication usually must be taken three or four times daily, so at least one dose must be taken away from home. People attempt to be private about taking their medications and/or develop "normal" pill accounts ("it's to help my digestion"). One woman's mother told her to take medications regularly, as she would for any other sickness:

> When I was younger it didn't bother me too bad. But as I got older, it would tend to bother me some. Whether it was, y'know, maybe somebody seeing me or somethin', I don't know. But it did.

Most people develop skills to minimize potential stigmatization from taking pills in public.

On occasion, stopping medications is an attempt to vacate the stigmatized status of epileptic. One respondent wrote us a letter describing how she tried to get her mother to accept her by not taking her medications. She wrote:

> This is going to sound real dumb, but I can't help it. My mother never accepted me when I was little because I was "different." I stopped taking my medication in an attempt to be normal and accepted by her. Now that I know I need medication it's like I'm completely giving up trying to be "normal" so mom won't be ashamed of me. I'm going to accept the fact that I'm "different" and I don't really care if mom gives a damn or not.

Taking medications in effect acknowledges this "differentness."

It is, of course, more difficult to hide the meaning of medications from one's self. Taking medication is a constant reminder of having epilepsy. For some it is as if the medication itself represents the stigma of epilepsy. The young social worker quoted earlier felt if she could stop taking her medications she would no longer be an epileptic. A young working woman summed up succinctly why avoiding medications would be avoiding stigma: "Well, at least I would not be . . . generalized and classified in a group as being an epileptic."

Practical Practice

Self-regulators spoke often of how they changed the dose or regimen of medication in an effort to reduce the risk of having a seizure, particularly during "high stress" situations. Several respondents who were students said they take extra medications during exam periods or when they stay up late studying. A law student who had not taken his medication for 6 months took some before his law school exams: "I think it increases the chances [seizures] won't happen." A woman who often participated in horse shows said she "usually didn't pay attention" to her medication in practice but takes extra when she doesn't get the six to eight hours of sleep she requires: "I'll wake up and take two capsules instead of one . . . and I'll generally take it like when we're going to horse shows. I'll take it pretty consistently." Such uses of medication are common ways of trying to forestall "possible trouble."

People with epilepsy changed their medication practice for practical ends in two other kinds of circumstances. Several reported they took extra medication if they felt a "tightening" or felt a seizure coming on. Many people also said they did not take medications if they were going to drink alcohol. They believed that medication (especially Phenobarbital) and alcohol do not mix well.

In short, people change their medication practice to suit their perceptions of social environment. Some reduce medication to avoid potential problems from mixing alcohol and drugs. Others reduce it to remain "clear-headed" and "alert" during "important" performances (something of a "Catch-22" situation). Most, however, adjust their medications practically in an effort to reduce the risk of seizures.

CONCLUSION: ASSERTING CONTROL

Regulating medication represents an attempt to assert some degree of control that appears at times to be completely beyond control. Loss of control is a significant concern for people with epilepsy. While medical treatment can increase both the sense and the fact of control over epilepsy, and information control can limit stigmatization, the regulation of medications is one way people with epilepsy struggle to gain some personal control over their condition.

Medication practice can be modified on several different grounds. Side effects that make managing everyday social interaction difficult can lead to the reduction or termination of medication. People will change their medication practice, including stopping altogether, in order to "test" for the existence or "progress" of the disorder. Medication may be altered to control the perceived level of dependence, either on the drugs themselves or on those who "push" them to adhere to a particular medication practice. Since the medication can represent the stigma potential of epilepsy, both literally and symbolically, altering medication practice can be a form of destigmatization. And finally, many people modify their medication practice in anticipation of specific social circumstances, usually to reduce the risk of seizures.

It is difficult to judge how generalizable these findings are to other illnesses. Clearly, people develop medication practices whenever they must take medications regularly. This is probably most true for long-term chronic illness where medication becomes a central part of everyday life, such as diabetes, rheumatoid arthritis, hypertension and asthma. The degree and amount of self-regulation may differ among illnesses—likely to be related to symptomatology, effectiveness of medications and potential of stigma—but I suspect most of the meanings of medications described here would be present among sufferers of any illness that people must continually manage.

In sum, we found that a large proportion of the people with epilepsy we interviewed said they themselves regulate their medication. Medically centered compliance research presents a skewed and even distorted view of how and why patients manage medication. From the perspective of the person with epilepsy, the issue is more clearly one of responding to the meaning of medications in everyday life than "compliance" with physicians' orders and medical regimens. Framing the problem as self-regulation rather than compliance allows us to see modifying medication practice as a vehicle for asserting some control over epilepsy. One consequence of such a reframing would be to reexamine the value of achieving "compliant" behavior and to rethink what strategies might be appropriate for achieving greater adherence to prescribed medication regimens.

ACKNOWLEDGMENT

My thanks and appreciation to Joseph W. Schneider, my co-investigator in the epilepsy research, for his insightful comments on an earlier version of this paper. This research was supported in part by grants from the Drake University Research Council, the Epilepsy Foundation of America and the National Institute of Mental Health (MH 30818-01).

Notes

1. Two previous studies of epilepsy which examine the patients' perspective provide parallel evidence for the significance of developing such an approach in the study of "noncompliance" (see [26] and [27]).

2. Reports in the medical literature indicate that noncompliance with epilepsy regimens is considered a serious problem [28–32]. One study reports that 40% of patients missed the prescribed medication dose often enough to affect their blood-level medication concentrations [33]; an important review article estimates noncompliance with epilepsy drug regimens between 30 and 40%, with a range from 20 to 75% [34]. Another study suggests that noncompliant patients generally had longer duration of the disorder, more complicated regimens and more medication changes [35]. Attempts to increase epilepsy medication compliance include improving doctor–patient communication, incorporating patients more in treatment programs, increasing patient knowledge and simplifying drug regimens. Since noncompliance with anti-convulsant medication regimens is deemed the most frequent reason why patients suffer recurrent seizures [30], some researchers suggest, "If the patient understands the risks of stopping medication, he *will not stop*" [36]. Yet there also have been reports of active noncompliance with epilepsy medications [37]. In sum, epilepsy noncompliance studies are both typical of and reflect upon most other compliance research. In this sense, epilepsy is a good example for developing an alternative approach to understanding how people manage their medications.

3. These are reported side effects. They may or may not be drug related, but our respondents attribute them to the medication.

References

1. Haynes R. B., Taylor D. W. and Sackett D. L. (Eds) *Compliance in Health Care*. Johns Hopkins University Press, Baltimore, 1979.

2. Davis M. Variations in patients' compliance with doctor's advice: an empirical analysis of patterns of communication. *Am J. Publ. Hlth* 58, 272, 1968.

3. Hulka B. S., Kupper L. L., Cassel J. LC. and Barbineau R. A. Practice characteristics and quality of primary medical care: the doctor–patient relationship. *Med Care* 13, 808–820, 1975.

4. Christenson D. B. Drug-taking compliance: a review and synthesis. *Hlth. Serv. Res.* 6, 171–187, 1978.

5. Sackett D. L. and Snow J. C. The magnitude of compliance and non-compliance. In *Compliance in Health Care* (Edited by Haynes R. B. *et al.*), pp. 11–22. Johns Hopkins University Press, Baltimore, 1979.

6. Sackett D. L. and Haynes R. B. (Eds.) *Compliance with Therapeutic Regimens.* Johns Hopkins University Press, Baltimore, 1976.

7. DiMatteo M. R. and DiNicola D. D. *Achieving Patient Compliance.* Pergamon Press, New York, 1982.

8. Hingson R., Scotch N. A., Sorenson J. and Swazey J. P. In Sickness and in Health: Social Dimensions of Medical Care. C. V. Mosby, St. Louis, 1981.

9. Haynes R. B. Determinants of compliance: the disease and the mechanics of treatment. In *Compliance in Health Care* (Edited by Haynes R. B. *et al.*), pp. 49–62. Johns Hopkins University Press, Baltimore, 1979.

10. Garrity T. F. Medical compliance and the clinician–patient relationship: a review. *Soc. Sci. Med.* 15E, 215–222, 1981.

11. Svarstad B. L. Physician–patient communication and patient conformity with medical advice. In *Growth of Bureaucratic Medicine* (Edited by Mechanic D.), pp. 220–238. Wiley, New York, 1976.

12. Francis V., Korsch B. and Morris M. Gaps in doctor–patient communication: patients' response to medical advice. *New Engl. J. Med.* 280, 535, 1969.

13. Korsch B., Gozzi E. and Francis V. Gaps in doctor– patient communication I. Doctor–patient interaction and patient satisfaction. *Pediatrics* 42, 885, 1968.

14. Becker M. H. and Maiman L. A. Sociobehavioral determinants of compliance with health and medical care recommendations. *Med Care* 13, 10–24.

15. Becker M. H. Sociobehavioral determinants of compliance. In *Compliance With Therapeutic Regimens* (Edited by Sackett D. L. and Haynes R. B.), pp. 40–50.

Johns Hopkins University Press, Baltimore, 1976.

16. Becker M. H., Maiman L. A., Kirscht J. P., Haefner D. L., Drachman R. H. and Taylor D. W. Patient perceptions and compliance: recent studies of the health belief model. In *Compliance in Health Care* (Edited by Haynes, R. B. *et al.*), pp. 79–109. Johns Hopkins University Press, Baltimore, 1979.

17. Berkanovic E. The health belief model and voluntary health behavior. Paper presented to Conference on Critical issues in Health Delivery Systems, Chicago, 1977.

18. Parsons T. *The Social System.* Free Press, Glencoe, 1951.

19. Stimson G. V. Obeying doctor's orders: a view from the other side. *Soc. Sci. Med.* 8, 97–104, 1974.

20. Arluke A. Judging drugs: patients' conceptions of therapeutic efficacy in the treatment of arthritis. *Hum. Org.* 39, 84–88, 1980.

21. Hayes-Battista D. E. Modifying the treatment: patient compliance, patient control and medical care. *Soc. Sci. Med.* 10, 233–238, 1976.

22. Zola I. K. Structural constraints in the doctor– patient relationship: the case of non-compliance. In *The Relevance of Social Science for Medicine* (Edited by Eisenberg L. and Kleinman A.), pp. 241–252. Reidel, Dordrecht, 1981.

23. Strauss A. and Glaser B. *Chronic Illness and the Quality of Life,* pp. 21–32. C. V. Mosby, St. Louis, 1975.

24. Schneider J. and Conrad P. *Having Epilepsy: The Experience and Control of Illness.* Temple University Press, Philadelphia, 1983.

25. Glaser B. and Strauss A. *The Discovery of Grounded Theory.* Aldine, Chicago, 1967.

26. West P. The physician and the management of childhood epilepsy. In *Studies in Everyday Medicine* (Edited by Wadsworth M. and

Robinson D.), pp. 13–31. Martin Robinson, London, 1976.

27. Trostle J. *et al.* The logic of non-compliance: management of epilepsy from a patient's point of view. *Cult. Med. Psychiat.* 7, 35–56, 1983.

28. Lund M., Jurgensen R. S. and Kuhl V. Serum diphenylhydantoin in ambulant patients with epilepsy. *Epilepsia* 5, 51–58, 1964.

29. Lund M. Failure to observe dosage instructions in patients with epilepsy. *Acta Neurol. Scand.* 49, 295–306, 1975.

30. Reynolds E. H. Drug treatment of epilepsy. *Lancet* II, 721–725, 1978.

31. Browne T. R. and Cramer I. A. Antiepileptic drug serum concentration determinations. In *Epilepsy: Diagnosis and Management* (Edited by Browne T. R. and Feldman R. G.). Little, Brown, Boston, 1982.

32. Pryse-Phillips W., Jardine F. and Bursey F. Compliance with drug therapy by epileptic patients. *Epilepsia* 23, 269–274, 1982.

33. Eisler J. and Mattson R. H. Compliance with anticonvulsant drug therapy. *Epilepsia* 16, 203, 1975.

34. The Commission for the Control of Epilepsy and Its Consequences. The literature on patient compliance and implications for cost-effective patient education programs with epilepsy. In *Plan for Nationwide Action on Epilepsy,* Vol. II, Part 1, pp. 391–415. U.S. Government Printing Office, Washington, DC, 1977.

35. Bryant S. G. and Ereshfsky L. Determinants of compliance in epileptic conditions. *Drug Intel. Clin. Pharmac.* 15, 572–577, 1981.

36. Norman S. E. and Browne T. K. Seizure disorders. *Am. J. Nurs.* 81, 893, 1981.

37. Desei B. T., Reily T. L., Porter R. J. and Penry J. K. Active non-compliance as a cause of uncontrolled seizures. *Epilepsia* 19, 447–452, 1978.

38. Schneider J. and Conrad P. In the closet with illness: epilepsy, stigma potential and information control. *Soc. Probl.* 28, 32–44, 1980.

BEING-IN-DIALYSIS

The Experience of the Machine–Body for Home Dialysis Users

Rhonda Shaw

INTRODUCTION

Quality of life for people receiving dialysis treatment is increasingly focused on approaches to self-care that account for the experiences and viewpoints of dialysis patients themselves (Calvey and Mee, 2011; Clarkson and Robinson, 2010; Giles, 2003, 2005; Polaschek, 2003, 2006). The aim of this article is to contribute to the literature on renal replacement therapy and home dialysis from the patient's perspective and to investigate the experience of being-in-dialysis as an intercorporeal relation between self and other, technology and world. This entails examining how dialysis patients experience the home dialysis machine in relation to the organisation of their daily lives and how they make sense of changes to their identities in the process of receiving renal replacement therapy.

People using therapeutic technologies such as dialysis experience chronic renal failure and require long-term treatment for their condition. The two main treatment options available for patients are haemodialysis (HD) and continuous ambulatory peritoneal dialysis (CAPD) or automatic peritoneal dialysis (APD). In New Zealand, peritoneal dialysis (PD) is a self-management procedure that is not commonly undertaken in the hospital environment and must be done every day. CAPD is carried out four times a day and each exchange typically takes about 30–40 minutes. APD is done daily, usually at night for between 8 and 10 hours. HD requires a machine and an artificial kidney and is typically performed three to five times a week for 3–5 hours a time. HD treatment can be undertaken in-centre at a hospital, in a satellite base set-up closer to patients' homes and in home settings.

Being-in-Dialysis: The Experience of the Machine–Body for Home Dialysis Users, Rhonda Shaw in *Health, 19*(3), 2015, pp. 229–244. With permission from SAGE Publications, Inc.

New Zealand and Australia lead the world in rates of home dialysis therapy use (Agar, 2008; Harwood and Leitch, 2006; Lynn and Buttimore, 2005; Marshall et al., 2011). In the first decades of dialysis, a strong home programme philosophy led to the implementation of home dialysis policy in many regional hospital units throughout New Zealand. With on-going programme infrastructure support, plus a light spread of population throughout the country, home dialysis in New Zealand, and in Australia, proved to be the most effective modality from a health management perspective (Lynn and Buttimore, 2005). In comparison, home dialysis rates in the United Kingdom (Cases et al., 2011) and the United States are low. According to Courts (2000), rates are low in the United States due to Medicare funding provision for in-centre HD and disincentives for home HD, research indicating stresses with home HD and high costs associated with training and 'on-call' HD assistance.

THEORETICAL APPROACH

Health and medical technologies associated with renal replacement therapies have been interpreted in various ways in the social sciences (see Kierans, 2010; Timmermans and Berg, 2003). In this article, I focus primarily on the relation between technology, culture and the micro-level experience of dialysis patients in terms of what social theorists describe as hybrid embodiment and cyborg identity. The aim is to establish whether the concept of the machine–body enhances our understanding of the experience of dialysis patients as they manage disruptions to bodily integrity, due to end-stage renal failure. Like Giles's (2003, 2005) earlier exploratory study, the phenomenological themes of lived body (corporeality), lived time (temporality), lived space (spatiality) and lived relation (relationality) to the other (Van Manen, 1990) frame the discussion of dialysis patients' relation to renal prosthetic therapy and the kidney machine. The phrase 'being-in-dialysis' refers to Heidegger's (2008) notion of being-in-the-world. This notion is examined in relation to the relevance of the concept of

the machine–body for the lived experience of people who rely on receiving dialysis treatment to sustain life. A key objective of the article is to test this theoretical framing against dialysis patients' accounts of their embodied subjectivity and, regardless of terminology-fit, to document their perceptions of the body-in-dialysis in the course of their everyday lives.

One of the most well-known articulations of the machine–body in the social sciences is the concept of the cyborg. The term entered academic vernacular during the 1990s, when Donna Haraway (1990) defined it as 'a cybernetic organism, a hybrid of machine and organism, a creature of social reality as well as a creature of fiction' (p. 191). In a cyborg human–machine hybrid, machine parts become replacements in the body integrating or supplementing natural bodily functions to normalise or enhance the body's biological and physiological potential. Haraway's view was that processes of cyborgification had become so pervasive that the intermingling of humans with machines not only transformed the way we use our bodies to do things and move through space but also generated new kinds of subjectivity beyond the control of individuals subject to the technologies they relied upon. Although critics maintain that human being has always been mediated by technological and cultural processes, it is nonetheless agreed that prosthetic life is on the rise. The population utilising therapeutic technologies such as dialysis machines to purify their blood, for example, and those on waiting lists anticipating kidney transplantation continues to grow. There are currently more than 2500 New Zealanders on dialysis and the number requiring renal replacement therapy rises at a rate of 5 per cent per year on average (Pidgeon, 2012), with much of this growth attributable to the increase in Type II diabetes and improved survival rates for renal patients.

To explore the experience of the machine–body and cyborg identity for patients on dialysis treatment, the following discussion is structured around observations derived from philosophical phenomenology. The value of phenomenology for understanding lived experience is that it recognises the social and cultural characteristics of embodied existence and being-in-the-world. A key insight is that body and self are inextricably connected with objects, other human beings and technologies, and these technologies are not limited to tools and instruments. In the medical context they include, 'drugs, devices, and medical and surgical procedures used in medical care and the organizational and supportive systems within which such care is provided' (Gabe et al., 2006: 145). Because our bodies are the medium through which we understand and experience the world, modifications to the body that control or disrupt its integrity during organ transfer processes or renal replacement therapies (e.g. the loss of body parts and/or the relocation of foreign body parts in others or the permanent or semi-permanent connection of the body to a prosthetic device) effect peoples' sense of self and identity. In short, as Shildrick et al. (2009) state, corporeal changes to one's body effect psychosocial changes to the self.

People with end-stage renal failure report lower quality of life compared to the general population (Timmers et al., 2008). In addition to a loss of self-concept and self-esteem due to reduced workforce participation and less participation in sport, social and leisure activities, they are acutely and persistently aware of the importance of their bodies in everyday life. Constant attentiveness to their bodily state, brought about by specific illness events, bodily change and vulnerability shifts the way they experience their body and its functioning, often disrupting practical engagement and activity in the world. At the centre of the patient experience, as Hagren et al. (2005) note, is the 'lifeline' role played by the dialysis machine: it is a tool connected to the body and relied upon to sustain life as it simultaneously restricts and delimits patients' freedom. The dialysis machine literally implicates all aspects of the patient's life, from reliance on other medications and supplements that must be taken in conjunction with dialysis therapy, to diet and fluid intake, work, leisure and pleasure, travel, sex and relationships. A core existential theme for renal patients is thus how to adapt and incorporate being-in-dialysis as a machine–body.

Kierans (2010) points out that successful incorporation of the machine into practical everyday life and life projects depends on an array of interconnected factors such as socio-cultural worldviews, health and bioethical legislation, district health board policies and resource allocation, institutional rules and regulations, diagnostic methods, technical procedures and pharmaceuticals, and health practitioner and patient decision-making. If dialysis patients experience the distinction between their sense of self, body and the machine as minimal, then dialysis is seen as relatively manageable, and the dialysis machine becomes what Heidegger (2008) calls a ready-to-hand tool; cohesively integrated into the dialysing patients' attitude towards his or her lifeworld. However, if the machine cannot be connected perceptually to the patient's body, or if it breaks down, then they are more likely to see the machine as a 'thing' or present-at-hand object. If this occurs, dialysis therapy is experienced as alienating and estranging, and is expressed in terms of objectification and disembodiment rather than care of self. The relevance of Heidegger's discussion of attitudes toward things in the world for this article is to ask how the experience of receiving dialysis treatment is psychosocially represented and lived by the dialysis patient, and how patients articulate the experience of being a machine–body or cyborg subject in meaningful ways. The data themes that follow are framed so as to illustrate and explore these theoretical questions.

METHODS

This article reports data from 24 in-depth face-to-face interviews and field notes from two connected research projects, a key component of which entailed investigating perceptions of renal replacement therapy for individuals experiencing end-stage renal failure. Both studies were granted research ethics approval (MEC/08/03/027; MEC/11/EXP/089). The interviews for Study 1 were undertaken between 2009 and 2012, with 17 kidney transplant recipients, 14 of whom received dialysis treatment, as well as 1 kidney donor who was receiving dialysis treatment and awaiting transplantation at the time of interview. Interviews for Study 2 involved talking with six dialysis patients. These data were gathered during 2012 as part of a study on kidney health. Kidney transplantation was not an option for one woman in this group who had cancer. In the combined studies, all but two study participants were on home dialysis (see Table 16.1). One woman from Study 1 received HD in a hospital unit for 3 months and one man from Study 1 received HD for 5 months. Four participants received initial HD treatment in hospital units but then dialysed at home, specifying this as a preferred option.

Study participants' ages ranged between 26 and 75 years at the time of interview, with the majority clustered around the 40–55 (seven participants), 55–65 (seven participants) and 65–75 (seven participants) age bands.

Participants were self-selected adults from all over New Zealand, independently recruited through advertisements placed in national media associated with organ transplantation and by a snowballing technique. The advertisements requested people who had been involved in making decisions about organ donation and those who had experience of organ transplantation and/or dialysis treatment. Prospective participants were sent an information sheet explaining the nature of the study and the purpose of the interviews, which were undertaken

TABLE 16.1 ■ Type of Dialysis Modality

	Male	Female	Total
Study 1			
PD only	3	1	4
HD only	8	2	10
Pre-emptive transplant	3	1	4
Total	14	4	18
Study 2			
PD only	2	1	3
PD and HD		3	3
Total	2	4	6

PD: peritoneal dialysis; HD: haemodialysis.

in people's homes or in a location convenient to research participants. Participants' carers, spouses or partners were often present for the interview, which lasted between 1½ and 2½ hours. Field notes were written up on the day of the interview and include data from conversations after the audio-tape had been turned off. Some participants insisted the interviewer inspect their home dialysis machines, and where they dialysed. On several occasions, post-interview discussions were lengthy. The interviews were audio-taped with participants' consent and transcribed verbatim. Following conventions of contemporary qualitative research, transcripts were sent to participants for validation and editing and then amended accordingly. To protect confidentiality, study participants have been given pseudonyms. The abbreviation 'M' or 'F' in the interview extracts refers to 'Male' or 'Female' and the number following the letter indicates the order in which the interviews were conducted. The interviews with kidney recipients and dialysis patients were narrative and began with explanations of illness onset, physical symptoms and mishaps. Participants' stories were recounted largely uninterrupted. Reflections on participants' experience and self-understandings as well as discussion about explicitly ethical and ontological issues were constructed dialogically with the author in the interview situation.

The aim of the study was to obtain an information-rich sample that described the phenomenon of organ transfer and being-in-dialysis in depth. Sample size for qualitative research that is phenomenologically nuanced is typically small: Polkinghorne (in Creswell, 2007) recommends between 5 and 25 interviews, Kuzel (1992) suggests 6–8 interviews for a homogeneous sample and Smith (2004) encourages idiographic description with one single case. The sample size of this study is at the upper end of these guidelines and rests on the researcher's judgment that the collection of more data would not have shed new light on the study phenomena. Thematic analysis was used to manually process the research data due to applicability as a broad method for identifying and categorising common themes across a range of theoretical perspectives and epistemological approaches, particularly phenomenology

(Braun and Clarke, 2006; Guest et al., 2012). The part of the data corpus examined in this article pertains to a theoretical interest in participants' experience of the impact of dialysis treatment on their everyday lives. The themes for the data set are structurally linked to the phenomenological constructs of spatiality, temporality, corporeality and relationality. The data are organised around the sub-themes of decision-making about dialysis treatment, the practicalities of everyday life on dialysis, the physical experience of being-in-dialysis and existence and identity in relation to the dialysis machine. The results and discussion sections of this article have been integrated subsequently and implications of the study for policy and practice have been emphasised. The significance of dialysis treatment for the lives of participants' carers and other family members, the theme of relationality, is discussed elsewhere.

STUDY DATA AND DISCUSSION: TIME, MOBILITY AND SPACE

In line with the literature (Al-Arabi, 2006; Bayhakki and Hatthakit, 2012; Calvey and Mee, 2011; Clarkson and Robinson, 2010; Hagren et al., 2001, 2005; Moran et al., 2009; Polaschek, 2003), the most significant issues for participants in this study concerned the physical and psychosocial limitations of being-in-dialysis, elaborated next in terms of restrictions on time, space and lifestyle.

Many study participants talked about the differences they perceived between hospital HD, home HD and PD in terms of autonomy and dependence: as either freeing them up or limiting them time-wise and enabling them to participate in life or limiting them as a 'physical shackle' (Bayhakki and Hatthakit, 2012: 297). Participants generally agreed that while dialysis therapy sustained life, it also limited what they referred to as 'lifestyle'. The belief that dialysis therapy was a limitation on time and lifestyle was baldly stated by M2 who commented that there is 'no life on dialysis'. Participants

concurred that dialysis was all-consuming, yet also affirmed M15's view that 'you dialyse to live, not live to dialyse'. In the absence of kidney transplantation as an option, the participants agreed that although dialysis took a toll on their bodies health-wise, it was a lot better than not being on dialysis.

Views about the advantages and disadvantages of PD versus HD as an intrusion on time varied. M4 described PD as compartmentalising life 'in four hour blocks' but graciously conceded that it made 'life as normal as possible' since it gave him mobility and the freedom to travel overseas on holidays and go to work in a way he maintained HD could not. The belief that PD enabled independence was also confirmed by M10, M5 and F3. F3 said she was able to hold down a full-time job with PD by dialysing in the car at work, although she expressed caution with this practice around ensuring hygiene and safe disposal of wastes. For her, an additional benefit of PD was that it reduced the risk of transmitting infection associated with access to blood and blood products.

Study 2 participants felt similarly about the benefits of PD versus HD. F5 stated emphatically that she did not like HD, a comment corroborated in a separate interview by her mother from whom she had received a kidney. As F5 put it, 'You can't keep going into HD every two days: how long can you do that for? You kind of need some kind of life back so that's when we looked at [CAPD]'. Although there were numerous complications effecting F8's renal therapy, she recalled her realisation that HD 'didn't suit my lifestyle at all':

> I can't deal with the rest on my life on Haemo and that was the first time that I'd really thought seriously about transplant. Up until then I thought it was too big an ask, you know; to ask someone for an organ so I just had not considered it.

F8 and her partner likened hospital HD to an 'assembly line'; 'short of resources and staff and whatever; it's just like pushing more people into a crowded room'. As F8 said, 'It's terrible being in the hospital dialysis unit because that's where all the really sick people go. And people can't look after themselves and it is just depressing'. F4's husband also commented, 'You were given a time to attend and you had to fit with that'. Like F8 who made an affirmative decision to go onto PD, F6 also commented that PD enabled her to get on with life. Confirming other studies (Cases et al., 2011; Courts, 2000; Courts and Boyette, 1998; Delgado et al., 2010), the benefits of dialysing at home compared with hospital HD were emphasised by participants. For F6, hospital HD was not an option she was keen to consider since it would constrain her ability to do things. As she puts it,

> By the time I get there, have a whole day of my blood change, then get home, I will be out of my house for eight hours every second day. I can't live like that, I've got life to get on with, I've got a business to run and I've got things to do, I can't be doing that.

M15 and his wife, who donated him a kidney, were of the same mind about the time commitment with hospital HD, and the lengthy travel time to and from home. M12 said home HD fitted his particular work regime better than PD, which would have to be done four times a day. For him, home HD could be done any time of the day (morning, afternoon or evening) and, as the machine could be moved around, it gave him flexibility. Although a mother from Study 2 was sure HD was a worse option for her son, she also commented that doing PD every night for 8 hours for a young man constrained his lifestyle. Not only could he not go out and 'have a drink with his mates', sleeping with his girlfriend was also off limits due to self-care requirements to be vigilant about sleep, hygiene and avoiding infection. When this young man reflected on his embodied predicament, it made him feel 'helpless and hopeless'. F5, also in her 20s, commented on trying to make the most of dialysis: 'otherwise it's very easy [. . .] to end up in a cycle of depression'. She felt similarly about hygiene and the possibilities of contracting life-threatening peritonitis, saying, 'I'm very conscious of keeping everything clean and that means keeping everybody away. I have turfed

the husband out and sleep in my own bedroom [laughter]'.

The ability to travel as an integral part of participants' lifestyle was a recurring motif in the interviews, reflecting unspoken assumptions about mobility as a stratifying factor linked to social class. Participants were nonetheless pragmatic about this aspect of their lives, indicating that it required considerable effort, planning and resources to organise. Most participants had positive experiences of temporarily dialysing in hospitals around New Zealand and overseas because they organised their treatment options well in advance of travel. As M11 said,

> You can [travel on dialysis] but it takes an awful lot of arranging and it's pretty restricted in where you can go. I've known people going to Australia and the UK, but you've got to get all your dialysis days arranged before you go and it can take a lot of effort for the dialysis staff who do most of it for you.

The upshot for participants who want mobility is that they must rely not only on their own resources but also on a network of caring relationships in different locations in order to construct the experience of 'normality'. This might entail enduring discomfort, as M12 notes, 'The only real hurdle with travel [was] that you had to ensure, or you could go, I could go four days or maybe five days if I pushed it, without dialysing'.

For New Zealanders, travel to the Pacific Islands, a favoured holiday destination was even more difficult. They spoke of exorbitant costs associated with freighting PD gear to destinations, and this was especially problematic for those using HD, with resource restrictions severely limiting options. Most Pacific Islands do not have HD capacity on-island due to cost and staffing requirements or, if they do, capacity is minimal (see Wilson, 2011). Although people talked about going to some of these places as achievable despite being a 'major expedition', they also expressed worry about the cleanliness of environments away from home.

These concerns did not deter travel altogether. Unlike other studies in which patients explicitly noted travel restrictions (e.g. Calvey and Mee, 2011; Clarkson and Robinson, 2010), the ability to travel and to participate in normal activities was discussed by participants in this study as liberating. F4 in Study 2 mentioned how much she appreciated PD because 'we go away for weekends all the time'. Likewise, F2 talked about being able to access a Kidney Society dialysis camper van and go on holiday:

> You can go wherever you like and just go to a camping ground and hook-up and have a few adventures. . . . You know you feel like a normal person when you can, don't have to, um, hook-up at a certain place, at a certain time, you can hook-up where you are. That's if the water pressure in the camping ground is all right.

M12's wife also noted the freeing ability to travel where access to dialysis machines was available:

> The dialysis cruise was great because it meant that, um, we could go away and still have a holiday, but I didn't worry his dialysis at all. I sat on the deck and had alcoholic coffees in the middle of the afternoon and went to the casino. This was excellent, all the time he was down in the bowels of the ship being dialysed.

All but four participants received kidney transplants, so the discussion around dialysis treatment was related to quality of life post transplantation. Congruent with the literature (Calvey and Mee, 2011; Hagren et al., 2001; Polaschek, 2003), it was to be expected that the research participants would talk about kidney transplantation as 'freedom from dialysis'. To illustrate, M10 commented,

> Well, I guess, particularly for people on dialysis it's a huge lifestyle change. It's an extraordinary change of a lifestyle which is pretty awful, to be tied to a dialysis machine

where quality of life is pretty awful. So, there's this immediate and extraordinary change of life. Because mine was a pre-emptive transplant I was never that badly affected. So, there wasn't this dramatic improvement. But for those who are on dialysis it's this extraordinary change of life.

Similarly, M1 said transplantation 'freed' him:

> From being chained to a machine every second day . . . You can rationalise the time, and I could arrange my job around it, but essentially every second day is defined for you. Um, and that of course, I travelled through Australia while I was on dialysis, but having to find a hospital every second day, particularly when you're in strange cities, yeah, that was pretty taxing too.

M12 also talked about kidney transplantation as life-changing after being-in-dialysis:

> I suppose to me it was a life changing thing, so I'm totally appreciative of, and I mean that's the reality. I suppose words can't really say how much it really means to you because for us it gave us back 18 hours a week which we didn't have. It also gave us the freedom to travel. We still didn't let it restrict our lives. Because we used to travel to Australia, or even to Dunedin, so we used to do our travel.

One of the drawbacks of home HD and PD participants talked about related to space, finding space to store equipment, not having enough of it and disposing of a large amount of waste (see also Agar, 2008). Listening to people talk, it was clear that the home was transformed into a mini-hospital environment, such that participants had to consider the organisation and layout of space to accommodate the dialysis machine and medical supplies. Virtually, all participants mentioned the space 'all the stuff takes up' (F6). As F6 said of the dialysing equipment,

It has to be stored at a certain temperature and it has to be out of the weather and all that sort of thing, so, it's the garage that's a place it can be, and the fact that the machine takes space up in my bedroom.

The partners of several women participants commented on the weight of the boxes and bags of fluid: 'Ten or twelve kg depending on what you are doing' (F4's husband). F8's partner commented on the difficulty lifting boxes when they have no handles and that this was a serious issue because 'a renal patient is not able to lug twelve kilos'. M15 said, 'I receive 87 of those [boxes] every month; where am I supposed to put them?' 'Every wardrobe was full . . . the kids used to have a bedroom and they'd fill the wall', informed his wife. M15 added, '[They] built a big wall around their drum kit [drum set] to actually stop the noise of the drum kit. . . . The only problem is the wall would slowly come down during the month'.

CORPOREALITY AND THE MACHINE–BODY

It is important to note how different modalities affect participants' sense of self in relation to how they manage their respective care regimes. The benefits of dialysis treatment were sometimes discussed by participants in language pertaining to physicality and gendered embodiment. Three women dialysis patients from Study 2 (F4, F5 and F8) pointed out that PD was their preferred treatment option and suited their body type. They remarked that due to their small (female) frames, HD was too aggressive and harsh, leaving them 'washed out' and drained of energy. As a benefit, the physical and emotional 'peaks and troughs' characteristic of HD were not experienced with PD for these participants. Contrastingly, several men in Study 1 alluded to the gender of the HD machine as feminine. This nomenclature could be interpreted as in keeping with the cultural connection between technological competence and men using and controlling machines (Wajcman, 2004).

Other studies (Courts, 2000; Courts and Boyette, 1998; Levy, 1981, 2000) indicate psychosocial losses associated with HD that challenge lifestyle and self-image, including employment constraints, loss of social status, family role and male sexual dysfunction (Levy, 1981, 2000). Although these losses can lead to anxiety around self-concept, M7 described his relation to home HD therapy in keeping with his masculine sense of self as active and adventurous. As he puts it,

> There's something a bit macho about being a hemodialysis patient anyway: we were the real tough boys, the blood and thunder operators. None of this feminine stuff, of sticking a needle in your stomach and walking around with it and letting it happen. We were under blood spills and exciting things like that.

Here, M7 alludes to taking an active role in facilitating his own treatment, despite what appears to be dependence on a machine. Unlike PD which he derides as a passive therapy, M7 identifies with HD as a treatment modality because it contains an element of risk: there is something thrilling about operating the haemo machine. M2, who also trained to do home HD, conveyed a similar sentiment about the capacity of HD to restore a sense of agency. He reckoned, 'You make every cock-up [a blunder] known to man, doing it yourself, but that's all right, blood on the floor a few times . . . [laughter]'.

Learning how to use home dialysis machines proved challenging for these patients; integrating the technology was an accomplishment and tended to bolster self-esteem. Several participants personalised their dialysis machines, a phenomenon also discussed by Giles (2005). F4 remarked that 'the machine misbehaves', and although each machine looked 'exactly the same', each seemed to have a different temperament. Some participants referred to their machine by name, especially the male HD patients from Study 1 for whom the machine, while 'active', was feminised. M7 described having an intimate relation with his dialysis machine:

They moved a machine into my house with special plumbing, which I came to name 'Lola' because Lola, I always thought, was a very intelligent drag queen basically. She sucked my blood three times a week, she kept me alive and I could keep thinking about that song by the Kinks because she used to control my life for six years. But I learnt to respect her; she was a really intelligent animal.

The discussions with Study 1 participants prompted the interviewer to ask Study 2 participants about whether they, too, named their machines. F4 responded to this line of questioning, saying,

Name? Yeah, no, I've never done that, never called the machine. . . . [Partner says, 'Well, you call it. . . . '] I've called it a bastard—when it beeps at me [laughter]. . . . But no, I haven't, I haven't really personified the machine in that sense at all really.

For some participants, there was no need to name the machine as an entity distinct from the self. In a joint husband and wife interview from Study 1, M3 was matter-of-fact about the machine as simply part of his life. For him, the machine was unambiguously 'ready-to-hand', saying 'It's just, it's my life', to which his wife responded, 'He's got me; he doesn't have to name his machine [laughs]. I'm the machine'. This expression of dialysis therapy as incorporated into one's life and as part of embodied identity reveals the contradiction between people's experience of the dialysis machine as both alienating and non-objectifying. This is confirmed by a participant from another New Zealand study who described their dialysis machine as, 'a security blanket . . . when they took it out after having my transplant it was like having my arm cut off, losing your pet' (Polaschek, 2003: 49).

One participant talked about learning how to skilfully operate her dialysis equipment as ready-to-hand while describing the machine in an exasperated manner as controlling her life. Her negotiated relation to the machine was ambivalent, as the following quotations show:

It took a little while of course, as you know, to get used to how to handle the machine. I am and still am totally computer illiterate and this is all run on the computer so it was something very alien to me to learn how to use this, and they're all very impressed with the way I know what to do with it and if it gets a little hiccup or something, I know how to handle that. (F6)

Although F6 used her 'kiwi ingenuity' to adjust the dialysing equipment, like tying some of the lines down so they did not flap around and become loose during the night, she also stated,

I do not like something else taking over me. I'm not in control. And the slogan is 'you are in control', you do what you like and the machine follows along. . . . But it's not that way. The machine actually takes over your life; you know that your life depends on that machine. . . . I don't appreciate it at all. . . . No, nobody tells me that I'm going to learn to have a machine take over my life and this is my attitude to this one, this is why I want the transplant. Get off this machine. It's looking after me fine, but get off it, I don't want to be taken over by a machine. This is 1984, or whatever it is. . . . And yet I have to say 'thank god for it' because I certainly wouldn't be alive today and I am not prepared to die. It is not on my agenda, no. I am going to live forever; I've got too much to do. There is too much going on out there. I've got to see my grandchildren grow up. I've got to get on with life out there and do things.

F6's reference to the dystopian science fiction novel *Nineteen Eighty-Four* captures the ambivalence participants felt about maintenance dialysis; optimistically couching it as a technology of hope (Franklin, 1997) that extends life expectancy, while reluctantly acknowledging the requirement to 'capitulate to the confines of a fabricated life' (Bevan, 2000: 442). There is a tension here, as Heidegger remarks, between mastering the technology by getting it 'intelligently in hand' and the technology taking over. Dialysis patients who experience quality of life get beyond dehumanisation by the machine because they are willing and able to adhere to a dialysis self-care regimen (see Agar, 2008; Allen et al., 2011; Cases et al., 2011). This requires a combination of factors, including concordance with health professionals, adequate education, mastering medical terminology, understanding the rules of illness management, exercising self-surveillance, resourcefulness and the application of know-how to individual circumstances. They also adopt a dynamic relation to the technologies they encounter.

For F6, hope is premised on the future-orientated desire to 'watch her grandchildren grow up'. Like Rittman et al.'s (1993) study, participants in the present project were also self-consciously engaged in a potentiality-for-being (Heidegger, 2008). Almost all talked about contributing in various ways to their community, by giving back to society post transplant, thus conveying engagement with life's activities (Shaw, 2012). As with F6's quotation above, several participants expressed being there in existential terms. Their ethic of self-care included 'not letting your illness become you' (F4) and 'getting past being the sick person . . . outside of your kidney issues and outside of your transplant' (F5). F5 reflected,

> Once I got home and started to get a bit better and I was able to become me again, I realised that the little things just weren't worth getting worried about. . . . You kind of spend so much time getting caught up in the day-to-day of Monday to Friday and all the rest of it and not having a Monday or a Friday for so long. You kind of say, 'oh, yay, it's Friday', or 'god, it's Monday', but when you don't have that it's amazing how much you want it.

For F4,

> I think being seriously ill gives you a different perspective. It's like anything, anything you do. Like you know, when you first have a baby, I mean you go home after being in hospital with a real baby and you're like going. . . .

> [Husband: Who gave us this? [laughter] How come I'm allowed to do this? Where are the instructions?] You know your whole life is changed from that point, it's never, ever the same and it wouldn't matter what happened, your life completely changes, and you, you occasionally might resent it when you're tired and grumpy or the baby's up at 3.00 am but you never really resent it because it's a new phase. And in some ways I feel like that about being ill. You know I can resent it, but it's still actually given me a perspective on living that maybe I didn't have. It does make you think about dying and therefore you think about living.

For this participant, the topic of death was viewed existentially (see also Calvey and Mee, 2011). Like others in the study, she spoke about being ill and dying as an opportunity to accept her own finality and rise to the challenge of living. The realisation that time is limited gave her a renewed sense of responsibility for her own life and a determination to live fully.

CONCLUSION

Study data suggest that the notion of the machine–body contributes to an understanding of the lived experience of being-in-dialysis as mediated by technological factors. In line with other investigations, the relationship between dialysis patients and the machine is described as ambivalent. Dialysing in the hospital setting is characterised by study participants who had experience of this modality as negative. There was agreement that hospital dialysis results in a loss of personal autonomy and reduced lifestyle flexibility compared with the option of home HD or PD. However, although those using home dialysis were able to take responsibility for their self-management, they were nonetheless dependent on and controlled by the dialysis machine for their continued survival. Living with a home dialysis machine required forethought, planning and reorganisation of lived space and time. For renal patients, being-in-dialysis entails successfully and sometimes reluctantly incorporating medical technology into their life, while simultaneously retaining a sense of hope for the possibility of a future transplant. Participants were therefore not prepared to be overcome by the practicalities of 'being caught up in the day-to-day of Monday to Friday' of their crisis situation. Rather, they made an effort to live deliberately, consciously deciding on a dialysis therapy that suited their lifestyle in order to get on with the business of living and interact with the world.

Access to material resources such as disposable income and adequate housing afforded study participants opportunities not available to New Zealand dialysis patients from lower socio-economic backgrounds. Given the rising rate of end-stage renal disease for Māori and Pasifika peoples, who are over-represented in socio-economically disadvantaged groups, this is significant. Home HD is easier to access for patients who own their own homes and travel is an option for those who can afford it. Hidden costs, associated with storage of dialysis equipment and disposal requirements, also need to be taken into account. Given the geographical isolation of New Zealand patients in some regions and unsuitable housing situations for independent dialysis, a number of District Health Boards have set up staffed satellite units and dialysis houses without staff, to allow better quality of life for patients living in these regions. Additionally, since 2011, four new and expanded dialysis centres have been set up throughout New Zealand's North Island. Further research with diverse population samples around perceptions of dialysis use in these settings would enhance understanding of New Zealanders' experiences of being-in-dialysis.

Study participants did not use the term cyborg to describe their hybrid identity, but Heidegger's notion of technological apparatuses as ready-to-hand or present-at-hand fits their experience in relation to the self-management of their therapy when applied to the dialysis machine. The more independence participants had, the more integrated their positive lived experience with the various dialysis treatment modalities. Although being-in-dialysis is not a cure for end-stage renal failure, having access to equipment at home presented both a positive learning challenge for numerous participants as well as enabling a measure of self-control over their own lives. At the same time, participants recognised that renal replacement therapy, including the hoped-for kidney transplant, did not represent a miraculous end point in the experience of technological and medical intervention. Kidney transplantation, as participants noted, comes with its own set of intervening iatrogenic regimens making future-oriented projects uncertain while intensifying the urgency to live fully in the present. Contrary to popular opinion, renal replacement therapy saves lives, but the extent to which life is fully restored remains moot for renal patients. Sadly, several dialysis patients in the study died while awaiting transplantation.

Returning to the definition of medical technologies cited earlier (Gabe et al., 2006), the benefits of home HD depend very much on collaborative decision-making models that integrate medical expertise and patients' experience, as well as the support of partners and other family members. A comprehensive phenomenological account of being-in-dialysis, both in home and hospital settings, thus necessitates discussion of patients' lived relation to others as caregivers and the work attached to the bodies of those who are cared for. Successful renal therapy from a patient perspective also depends on perceptions of the dialysis machine as actively mediating identity, rather than a device or tool to be mastered.

References

Agar JWM (2008) Home hemodialysis in Australia and New Zealand: Practical problems and solutions. *Hemodialysis International* 12: 526–532.

Al-Arabi S (2006) Quality of life: Subjective descriptions of challenges to patients with end stage renal disease. *Nephrology Nursing Journal* 33(3): 285–292.

Allen D, Wainwright M and Hutchinson T (2011) 'Non-compliance' as illness management: Hemodialysis patients' descriptions of adversarial patient-clinician interactions. *Social Science & Medicine* 73: 129–134.

Bayhakki and Hatthakit U (2012) Lived experiences of patients on hemodialysis: A meta-synthesis. *Nephrology Nursing Journal* 39(4): 295–304.

Bevan MT (2000) Dialysis as 'deus ex machina': A critical analysis of haemodialysis. *Journal of Advanced Nursing* 31(2): 437–443.

Braun V and Clarke V (2006) Using thematic analysis in psychology. *Qualitative Research in Psychology* 3: 77–101.

Calvey D and Mee L (2011) The lived experience of the person dependent on haemodialysis. *Journal of Renal Care* 37(4): 201–207.

Cases A, Dempster M, Davies M, et al. (2011) The experience of individuals with renal failure participating in home haemodialysis: An interpretative phenomenological analysis. *Journal of Health Psychology* 16(6): 884–894.

Clarkson KA and Robinson K (2010) Life on dialysis: A lived experience. *Nephrology Nursing Journal* 37(1): 29–35.

Courts NF (2000) Psychosocial adjustment of patients on home hemodialysis and their dialysis partners. *Clinical Nursing Research* 9(2): 177–190.

Courts NF and Boyette BG (1998) Psychosocial adjustment of males on three types of dialysis. *Clinical Nursing Research* 7(1): 47–63.

Creswell JW (2007) *Qualitative Inquiry & Research Design: Choosing among Five Approaches*. Thousand Oaks, CA: SAGE.

Delgado CEY, Delgado FLY, Betancourt MLV, et al. (2010) A qualitative study of patient's perceptions of a preventive renal programme in Colombia 2008. *Chronic Illness* 6: 252–262.

Franklin S (1997) *Embodied Progress: A Cultural Account of Assisted Conception*. London: Routledge.

Gabe J, Bury M and Elston MA (2006) *Key Concepts in Medical Sociology*. London: SAGE.

Giles S (2003) Transformations: A phenomenological investigation into the life-world of home haemodialysis. *Social Work in Health Care* 38(2): 29–50.

Giles S (2005) Struggles between the body and machine: The paradox of living with a home haemodialysis machine. *Social Work in Health Care* 41(2): 19–35.

Guest G, MacQueen KM and Namey EE (2012) *Applied Thematic Analysis*. Los Angeles, CA: SAGE.

Hagren B, Pettersen I-M, Severinsson E, et al. (2001) The haemodialysis machine as a lifeline: Experiences of suffering from end-stage renal disease. *Journal of Advanced Nursing* 34(2): 196–202.

Hagren B, Pettersen I-M, Severinsson E, et al. (2005) Maintenance haemodialysis: Patients' experiences of their life situation. *Journal of Clinical Nursing* 14: 294–300.

Haraway D (1990) A manifesto for cyborgs: Science, technology, and socialist feminism in the 1980s. In: Nicholson L (ed.) *Feminism/Postmodernism*. New York: Routledge, pp. 190–233.

Harwood L and Leitch R (2006) Home dialysis therapies. *Nephrology Nursing Journal* 33(1): 46–59.

Heidegger M (2008) *Being and Time* (trans. J Macquarrie and E Robinson). New York: Harper Perennial.

Kierans C (2010) Transplantation, organ donation and (in)human experience: Re-writing boundaries through embodied perspectives on kidney failure. In: Ettore E (ed.) *Culture, Bodies and the Sociology of Health*. Surrey: Ashgate, pp. 21–43.

Kuzel A (1992) Sampling in qualitative inquiry. In: Crabtree B and Miller W (eds) *Doing Qualitative Research*. Newbury Park, CA: SAGE, pp. 31–44.

Levy NB (1981) Psychological reactions to machine dependency: Hemodialysis. *Psychiatric Clinics of North America* 4(2): 351–363.

Levy NB (2000) Psychiatric considerations in the primary medical care of the patient with renal failure. *Advances in Renal Replacement Therapy* 7(3): 231–238.

Lynn KL and Buttimore AL (2005) Future of home haemodialysis in Australia and New Zealand. *Nephrology* 10: 231–233.

Marshall MR, Hawley CM, Kerr PG, et al. (2011) Home hemodialysis and mortality risk in Australian and New Zealand Populations. *American Journal of Kidney Diseases* 58(5): 782–793.

Moran A, Scott PA and Darbyshire P (2009) Existential boredom: The experience of living on haemodialysis therapy. *Medical Humanities* 35: 70–75.

Pidgeon G (2012) New Zealand dialysis and transplantation audit 2010. National Renal Advisory Board. Available at: http://www.moh.govt.nz/nrab (accessed 27 November 2012).

Polaschek N (2003) Living on dialysis: Concerns of clients in a renal setting. *Journal of Advanced Nursing* 41(1): 44–52.

Polaschek N (2006) Managing home dialysis: The client perspective on independent treatment. *Renal Society of Australasia Journal* 2(3): 53–63.

Rittman M, Northsea C, Hausauer N, et al. (1993) Living with renal failure. *ANNA Journal* 20(3): 327–332.

Shaw R (2012) Thanking and reciprocating under the New Zealand organ donation system. *Health: An Interdisciplinary Journal for the Social Study of Health, Illness and Medicine* 16(3): 298–313.

Shildrick M, McKeever P, Abbey S, et al. (2009) Troubling dimensions of heart transplantation. *Medical Humanities* 35: 35–38.

Smith JA (2004) Reflecting on the development of interpretative phenomenological analysis and its contribution to qualitative research in psychology. *Qualitative Research in Psychology* 1: 39–54.

Timmermans S and Berg M (2003) The practice of medical technology. *Sociology of Health & Illness* 25: 97–114.

Timmers L, Thong M, Dekker FW, et al. (2008) Illness perceptions in dialysis patients and their association with quality of life. *Psychology & Health* 23(6): 679–690.

Van Manen M (1990) *Researching Lived Experience: Human Science for an Action Sensitive Pedagogy*. Albany, NY: State University of New York Press.

Wajcman J (2004) *TechnoFeminism*. Malden, MA: Polity Press.

Wilson C (2011) *Cost-benefit study of the feasibility of providing dialysis in the Cook Islands*. S.l.: Eve Bay Resarch.

THE SOCIAL ORGANIZATION OF MEDICAL CARE

In Part II, we turn from the production of disease and illness to the social organizations created to treat it. Here, we begin to examine the institutional aspects of health and illness in the medical care system. We look at the social organization of medical care historically, structurally, and, finally, interactionally. We seek to understand how this complex system operates and how its particular characteristics have contributed to the current health care situation.

THE RISE AND FALL OF
THE DOMINANCE OF MEDICINE

Physicians have a professional monopoly on medical practice in the United States. They have an exclusive, state-supported right, manifested in the licensing of physicians, to medical practice. With their licenses, physicians can legally do what no one else can, including cutting into the human body. While in recent years this monopoly has been challenged around the edges—for example, with the development of nurse practitioners and the greater acceptance of chiropractors—physicians still maintain much of the monopoly on medical practice.

Until the latter part of the nineteenth century, various groups and individuals (e.g., homeopaths, midwives, botanical doctors) competed for "medical turf." By the second decade of the twentieth century, virtually only medical doctors (MDs) had the legal right to practice medicine in this country. One might suggest that physicians achieved their exclusive rights to the nation's medical territory because of their superior scientific and clinical achievements, a line of reasoning that suggests physicians demonstrated superior healing and curative skills, and the government therefore supported their rights against less effective healers and quacks. But this seems not to have been the case. As we noted earlier, most of the improvement in the health status of the population resulted from social changes, including better nutrition, sanitation, and a rising standard of living, rather than from the interventions of clinical medicine. Medical techniques were in fact rather limited, often even dangerous, until the early twentieth century. As L. J. Henderson observed, "Somewhere between 1910 and 1912 in this country, a random patient, with a random disease, consulting a doctor chosen at random, had, for the first time in the history of mankind, a better than fifty-fifty chance of profiting from the encounter" (Blumgart 1964).

The success of the American Medical Association in consolidating its power was central to securing a monopoly for MDs. By virtue of their monopoly over medical practice, physicians have exerted an enormous influence over the entire field of medicine, including the right to define what constitutes disease and how to treat it. Freidson's (1970a, 251) observation is still valid: "The medical profession has first claim to jurisdiction over the label of illness and *always* to how it can be attached, irrespective of its capacity to deal with it effectively." It takes a doctor to legitimize a condition as an illness, and conversely, anything that is officially termed an illness routinely is considered within the realm of the medical profession.

Physicians also gained "professional dominance" over the organization of medical services in the United States (Freidson 1970b). This monopoly gave the medical profession functional autonomy and a structural insulation from outside evaluations of medical practice. In addition, professional dominance includes not only the exclusive right to treat disease but also the right to limit and evaluate the performance of most other medical care workers. Finally, the particular vision of medicine that became institutionalized included a "clinical mentality" (Freidson 1970a) that focused on medical responsibility to *individual* patients rather than to the community or public.

In the first selection, "Professionalization, Monopoly, and the Structure of Medical Practice," Peter Conrad and Joseph W. Schneider present a brief review of the historical development of this medical monopoly. They examine the case of abortion in the nineteenth century to highlight how specific medical interests were served by a physician-led crusade against abortion. By successfully outlawing abortion and institutionalizing their own professional ethics, "regular" physicians were able to effectively eliminate some of their competitors and secure greater control of the medical market.

Richard W. Wertz and Dorothy C. Wertz expand on this theme of monopolization and professional dominance in "Notes on the Decline of Midwives and the Rise of Medical Obstetricians."

They investigate the medicalization of childbirth historically and the subsequent decline of midwifery in this country. Female midwifery, which continues to be practiced in most industrialized and developing countries, was virtually eliminated in the United States. The authors show that it was not merely professional imperialism that led to the exclusion of midwives (although this played an important role) but also a subtle and profound sexism within and outside the medical profession. They postulate that the physicians' monopolization of childbirth resulted from a combination of a change in middle-class women's views of birthing, physicians' economic interests, and the development of sexist notions that suggested women weren't suitable for attending births. Physicians became increasingly interventionist in their childbirth practice partly due to their training (they felt they had to "do" something) but also due to their desire to use instruments "to establish a superior status" and treat childbirth as an illness rather than a natural event. In recent years, we have seen the reemergence of nurse midwives, but their work is usually limited to hospitals under medical dominance (Rothman 1982). Also, there are currently a small number of "lay" midwives whose practice is limited to states where it is recognized and legal, and thus outside of medical control (see Sullivan and Weitz 1988; Tritten 2010).

Physicians' professional dominance has been decreasing in the past three decades. Richard Scott and his colleagues (Mandel and Scott 2010) point to the expansion of federal responsibility (Medicare and Medicaid) and managed care (corporatized health care and specialized health care systems) as key to the erosion of professional dominance. Physicians had to be accountable to these organizations. Others have argued that the rise of corporate and bureaucratic medicine, the emphasis on cost containment by third-party payers, the complexity of medical technology, and the dramatic increase in malpractice suits have left the medical profession feeling besieged (Stoeckle 1988). There is evidence that professional sovereignty is declining and commercial interest in the health sector is increasing. One analyst has suggested that this is partly due to the actual surplus of doctors in this country and the increasing power of third parties in financing medicine (Starr 1982), although this surplus is now manifested mostly in highly specialized (and thus expensive) physicians as opposed to a shortage of primary care physicians. In the current medical environment, professional dominance is clearly changing and is reshaping the influence and authority over medical care. Although medicine maintains some of its monopoly, its dominance over the health care system has clearly declined.

In the third article, "The End of the Golden Age of Doctoring," John B. McKinlay and Lisa D. Marceau point to many of the social factors involved in the erosion of professional dominance and the rise of corporate dominance in the twenty-first century. They analyze eight interrelated factors that contributed to the decline of the "golden age of doctoring." It is clear that these changes have profoundly altered the medical profession and doctoring in the current era.

Donald W. Light, in the fourth selection, "Countervailing Power: The Changing Character of the Medical Profession in the United States," posits a changing balance of power among professions and related social institutions. "The notion of countervailing powers locates professions within a field of institutional and cultural forces in which one party may gain dominance by subordinating the needs of significant other parties, who, in time, mobilize to counter this dominance" (Hafferty and Light 1995, 135). In American society, professional medicine historically dominated health care, but we now see "buyers" (e.g., corporations who pay for employees' medical insurance, along with other consumers); "providers" (e.g., physicians, hospitals, HMOs, nursing homes, and other medical care providers); and "payers" (e.g., insurance companies and governments) all vying for power and influence over medical care. This changes the nature of professional power and dominance. Light points out that as medical care evolves into a more buyer-driven system, fundamental tenets of professionalism— including physicians' autonomy over their work and their monopoly over knowledge—are thrown into question. Currently, physicians certainly maintain aspects of their dominance and sovereignty, but it is clearly a situation undergoing dynamic changes. One can ask: How has professional authority fared under the 2010 health reform passed under the Obama administration (see Pescosolido, Tuch, and Martin 2001; Timmermans and Oh 2010)? How will attempts by the Trump administration and Republican-controlled Congress to repeal Obamacare affect power in medicine?

In the twenty-first century, we are increasingly finding aspects of the medical profession either creating or clashing with medical markets, including the health insurance industry, competing hospitals, the pharmaceutical industry, and the growing business of medicine. With the increasing dominance of market-oriented values, historical trust in physicians has eroded. Since 2000, however, "organized professional bodies have mounted campaigns to restore their professionalism and lost trust" (Light 2010, 270). This has occurred along with the increasing commercialization of medicine in terms of for-profit medical care, increasing medical markets for cosmetic surgery, and the increased power of third-party payers, such as health insurance (Conrad and Leiter 2004).

References

Blumgart, H. L. 1964. "Caring for the Patient." *New England Journal of Medicine* 270: 449–56.

Conrad, Peter, and Valerie Leiter. 2004. "Medicalization, Markets and Consumers" *Journal of Health and Social Behavior* 45, extra issue: 158–76.

Freidson, Eliot. 1970a. *Profession of Medicine.* New York: Dodd, Mead.

———. 1970b. *Professional Dominance.* Chicago: Aldine.

Hafferty, Fredric W., and Donald W. Light. 1995. "Professional Dynamics and the Changing Nature of Medical Work." *Journal of Health and Social Behavior* extra issue: 132–153.

Light, Donald W. 2010. "Health Care Professions, Markets and Countervailing Powers." In *Handbook of Medical Sociology,* 6th edition, edited by Chloe Bird, Peter Conrad, Allen Fremont, and Stefan Timmermans, 270–89. Nashville, TN: Vanderbilt University Press.

Mandel, Peter, and W. Richard Scott. 2010. "Institutional Change and the Organization of Health Care." In *Handbook of Medical Sociology,* 6th edition, edited by Chloe Bird, Peter Conrad, Allen Fremont, and Stefan Timmermans, 49–69. Nashville, TN: Vanderbilt University Press.

Pescosolido, Bernice A., Steven A. Tuch, and Jack K. Martin. 2001. "The Profession of Medicine and the Public: Examining Americans' Changing Confidence in Physician Authority from the Beginning of the 'Health Care Crisis' to the Era of Health Care Reform." *Journal of Health and Social Behavior* 42: 1–16.

Rothman, Barbara Katz. 1982. *In Labor.* New York: Norton.

Starr, Paul. 1982. *The Social Transformation of American Medicine.* New York: Basic Books.

Stoeckle, John D. 1988. "Reflections on Modern Doctoring." *Milbank Quarterly* 66(Suppl. 2): 76–91.

Sullivan, Deborah A., and Rose Weitz. 1988. *Labor Pains: Modern Midwives and Home Birth.* New Haven: Yale University Press.

Timmermans, Stefan, and Hyeyoung Oh. 2010. "The Continued Social Transformation of the Medical Profession." *Journal of Health and Social Behavior* 51: S94–S106.

Tritten, Jan. 2010. *Birth Wisdom.* American Digital Services. Kindle edition.

PROFESSIONALIZATION, MONOPOLY, AND THE STRUCTURE OF MEDICAL PRACTICE

Peter Conrad and Joseph W. Schneider

...Medicine has not always been the powerful, prestigious, successful, lucrative, and dominant profession we know today. The status of the medical profession is a product of medical politicking as well as therapeutic expertise. This discussion presents a brief overview of the development of the medical profession and its rise to dominance.

EMERGENCE OF THE MEDICAL PROFESSION: UP TO 1850

In ancient societies, disease was given supernatural explanations, and "medicine" was the province of priests or shamans. It was in classical Greece that medicine began to emerge as a separate occupation and develop its own theories, distinct from philosophy or theology. Hippocrates, the great Greek physician who refused to accept supernatural explanations or treatments for disease, developed a theory of the "natural" causes of disease and systematized all available medical knowledge. He laid a basis for the development of medicine as a separate body of knowledge. Early Christianity depicted sickness as punishment for sin, engendering new theological explanations and treatments. Christ and his disciples believed in the supernatural causes and cures of disease. This view became institutionalized in the Middle Ages, when the Church dogma dominated theories and practice of medicine and priests were physicians. The Renaissance in Europe brought a renewed interest in ancient Greek medical knowledge. This marked the beginning of a drift toward natural explanations of disease and the emergence of medicine as an occupation separate from the Church (Cartwright, 1977).

But European medicine developed slowly. The "humoral theory" of disease developed by Hippocrates dominated medical theory and practice until well into the 19th century. Medical diagnosis was impressionistic and often inaccurate, depicting conditions in such general terms as "fevers" and "fluxes." In the 17th century, physicians relied mainly on three techniques to determine the nature of illness: what the patient said about symptoms; the physician's own observations of signs of illness and the patient's appearance and behavior; and more rarely, a manual examination of the body (Reiser, 1978, p. 1). Medicine was by no means scientific, and "medical thought involved unverified doctrines and resulting controversies" (Shryock, 1960, p. 52). Medical practice was a "bedside medicine" that was patient oriented and did not distinguish the illness from the "sick man" (Jewson, 1976). It was not until Thomas Sydenham's astute observations in the late 17th century that physicians could begin to distinguish between the patient and the disease. Physicians possessed few treatments that worked regularly, and many of their treatments actually worsened the sufferer's condition. Medicine in colonial America inherited this European stock of medical knowledge.

Colonial American medicine was less developed than its European counterpart. There were no medical schools and few physicians, and because of the vast frontier and sparse population, much medical care was in effect self-help. Most American physicians were educated and trained by apprenticeship; few were university trained. With the exception of surgeons, most were undifferentiated practitioners. Medical practices were limited. Prior to the revolution, physicians did not commonly attend births; midwives, who were not seen as part of the medical establishment, routinely attended birthings (Wertz and Wertz, 1977). William Rothstein (1972) notes that "American colonial medical practice, like European practice of the period, was characterized by the lack of any substantial body of usable scientific knowledge" (p. 27). Physicians, both educated and otherwise, tended to treat their patients

pragmatically, for medical theory had little to offer. Most colonial physicians practiced medicine only part-time, earning their livelihoods as clergymen, teachers, farmers, or in other occupations. Only in the early 19th century did medicine become a full-time vocation (Rothstein, 1972).

The first half of the 19th century saw important changes in the organization of the medical profession. About 1800, "regular," or educated, physicians convinced state legislatures to pass laws limiting the practice of medicine to practitioners of a certain training and class (prior to this nearly anyone could claim the title "doctor" and practice medicine). These state licensing laws were not particularly effective, largely because of the colonial tradition of medical self-help. They were repealed in most states during the Jacksonian period (1828–1836) because they were thought to be elitist, and the temper of the times called for a more "democratic" medicine.

The repeal of the licensing laws and the fact that most "regular" (i.e., regularly educated) physicians shared and used "a distinctive set of medically invalid therapies, known as 'heroic' therapy," created fertile conditions for the emergence of *medical sects* in the first half of the 19th century (Rothstein, 1972, p. 21). Physicians of the time practiced a "heroic" and invasive form of medicine consisting primarily of such treatments as bloodletting, vomiting, blistering, and purging. This highly interventionist, and sometimes dangerous, form of medicine engendered considerable public opposition and resistance. In this context a number of medical sects emerged, the most important of which were the homeopathic and botanical physicians. These "irregular" medical practitioners practiced less invasive, less dangerous forms of medicine. They each developed a considerable following, since their therapies were probably no less effective than those of regulars practicing heroic medicine. The regulars attempted to exclude them from practice; so the various sects set up their own medical schools and professional societies. This sectarian medicine created a highly *competitive* situation for the regulars (Rothstein, 1972). Medical sectarianism, heroic therapies, and ineffective treatment contributed to the low status and lack of prestige of early 19th-century medicine. At this time, medicine was neither a prestigious occupation nor an important economic activity in American society (Starr, 1977).

The regular physicians were concerned about this situation. Large numbers of regularly trained physicians sought to earn a livelihood by practicing medicine (Rothstein, 1972, p. 3). They were troubled by the poor image of medicine and lack of standards in medical training and practice. No doubt they were also concerned about the competition of the irregular sectarian physicians. A group of regular physicians founded the American Medical Association (AMA) in 1847 "to promote the science and art of medicine and the betterment of public health" (quoted in Coe, 1978, p. 204). The AMA also was to set and enforce standards and ethics of "regular" medical practice and strive for exclusive professional and economic rights to the medical turf.

The AMA was the crux of the regulars' attempt to "professionalize" medicine. As Magali Sarfatti Larson (1977) points out, professions organize to create and control *markets.* Organized professions attempt to regulate and limit the competition, usually by controlling professional education and by limiting licensing. Professionalization is, in this view, "the process by which producers of special services sought to constitute *and control* the market for their expertise" (Larson, 1977, p. xvi). The regular physicians and the AMA set out to consolidate and control the market for medical services. As we shall see in the next two sections, the regulars were successful in professionalization, eliminating competition and creating a medical monopoly.

CRUSADING, DEVIANCE, AND MEDICAL MONOPOLY: THE CASE OF ABORTION

The medical profession after the middle of the 19th century was frequently involved in various activities that could be termed social reform. Some of these reforms were directly related to health and illness and medical work; others were peripheral to the manifest medical calling of preventing illness and healing the sick. In these reform movements, physicians became medical crusaders, attempting to influence public morality and behavior. This medical crusading often led physicians squarely into the moral sphere, making them advocates for moral positions that had only peripheral relations to medical practice. Not infrequently these reformers sought to change people's values or to impose a set of particular values on others. . . . We now examine one of the more revealing examples of medical crusading: the criminalization of abortion in American society.[1]

Most people are under the impression that abortion was always defined as deviant and illegal in America prior to the Supreme Court's landmark decision in 1973. This, however, is not the case. American abortion policy, and the attendant defining of abortion as deviant, were specific products of medical crusading. Prior to the Civil War, abortion was a common and largely legal medical procedure performed by various types of physicians and midwives. A pregnancy was not considered confirmed until the occurrence of a phenomenon called "quickening," the first perception of fetal movement. Common law did not recognize the fetus before quickening in criminal cases, and an unquickened fetus was deemed to have no living soul. Thus most people did not consider termination of pregnancy before quickening to be an especially serious matter, much less murder. Abortion before quickening created no moral or medical problems. Public opinion was indifferent, and for the time it was probably a relatively safe medical procedure. Thus, for all intents and purposes, American women were free to terminate their pregnancies before quickening in the early 19th century. Moreover, it was a procedure relatively free of the moral stigma that was attached to abortion in this century.

After 1840 abortion came increasingly into public view. Abortion clinics were vigorously and openly advertised in newspapers and magazines. The advertisements offered euphemistically couched services for "women's complaints," "menstrual blockage," and "obstructed menses." Most contemporary observers suggested that more and more women were using these services. Prior to 1840 most abortions were performed on the unmarried and desperate of the "poor and unfortunate classes." However, beginning about this time, significantly increasing numbers of middle- and upper-class white, Protestant, native-born women began to use these services. It is likely they either wished to delay childbearing or thought they already had all the children they wanted (Mohr, 1978, pp. 46–47). By 1870 approximately one abortion was performed for every five live births (Mohr, 1978, pp. 79–80).

Beginning in the 1850s, a number of physicians, especially moral crusader Dr. Horatio Robinson Storer, began writing in medical and popular journals and lobbying in state legislatures about the danger and immorality of abortion. They opposed abortion before and after quickening and under Dr. Storer's leadership organized an aggressive national campaign. In 1859 these crusaders convinced the AMA to pass a resolution condemning abortion. Some newspapers, particularly *The New York Times,* joined the antiabortion crusade. Feminists supported the crusade, since they saw abortion as a threat to women's health and part of the oppression of women. Religious leaders, however, by and large avoided the issue of abortion, either they didn't consider it in their province or found it too sticky an issue to discuss. It was the physicians who were the guiding force in the antiabortion crusade. They were instrumental in convincing legislatures to pass state laws, especially between 1866 and 1877, that made abortion a criminal offense.

Why did physicians take the lead in the antiabortion crusade and work so directly to have abortion defined as deviant and illegal? Undoubtedly they believed in the moral "rightness" of their cause. But social historian James Mohr (1978) presents two more subtle and important reasons for the physicians' antiabortion crusading. First, concern was growing among medical people and even among some legislators about the significant drop in birthrates. Many claimed that abortion among married women of the "better classes" was a major contributor to the declining birthrate. These middle- and upper-class men (the physicians and legislators) were aware of the waves of immigrants arriving with large families and were anxious about the decline in production of native American babies. They were deeply

afraid they were being betrayed by their own women (Mohr, 1978, p. 169). Implicitly the antiabortion stance was classist and racist; the anxiety was simply that there would not be enough strong, native-born, Protestant stock to save America. This was a persuasive argument in convincing legislators of the need of antiabortion laws.

The second and more direct reason spurring the physicians in the antiabortion crusade was to aid their own nascent professionalization and create a monopoly for regular physicians. . . . The regulars had formed the AMA in 1847 to promote scientific and ethical medicine and combat what they saw as medical quackery. There were, however, no licensing laws to speak of, and many claimed the title "doctor" (e.g., homeopaths, botanical doctors, eclectic physicians). The regular physicians adopted the Hippocratic oath and code of ethics as their standard. Among other things, this oath forbids abortion. Regulars usually did not perform abortions; however, many practitioners of medical sects performed abortions regularly, and some had lucrative practices. Thus for the regular AMA physicians the limitation of abortion became one way of asserting their own professional domination over other medical practitioners. In their crusading these physicians had translated the social goals of cultural and professional dominance into moral and medical language. They lobbied long and hard to convince legislators of the danger and immorality of abortion. By passage of laws making abortion criminal any time during gestation, regular physicians were able to legislate their code of ethics and get the state to employ sanctions against their competitors. This limited these competitors' markets and was a major step toward the regulars' achieving a monopolization of medical practice.

In a relatively short period the antiabortion crusade succeeded in passing legislation that made abortion criminal in every state. A by-product of this was a shift in American public opinion from an indifference to and tolerance of abortion to a hardening of attitudes against what had until then been a fairly common practice. The irony was that abortion as a medical procedure probably was safer at the turn of the 20th century than a century before, but it was defined and seen as more dangerous. By 1900 abortion was not only illegal but deviant and immoral. The physicians' moral crusade had successfully defined abortion as a deviant activity. This definition remained largely unchanged until the 1973 Supreme Court decision, which essentially returned the abortion situation to its pre-1850 condition. . . .

GROWTH OF MEDICAL EXPERTISE AND PROFESSIONAL DOMINANCE

Although the general public's dissatisfaction with heroic medicine remained, the image of medicine and what it could accomplish was improving by the middle of the 19th century. There had been a considerable reduction in the incidence and mortality of certain dread diseases. The plague and leprosy had nearly disappeared. Smallpox, malaria, and cholera were less devastating than ever before. These improvements in health engendered optimism and increased people's faith in medical practice. Yet these dramatic "conquests of disease" were by and large *not* the result of new medical knowledge or improved clinical medical practice. Rather, they resulted from changes in social conditions: a rising standard of living, better nutrition and housing, and public health innovations like sanitation. With the lone exception of vaccination for smallpox, the decline of these diseases had nearly nothing to do with clinical medicine (Dubos, 1959; McKeown, 1971). But despite lack of effective treatments, medicine was the beneficiary of much popular credit for improved health.

The regular physicians' image was improved well before they demonstrated any unique effectiveness of practice. The AMA's attacks on irregular medical practice continued. In the 1870s the regulars convinced legislatures to outlaw abortion and in some states to restore licensing laws to restrict medical practice. The AMA was becoming an increasingly powerful and authoritative voice representing regular medical practice.

But the last three decades of the century saw significant "breakthroughs" in medical knowledge and treatment. The scientific medicine of the regular physicians was making new medical advances. Anesthesia and antisepsis made possible great strides in surgical medicine and improvements in hospital care. The bacteriological research of Koch and Pasteur developed the "germ theory of disease," which had important applications in medical practice. It was the accomplishments of surgery and bacteriology that put medicine on a scientific basis (Freidson, 1970a, p. 16). The rise of scientific medicine marked a death knell for medical sectarianism (e.g., the homeopathic physicians eventually joined the regulars). The new laboratory sciences provided a way of testing the theories and practices of various sects, which ultimately led to a single model of medical practice. The well-organized regulars were able to legitimate their form of medical practice and support it with "scientific" evidence.

With the emergence of scientific medicine, a unified paradigm, or model, of medical practice developed. It was based, most fundamentally, on viewing the body as a machine (e.g., organ malfunctioning) and on the germ theory of disease (Kelman, 1977). The "doctrine of specific etiology" became predominant: each disease was caused by a specific germ or agent. Medicine focused solely on the internal environment (the body), largely ignoring the external environment (society) (Dubos, 1959). This paradigm proved fruitful in ensuing years. It is the essence of the "medical model." . . .

The development of scientific medicine accorded regular medicine a convincing advantage in medical practice. It set the stage for the achievement of a medical monopoly by the AMA regulars. As Larson (1977) notes, "Once scientific medicine offered sufficient guarantees of its superior effectiveness in dealing with disease, the rate willingly contributed to the creation of a monopoly by means of registration and licensing" (p. 23). The new licensing laws created regular medicine as a *legally enforced monopoly of practice* (Freidson, 1970b, p. 83). They virtually eliminated medical competition.

The medical monopoly was enhanced further by the Flexner Report on medical education in 1910. Under the auspices of the Carnegie Foundation, medical educator Abraham Flexner visited nearly all 160 existing medical schools in the United States. He found the level of medical education poor and recommended the closing of most schools. Flexner urged stricter state laws, rigid standards for medical education, and more rigorous examinations for certification to practice. The enactment of Flexner's recommendations effectively made all nonscientific types of medicine illegal. It created a near total AMA monopoly of medical education in America.

In securing a monopoly, the AMA regulars achieved a unique professional state. Medicine not only monopolized the market for medical services and the training of physicians, it developed an unparalleled "professional dominance." The medical profession was *functionally autonomous* (Freidson, 1970b). Physicians were insulated from external evaluation and were by and large free to regulate their own performance. Medicine could define its own territory and set its own standards. Thus, Eliot Freidson (1970b) notes, "while the profession may not everywhere be free to control the *terms* of its work, it is free to control the *content* of its work" (p. 84).

The domain of medicine has expanded in the past century. This is due partially to the prestige medicine has accrued and its place as the steward of the "sacred" value of life. Medicine has sometimes been called on to repeat its "miracles" and successful treatments on problems that are not biomedical in nature. Yet in other instances the expansion is due to explicit medical crusading or entrepreneurship. This expansion of medicine, especially into the realm of social problems and human behavior, frequently has taken medicine beyond its proven technical competence (Freidson, 1970b). . . .

The organization of medicine has also expanded and become more complex in this century. In the next section we briefly describe the structure of medical practice in the United States.

STRUCTURE OF MEDICAL PRACTICE

Before we leave our discussion of the medical profession, it is worthwhile to outline some general features of the structure of medical practice that have contributed to the expansion of medical jurisdiction.

The medical sector of society has grown enormously in the 20th century. It has become the second largest industry in America. There are about 350,000 physicians and over 5 million people employed in the medical field. The "medical industries," including the pharmaceutical, medical technology, and health insurance industries, are among the most profitable in our economy. Yearly drug sales alone are over $4.5 billion. There are more than 7000 hospitals in the United States with 1.5 million beds and 33 million inpatient and 200 million outpatient visits a year (McKinlay, 1976).

The organization of medical practice has changed. Whereas the single physician in "solo practice" was typical in 1900, today physicians are engaged increasingly in large corporate practices or employed by hospitals or other bureaucratic organizations. Medicine in modern society is becoming bureaucratized (Mechanic, 1976). The power in medicine has become diffused, especially since World War II, from the AMA, which represented the individual physician, to include the organizations that represent bureaucratic medicine: the health insurance industry, the medical schools, and the American Hospital Association (Ehrenreich and Ehrenreich, 1970). Using Robert Alford's (1972) conceptualizations, corporate rationalizers have taken much of the power in medicine from the professional monopolists.

Medicine has become both more specialized and more dependent on technology. In 1929 only 25 percent of American physicians were fulltime specialists; by 1969 the proportion had grown to 75 percent (Reiser, 1978). Great advances were made in medicine, and many were directly related to technology: miracle medicines like penicillin, a myriad of psychoactive drugs, heart and brain surgery, the electrocardiograph, CAT scanners, fetal monitors, kidney dialysis machines, artificial organs, and transplant surgery, to name but a few. The hospital has become the primary medical workshop, a center for technological medicine.

Medicine has made a significant economic expansion. In 1940, medicine claimed about 4 percent of the American gross national product (GNP); today it claims about 9 percent, which amounts to more than $150 billion. The causes for this growth are too complex to describe here, but a few factors should be noted. American medicine has always operated on a "fee-for-service" basis, that is, each service rendered is charged and paid for separately. Simply put, in a capitalist medical system, the more services provided, the more fees collected. This not only creates an incentive to provide more services but also to expand these medical services to new markets. The fee-for-service system may encourage unnecessary medical care. There is some evidence, for example, that American medicine performs a considerable amount of "excess" surgery (McCleery and Keelty, 1971); this may also be true for other services. Medicine is one of the few occupations that can create its own demand. Patients may come to physicians, but physicians tell them what procedures they need. The availability of medical technique may also create a demand for itself.

The method by which medical care is paid for has changed greatly in the past half-century. In 1920 nearly all health care was paid for directly by the patient-consumer. Since the 1930s an increasing amount of medical care has been paid for through "third-party" payments, mainly through health insurance and the government. About 75 percent of the American population is covered by some form of medical insurance (often only for hospital care). Since 1966 the government has been involved directly in financing medical care through Medicare and Medicaid. The availability of a large amount of federal money, with nearly no cost controls or regulation of medical practice, has been a major factor fueling our current medical "cost crisis." But the ascendancy of third-party payments has affected the expansion of medicine in another way: more and more human problems become defined as "medical problems" (sickness) because that is the only way insurance programs will "cover" the costs of services. . . .

In sum, the regular physicians developed control of medical practice and a professional dominance with nearly total functional autonomy. Through professionalization and persuasion concerning the superiority of their form of medicine, the medical profession (represented by the AMA) achieved a legally supported monopoly of practice. In short, it cornered the medical market. The medical profession has succeeded in both therapeutic and economic expansion. It has won the almost exclusive right to reign over the kingdom of health and illness, no matter where it may extend.

Note

1. We rely on James C. Mohr's (1978) fine historical account of the origins and evolution of American abortion policy for data and much of the interpretation in this section.

References

Alford, R. The political economy of health care: dynamics without change. *Politics and Society,* 1972, 2 (2), 127–64.

Cartwright, F. F. *A Social History of Medicine.* New York: Longman, 1977.

Coe, R. *The Sociology of Medicine.* Second edition. New York: McGraw-Hill, 1978.

Dubos, R. *Mirage of Health.* New York: Harper and Row, 1959.

Ehrenreich, B., and Ehrenreich, J. *The American Health Empire.* New York: Random House, 1970.

Freidson, E. *Profession of Medicine.* New York: Dodd, Mead, 1970a.

Freidson, E. *Professional Dominance.* Chicago: Aldine, 1970b.

Jewson, N. D. The disappearance of the sick-man from medical cosmology, 1770–1870. *Sociology,* 1976, 10, 225–44.

Kelman, S. The social nature of the definition of health. In V. Navarro, *Health and Medical Care in the U.S.* Farmingdale, N.Y.: Baywood, 1977.

Larson, M. S. *The Rise of Professionalism.* Berkeley: California, 1977.

McCleery, R. S., and Keelty, L. T. *One Life-One Physician: An Inquiry into the Medical Profession's Performance in Self-regulation.* Washington, D.C.: Public Affairs Press, 1971.

McKeown, T. A historical appraisal of the medical task. In G. McLachlan and T. McKeown (eds.), *Medical History and Medical Care: A Symposium of Perspectives.* New York: Oxford, 1971.

McKinlay, J. B. The changing political and economic context of the physician-patient encounter. In E. B. Gallagher (ed.), *The Doctor-Patient Relationship in the Changing Health Scene.* Washington, D.C.: U.S. Government Printing Office, 1976.

Mechanic, D. *The Growth of Bureaucratic Medicine.* New York: Wiley, 1976.

Mohr, J. C. *Abortion in America.* New York: Oxford, 1978.

Reiser, S. J. *Medicine and the Reign of Technology.* New York: Cambridge, 1978.

Rothstein, W. G. *American Physicians in the Nineteenth Century: From Sects to Science.* Baltimore: Johns Hopkins, 1972.

Shryock, R. H. *Medicine and Society in America: 1660–1860.* Ithaca, N.Y.: Cornell, 1960.

Starr, P. Medicine, economy and society in nineteenth-century America. *Journal of Social History,* 1977, 10, 588–607.

Wertz, R., and Wertz, D. *Lying-In: A History of Childbirth in America.* New York: Free Press, 1977.

18

NOTES ON THE DECLINE OF MIDWIVES AND THE RISE OF MEDICAL OBSTETRICIANS

Richard W. Wertz and Dorothy C. Wertz

. . .The Americans who were studying medicine in Great Britain [in the late eighteenth century] discovered that men could bring the benefits of the new midwifery to birth and thereby gain income and status. In regard to the unresolved question of what medical arts were appropriate, the Americans took the view of the English physicians, who instructed them that nature was usually adequate and intervention often dangerous. From that perspective they developed a model of the new midwifery suitable for the American situation.

From 1750 to approximately 1810 American doctors conceived of the new midwifery as an enterprise to be shared between themselves and trained midwives. Since doctors during most of that period were few in number, their plan was reasonable and humanitarian and also reflected their belief that, in most cases, natural processes were adequate and

the need for skilled intervention limited, though important. Doctors therefore envisaged an arrangement whereby trained midwives would attend normal deliveries and doctors would be called to difficult ones. To implement this plan, Dr. Valentine Seaman established a short course for midwives in the New York (City) Almshouse in 1799, and Dr. William Shippen began a course on anatomy and midwifery, including clinical observation of birth, in Philadelphia. Few women came as students, however, but men did, so the doctors trained the men to be man-midwives, perhaps believing, as Smellie had contended, that the sex of the practitioner was less important than the command of new knowledge and skill.[1]

As late as 1817, Dr. Thomas Ewell of Washington, D.C., a regular physician, proposed to establish a school for midwives, connected with a hospital,

Notes on the Decline of Midwives and the Rise of Medical Obstetricians, Richard W. Wertz and Dorothy C. Wertz in *Lying In: A History of Childbirth in America*. Copyright 1989, Yale University Press. Reprinted with permission of the publisher.

similar to the schools that had existed for centuries in the great cities of Europe. Ewell sought federal funding for his enterprise, but it was not forthcoming, and the school was never founded. Herein lay a fundamental difference between European and American development of the midwife. European governments provided financial support for medical education, including the training of midwives. The U.S. government provided no support for medical education in the nineteenth century, and not enough of the women who might have aspired to become midwives could afford the fees to support a school. Those who founded schools turned instead to the potentially lucrative business of training the many men who sought to become doctors.[2]

Doctors also sought to increase the supply of doctors educated in America in the new midwifery and thus saw to it that from the outset of American medical schools midwifery became a specialty field, one all doctors could practice.

The plans of doctors for a shared enterprise with women never developed in America. Doctors were unable to attract women for training, perhaps because women were uninterested in studying what they thought they already knew and, moreover, studying it under the tutelage of men. The restraints of traditional modesty and the tradition of female sufficiency for the management of birth were apparently stronger than the appeal of a rationalized system for a more scientific and, presumably, safer midwifery system.

Not only could doctors not attract women for training in the new science and arts, but they could not even organize midwives already in practice. These women had never been organized among themselves. They thought of themselves as being loyal not primarily to an abstract medical science but to local groups of women and their needs. They reflected the tradition of local self-held empiricism that continued to be very strong in America. Americans had never had a medical profession or medical institutions, so they must have found it hard to understand why the European-trained doctors wished to organize a shared, though hierarchical, midwifery enterprise. How hard it was would be shown later, when doctors sought to organize

themselves around the new science of midwifery, in which they had some institutional training. Their practice of midwifery would be governed less by science and professional behavior than by empirical practice and economic opportunity.

In the years after 1810, in fact, the practice of midwifery in American towns took on the same unregulated, open-market character it had in England. Both men and women of various degrees of experience and training competed to attend births. Some trained midwives from England immigrated to America, where they advertised their ability in local newspapers.[3] But these women confronted doctors trained abroad or in the new American medical schools. They also confronted medical empirics who presented themselves as "intrepid" man-midwives after having imbibed the instrumental philosophy from Smellie's books. American women therefore confronted a wide array of talents and skills for aiding their deliveries.

Childbirth in America would not have any neat logic during the nineteenth century, but one feature that distinguished it from childbirth abroad was the gradual disappearance of women from the practice of midwifery. There were many reasons for that unusual development. Most obvious was the severe competition that the new educated doctors and empirics brought to the event of birth, an event that often served as entrance for the medical person to a sustained practice. In addition, doctors lost their allegiance to a conservative view of the science and arts of midwifery under the exigencies of practice; they came to adopt a view endorsing more extensive interventions in birth and less reliance upon the adequacy of nature. This view led to the conviction that a certain mastery was needed, which women were assumed to be unable to achieve.

Women ceased to be midwives also because of a change in the cultural attitudes about the proper place and activity for women in society. It came to be regarded as unthinkable to confront women with the facts of medicine or to mix men and women in training, even for such an event as birth. As a still largely unscientific enterprise, medicine took on the cultural attributes necessary for it to survive, and the Victorian culture found certain roles unsuitable for women. Midwives also disappeared because they had not been organized and had never developed any leadership. Medicine in America may have had minimal scientific authority, but it was beginning to develop social and professional organization and leadership; unorganized midwives were an easy competitive target for medicine. Finally, midwives lost out to doctors and empirics because of the changing tastes among middle- and upper-class women; for these women, the new midwifery came to have the promise of more safety and even more respectability.[4]

Midwives therefore largely ceased to attend the middle classes in America during the nineteenth century. Except among ethnic immigrants, among poor, isolated whites, and among blacks, there is little significant evidence of midwifery. This is not to say that there were no such women or that in instances on the frontier or even in cities when doctors were unavailable women did not undertake to attend other women. But educated doctors and empirics penetrated American settlements quickly and extensively, eager to gain patients and always ready to attend birth. The very dynamics of American mobility contributed to the break-up of those communities that had sustained the midwives' practices.

Because of continued ethnic immigration, however, by 1900 in many urban areas half of the women were still being delivered by immigrant midwives. The fact that ethnic groups existed largely outside the development of American medicine during the nineteenth century would pose a serious problem in the twentieth century.

Native-born educated women sought to become doctors, not midwives, during the nineteenth century. They did not want to play a role in birth that was regarded as inferior and largely nonmedical— the midwife's role—but wished to assume the same medical role allowed to men.

It is important to emphasize, however, that the disappearance of midwives at middle- and upper-class births was not the result of a conspiracy between male doctors and husbands. The choice of medical attendants was the responsibility of women, upon whom devolved the care of their

families' health. Women were free to choose whom they wished. A few did seek out unorthodox practitioners, although most did not. But as the number of midwives diminished, women of course found fewer respectable, trained women of their own class whom they might choose to help in their deliveries.

In order to understand the new midwifery [i.e. medical obstetrics], it is necessary to consider who doctors were and how they entered the medical profession. The doctors who assumed control over middle-class births in America were very differently educated and organized from their counterparts in France or England. The fact that their profession remained loosely organized and ill-defined throughout most of the nineteenth century helps to explain their desire to exclude women from midwifery, for often women were the only category of people that they could effectively exclude. Doctors with some formal education had always faced competition from the medical empirics—men, women, and even freed slaves—who declared themselves able to treat all manner of illnesses and often publicly advertised their successes. These empirics, called quacks by the orthodox educated doctors, offered herbal remedies or psychological comfort to patients. Orthodox physicians objected that the empirics prescribed on an individual, trial-and-error basis without reference to any academic theories about the origins and treatment of disease. Usually the educated physician also treated his patients empirically, for medical theory had little to offer that was practically superior to empiricism until the development of bacteriology in the 1870s. Before then there was no convincing, authoritative, scientific nucleus for medicine, and doctors often had difficulty translating what knowledge they did have into practical treatment. The fundamental objection of regular doctors was to competition from uneducated practitioners. Most regular doctors also practiced largely ineffective therapies, but they were convinced that their therapies were better than those of the empirics because they were educated men. The uneducated empirics enjoyed considerable popular support during the first half of the nineteenth century because their therapies were as often successful as the therapies of the regulars, and sometimes less strenuous. Like the empirics, educated doctors treated patients rather than diseases and looked for different symptoms in different social classes. Because a doctor's reputation stemmed from the social standing of his patients, there was considerable competition for the patronage of the more respectable families.

The educated, or "regular," doctors around 1800 were of the upper and middle classes, as were the state legislators. The doctors convinced the legislators that medicine, like other gentlemen's professions, should be restricted to those who held diplomas or who had apprenticed with practitioners of the appropriate social class and training. State licensure laws were passed, in response to the Federalist belief that social deference was due to professional men. The early laws were ineffectual because they did not take into account the popular tradition of self-help. People continued to patronize empirics. During the Jacksonian Era even the nonenforced licensing laws were repealed by most states as elitist; popular belief held that the practice of medicine should be "democratic" and open to all, or at least to all men.[5]

In the absence of legal control, several varieties of "doctors" practiced in the nineteenth century. In addition to the empirics and the "regular" doctors there were the sectarians, who included the Thomsonian Botanists, the Homeopaths, the Eclectics, and a number of minor sects of which the most important for obstetrics were the Hydrotherapists.

The regular doctors can be roughly divided into two groups: the elite, who had attended the better medical schools and who wrote the textbooks urging "conservative" practice in midwifery; and the great number of poorly educated men who had spent a few months at a proprietary medical school from which they were graduated with no practical or clinical knowledge. (Proprietary medical schools were profit-making schools owned by several local doctors who also taught there. Usually such schools had no equipment or resources for teaching.) In the eighteenth century the elite had had to travel to London, or more often Edinburgh, for training. In 1765, however, the Medical College of Philadelphia was founded, followed by King's College (later Columbia) Medical School in 1767 and Harvard in 1782. Obstetrics, or "midwifery," as it was then called, was

the first medical specialty in those schools, preceding even surgery, for it was assumed that midwifery was the keystone to medical practice, something that every student would do after graduation as part of his practice. Every medical school founded thereafter had a special "Professor of Midwifery." Among the first such professors were Drs. William Shippen at Philadelphia, Samuel Bard at King's College, and Walter Channing at Harvard. In the better schools early medical courses lasted two years; in the latter half of the nineteenth century some schools began to increase this to three, but many two-year medical graduates were still practicing in 1900.

A prestigious medical education did not guarantee that a new graduate was prepared to deal with patients. Dr. James Marion Sims, a famous nineteenth-century surgeon, stated that his education at Philadelphia's Jefferson Medical College, considered one of the best in the country in 1835, left him fitted for nothing and without the slightest notion of how to treat his first cases.[6] In 1850 a graduate of the University of Buffalo described his total ignorance on approaching his first obstetrical case:

> I was left alone with a poor Irish woman and one crony, to deliver her child . . . and I thought it necessary to call before me every circumstance I had learned from books—I must examine, and I did—But whether it was head or breech, hand or foot, man or monkey, that was defended from my uninstructed finger by the distended membranes, I was as uncomfortably ignorant, with all my learning, as the foetus itself that was making all this fuss.[7]

Fortunately the baby arrived naturally, the doctor was given great praise for his part in the event, and he wrote that he was glad "to have escaped the commission of murder."

If graduates of the better medical schools made such complaints, those who attended the smaller schools could only have been more ignorant. In 1818 Dr. John Stearns, President of the New York Medical Society, complained, "With a few honorable exceptions in each city, the practitioners are ignorant, degraded, and contemptible."[8] The American Medical Association later estimated that between 1765 and 1905 more than eight hundred medical schools were founded, most of them proprietary, money-making schools, and many were short-lived. In 1905 some 160 were still in operation. Neither the profession nor the states effectively regulated those schools until the appearance of the Flexner Report, a professional self-study published in 1910. The report led to tougher state laws and the setting of standards for medical education. Throughout much of the nineteenth century a doctor could obtain a diploma and begin practice with as little as four months' attendance at a school that might have no laboratories, no dissections, and no clinical training. Not only was it easy to become a doctor, but the profession, with the exception of the elite who attended elite patients, had low standing in the eyes of most people.[9] . . .

. . .Nineteenth-century women could choose among a variety of therapies and practitioners. Their choice was usually dictated by social class. An upper-class woman in an Eastern city would see either an elite regular physician or a homeopath; if she were daring, she might visit a hydropathic establishment. A poor woman in the Midwest might turn to an empiric, a poorly educated regular doctor, or a Thomsonian botanist. This variety of choice distressed regular doctors, who were fighting for professional and economic exclusivity. As long as doctors were organized only on a local basis, it was impossible to exclude irregulars from practice or even to set enforceable standards for regular practice. The American Medical Association was founded in 1848 for those purposes. Not until the end of the century, however, was organized medicine able to re-establish licensing laws. The effort succeeded only because the regulars finally accepted the homeopaths, who were of the same social class, in order to form a sufficient majority to convince state legislators that licensing was desirable.

Having finally won control of the market, doctors were able to turn to self-regulation, an ideal adopted by the American Medical Association in 1860 but not put into effective practice until after 1900. Although there had been progress in medical science and in the education of the elite and the specialists during the nineteenth century, the average doctor was still woefully undereducated. The Flexner Report in 1910 revealed that 90 percent of doctors were then without a college education and that most had attended substandard medical schools.[10] Only after its publication did the profession impose educational requirements on the bulk of medical practitioners and take steps to accredit medical schools and close down diploma mills. Until then the average doctor had little sense of what his limits were or to whom he was responsible, for there was often no defined community of professionals and usually no community of patients.

Because of the ill-defined nature of the medical profession in the nineteenth century and the poor quality of medical education, doctors' insistence on the exclusion of women as economically dangerous competitors is quite understandable. As a group, nineteenth-century doctors were not affluent, and even their staunchest critics admitted that they could have made more money in business. Midwifery itself paid less than other types of practice, for many doctors spent long hours in attending laboring women and later had trouble collecting their fees. Yet midwifery was a guaranteed income, even if small, and it opened the way to family practice and sometimes to consultations involving many doctors and shared fees. The family and female friends who had seen a doctor "perform" successfully were likely to call him again. Doctors worried that, if midwives were allowed to deliver the upper classes, women would turn to them for treatment of other illnesses and male doctors would lose half their clientele. As a prominent Boston doctor wrote in 1820, "If female midwifery is again introduced among the rich and influential, it will become fashionable and it will be considered indelicate to employ a physician."[11] Doctors had to eliminate midwives in order to protect the gateway to their whole practice.

They had to mount an attack on midwives, because midwives had their defenders, who argued that women were safer and more modest than the new man-midwives. For example, the *Virginia Gazette* in 1772 carried a "LETTER on the present State of MIDWIFERY," emphasizing the old idea that "Labour is Nature's Work" and needs no more art than women's experience teaches, and that it was safer when women alone attended births.

> It is a notorious fact that more Children have been lost since Women were so scandalously indecent as to employ Men than for Ages before that Practice became so general. . . . [Women midwives] never dream of having recourse to Force; the barbarous, bloody Crochet, never stained their Hands with Murder. . . . A long unimpassioned Practice, early commenced, and calmly pursued is absolutely requisite to give Men by Art, what Women attain by Nature.

The writer concluded with the statement that men-midwives also took liberties with pregnant and laboring women that were "sufficient to taint the Purity, and sully the Chastity, of any Woman breathing." The final flourish, "True Modesty is incompatible with the Idea of employing a MANMIDWIFE," would echo for decades, causing great distress for female patients with male attendants. Defenders of midwives made similar statements throughout the first half of the nineteenth century. Most were sectarian doctors or laymen with an interest in women's modesty.[12] No midwives came forward to defend themselves in print.

The doctors' answer to midwives' defenders was expressed not in terms of pecuniary motives but in terms of safety and the proper place of women. After 1800 doctors' writings implied that women who presumed to supervise births had overreached their proper position in life. One of the earliest American birth manuals, the *Married Lady's Companion and Poor Man's Friend* (1808), denounced the ignorance of midwives and urged them to "submit to their station."[13]

Two new convictions about women were at the heart of the doctors' opposition to midwives: that women were unsafe to attend deliveries and that no "true" woman would want to gain the knowledge and skills necessary to do so. An anonymous pamphlet, published in 1820 in Boston, set forth these convictions along with other reasons for excluding midwives from practice. The author, thought to have been either Dr. Walter Channing or Dr. Henry Ware, another leading obstetrician, granted that women had more "passive fortitude" than men in enduring and witnessing suffering but asserted that women lacked the power to act that was essential to being a birth attendant:

> They have not that power of action, or that active power of mind, which is essential to the practice of a surgeon. They have less power of restraining and governing the natural tendencies to sympathy and are more disposed to yield to the expressions of acute sensibility . . . where they become the principal agents, the feelings of sympathy are too powerful for the cool exercise of judgment.[14]

The author believed only men capable of the attitude of detached concern needed to concentrate on the techniques required in birth. It is not surprising to find the author stressing the importance of interventions, but his undervaluing of sympathy, which in most normal deliveries was the only symptomatic treatment necessary, is rather startling. Clearly, he hoped to exaggerate the need for coolness in order to discountenance the belief of many women and doctors that midwives could safely attend normal deliveries.

The author possibly had something more delicate in mind that he found hard to express. He perhaps meant to imply that women were unsuited because there were certain times when they were "disposed to yield to the expressions of acute sensibility." Doctors quite commonly believed that during menstruation women's limited bodily energy was diverted from the brain, rendering them, as doctors phrased it, idiotic. In later years another Boston doctor, Horatio Storer, explained why he thought women unfit to become surgeons. He granted that exceptional women had the necessary courage, tact, ability, money, education, and patience for the career but argued that, because the "periodical infirmity of their sex . . . in every case . . . unfits them for any responsible effort of mind," he had to oppose them. During their "condition," he said, "neither life nor limb submitted to them would be as safe as at other times," for the condition was a "temporary insanity," a time when women were "more prone than men to commit any unusual or outrageous act."[15]

The author of the anonymous pamphlet declared that a female would find herself at times (i.e., during menstruation) totally unable to manage birth emergencies, such as hemorrhages, convulsions, manual extraction of the placenta, or inversion of the womb, when the newly delivered organ externally turned itself inside out and extruded from the body, sometimes hanging to the knees. In fact, an English midwife, Sarah Stone, had described in 1737 how she personally had handled each of these emergencies successfully. But the author's readers did not know that, and the author himself could have dismissed Stone's skill as fortuitous, exercised in times of mental clarity.[16]

The anonymous author was also convinced that no woman could be trained in the knowledge and skill of midwifery without losing her standing as a lady. In the dissecting room and in the hospital a woman would forfeit her "delicate feelings" and "refined sensibility"; she would see things that would taint her moral character. Such a woman would "unsex" herself, by which the doctors meant not only that she would lose her standing as a "lady" but also, literally, that she would be subject to physical exertions and nervous excitements that would damage her female organs irreparably and prevent her from fulfilling her social role as wife and mother.[17]. . .

. . . The exclusion of women from obstetrical cooperation with men had important effects upon the "new practice" that was to become the dominant tradition in American medical schools. American obstetric education differed significantly from training given in France, where the principal maternity hospitals trained doctors clinically alongside student midwives. Often the hospital's midwives, who supervised all normal births, trained the doctors in normal deliveries. French doctors never lost touch with the conservative tradition that said "Dame Nature is the best midwife." In America, where midwives were not trained at all and medical education was sexually segregated, medicine turned away

from the conservative tradition and became more interventionist.

Around 1810 the new midwifery in America appears to have entered a new phase, one that shaped its character and problems throughout the century. Doctors continued to regard birth as a fundamentally natural process, usually sufficient by itself to effect delivery without artful assistance, and understandable mechanistically. But this view conflicted with the exigencies of their medical practice, which called upon them to demonstrate skills. Gradually, more births seemed to require aid.

Young doctors rarely had any clinical training in what the theory of birth meant in practice. Many arrived at birth with only lectures and book learning to guide them. If they (and the laboring patient) were fortunate, they had an older, experienced doctor or attending woman to explain what was natural and what was not. Many young men were less lucky and were embarrassed, confused, and frightened by the appearances of labor and birth. Lacking clinical training, each had to develop his own sense of what each birth required, if anything, in the way of artful assistance; each had to learn the consequence of misdirected aids.[18]

If the doctor was in a hurry to reach another patient, he might be tempted to hasten the process along by using instruments or other expedients. If the laboring woman or her female attendants urged him to assist labor, he might feel compelled to use his tools and skills even though he knew that nature was adequate but slow. He had to use his arts because he was expected to "perform." Walter Channing, Professor of Midwifery at Harvard Medical School in the early nineteenth century, remarked about the doctor, in the context of discussing a case in which forceps were used unnecessarily, that he "must do something. He cannot remain a spectator merely, where there are too many witnesses and where interest in what is going on is too deep to allow of his inaction." Channing was saying that, even though well-educated physicians recognized that natural processes were sufficient and that instruments could be dangerous, in their practice they also had to appear to *do* something for their patient's symptoms, whether that entailed giving a drug to alleviate pain or shortening labor by using the forceps. The doctor could not appear to be indifferent or inattentive or useless. He had to establish his identity by doing something, preferably something to make the patient feel better. And if witnesses were present there was perhaps even more reason to "perform." Channing concluded: "Let him be collected and calm, and he will probably do little he will afterwards look upon and regret."[19]

If educated physicians found it difficult in practice to appeal before their patients to the reliability of nature and the dangers of instruments, one can imagine what less confident and less competent doctors did with instruments in order to appear useful. A number of horror stories from the early decades of the century have been retailed by men and women who believed that doctors used their instruments unfairly and incompetently to drive midwives from practice.[20] Whatever the truth may be about the harm done, it is easy to believe that instruments were used regularly by doctors to establish their superior status.

If doctors believed that they had to perform in order to appear useful and to win approval, it is very likely that women, on the other hand, began to expect that more might go wrong with birth processes than they had previously believed. In the context of social childbirth, which . . . meant that women friends and kin were present at delivery, the appearance of forceps in one birth established the possibility of their being used in subsequent births. In short, women may have come to anticipate difficult births whether or not doctors urged that possibility as a means of selling themselves. Having seen the "best," perhaps each woman wanted the "best" for her delivery, whether she needed it or not.

Strange as it may sound, women may in fact have been choosing male attendants because they wanted a guaranteed performance, in the sense of both guaranteed safety and guaranteed fashionableness. Choosing the best medical care is itself a kind of fashion. But in addition women may have wanted a guaranteed audience, the male attendant, for quite specific purposes; namely, they may have wanted a representative male to see their pain and suffering in order that their femininity might be established and

their pain verified before men. Women, then, could have had a range of important reasons for choosing male doctors to perform: for themselves, safety; for the company of women, fashion; for the world of men, femininity.

So a curious inconsistency arose between the principle of noninterference in nature and the exigencies of professional practice. Teachers of midwifery continued to stress the adequacy of nature and the danger of instruments. Samuel Bard, Dean of King's College Medical School, wrote a text on midwifery in 1807 in which he refused even to discuss forceps because he believed that interventions by unskilled men, usually inspired by Smellie's writings, were more dangerous than the most desperate case left to nature. Bard's successors made the same points in the 1830s and 1840s. Dr. Chandler Gilman, Professor of Obstetrics at the College of Physicians and Surgeons in New York from 1841 to 1865, taught his students that "Dame Nature is the best midwife in the world. . . . Meddlesome midwifery is fraught with evil. . . . The less done generally the better. Non-interference is the cornerstone of midwifery."[21] This instruction often went unheeded, however, because young doctors often resorted to instruments in haste or in confusion, or because they were poorly trained and unsupervised in practice, but also, as we have indicated, because physicians, whatever their state of knowledge, were expected to do something.

What they could do—the number of techniques to aid and control natural processes—gradually increased. In 1808, for example, Dr. John Stearns of upper New York State learned from an immigrant German midwife of a new means to effect the mechanics of birth. This was ergot, a powerful natural drug that stimulates uterine muscles when given orally. Ergot is a fungus that grows on rye and other stored grains. It causes powerful and unremitting contractions. Stearns stressed its value in saving the doctor's time and in relieving the distress and agony of long labor. Ergot also quickens the expulsion of the placenta and stems hemorrhage by compelling the uterus to contract. Stearns claimed that ergot had no ill effects but warned that it should be given only after the fetus was positioned for easy delivery, for it induced an incessant action that left no time to turn a child in the birth canal or uterus.

There was in fact no antidote to ergot's rapid and uncontrollable effects until anesthesia became available in later decades. So if the fetus did not move as expected, the drug could cause the uterus to mold itself around the child, rupturing the uterus and killing the child. Ergot, like most new medical arts for birth, was a mix of danger and benefit. Critics of meddlesome doctors said that they often used it simply to save time. However true that was, ergot certainly fitted the mechanistic view of birth, posed a dilemma to doctors about wise use, and enlarged the doctors' range of arts for controlling birth. Doctors eventually determined that using ergot to induce labor without an antidote was too dangerous and limited its use to expelling the placenta or stopping hemorrhage.[22]

Despite the theory of the naturalness of birth and the danger of intervention, the movement in midwifery was in the opposite direction, to less reliance on nature and more reliance on artful intervention. The shift appeared during the 1820s in discussions as to what doctors should call themselves when they practiced the new midwifery. "Male-midwife," "midman," "manmidwife," "physician man-midwife," and even "androboethogynist" were terms too clumsy, too reminiscent of the female title, or too unreflective of the new science and skill. "Accoucheur" sounded better but was French. The doctors of course ignored Elizabeth Nihell's earlier, acid suggestion that they call themselves "pudendists" after the area of the body that so interested them. Then an English doctor suggested in 1828 that "obstetrician" was as appropriate a term as any. Coming from the Latin meaning "to stand before," it had the advantage of sounding like other honorable professions, such as "electrician" or "geometrician," in which men variously understood and dominated nature.[23]

The renaming of the practice of midwifery symbolized doctors' new sense of themselves as professional actors. In fact, the movement toward greater dominance over birth's natural processes cannot be understood unless midwifery is seen in the context of general medical practice. In that

perspective, several relations between midwifery and general practice become clearly important. In the first place, midwifery continued during the first half of the nineteenth century to be one of the few areas of general practice where doctors had a scientific understanding and useful medical arts. That meant that practicing midwifery was central to doctors' attempts to build a practice, earn fees, and achieve some status, for birth was one physical condition they were confident they knew how to treat. And they were successful in the great majority of cases because birth itself was usually successful. Treating birth was without the risk of treating many other conditions, but doctors got the credit nonetheless.

In the second place, however, birth was simply one condition among many that doctors treated, and the therapeutic approach they took to other conditions tended to spill over into their treatment of birth. For most physical conditions of illness doctors did not know what processes of nature were at work. They tended therefore to treat the patient and the patient's symptoms rather than the processes of disease, which they did not see and were usually not looking for. By treating his or her symptoms the doctors did something for the patient and thereby gained approbation. The doctors' status came from pleasing the patients rather than from curing diseases. That was a risky endeavor, for sometimes patients judged the treatment offered to relieve symptoms to be worthless or even more disabling than the symptoms themselves. But patients expected doctors to do something for them, an expectation that carried into birth also. So neither doctors nor patients were inclined to allow the natural processes of birth to suffice.

There is no need to try to explain this contradiction by saying that doctors were ignorant, greedy, clumsy, hasty, or salacious in using medical arts unnecessarily (although some may have been), for the contradiction reflects primarily the kind of therapy that was dominant in prescientific medicine.

The relations between midwifery and general medical practice become clearer if one considers what doctors did when they confronted a birth that did not conform to their understanding of birth's natural processes. Their mechanistic view could not explain such symptoms as convulsions or high fevers, occasionally associated with birth. Yet doctors did not walk away from such conditions as being mysterious or untreatable, for they were committed to the mastery of birth. Rather, they treated the strange symptoms with general therapies just as they might treat regular symptoms of birth with medical arts such as forceps and ergot.

Bloodletting was a popular therapy for many symptoms, and doctors often applied it to births that seemed unusual to them. If a pregnant woman seemed to be florid or perspiring, the doctor might place her in a chair, open a vein in her arm, and allow her to bleed until she fainted. Some doctors bled women to unconsciousness to counter delivery pains. A doctor in 1851 opened the temporal arteries of a woman who was having convulsions during birth, "determined to bleed her until the convulsion ceased or as long as the blood would flow." He found it impossible to catch the blood thrown about during her convulsions, but the woman eventually completed her delivery successfully and survived. Bloodletting was also initiated when a woman developed high fever after delivery. Salmon P. Chase, Lincoln's Secretary of the Treasury and later Chief Justice, told in his diary how a group of doctors took 50 ounces of blood from his wife to relieve her fever. The doctors gave careful attention to the strength and frequency of her pulse, debating and deliberating upon the meaning of the symptom, until finally Mrs. Chase died.[24]

For localized pain, doctors applied leeches to draw out blood from the affected region. A distended abdomen after delivery might merit the application of twelve leeches; a headache, six on the temple; vaginal pain also merited several.[25]

Another popular therapy was calomel, a chloride of mercury that irritated the intestine and purged it. A woman suffering puerperal fever might be given extended doses to reduce swelling by purging her bodily contents. If the calomel acted too violently, the doctors could retard it by administering opium. Doctors often gave emetics to induce vomiting when expectant women had convulsions, for they speculated that emetics might be specifics for hysteria or other nervous diseases causing convulsions.

An expectant or laboring woman showing unusual symptoms might be subjected to a battery of such agents as doctors sought to restore her symptoms to a normal balance. In a famous case in Boston in 1833 a woman had convulsions a month before her expected delivery. The doctors bled her of 8 ounces and gave her a purgative. The next day she again had convulsions, and they took 22 ounces of blood. After 90 minutes she had a headache, and the doctors took 18 more ounces of blood, gave emetics to cause vomiting, and put ice on her head and mustard plasters on her feet. Nearly four hours later she had another convulsion, and they took 12 ounces, and soon after, 6 more. By then she had lapsed into a deep coma, so the doctors doused her with cold water but could not revive her. Soon her cervix began to dilate, so the doctors gave ergot to induce labor. Shortly before delivery she convulsed again, and they applied ice and mustard plasters again and also gave a vomiting agent and calomel to purge her bowels. In six hours she delivered a stillborn child. After two days she regained consciousness and recovered. The doctors considered this a conservative treatment, even though they had removed two-fifths of her blood in a two-day period, for they had not artificially dilated her womb or used instruments to expedite delivery.[26]

Symptomatic treatment was intended not simply to make the patient feel better—often the treatment was quite violent, or "heroic"—but to restore some balance of healthy appearances. Nor were the therapies given to ailing women more intrusive or different from therapies given to suffering men. The therapies were not, in most instances, forced upon the patients without their foreknowledge or consent. People were often eager to be made healthy and willing to endure strenuous therapies to this end. Doctors did believe, however, that some groups of people were more susceptible to illness than others and that different groups also required, or deserved, different treatments.

These views reflected in large part the doctors' awareness of cultural classifications of people; in other words, the culture's position on the relative social worth of different social classes influenced doctors' views about whose health was likely to be endangered, how their endangered health affected the whole society, and what treatments, if any, were suitable. For birth this meant, for example, that doctors believed it more important for them to attend the delivery of children by middle- and upper-class women than the delivery of children by the poor. It meant that doctors expected "fashionable" women to suffer more difficult deliveries because their tight clothing, rich diet and lack of exercise were unhealthy and because they were believed to be more susceptible to nervous strain. It also meant that doctors thought it fitting for unmarried and otherwise disreputable mothers not to receive charitable care along with other poor but respectable women.

There is abundant evidence that doctors came to believe in time that middle- and upper-class women typically had more difficult deliveries than, for example, farm women. One cannot find an objective measure of the accuracy of their perception, nor, unfortunately and more to the point, can one find whether their perception that some women were having more difficult deliveries led doctors consistently to use more intervention in attending them than in attending poorer women with normal deliveries. Doctors' perception of the relative difficulty of deliveries was part of their tendency to associate different kinds of sickness with different social classes. They expected to find the symptoms of certain illnesses in certain groups of people, and therefore looked for those particular symptoms or conditions. In the nineteenth century upper-class urban women were generally expected to be sensitive and delicate, while farm women were expected to be robust. Some doctors even believed that the evolutionary result of education was to produce smaller pelves in women and larger heads in babies, leading to more difficult births among civilized women. There is no evidence that these beliefs were medically accurate. Whether a doctor considered a patient "sick" or "healthy" depended in part upon class-related standards of health and illness rather than on objective scientific standards of sickness.

Treatment probably varied according to the doctor's perception of a woman's class and individual character. At some times and places the treatment given probably reflected the patient's class as much as

her symptoms. Thus some doctors may have withheld the use of instruments from their upper-class patients in the belief that they were too fragile to undergo instrumental delivery. The same doctors may have used instruments needlessly on poor patients, who were considered healthy enough to stand anything, in order to save the doctor's time and permit him to rush off to the bedside of a wealthier patient. On the other hand, some doctors may have used instruments on the upper-class women in order to shorten labor, believing that they could not endure prolonged pain or were too weak to bring forth children unassisted, and also in order to justify higher fees. The same doctors may have withheld forceps from poor women whom they considered healthy enough to stand several days of labor. Unfortunately, there is no way of knowing exactly how treatments differed according to class, for very few doctors kept records of their private patients. The records now extant are for the small number of people, perhaps 5 percent of the population, who were treated in hospitals in the nineteenth century. Only poor women, most unmarried, delivered in hospitals, so the records do not cover a cross-section of classes. These hospital records do indicate a large number of instrumental deliveries and sometimes give the reasons as the patient's own "laziness" or "stupidity" in being unable to finish a birth. It is likely that doctors' expectations of lower-class performance are reflected here. Hospital records also reflect the use of poor patients for training or experimentation, another reason for a high incidence of instrumental deliveries.

The fact that doctors' tendency to classify patients according to susceptibility did not lead to consistent differences in treatment is an important indication that they were not merely slavish adherents to a mechanistic view of nature or to cultural and class interests. Doctors were still treating individual women, not machines and not social types. The possibility of stereotypical classification and treatment, however, remained a lively threat to more subtle discernments of individual symptoms and to truly artful applications of treatment in birth.

At the same time, it was possible that patients would find even unbiased treatments offensively painful, ineffective, and expensive, or would doubt that the doctor had a scientific reason for giving them. Such persons could seek other treatments, often administered by laypeople or by themselves. Yet those treatments, including treatments for birth, were also directed toward symptoms. At a time when diseases were unrecognized and their causes unknown, the test of therapy was the patient's whole response, not the curing of disease. So patients who resented treatments as painful, ineffective, or officious rejected the doctor and the treatments. A woman who gave birth in Ohio in 1846 recalled that the doctor bled her and then gave her ergot even though the birth was proceeding, in her view, quite normally. She thought he was simply drunk and in a hurry and angrily judged him a "bad man."[27]

The takeover of birth by male doctors in America was an unusual phenomenon in comparison to France and England, where traditional midwifery continued as a much more significant part of birth. Practice developed differently in America because the society itself expanded more rapidly and the medical profession grew more quickly to doctor in ever new communities. American mobility left fewer stable communities than in France or England, and thus networks of women to support midwives were more often broken. The standards of the American medical profession were not so high or so strictly enforced as standards in other countries, and thus there were both more "educated" doctors and more self-proclaimed doctors in America to compete with midwives. So American midwives disappeared from view because they had less support from the stable communities of women and more competition from male doctors.

The exclusion of women from midwifery and obstetrics had profound effects upon practice. Most obviously, it gave obstetrics a sexist bias; maleness became a necessary attribute of safety, and femaleness became a condition in need of male medical control. Within this skewed view of ability and need, doctors found it nearly impossible to gain an objective view of what nature could do and what art should do, for one was identified with being a woman and the other with being a man.

The bias identified functions, attributes, and prerogatives, which unfortunately could become compulsions, so that doctors as men may have often felt that they had to impose their form upon the processes of nature in birth. Obstetrics acquired a basic distortion in its orientation toward nature, a confusion of the need to be masterful and even male with the need for intervention.

Samuel Bard, one of the few doctors to oppose the trend, remarked that the young doctor, too often lacking the ability to discriminate about natural processes, often became alarmed for his patient's safety and his own reputation, leading him to seek a speedy instrumental delivery for both. A tragedy could follow, compounded because the doctor might not even recognize that he had erred and might not, therefore, learn to correct his practice. But doctors may also have found the "indications" for intervention in their professional work—to hurry, to impress, to win approval, and to show why men rather than women should attend births.

The thrust for male control of birth probably expressed psychosexual needs of men, although there is no basis for discussing this historically. The doctor appears to history more as a ritualistic figure, a representative man, identifying and enforcing sexual roles in critical life experiences. He also provided, as a representative scientist, important rationalizations for these roles, particularly why women should be content to be wives and mothers, and, as a representative of dominant cultural morality, determined the classifications of women who deserved various kinds of treatment. Thus the doctor could bring to the event of birth many prerogatives that had little to do with aiding natural processes, but which he believed were essential to a healthy and safe birth.

Expectant and laboring women lost a great deal from the exclusion of educated female birth attendants, although, of course, they would not have chosen men if they had not believed men had more to offer, at least in the beginning decades of the century. Eventually there were only men to choose. Although no doubt doctors were often sympathetic, they could never have the same point of view as a woman who had herself borne a child and who might be more patient and discerning about birth processes. And female attendants would not, of course, have laid on the male prerogatives of physical and moral control of birth. . . .

References

1. Valentine Seaman, *The Midwives' Monitor and Mother's Mirror* (New York, 1800); Lewis Scheffey, "The Early History and the Transition Period of Obstetrics and Gynecology in Philadelphia," *Annals of Medical History*, Third Series, 2 (May, 1940), 215–224.

2. John B. Blake, "Women and Medicine in Antebellum America," *Bulletin of the History of Medicine* 34, No. 2 (March-April 1965): 108–109; see also Dr. Thomas Ewell, *Letters to Ladies* (Philadelphia, 1817) pp. 21–31.

3. Julia C. Spruill, *Women's Life and Work in the Southern Colonies* (New York: Norton, 1972), pp. 272–274; Jane Bauer Donegan, "Midwifery in America, 1760–1860: A Study in Medicine and Morality." Unpublished Ph.D. dissertation, Syracuse University, 1972, pp. 50–52.

4. Alice Morse Earle (ed.), *Diary of Anna Green Winslow, a Boston Schoolgirl of 1771* (Detroit: Singing Tree Press, 1970), p. 12 and n. 24.

5. William G. Rothstein, *American Physicians in the Nineteenth Century: From Sects to Science* (Baltimore: Johns Hopkins Press, 1970), pp. 47–49.

6. J. Marion Sims, *The Story of My Life* (New York, 1888), pp. 138–146.

7. *Buffalo Medical Journal* 6 (September, 1850): 250–251.

8. John Stearns, "Presidential Address," *Transactions of the New York State Medical Society* 1:139.

9. Sims, *Story of My Life*, pp. 115–116.

10. Abraham Flexner, *Medical Education in the United States and Canada: A Report to the Carnegie Foundation for the Advancement of Teaching* (New York, 1910).

11. Anonymous, *Remarks on the Employment of Females as Practitioners in Midwifery*, 1820, pp. 4–6. See also Samuel Gregory, *Man-Midwifery Exposed and Corrected* (Boston, 1848) pp. 13, 49; Donegan, "Midwifery in America," pp. 73–74, 240; Thomas Hersey, *The Midwife's Practical Directory; or, Woman's Confidential Friend* (Baltimore, 1836), p. 221; Charles Rosenberg, "The Practice of Medicine in New York a Century Ago," *Bulletin of the History of Medicine* 41 (1967):223–253.

12. Spruill, *Women's Life and Work*, p. 275; Gregory, *Man-Midwifery Exposed*, pp. 13, 28, 36.

13. Samuel K. Jennings, *The Married Lady's Companion and Poor Man's Friend* (New York, 1808), p. 105.

14. Anonymous, *Remarks*, p. 12.

15. Horatio Storer, M.D., *Criminal Abortion* (Boston, 1868), pp. 100–101*n*.

16. Sarah Stone, *A Complete Practice of Midwifery* (London, 1737).

17. Anonymous, *Remarks*, p. 7.

18. Harold Speert, M.D., *The Sloane Hospital Chronicle* (Philadelphia: Davis, 1963), pp. 17–19; Donegan, "Midwifery in America," p. 218.

19. Walter Channing, M.D., *A Treatise on Etherization in Childbirth, Illustrated by 581 Cases* (Boston, 1848), p. 229.

20. Gregory, *Man-Midwifery Exposed*, pp. 13, 28, 36; Hersey, *Midwife's Practical Directory*, p. 220; Wooster Beach, *An Improved System of Midwifery Adapted to the Reformed Practice of Medicine . . .* (New York, 1851), p. 115.

21. Speert, *Sloane Hospital Chronicle*, pp. 31–33, 77–78.

22. Palmer Findlay, *Priests of Lucina: The Story of Obstetrics* (Boston, 1939), pp. 220–221.

23. Elizabeth Nihell, *A Treatise on Art of Midwifery: Setting Forth Various Abuses Therein, Especially as to the Practice with Instruments* (London, 1760), p. 325; Nicholson J. Eastmen and Louis M. Hellman, *Williams Obstetrics,* 13th Ed. (New York: Appleton-Century-Crofts, 1966), p. 1.

24. Rothstein, *American Physicians,* pp. 47–49.

25. *Loc. cit.*

26. Frederick C. Irving, *Safe Deliverance* (Boston, 1942), pp. 221–225.

27. Harriet Connor Brown, *Grandmother Brown's Hundred Years, 1827–1927* (Boston, 1929), p. 93.

THE END OF THE
GOLDEN AGE OF DOCTORING

John B. McKinlay and Lisa D. Marceau

If we want things to stay as they are, things will have to change.

—Giuseppe di Lampedusa (1)

There are striking similarities between the rise and fall of religious monasticism during the Middle Ages and the rise and still continuing decline of professionalism around the turn of the 21st century. During the medieval period, groups of monks (religious orders) clustered together in functionally dependent units (monasteries), eschewed worldly interests (commerce), and professed through values, beliefs, and actions their adherence to another world. Monks considered themselves "called" to their special vocation and embarked on a period of sacrifice and training as novices, during which they learned appropriate forms of behavior and an unquestioning deference to a special body of revealed knowledge.

Secrecy, elaborate rituals, special costumes, and an exclusive brotherly devotion to others in their religious order (the brotherhood) insulated them from surrounding worldly corruption. They occupied a special position in the social order and enjoyed a protected status as moral arbiters of all that was good and evil. Civilian authorities (wealthy landowners, royalty, or local governments) generally left them to their own devices or used them to legitimate worldly activities (e.g., unfair taxation, repression, exploitation).

Viewed simplistically as a contest between two competing worldviews (monasticism versus civilian authorities) it is now clear who won. Macroeconomic

The End of the Golden Age of Doctoring, John B. McKinlay and Lisa D. Marceau in *International Journal of Health Services*, 32(2), 379–416, 2002. With permission from SAGE Publications, Inc.

forces transforming the surrounding society made monasteries increasingly untenable economic units. Increasingly considered anachronistic and out of touch, the once powerful monasteries eventually declined. While a few continued to cling to the traditional order, most were swept away with social and economic change. Rigid adherence to an idealized worldview precluded strategic economic and political alliances that might have halted or forestalled their inexorable decline. From our historical vantage point at the beginning of the 21st century, sociologists of religion can look back and examine the rise and fall of medieval monasticism: with appropriate intellectual distance, we can now understand how religious orders acquired and maintained their special position in society, the functions they performed for other established elites, and how their insulated existence eventually led to their decline.

Present-day observers are just too close to late 20th and early 21st century changes in U.S. medical care to enjoy the vantage point of, say, a contemporary historian reviewing medieval societal changes. Not enough time has elapsed for the full social consequences of the late capitalist transformation of U.S. health care to completely unfold. Still, there are remarkable parallels between the rise and fall of monasticism and the rise and continuing fall of professionalism. Inevitably, modern-day commentators are prisoners of the proximate-being so involved in the phenomenon of interest, it is difficult to assume the distance necessary to appreciate the underlying causes and likely consequences of the subject of our inquiry. To understand the consequences of the industrial revolution as it finally caught up with medicine, we can observe effects produced by its earlier impact on other industrial sectors (like farming, banking, and transportation).

Over a decade ago, the first author and a colleague (Dr. John Stoeckle) argued that the corporatization of medical care was transforming the U.S. medical workplace and profoundly altering the everyday work of the doctors (2). We questioned the adequacy of the prevailing view of professionalism (Freidson's notion of professional dominance) and proposed an alternative view more informed

by current developments in the U.S. medical care marketplace (2–4). Our work explicitly repudiated "doctor bashing," a popular sport among social scientists at the time, in favor of a theoretically grounded political-economic explanation (historic changes in the mode of medical care production) of the demise of doctoring. It produced a fierce reaction among many physicians and some medical sociologists. We probably added fuel to the flames by initially employing the Marxist notion of proletarianization—a term eventually abandoned in favor of a less threatening term like "corporatization." That much of the reaction resulted from the term "proletarianization" is evident from the fact that nothing else in the paper was changed— not one argument or datum. While strenuously rejecting the claim that doctors were being slowly "proletarianized," many agreed that doctors were indeed being "corporatized." Apparently it was the word "proletarianized" and what it implied that was objectionable, not our underlying thesis. In our view, it was important that the thesis not be dismissed because of a single word (5–7).

While some could not accept the notion of corporatization (or proletarianization) back in the 1980s, there is hardly an objection today (8). In just 25 years, U.S. health care has been historically transformed—from a predominantly fee-for-service system controlled by dominant professionals to a corporatized system dominated by increasingly concentrated and globalized financial and industrial interests (9). Dudley and Luft (10) believe U.S. health care has experienced "a sea change in the past two decades—not just in the financing of health insurance, but also in the way medicine is practiced." With the golden age of medicine now almost behind us, doctors are huddling in their monasteries (hospitals and medical centers) powerlessly awaiting the next corporate onslaught. One unanticipated consequence of the Clinton administration's failed attempt at health care reform in 1994 was to further dissipate the power of doctors and coalesce opposing economic interests (especially the private insurance, pharmaceutical, and hospital sectors) against progressive change.

Professionalism can be defined as a system of values and beliefs and behavior (concerning how things ought to be done) resulting from dedicated commitment usually following a prolonged period of training. Adherents to this system (professionals) have enjoyed a privileged position and status in society, and their activities have typically been protected or sanctioned by the state. Professional activities were often insulated from observability by secrecy, protective subordinates, and impregnable institutions (11). An ethos of professional collegiality and confidentiality (the brotherhood) was hardly conducive to public scrutiny. From such a viewpoint and for much of the 20th century, professionalism was a powerful social force—it encouraged adherents to behave "ethically" and promoted unquestioning trust among the public (*credat emptor*); it institutionalized the conflict within organizations, between bureaucratic authority (based on tenure in a position in a hierarchy) and professional authority (based on a body of knowledge and technical expertise) and worked against dialectical change; it allowed rapacious interests to disguise their activities in good intentions and a transparent beneficence.

The recent (late 20th and early 21st century) decline of the medical profession and of professionalism as a social force undoubtedly results from many different social influences—at least eight of varying importance are discussed in this article. For convenience we organize them into extrinsic factors (which appear outside the control of the profession) and intrinsic factors (which may be amenable to change by the profession itself). Major *extrinsic factors* are (*a*) the changing nature of the state and loss of its partisan support for doctoring; (*b*) the bureaucratization (corporatization) of doctoring; (*c*) the emerging competitive threat from other health care workers; (*d*) the consequences of globalization and the information revolution; (*e*) the epidemiologic transition and changes in public conceptions of the body; and (*f*) changes in the doctor-patient relationship and the erosion of patient trust. Major *intrinsic factors* are (*g*) the weakening of physicians' or market position through oversupply; and

(*h*) the fragmentation of the physicians' union (the American Medical Association, AMA).

SHIFTING ALLEGIANCE OF THE STATE

Various studies have described the important role of the state (local and national government structures) as a sponsor for professionalism generally and as a protector of doctoring in particular. The rise of the medical profession during the 20th century was powerfully reinforced by government action (9, 12–16). The state served a legitimating function for many professional activities, accorded select groups (e.g., physicians and attorneys) a monopolistic position and privileged status, and served as a guarantor of their profits (through programs like Medicare and Medicaid). Hardly neutral with respect to the medical profession, the state has through political and legal means unabashedly advanced professional interests and disposed of perceived threats to professional dominance (13, 17, 18). For its rise during the 20th century, the medical profession (among other privileged interest groups) achieved much for which the state can be thanked. Figure 19.1 depicts principal sources of support for the medical profession in the United States during much of the 20th century (with government and the AMA as mainstay institutional supports).

While there is extensive discussion in the social sciences around the changing structure, functioning, and power of the state, this has yet to feature prominently in the major theories of professionalism or in the debate on the decline of professionalism, despite the state's recognized influence on all health-related activities (the nature and financing of our health care system, the power of medical professionals, the legitimation of competing interests, and the level of support for social policies affecting doctoring). The future of the medical profession and the nature of doctoring in the 21st century will depend on, more than any other influence, the changing nature and support of the state (19, 20). We devote more emphasis to this than any other factor.

FIGURE 19.1 ■ Sources of Support for Doctoring in the Middle of the 20th Century

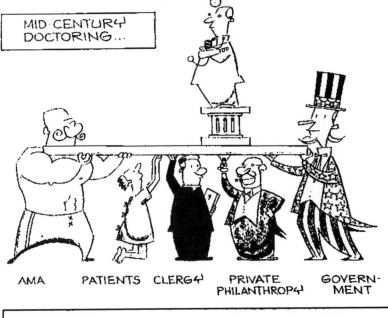

MID·CENTURY DOCTORING...

AMA   PATIENTS   CLERGY   PRIVATE PHILANTHROPY   GOVERN-MENT

HAD MANY INSTITUTIONAL SUPPORTS

The "state" can be viewed organizationally as the "apparatus of government in its broadest sense: that is, as that set of institutions that are recognizably 'public' in that they are responsible for the collective organization of social existence and are funded at the public's expense" (21, p. 84). Most observers view the state as consisting of a wide range of institutions, including the government or legislature (which passes laws), the bureaucracy or civil service (which implements government decisions), the courts and police (which are responsible for law enforcement), and the armed forces (whose job it is to protect the state from external threats). Included under this broad definition are such institutions as welfare services, the education system, and the health care establishment (22).

As far as the United States is concerned—as evidenced by the attempt at health care reform in 1994 (23), the defeat of anti-tobacco legislation (24), and the rapid evolution of managed care—the state

appears to have lost some of its ability, or willingness, to act on behalf of and protect the profession's interests. Figure 19.2 depicts the way in which, in the United States during the last decades of the 20th century, the state shifted its primary allegiance from the profession's interests to often conflicting private interests. Such a shift will shape the content and sociopolitical context of doctoring during the new millennium (25).

While there are numerous theories of the state, for the purpose of this discussion of the decline of professionalism and the medical profession, it may be useful to distinguish just three general viewpoints.

1. The *Marxist perspective,* which has never been predominant in the United States, views the state as partisan—maintaining the class system by either subordinating certain groups (e.g., racial and ethnic minorities and women) or dissipating class conflict. According to this view, the state cannot be

FIGURE 19.2 ■ Sources of Support for Doctoring in the Early 21st Century

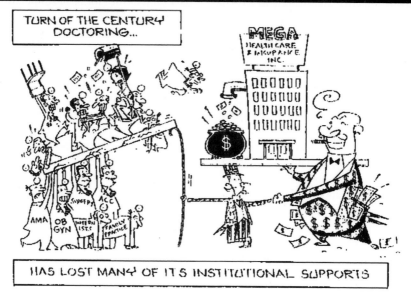

understood separately from the prevailing economic structure of society. Here we have a clear alternative to the popular pluralist view of the state and neutral arbiter or umpire of competing countervailing interests. The Marxist theory of the state has undergone considerable debate and revision, especially with contributions from Gramsci (26), Mosca (27), Miliband (28), Poulantzas (29), Mills (30), and more recently Jessop (31). Neomarxists, while attempting to remain faithful to the classical ideas of Marx, have generally abandoned the idea that the state is merely a reflection of the class system. The original two-class model is now recognized as simplistic, and Poulantzas (29) has identified significant divisions within the ruling elite (e.g., between financial and industrial (manufacturing) capital). Neomarxists have also tried to provide an alternative to the mechanistic and simplistic views of traditional Marxism (often incurring the wrath of the orthodox in the process) and to move beyond crude economic determinism. Jessop (32), for example, views the state not as an instrument wielded by a dominant group but as "the crystallization of political strategies," a dynamic entity that reflects the

balance of power within society at any given time, and thus reflects the outcome of an ongoing hegemonic struggle. Current developments with respect to globalization (the subordination of national governments to supranational organizations and agencies) appear to give the Marxist theory of the state increasing currency.

2. The *pluralist perspective,* with origins traceable to the 17th century liberalism of Thomas Hobbes and John Locke and more recently the work of John Rawls (33), views the state as a neutral body that arbitrates between competing interests in society. There is an often unacknowledged assumption of neutrality—the government sets the rules and acts as an umpire or referee in society. It is viewed as acting in the interest of *all* citizens and therefore as representing the common good or public interest. Many pluralists embrace a constant sum concept of power (there is a fixed amount of power that is widely and evenly dispersed) and view the state as having no interest of its own that is separate from society. Heywood (21) identifies two assumptions underlying the pluralist theory of the state: (*a*) the state is effectively subordinated to

government (nonelected state bodies such as the civil service are strictly impartial and subjects to the legitimate authority of their political masters); and (*b*) the democratic process is effective and meaningful (party competition and interest-group activity ensure the government remains responsive to public will). With the work of Dahl (34), Lindblom (35), Marsh (36), and Galbraith (37), among others, it is now recognized that the traditional pluralist theory of the state requires some revision, especially to take account of modernizing trends such as globalization and the emergence of postindustrial society. Neopluralists view Western democracies as "deformed polyarchies," in which major multinational corporations and globalized interests now exert disproportionate influence (21). The medical profession thrived during the latter half of the 20th century under a pluralist state (it was a dominant interest group with widespread public support). The theory of countervailing powers advanced by Mechanic (38) and Light (39) in their discussion of the medical profession appears to rest on a now outmoded pluralist view of the state. Historical developments have left these theories (and especially Freidson's notion (40) of professional dominance) with little explanatory currency. Professional powers appear, incidentally, to have countervailed little in the context of changes in the National Health Service in Britain (41).

3. The *New Right perspective* is a recent powerful reaction against the view of the state as "leviathan"—a self-serving monster intent on its own expansion and aggrandizement (21). The two perspectives discussed so far (pluralist and Marxist) have been termed "society centered"—the state and its actions are shaped by external forces in society as a whole. Pluralism views the state's actions as determined by the democratic will of the people; Marxist theory sees its actions as shaped by the interests of an increasingly concentrated cluster of powerful institutions and individuals. Clearly, society can and does influence the structure and functioning of the state, but obviously the reverse can also occur. This possibility has given rise to what are termed "state-centered" approaches to the theory of power and modern society (22). These approaches (and the New Right is but one of them) view the state as acting independently, or autonomously, to shape social

behavior. Nordlinger (42) suggests that state itself has acquired three forms of autonomy: (*a*) when the state has preferences that differ from those of major groups in society and implements its preferred policies despite pressure for it not to do so; (*b*) when the state is able to persuade opponents of its policies to change their mind and support the government; and (*c*) when the state follows policies that are supported, or at least not opposed, by the public or powerful interest groups in society (22).

The New Right perspective, which appears to be on the ascendance in the United States, is distinguished by its strong laissez-faire attitude and antipathy toward state intervention in economic and social life (even medical care). Its proponents argue that the state should retreat from responsibility for medical care (and protection of doctoring) and let market forces prevail. Rooted in a radical form of individualism and exemplified in the writings of Robert Nozick (43), the New Right considers the state a parasitic growth that threatens individual liberty and even economic development. The New Right perspective has been described as follows (21, p. 91):

> In this view, the state, instead of being as pluralists suggest, an impartial umpire or arbiter, is an overbearing "nanny," desperate to interfere or meddle in every aspect of human existence.... [The] state pursues interests that are separate from those of society (setting it apart from Marxism), and ... those interests demand an unrelenting growth in the role or responsibilities of the state itself.... [The] twentieth century tendency towards state intervention reflects not popular pressure for economic and social security, or the need to stabilize capitalism by ameliorating class tensions, but rather the internal dynamics of the state.

Figure 19.3 summarizes the three perspectives on the modern state.

To most political scientists, the three perspectives identified and discussed here will be a gross simplification of the complex debate occurring over several decades. Since each viewpoint has its own philosophical tradition, efforts to integrate

FIGURE 19.3 ■ Theories of the Modern State

Marxist	Pluralist	New Right
Beholden to and acts on behalf of **dominant economic interests** (classes) in society.	A **neutral body** balancing competing interests in service of the public to which it is responsible.	A **self-serving entity** intent on its own expansion and aggrandizement.
Medical care should help eliminate inequalities and protect the health of disadvantaged groups.	Medical care system should be balanced and protect the interests of all groups and individuals. The state as weather vane, blown in whatever direction the public dictates.	Medical care should be predominantly private and health an individual responsibility. Government should have minimal involvement.

them creatively so as to achieve some overall theoretical synthesis will remain an elusive task. The appropriateness of any theory of the state probably varies *among* countries, although with globalization this may be changing. The role of the state may also change over time *within* a particular country: *in the United States we are witnessing a move from a pluralist to a New Right state.* New society programs (e.g., Medicare and Medicaid) were formulated and implemented during a more liberal pluralist era—the nature of the state then made them possible. Efforts at health care reform in the United States failed in large part because of a well-orchestrated assault on the leviathan state (as Big Government, increased taxation, public dependency, and curtailed freedoms) (23). Likewise, the ability of the New Right (in combination with the business community) to portray physicians as greedy and willing participants in fraud (overbilling for services) has implications for regulation and public trust. The encroachment of the state even on the once-sacred physician-patient relationship (through "gag rules" and court opinions) is discussed later.

The medical profession thrived during the era of the pluralist state: as a major public interest group with considerable public support, the umpire invariably ruled in its favor. Writing in the context of Britain, but with application to the U.S. scene, Klein (44) describes "the politics of the double bed," referring to the way doctors in the United Kingdom were directly involved in policy decisions affecting their activities. While the state (government) is often

viewed as an unchanging entity, it is now clear that a subtle change occurred during the last decades of the 20th century: the state is transitioning from a pluralist to an antileviathan New Right viewpoint. Commentators have discussed the transition from a Fordist to a post-Fordist state and what this portends for the medical profession (45–48). Farrell's recent biography (49) of U.S. House Speaker Tip O'Neill describes the nature and focus of government during the late 20th century, ending with a presidential declaration during a State of the Union address that "the era of big government is over." This now dominant New Right perspective has resulted in an important shift in the primary allegiance of the state—from protecting the interests of the medical profession to advancing the interests of the financial and industrial owners of an ever more corporatized U.S. health care system. Figure 19.2 depicts the changes in institutional support for doctoring, with the state shifting its principal allegiance to other interests.

A recent discussion of the implications of the 2000 election for health care in the United States concludes that (50):

> the election of Bush as president has brought a different focus and tone to health policy. . . . Clinton advocated a larger federal role. . . . President Bush has a very different view of the government's role in health care. He emphasizes individual responsibility in making decisions about health care and paying for it, as well as the positive role of the private

market place. Bush also believes that local charities should be encouraged to provide needed health care services, that state governments should assume the primary role in many areas of health care policy, and that the federal role should be smaller.

Partisan protection of professional prerogatives now appears secondary to the advancement of global corporate interests. Whereas previously, the state enacted legislation designed to protect physicians, nowadays the New Right state's protective cloak is first used to cover the corporate interests that now determine the structure and content of U.S. health care. Rather than setting the rules and acting as a neutral umpire as Light (51) envisages it, the emerging New Right state is now on the side of and in the service of multinational financial and industrial interests. The gradual shift in the state's principal allegiance (from the medical profession to the corporation and especially its owners) has fostered the erosion of professionalism, leaving the medical profession with little more than ostensible support (see Figure 19.3). Just as the state was important in the earlier rise of the medical profession, so too has its recent protection of corporate interests left the medical profession without a significant source of support, thereby threatening the profession's special position and status. Zola (52) traced the origins of the earlier, special position of physicians as agents of social control to the sponsorship they derived from the state (see also 14). Much of this is now eroding as the state comes increasingly under the control of new global masters. While the decline of the medical profession appears to be a global phenomenon, there is presently no universal explanation for this, but many complex reasons that differ from country to country (53).

BUREAUCRATIZATION (CORPORATIZATION) OF DOCTORING

Using data from the AMA's Socioeconomic Monitoring System (a series of periodic nationally representative samples of the entire U.S. physician

population), Kletke and his colleagues (54, 55) report dramatic changes in the nature of physician employment (type of work arrangement) from 1983 to 1997. Between these years, the proportion of patient-care physicians working as employees (with no ownership interest in their practice) rose from 24 to 43 percent, an increase of 19 percentage points (Figure 19.4). Also during this period, the proportion of physician's in *self-employed solo practices* (one-physician practices with an ownership interest) fell from 40 to 26 percent. The proportion of physicians in *self-employed group practices* (multiple-physician practices with an ownership interest) fell from 35 to 31 percent. Kletke and colleagues (54, 55) note that these trends are accelerating—most of them occurring during the latter part of the study period. Moreover, these trends are especially evident among younger physicians (Figure 19.5). Among newly practicing doctors (0 to 5 years in practice), the proportion who were salaried employees increased from 37 to 66 percent between 1983 and 1997. The authors conclude: "These trends are pervasive throughout the patient care physician population, occurring for both male and female physicians, for U.S. medical graduates and international medical graduates, for all specialty groups, and in most parts of the country. . . . That these changes have been especially pronounced among younger physicians suggests that their impact on the delivery of medical care will continue long into the future" (55, p. 559). Under late 20th century bureaucratized medicine, physicians are *required* (there are now few practice options) to participate in assembly-line medicine. Stoeckle (56) described "working on the factory floor with an M.D. degree." Speedup of the medical care production process (physicians are "permitted" six to eight minutes with a patient) occurs continuously under the guise of efficiency, or even clinical appropriateness. A report recently suggested that the length of the doctor-patient encounter has not shortened under managed care (57), but its methodology has limitations and its findings differ from the everyday experience of many practicing doctors on the medical care production line. While originally motivated by concern over the quality of care, clinical practice

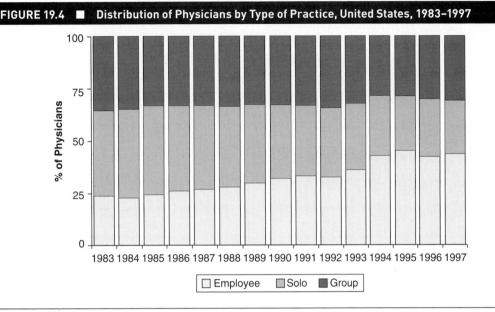

FIGURE 19.4 ■ Distribution of Physicians by Type of Practice, United States, 1983–1997

Source: Kletke et al. (54) and personal communication, 1998.

guidelines are welcomed by corporatized medicine and serve to curtail extraneous and costly procedures and to streamline the production process (58). The reward structure for physicians is increasingly tied to exemplary performance of the bureaucratic employee role (the number and types of diagnoses, referrals to other specialties, throughput of patients per practice session). Toward the end of the 20th century, Taylorism appears to have finally caught up with American medical care (59, 60).

Of special concern to some "old-time" doctors is the absence of any real professional resistance to worrisome bureaucratic encroachments. The loss of administrative and economic autonomy is understandable and even tolerable; but for many physicians, the loss of clinical autonomy is especially troubling (61, 62). Where they should actually practice (selective contracting) and how much they should be paid are now largely determined by others; but having others determine *how* they should practice (the technical content of care) is just too much (63–65). Sophisticated data-management systems can now track the minutest aspects of care; these systems appear to exist as much to

monitor the productivity and costs incurred by providers as to monitor any beneficial clinical outcomes (66). Increasingly, the treatment regimen is formulated before a live case actually presents for medical care. Prior approval is often required from a non–medically qualified reviewer at some geographically distant corporate headquarters before a final decision can be made. The choice of treatment (e.g., which medication can be prescribed) is often determined by what is allowed by a patient's health insurance or by the physician's employer. All clinical actions are scrutinized on a regular basis, and deviant practice behavior is highlighted and corrective steps taken to ensure future conformity with overall practice norms. Older recalcitrant or unproductive practitioners can easily be replaced with younger physicians (oversupply is discussed later) or replaced by less expensive nonphysician clinicians (also described later). As one chief of medicine recently remarked to us, "I listen to all these complaints from the doctors and ask myself, 'But where are they going to go?'" In order to get along under corporatized medicine, it appears that most physicians, for understandable reasons, must be willing to go along.

FIGURE 19.5 ■ **Distribution of Young Physicians (Five or Fewer Years of Practice) by Type of Practice, United States, 1983–1997**

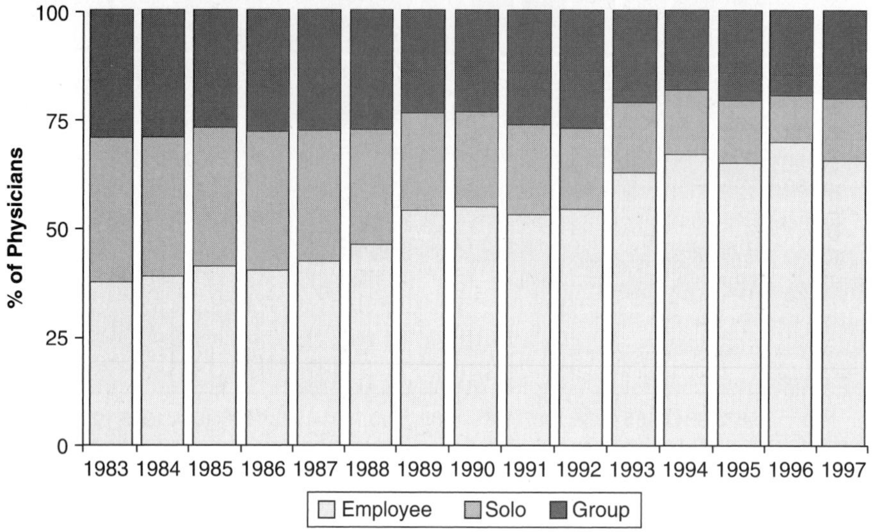

Source: Kletke et al. (54).

AN INCREASINGLY CROWDED PLAYING FIELD

During much of the 20th century, physicians gained a privileged position as the principal providers of medical services in the U.S.: the term "monopoly" has been used to characterize their unique situation and behavior (13). Of the many factors that contributed to the emergence of "the golden age" of doctoring, clearly the most influential was the highly supportive action taken by a generally partisan pluralist state described earlier (9, 12–14, 40). First, early in the century the legitimacy of the medical profession was established through *state licensing and regulations*—no other group of health care providers could legitimately perform certain tasks. If there were exceptions for particular groups, they had to work under the direct supervision of physicians. Second, during the middle of the 20th century, *third-party reimbursement* enhanced the economic position of the medical profession—they could bill for almost anything and solely determined what was appropriate

treatment. Through programs like Medicaid and Medicare (which reimbursed a physician's full costs), the state acted as both an underwriter and a guarantor of professional profits. Third, with considerable support for medical education from government, the medical profession strengthened its position by *training new physicians* in numbers that eclipsed other medically related discipline.

Physicians had the medical playing field to themselves for most of the 20th century, but the last several decades witnessed the arrival of a group of ever more powerful and legitimate new players who are threatening the physician's traditional game. Nonphysician clinicians (NPCs) are responsible for increasing amounts of the medical care that was previously provided almost exclusively by physicians (9, 67–73). With increasing numbers and improvement of their position, NPCs appear to be using the same political game plan that physicians used to secure this special status so successfully in earlier times (70, 74–77).

Cooper and his colleagues (72, 74) have projected the future likely workforce of NPCs and what their rapid increase portends for physicians. Most NPCs are within ten different medical and surgical specialties, which can be classified into three broad groups: (*a*) *the traditional disciplines*—nurse practitioners (NPs), certified nurse-midwives (CNMs), and physician assistants (PAs); (*b*) *the alternative or complementary providers*—chiropractors, naturopaths, acupuncturists, and practitioners of herbal medicine; and (*c*) *specialty disciplines*—optometrists, podiatrists, certified registered nurse anesthetists (CRNAs), and clinical nurse specialists (CNSs).

Through statutes and regulations, states have granted extensive practice prerogatives to *all* the NPCs listed previously. The most important of these prerogatives is licensure, which has established the right of these disciplines to practice (although it does not yet assure their autonomy as providers). There are marked differences in the practice prerogatives that states grant to NPCs in the various disciplines. For most disciplines, the magnitude of the prerogative correlates with the number of NPCs in each state. In some states, "practice prerogatives [have] authorized a high degree of autonomy and a broad range of authority to provide discrete levels of uncomplicated primary and specialty care" (72, p. 795).

Late 20th century changes in the organization and financing of health care (especially the emergence of profit-driven corporatized care) enhanced the labor market position of NPCs. For a profit-driven organization, the growth of NPCs offers an opportunity to hire appropriate replacements for a physician. Studies comparing the performance of NPCs and physicians show that there are few differences in any clinical outcome, but NPCs are considerably less expensive and patients often prefer the quality of care they offer. Lower costs and customer satisfaction are imperatives in the new medical marketplace.

With respect to the likely magnitude of the threat to physicians posed by NPCs, the aggregate number of NPCs graduating annually in the ten disciplines listed earlier doubled between 1992 and 1997, and a further increment of 20 percent is projected for 2001 (72). The supply of NPCs is expected to grow from 228,000 in 1995 to 384,000 in 2005, and is

likely to continue to expand at a similar rate thereafter. Figures 19.6, 19.7, and 19.8 depict the projected increase in the three broad groups of competing medical care providers.

Competition on the medical playing field is likely to become increasingly intense, especially given the existing oversupply of physicians combined with the national desire to contain health care costs. The size of the overall pie is unlikely to increase, and larger numbers of ever more powerful disciplines are competing for a piece of it. Grumbach and Coffman consider the emerging situation as subject to "Evans Law of Economic Identity" (78), which they describe as follows (79, pp. 825–826):

> . . . total expenditures on professional health care services are by definition equal to the total number of services provided multiplied by the price of each service, which are in turn equal to the total number of persons

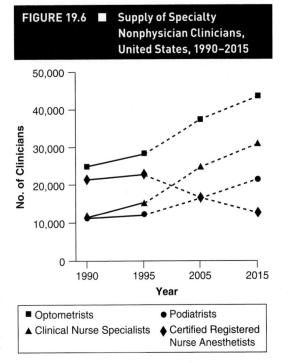

FIGURE 19.6 ■ Supply of Specialty Nonphysician Clinicians, United States, 1990–2015

■ Optometrists   ● Podiatrists
▲ Clinical Nurse Specialists   ◆ Certified Registered Nurse Anesthetists

Source: Cooper et al. (72).

earning incomes in health care multiplied by the income of each person. If the supply of health care workers increases and income per worker remains constant, then health expenditures also will increase. To increase the supply of workers without increasing overall costs, either incomes per worker must diminish or new workers must displace other workers. . . . [This] implies either a substantial growth in expenditures for payment of these practitioners or rivalry among physicians and NPCs to protect incomes and jobs in a financially constrained system.

Commenting on the growth of NPCs in relation to the likely supply of physicians over the next decade, Cooper observes (69, p. 1542):

When assessed in terms of physician equivalent effort, the number of NPCs will increase from 51 per 100,000 in 1994, a level equal to 25 percent of patient care physicians, to 84 per 100,000 in 2010, which is equal to 34 percent of the physician workforce in 2010. The incremental increase of NPCs between 1994 and 2010, expressed as physician equivalents, is 33 percent, which is identical to the increment of physician supply that is projected during the same period. . . . [The] the order of magnitude of the projected growth in their numbers is large in proportion to any estimate of physician surpluses. Moreover, there does not appear to be the capacity to absorb both the increased numbers of physicians that have been projected and a parallel workforce of NPCs of this magnitude.

The recent rapid increase in the number of physicians and other health workers is already creating intradisciplinary (between physicians) and interdisciplinary (between physician and nonphysician clinicians) rivalries. Several observers have noted a decline of intradisciplinary courtesy and reciprocity. Some doctors are barely hanging on, while others are reported to be abandoning a sinking ship (Figure 19.9). All of this is to emphasize that much of the debate over medical workforce trends

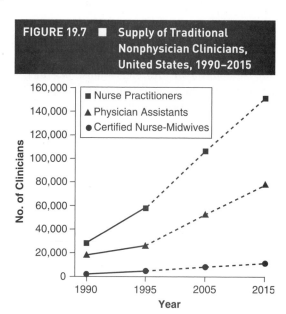

FIGURE 19.7 ■ Supply of Traditional Nonphysician Clinicians, United States, 1990–2015

Source: Cooper et al. (72).

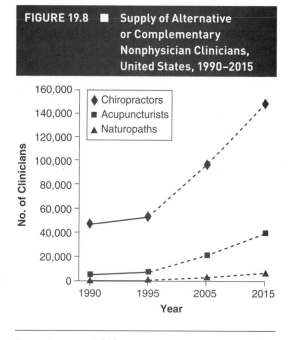

FIGURE 19.8 ■ Supply of Alternative or Complementary Nonphysician Clinicians, United States, 1990–2015

Source: Cooper et al. (72).

(oversupply versus undersupply) and their likely consequences appears to be without (political or economic) context or background (80). Discussion of

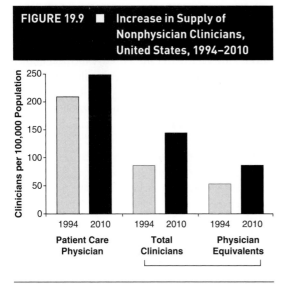

FIGURE 19.9 ■ Increase in Supply of Nonphysician Clinicians, United States, 1994–2010

Note: The actual the supply of physicians in 2010, 224 per 100,000, and the actual number of nurse practitioners in 2010, 140,000, were slightly lower than predicted while the actual number of physician assistants was slightly higher than predicted (83,600 versus 78,000). The number of specialty non-physician clinicians was lower than predicted (about 10,000 lower for optometrists and 7,000 lower for podiatrists). The biggest discrepancy was for the supply of chiropractors: about 150,000 were projected but there were just 52,600 in 2010 (www.bls.gov/ooh/Healthcare).

the intrinsic threat to doctoring resulting from statistical oversupply appears myopic and overlooks the even more significant extrinsic threats presented by macroeconomic changes in the surrounding society (e.g., corporatization and the trend to employee status, the changing nature and shifting allegiance of the state, and the erosion of patients' trust). Beneath the threat to doctoring that accompanies statistical oversupply and competition lie even more significant social trends that are undermining the position of physicians in the division of medical labor and the status of doctoring in the surrounding society.

GLOBALIZATION AND THE INFORMATION REVOLUTION

Globalization and the information revolution are also phenomena with potential to alter the social position of doctors worldwide. While globalization

may appear only to concern abstract phenomena at the level of nation states and macroeconomics that have little bearing on behavior at the local level (e.g., currency and market fluctuations in one geographic region can force governments in far-off regions to dramatically change local economic policy), nothing could be further from the truth: "it is the very dynamic of globalization that its dimensions operate *both* at the global and local level *at the same time*" (81, p. 55). Giddens observes: "It is wrong to think of globalization as just concerning the big system, like the world financial order. Globalization isn't only about what is 'out there,' remote and far away from the individual. It is an 'in here' phenomena too, influencing intimate and personal aspects of our lives" (82, p. 30). The implications of globalization and the information revolution at the local level for the organization and delivery of health care, for the social position of doctors, and for the content of medical work (doctoring) have received little attention and remain poorly understood.

The term "globalization" refers to the emerging consciousness of the world as a single place and the accompanying process whereby geographically disparate social systems are becoming linked so as to assume a worldwide scale. Modern electronic communications (especially the Internet) provide the lifeblood for emerging global bodies. Globalization is being institutionalized through the activities of transnational corporations and the formation of supranational agencies like the World Bank, the World Trade Organization, and the World Health Organization. Regional affiliations between countries (e.g., the North American Free Trade Agreement and the European Union), which may be termed "intermediate globalization," may eventually result in the formation of worldwide structures. There are several ways in which their activities affect the social position of doctors and the everyday value of doctoring.

Much of the power and position of the medical profession has been traced to the protective activities of professional associations (the doctors' union), often manifest through locally powerful medical societies. As described elsewhere, professional associations like the AMA in the United States and the British Medical Association in Great Britain have exerted considerable influence on the state, shaping legislation affecting their prerogatives. Policies promulgated by supranational organizations and agreements between governments are marginalizing once powerful national and local professional associations, limiting their ability to control licensure and training and shape legislation so as to benefit their constituency. NAFTA is a reciprocal agreement between the United States of America, Mexico, and Canada that provides for the free-trade movement of physicians and other professionals between these three countries. It is expected that other countries will be added to NAFTA in the near future. Similarly, the interests of professional associations in the member countries of the European Union are now subordinated to legislation emanating from Brussels. Despite the local training and licensing requirement of local medical interests, employment mobility of physicians between countries linked through global structures is increasingly common. Illustrative are perhaps the recent reports of South African doctors being lured to work in Canada. South Africa's foreign minister and its ambassador to Canada have said it is unethical for the West to lure doctors from the developing world, which already has too few doctors and struggles to provide medical care for millions of impoverished people and to cope with epidemics such as AIDS and tuberculosis. According to some estimates, 1,500 South African doctors are now working in Canada. Apparently, the president of the Saskatchewan Medical Association (a South African) was able to stand before a group at the association's annual golf tournament last year and tell a joke in Afrikaans (83).

Increasingly widespread use of the Internet, while empowering patients by providing valuable health information, also may have the unanticipated consequence of undermining key aspects of physician authority. For much of the 20th century, the medical profession seemed to exemplify the adage "knowledge is power." Possession of a body of purportedly scientific knowledge about the human body and various methods to possibly prolong life, avoid death, and alleviate suffering contributed to the privileged position of doctors in the social order (described later). Acquisition of technical expertise

through prolonged training (professional socialization) was considered a defining characteristic (attribute) of any profession (84). Public access to this highly valued and authoritative medical knowledge was possible only through consultation, usually face-to-face, with a certified (licensed) physician. Any other source of health information was considered suspect and lacking in scientific legitimacy. The ready availability of sophisticated medical information to anyone with Internet access is increasing levels of public medical knowledge, interposing a lay electronic help-seeking system, and changing the structure and content of the doctor-patient relationship.

In contrast with earlier times, newly empowered patients now enter the doctor-patient encounter with (a) considerable *up-to-date information* concerning a medical condition and possible types of diagnoses and (b) industry-generated *requests* for specific tests or treatments ("ask your doctor about . . .") and expectations concerning what ought to occur during the encounter. And (c), subsequent to the encounter, patients now use the Internet to *informally evaluate* the appropriateness of particular treatments and procedures received. The timing of a Web search appears to depend on the person for whom health information is being sought: if for someone else, it usually occurs after a doctor's visit; if for oneself, it tends to occur before a doctor's visit, presumably to see what the diagnosis might be (85).

Physician behavior around the mid-20th century was described as "insulated from observability" (11). Doctors tended to act as independent agents, free from administrative oversight with little formal accountability. As professionals, and again with the acquiescence of the state, doctors acquired a legally sanctioned privilege accorded few occupations—self-regulation. Probably because doctors could "bury their mistakes," professional misconduct appeared to be a rare event, and whenever oversight or investigation was required, it was conducted in closed-door sessions involving only selected members of the profession. With the changes in physician employment described in this article (corporatization), the computerization of medical records, and the online availability of data on the comparative performance of medical facilities and particular practitioners, the everyday work situation of doctors is changing dramatically.

Computerized information systems can now capture minute aspects of the clinical encounter (e.g., length of visit, tests ordered, referrals made, prescriptions written, clinical outcomes, patient satisfaction, and costs incurred). Particular providers are now easily compared with each other in terms of patient throughput, productivity, and patient satisfaction, and their performance assessed against officially agreed upon standards of care (practice guidelines). Legal actions against providers for alleged malpractice were once largely based on the testimony (memory) of the parties involved, or required plaintiffs to find a doctor willing to testify against one of their own. Nowadays, the computerized medical record provides an independent contemporaneous record of everything that is done (or not done) during a doctor-patient encounter, and it constitutes evidence thought to be superior to the memory of self-interested parties. Anyone can now go online to acquire previously private information on particular providers: their age, educational background, employment history, and the frequency and success of any legal actions. Through the use of the Web, patients today can enter the doctor-patient relationship with up-to-date information on any medical condition, informed expectations about what constitutes appropriate practice, and considerable information on the personal biography of their provider.

Globalization is also having more subtle effects on the position of doctors and the work of doctoring around the world. During the 18th and 19th centuries, British imperialism involved more than only the export of industrial production and products through colonization. Anglo-Saxon culture was also exported. So, too, globalization involves more than just the production, distribution, and exchange of tangible commodities on a worldwide scale. It also involves the development of a worldwide common culture of values, images, and assumptions as to what is modern, stylish, right or wrong, and ideal. For example, a multibillion-dollar diet industry in the United States produces and distributes both pills and diet supplements *and* a demand-producing image of the ideal body (the so-called "tyranny of thinness"). New electronic forms of communication (especially films, television, and the Internet) are greatly facilitating this process.

Transnational corporations involved in the globalization of medicine (pharmaceuticals, services, medical insurance, and biotechnology) generate local demand for services, which indigenous systems are simply unable or unprepared to meet, often widening existing health disparities. In most countries it is usually those who can afford to pay, those who have access to private health care facilities, who receive the benefits of globalized medicine. For the medical profession, being "up to date" or "cutting edge" is highly valued around the world. This usually entails using the latest Western approaches and equipment. In developing countries, scarce resources are often consumed by the latest high-tech equipment and specialties, diverting resources from equipment that is culturally more appropriate, disfiguring indigenous health systems, and disrupting local patterns of medical care. The field of international health is replete with examples of the often unanticipated disfiguring consequences for indigenous systems of globalized health care.

The globalization of medical culture also fosters division within local health care systems. Patients may prefer providers who appear more cosmopolitan, who have "been abroad" and studied at prestigious Western (usually U.S.) medical institutions. Many academic centers now offer distance learning courses for providers in the developing world. The work and status of traditional and indigenous providers, whose orientation is more toward local culture and medical needs, is therefore devalued. Social status within the profession often derives from how Westernized a provider is (educational background, linkage to overseas institutions, regular participation in international symposia), not from the esteem that derives from effectively managing local medical problems. Local medical care systems and the social position of doctors around the world are being insidiously eroded as much by the globalization of Western medical culture as by the globalization of medical care production (manufactured goods and services).

THE EPIDEMIOLOGIC TRANSITION AND CHANGING CONCEPTS OF THE BODY

Sociologists have been engaged for decades in a lively debate on the conceptualization and measurement of occupational status or prestige, and much appears to depend upon the theoretical framework employed (this determines which criteria are given priority) and the purpose for which an occupational classification is developed (the interests of academic researchers and government officials are sometimes at odds). A large body of sociological work on the profession can be reduced to two main schools of thought (although most purists would reject any such simplification): one view (advanced by functionalists) emphasizes the value of "the" professions to society; the other view (advanced by critical theorists and social constructionists) emphasizes the power and self-interest of the professions and the value of their activities to the advancement of their own social position. Both viewpoints may contribute to understanding the changing social position of any occupation. The prestige of any occupation depends to some extent on its contribution to what is valued in any society (e.g., health, the prolongation of life, and the reduction of suffering). There have been changes over time in both the nature of disease and the ability of medical care providers to beneficially alter the natural course of illnesses. Little attention has been devoted to how such epidemiologic changes relate to the changing social position of doctors.

Patterns of mortality, morbidity, and disability obviously change over time: just as each historical epoch has its own predominant form of production (agricultural, industrial, informational), so too does it have its own predominant form of illness (86). Omran (87) suggested that changes in patterns of disease and death can be characterized as moving through three distinct phases. The *age of pestilence and famine* characterizes premodern and preindustrial societies. It was characterized by high mortality

associated with environmental exposure and accidents and conflict. Total life expectancy was only 20 to 40 years. During the *age of receding pandemics,* improvements in housing, sanitation, and nutrition and public health activities resulted in a decline in deaths from infectious and parasitic diseases. Specific medical measures contributed little to the decline in the diseases (88–91). People began to survive into older age, when they were more likely to die from chronic degenerative diseases. Life expectancy increased to about 50 years. Equilibrium in mortality characterizes the *age of degenerative and human-made diseases.* Overall mortality rates continued to drop and life expectancy increased to about 70 years. A small number of chronic conditions (heart disease, cancer, and stroke) were major contributors to mortality, and (with the exception of cancer) these began an unexpected rapid decline beginning in the mid-1960s. It is common to attribute these improvements to secular changes in lifestyles and improvements in medical care, although the evidence for this remains somewhat inconclusive.

Olshansky and Ault (92) propose a fourth stage of epidemiologic transition, which they term the *age of delayed degenerative diseases.* During this stage the major causes of death remained unchanged, but they became more concentrated in the older age groups. There is evidence that while people may be living longer, they are experiencing increasing periods of disability (93). Palliative care has become an important component of modern medical practice. A fifth stage now appears to be emerging, which can be termed the *age of globalized health threats.* This stage is characterized by (*a*) the emergence of new infectious diseases and the reemergence of old (but newly resistant) foes (e.g., TB and malaria); and (*b*) the emergence of worldwide environmental threats (e.g., pollution, ozone depletion, bioterrorism) (94–96). While these threats have similarities with those of earlier stages, they differ in at least two respects: their global impact and the rapidity of their transmission. With respect to TB for example, the WHO estimates that *Mycobacterium tuberculosis* now infects some two billion people: one in every three worldwide. Approximately 10 percent of these carriers develop the disease and become infectious to an average of 10 to 15 other people. Globally, TB is now the fifth largest cause of death and the major cause of death for women. It is estimated that by 2020 there will be one billion new cases and around 70 million deaths. This new globalized threat of (often drug-resistant) TB obviously requires a globalized public health response—like the Global Alliance for TB Drug Development, involving governments, supranational agencies, transnational corporations, and major philanthropic organizations. Similarly, these emerging worldwide environmental threats will require new forms of sociopolitical intervention as part of a global public health strategy for the 21st century. It is clear that one-on-one curative interventions by health providers (e.g., physicians) will have little impact during the Age of Globalized Health Threats.

The social position of healer in society, only recently termed "the doctor," appears to have changed as the nature of the threat to health has changed over time. Although the evidence is fragmentary, it appears there was little role for a healer during the age of pestilence and famine. During and following the industrial revolution, with its air, water, food, and vector borne diseases, the afflicted either died (in accordance with the will of God) or quickly recovered (as a result of the intervention of a physician). In other words, doctors were perceived to be effective when people survived; failure was attributed to the will of God. Doctoring reached its zenith during the age of degenerative and human-made diseases, when pharmaceuticals and surgery were considered effective cures against the major conditions (heart disease, cancer, and stroke) of the modern era. Curing appears to have been supplanted by caring and palliative measures during the age of delayed degenerative diseases. Much of the focus of doctoring has now shifted to regular monitoring of presently incurable conditions (diabetes, hypertension, asthma, arthritis, cancer) and to improving the quality of life. Curing is commonly thought to be a more glamorous and valued activity than caring. Moreover, caring may be more appropriately performed by the many other providers (discussed previously) now considered to be equal

partners with physicians on the health care team. The emerging threats to health that accompany globalization will likely require entirely different types of interventions, of a more sociopolitical nature.

Several other cultural phenomena have contributed to the erosion of the doctor's social position in the United States. First, increased public access to medical knowledge has resulted in some demystification of the body. The understanding of illness and disease has moved from the metaphysically inexplicable (which once gave providers almost priestly functions) and been reduced to biophysiologic functions. Second, the body is increasingly viewed as a machine that requires regular calibration (weight and diet control) and preventive maintenance (annual physicals). Defective parts like hearts, liver, kidneys, knees, or hips that deteriorate through excessive mileage (aging) are now able to be replaced. Doctoring now shares many similarities with the work of skilled car mechanics. Third, responsibility for personal health has shifted from paternalistic medical care providers: people are now viewed as personally responsible for their own health. Self-care (weight, exercise, diet, stress, self-examination) is beginning to assume the status of a moral obligation. Diagnoses of many medical conditions (diabetes, hypertension, pregnancy, some cancers) can now be made at the kitchen table. Computer-assisted diagnosis and the filling of prescriptions is now possible via the Internet, often rendering a face-to-face encounter with a doctor unnecessary. While such phenomena are increasingly marginalizing the doctor and are a source of some concern for the medical profession, they are often viewed by physician employers as welcome developments likely to reduce costs.

FROM RELATIONSHIP TO ENCOUNTER—THE EROSION OF PATIENTS' TRUST

Macrolevel changes in the content and organization of doctoring and the accompanying decline in the social position and status of doctors bring microlevel changes to the doctor-patient relationship. A measure of the change in this relationship lies in the words now used to describe it: "doctor" has become "provider," the "patient" has become a "client," and the "relationship" is now an "encounter." Recognizing that profound changes are occurring, we have suggested elsewhere the need for new, third-generation studies of the doctor-patient relationship (97). First-generation studies focused on the influence of patients' attributes (age, race, social class, gender, physical attractiveness, and so forth) on the doctor-patient relationship and clinical decision-making. Second-generation studies brought a shift in focus to the characteristics of physicians/providers (age or clinical experience, gender, race/ethnicity, medical specialty). These two types

of study tend to employ a closed-system model of the doctor-patient encounter—the exchange is viewed as occurring in a sociological vacuum (a patient interacting with a physician). Our proposed third-generation studies recognize the increasing intrusion of social, economic, and organizational influences on the structure and content of the encounter. Table 19.1 summarizes some differences in the doctor-patient relationship from the mid-20th century to the early 21st century.

During the middle years of the 20th century, physicians acquired a widely discussed position of professional dominance (12, 40), and the doctor-patient relationship was depicted as "asymmetric." While commentators questioned the role of physicians as "medical imperialists" and "agents of social

TABLE 19.1 ■ Some Differences in the Doctor-Patient Relationship From Mid to Late 20th Century		
	Mid 20th Century	**Late 20th Century**
Terminology	Doctor-patient relationship	Client-provider encounter
The state (government) and insurance companies	Recognizes sanctity of "the" relationship	Intrudes on the encounter (e.g., gag rules)
Ownership	Patient is "owned" by the doctor	Client is "owned" by provider's employer
Reference group	Independent physician works for the patient (sole practitioner)	Salaried provider works for an employer
Duration of relationship	Continuity of care (often over many years)	Discontinuity of care (changes with employer and medical staff)
Length of encounter	15–20 minutes	6–8 minutes
Power	Doctor in control (patient has few options)	Client more in control (able to "shop around")
Trust	*Credat emptor*	*Caveat emptor*
Treatment options	Physician does what the patient requests/needs	Provider does what organizational policy permits
Reimbursement	Physician rewarded for doing more (fee-for-service)	Provider rewarded for doing less (salaried employee)
Confidentiality	Held to be inviolable	Threatened by the number of parties involved and computerized medical records.

control," still doctors were generally considered to be on the patient's side. There was a coincidence of interest between physicians (who, through autonomous practice on behalf of patients, maximized their income) and patients (who cooperated with their doctor in order to get well). *Credat emptor* was considered an appropriate motto and a necessary condition for an effective encounter (98, 99).

Even the once cherished privacy of the physician-patient relationship is under attack. State encroachment on the relationship is evident in the "gag rule" prohibiting doctors in federally funded clinics from speaking about abortion with their patients. This rule, and the supporting Supreme Court opinion in *Rust* v. *Sullivan*, permitted increased governmental control over physicians' speech (100, 101). Testifying before Congress, an AMA representative considered the gag rule would "denigrate the integrity of the doctor-patient relationship and force health care professionals to violate established standards of medical care and professional ethics" (102).

With the phenomenal growth of corporatized medical care the average physician's administrative, economic, and even clinical autonomy has been challenged. Professional dominance has been supplanted by bureaucratic dominance, with the resulting appearance of a conflict of interest for physicians. Physicians now find themselves between a rock and a hard place: there is evidence that many must employ manipulative "covert advocacy" tactics so that patients can receive care that physicians perceive as essential (103). Essentially they must do the wrong thing (lie) to achieve the right outcome (their preferred medical treatment). It is not unreasonable to ask whether physicians are still able to serve the interests of their patients or are required to advance the interests of their employers (104). Physicians have even been referred to as "double agents" (105). Profound changes in the structure and content of late 20th century medical care appear to be eroding the trust that is thought to be a crucial ingredient in the doctor-patient relationship (106–110). Kao and colleagues (104) show that the method of physician payment is related to the level of patients trust.

While usually confined to other market transactions (like auto repair, insurance, and the purchase of real estate), the motto *caveat emptor* is now increasingly invoked in the context of the corporate provider-client encounter.

WEAKENING OF MARKET POSITION THROUGH OVERSUPPLY

Much of the decline of modern doctoring can be attributed to influences outside the control of the profession: such *extrinsic factors,* as discussed previously, include the bureaucratization of medical care and the decline in public trust, profit-driven corporatization, the erosion of state sponsorship, and the competition presented by other health workers. There are, however, factors *intrinsic* to the medical profession (and certainly under its control) that also are undermining its privileged social position. Of the intrinsic factors, the most important is almost certainly the weakening of physicians' own labor market position by physician oversupply and unwillingness to curtail the overproduction of new medical graduates.

For several decades numerous reports have warned of a looming physician surplus; these worrisome projections are now a reality for the medical profession (111–117). More than 20 years ago (in 1976) it was predicted that by 1990 there would be a surplus of 70,000 active physicians (a 13 percent surplus) and that by 2000 this would increase to 145,000 (22 percent surplus) (111). Weiner (77) projected a surplus of 165,000 physicians (28 percent of practicing physicians) by 2000. He subsequently revised his projected surplus to an oversupply of 270,000 physicians (39 percent of all patient-care physicians) by 2000 (118). These and numerous other projections (and the devil is in the assumptions on which they are based) are the subject of intense debate (119). Despite some disagreement over whether a *national* physician surplus exists there is little doubt that oversupply presents a serious problem in some geographic areas (112, 120–126). The Boston–Washington corridor, for example, accounts for much of the projected surplus (20 percent). One commentator thinks that a decrease of 25,000 physicians (40 percent) and 16,000 residents (40 percent) is necessary to bring this region to the national norm: "it is unlikely that in the near term this region could absorb more physicians per capita than now exist" (69, p. 1541). In the context of national oversupply, there are of course other areas of the country with alarming health inequalities that continue to be severely underdoctored. The most valuable national data on physician supply and demand and their likely consequences for modern doctoring are presented by Cooper (69), who suggests that supply may exceed demand by up to 62,000 physicians (8 percent) through 2010 (see note, p. 245). Cooper predicts that a small deficit may occur by 2020, when the growth rate of physicians is projected to be less than the growth rate of U.S. population (Figure 19.10).

The debate over likely trends will no doubt continue, with different constituencies presenting different scenarios. Practicing physicians are already feeling the squeeze and suggesting that the production of medical graduates should be carefully monitored. But the medical education establishment is required to increase the production of medical graduates to justify earlier massive investments in institutional development. No medical school is likely to close its doors in the foreseeable future (the supply of student applicants will continue to exceed the number of available places). If oversupply is a likely scenario, then the medical profession appears to be on a self-destructive course. In our view there is clearly an overproduction of physicians. But current proposals to address the problem, like encouraging specialty and geographic redistribution and some constraints on international medical graduates, appear inadequate and are unlikely to be effective (127, 128). One high-level meeting on this subject (the Trilateral Physician Workforce Conference, held in 1996) concluded that the difficulty of translating the results of workforce research into public policy is more pronounced in the United States than elsewhere (e.g., Canada and the United Kingdom) and that the situation in the United States suffers from "paralysis by analysis" (129).

Until quite recently, a medical degree guaranteed full employment immediately upon graduation from a reputable medical school. Physician unemployment is still rare, but *under* employment appears to be quite common (more than other occupations, physicians are able to supplement their income with

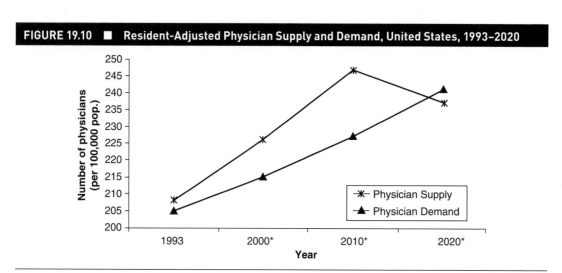

FIGURE 19.10 ■ **Resident-Adjusted Physician Supply and Demand, United States, 1993–2020**

Source: Cooper (69).

See Note at bottom of Figure 19.9 for actual supply of physicians in 2010.

non-patient-care activities). Miller and her colleagues (126) reported that one-quarter of newly trained physicians experienced difficulty finding appropriate employment; 67 percent obtained clinical practice positions in their specialties.

Through an inability to even acknowledge let alone control their own worrisome overproduction, physicians appear determined to continue along the path of their own demise—very much like lemmings inexplicably self-destructing into the Arctic Ocean. This erosion of labor market position is, of course, exacerbated by trends in the growth of other health workers as described earlier.

THE DOCTORS' UNION— DIVIDE AND CONQUER

During much of the 20th century, the special position of physicians and the state-supported prerogatives they acquired were engineered and advanced by an ever more powerful union—the American Medical Association. During mid-century, the support or opposition of the AMA determined the success or failure of major national legislation. There was no greater prize for aspiring politicians than some form of support or even endorsement from the AMA. Medical specialization, however, splintered the once unified posture of the AMA. Medical specialization, however, splintered the once unified posture of the AMA; specialty-based societies (unions) replaced the increasingly distant AMA as the primary reference group of many physicians. For example, cardiologists joined the American College of Cardiology and internists joined the Society for General Internal Medicine. These memberships were instead of rather than in addition to membership in the AMA. While the AMA was a dominant institutional force around the middle of the 20th century, probably as influential as the state itself in advancing the prerogatives of "the" profession (Figure 19.1), its influence today is shared with often rival specialist medical societies (Figure 19.2). Its power now appears no greater than that exerted by competing state or specialist societies, and a coincidence of interests cannot be assumed.

Membership in the AMA was never compulsory, but during the middle of the 20th century nearly all physicians joined and paid their dues. It is safe to assume that most physicians still belong to some professional association (or union), but nowadays membership in the AMA is deemed unnecessary by more than half of U.S. physicians. Figure 19.11 shows that at the turn of the 20th century the United States had an estimated 800,000 active physicians, but membership in the AMA had slipped to well under 300,000 (only 40 percent of the nation's doctors).

Particularly disturbing for the AMA is the tendency for younger physicians or new medical graduates not to become members. In other words, the current membership is declining and aging. Previously unheard of divisions within the AMA are now also apparent: an upstart challenge (by Raymond Scaletter) to the usually well-choreographed installation of an heir apparent (Thomas Reardon) reflected discontent within this once unified pressure group (130). A decision by the AMA in 1997 to enter into an exclusive trademark licensing agreement with Sunbeam Products, Inc., created turmoil within the organization over the relationship of business and professionalism and particularly disturbed the leadership because it became public: it caused "wrenching public adversity" and "horrendous and well publicized difficulty" (131–133).

The AMA's declining influence on national public policy was evident during the 1994 debate over health care reform—its submission at one early point was given no more time or weight than those of other labor unions and public interest groups. Through its political arm, the American Medical Political Action Committee (AMPAC), the AMA is obviously still a powerful professional interest group—it remains one of the highest-spending lobbying group in the United States (100). Its positions on major issues such as smoking, domestic violence, teen pregnancies, handguns, and the distorting influences of commercialism on medical care are consonant with a majority of public opinion. But the influence of the AMA does appear to have diminished; nowhere is this more evident than in its ability to withstand the movement toward managed care and the corrosive effect of commercialism on professional behavior.

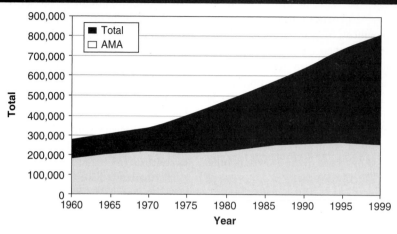

FIGURE 19.11   ■   **Physicians in the United States and Membership in the AMA, 1960–1999**

Source: AMA Physician Masterfile 2000.

Fragmentation of physicians into specialist societies and internal dissention within the AMA itself have created a divide-and-conquer opportunity for both private business interests and the state. Groups of physicians with particular specialty interests can be pitted against each other to achieve an outcome that is sometimes not in the overall or long-term interest of the profession.

CONCLUSION

We have argued in this article that late capitalist changes in the ownership and organization of U.S. health care are eroding the ethos of professionalism, reducing the social status of doctors, and transforming the nature of everyday medical work (doctoring). To underscore the historic magnitude of these changes, we draw parallels with the rise and fall of religious monasticism during the Middle Ages. In just 25 years, U.S. medical care has been transformed from a mainly fee-for-service system controlled by dominant professionals to a corporatized system dominated by increasingly concentrated and globalized financial and industrial interests. Present-day observers are, however, too close to late 20th and early 21st century

changes in U.S. medical care to enjoy the vantage point of, say, a modern-day historian studying medieval monasticism. Recognizing the increasing threat to professionalism and doctoring, some commentators have recommended what may be termed intermediate solutions (e.g., more emphasis on a new professional ethic during an already overcrowded medical school curriculum, interventions to increase patients' trust, unionization of discontented doctors, and even a patients' bill of rights). In the context of the global macroeconomic forces now transforming U.S. medical care, such proposals, while well intentioned, appear unfortunately naive.

Freidson (134) has recently made revisions to his earlier work on professional dominance. While recognizing profound changes, he continues to look *inside medicine* to understand the changing status of doctors (training, specialized knowledge, and "the soul of professionalism") rather than *outside medicine*, at more influential surrounding macroeconomic circumstances. He misinterprets and dismisses attempts to look at these latter factors as ideologically inspired attacks and simply shibboleths rather than efforts to understand the more fundamental reasons for the historical decline of doctoring.

We argue that the recent (late 20th century and early 21st century) erosion of professionalism and decline of the medical profession result from many different social influences—at least eight of varying importance are discussed in this article. For convenience we organized these into *extrinsic factors* (six of which appear to be outside the control of the profession) and *intrinsic factors* (two of which may be amenable to change by the medical profession itself). The major extrinsic factors are:

- The changing nature of the U.S. state (from pluralist to New Right) and loss of historically important institutional support for doctoring.

- The bureaucratization (corporation) of doctoring and consequent loss of professional autonomy.

- The emerging competitive threat from other health care workers who provide an opportunity for profit-driven owners to replace doctors with appropriately trained workers at cheaper labor rates.

- Globalization and the information revolution, which are subordinating national and local medical societies, stripping doctors of their monopoly on medical knowledge, and permitting the monitoring of the minutest aspects of the doctor's everyday behavior.

- The epidemiologic transition (to palliative care and global health threats), changing concept of the body (a well-maintained machine), and routinization of the doctor's charisma as an agent of life or death.

- Changes in the nature of the doctor-patient relationship and the erosion of patients' trust, which are corroding the esteem in which the profession is held.

Two intrinsic factors are:

- The weakening of physicians' labor market position through oversupply.

- The continuing fragmentation of the once powerful physicians' union (AMA) through specialty and subspecialty differentiation.

This article is *not* an attempt to assess the strengths and weaknesses of the competing theories of professionalism (dominance, corporatization, deprofessionalism). Its purpose, rather, is to describe the historic magnitude of the changes in the financing and organization of U.S. medical care and their implications for professionalism, the social position of doctors, and the everyday work of doctoring. Just as medieval monks were considered increasingly anachronistic and out of touch, hoping that macroeconomic secular changes in the surrounding society would pass them by, so too do some contemporary observers of medicine cling to the hope that things will eventually get better. With the golden age of medicine now almost behind us, doctors are huddling in their monasteries (hospitals and medical centers) powerlessly awaiting the next corporate onslaught. It is unlikely that the laity (the public) will rise up and save the church (hospital organizations) and the monks (the doctors). In other words, it is unlikely that any actions taken by the institution of medicine—health care organizations, the training and mobilization of doctors— or public protest will have any major effects, given the momentum already in motion. Our only hope probably lies in some form of government action (some fundamental reorganization of the health system to protect the profession and the public). Given the shift in the state's allegiance to the interests that are behind the recent changes in U.S. medical care, whose consequences for doctors we wish to mitigate, that unfortunately must be considered false hope.

ACKNOWLEDGMENTS

Our appreciation to Drs. John Stoeckle (Harvard Medical School), Lee Strunin (Boston University School of Public Health), and Paul Cleary (Harvard Medical School), who provided helpful comments. Nationally syndicated cartoonist Mark Tonra provided valuable assistance with the illustrations.

References

1. di Lampedusa, G. *The Leopard.* Parthenon Books, New York, 1960.

2. McKinlay, J. B., and Stoeckle, J. D. Corporatization and the social transformation of doctoring. *Int. J. Health Serv.* 18: 191–205, 1988.

3. McKinlay, J. B., and Arches, J. Towards the proletarianization of physicians. *Int. J. Health Serv.* 15: 161–195, 1985.

4. McKinlay, J. B. The business of good doctoring or doctoring as good business: Reflections on Freidson's view of the medical game. *Int. J. Health Serv.* 8: 459–488, 1978.

5. Navarro, V. Professional dominance or proletarianization? Neither. *Milbank Q.* 66(Suppl. 2): 57–75, 1989.

6. Coburn, D. Canadian medicine: Dominance or proletarianization? *Milbank Q.* 66(Suppl. 2): 92–116, 1988.

7. Scarpachi, J. L. Physician proletarianization and medical care restructuring in Argentina and Uruguay. *Econ. Geography* 6: 362–377, 1990.

8. Wolinsky, F. D. The professional dominance, deprofessionalization, proletarianization and corporatization perspectives: An overview and synthesis. In *The Changing Medical Profession: An International Perspective,* edited by F. W. Hafferty and J. B. McKinlay. Oxford University Press, New York, 1993.

9. Starr, P. *The Social Transformation of American Medicine.* Basic Books, New York, 1982.

10. Dudley, R. A., and Luft, H. S. Managed care in transition. *N. Engl. J. Med.* 344(14): 1087–1091, 2001.

11. Coster, R. L. Insulation from observability and types of social conformity. *Am. Sociol. Rev.* 25: 28–39, February 1961.

12. Freidson, E. *Profession of Medicine.* Dodd, Mead, New York, 1970.

13. Berlant, J. L. *Profession and Monopoly.* University of California Press, Berkeley, 1975.

14. Johnson, T. The state and the professions: Peculiarities of the British. In *Social Class and the Division of Labour,* edited by A. Giddens and G. Mackenzie. Cambridge University Press, Cambridge, 1982.

15. Coburn, D., Torrance, G. M., and Kaufert, J. M. Medical dominance in Canada in historical perspective: The rise and fall of medicine. *Int. J. Health Serv.* 13: 407–432, 1983.

16. Willis, E. *Medical Dominance: The Division of Labour in Australian Health Care.* George Allen and Unwin, Sydney, 1983.

17. Alford, R. *Health Care Politics: Ideological and Interest Group Barriers to Reform.* University of Chicago Press, Chicago, 1975.

18. McKinlay, J. B. On the professional regulation of change. In *Professionalism and Social Change,* edited by P. J. Halmos, pp. 61–84. Sociological Review Monographs, Vol. 20. University of Keele, Keele, U.K., 1973.

19. Fougere, G. Struggling for control: The state and the medical profession in New Zealand. In *The Changing Medical Profession: An International Perspective,* edited by F. W. Hafferty and J. B. McKinlay, pp. 115–123. Oxford University Press, New York, 1993.

20. Krause, E. A. *Death of Guilds, Professions, States, and the Advance of Capitalism, 1930 to the Present.* Yale University Press, New Haven, Conn., 1996.

21. Heywood, A. *Politics.* Macmillan, London, 1997.

22. Haralambos, M., and Holborn, M. *Sociology Themes and Perspectives,* Ed. 4. Collins Educational, London, 1995.

23. Skocpol, T. *Boomerang—Health Care Reform and the Turn against Government.* North, New York, 1997.

24. McKinlay, J. B., and Marceau, L. D. Value for Money in the Battle for the Public Health. Paper presented at the National Institutes of Health, November 6, 1998.

25. Coburn, D. State authority, medical dominance, and trends in the regulation of the health professions: The Ontario case. *Soc. Sci. Med.* 37(2): 129–138, 1993.

26. Gramsci, A. *Selections from the Prison Notebooks,* edited by Q. Hoare and G. Nowell-Smith. International Publishing, Chicago, 1971.

27. Mosca, G. *The Ruling Class,* translated by A. Livingstone. McGraw-Hill, New York, 1939 [1896].

28. Miliband, R. *The State in Capitalist Society.* Weidenfeld and Nicolson, London, 1969.

29. Poulantzas, N. *Political Power and Social Classes.* New Left Books, London, 1968.

30. Mills, C. W. *The Power Elite.* Oxford University Press, New York, 1956.

31. Jessop, B. *State Theory: Putting Capitalist States in Their Place.* Polity Press, Oxford, 1990.

32. Jessop, B. *The Capitalist State.* Martin Robertson, Oxford, 1982.

33. Rawls, J. *A Theory of Justice.* Oxford University Press, Oxford, 1971.

34. Dahl, R. *Modern Political Analysis,* Ed. 4. Prentice-Hall, Englewood Cliffs, N.J., 1984.

35. Lindblom, C. *Politics and Markets.* Basic Books, New York, 1977.

36. Marsh, D. (ed.). *Pressure Politics.* Junction Books, London, 1983.

37. Galbraith, J. K. *The Culture of Contentment.* Sinclair Stevenson, London, 1992.

38. Mechanic, D. Sources of countervailing power in medicine. *J. Health Polit. Policy Law* 16: 485, 1991.

39. Light, D. Professionalism as a countervailing power. *J Health Polit. Policy Law* 16: 499–506, 1991.

40. Freidson, E. *Professional Dominance: The Social Structure of Medical Care.* Aldine, Chicago, 1970.

41. Harrison, S., and Pollitt, C. *Controlling Health Professionals: The Future of Work and Organisation in the NHS.* Open University Press, Buckingham, U.K., 1994.

42. Nordlinger, E. *On the Autonomy of the Democratic State.* Harvard University Press, Cambridge, 1981.

43. Nozick, R. *Anarchy, State, and Utopia.* Basil Blackwell, Oxford, 1974.

44. Klein, R. The state and the profession: The politics of the double bed. *BMJ* 301: 701–702, 1990.

45. Barnett, J. R., Barnett, P., and Kearns, R. A. Declining professional dominance? Trends in the proletarianisation of primary care in New Zealand. *Soc. Sci. Med.* 46(2): 193–207, 1998.

46. Mohan, J. *A National Health Service? The Restructuring of Health Care in Britain since 1979.* Macmillan, Basingstoke, U.K., 1995.

47. Twaddle, A. C. Health system reforms: Toward a framework for international comparisons. *Soc. Sci. Med.* 43: 637–654, 1996.

48. Burrows, R., and Loader, B. (eds.). *Towards a Post Fordist Welfare State.* Routledge, London, 1994.

49. Farrell, J. A. *Tip O'Neill and the Democratic Century.* Little, Brown, Boston, 2001.

50. Blendon, R. J., et al. The implications of 2000 election. *N. Engl. J. Med.* 344(9): 679–684, 2001.

51. Light, D. Comparative models of "health care" systems. In *The Sociology of Health and Illness,* edited by P. Conard and R. Kern. St. Martin's Press, New York, 1994.

52. Zola, I. K. Medicine as an institution of social control. *Sociol. Rev.* 204(4): 487–504, 1972.

53. Hafferty, F., and McKinlay, J. B. (eds.). *The Changing Medical Profession: An International Perspective.* Oxford University Press, New York, 1993.

54. Kletke, P. R., Emmons, D. W., and Gillis, K. D. Current trends in physicians' practice arrangements: From owners to employees. *Journal of the American Medical Association* 276(7): 555–560, 1996.

55. Kletke, P. R. The changing proportion of employee physicians: Evidence of new trends. *AHSR FHSR Annual Meeting Abstracts* 11: 68–69, 1994.

56. Stoeckle, J. D. Working on the factory floor. *Ann. Intern. Med.* 107(2): 250–251, 1987.

57. Mechanic, D. Managed care and the imperative for a new professional ethic. *Health Aff. (Millwood)* 19(5): 100–111, 2000.

58. Sandrick, K. Out in front: Managed care helps push clinical guidelines forward. *Hospitals* 67: 30–31, 1993.

59. Bodenheimer, T., and Grumbach, K. The reconfiguration of US medicine. *Journal of the American Medical Association* 274: 85–90, 1995.

60. Hunter, D. J. From tribalism to corporatism: The managerial challenge to medical dominance. In *Challenging Medicine,* edited by J. Gabe, D. Kelleher, and G. Williams, pp. 1–22. Routledge, London, 1994.

61. Burdi, M. D., and Baker, L. C. Physicians' perceptions of autonomy and satisfaction in California. *Health Aff. (Millwood).* July–August 1999, pp. 134–135.

62. Kassirer, J. P. Doctor discontent. *N. Engl. J. Med.* 339(21): 1543, 1998.

63. O'Connor, S. J., and Lanning, J. A. The end of autonomy? Reflections on the post-professional physician. *Health Care Manag. Rev.* 17(63): 63–72, 1992.

64. Calnan, M., and Williams, S. Challenges to professional autonomy in the United Kingdom? The perceptions of general practitioners. *Int. J. Health Serv.* 25: 219–241, 1995.

65. Rappolt, S. G. Clinical guidelines and the fate of medical autonomy in Ontario. *Soc. Sci. Med.* 4: 977–987, 1997.

66. Feinglass, J., and Salmon, J. W. Corporatization of medicine: The use of medical management information systems to increase the clinical productivity of physicians. *Int. J. Health Serv.* 20: 233–252, 1990.

67. Brennan, T., and Berwick, D. *Regulation, Markets, and the Quality of American Health Care.* Jossey-Bass, San Francisco, 1996.

68. Cooper, R. A., and Stoflet, S. J. Trends in the education and practice of alternative medicine clinicians. *Health Aff. (Millwood)* 15: 226–238, 1996.

69. Cooper, R. A. Perspectives on the physician workforce to the year 2020. *Journal of the American Medical Association* 274(19): 1534–1543, 1995.

70. Osterweis, M., et al. (eds.). *The US Health Workforce: Power, Politics, and Policy.* Association of Academic Health Centers, Washington, D.C., 1996.

71. Safreit, B. J. Impediments to progress in health care workforce policy. *Inquiry* 31: 310–317, 1994.

72. Cooper, R. A., Laud, P., and Dietrich, C. L. Current and projected workforce of nonphysician clinicians. *Journal of the American Medical Association* 280(9): 788–794, 1998.

73. Jones, P. E., and Cawley, J. F. Physician assistants and health system reform: Clinical capabilities, practice activities and potential roles. *JAMA* 271(16): 1266–1272, 1994.

74. Cooper, R. A., Henderson, T., and Dietrich, C. L. Roles of nonphysician clinicians as autonomous providers of patient care. *Journal of the American Medical Association* 280(9): 795–802, 1998.

75. Lohr, K. N., Vaneslow, N. A., and Detmer, D. E. *The Nation's Physician Workforce: Options for Balancing Supply and Requirements.* National Academy Press, Washington, D.C., 1996.

76. Cohen, J. J., and Todd, J. S. Association of American Medicine Colleges and American Medical Association joint statement on physician workforce planning and graduate medical education reform policies. *Journal of the American Medical Association* 272: 712, 1994.

77. Weiner, J. P. Forecasting the effects of health reform on US physician workforce requirement: Evidence from HMO staffing patterns. *Journal of the American Medical Association* 272: 222–230, 1994.

78. Evans, R. G. Going for the gold: The redistributive agenda behind market based health care reform. *J. Health Polit. Policy Law* 22: 427–465, 1997.

79. Grumbach, K., and Coffman, J. Physician and nonphysician clinicians: Complements or competitors. *JAMA* 280(9): 825–826, 1998.

80. Greenberg, L., and Cultice, J. M. Forecasting the need for physicians in the United States: The health resources and services administration's physician requirements model. *Health Serv. Res.* 313(6): 723–737, 1997.

81. Bilton, T., et al. *Introducing Sociology,* Ed. 3. Macmillan, London, 1997.

82. Giddens, A. *Consequences of Modernity.* Stanford University Press, Stanford, Calif., 1990.

83. Swarns, R. L. West lures its doctors; South Africa fights back. *New York Times,* February 11, 2001.

84. Goode, W. J. Encroachment, charlatanism, and the emerging profession: Psychology, sociology, and medicine. *Am. Sociol. Rev.* 25: 902–914, 1960.

85. Fox, S., and Rainie, L. The online healthcare revolution: How the Web helps Americans take better care of themselves. November 26, 2000. www.pewinternet.org.

86. Fitzpatrick, R. M. Society and changing patterns of disease. In *Sociology as Applied to Medicine,* Ed. 3, edited by G. Scambler, pp. 3–17. Bailliere Tindall, London, 1991.

87. Omran, A. R. Epidemiologic transition: A theory of the epidemiology of population change. *Milbank Q.* 49: 309–338, 1971.

88. McKeown, T. The direction of medical research. *Lancet* 2(8155): 1281–1284, 1979.

89. Powles, J. On the limits of modern medicine. In *The Challenges of Community Medicine,* edited by R. L. Kane, pp. 89–122. Springer, New York, 1974.

90. Dubos, R. *Mirage of Health.* Harper and Row, New York, 1959.

91. McKinlay, J., and McKinlay, S. The questionable contribution of medical measures to the decline of mortality in the United States in the twentieth century. *Milbank Mem. Fund Q. Health Society* 55(3): 405–428, 1977.

92. Olshansky, S. D., and Ault, A. B. The fourth stage of the epidemiologic transition: The age of delayed degenerative diseases. *Milbank Q.* 64(3): 355–391, 1986.

93. McKinlay, J., McKinlay, S., and Beaglehole, R. Trends in death and disease and the contribution of medical measures. In *Handbook of Medical Sociology,* Ed. 4, edited by H. Freeman and S. Levine. Prentice-Hall, Englewood Cliffs, N.J., 1989.

94. McMichael, A. J., et al. (eds.). *Climate Change and Human Health—An Assessment Prepared by a Task Group on Behalf of the WHO, WMO, and UNEP.* WHO/EHG/96.7. WHO, Geneva, 1996.

95. Kovats, S., et al. Climate change and human health in Europe. *BMJ* 318: 1682–1685, 1999.

96. Githeko, A. K., et al. Climate change and vector borne diseases: A regional analysis. *Bull. World Health Organ.* 78: 1136–1147, 2000.

97. McKinlay, J. B., and Marceau, L. D. U.S. public health and the 21st century: Diabetes mellitus. *Lancet* 356: 757–761, 2000.

98. Thom, D. H., and Campbell, B. Patient-physician trust: An exploratory study. *J. Fam. Pract.* 44: 169–176, 1997.

99. Leopold, N., Cooper, M., and Clancy, C. Sustained partnership in primary care. *J. Fam. Pract.* 42: 129–137, 1996.

100. Sharfstein, J. M., and Sharfstein, S. S. Campaign contributions from the American Medical Political Action Committee to members of Congress. *N. Engl. J. Med.* 330(1): 32–37, 1994.

101. Sugarman, J., and Powers, M. How the doctor got gagged: The disintegrating right of privacy in the physician-patient relationship. *Journal of the American Medical Association* 266: 3323–3327, 1991.

102. Scalettar, R. Public Health Services Act, Title X Family Planning Regulations, Statement of the American Medical Association to the Subcommittee on Health and the Environment, Energy and Commerce Committee, United States House of Representatives, March 30, 1992. AMA, Chicago, 1992.

103. Wynia, M. K., et al. Physician manipulation of reimbursement rules for patients. *Journal of the American Medical Association* 283(14): 1858–1865, 2000.

104. Kao, A. C., et al. Patients' trust in their physician. *J. Gen. Intern. Med.* 13: 681–686, 1998.

105. Shortell, S. M., et al. Physicians as double agents: Maintaining trust in an era of multiple accountabilities. *Journal of the American Medical Association* 280(12): 1102–1108, 1998.

106. Gray, B. H. Trust and trustworthy care in the managed care era. *Health Aff. (Millwood)* 16: 34–49, 1995.

107. Mechanic, D., and Schlesinger, M. The impact of managed care on patients' trust in medical care and their physicians. *Journal of the American Medical Association* 275: 1693–1697, 1996.

108. Crawshaw, R., Rogers, D. E., and Pellegrino, E. D. Patient-physician covenant. *Journal of the American Medical Association* 273: 1553, 1995.

109. Mechanic, D. Changing medical organization and the erosion of trust. *Milbank Q.* 74: 171–189, 1996.

110. Emanuel, E. J. Managed competition and the patient-physician relationship. *N. Engl. J. Med.* 329: 879, 1993.

111. U.S. Department of Health and Human Services. *Report of the Graduate Medical Education National Advisory Committee: Summary Report.* US DHHS, HAS 81-651. Washington, D.C., 1981.

112. Council on Graduate Medical Education. *Fourth Report: Recommendations to Improve Access to Health Care through Physician Workforce Reform.* U.S. Dept. of Health and Human Services, Rockville, Md., 1994.

113. Gamliel, S., et al. Managed care on the march: Will physicians meet the challenge? *Health Aff. (Millwood)* 14: 131–142, 1995.

114. Tarlov, A. R. The rising supply of physicians and the pursuit of better health. *J. Med. Educ.* 63: 94–107, 1988.

115. Tarlov, A. R. The increasing supply of physicians, the changing structure of the health services system and the future practice of medicine. *N. Engl. J. Med.* 308: 1235–1244, 1983.

116. Physician Payment Review Commission. Training physicians to meet the nation's needs. In *Annual Report to Congress 1992*, Chapt. 11. Washington, D.C., 1992.

117. Physician Payment Review Commission. The changing labor market for physicians. In *Annual Report to Congress 1995*, Chapt. 14. Washington, D.C., 1995.

118. Weiner, J. P. *Assessing Current and Future US Physician Requirements Based on HMO Staffing Rates: A Synthesis of New Sources of Data and Forecasts for the Years 2000 and 2020.* HRSA 94-576 (P). U.S. Dept. of Health and Human Services, Bureau of Health Professions, Washington, D.C., 1995.

119. Tarlov, R. A. Estimating physician workforce requirements: The devil is in the assumptions. *Journal of the American Medical Association* 274(19): 1558–1560, 1995.

120. Institute of Medicine. *The Nation's Physician Workforce: Options for Balancing Supply Requirements.* National Academy Press, Washington, D.C., 1996.

121. Pew Health Professions Commission. *Critical Challenges: Revitalizing the Health Professions for the Twenty-first Century.* University of California, San Francisco, Center for the Health Professions, San Francisco, 1995.

122. Council on Graduate Medical Education. *Tenth Report: Physician Distribution and Health Care Challenges in Rural and Inner-City Areas.* U.S. Dept. of Health and Human Services, Rockville, Md., 1998.

123. Bureau of Health Professions. *Seventh Report to the President and Congress on the Status of Health Personnel in the United States.* National Academy Press, Washington, D.C., 1996.

124. Ginsburg, J. A. The physician workforce and financing of graduate medical education. *Ann. Intern. Med.* 128: 142–148, 1998.

125. Reinhardt, U. W. Planning the nation's health workforce: Let the market in. *Inquiry* 31: 250–263, 1994.

126. Miller, R. S., et al. Employment seeking experiences of resident physicians completing training during 1996. *Journal of the American Medical Association* 280(9): 777–783, 1998.

127. Fox, D. M. From piety to platitudes to pork: The changing politics of health workforce policy. *J. Health Polit. Policy Law* 21: 825–853, 1996.

128. Foreman, S. Managing the physician workforce: Hands off, the market is working. *Health Aff. (Millwood)* 15: 243–249, 1996.

129. Stoddard, J., Sekscenski, E., and Weiner, J. The physician workforce: Broadening the search for solutions. *Health Aff. (Millwood)* 17(1): 252–257, 1998.

130. Goldstien, A. AMA rejects leadership challenge. *Washington Post,* June 23, 1997.

131. The AMA's appliance sale (editorial). *New York Times,* August 14, 1997.

132. Auctioning a seal of approval (editorial). *Washington Post,* August 20, 1997.

133. Kassirer, J. P., and Angell, M. The high price of product endorsement. *N. Engl. J. Med.* 337: 700–701, 1997.

134. Freidson, E. *Professionalism: The Third Logic.* University of Chicago Press, Chicago, 2001.

COUNTERVAILING POWER

The Changing Character of the Medical Profession in the United States

Donald W. Light

The medical profession appears to be losing its autonomy even as its sovereignty expands. With the more frequent use of physician profiling and other comparative measures of performance, together with the ability of sophisticated programmers to capture the decision-making trees of differential diagnosis on computers so well that they can check out and improve the performance of practitioners, theories of professionalism that rest on autonomy as their cornerstone need to be reconstructed from the ground up (Light 1988).

Although physicians play a central role in developing tools for scrutinizing the core of professional work, they work for purchasers who use them for the external measure of quality and cost-effectiveness. Thus, not only autonomy but also the monopoly over knowledge as the foundation of professionalism

is thrown into question. The computerized analysis of practice patterns and decision making, together with the growth of active consumerism, constitute deprofessionalization as a trend (Haug 1973; Haug and Lavin 1983). Patients, governments, and corporate purchasers are taking back the cultural, economic, and even technical authority long granted to the medical profession.

The sovereignty of the profession nevertheless is growing. Evan Willis (1988) was the first to distinguish between autonomy over one's work and sovereignty over matters of illness. The sovereignty of medicine expands with advances in pharmacology, molecular biology, genetics, and diagnostic tools that uncover more and more pathology not known before. Although chronicity is the residue of cure and the growing proportion of insoluble problems is providing a new legitimacy to nonmedical forms of healing, care, and therapy, no other member of the illness trade has a knowledge and skill base that is expanding so rapidly as is the physician's.

This chapter describes the changes in the American medical profession over the past two decades and outlines the concept of countervailing power as a useful way to understand the profession's relations with the economy and the state.

SOME LIMITATIONS OF CURRENT CONCEPTS

In the special issue of the *Milbank Quarterly* . . . Sol Levine and I reviewed the concepts of professional dominance, deprofessionalization, proletarianization, and corporatization (Light and Levine 1988). Each has its truth and limitations. Each captures in its word one characteristic and trend, but this means that each mistakes the part for the whole and for the future. One set predicts the opposite of the other, yet neither can account for reversals. This is best illustrated by the oldest concept among them, professional dominance.

Professional dominance captured in rich complexity the clinical and institutional grip that the profession had over society in the 1960s, a formulation that supplanted Parsons' benign and admiring theoretical reflections of the 1940s and 1950s (Freidson 1970a, 1970b; Light 1989). But the concept of professional dominance cannot account for decline; dominance over institutions and resources leads only to still more dominance. As the very fruits of dominance itself weakened the profession from within and prompted powerful changes from without, the concept has become less useful. In its defense, Freidson (1984, 1985, 1986, 1989) has been forced to retreat from his original concept of dominance, by which he meant control over the cultural, organizational, economic, and political dimensions of health care, to a much reduced concept that means control over one's work and those involved in it. Even that diminution to the pre-Freidson concept of professionalism may not stand, given the fundamental challenges to autonomy.

Space precludes reiterating the limitations of the other concepts, but it is worth noting the danger of conflating many by-products of professional dominance after World War II (such as increasing complexity, bureaucratization, and rationalization) with recent efforts by investors to corporatize medicine and by institutional payers such as governments and employers to get more effective health care for less money. The concept of corporatization in particular includes five dimensions that characterize medical work today as segmented and directed by the administrators of for-profit organizations that control the facilities, the technology used, and the remuneration of the physician-workers (McKinlay 1988). As the empirical part of this chapter shows, this characterization is not typical and does not capture the complex relations between doctors and corporations.

THE CONCEPT OF COUNTERVAILING POWERS

Sociology needs a concept or framework that provides a way of thinking about the changing relations over time between the profession and the major institutions with which it interacts. The concept of countervailing powers builds on the work of Johnson (1972) and Larson (1977), who analyzed such relations with a dynamic subtlety not found elsewhere. Montesquieu (de Secondat Montesquieu 1748) first developed the idea in his treatise about the abuses of absolute power by the state and the need for counterbalancing centers of power. Sir James Steuart (1767) developed it further in his ironic observations of how the monarchy's promotion of commerce to enhance its domain and wealth produced a countervailing power that tempered the absolute power of the monarchy and produced a set of interdependent relationships. One might discern a certain analogy to the way in which the American medical profession encouraged the development of pharmaceutical and medical supply companies within the monopoly markets it created to protect its own autonomy. They enriched the profession and extended its power, but increasingly on their terms.

The concept of countervailing powers focuses attention on the interactions of a few powerful actors in a field in which they are inherently interdependent yet distinct. If one party is dominant, as the American medical profession has been, its dominance is contextual and likely to elicit countermoves eventually by other powerful actors in an effort not to destroy it but to redress an imbalance of power. "Power on one side of a market," wrote John Kenneth Galbraith (1956: 113) in his original treatise on the dynamics of countervailing power in oligopolistic markets, "creates both the need for, and the prospect of reward to the exercise of countervailing power from the other side." In states where the government has played a central role in nurturing professions within the state structure but has allowed the professions to establish their own institutions and power base, the professions and the state go through phases of harmony and discord in which countervailing actions emerge. In states where the medical profession has been largely suppressed, we now see their rapid reconstitution once governmental oppression is lifted.

Countervailing moves are more difficult to accomplish and may take much longer when political and institutional powers are involved than in an economic market. Nevertheless, dominance tends to produce imbalances, excesses, and neglects that anger other countervailing (latent) powers and alienate the larger public. These imbalances include internal elaboration and expansion that weaken the dominant institution from within, a subsequent tendency to consume more and more of the nation's wealth, a self-regarding importance that ignores the concerns of its clients or subjects and institutional partners, and an expansion of control that exacerbates the impact of the other three. Other characteristics of a profession that affect its relations with countervailing powers are the degree and nature of competition with adjacent professions, about which Andrew Abbott (1988) has written with such richness, the changing technological base of its expertise, and the demographic composition of its membership.

As a sociological concept, countervailing powers is not confined to buyers and sellers; it includes a handful of major political, social, and other economic groups that contend with each other for legitimacy, prestige, and power, as well as for markets and money. Deborah Stone (1988) and Theodore Marmor with Jonathan Christianson (1982) have written insightfully about the ways in which countervailing powers attempt to portray benefits to themselves as benefits for everyone or to portray themselves as the unfair and damaged victims of other powers (particularly the state), or to keep issues out of public view. Here, the degree of power consists of the ability to override, suppress, or render as irrelevant the challenges by others, either behind closed doors or in public.

Because the sociological concept of countervailing powers recognizes several parties, not just buyers and sellers, it opens the door to alliances between two or more parties. These alliances, however, are often characterized by structural ambiguities, a term based on Merton and Barber's (1976) concept of sociological ambivalence that refers to the crosscutting pressures and expectations experienced by an institution in its relations with other institutions (Light 1983:345–46). For example, a profession's relationships to the corporations that supply it with equipment, materials, and information technology both benefit the profession and make it dependent in uneasy ways. The corporations can even come to control professional practices in the name of quality. Alliances with dominant political parties (Krause 1988; Jones 1991) or with governments are even more fraught with danger. The alliance of the German medical profession with the National Socialist party, for example, so important to establishing the party's legitimacy, led to a high degree of governmental control over work and even the professional knowledge base (Jarausch 1990; Light, Liebfried, and Tennstedt 1986).

COUNTERVAILING POWERS IN AMERICAN MEDICINE

In the case of the American medical profession, concern over costs, unnecessary and expensive procedures, and overspecialization grew during the

1960s to the "crisis" announced by President Richard Nixon, Senator Edward Kennedy, and many other leaders in the early 1970s. President Nixon attempted to establish a national network of health maintenance organizations (HMOs) bent on efficiency and cost-effectiveness. He and the Congress created new agencies to regulate the spending of capital, the production of new doctors, and even the practice of medicine through institutionalized peer review. All of these were done gingerly at first, in a provider-friendly way. When, at the end of the 1970s, little seemed to have changed, the government and corporations launched a much more adversarial set of changes, depicted in Table 20.1. The large number of unnecessary procedures, the unexplained variations in practice patterns, the unclear answers to rudimentary questions about which treatments were most

cost-effective, and the burgeoning bills despite calls for self-restraint had eroded the sacred trust enjoyed by the profession during the golden era of medicine after World War II. To some degree, the dominance of the medical profession had been allowed on the assumption that physicians knew what they were doing and acted in the best interests of society. Unlike the guilds of earlier times, however, the medical profession had failed to exercise controls over products, practices, and prices to ensure uniformly good products at fair prices.

The reassertion of the payers' latent countervailing powers called for a concentration of will and buying power that was only partially achieved. Larger corporations, some states, and particularly the federal government changed from passively paying bills submitted by providers to scrutinizing bills and

TABLE 20.1 ■ Axes of Change in the American Health Care System

Dimensions	Provider Driven	Buyer Driven
Ideological	Sacred trust in doctors	Distrust of doctors' values, decisions, even competence
Economic	Carte blanche to do what seems best; power to set fees; incentives to specialize, develop techniques Informal array of cross-subsidizations for teaching, research, charity care, community services	Fixed prepayment or contract with accountability for decisions and their efficacy Elimination of "cost shifting"; pay only for services contracted
Political	Extensive legal and administrative power to define and carry out professional work without competition and to shape the organization and economics of medicine	Minimal legal and administrative power to do professional work but not shape the organization and economics of services
Clinical	Exclusive control of clinical decision making Emphasis on state-of-the-art specialized interventions; disinterest in prevention, primary care, and chronic care	Close monitoring of clinical decisions— their cost and their efficacy Emphasis on prevention, primary care, and functioning; minimize high-tech and specialized interventions
Technical	Political and economic incentives to develop new technologies in protected markets	Political and economic disincentives to develop new technologies
Organizational	Cottage industry	Corporate industry
Potential disruptions and dislocations	Overtreatment; iatrogenesis; high cost; unnecessary treatment; fragmentation; depersonalization	Undertreatment; cuts in services; obstructed access; reduced quality; swamped in paperwork

organizing markets for competitive contracts that covered a range of services for a large pool of people. The health insurance industry, originally designed to reimburse hospitals and doctors, was forcefully notified that it must serve those who pay the premiums or lose business. Today, thousands of insurance sales representatives are now agents of institutional buyers, and insurance companies have developed a complex array of managed care products. Hundreds of utilization management companies and entire divisions of insurance companies devoted to designing these products have arisen (Gray and Field 1989: Ch. 3).

These changes have produced analogous changes among providers: more large groups, vertically integrated clinics, preferred provider organizations (PPOs), health maintenance organizations (HMOs), and hospital-doctor joint ventures. When the federal government created and implemented a national schedule of prospective payments for hospital expenses, termed diagnosis related groups (DRGs), doctors and health care managers countered by doing so much more business outside the DRG system that they consumed nearly all the billions saved on inpatient care. Congress more than ever now regards doctors as the culprits, and it has countered by instituting a fee schedule based on costs. In response, the specialties affected have joined hands in a powerful political countermove designed to water down the sharp reductions in the fee schedule for surgeons and technology-based specialists (like radiologists).

Thus, although the buyers' revolt depicted in Table 20.1 spells the end of dominance, it by no means spells the end to professional power. Closely monitored contracts or payments, corporate amalgamation, and significant legal changes to foster competition are being met by responses that the advocates of markets, as the way to make medicine efficient, did not consider. Working together (or, as the other side terms it, collusion), appropriate referrals (known as cost shifting to somebody else's budget), market segmentation, market expansion, and service substitution are all easier and often more profitable than trying to become more efficient, particularly when the work is complex, contingent, and uncertain (Light 1990). Moreover, most inefficiencies in medicine are embedded in organizational structures, professional habits,

and power relations so that competitive contracting is unlikely to get at them (Light 1991).

On the buyers' side, the majority of employers and many states have still not been able to take concerted action, much less combine their powers. The utilization management industry has produced a bewildering array of systems and criteria, which are adjusted to suit the preferences of each employer-client. The Institute of Medicine (IOM) study on the subject states that the Mayo Clinic deals with a thousand utilization review (UR) plans (Gray and Field 1989: 59), and large hospitals deal with one hundred to two hundred of them. Who knows which are more "rational" or effective? Moreover, the countervailing efforts of institutional buyers rest on a marshland of data. "Studies continue to document," states the IOM report, "imprecise or inaccurate diagnosis and procedure coding, lack of diagnostic codes on most claim forms, only scattered documentation about entire episodes of treatment or illness, errors and ambiguities in preparation and processing of claims data, and limited information on patient and population characteristics" (Gray and Field 1989:48).

In spite of this morass, a profound restructuring of incentives, payments, and practice environments is beginning to take place, and more solid, coordinated data are rapidly being accumulated. The threat of denial, or of being dropped as a high-cost provider in a market, has probably reduced treatments but in the process increased diagnostic services and documentation, a major vehicle for the expansion of medical sovereignty. Accountability, then, may be the profession's ace card as governments and institutional buyers mobilize to make the profession accountable to their concerns.

CHANGING PRACTICE PATTERNS

Cost and Income

If the first round in the struggle to control rising medical expenditures consisted of tepid and unsuccessful efforts to regulate capital and services in the 1970s, then providers again emerged as the winners of the second round in the 1980s. They expanded services, took market share away from hospitals, packaged services to the most attractive market niches, featured numerous products developed by the highly profitable companies specializing in new medical technology, and advertised vigorously. Eye centers, women's centers, occupational medicine clinics, ambulatory surgical centers, imaging centers, detoxification programs: these and other enterprises caused medical expenditures to rise from $250 billion in 1980 to about $650 billion in 1990. This equals 12 percent of the nation's entire gross national product (GNP), one-third higher than the average for Western Europe. There seems to be no way to avoid health expenditures' rising to 16 percent of GNP by 1995.

At the level of personal income, many physicians tell anyone who will listen that one can no longer make "good money" in medicine, but the facts are otherwise. From 1970 to about 1986, their average income stayed flat after inflation, but since then it has been rising. The era of cost containment and dehospitalization has actually been an opportunity for market expansion. Although physicians' market share of national health expenditures declined from 20 to 17 percent as hospitals' share rose between 1965 and 1984, it has climbed back up to 19 percent since then (Roback, Randolph, and Seidman 1990: Table 105). The profession appears thoroughly commercialized (Potter, McKinlay, and D'Agostino 1991), doing more of what pays more and less of what pays less. Although the profession likes to think it was more altruistic in the golden era of medicine after World War II, this was a time when physicians' incomes rose most rapidly and when it controlled insurance payment committees.

In addition, the range of physicians' incomes has spread. For example, surgeons earned 40 percent more than general practitioners in 1965 but 57 percent more in 1985 (Statistical Abstract 1989). As of 1989, surgeons earned on average $200,500 after expenses but before taxes, while family or general practitioners earned $95,000. All specialties averaged a sixty-hour week. Beleaguered obstetricians, even after their immense malpractice premiums, are doing well. They netted $194,300, up $14,000 from 1988, which was up $17,500 from 1987.

Despite the success so far of the profession in generating more demand, services, and income, the tidal force of population growth is against them. The number of physicians increased from 334,000 in 1970 to 468,000 in 1980 to 601,000 in 1990. By the year 2000, there will be about 722,000 physicians (Roback, Randolph, and Seidman 1990: Table 88). Although about 8.5 percent are inactive or have unknown addresses, the number of physicians in America is growing rapidly nevertheless, as it is in many European countries. There is no slowdown in sight, given the number of doctors graduating from medical schools and the nation's ambivalence about reducing the influx of foreign-trained doctors, many of whom are American born. In fact, between 1970 and 1989, foreign-trained doctors increased 126 percent compared to a 72 percent increase in American-trained doctors, and they constituted 130,000 of the 601,000 doctors in 1990 (Roback, Randolph, and Seidman 1990). As a result, the number of persons per physician is steadily dropping, from around 714 people per doctor thirty years ago to about 417 today and 370 in the year 2000. Will 370 men, women, and children be enough to maintain the average doctor in the style to which he or she is accustomed about five and a half times the average income in the face of countervailing forces? And how will the gross imbalance between the number of specialists and the need for their services play itself out? Today we have what could be called the 80-20 inversion: 80 percent of the doctors are specialists, but only about 20 percent or fewer of the nation's patients have problems warranting the attention of a specialist. Nearly all growth depends on an increasing number of subspecialties in medicine and surgery, and there are now about two hundred specialty societies, many not officially recognized but vying for legitimacy and a market niche (Abbott 1988). Thus, the rapid growth of physicians and their specialty training has set the stage for sharp clashes between countervailing powers.

Trends in the Organization of Practice

The post-Freidson era, from 1970 to the late 1980s, saw a steady trend of dehospitalization and a long-term shift back to office-based care. Most doctors (82%) are involved in patient care, and despite all the talk today about physician-executives, the data show no notable uptrend in numbers (Roback, Randolph, and Seidman 1990: Table A-2). Office-based practice has been rising slowly since 1975 (from 55% to 58.5%), and full-time hospital staff has declined from 10.4 to 8.5 percent in the same period. Hospital-based practice still makes up 23.6 percent of all practice sites because of all the residents and fellows in training. These data underscore the immense role that medical education, practically an industry in itself, plays in staffing and supporting hospital-based practice. The total number of residents has grown since 1970 by 60 percent, and they are a major source of cheap labor. They grew in use during the golden age of reimbursement, and curtailment of the workweek from 100 hours to 80 or fewer is already raising costs.

An increasing number of the 58 percent of doctors practicing in offices (that is, not a hospital or institution) do so in groups. Since the mid-1960s, when private and public insurance became fully established and funded expansion with few restraints, more and more doctors have combined into groups and formed professional corporations. The motives appear largely to have been income and market share. There were 4,300 groups in 1965 (11% of all nonfederal physicians), 8,500 in 1975, and 16,600 in 1988 (30%, or 156,000) (Havlicek 1990: Ch. 8). Supporting this emphasis on economic rather than service motives, an increasing percentage have been single specialty groups, up from 54 percent in 1975 to 71 percent in 1988. They tend to be small, from an average of 5 in 1975 to 6.2 in 1988, and their purpose seems largely to share the financing of space, staff, and equipment and to position themselves for handling larger specialty contracts from institutional buyers.

The future of groups will be affected by demands of the buyers' market. For example, almost all fee-for-service care now is managed by having an array of monitoring activities and cost-containment programs. These complex and expensive controls favor larger groups, and Havlicek (1990:8–38) believes we will see more mergers than new groups in the 1990s. He also suspects there will be more cooperative efforts with hospitals, which have more capital and staff but are subject to more cost controls.

Capitalist Professionals

An important, perhaps even integral, part of the rapid expansion of groups since the mid-1970s has involved doctors' investing in their own clinical laboratories (28% of all groups), radiology laboratories (32%), electrocardiological laboratories (28%), and audiology laboratories (16%). (Additionally, 40 percent of all office-based physicians have their own laboratories.) The larger the group is, the more likely it owns one or more of these facilities. For example, 23 percent of three-person groups own clinical laboratories and 78 percent of all groups with seventy-six to ninety-nine doctors. Large groups also own their own surgical suites: from 15 percent of groups with sixteen to twenty-five people to 41 percent of groups ranging from seventy-six to ninety-nine physicians. The hourly charges are very attractive (Havlicek 1990).

Growth of HMOs, PPOs, and Managed Care

The countervailing power of institutional buyers has forced practitioners to reorganize into larger units of health care that can manage the costs and quality of the services rendered. Health maintenance organizations, first developed in the 1920s, became the centerpiece of President Nixon's 1971 reforms to make American health care efficient and affordable. Medical lobbies fought the reform; when they saw it would pass, they weighed it down with requirements and restrictions. By 1976, there were 175 HMOs with 6 million members, half of them in just six HMOs that had built a solid reputation for good, coordinated care (Gruber, Shadle, and Polich 1988). Among them, PruCare and U.S. Health Care represented the new wave of expansion: national systems of HMOs run by insurers as a key "product" to sell to employers for cost containment or run by investors for the same purpose. Moreover, most of the new HMOs consisted of networks of private practitioners linked by part-time contracts rather than a core dedicated staff.

By December 1987, there were 650 HMOs with about 29 million members. Both Medicare and Medicaid revised terms to favor these groups as a way to moderate costs, as did many revised benefit plans by corporations. HMOs keep annual visits per person down to 3.8 and hospital inpatient bed-days down to 438 per thousand enrollees, well below the figures for autonomous, traditional care (Hodges, Camerlo, and Gold 1990). There were now forty-two national firms, and they enrolled half the total. The proportion of these firms that use networks of independent practitioners rose from 40 percent in 1980 to 62 percent in 1987. To increase their attractiveness, new hybrid HMOs were beginning to form that allowed members to get services outside the HMO's list of physicians if they paid a portion of the bill.

Preferred provider organizations come in many varieties, but all essentially consist of groups of providers who agree to give services at a discount. Employers then structure benefits to encourage employees to use them. For example, they offer to pay all of the fees for PPO providers but only 80 percent of fees from other doctors.

PPOs became significant by the mid-1980s, and by 1988 they had 20 million enrollees (Rice, Gabel, and Mick 1989). This figure is only approximate because patterns of enrollment are constantly changing. Perhaps more reliable are data from employers, who say that 13 to 15 percent of all employees and half their dependents are covered by PPOs (Sullivan and Rice 1991). Increasingly insurers are using PPOs as a managed care product, and they are forming very large PPOs in the range of 200,000 enrollees each with 100 to 200 hospitals and 5,000 to 15,000 physicians involved in their systems. From the other side, physician group practices derive from 13 to 30 percent of their income from PPOs as group size increases. Besides volume discounts on fees, half to three-quarters of the PPOs use physician profiling (to compare the cost-effectiveness of different doctors), utilization review, and preselection of cost-effective providers.

In response to the "buyers' revolt" and the growth of HMOs and PPOs, a growing number of traditional, autonomous, fee-for-service practices have taken on the same techniques of managed care:

preadmission review, daily concurrent review to see if inpatients need to stay another day, retrospective review of hospitalized cases, physician profiling to identify high users of costly services, and case management of costly, complex cases. By 1990, the most thorough study of all small, medium, and large employers, including state and local governments, found that only 5 percent of all employees and their families now have traditional fee-for-service physicians without utilization management (Sullivan and Rice 1991).

CONCLUSION

The countervailing power of institutional buyers certainly ends the kind of dominance the medical profession had in 1970, but by no means does it turn doctors into mere corporatized workers. The medical profession's relations with capital are now quite complex. Physicians are investing heavily in their own buildings and equipment, spurred by a refocus of the medical technology industry on office or clinic-based equipment that will either reduce costs or generate more income. Employers and their agents (insurance companies, management companies) are using their oligopolistic market power to restructure medical practice into managed care systems, but physicians have many ways to make those systems work for them. Hospitals are using their considerable capital to build facilities and buy equipment that will attract patients and their physicians, whom they woo intensively.

The state is by far the largest buyer and has shown the greatest resolve to bring costs under control. The federal government has pushed through fundamental changes to limit how much it pays hospitals and doctors. Each year brings more stringent or extensive measures. At the same time, the state faces a societal duty to broaden benefits to those not insured and to deepen them to cover new technologies or areas of treatment. And the state is itself a troubled provider through its Veterans Administration health care system and its services to special populations.

Both buyers and providers constantly attempt to use the legal powers of the state to advance their interests. Thus, regulation is best analyzed from this perspective as a weapon in the competition between countervailing powers rather than as an alternative to it. At the same time, competition itself is a powerful form of regulation (Leone 1986). However, Galbraith warned that the self-regulating counterbalance of contending powerblocs works poorly if demand is not limited, because it undermines the bargaining power of the buyers of the agents. This is another basic reason why institutional buyers are, so far, losing.

In response, buyers and the state are using other means besides price and contracts to strengthen their hand. Even as providers keep frustrating the efforts of institutional buyers through "visit enrichment," more bills, and higher incomes, a fundamental change has taken place. The game they are winning (at least so far) has ceased to be their game. Most of the terms are being set by the buyers.

The paradox of declining autonomy and growing sovereignty indicates a larger, more fundamental set of countervailing powers at work than simply the profession and its purchasers. As the dynamic unfolds, capitalism comes face to face with itself, for driving the growing sovereignty or domain of medicine is the medical-industrial complex, perhaps the most successful and largest sector of the entire economy. It is Baxter-Travenol or Humana versus General Motors or Allied Signal, with each side trying to harness the profession to its purposes. Different parts of the profession participate in larger institutional complexes to legitimate their respective goals of "the best medicine for every sick patient" and "a healthy, productive work force at the least cost." The final configuration is unclear, but the concept of professionalism as a countervailing power seems most clearly to frame the interactions.

References

Abbott, A. 1988. *The System of Professions: An Essay on the Division of Expert Labor.* Chicago: University of Chicago Press.

de Secondat Montesquieu, C. L. 1748. *De l'Esprit des Loix.* Geneva: Barillot & Sons.

Freidson, E. 1970a. *Professional Dominance: The Social Structure of Medical Care.* Chicago: Aldine.

Freidson, E. 1970b. *Profession of Medicine: A Study of the Sociology of Applied Knowledge.* New York: Dodd, Meed.

Freidson, E. 1984. The Changing Nature of Professional Control. *Annual Review of Sociology* 10:1–20.

Freidson, E. 1985. The Reorganization of the Medical Profession. *Medical Care Review* 42:11–35.

Freidson, E. 1986. *Professional Powers: A Study of the Institutionalization of Formal Knowledge.* Chicago: University of Chicago Press.

Freidson, E. 1989. Industrialization or Humanization? In *Medical Work in America.* New Haven: Yale University Press.

Galbraith, J. K. 1956. *American Capitalism: The Concept of Countervailing Power.* Boston: Houghton Mifflin.

Gray, B. H., and M. J. Field, eds. 1989. *Controlling Costs and Changing Patient Care: The Role of Utilization Management.* Washington, D.C.: Institute of Medicine, National Academy Press.

Gruber, L. R., M. Shadle, and C. L. Politch. 1988. From Movement to Industry: The Growth of HMOs. *Health Affairs* 7(3):197–298.

Haug, M. R. 1973. Deprofessionalization: An Alternative Hypothesis for the Future. *Sociological Review Monograph* 20:195–211.

Haug, M. R., and B. Lavin. 1983. *Consumerism in Medicine: Challenging Physician Authority.* Beverly Hills: Sage.

Havlicek, P. L. 1990. *Medical Groups in the U.S.: A Survey of Practice Characteristics.* Chicago: American Medical Association.

Hodges, D., K. Camerlo, and M. Gold. 1990. *HMO Industry Profile.* Vol. 2: *Utilization Patterns, 1988.* Washington, D.C.: Group Health Association of America.

Jarausch, K. H. 1990. *The Unfree Professions: German Lawyers, Teachers, and Engineers, 1900–1950.* New York: Oxford University Press.

Johnson, T. J. 1972. *Professions and Power.* London: Macmillan.

Jones, A., ed. 1991. *Professions and the State: Expertise and Autonomy in the Soviet Union and Eastern Europe.* Philadelphia: Temple University Press.

Krause, E. A. 1988. Doctors, Partitocrazia, and the Italian State. *Milbank Quarterly* 66(Suppl. 2): 148–66.

Larson, M. S. 1977. *The Rise of Professionalism: A Sociological Analysis.* Berkeley: University of California Press.

Light, D. W. 1983. The Development of Professional Schools in America. In *The Transformation of Higher Learning, 1860–1930,* ed. K. H. Jarausch, 345–66. Chicago: University of Chicago Press.

Light, D. W. 1988. Turf Battles and the Theory of Professional Dominance. *Research in the Sociology of Health Care* 7:203–25.

Light, D. W. 1989. Social Control and the American Health Care System. In *Handbook of Medical Sociology,* ed. H. E. Freeman and S. Levine, 456–74. Englewood Cliffs, N.J.: Prentice-Hall.

Light, D. W. 1990. Bending the Rules. *Health Services Journal* 100(5222):1513–15.

Light, D. W. 1991. Professionalism as a Countervailing Power. *Journal of Health Politics, Policy and Law* 16:499–506.

Light, D. W., and S. Levine. 1988. The Changing Character of the Medical Profession: A Theoretical Overview. *Milbank Quarterly* 66(Suppl. 2): 10–32.

Light, D. W., S. Liebfried, and F. Tennstedt. 1986. Social Medicine vs. Professional Dominance: the German Experience. *American Journal of Public Health* 76(1):78–83.

Marmor, T. R., and J. B. Christianson. 1982. *Health Care Policy: A Political Economy Approach.* Beverly Hills: Sage.

Merton, R. K. and B. Barber, eds. 1976. Sociological Ambivalence. In *Sociological Ambivalence and Other Essays.* New York: Free Press.

Potter, D. A., J. B. McKinlay, and R. B. D'Agostino. 1991. *Understanding How Social Factors Affect Medical Decision Making: Application of a Factorial Experiment.* Watertown, Mass.: New England Research Institute.

Rice, T., J. Gabel, and S. Mick. 1989. *PPOS: Bigger, Not Better.* Washington, D.C.: HIAA Research Bulletin.

Roback, G., L. Randolph, and S. Seidman. 1990. *Physician Characteristics and Distribution in the U.S.* Chicago: American Medical Association.

Statistical Abstract of the United States. 1989. Washington, D.C.: Department of Commerce.

Steuart, J. 1767. *Inquiry into the Principles of Political Economy,* vol. 1. London: A. Miller and T. Cadwell.

Stone, D. A. 1988. *Policy Paradox and Political Reason.* Glenview, Ill.: Scott, Foresman.

Sullivan, C., and T. Rice. 1991. The Health Insurance Picture in 1990. *Health Affairs* 10(2):104–15.

Willis, E. 1988. Doctoring in Australia: A View at the Bicentenary. *Milbank Quarterly* 66(Suppl 2): 167–81.

OTHER PROVIDERS IN AND OUT OF MEDICINE

When we talk about medicine, we frequently think about doctors, or maybe doctors and nurses. But the number of people employed in medical care goes far beyond the 713,800 practicing physicians and 2.96 million registered nurses (RNs) in the United States in 2016, and it continues to grow (Bureau of Labor Statistics 2017a). Today, 6.5 million people work as health care practitioners or technicians, and another 3.6 million work in health care support occupations, such as home health aides and medical assistants (Bureau of Labor Statistics 2017a), not to mention the health care administrators and medical billing staff employed in many health care settings. Between 2016 and 2026, employment in health care occupations is projected to grow by 18 percent, adding 2.3 million jobs (Bureau of Labor Statistics 2017b).

In the 1950s, policy analysts predicted a physician shortage; in the 1980s, some scholars predicted a physician surplus (Starr 1982), and recently, some are predicting a shortage while others are predicting a surplus (U.S. Department of Health and Human Services 2008). Today, both shortages and surpluses can be found depending on where one looks. There are shortages of primary care physicians and surpluses of many subspecialists; there are shortages of OB/GYNs in some geographic areas and surpluses of cosmetic surgeons in others. Furthermore, many rural areas and inner cities are still designated as underserved because of the paucity of physicians practicing in them. Nurse practitioners and physician assistants are increasingly filling gaps in primary care, and those professions are expected to grow by 30% or more over the next decade (Bureau of Labor Statistics 2017b).

Whereas in the past there was general agreement about a future shortage of RNs, currently some states are projected to have shortages (e.g., California), while others are expected to have surpluses (e.g., Florida) in the future (U.S. Department of Health and Human Services 2017). Retirement of older nurses was thought to contribute to projected shortages in U.S. health care right about now, but many registered nurses are delaying retirement, and there has been a surge of new entrants into the field (Auerbach, Buerhaus, and Staiger 2011, 2014). Therefore, the long-projected RN shortage has merely been pushed off temporarily. There are complicated reasons for the projected nursing shortage, including fewer women choosing nursing as a career, a greater need for nurses in an aging population, serious job burnout and dissatisfaction with the profession (Aiken et al. 2001), and a shortage of nurses with graduate degrees to teach the next generation (American Association of Colleges of Nursing 2017). Increasing bureaucratic pressures on hospital nurses, especially in the context of managed care, fuels job dissatisfaction, as it keeps nurses from doing what brought them to the profession—caring for patients (Weinberg 2003).

In our first selection in this section, "A Caring Dilemma: Womanhood and Nursing in Historical Perspective," Susan Reverby traces the emergence of nursing, focusing in particular on how "caring as a duty" was connected to the fact that women were doing the caring. In women, medical administrators could find a caring, disciplined, and cheap labor force. Reverby shows how the dilemmas nurses faced and the struggles they engaged in to improve their image, stature, and authority were shaped by the gender stratification of society. She argues that this historical past is reflected in nursing's current position in the health care hierarchy and its continuing dilemmas.

One place the health care work force has expanded is in the growth and acceptance of complementary and alternative medicine (CAM). The term *alternative medicine* encompasses a wide range of practitioners from esoteric disciplines like "crystal healing" or "zone therapy" to now widely available treatments like acupuncture and chiropractic. CAM has grown enormously in the past three decades and is increasingly used and accepted by patients and providers of American health care. There is a growing body of research suggesting that some types of CAM have considerable treatment efficacy (Goldstein 2002), and the National Center for Complementary and Alternative Medicine, a part of the National Institutes of Health, now funds efficacy research on CAM. The effort to bring CAM into mainstream medical practice is sometimes called the *development of integrated medicine.*

In the second selection, "From Quackery to Complementary Medicine: The American Medical Profession Confronts Alternative Therapies," Terri A. Winnick traces the medical profession's changing relationship to alternative medicine. Examining five prestigious medical journals from 1965 to 1999, Winnick shows how the medical profession responded to the growth of CAM. She identifies three major phases: condemnation, reassessment, and integration, each occurring in a particular time period. This analysis reflects an evolutionary process of professionalization, which is driven in part by consumers, alternative practitioners, and finally the medical profession itself. It is of interest to ask how far this integration will progress, and what might be continued barriers to full acceptance.

References

Aiken, L. H., S. P. Clarke, D. M. Sloane, J. A. Sochalski, R. Busse, H. Clarke, P. Giovannetti, J. Hunt, A. M. Rafferty, and J. Shamian. 2001. "Nurses' Reports of Hospital Quality of Care and Working Conditions in Five Countries." *Health Affairs* 20 (3): 43–53.

American Association of Colleges of Nursing. 2017. *Nursing Faculty Shortage.* Accessed November 22, 2017. http://www.aacnnursing.org/News-Information/Fact-Sheets/Nursing-Faculty-Shortage.

Auerbach, David I., Peter I. Buerhaus, and Douglas O. Staiger. 2011. "Registered Nurse Supply Grows Faster Than Projected Amid Surge in New Entrants ages 23–26." *Health Affairs* 30 (12): 2286–92.

Auerbach, David I., Peter I. Buerhaus, and Douglas O. Staiger. 2014. "Registered Nurses Are Delaying Retirement, a Shift That Has Contributed to Recent Growth in the Nurse Workforce." *Health Affairs* 33 (8): 1474–80.

Bureau of Labor Statistics, U.S. Department of Labor. 2017a. *May 2016 National Industry-Specific Occupational Employment and Wage Estimates.* Accessed November 22, 2017. https://www.bls.gov/oes/current/naics2_62.htm#29-0000.

Bureau of Labor Statistics, U.S. Department of Labor. 2017b. *Occupational Outlook Handbook.* Accessed November 22, 2017. https://www.bls.gov/ooh/healthcare/home.htm.

Goldstein, Michael S. 2002. "The Emerging Socioeconomic and Political Support for Alternative Medicine in the United States." *The Annals of the Academy of Political and Social Science* 583 (September): 44–63.

Starr, Paul. 1982. *The Social Transformation of American Medicine.* New York: Basic Books.

U.S. Department of Health and Human Services, Health Resources and Service Administration. 2017. *Supply and Demand Projections of the Nursing Workforce: 2014–2020.* Accessed November 22, 2017. https://bhw.hrsa.gov/sites/default/files/bhw/nchwa/projections/NCHWA_HRSA_Nursing_Report.pdf.

U.S. Department of Health and Human Services, Health Resources and Service Administration. 2008. *The Physician Workforce: Projections and Research Into Current Issues Affecting Supply and Demand.* Accessed February 8, 2012. https://bhw.hrsa.gov/sites/default/files/bhw/nchwa/projections/physiciansupplyissues.pdf.

Weinberg, Dana Beth. 2003. *Code Green: Money-Driven Hospitals and the Dismantling of Nursing.* Ithaca, NY: Cornell University Press.

A CARING DILEMMA

Womanhood and Nursing in Historical Perspective

Susan Reverby

"Do not undervalue [your] particular ability to care," students were reminded at a recent nursing school graduation.[1] Rather than merely bemoaning yet another form of late twentieth-century heartlessness, this admonition underscores the central dilemma of American nursing: The order to care in a society that refuses to value caring. This article is an analysis of the historical creation of that dilemma and its consequences for nursing. To explore the meaning of caring for nursing, it is necessary to unravel the terms of the relationship between nursing and womanhood as these bonds have been formed over the last century.

THE MEANING OF CARING

Many different disciplines have explored the various meanings of caring.[2] Much of this literature, however, runs the danger of universalizing caring as an element in female identity, or as a human quality, separate from the cultural and structural circumstances that create it. But as policy analyst Hilary Graham has argued, caring is not merely an identity; it is also work. As she notes, "Caring touches simultaneously on who you are and what you do."[3] Because of this duality, caring can be difficult to define and even harder to control. Graham's analysis moves beyond seeing caring as a psychological trait; but her focus is primarily on women's unpaid labor in the home. She does not fully discuss how the forms of caring are shaped by the context under which they are practiced. Caring is not just a subjective and material experience; it is a historically created one. Particular circumstances, ideologies, and power relations thus create the conditions under which caring can occur, the forms it

A Caring Dilemma: Womanhood and Nursing in Historical Perspective, Susan Reverby in *Nursing Research*, *36*(1), 5–11, 1987. With permission from Wolters Kluwer Health, Inc.

will take, the consequences it will have for those who do it.

The basis for caring also shapes its effect. Nursing was organized under the expectation that its practitioners would accept a duty to care rather than demand a right to determine how they would satisfy this duty. Nurses were expected to act out of an obligation to care, taking on caring more as an identity than as work, and expressing altruism without thought of autonomy either at the bedside or in their profession. Thus, nurses, like others who perform what is defined as "women's work" in our society, have had to contend with what appears as a dichotomy between the duty to care for others and the right to control their own activities in the name of caring. Nursing is still searching for what philosopher Joel Feinberg argued comes prior to rights, that is, being "recognized as having a claim on rights."[4] The duty to care, organized within the political and economic context of nursing's development, has made it difficult for nurses to obtain this moral and, ultimately, political standing.

Because nurses have been given the duty to care, they are caught in a secondary dilemma: forced to act as if altruism (assumed to be the basis for caring) and autonomy (assumed to be the basis for rights) are separate ways of being. Nurses are still searching for a way to forge a link between altruism and autonomy that will allow them to have what philosopher Larry Blum and others have called "caring-with-autonomy," or what psychiatrist Jean Baker Miller labeled "a way of life that includes serving others without being subservient."[5] Nursing's historical circumstances and ideological underpinnings have made creating this way of life difficult, but not impossible, to achieve.

CARING AS DUTY

A historical analysis of nursing's development makes this theoretical formulation clearer. Most of the writing about American nursing's history begins in the 1870s when formal training for nursing was introduced in the United States. But nursing did not

appear de novo at the end of the nineteenth century. As with most medical and health care, nursing throughout the colonial era and most of the nineteenth century took place within the family and the home. In the domestic pantheon that surrounded "middling" and upper-class American womanhood in the nineteenth century, a woman's caring for friends and relatives was an important pillar. Nursing was often taught by mother to daughter as part of female apprenticeship, or learned by a domestic servant as an additional task on her job. Embedded in the seemingly natural or ordained character of women, it became an important manifestation of women's expression of love of others, and was thus integral to the female sense of self.[6] In a society where deeply felt religious tenets were translated into gendered virtues, domesticity advocate Catharine Beecher declared that the sick were to be "commended" to a "woman's benevolent ministries."[7]

The responsibility for nursing went beyond a mother's duty for her children, a wife's for her husband, or a daughter's for her aging parents. It attached to all the available female family members. The family's "long arm" might reach out at any time to a woman working in a distant city, in a mill, or as a maid, pulling her home to care for the sick, infirm, or newborn. No form of women's labor, paid or unpaid, protected her from this demand. "You may be called upon at any moment," Eliza W. Farrar warned in *The Young Lady's Friend* in 1837, "to attend upon your parents, your brothers, your sisters, or your companions."[8] Nursing was to be, therefore, a woman's duty, not her job. Obligation and love, not the need of work, were to bind the nurse to her patient. Caring was to be an unpaid labor of love.

THE PROFESSED NURSE

Even as Eliza Farrar was proffering her advice, pressures both inward and outward were beginning to reshape the domestic sphere for women of the then-called "middling classes." Women's obligations and work were transformed by the expanding industrial economy and changing cultural assumptions. Parenting took on increasing importance as notions of "moral mothering" filled the domestic arena and other productive labor entered the cash nexus. Female benevolence similarly moved outward as women's charitable efforts took increasingly institutional forms. Duty began to take on new meaning as such women were advised they could fulfill their nursing responsibilities by managing competently those they hired to assist them: Bourgeois female virtue could still be demonstrated as the balance of labor, love, and supervision shifted.[9]

An expanding economy thus had differing effects on women of various classes. For those in the growing urban middle classes, excess cash made it possible to consider hiring a nurse when circumstances, desire, or exhaustion meant a female relative was no longer available for the task. Caring as labor, for these women, could be separated from love.

For older widows or spinsters from the working classes, nursing became a trade they could "profess" relatively easily in the marketplace. A widow who had nursed her husband till his demise, or a domestic servant who had cared for an employer in time of illness, entered casually into the nursing trade, hired by families or individuals unwilling, or unable, to care for their sick alone. The permeable boundaries for women between unpaid and paid labor allowed nursing to pass back and forth when necessary. For many women, nursing thus beckoned as respectable community work.

These "professed" or "natural-born" nurses, as they were known, usually came to their work, as one Boston nurse put it, "laterly" when other forms of employment were closed to them or the lack of any kind of work experience left nursing as an obvious choice. Mehitable Pond Garside, for example, was in her fifties and had outlived two husbands and her children could not, or would not, support her when she came to Boston in the 1840s to nurse. Similarly Alma Frost Merrill, the daughter of a Maine wheelwright, came to Boston in 1818 at nineteen to become a domestic servant. After years as a domestic and seamstress, she declared herself a nurse.[10]

Women like Mehitable Pond Garside and Alma Frost Merrill differed markedly from the Sairy Gamp

character of Dickens' novel, *Martin Chuzzlewit*. Gamp was portrayed as a merely besotted representative of lumpen-proletarian womanhood, who asserted her autonomy by daring to question medical diagnosis, to venture her own opinions (usually outrageous and wrong) at every turn, and to spread disease and superstition in the name of self-knowledge. If they were not Gamps, nurses like Garside and Merrill also were not the healers of some more recent feminist mythology that confounds nursing with midwifery, praising the caring and autonomy these women exerted, but refusing to consider their ignorance.[11] Some professed nurses learned their skills from years of experience, demonstrating the truth of the dictum that "to make a kind and sympathizing nurse, one must have waited, in sickness, upon those she loved dearly."[12] Others, however, blundered badly beyond their capabilities or knowledge. They brought to the bedside only the authority that their personalities and community stature could command: Neither credentials nor a professional identity gave weight to their efforts. Their womanhood, and the experience it gave them, defined their authority and taught them to nurse.

THE HOSPITAL NURSE

Nursing was not limited, however, to the bedside in a home. Although the United States had only 178 hospitals at the first national census in 1873, it was workers labeled "nurses" who provided the caring. As in home-based nursing, the route to hospital nursing was paved more with necessity than with intentionality. In 1875, Eliza Higgins, the matron of Boston's Lying-In Hospital, could not find an extra nurse to cover all the deliveries. In desperation, she moved the hospital laundress up to the nursing position, while a recovering patient took over the wash. Higgins' diaries of her trying years at the Lying-In suggest that such an entry into nursing was not uncommon.[13]

As Higgins' reports and memoirs of other nurses attest, hospital nursing could be the work of devoted women who learned what historian Charles Rosenberg has labeled "ad hoc professionalism," or the temporary and dangerous labor of an ambulatory patient or hospital domestic.[14] As in home-based nursing, both caring and concern were frequently demonstrated. But the nursing work and nurses were mainly characterized by the diversity of their efforts and the unevenness of their skills.

Higgins' memoirs attest to the hospital as a battleground where nurses, physicians, and hospital managers contested the realm of their authority. Nurses continually affirmed their right to control the pace and content of their work, to set their own hours, and to structure their relationships to physicians. Aware that the hospital's paternalistic attitudes and practices toward its "inmates" were attached to the nursing personnel as well, they fought to be treated as workers, "not children," as the Lying-In nurses told Eliza Higgins, and to maintain their autonomous adult status.[15]

Like home-based nursing, hospital nurses had neither formal training nor class status upon which to base their arguments. But their sense of the rights of working-class womanhood gave them authority to press their demands. The necessity to care, and their perception of its importance to patient outcome, also structured their belief that demanding the right to be relatively autonomous was possible. However, their efforts were undermined by the nature of their onerous work, the paternalism of the institutions, class differences between trustees and workers, and ultimately the lack of a defined ideology of caring. Mere resistance to those above them, or contending assertions of rights, could not become the basis for nursing authority.

THE INFLUENCE OF NIGHTINGALE

Much of this changed with the introduction of training for nursing in the hospital world. In the aftermath of Nightingale's triumph over the British Army's medical care system in the Crimea, similar attempts by American women during the Civil War, and the need to find respectable work for daughters of the middling classes, a model and support for nursing

reform began to grow. By 1873, three nursing schools in hospitals in New York, Boston, and New Haven were opened, patterned after the Nightingale School at St. Thomas' Hospital in London.

Nightingale had envisioned nursing as an art, rather than a science, for which women needed to be trained. Her ideas linked her medical and public health notions to her class and religious beliefs. Accepting the Victorian idea of divided spheres of activity for men and women, she thought women had to be trained to nurse through a disciplined process of honing their womanly virtue. Nightingale stressed character development, the laws of health, and strict adherence to orders passed through a female hierarchy. Nursing was built on a model that relied on the concept of duty to provide its basis for authority. Unlike other feminists of the time, she spoke in the language of duty, not rights.

Furthermore, as a nineteenth-century sanitarian, Nightingale never believed in germ theory, in part because she refused to accept a theory of disease etiology that appeared to be morally neutral. Given her sanitarian beliefs, Nightingale thought medical therapeutics and "curing" were of lesser importance to patient outcome, and she willingly left this realm to the physician. Caring, the arena she did think of great importance, she assigned to the nurse. In order to care, a nurse's character, tempered by the fires of training, was to be her greatest skill. Thus, to "feminize" nursing, Nightingale sought a change in the class-defined behavior, not the gender, of the work force.[16]

To forge a good nurse out of the virtues of a good woman and to provide a political base for nursing, Nightingale sought to organize a female hierarchy in which orders passed down from the nursing superintendent to the lowly probationer. This separate female sphere was to share power in the provision of health care with the male-dominated areas of medicine. For many women in the Victorian era, sisterhood and what Carroll Smith-Rosenberg has called "homosocial networks" served to overcome many of the limits of this separate but supposedly equal system of cultural division.[17] Sisterhood, after all, at least in its fictive forms, underlay much of the female power that grew out of women's culture in the nineteenth century. But in nursing, commonalities of the gendered experience could not become the basis of unity since hierarchical filial relations, not equal sisterhood, lay at the basis of nursing's theoretical formulation.

Service, Not Education

Thus, unwittingly, Nightingale's sanitarian ideas and her beliefs about womanhood provided some of the ideological justification for many of the dilemmas that faced American nursing by 1900. Having fought physician and trustee prejudice against the training of nurses in hospitals in the last quarter of the nineteenth century, American nursing reformers succeeded only too well as the new century began. Between 1890 and 1920, the number of nursing schools jumped from 35 to 1,775, and the number of trained nurses from 16 per 100,000 in the population to 141.[18] Administrators quickly realized that opening a "nursing school" provided their hospitals, in exchange for training, with a young, disciplined, and cheap labor force. There was often no difference between the hospital's nursing school and its nursing service. The service needs of the hospital continually overrode the educational requirements of the schools. A student might, therefore, spend weeks on a medical ward if her labor was so needed, but never see the inside of an operating room before her graduation.

Once the nurse finished her training, however, she was unlikely to be hired by a hospital because it relied on either untrained aides or nursing student labor. The majority of graduate nurses, until the end of the 1930s, had to find work in private duty in a patient's home, as the patient's employee in the hospital, in the branches of public health, or in some hospital staff positions. In the world of nursing beyond the training school, "trained" nurses still had to compete with the thousands of "professed" or "practical" nurses who continued to ply their trade in an overcrowded and unregulated marketplace. The title of nurse took on very ambiguous meanings.[19]

The term, "trained nurse," was far from a uniform designation. As nursing leader Isabel Hampton Robb lamented in 1893, "the title 'trained nurse' may mean then anything, everything, or next to nothing."[20]

The exigencies of nursing acutely ill or surgical patients required the sacrifice of coherent educational programs. Didactic, repetitive, watered-down medical lectures by physicians or older nurses were often provided for the students, usually after they finished ten to twelve hours of ward work. Training emphasized the "one right way" of doing ritualized procedures in hopes the students' adherence to specified rules would be least dangerous to patients.[21] Under these circumstances, the duty to care could be followed with a vengeance and become the martinet adherence to orders.

Furthermore, because nursing emphasized training in discipline, order, and practical skills, the abuse of student labor could be rationalized. And because the work force was almost entirely women, altruism, sacrifice, and submission were expected, encouraged, indeed, demanded. Exploitation was inevitable in a field where, until the early 1900s, there were no accepted standards for how much work an average student should do or how many patients she could successfully care for, no mechanisms through which to enforce such standards. After completing her exhaustive and depressing survey of nursing training in 1912, nursing educator M. Adelaide Nutting bluntly pointed out: "Under the present system the school has no life of its own."[22] In this kind of environment, nurses were trained. But they were not educated.

Virtue and Autonomy

It would be a mistake, however, to see the nursing experience only as one of exploitation and the nursing school as a faintly concealed reformatory for the wayward girl in need of discipline. Many nursing superintendents lived the Nightingale ideals as best they could and infused them into their schools. The authoritarian model could and did retemper many women. It instilled in nurses idealism and pride in their skills, somewhat differentiated the trained nurse from the untrained, and protected and aided the sick and dying. It provided a mechanism for virtuous women to contribute to the improvement of humanity by empowering them to care.

For many of the young women entering training in the nineteenth and early twentieth centuries, nursing thus offered something quite special: both a livelihood and a virtuous state. As one nursing educator noted in 1890: "Young strong country girls are drawn into the work by the glamorer [sic] thrown about hospital work and the halo that sanctifies a Nightingale."[23] Thus, in their letters of application, aspiring nursing students expressed their desire for work, independence, and womanly virtue. As with earlier, nontrained nurses, they did not seem to separate autonomy and altruism, but rather sought its linkage through training. Flora Jones spoke for many such women when she wrote the superintendent of Boston City Hospital in 1880, declaring, "I consider myself fitted for the work by inclination and consider it a womanly occupation. It is also necessary for me to become self-supporting and provide for my future."[24] Thus, one nursing superintendent reminded a graduating class in 1904: "You have become self-controlled, unselfish, gentle, compassionate, brave, capable in fact, you have risen from the period of irresponsible girlhood to that of womanhood."[25] For women like Flora Jones, and many of nursing's early leaders, nursing was the singular way to grow to maturity in a womanly profession that offered meaningful work, independence, and altruism.[26]

Altruism, Not Independence

For many, however, as nursing historian Dorothy Sheahan has noted, the training school, "was a place where . . . women learned to be girls."[27] The range of permissible behaviors for respectable women was often narrowed further through training. Independence was to be sacrificed on the altar of altruism. Thus, despite hopes of aspiring students and promises of training school superintendents, nursing rarely united altruism and autonomy. Duty remained the basis for caring.

Some nurses were able to create what they called "a little world of our own." But nursing had neither the financial nor the cultural power to create the separate women's institutions that provided so much of the basis for women's reform and rights efforts.[28] Under these conditions, nurses found it difficult to make the collective transition out of a woman's culture of obligation into an activist assault on the structure and beliefs that oppressed them. Nursing

remained bounded by its ideology and its material circumstances.

THE CONTRADICTIONS OF REFORM

In this context, one begins to understand the difficulties faced by the leaders of nursing reform. Believing that educational reform was central to nursing's professionalizing efforts and clinical improvements, a small group of elite reformers attempted to broaden nursing's scientific content and social outlook. In arguing for an increase in the scientific knowledge necessary in nursing, such leaders were fighting against deep-seated cultural assumptions about male and female "natural" characteristics as embodied in the doctor and nurse. Such sentiments were articulated in the routine platitudes that graced what one nursing leader described as the "doctor homilies" that were a regular feature at nursing graduation exercises.[29]

Not surprisingly, such beliefs were professed by physicians and hospital officials whenever nursing shortages appeared, or nursing groups pushed for higher educational standards or defined nursing as more than assisting the physician. As one nursing educator wrote, with some degree of resignation after the influenza pandemic in 1920: "It is perhaps inevitable that the difficulty of securing nurses during the last year or two should have revived again the old agitation about the 'overtraining' of nurses and the clamor for a cheap worker of the old servant–nurse type."[30]

First Steps Toward Professionalism

The nursing leadership, made up primarily of educators and supervisors with their base within what is now the American Nurses' Association and the National League for Nursing, thus faced a series of dilemmas as they struggled to raise educational standards in the schools and criteria for entry into training, to register nurses once they finished their training, and to gain acceptance for the knowledge base and skills of the nurse. They had to exalt the womanly character, self-abnegation, and service ethic of nursing while insisting on the right of nurses to act in their own self-interest. They had to demand higher wages commensurate with their skills, yet not appear commercial. They had to simultaneously find a way to denounce the exploitation of nursing students, as they made political alliances with hospital physicians and administrators whose support they needed. While they lauded character and sacrifice, they had to find a way to measure it with educational criteria in order to formulate registration laws and set admission standards. They had to make demands and organize, without appearing "unlady-like." In sum, they were forced by the social conditions and ideology surrounding nursing to attempt to professionalize altruism without demanding autonomy.

Undermined by Duty

The image of a higher claim of duty also continually undermined a direct assertion of the right to determine that duty. Whether at a bedside, or at a legislative hearing on practice laws, the duty to care became translated into the demand that nurses merely follow doctors' orders. The tradition of obligation almost made it impossible for nurses to speak about rights at all. By the turn of the century necessity and desire were pulling more young women into the labor force, and the women's movement activists were placing rights at the center of cultural discussion. In this atmosphere, nursing's call to duty was perceived by many as an increasingly antiquated language to shore up a changing economic and cultural landscape. Nursing became a type of collective female grasping for an older form of security and power in the face of rapid change. Women who might have been attracted to nursing in the 1880s as a womanly occupation that provided some form of autonomy, were, by the turn of the century, increasingly looking elsewhere for work and careers.

A DIFFERENT VISION

In the face of these difficulties, the nursing leadership became increasingly defensive and turned on its own rank and file. The educators and supervisors who comprised leadership lost touch with the pressing concern of their constituencies in the daily work world of nursing and the belief systems such nurses continued to hold. Yet many nurses, well into the twentieth century, shared the nineteenth-century vision of nursing as the embodiment of womanly virtue. A nurse named Annette Fiske, for example, although she authored two science books for nurses and had an M.A. degree in classics from Radcliffe College before she entered training, spent her professional career in the 1920s arguing against increasing educational standards. Rather, she called for a reinfusion into nursing of spirituality and service, assuming that this would result in nursing's receiving greater "love and respect and admiration."[31]

Other nurses, especially those trained in the smaller schools or reared to hold working-class ideals about respectable behavior in women, shared Fiske's views. They saw the leadership's efforts at professionalization as an attempt to push them out of nursing. Their adherence to nursing skill measured in womanly virtue was less a conservative and reactionary stance than a belief that seemed to transcend class and educational backgrounds to place itself in the individual character and workplace skills of the nurse. It grounded altruism in supposedly natural and spiritual, rather than educational and middle-class, soil. For Fiske and many other nurses, nursing was still a womanly art that required inherent character in its practitioners and training in practical skills and spiritual values in its schools. Their beliefs about nursing did not require the professionalization of altruism, nor the demand for autonomy either at the bedside or in control over the professionalization process.

Still other nurses took a more pragmatic viewpoint that built on their pride in their work-place skills and character. These nurses also saw the necessity for concerted action, not unlike that taken by other American workers. Such nurses fought against what one 1888 nurse, who called herself Candor, characterized as the "missionary spirit . . . [of] self-immolation" that denied that nurses worked because they had to make a living.[32] These worker-nurses saw no contradiction between demanding decent wages and conditions for their labors and being of service for those in need. But the efforts of various groups of these kinds of nurses to turn to hours' legislation, trade union activity, or mutual aid associations were criticized and condemned by the nursing leadership. Their letters were often edited out of the nursing journals, and their voices silenced in public meetings as they were denounced as being commercial, or lacking in proper womanly devotion.[33]

In the face of continual criticism from nursing's professional leadership, the worker-nurses took on an increasingly angry and defensive tone. Aware that their sense of the nurse's skills came from the experiences of the work place, not book learning or degrees, they had to assert this position despite continued hostility toward such a basis of nursing authority.[34] Although the position of women like Candor helped articulate a way for nurses to begin to assert the right to care, it did not constitute a full-blown ideological counterpart to the overwhelming power of the belief in duty.

The Persistence of Dilemmas

By midcentury, the disputes between worker-nurses and the professional leadership began to take on new forms, although the persistent divisions continued. Aware that some kind of collective bargaining was necessary to keep nurses out of the unions and in the professional associations, the ANA reluctantly agreed in 1946 to let its state units act as bargaining agents. The nursing leadership has continued to look at educational reform strategies, now primarily taking the form of legislating for the B.S. degree as the credential necessary for entry into nursing practice, and to changes in the practice laws that will allow increasingly skilled nurses the autonomy and status they deserve. Many nurses have continued to be critical of this educational strategy, to ignore the professional associations, or to leave nursing altogether.

In their various practice fields nurses still need a viable ideology and strategy that will help them adjust to the continual demands of patients and an ever more bureaucratized, cost-conscious, and rationalized work setting. For many nurses it is still, in an ideological sense, the nineteenth century. Even for those nurses who work as practitioners in the more autonomous settings of health maintenance organizations or public health offices, the legacy of nursing's heritage is still felt. Within the last two years, for example, the Massachusetts Board of Medicine tried to push through a regulation that health practitioners acknowledge their dependence on physicians by wearing a badge that identified their supervising physician and stated that they were not doctors.

Nurses have tried various ways to articulate a series of rights that allow them to care. The acknowledgment of responsibilities, however, so deeply ingrained in nursing and American womanhood, as nursing school dean Claire Fagin has noted, continually drown out the nurse's assertion of rights.[35]

Nurses are continuing to struggle to obtain the right to claim rights. Nursing's educational philosophy, ideological underpinnings, and structural position have made it difficult to create the circumstances within which to gain such recognition. It is not a lack of vision that thwarts nursing, but the lack of power to give that vision substantive form.[36]

BEYOND THE OBLIGATION TO CARE

Much has changed in nursing in the last forty years. The severing of nursing education from the hospital's nursing service has finally taken place, as the majority of nurses are now educated in colleges, not hospital-based diploma schools. Hospitals are experimenting with numerous ways to organize the nursing service to provide the nurse with more responsibility and sense of control over the nursing care process. The increasingly technical and machine-aided nature of hospital-based health care has made nurses feel more skilled.

In many ways, however, little has changed. Nursing is still divided over what counts as a nursing skill, how it is to be learned, and whether a nurse's character can be measured in educational criteria. Technical knowledge and capabilities do not easily translate into power and control. Hospitals, seeking to cut costs, have forced nurses to play "beat the clock" as they run from task to task in an increasingly fragmented setting.[37]

Nursing continues to struggle with the basis for, and the value of, caring. The fact that the first legal case on comparable worth was brought by a group of Denver nurses suggests nursing has an important and ongoing role in the political effort to have caring revalued. As in the Denver case, contemporary feminism has provided some nurses with the grounds on which to claim rights from their caring.[38]

Feminism, in its liberal form, appears to give nursing a political language that argues for equality and rights within the given order of things. It suggests a basis for caring that stresses individual discretion and values, acknowledging that the nurses' right to care should be given equal consideration with the physician's right to cure. Just as liberal political theory undermined more paternalistic formulations of government, classical liberalism's tenets applied to women have much to offer nursing. The demand for the right to care questions deeply held beliefs about gendered relations in the health care hierarchy and the structure of the hierarchy itself.

Many nurses continue to hope that with more education, explicit theories to explain the scientific basis for nursing, new skills, and a lot of assertiveness training, nursing will change. As these nurses try to shed the image of the nurse's being ordered to care, however, the admonition to care at a graduation speech has to be made. Unable to find a way to "care with autonomy" and unable to separate caring from its valuing and basis, many nurses find themselves forced to abandon the effort to care, or nursing altogether.

ALTRUISM WITH AUTONOMY

These dilemmas for nurses suggest the constraints that surround the effectiveness of a liberal feminist

political strategy to address the problems of caring and, therefore, of nursing. The individualism and autonomy of a rights framework often fail to acknowledge collective social need, to provide a way for adjudicating conflicts over rights, or to address the reasons for the devaluing of female activity.[39] Thus, nurses have often rejected liberal feminism, not just out of their oppression and "false consciousness," but because of some deep understandings of the limited promise of equality and autonomy in a health care system they see as flawed and harmful. In an often inchoate way, such nurses recognize that those who claim the autonomy of rights often run the risk of rejecting altruism and caring itself.

Several feminist psychologists have suggested that what women really want in their lives is autonomy with connectedness. Similarly, many modern moral philosophers are trying to articulate a formal modern theory that values the emotions and the importance of relationships.[40] For nursing, this will require the creation of the conditions under which it is possible to value caring and to understand that the empowerment of others does not have to require self-immolation. To achieve this, nurses will have both to create a new political understanding for the basis of caring and to find ways to gain the power to implement it. Nursing can do much to have this happen through research on the importance of caring on patient outcome, studies of patient improvements in nursing settings where the right to care is created, or implementing nursing control of caring through a bargaining agreement. But nurses cannot do this alone. The dilemma of nursing is too tied to society's broader problems of gender and class to be solved solely by the political or professional efforts of one occupational group.

Nor are nurses alone in benefiting from such an effort. If nursing can achieve the power to practice altruism with autonomy, all of us have much to gain. Nursing has always been a much conflicted metaphor in our culture, reflecting all the ambivalences we give to the meaning of womanhood.[41] Perhaps in the future it can give this metaphor and, ultimately, caring, new value in all our lives.

Notes

This selection is based on the author's book, *Ordered to Care: The Dilemma of American Nursing,* published in 1987 by Cambridge University Press, New York.

1. Gregory Witcher, "Last Class of Nurses Told: Don't Stop Caring," *Boston Globe,* May 13, 1985, pp. 17–18.

2. See, for examples, Larry Blum et al., "Altruism and Women's Oppression," in *Women and Philosophy,* eds. Carol Gould and Marx Wartofsy (New York: G.P. Putnam's, 1976), pp. 222–247; Nel Noddings, *Caring.* Berkeley: University of California Press, 1984; Nancy Chodorow, *The Reproduction of Mothering.* Berkeley: University of California Press, 1978; Carol Gilligan, *In a Different Voice.* Cambridge: Harvard University Press, 1982; and Janet Finch and Dulcie Groves, eds., *A Labour of Love, Women, Work and Caring.* London and Boston: Routledge, Kegan Paul, 1983.

3. Hilary Graham, "Caring: A Labour of Love," in *A Labour of Love,* eds. Finch and Groves, pp. 13–30.

4. Joel Feinberg, *Rights, Justice and the Bounds of Liberty* (Princeton: Princeton University Press, 1980), p. 141.

5. Blum et al., "Altruism and Women's Oppression," p. 223; Jean Baker Miller, *Toward a New Psychology of Women* (Boston: Beacon Press, 1976), p. 71.

6. Ibid; see also Iris Marion Young, "Is Male Gender Identity the Cause of Male Domination," in *Mothering: Essays in Feminist Theory,* ed. Joyce Trebicott (Totowa, NJ: Rowman and Allanheld, 1983), pp. 129–146.

7. Catherine Beecher, *Domestic Receipt-Book* (New York: Harper and Brothers, 1846) p. 214.

8. Eliza Farrar, *The Young Lady's Friend By a Lady* (Boston: American Stationer's Co., 1837), p. 57.

9. Catherine Beecher, *Miss Beecher's Housekeeper and Healthkeeper.* New York: Harper and Brothers, 1876; and Sarah Josepha Hale, *The Good Housekeeper.* Boston: Otis Brothers and Co., 7th edition, 1844. See also Susan Strasser, *Never Done: A History of Housework.* New York: Pantheon, 1982.

10. Cases 2 and 18, "Admissions Committee Records," Volume I, Box 11, Home for Aged Women Collection, Schlesinger Library, Radcliffe College, Cambridge, Mass. Data on the nurses admitted to the home were also found in "Records of Inmates, 1858–1901," "Records of Admission, 1873–1924," and "Records of Inmates, 1901–1916," all in Box 11.

11. Charles Dickens, *Martin Chuzzlewit.* New York: New American Library, 1965, original edition, London: 1865; Barbara Ehrenreich and Deirdre English, *Witches, Nurses, Midwives: A History of Women Healers.* Old Westbury: Glass Mountain Pamphlets, 1972.

12. Virginia Penny, *The Employments of Women: A Cyclopedia of Women's Work* (Boston: Walker, Wise, and Co., 1863), p. 420.

13. Eliza Higgins, Boston Lying-In Hospital, *Matron's Journals,* 1873–1889, Volume I, January 9, 1875, February 22, 1875, Rare Books Room, Countway Medical Library, Harvard Medical School, Boston, Mass.

14. Charles Rosenberg, "'And Heal the Sick': The Hospital and the Patient in 19th Century America," *Journal of Social History* 10 (June 1977):445.

15. Higgins, *Matron's Journals,* Volume II, January 11, 1876, and July 1, 1876. See also a parallel discussion of male artisan behavior

in front of the boss in David Montgomery, "Workers' Control of Machine Production in the 19th Century," *Labor History* 17 (Winter 1976):485–509.

16. The discussion of Florence Nightingale is based on my analysis in *Ordered to Care*, chapter 3. See also Charles E. Rosenberg, "Florence Nightingale on Contagion: The Hospital as Moral Universe," in *Healing and History*, ed. Charles E. Rosenberg. New York: Science History Publications, 1979.

17. Carroll Smith-Rosenberg, "The Female World of Love and Ritual," *Signs: Journal of Women in Culture and Society* 1 (Autumn 1975):1.

18. May Ayers Burgess, *Nurses, Patients and Pocketbooks*. New York: Committee on the Grading of Nursing, 1926, reprint edition (New York: Garland Publishing Co, 1985), pp. 36–37.

19. For further discussion of the dilemmas of private duty nursing, see Susan Reverby, "'Neither for the Drawing Room nor for the Kitchen': Private Duty Nursing, 1880–1920," in *Women and Health in America,* ed. Judith Walzer Leavitt. Madison: University of Wisconsin Press, 1984, and Susan Reverby, "'Something Besides Waiting': The Politics of Private Duty Nursing Reform in the Depression," in *Nursing History: New Perspectives, New Possibilities*, ed. Ellen Condliffe Lagemann. New York: Teachers College Press, 1982.

20. Isabel Hampton Robb, "Educational Standards for Nurses," in *Nursing of the Sick 1893* (New York: McGraw-Hill, 1949), p. 11. See also Janet Wilson James, "Isabel Hampton and the Professionalization of Nursing in the 1890s," in *The Therapeutic Revolution*, eds. Morris Vogel and Charles E. Rosenberg. Philadelphia: University of Pennsylvania Press, 1979.

21. For further discussion of the difficulties in training, see JoAnn Ashley, *Hospitals,*

Paternalism and the Role of the Nurse. New York: Teachers College Press, 1976, and Reverby, *Ordered to Care,* chapter 4.

22. *Educational Status of Nursing*, Bureau of Education Bulletin Number 7, Whole Number 475 (Washington, D.C.: Government Printing Office, 1912), p. 49.

23. Julia Wells, "Do Hospitals Fit Nurses for Private Nursing," *Trained Nurse and Hospital Review* 3 (March 1890):98.

24. Boston City Hospital (BCH) Training School Records, Box 4, Folder 4, Student 4, February 14, 1880, BCH Training School Papers, Nursing Archives, Special Collections, Boston University, Mugar Library, Boston, Mass. The student's name has been changed to maintain confidentiality.

25. Mary Agnes Snively, "What Manner of Women Ought Nurses To Be?" *American Journal of Nursing* 4 (August 1904):838.

26. For a discussion of many of the early nursing leaders as "new women," see Susan Armeny, "'We Were the New Women': A Comparison of Nurses and Women Physicians, 1890–1915." Paper presented at the American Association for the History of Nursing Conference, University of Virginia, Charlottesville, Va., October 1984.

27. Dorothy Sheahan, "Influence of Occupational Sponsorship on the Professional Development of Nursing." Paper presented at the Rockefeller Archives Conference on the History of Nursing, Rockefeller Archives, Tarrytown, NY, May 1981, p. 12.

28. Estelle Freedman, "Separatism as Strategy: Female Institution Building and American Feminism, 1870–1930," *Feminist Studies* 5 (Fall 1979):512–529.

29. Lavinia L. Dock, *A History of Nursing*, volume 3 (New York: G.P. Putnam's, 1912), p. 136.

30. Isabel M. Stewart, "Progress in Nursing Education during 1919," *Modern Hospital* 14 (March 1920):183.

31. Annette Fiske, "How Can We Counteract the Prevailing Tendency to Commercialism in Nursing?" *Proceedings of the 17th Annual Meeting of the Massachusetts State Nurses' Association,* p. 8, Massachusetts Nurses Association Papers, Box 7, Nursing Archives.

32. Candor, "Work and Wages," Letter to the Editor, *Trained Nurse and Hospital Review* 2 (April 1888):167–168.

33. See the discussion in Ashley, *Hospitals, Paternalism and the Role of the Nurse,* pp. 40–43, 46–48, 51, and in Barbara Melosh, *"The Physician's Hand": Work Culture and Conflict in American Nursing* (Philadelphia: Temple University Press, 1982), passim.

34. For further discussion see Susan Armeny, "Resolute Enthusiasts: The Effort to Professionalize American Nursing, 1880–1915." PhD dissertation, University of Missouri, Columbia, Mo., 1984, and Reverby, *Ordered to Care,* chapter 6.

35. Feinberg, *Rights,* pp. 130–142; Claire Fagin, "Nurses' Rights," *American Journal of Nursing* 75 (January 1975):82.

36. For a similar argument for bourgeois women, see Carroll Smith-Rosenberg, "The New Woman as Androgyne: Social Disorder and Gender Crisis," in *Disorderly Conduct* (New York: Alfred Knopf, 1985), p. 296.

37. Boston Nurses' Group, "The False Promise: Professionalism in Nursing," *Science for the People* 10 (May/June 1978):20–34; Jennifer Bingham Hull, "Hospital Nightmare: Cuts in Staff Demoralize Nurses as Care Suffers," *Wall Street Journal,* March 27, 1985.

38. Bonnie Bullough, "The Struggle for Women's Rights in Denver: A Personal Account," *Nursing Outlook* 26 (September 1978): 566–567.

39. For critiques of liberal feminism see Allison M. Jagger, *Feminist Politics and Human Nature* (Totowa, NJ: Rowman and Allanheld, 1983), pp. 27–50, 173, 206; Zillah Eisenstein, *The Radical Future of Liberal Feminism.* New York and London: Longman, 1981; and Rosalind Pollack Petchesky, *Abortion and Women's Choice* (Boston: Northeastern University Press, 1984), pp. 1–24.

40. Miller, *Toward A New Psychology;* Jane Flax, "The Conflict Between Nurturance and Autonomy in Mother-Daughter Relationships and within Feminism," *Feminist Studies* 4 (June 1978):171–191; Blum et al., "Altruism and Women's Oppression."

41. Claire Fagin and Donna Diers, "Nursing as Metaphor," *New England Journal of Medicine* 309 (July 14, 1983): 116–117.

22

FROM QUACKERY TO "COMPLEMENTARY" MEDICINE

The American Medical Profession Confronts Alternative Therapies

Terri A. Winnick

Medical practices outside the orthodoxy can be referred to and defined in a number of ways. While some still call them "quackery" (Barrett and Jarvis 1993; Dawkins 2003) or, less derisively, "unorthodox" or "unconventional" therapies, the current custom among researchers is to refer to treatments such as acupuncture, chiropractic, homeopathy, naturopathy, and herbal remedies collectively as "complementary and alternative medicine" or CAM. The term CAM acknowledges both their disjuncture or lack of "conformity with the standards of the medical community" (Eisenberg et al. 1993:246), and the simultaneous growth of public acceptance and their integration into conventional treatment regimens.

Almost half of Americans have tried some type of CAM. Visits to CAM practitioners have eclipsed visits to primary care physicians, with expenditures for these treatments in 1997 estimated at approximately $27 billion (Eisenberg et al. 1989). Articles on CAM referenced in Medline in 1996 represented about 10 percent of scientific articles in the medical literature (Barnes et al. 1999). In November 1998, an entire issue of the *Journal of the American Medical Association* (*JAMA*) was dedicated to CAM, and included several articles presenting the results of randomized controlled trials. As Michael S. Goldstein (1999) cogently observes, CAM "has taken on a significant and growing presence in America" (p. 8).

This article examines the medical profession's reaction to CAM in general, with a focus on the last three and a half decades of the twentieth century, and on the strategies used during that period to block, control, and finally manage the threat that CAM posed. To supply the historical context for this discussion, I first briefly review the nineteenth-century conflict between a medical sect known as "allopathy" (or "regular" medicine) and competing sects such as homeopathy, eclecticism, osteopathy, and others. I show how the ultimate outcome of the struggle between these groups was the development of a state-sanctioned medical monopoly. I then draw upon theories of professionalization in order to explain professional dominance as a political achievement, enabled by optimum structural arrangements that favored regular medicine over competing paradigms of care, that in fact contributed to the demise or marginalization of competing groups. I then consider the meaning of these competing groups' reemergence in terms of professional dominance, and use the medical profession's confrontation with CAM as a lens with which to view continued professional evolution. The analysis of the medical profession's response to CAM is presented in three stages, distinct in the type of strategies that were employed in order to sustain dominance. Stage one involved obstructionism and attempts to enlist institutional allies. Stage two involved reassessment, reorganization, and coming to terms with CAM's popularity. In the third stage CAM therapies were drawn into the medical mainstream and controlled through exposure to scientific scrutiny and adoption by regular practitioners. Future relations between the medical profession and CAM are also considered.

Data are gleaned from coverage of CAM in five of the most prestigious medical journals between 1965 and 1999, a period of intense reorganization within medicine. A sample of the editorials, features, and scientific articles contained in this literature are content-analyzed in order to gain a deeper understanding of the opinions, concerns, and policy suggestions made by editors and other writers who chose to submit documents for the edification of their peers. While not necessarily reflecting the typical practitioner's point of view, this discourse portrays professional concerns at high levels of influence.

HISTORICAL CONTEXT

Allopaths, or regular doctors, were one of a number of medical sects vying for professional dominance throughout the nineteenth century. The term "allopath" was coined by Samuel Hahnemann, the founder of a competing medical sect known as homeopathy, to differentiate physicians who subscribed to a homeopathic philosophy from those who did not (Kaufman 1971). Where homeopaths treated illness by prescribing an infinitesimal dose of a substance that could provoke similar symptoms in a well person in order to stimulate the body's immune response, allopaths were more likely to treat illness with "heroic" measures such as bleeding, blistering, and purging with emetics or strong laxatives. Other sects, such as the Thomsonians (later called the eclectics) and naturopaths favored botanical remedies, while osteopaths introduced spinal manipulation (Rothstein 1972). A number of other treatments were also practiced, among them mesmerism, hydrotherapy, and finally chiropractic, a sect founded in the last years of the nineteenth century (Wardwell 1994).

Regular practitioners insisted that their philosophy alone was based on science, even though their practices at that time were no more scientific than their competitors. What mattered, however, was their *claim* to science, which, as Wolpe (1999) points out, allowed allopathy or regular medicine to "create a monopoly over definitions of what is scientific" (p. 224). As the sole arbiter of science, regular medicine was able to blithely dismiss competing philosophies and treatments as unscientific. More importantly, they were also able to align themselves with the state and seek its protection over their work. The state, persuaded by the profession to act in the public interest, limited funding of medical education to regular schools, and passed licensing laws restricting "irregular" practice (Pescosolido and Boyer 2001). Bolstered by these favorable institutional arrangements, regular medicine professionalized rapidly, building schools, hospitals, and a strong professional organization (Wolpe 1999). By the early part of the twentieth century, regular medicine had managed to gain monopolistic control over medical practice (Starr 1982) and to maintain this dominant position up until the 1960s, a period known as "the era of professional dominance" (Freidson 1970) or, more descriptively, as "the golden age of doctoring" (McKinlay and Marceau 2002; Pescosolido and Boyer 2001).

While some practitioners, such as hydrotherapists and midwives, either fell out of favor or were legislated nearly out of existence (Gevitz 1988; Wertz and Wertz 1989), eclectics, homeopaths, and osteopaths merged with regular medicine. They merged because their philosophies by century's end had converged to where they were nearly indistinguishable, given that regular medicine had abandoned "heroic" treatments for more scientifically-based treatments and integrated many of their competitors' approaches. Each of these sects also shared a mutual desire to enhance power through unification under the increasingly powerful umbrella of the American Medical Association (AMA) (Rothstein 1972).

Chiropractic was a late-nineteenth-century upstart, begun in 1895 by D. D. Palmer who believed that all illness was caused by a misalignment of the spine. Chiropractic offered a genuine alternative to the emerging orthodoxy. Unlike other medical sects whose philosophies had become more congruent with regular medicine, chiropractic was not folded into the AMA, nor did it disappear. Although certainly marginalized by the dominant profession, chiropractors survived by serving patients of lower-status who were often dissatisfied, and hence troublesome and time-consuming, while at the same time providing justification for regular medicine's claims to superiority (Firman and Goldstein 1975). By the 1970s, chiropractors had managed to establish for themselves a limited but independent profession with its own system of education, licensing, and inclusion in government-funded health insurance. Other CAM groups, notably acupuncturists, naturopaths, homeopaths, and massage therapists, have recently begun to follow suit. Regular medicine retains its

dominant position, but within the last few decades there has been a resurgence of unconventional treatments and practitioners.

In the analysis presented here, I illustrate the ways in which the medical profession responded to CAM. Their first reaction involved condemnation and attempts to obstruct CAM. Failing that, their next response was reassessment, where they struggled to come to terms with CAM and its growing popularity. Next came integration, where they found a way to work around and with CAM. In doing so, the profession finally moved beyond the threat that CAM posed and emerged, secure in their dominant position. Each phase was an adaptive response to the challenges that the medical profession faced, each adaptive response employed strategies suited to the climate of the medical marketplace at that time, and each strategy was intended to help the dominant profession sustain its position.

One way to enhance our understanding of professional change processes is to examine what is said about CAM within the professional literature. This literature (medical journals) reflects the official view of the profession. In this capacity, the journals have the potential, and often the mission, to educate and direct their readers. The critical role of journals in influencing medical practitioners makes journals an ideal venue from which to better understand the response of the medical profession to the rise of CAM, as well as the utility of the strategies the profession adopted to deal with the threat that CAM posed.

DATA AND METHODS

The data set consists of citations for all documents on CAM published in five top general medical journals (*JAMA, the New England Journal of Medicine, the American Journal of Medicine, Annals of Internal Medicine,* and *Archives of Internal Medicine*) over a 35-year period (1965–1999). These journals are among the most prestigious, widely read, and influential medical journals in the United States (Garfield 1999).[1] They are likely to be of continuing general interest to a broad spectrum of practicing physicians. The period from 1965 to 1999 was chosen because it represents a period of substantial change within medicine. During this time, "the golden age of doctoring" drew to a close, "the health care crisis" ensued, and "the era of managed care" commenced, with all the concomitant changes (Pescosolido and Boyer 2001). These changes provide a frame of reference in these analyses, following the premise that historical landmarks are important to consider in time-ordered analyses (Griffin and Isaac 1992; Isaac and Griffin 1989).

Citations were collected from two main sources: *Medline* databases and the *Cumulated Index Medicus*. In order to be as comprehensive as possible, CAM was broadly defined, and categories searched were: acupuncture, alternative medicine, amygdalin (Laetrile), ayurvedic, Chinese herbal drugs, chiropractic, herbs, herbal medicine, holistic health, homeopathy, indigenous health services, Oriental medicine, primitive (later traditional) medicine, midwifery naturopathy, and quackery.[2] These categories satisfy the criteria established by David M. Eisenberg and associates (1993) as treatments outside the purview of conventional medicine and capture temporal trends in interest and changes in nomenclature.[3] Citations for all types of documents (i.e., scientific articles, editorials, commentaries, news reports and other features, letters, and replies) were included. Together these journals furnished approximately 700 separate citations for documents on CAM ($N = 699$). These citations were listed sequentially, counted, and plotted by year in order to examine the overall trend in coverage (see Figure 22.1).

FINDINGS

Trends in the Amount and Nature of Attention to CAM

Coverage of CAM varied over time and across modality. Figure 22.1 displays the trend in the total number of citations for documents on CAM in these five journals ($N = 699$) between 1965 and 1999. This figure shows a steady stream of attention to CAM throughout the period, with the most notable and dramatic increase occurring during the 1990s when the Office of Alternative Medicine (OAM) was established, powerfully legitimating these remedies, and patient utilization of CAM surged (Eisenberg et al. 1998). Figure 22.2 partially disaggregates the overall trend by displaying trends in citations over time for the four CAM modalities most frequently discussed in the subsample ($n = 102$) selected for content analysis. This figure illustrates that when broken down by modality, this attention is relatively specific and periodic in nature, with interest corresponding to structurally important historical events.

Rising interest in chiropractic during the late 1960s and early 1970s corresponds to the licensure of chiropractic in the final three uncommitted states and inclusion in Medicare and Medicaid during that period. The amount of attention persists to a lesser degree throughout the 1980s as the *Wilk v. American Medical Association* (AMA) anti-trust suit went through a series of appeals before it was finally decided in favor of chiropractors in 1987.[4] The *Wilk* case marked the end of an AMA policy banning interprofessional relationships and an official shift in attitude toward these competitors (Dossey and Swyers 1994; Johnson 1988; Wardwell 1992). Attention to Chinese (then called "Oriental") medicine developed in the early 1970s, coinciding with the publicity surrounding the opening of political relations with China, and it remained fairly steady throughout the period examined. Interest in Laetrile treatment for cancer was quite discontinuous, with a surge of attention arising during the late 1970s and early 1980s, and no discussion thereafter. Interest in herbal medicine was not particularly strong during the early period, but rapidly increased during the 1990s, after the Food and Drug Administration (FDA) condoned the marketing of over-the-counter herbal medications as dietary supplements beneficial to specific health ailments. Note that discussion of all modalities except Laetrile treatment rises sharply following the establishment of the OAM in 1992. As Figures 21.1 and 21.2 demonstrate, increased coverage of CAM corresponded to structural events. As the content analysis will show, these events helped shape the profession's response.

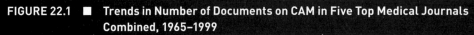

FIGURE 22.1 ■ **Trends in Number of Documents on CAM in Five Top Medical Journals Combined, 1965–1999**

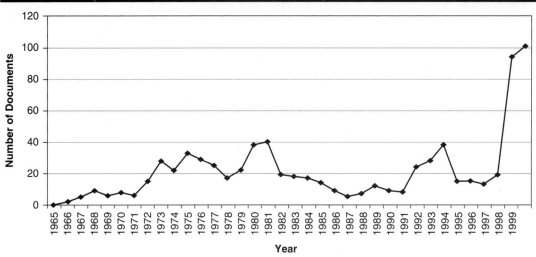

FIGURE 22.2 ■ **Trends in Coverage of Four Most Frequently Discussed CAM Modalities (1965–1999)**

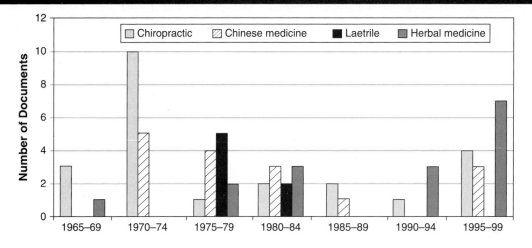

CONTENT ANALYSIS

An examination of the content of the documents reveals a qualitative difference between the types of articles published in the beginning of the period and those published near the end. As displayed in Table 22.1, early readers of these journals primarily learned about CAM through editorials, while later readers received information from a number of sources, including scientific reports. Another notable difference is that of tone quality. While tone is a stylistic artifact of the type of article written, differences exceed obvious stylistic dissimilarities between editorials and scientific reports. Articles written in

TABLE 22.1 ■ Distribution of Editorials, Scientific Research Articles, and Other Types of Articles Among the Sample of Documents on CAM in Five Top Medical Journals, 1965–1999

	Editorials and Commentaries		Scientific Research Articles		Other Types of Articles[a]		Total Sample	
Year	n	%	n	%	n	%	n	%
1965–1969	5	62.5	0	23.8	3	37.5	8	100
1970–1974	14	82.5	0	6.3	3	17.6	17	100
1975–1979	10	47.6	5	12.5	6	28.6	21	100
1980–1984	8	50.0	1	25.9	7	43.8	16	100
1985–1989	2	40.0	0	13.7	3	60.0	5	100
1990–1994	3	37.5	1		4	50.0	8	100
1995–1999	9	33.3	7		11	40.7	27	100
1965–1999	51	50	14		37	36.3	102	100

[a]Other types of articles include case studies, reports, features such as "Law in Medicine," "Medicine Abroad," and "When Friends or Patients Ask About. . . ."

the early period employ a bitingly negative, almost combative tone, while later articles discuss CAM with objective disinterest.

In the next sections, data from the content analysis are presented. Each section describes a relatively distinct phase in the relations between the medical profession and CAM. These phases somewhat overlap with the periods identified by Pescosolido and Boyer (2001) as periods when the medical profession was beset by challenges on other fronts. As gleaned from these documents, during each phase, the medical profession responded in a different way to CAM, with the response related to the shifting structural milieu. Each phase is roughly demarcated by time, tone, and focus. The first phase, *condemnation,* lasted from the mid-1960s through the early 1970s, coinciding with the golden age of doctoring. In this phase, spokespersons for the profession were arrogant and insulting, expressing sharp disapproval of these therapies, exaggerating their risks, and making preposterous the idea of anyone using these treatments. In the next phase, *reassessment,* during the period of health care crisis from the mid-1970s through the early 1990s, authors were more introspective. Spokespersons for the profession examined relations with patients and shortcomings in treatment in an effort to

understand the public's attraction to this phenomenon, an attraction confirmed by utilization studies attesting to the popularity of CAM. The last phase, *integration,* during the era of managed care that lasted throughout the 1990s, saw a shift toward greater tolerance of CAM in a more pluralistic medical marketplace. Content analyses reveal a general abandonment of efforts to outlaw or regulate CAM by legal means. Physicians were encouraged to "work around" CAM by becoming knowledgeable enough to help guide and manage patients using these therapies. Scientific testing, facilitated by the establishment of the OAM, became the predominant means of control.

THE CONDEMNATION PHASE

In articles published in these journals in the late 1960s and early 1970s, CAM and chiropractic were all but synonymous. Although these journals featured some articles on indigenous medicine, and often heralded indigenous practitioners for delivering at least rudimentary health care to remote populations abroad (Sidell 1968), there is little evidence that they were regarded as a threat. In this sample, Chinese medicine or acupuncture was written about as something practiced by the Chinese—in China (Sidell 1972, 1975)—and when discussed as a treatment modality, largely was dismissed (Gaw, Chang, and Shaw 1975; Lee et al. 1975). Chiropractic, however, was a different story. In days when treatment with acupuncture needles was still astonishing Western observers, chiropractors were rapidly becoming entrenched within the medical marketplace and constituting a genuine threat. Marginalized by the AMA since the late nineteenth century, chiropractors had achieved licensing in all 50 states and Medicaid reimbursement by the early 1970s, and were on the cusp of being included in Medicare and some private insurance plans (Wardwell 1992). Since, as Susan Olzak (1992) has shown, conflicts between more and less dominant groups intensify only as less dominant groups grow stronger, it is logical that chiropractic would be seen in a different light, for chiropractors as a group were stronger and better organized than other types of CAM.

Condemnation spiked with ridicule was the first tactic in the strategy aimed at eliminating CAM. Authors used words like "quackery" and "dangerous cult," especially when referring to chiropractic, and explicitly claimed that these practices were harmful. In an editorial with the unequivocal title "Chiropractic CONDEMNED," the author (JAMA 1969) reminded readers that, according to the official policy statement of the AMA, "chiropractic constitutes a hazard to rational health care in the United States" (p. 352). Another author (Casterline 1972) suggested somewhat facetiously that since chiropractic treatment and smoking cigarettes were equally hazardous, chiropractors should be required to post warnings in their offices similar to the warnings posted on packages of cigarettes:

> Warning: The Department of Health, Education and Welfare Has Determined That the Chiropractic Method (Unscientific Cultism) is Dangerous to Your Health. (p. 1009)

But the mocking carried an underlying theme of danger, allowing one spokesperson for the profession

(JAMA 1969) to frame his or her concern in terms of "protect[ing] the public health" (p. 352).

The second tactic consisted of issuing dire warnings aimed at practitioners who would then "forcefully [bring them] to the attention of the healthcare consumer and those in government responsible for the laws" (Wilbur 1971:1307), in order to scare the public away from these treatments. Readers of these journals learned that 12 persons suffered strokes "related to chiropractic manipulation" (Miller and Burton 1974:190), and a legal expert twice (Holder 1972, 1973) discussed the criminal liability a physician might face in the event a patient dies at the hands of a chiropractor. Although dire warnings primarily centered on spinal manipulation in this sample, other types of non-conventional treatment were also deemed extremely hazardous, if not deadly.[5] Within these pages Paul Sherlock and Edmond O. Rothschild (1967) reported that the Zen macrobiotic diet was a "threat to life" based upon the case of one strict adherent who developed "classic manifestations of scurvy and severe folic acid deficiency" (p. 130) as a result. Chelation therapy for arteriosclerosis was deemed experimental and potentially dangerous (Soffer 1977), and Laetrile was disparaged as an ineffective, potentially deadly drug, one that hastens a cancer patient's inevitable demise (Sadoff, Fuchs, and Hollander 1978).[6] That CAM would replace conventional (or "appropriate") treatment was another peril frequently mentioned (JAMA 1969:352). The hazard to the patient was that he or she would avoid conventional treatment in the early, treatable stages of a serious or life-threatening disease, choosing instead to self-medicate or frequent a CAM practitioner, and only turn to conventional care when terminally ill (Sherlock and Rothschild 1967; Soffer 1977; Wilbur 1971).

However likely or unlikely the risks described, they supplied justification for the third tactic: political action. As one author (JAMA 1972) reminded readers, the AMA in its history had "successfully dealt with secret-formula nostrums," had "put diploma mills out of business," and would now to do everything in its power to "expose the charlatanism of chiropractic" (p. 914) and to hinder their professional progress.

As gleaned from the content of these documents, during the late 1960s members of the AMA persuaded Congress to order the U.S. Department of Health, Education, and Welfare to investigate chiropractic. The outcome of this investigation was a report, described approvingly by the author (JAMA 1969) as a "devastating indictment of chiropractic" (p. 352), recommending that Medicare coverage not extend to chiropractic service. This report prompted calls for task forces to lobby for a "legislative amendment" to rescind Medicaid coverage of chiropractic in states with these benefits already in place and to prohibit Medicare benefits entirely (JAMA 1970:1481). Other initiatives included "an orderly program for withdrawal of chiropractic licenses" (Sabatier 1969:1712), or, failing that, licenses made contingent upon chiropractors having met "the same standards of education and training as those licensed to practice medicine" (Casterline 1972:1009).

It is not surprising that the medical profession, long accustomed to state protection of its monopoly on practice, would call upon the state to defend that monopoly. The intensity of the mobilization and the concerted effort to marshal support from multiple directions, however, demonstrates that more than the monopoly of medical care provision was at stake. Also at stake was the monopoly on third-party reimbursement that the medical profession had enjoyed previously. Indeed, gauged by the tone quality of these documents, one may surmise that the most distressing event in the entire period examined was that chiropractors had achieved third-party support, with the most contentious issue being the inclusion of chiropractic benefits in Medicaid and Medicare.

Arguments against inclusion were framed in terms of fiscal responsibility and concern that Medicare not be overwhelmed or unduly burdened (Wilbur 1971). A 1971 JAMA editorial (JAMA 1971) bemoaned the waste of tax dollars for compensation of "worthless and morally dangerous" (p. 959) treatments as well as the vast increases in federal spending that the inclusion of chiropractic benefits would entail. Ironically, the concerns articulated in these writings mirrored the health care crisis in which the medical profession itself was becoming

entrenched, and echoed public concerns during that same period about medical care in general, concerns that were prompting profound changes in the structure of health care financing. In both public and private sectors, health care financing was being radically overhauled. In addition to government-sponsored plans, new forms of financing, such as health maintenance organizations (HMOs), were being developed and introduced (Mayer and Mayer 1985). One editorialist (Huth 1975) acknowledged that it was "particularly galling" that "a healing cult without scientific validation is legitimated by a fiat" at a time when the medical profession "finds itself under potential threat of policing its services by a central bureaucracy" (p. 843).[7]

What had to be even more "galling" was the fact that none of the strategies outlined earlier accomplished the profession's aims. Chiropractors retained practice rights in all 50 states. In 1972, Congress included chiropractic in Medicare as well as Medicaid, bringing the medical profession's monopoly on third-party support to an end. In 1974, the U.S. Office of Education began accrediting chiropractic colleges. In 1976, chiropractors brought an antitrust suit against the AMA. *Wilk v. AMA* was initially unsuccessful, but ultimately was decided for the plaintiffs on appeal in 1987. In 1985, chiropractors won their first hospital privileges (Wardwell 1992).

Although the medical profession failed in its attempt to eradicate chiropractic or to exclude chiropractors from third-party coverage, it did succeed in gaining control of the practice of acupuncture. Acupuncture was controlled not by a campaign to discredit it but by restricting the practice to MDs or healers under medical supervision and by limiting acupuncture treatment to pain relief rather than a program of general health maintenance, effectively checking the development of another competing professional group (Curran 1974; Saks 1995; Wolpe 1985).[8] The medical profession also countered the challenge from midwives (although not a topic in this sample) that arose during the same period by certifying practitioners as nurse-midwives and placing them under supervisory control (Davis-Floyd 1992; Wertz and Wertz 1989; Winnick 2004). The likely lesson learned by the medical profession was that tactics of ridicule in exaggerating risks and summoning the state, so clearly articulated in the pages of these journals, do not guarantee and safeguard professional dominance. In fact, they may even achieve the opposite result. The tactics described earlier in all likelihood prompted the federal judge to rule in *Wilk* that the AMA indeed had "conspired to intentionally harm the chiropractic profession" (Dossey and Swyers 1994: xlv). This decision forced the AMA to rewrite its code of ethics regarding association and referral to non-physician providers (Johnson 1988).

THE REASSESSMENT PHASE

Beginning in the mid-1970s and continuing throughout the 1980s into the early 1990s, articles on CAM shifted in focus and in tone. CAM no longer remained synonymous with chiropractic, but broadened in scope, encompassing herbal remedies, acupuncture, and, briefly, Laetrile treatments as topics in these documents. The caustic tone of decades past gave way, and CAM received more even and measured discussion. As evinced from the documents analyzed during this period, this phase was characterized by a time of deep introspection within the medical profession. These writings reveal the authors' struggle to understand a number of issues—patient satisfaction, limitations in conventional treatment, the increasing popularity of CAM treatments, and the interconnection of these factors defining the current crisis in health care. In this process they gained an enhanced awareness of the appeal to CAM patients and practitioners, and a more realistic view of their place in a more pluralistic, consumer-centered medical marketplace.

One feature that stands out in the writing of this period is the discovery of the patient. Patient satisfaction had hitherto not been a pressing concern and, in fact, was not mentioned at all in the literature sampled during the first ten years. One explanation may have been that the medical profession's monopoly on practice permitted consumers

very little discretion in medical options (Pescosolido 1982). Consumers could be taken for granted, and this insouciance is evident in the early articles in the sample. But as choices in medical treatment kept expanding, consumers finally came into focus and authors began reflecting upon the quality of the doctor–patient relationship. One author (Cranshaw 1978) drew comparisons between conventional and CAM practitioners. He observed, "Where I saw zeal in the barefoot physician [of China], I see difference—perhaps indifference, in the white coated physician . . . Our medical education is notorious for being four years of training that leaves too many young people bereft of compassionate imagination and altruistic ideals," and he challenged Western physicians to learn from practitioners of Chinese medicine how to "listen to and speak to patients as human beings" (p. 2259).

An emerging topic in this period was the nascent "whole patient" or "holistic" movement, which incorporated psychological and spiritual approaches (and later CAM) to healing. One advocate of this approach (Cassileth 1982a) criticized the "biomedically proficient, highly specialized profession lacking a 'whole patient' perspective and often blind to the patient's emotional needs" (p. 1087). Another proponent (Schwartz 1991) lamented that physicians "have lost their humanity and become simply mechanics" (p. 3064). Roy W. Menninger (1976) found the rise of medical specialization especially alienating: "Too many patients . . . receive only partial help which leaves a significant segment of their person undealt with; they remain unsatisfied, and sometimes disappointed and resentful" (p. 603). Drawing connections between expanding specialization and CAM, he observed that specialization "has left a great vacuum into which new approaches [focusing on health, growth fulfillment, self-actualization, and other non-pathology-oriented objectives] have rapidly moved" (p. 604) and to which patients were increasingly turning.

Some acknowledged the connections, but resented and found manipulative CAM practitioners who capitalized on patients' desire for an improved doctor–patient relationship. As Edward W. Campion (1993) wryly noted, "Consumers . . . seek out unconventional healers because they think their problem will be taken seriously. They receive the benefit of time and attention, with invitations to return often" (p. 282). Yet the point made is fairly clear: interest in keeping patients satisfied increased as interest in CAM and visits to CAM practitioners increased. CAM's presence reminded physicians that medicine had indeed become what Elliot Freidson (1970) called a "consulting profession"; that is, its livelihood was ultimately dependent on the support of its clientele, a fact made more compelling in a newly competitive marketplace.

During this phase, physicians also examined shortcomings of conventional treatment, an appraisal thrust upon them by the popularity of Laetrile, an anti-cancer drug roundly condemned by the medical profession, but eagerly sought after by patients (Newell 1978).[9] Laetrile presented a unique challenge. It arose as a heresy within conventional medicine, but enjoyed judicial and legislative support (Jukes 1976).[10] In the next section, I will discuss how the medical profession relied on a scientific study to disillusion physicians about this treatment. The importance of Laetrile in the present section of this article is its role in bringing to light facts previously ignored in this literature: that limitations in conventional treatment exist, that these limitations were causing a crisis in public confidence, and that at least some orthodox physicians were becoming open to exploring treatments outside the biomedical paradigm.

Prior to 1975, only one article in the sample contained an acknowledgment of conventional medicine's inability to cure every illness. During the late 1970s and early 1980s in articles chronicling the medical profession's struggle to suppress Laetrile treatment, most of the articles did. In author Kenneth Gardner's (1980) view, Laetrile reminded physicians that there remained "an enduring market for quack cures" because a relationship existed between CAM and "diseases that are chronic, debilitating and potentially fatal." He added, "Unorthodox remedies exist, in part, because of science . . . Understandably, suffering persons turn elsewhere when medical researchers tell them, 'We don't know the cause. We can offer no cure or lasting relief'" (p. 503).

Reflections on medicine's shortcomings continued into the 1990s. Marcia Angell and Jerome P. Kassirer (1998) noted the irony of a "reversion to irrational approaches . . . even while scientific medicine is making some of its most dramatic advances" (p. 840). They laid part of the blame on the "often harried and impersonal care delivered by conventional physicians, as well as the harsh treatments necessary for life-threatening conditions" (p. 840). Campion (1993) observed, "Though Americans want all that modern medicine can deliver, they also fear it. They resent the way visits to physicians quickly lead to pills, tests and technology. Most now know of iatrogenic disasters from medicine gone wrong" (p. 282). Andrew Weil, an MD and a well-known advocate for CAM, pointed out that consumers who embrace CAM are often "patients who have been through conventional medicine, often many times over, have been tested to death, have tried many conventional therapies, and have found that they haven't worked or have caused harm, or both, and it is that what motivates them to look for other kinds of treatment" (quoted in Dalen 1999:2125). Laetrile exposed the crisis in public confidence in conventional medicine, and put MDs on the defensive. Barrie R. Cassileth (1982b) observed that physicians found they had to defend themselves against "timeworn conspiracy dogma, which states that the medical system, the Food and Drug Administration, and the federal government withhold true cures from the public . . . in order to further the Establishment's economic interests" (p. 1482).

By the early 1990s, medical researchers began offering empirical evidence of the public's growing acceptance of CAM. Eisenberg and associates (1993) conducted a national telephone survey of 1,539 adults in 1990 and discovered widespread use of CAM among the general public. This research quantified prevalence of use, identified the demographic group most likely to utilize these treatments, and put dollar figures on public expenditures on CAM. A follow-up study (Eisenberg et al. 1998) found utilization and expenditures on CAM had increased substantially. A wave of other studies (Astin 1998; Drivdah and Miser 1998; Druss and Rosenheck 1999; Elder, Gillcrist, and Minz 1997;

Fairfield et al. 1998) confirmed these findings. Campion (1993) lamented, "The public's expensive romance with alternative medicine is cause for our profession to worry" (p. 283).

THE INTEGRATION PHASE

Media coverage of CAM rose dramatically in the 1990s. Surging interest fed surging demand and vice versa, increasing the presence of CAM in American society (Goldstein 1999). Figure 22.1 shows that coverage within the medical press increased dramatically as well. Of the five top journals examined here, all increased coverage, save one, *The American Journal of Medicine.* Throughout the period, and even during the 1990s, the *AMA* managed to ignore CAM almost entirely.[11] Within the four journals that were actively engaged in following CAM, coverage was qualitatively different in this period than in the earlier years examined.

This period saw fewer editorial and more scientific CAM articles, including those describing the results of controlled trials. Interestingly, articles chosen for publication reported results that almost uniformly disparaged CAM treatments. In this sample, an herbal mixture known as PC-SPES produced adverse effects among prostate cancer patients (DiPaola et al. 1998); asthmatic children treated with spinal manipulation received no benefit from this therapy (Balon et al. 1998); acupuncture proved no more effective than placebo in reducing nicotine cravings (White, Resch, and Ernst 1998) or reducing pain in HIV-related neuropathies (Shlay et al. 1998); and an herbal anti-obesity agent failed to produce weight loss (Heymsfield et al. 1998). Yet articles, including editorials, were largely objective in their presentation, without ridicule or condemnation, in *JAMA*'s special issue devoted to CAM.

Authors also exhibited increased awareness that many patients had already integrated CAM into their health care regimens. Authors often cited results of utilization studies (Astin 1998; Eisenberg et al. 1993) that found that patients who used CAM or who frequented CAM practitioners did not tell their physicians for fear of being reproached

(Eisenberg et al. 1993). Frank A. Sonnenberg (1997) reminded readers of this surreptitious use and encouraged practitioners to present a nonjudgmental stance regarding CAM in order to encourage patients to confide in them. While readers of these journals were often urged to mount educational campaigns to inform patients about the dangers of these practices, they were also expected to continue to guide and direct patients, even in regard to the utilization of these therapies. Jeremy Sugarman and Larry Burk (1998) acknowledged that "physicians may feel pressured to learn about and prescribe beneficial alternative modalities" (p. 1624). They discussed how to go about acquiring training in these new methods of treatment, if for no other reason than to be knowledgeable enough about these treatments to work either with or around them in order to avoid hazardous interactions.

Another change during this phase was a shift away from a focus on the most threatening CAM modalities to a broader discussion of CAM in general. In these pages, as in the public arena, CAM was somewhat amorphous, or else the sheer quantity of healing approaches coming to light made it seem so. As Cassileth (1982b) perceptively observed, when one spoke of CAM, one spoke of "homeopathic and naturopathic beliefs, Indian and Oriental philosophy, and 19th century theories of intestinal purification . . . dietary regimens, detoxification, and internal cleansing, or mind control" (pp. 1482–83), without exhausting the list. CAM's lack of cohesive structure also made it difficult to control through traditional legal channels, for many CAM remedies "involve no agents that require FDA approval, and they consist of techniques that are self-administered or given by untrained professionals. Neither quasi-medical nor illegitimate, [they are] aspects of life style, beyond licensing or regulation" (p. 1483).

The articles published during the 1990s exhibited an understanding of the futility of control through traditional means. There was little talk of outlawing or eradicating CAM, though some authors (Angell and Kassirer 1998; Campion 1993; Gold and Cates 1980) did mount a campaign for increased surveillance and regulation of over-the-counter (OTC) herbal remedies. However, this endeavor failed in the pervasive deregulatory climate of the period. Instead, Congress substantially reduced the FDA's control over herbal medicine by making OTC herbal remedies (now called "diet supplements") exempt from FDA regulation. In addition, they were allowed to carry veiled treatment indications, which some authors (Angell and Kassirer 1998) referred to as "an art form of doublespeak" (p. 841).

The lesson of Laetrile and its successful control, however, was not lost on the profession. Documents from the period when Laetrile treatment was provoking strong concern (between 1978 and 1982) described a novel strategy, a large-scale clinical trial of Laetrile. The National Cancer Institute invited 385,000 physicians to submit cases where "bona fide, documented responses have occurred in association with Laetrile" (Newell 1978:217). Only 93 cases were submitted for review, 26 of which had data insufficient for evaluation. Data from the remaining 67 cases were combined and analyzed, and the results were published in *The New England Journal of Medicine* (Ellison, Byar, and Newell 1978). This research was held up as proof of Laetrile's fraudulence, and carried the caveat that physicians "must accept the associated liabilities" if they prescribed this "now established" toxic remedy (Moertel et al. 1982:206). Thereafter, discussion of Laetrile disappeared from these pages.[12] Its legal status and external support notwithstanding, Laetrile was felled by one meta-analysis establishing its lack of efficacy.

Studies to establish efficacy were not limited to CAM, of course. Evidence-based medicine emerged during this period of economic reform and fiscal responsibility as a method to evaluate the effectiveness of many treatments (Best and Glik 2000). Yet as evinced by the chorus that arose demanding more rigorous testing to determine if CAM therapies were—or were not—"scientifically valid," it seemed as if authors of these documents were beginning to grasp the significance of scientific testing as a means of control. After more than two decades of discussion and debate on the largely unsubstantiated merits of these therapies, controlled trials began in earnest in the late 1990s.

This approach was facilitated by the Office for the Study of Unconventional Medical Practices, later

called the Office of Alternative Medicine (OAM). This organizational body was established at the urging not of the medical profession, but of Congress, spearheaded by Iowa Senator Tom Harkin, chairman of the Senate Appropriations Subcommittee for Labor, Health, Human Services and Education. Harkin was a strong advocate of CAM, claiming that bee pollen had cured his allergies (Marshall 1994). Other incentives for the establishment of the OAM were Congressional concern over escalating costs for regular, high-technology medicine (Miles 1998) and public demand to learn more about these therapies (Marwick 1995).

The OAM was situated within the National Institute of Health (NIH), with an initial appropriation of $2 million (Marwick 1992). A committee of physicians, scientists, and CAM practitioners were given the challenge of evaluating CAM treatments. This daunting task became immediately problematic as biomedical scientists pushed for randomized controlled trials with an eye to mainstreaming useful treatments. CAM practitioners resisted this type of evaluation, claiming that these treatments are part of a larger system of healing that cannot be reduced to discrete biological components. Wayne Jonas, appointed in 1995 as the third director of the OAM, found ways to strike a balance between these competing groups with different knowledge paradigms and to fund research that, according to Goldstein (1999), was both "scientifically rigorous and contextually sensitive" (p. 181). Since 1998, the OAM has been elevated from a program office to a full center, now called the National Center for Complementary and Alternative Medicine (NCCAM), with a $50 million budget earmarked to support clinical trials and training (Jonas 1998; Marwick 1998).

For practitioners of CAM, the importance of this organization is hard to overestimate. It granted CAM "societal legitimacy, intellectual acceptance, and financial stability" (Goldstein 1999:184). The importance of this organization is equally hard for the medical profession to overestimate; it meant that evaluation of CAM could be conducted *on the medical profession's own terms* (Wolpe 1985). Given their greater cultural authority, it also meant that their assessments, whether positive or negative, would be given more weight. The OAM/NCCAM furnishes what one author (Gardner 1980) presciently sought: a system by which unorthodox remedies can be identified, investigated, and monitored," and where "*medical scientists . . .* take responsibility for the assessment of unorthodox cures" (p. 503; emphasis added). The mandate of the OAM to develop a repository of information for patients, practitioners, and policymakers and to facilitate the "discovery, development, and validation of potential treatments" (Berman and Larson 1994: x) allowed the regular profession to become the final arbiters of CAM's validity.

Scientific testing, facilitated by the OAM, soon replaced reliance on external legalistic control, which had a surprising effect. Interestingly, as the six clinical trials in the sample (described earlier) illustrate, finding CAM treatments ineffective had almost a paradoxical effect on the tone used to describe them. The authors became less caustic in their evaluations when they knew with some certainty that a therapy in question was inefficacious than when they only suspected it was so. The difference, of course, was that this time the profession was in control—handling, managing, and, most importantly, evaluating these therapies. With funds provided by the OAM, CAM treatments could be tested, and those demonstrating clinical efficacy could be mainstreamed into conventional practice. Or, as put more eloquently by Brian M. Berman and David B. Larson (1994), these treatments could be "added to the complementary wheel of alternatives currently available to patients and practitioners" (p. x). Those failing the test could be discredited, as Laetrile had been.

DISCUSSION

Optimum structural arrangements favoring regular medicine over other types of practice facilitated the medical profession's dominance. Structural changes in medicine over the last 30 or 40 years, such as relaxed medical regulation, consumerism, managed care, and the validation of ideas outside the biomedical paradigm, have not undermined the medical profession's supremacy. However, these changes

have affected the content and control of professional work, opened up opportunities for competitors, and forced the dominant profession to realign and reposition itself in a changing medical marketplace. This suggests that professionalization is an ongoing process, one that intensifies whenever structural supports shift or weaken (Bucher 1988). The literature examined here shows how the medical profession did, indeed, confront and struggle with the challenges CAM presented, but they also rebounded from whatever threat CAM might have posed. In the process, the profession underwent a period of refinement wherein continued professionalization involved, among other things, self-reflection, self-improvement, and adaptation.

These more recent developments suggest likely encroachment into these new approaches of treatment. One indicator that the medical profession may be gearing up to control or even "own" these new therapies is the relatively new trend in referencing CAM as "integrative" medicine, lending even greater support to the notion of continued professionalization. In a debate published in the *Archives of Internal Medicine* in 1999, holistic guru Andrew Weil predicted "integrative" medicine "is the future, not only because people want it, but because very powerful forces, operating both within science and outside of science, are moving us in this direction. Demand . . . is not just coming from customers . . . [but from] practitioners and members of the profession . . . [I]t is inevitable that we move in this direction" (quoted in Dalen 1999:2126).

Given these trends, the final stage in this struggle is likely to be cooptation. The medical profession will probably absorb many of today's CAM therapies, particularly remedies such as homeopathic or herbal remedies which can be dispensed as readily as prescription drugs. The medical profession, no doubt, will acquire this territory via application of "superior" medical knowledge, recasting CAM in terms compatible with the biomedical paradigm. Where these changes will lead is harder to predict. They may reverberate throughout the entire system, changing the medical profession's paradigm or the way medical service is delivered. CAM practitioners may be absorbed into the AMA (as was the case in the past for both homeopathy and osteopathy). CAM treatments may be absorbed into the biomedical paradigm and the practitioners abandoned (as was the case for acupuncture in the early 1970s). Although it is possible that the larger healing paradigms will be reduced to a handful of easily learned and executed treatments, as has already occurred with acupuncture (now mainly employed for pain relief), the persistence of incurable illness makes it less likely that they will be discarded entirely.

Politically, the interplay between the medical profession and CAM will continue to be important for both medicine and the sociology of medicine. Medicine should grow more sensitive to spiraling medical care costs and more concerned with doctor–patient relationships and patient satisfaction with treatment. These are issues cast in high relief by the popularity of these treatments, and further adjustments are likely. At the same time, they should benefit from exposure to new and novel approaches to healing outside the biomedical paradigm since they now have the tools to test and incorporate the most useful of these therapies into medical practice. For medical sociologists, the reemergence of CAM will continue to provide a unique opportunity to reexamine, refine, and reconceptualize ideas about professional development. They will continue to enjoy this unique opportunity to observe first-hand the "regulars" and "irregulars" entangled in conflict yet again, just as they were a century ago. At the

same time, the case of CAM compels medical sociologists to move beyond the professional dominance paradigm, updating and broadening theories of professional growth. Professionalization becomes not just an historical event, but an evolutionary process, one in which successful professions are sustained by their ability to adapt to changing structural conditions and to turn those changed circumstances to their favor (Bucher 1988; Light 2000).

Limitations of this research include its small sample size and its reliance on written artifacts from a nonrepresentative sample of physicians. Authors cited in this account represent the elite of the profession, those granted the position of spokespersons for the profession. To the degree that this is true, it is interesting in its own right, for it allows us to glimpse struggle at the highest level of influence. This research, however, does not represent the perspective of the ordinary medical doctor and should not be taken as such. Future research is needed to determine what that point of view may be, how the confrontation with CAM has played out with those on the front lines of treatment, and what adaptational strategies ordinary doctors may have employed within their own milieu. Future research should also examine the interplay between regular physicians and the nonphysician healers with whom they now share the medical marketplace, and the extent to which each may assist the other in ongoing professionalization.

Notes

1. These American journals consistently appeared among the top ten in terms of impact ranking in the *Science Citation Index*, in the volumes where impact rankings were published (1979, 1983, 1985, 1987, 1992, 1996, 1997, and 1998 issues).
2. Raw data for Pescosolido's (1982) unpublished dissertation were available for my use. These data consist of all citations for all published articles on CAM prior to 1980 in the *Cumulated Index Medicus* and the *Guide to Periodic Literature*. From these data, I drew all citations for the five journals used in this study. For later citations, I searched the annual *Cumulated Index Medicus* and also conducted overlapping *Medline* searches for any items that might have been overlooked over the entire 1965–1999 time period. I searched within the categories Pescosolido created and added any relevant

others within this genre. Since I only sampled from five rather conservative journals, not all categories were represented in the sample and some were only weakly represented (e.g., Ayervedic, midwifery, homeopathy, and naturopathy together composed only 7 percent of total citations).

3. "Alternative medicine" as a category was added in 1986. "Complementary medicine," a term currently in use, was not a separate category in the *Cumulated Index Medicus* during the time period observed.

4. In 1976, five chiropractors brought a civil antitrust suit against the AMA and several affiliated organizations. This suit was a reaction to aggressive tactics employed by the AMA to eliminate chiropractic as a profession. These tactics included a smear campaign and a policy stating that it would be unethical for MDs to associate with chiropractors. The court first found for the AMA in 1981, after they modified their code of ethics to permit association. Nonetheless, chiropractors appealed this decision, which was reversed in 1983 and finally settled in their favor in 1987. A federal judge ruled that the AMA and its affiliated organizations had indeed violated the Sherman Anti-Trust Act by conspiring to harm the chiropractic profession. The AMA was ordered to cease and desist its obstructive policies. The AMA appealed the decision to the U.S. Supreme Court, who declined to hear the case (Dossey and Swyers 1994; Wardwell 1992).

5. It is worth noting that most frequently warnings about CAM were presented as case histories (rather than as results of scientific research) in this sample.

6. Laetrile's action arises primarily from its chemical makeup as a cyanide compound. The reasoning behind its use, quite simply, was to "kill the cancer." The difficulty with this approach, however, is that the cyanide "diffuses and poisons the surrounding normal tissues . . . caus[ing] systemic poisoning" (Jukes 1976:1284).

7. The author of this editorial was referring to educational accreditation, not third-party reimbursement. In either case, chiropractic legitimacy is enhanced. The author notes the irony of competitors' gains at a time when allopathy was experiencing erosion of autonomy in the medical marketplace.

8. The documents sampled do not tell that story in detail. For a fascinating and detailed account of the how acupuncture was absorbed by the established medical profession, see Wolpe (1985).

9. Patients were strongly motivated to attain access to Laetrile. More than 43,000 citizens sent petitions to President Nixon demanding trials of Laetrile's anti-cancer properties (Jukes 1976:1284).

10. Developed in the 1950s by allopathic physician Dr. Ernest Krebs, Laetrile was the registered trade name for an old natural remedy, amygdalin. Derived from apricot pits, which contain cyanide, Laetrile's function was to treat malignancy by "kill[ing] the cancer." Laetrile presented a unique challenge, as there were no outside competitors to discredit, and appeals to governmental bodies were futile. Laetrile treatment was legal in 27 states, and its legitimacy had been affirmed by the U.S. Supreme Court (Jukes 1976:1284).

11. Of 699 citations in the full sample, only 12 were found in *The American Journal of Medicine*.

12. Laetrile use was controlled among U.S. physicians, but the therapy has not fallen out of use. Goldstein (1999) reports that Mexican clinics still offer Laetrile treatments.

References

Angell, Marcia and Jerome P. Kassirer. 1998. "Alternative Medicine—The Risks of Untested and Unregulated Remedies." *The New England Journal of Medicine* 339:839–41.

Astin, John A. 1998. "Why Patients Use Alternative Medicine." *Journal of the American Medical Association* 279:1548–53.

Balon, Jeffrey, Peter D. Aker, Edward R. Crowther, Clark Danielson, P. Gerald Cox, Denise O'Shaughnessy, Corinne Walker, Charles H. Goldsmith, Eric Duku, and Malcolm R. Sears. 1998. "A Comparison of Active and Simulated Chiropractic Manipulation as Adjunctive Treatment for Childhood Asthma." *The New England Journal of Medicine* 339:1013–20.

Barnes, J., N. C. Abbot, E. F. Harkness, and Edzard Ernst. 1999. "Articles on Complementary Medicine in the Mainstream Medical Literature: An Investigation on Medline." *Archives of Internal Medicine* 159:1721–25.

Barrett, Stephen and William T. Jarvis. 1993. *The Health Robbers: A Close Look at Quackery in America.* Buffalo, NY: Prometheus Books.

Berman, Brian M. and David B. Larson. 1994. "Preface." Pp. ix–x in *Alternative Medicine: Expanding Medical Horizons.* Washington, DC: U.S. Government Printing Office.

Best, Allen and Deborah Glik. 2000. "Research as a Tool for Integrative Health Service Reform." Pp. 239–54 in *Complementary and Alternative Medicine: Challenge and Change,* edited by Merrijoy Kelner, Beverly Wellman, Bernice Pescosolido, and Mike Saks. Amsterdam: Harwood Academic Publishers.

Bucher, Rue. 1988. "On the Natural History of Health Care Occupations." *Work and Occupations* 15:131–47.

Campion, Edward W. 1993. "Why Unconventional Medicine?" *The New England Journal of Medicine* 328:282–83.

Cassileth, Barrie R. 1982a. "Care of the Patient Revisited." *Archives of Internal Medicine* 142:1087–88.

———. 1982b. "Sounding Boards: After Laetrile, What?" *The New England Journal of Medicine* 306:1482–84.

Casterline, Ray L. 1972. "Unscientific Cultism: 'Dangerous to your Health!'" *Journal of the American Medical Association* 220:1009–10.

Cranshaw, Ralph. 1978. "A Lesson From Chinese Medicine: The Humanitarian Imperative." *Journal of the American Medical Association* 240:2257–59.

Curran, William J. 1974. "Acupuncture and the Practice of Medicine." *The New England Journal of Medicine* 291:1245–46.

Dalen, James E. 1999. "Is Integrative Medicine the Medicine of the Future?" *Archives of Internal Medicine* 159:2122–26.

Davis-Floyd, Robbie. 1992. *Birth as an American Rite of Passage.* Berkeley: University of California.

Dawkins, Richard. 2003. *A Devil's Chaplain. Reflections on Hope, Lies, Science, and Love.* Boston: Houghton-Mifflin.

DiPaola, Robert S., Huayan Zhang, George H. Lambert, Robert Meeker, Edward Licitra, Mohamed M. Rafi, Bao Ting Zhu, Heidi Spaulding, Susan Goodin, Michel B. Toledano, William N. Hait, and Michael A. Gallo. 1998. "Clinical and Biological Activity of an Estrogenic Herbal Combination (PC-SPEC) in Prostate Cancer." *The New England Journal of Medicine* 339:785–91.

Dossey, Larry and James P. Swyers. 1994. "Introduction." Pp. xxxvii–xlvii in *Alternative Medicine: Expanding Medical Horizons.* Washington, DC: U.S. Government Printing Office.

Drivdah, Christine and William F. Miser. 1998. "The Use of Alternative Health Care by a Family

Practice Population." *Journal of the American Board of Family Practice* 11:193–98.

Druss, Benjamin G. and Robert A. Rosenheck. 1999. "Association between Use of Unconventional Therapies and Conventional Medical Services." *JAMA* 282:651–56

Eisenberg, David M., Roger B. Davis, Susan L. Ettner, Scott Appel, Sonja Wilkey, Maria Van Rompay, and Ronald C. Kessler. 1998. "Trends in Alternative Medicine Use in the United States, 1990– 1997: Results of a Follow-up National Survey." *Journal of the American Medical Association* 280:1569–75.

Eisenberg, David M., Ronald C. Kessler, Cindy Foster, Frances E. Norlock, David R. Caulkins, and Thomas L. Delbanco. 1993. "Unconventional Medicine in the United States: Prevalence, Costs, and Patterns of Use." *The New England Journal of Medicine* 328:246–52.

Elder, Nancy C., Amy Gillcrist, and Rene Minz. 1997. "Use of Alternative Health Care by Family Practice Patients." *Archives of Family Medicine* 6:181–84.

Ellison, Neil M., David Byar, and Guy R. Newell. 1978. "Special Board on Laetrile: The NCI Laetrile Review." *The New England Journal of Medicine* 299:549–52.

Fairfield, Kathleen M., David Eisenberg, Roger Davis, Howard Libman, and Russell Phillips. 1998. "Patterns of Use, Expenditures, and Perceived Efficacy of Complementary and Alternative Therapies in HIV-Infected Patients." *Archives of Internal Medicine* 158:2257–64.

Firman, Gregory J. and Michael S. Goldstein. 1975. "The Future of Chiropractic: A Psychosocial View." *The New England Journal of Medicine* 293:639–42.

Freidson, Elliot. 1970. *Professional Dominance: The Social Structure of Medical Care.* New York: Atherton.

Gardner, Kenneth. 1980. "Hope, Quackery, and Orthodox Health Research." *Annals of Internal Medicine* 92:503.

Garfield, Eugene. 1999. "Journal Impact Factor: A Brief Review." *Canadian Medical Association Journal* 161:979–80.

Gaw, Albert C., Lenning W. Chang, and Lein-Chun Shaw. 1975. "Efficacy of Acupuncture on Osteoarthritic Pain." *New England Journal of Medicine* 293:375–78.

Gevitz, Norman. 1988. *Other Healers: Unorthodox Medicine in America.* Baltimore, MD: Johns Hopkins.

Gold, Julian and William Cates, Jr. 1980. "Herbal Abortifacients." *Journal of the American Medical Association* 243:1365–66.

Goldstein, Michael S. 1999. *Alternative Health Care: Medicine, Miracle, or Mirage.* Philadelphia: Temple University.

Griffin, Larry J. and Larry Isaac. 1992. "Recursive Regression and the Historical Use of Time in Time Series Analysis of Historical Process." *Historical Methods* 25:166–79.

Heymsfield, Steven B., David B. Allison, Joseph R. Vasselli, Angelo Pietrobelli, Debra Greenfield, and Christopher Nunez. 1998. "*Garcinia cambogia* (Hydroxycitric Acid) as a Potential Antiobesity Agents." *Journal of the American Medical Association* 280:1596–600.

Holder, Angela R. 1972. "Homicide by Quackery." *Journal of the American Medical Association* 222:1219–20.

———. 1973. "Physician's Records and the Chiropractor." *Journal of the American Medical Association* 224:1071–72.

Huth, E. J. 1975. "Chiropractic as 'Higher Learning.'" *Annals of Internal Medicine* 82:843.

Isaac, Larry W. and Larry J. Griffin. 1989. "Ahistoricism in Time-Series Analyses of

Historical Process: Critique, Redirection, and Illustrations from U.S. Labor History." *American Sociological Review* 54:873–90.

JAMA. 1969. "Chiropractic CONDEMNED." *Journal of the American Medical Association* 208:352.

_____. 1970. "Put Up or Shut Up." *Journal of the American Medical Association* 213:1481–82.

_____. 1971. "A Call to Arms." *Journal of the American Medical Association* 217:959.

_____. 1972. "Quackery Persists." *Journal of the American Medical Association* 221:914.

Johnson, Kirk B. 1988. "Statement from AMA's General Counsel." *Journal of the American Medical Association* 259:83.

Jonas, Wayne B. 1998. "What is the Office of Alternative Medicine and What Does It Do? A Commentary from OAM Director." *North Carolina Medical Journal* 59:148–50.

Jukes, Thomas H. 1976. "Laetrile for Cancer." *Journal of the American Medical Association* 236:1284–86.

Lee, Peter Ky, Thorkild W. Anderson, Jerome H. Modell, and Segundina A. Saga. 1975. "Treatment of Pain with Acupuncture." *Journal of the American Medical Association* 232:1133–35.

Light, Donald W. 2000. "The Medical Profession and Organizational Change: From Professional Dominance to Countervailing Power." Pp. 201–16 in *Handbook of Medical Sociology*, edited by C. Bird, P. Conrad, and A. M. Freemont. 5th ed. Upper Saddle River, NJ: Prentice Hall.

Marwick, Charles. 1992. "Congress Wants Alternative Medicine Studied: NIH Responds with Programs." *Journal of the American Medical Association* 268:957–58.

Marshall, Eliot. 1994. "The Politics of Alternative Medicine." *Science* 265:2000–2002.

Marwick, Charles. 1995. "Complementary Medicine Draws a Crowd." *JAMA* 274:106–7.

Marwick, Charles. 1998. "Alterations are Ahead at the OAM." *JAMA* 280:1553–54.

Mayer, Thomas R. and Gloria G. Mayer. 1985. "HMO's Origins and Development." *New England Journal of Medicine* 312:590–94.

McKinlay, John B. and Lisa D. Marceau. 2002. "The End of the Golden Age of Doctoring." *International Journal of Health Services* 32:379–416.

Menninger, Roy W. 1976. "Psychiatry 1976: Time for Holistic Medicine." *Annals of Internal Medicine* 84:603–4.

Miles, Mary C. 1998. "Expanding Medical Horizons: The National Institute of Health Office of Alternative Medicine." *Knowledge and Society* 11:87–105.

Miller, Robert G. and Robert Burton. 1974. "Stroke Following Chiropractic Manipulation of the Spine." *Journal of the American Medical Association* 229:189–90.

Moertel, Charles G., Thomas R. Fleming, Joseph Rubin, Larry K. Kvous, Gregory Sarna, Robert Koch, Violante E. Currie, Charles W. Young, Stephen E. Jones, and J. Paul Davignon. 1982. "A Clinical Trial of Amygdalin (Laetrile) in the Treatment of Human Cancer." *The New England Journal of Medicine* 306:201–6.

Newell, Guy R. 1978. "Clinical Evaluation of Laetrile: Two Perspectives." *The New England Journal of Medicine* 298:216–18.

Olzak, Susan. 1992. *Dynamics of Ethnic Competition and Conflict.* Stanford, CA: Stanford University.

Pescosolido, Bernice. 1982. "Medicine, Markets and Choice: The Social Organization of Decision-Making and Medical Care." Ph.D. dissertation, Department of Sociology, Yale University, New Haven, CT.

Pescosolido, Bernice A. and Carol A. Boyer. 2001. "The American Health Care System: Entering the Twenty-first Century with High Risk, Major Challenges, and Great Opportunities." Pp. 180–98 in *The Blackwell Companion to Medical Sociology,* edited by William C. Cockerham. Oxford: Blackwell.

Rothstein, William G. 1972. *American Physicians in the Nineteenth Century.* Baltimore: Johns Hopkins.

Sabatier, Joseph A. 1969. "At Your Own Risk: The Case Against Chiropractic." *Journal of the American Medical Association* 209:1712.

Sadoff, Leonard, Kaspar Fuchs, and Jonathan Hollander. 1978. "Rapid Death Associated with Laetrile Ingestion." *Journal of the American Medical Association* 239:1532.

Saks, Mike. 1995. *Professions and the Public Interest: Medical Power, Altruism and Alternative Medicine.* London: Routledge.

Schwartz, Stephen G. 1991. "Holistic Health: Seeking a Link Between Medicine and Metaphysics." *Journal of the American Medical Association* 266:3064.

Science Citation Index. 1979, 1983, 1985, 1987, 1992, 1996, 1997, 1998. Philadelphia, PA: Institute for Scientific Information.

Sherlock, Paul and Edmund O. Rothschild. 1967. "Scurvy Produced by a Zen Macrobiotic Diet." *Journal of the American Medical Association* 199:130–33.

Shlay, Judith C., Kathryn Chaloner, Mitchell B. Max, Bob Flaws, Patricia Reichelderfer, Deborah Went-worth, Shauna Hillman, Barbara Brizz, and David L. Cohn. 1998. "Acupuncture and Amitriptyline for Pain Due to HIV-Related Peripheral Neuropathy." *Journal of the American Medical Association* 280:1590–95.

Sidell, Victor W. 1968. "Feldshers and 'Feldsherism': The Role and Training of the Feldsher in the U.S.S.R." *The New England Journal of Medicine* 278:934–38.

——. 1972. "The Barefoot Doctors of the People's Republic of China." *The New England Journal of Medicine* 286:1292–99.

——. 1975. "Medical Care in the People's Republic of China." *Archives of Internal Medicine* 135:916–26.

Soffer, Alfred. 1977. "Chicken Soup or Laetrile— Which Would You Prescribe?" *Archives of Internal Medicine* 137:994–95.

Sonnenberg, Frank A. 1997. "Health Information on the Internet." *Archives of Internal Medicine* 157:151–52.

Starr, Paul. 1982. *The Social Transformation of American Medicine.* New York: Basic Books.

Sugarman, Jeremy and Larry Burk. 1998. "Physicians' Ethical Obligations Regarding Alternative Medicine." *JAMA* 280:1623–25.

Wardwell, Walter I. 1992. *Chiropractic: History and Evolution of a New Profession.* St. Louis, MO: Mosby Year Book.

Wardwell, Walter I. 1994. "Differential Evolution of the Osteopathic and Chiropractic Professions in the United States." *Perspectives in Biology and Medicine* 37:595–608.

Wertz, Richard W. and Dorothy C. Wertz. 1989. *Lying In: A History of Childbirth in America.* New Haven: Yale University.

White, Adrian R., Karl-Ludwig Resch, and Edzard Ernst. 1998. "Randomized Trial of Acupuncture for Nicotine Withdrawal Symptoms." *Archives of Internal Medicine* 158:2251–55.

Wilbur, Richard S. 1971. "What the Health-Care Consumer Should Know about Chiropractic." *Journal of the American Medical Association* 215:1307–9.

Winnick, Terri A. 2004. "Delivery: Gender and the Language of Birth." *Advances in Gender Research* 8:51–86.

Wolpe, Paul R. 1985. "The Maintenance of Professional Authority: Acupuncture and the American Physician." *Social Problems* 32:409–24.

_____. 1999. "Alternative Medicine and the AMA." Pp. 218–39 in The American Medical Ethics Revolution: How the AMA's Code of Ethics Has Transformed Physicians' Relationships to Patients, Professions, and Society, edited by R. B. Baker, A. L. Caplan, L. I. Emanuel, and S. R. Latham. Baltimore: Johns Hopkins.

PHARMACEUTICALIZATION

The pharmaceutical industry has grown enormously in the past few decades. As sociologist John Abraham (2010, 290) points out, "Between 1960 and the early 1980s, prescription drug sales were almost static as a percentage of GNP in most Western economies." Since the 1990s, medications like Prozac, Lipitor, OxyContin, and Viagra have had incredibly wide usage, and their brand names have become everyday terms in our culture. Blockbuster drugs like these bring in billions of dollars for the pharmaceutical companies. Since 1999 direct-to-consumer advertising (DTCA), especially on television, has expanded the markets for a range of medications. Virtually everyone recognizes the phrases "the little blue pill" and "ask your doctor if Viagra is right for you." Drug companies spend about 35 percent of their income on marketing and administration, much more than they spend on research for new drugs to treat diseases (Relman and Angell 2002). They are among the most profitable companies in the world.

There has been a considerable expansion of the role of the pharmaceutical industry in health care. As just one measure of this expansion, global pharmaceutical sales increased from $350 billion in 2000 to $700 billion in 2007 (Busfield 2010). In 2014, global pharmaceutical sales reached $1 trillion and continue to grow (https://www.statista.com/topics/1764/global-pharmaceutical-industry/). Without question, this expansion has resulted in some very effective and potent drugs that treat serious illnesses and improve individuals' lives. But it has also emphasized the commercial orientation of the pharmaceutical industry and called attention to the ways in which pharmaceutical companies promote their products.

Sociologists have developed the term *pharmaceuticalization*, which can be defined as "the process by which social, behavioral, or body conditions are treated, or deemed to be in need of treatment/interventions with pharmaceuticals" (Abraham 2010, 290). There are many aspects to pharmaceuticalization, including scientific research for drugs, promotion of pharmaceuticals for extant medical problems, promotion of existing medications for new or broadened health or body problems, or advertising drug solutions for a wide range of medical or nonmedical problems. In virtually all cases, this includes an expansion of pharmaceutical interventions for human problems.

In this section, we focus on the marketing and promotion of drugs by the pharmaceutical industry and the social impact on users and the wider culture. Many examples of the promotion of pharmaceuticals raise both sociological and ethical issues, such as the classic case of the anti-arthritis medication Vioxx a decade ago in which the drug companies knew the risk of the drug but didn't make the information public (Berenson et al. 2004). Among other recent cases, drug companies hired ghost writers to pen "scientific" articles for journals and paid researchers to put their name on articles that purposely presented the drug in a positive light, even if the evidence was more equivocal (Wilson 2008).

Creating and expanding markets are key goals in promoting pharmaceuticals. This raises sociological issues, such as the medicalization of life problems. One important case involves the drug Paxil, which entered a very crowded antidepressant market when it was introduced in 1992. The drug company GlaxoSmithKline (GSK) promoted a rather obscure (at that time) disorder—social anxiety disorder—with slogans such as "Imagine being allergic to people," and advertising copy like "Do you have difficulty speaking in public, or interacting at a cocktail party? If so, you may have social anxiety disorder. But there is no need to suffer. Paxil is the treatment" (Lane 2007). By 2006, Paxil, in large part due to its effective promotion, became one of the five bestselling antidepressants in the United States. But all was not well with Paxil despite its market success and potential therapeutic benefits. A jury later found that GSK had never adequately studied the adverse effects of Paxil and failed to warn doctors and patients about the drug's risk of birth defects. In 2010, GSK had to pay $1 billion to settle several lawsuits, which seems like a lot of money until it's compared with the $11.7 billion in Paxil sales (Bass 2008; Feeley 2010).

Although GSK had to work to create a market for a social anxiety drug, the situation with another well-known drug was different. Impotence, a man's inability to maintain an erection adequate for sexual intercourse, has been deemed a human problem since ancient times. Numerous treatments, both folk and medical, were offered over the centuries, but most were only mildly effective at best. Then along came Viagra, the first drug to successfully treat what is now called erectile dysfunction (ED). Viagra became a blockbuster drug, first promoted for the elderly and those with severe erectile problems caused by a medical condition (e.g., prostate cancer). Then, competitors' drugs hit the market, namely Levitra and Cialis, and because of this increased competition, all of the manufacturers had to look for ways to expand their ED markets. In short order, these drugs were promoted to younger men, men who worried about ED (but were not diagnosed), couples with sexual difficulties, and—less directly—to those who wanted to enhance their sexuality (Loe 2004). Drug companies didn't invent ED, but they certainly expanded the market.

In the first article, Peter Conrad and Valerie Leiter examine the promotion of ED drugs in "From Lydia Pinkham to Queen Levitra: Direct-to-Consumer Advertising and Medicalisation." The United States and New Zealand are the only two countries that allow prescription drugs to be advertised on television and any other broadcast media. In this article, Conrad and Leiter show how this kind of DTCA is reminiscent of nineteenth-century advertising of "patent medicines" (medical elixirs, often of questionable effectiveness) that were widely promoted to the public in newspapers and magazines. DTCA allows pharmaceutical companies to create a direct relationship with consumers, providing an important new strategy for expanding their markets and, as the authors point out, increasing the medicalization of human problems.

In the second selection, "Prescriptions and Proscriptions: Moralising Sleep Medications," Jonathan Gabe, Catherine M. Coveney, and Simon J. Williams studied cultural responses to the pharmaceuticalization of sleep medications. "Sleeping pills" have been around for a long time, although their use has become much more widespread. Sleeplessness (aka insomnia) is common and is widely treated, although there is some concern about overtreatment (Moloney, Konrad, and Zimmer 2011). Use of medications as sleep aids is controversial because of the risks of dependence, reported increase in mortality risks for long-term users, and other potential adverse effects. The authors used focus groups to explore the cultural meanings and collective views of the users of these prescription medications. They found that respondents used several repertoires about prescription sleep medication use that reflect distinct moral evaluations of these hypnotic-based sleeping aids. Thus, pharmaceuticalization is by no means culturally neutral, and these evaluations can impact social life.

(For a more general analysis of medicalization in other sectors of human life, see selections in the section titled "The Medicalization of American Society.")

References

Abraham, John. 2010. "The Sociological Concomitants of the Pharmaceutical Industry and Medications." In *Handbook of Medical Sociology*, 6th edition, edited by Chloe Bird, Peter Conrad, Allen Fremont, and Stefan Timmermans, 290–308. Nashville, TN: Vanderbilt University Press.

Bass, Alison. 2008. *Side Effects: A Prosecutor, a Whistle Blower and a Bestselling Antidepressant on Trial.* Chapel Hill, NC: Algonquin Books.

Berenson, Alex, Gardiner Harris, Barry Meier, and Andrew Pollack. 2004. "Despite Warnings, Drug Giant Took Long Path to Vioxx Recall," *New York Times,* November 14, 2004.

Busfield, Joan. 2010. "'Pill for Every Ill': Explaining the Expansion of Medicine Use." *Social Science and Medicine* 70: 934–41.

Feeley, Jef. 2010. "Glaxo Failed to Warn About Paxil Risks, Lawyer Says." *Bloomberg*, November 9, 2010. Accessed March 2012. https://www.bloomberg.com/news/articles/2010-11-09/glaxo-failed-to-warn-about-paxil-risks-lawyer-says-at-philadelphia-trial.

Lane, Christopher. 2007. *Shyness: How Normal Behavior Became a Sickness.* New Haven: Yale University Press.

Loe, Meika. 2004. *The Rise of Viagra: How the Little Blue Pill Changed Sex in America.* New York: NYU Press.

Moloney, Mairead E., Thomas R. Konrad, and Catherine R. Zimmer. 2011. "The Medicalization of Sleeplessness: A Public Health Concern." *American Journal of Public Health* 101 (8): 1429–32.

Relman, Arnold, and Marcia Angell. 2002. "How the Drug Industry Distorts Medicine and Politics." *New Republic* 227 (25): 27–41.

Wilson, Duff. 2008. "Drug Maker Said to Pay Ghostwriters for Journal Articles," *New York Times,* December 12, 2008.

FROM LYDIA PINKHAM TO QUEEN LEVITRA

Direct-to-Consumer Advertising and Medicalisation

Peter Conrad and Valerie Leiter

INTRODUCTION

The medicalisation of life problems has been occurring for well over a century (Conrad and Schneider 1992, Shorter 1992, Wertz and Wertz 1989) and may have increased in the past 30 years (Conrad 2005, 2007). Medicalisation occurs when previously non-medical problems are defined and treated as medical problems, usually in terms of illnesses or disorders, or when a medical intervention is used to treat the problem. In a recent article we argued that the push towards medicalisation comes more from the creation of medical markets than from professionals' desire to expand their jurisdiction (Conrad and Leiter 2004). Conrad (2005) has recently suggested that the shifting engines of medicalisation include biotechnology, managed care, and consumers.

In this paper we examine one strand of medicalisation over the last century and a half: the role of direct-to-consumer advertising (DTCA) in the medicalisation of life problems. To do this we compare patent medicine advertising with contemporary DTCA, highlighting the role of federal regulation of pharmaceuticals and advertising as a constraint on medicalisation during the 20th century. We rely primarily upon secondary data sources plus some primary Congressional documents on DTCA in our analyses. This historical comparison allows us to analyse current DTCA practices not as a new development, but as hearkening back to the patent medicine era, and to analyse the role that the medical profession played in creating and maintaining constraints on the advertisement of pharmaceuticals. Lydia E. Pinkham's Vegetable Compound was an exemplar of advertising in its time, and erectile dysfunction drugs, including Levitra, are exemplars of the contemporary DTCA era. History is often a great relativiser. By contrasting drugs that were promoted 130 years apart we seek to reflect more clearly on the potentials and pitfalls of DTCA in the 21st century.

PATENT MEDICINES IN THE 19TH CENTURY

It is important to recall the context of medicine in the 19th century. For example, in the US medicine was not a particularly prestigious profession, with often poorly trained practitioners and extremely limited medical knowledge. When the American Medical Association (AMA) was organised in 1847, among its goals were the improvement of the image of medicine and gaining control over the licensing of physicians (Freidson 1970). The public was ambivalent about the invasive and heroic medicine that most physicians offered, and hospitals were seen as places to go to die. In many communities in America there were no trained physicians, so self-help was an important alternative to medical care. One sector of medical care was so-called 'patent medicines'.

Medicines could be divided between 'ethical' drugs of known composition and patent drugs of undeclared composition. After the Civil War, there was a growing division between ethical drug firms and patent medicine firms (Spillane 2004). The ethical drug firms attempted to distance themselves from patent medicine firms and to align themselves with the fledgling medical profession by adopting the AMA code of not advertising directly to the public (Starr 1982). 'Indeed, the ethical firms took great pains to publicise the fact that they did not make direct advertising appeals

to the general public, but confined their sales pitches to persuading doctors and druggists of the superiority and reliability of their brands' (Spillane 2004: 2).

Patent medicines in the US originated in Britain and were imported until entrepreneurs discovered the potential domestic market (Young 1961). They were not actually patented but were proprietary drugs with secret or unlisted formulations, with a copyrighted trademark. Patent medicines were advertised directly to the public, encouraging consumers to medicalise everyday symptoms, such as being tired or nervous, through self-diagnosis and self-medication. By the 1850s 'the medicine taking habit was instilled by large usage in the American people. People wanted to take something and many doctors prescribed to demand' (Young 1961: 158). Patent medicines were advertised widely in Britain as well. For example, Thomas Holloway, a patent medicine merchant and later philanthropist, in 1880 spent 50,000 pounds, a great sum at the time, on advertising nostrums that made him wealthy but were later deemed to have little medicinal value (Harrison-Barbet 1994).

There were no limits on what manufacturers or sellers could claim; it was caveat emptor for consumers. At first, cure-alls of the snake oil variety were promoted but manufacturers soon discovered that marketing drugs for specific ailments was more profitable (Applegate 1998). Most of these nostrums were promoted with wildly excessive claims as cures for cancer or arthritis, remedies for baldness or small busts, or restorers of manhood. Almost any possible problem could yield to patent medicine cures.

Advertising for patent medicines went directly from the manufacturer to the consumer. The invention of cheap pulp paper for newsprint helped create an important route for patent medicine advertising. Nostrum advertising accounted for nearly one-third of profits in the newspaper business. 'In 1847, 2000 newspapers ran 11 million medicine ads' (Anderson 2000: 38). By the 1870s, a quarter of all advertising was for proprietary drugs. Dr. James C. Ayer pioneered saturation advertising for his best-selling Cherry Pectoral, by running ads in every newspaper in the US (Anderson 2000: 41).

Ads often emphasised symptoms most people experienced (*e.g.* fatigue, pains, indigestion, sleeplessness, headaches), contributing to a cultural medicalisation of life problems. These drug companies borrowed from the rising prestige of medicine while at the same time distancing themselves from doctors, advertising their treatments as cheaper, safer, less brutal and quicker. Nostrum advertisers 'recognised that nearly every man (sic) is vulnerable to the power of suggestion and sought to make him sick so they could make him well'. (Young 1961: 184). As one analyst suggests, 'Medicine manufacturers didn't collect orders and then fill them, as was the practice with other goods. Rather, they created a steady supply of the product, and then generated the demand' (Anderson 2000: 11). By the early 20th century Americans shelled out $75 million a year, which translates into $1.6 billion in current buying power for patent medicines (Crossen 2004: B1). Patent medicines were at their zenith at the turn of the century, with over 28,000 nostrums, few as successful or well known as Lydia E. Pinkham's Vegetable Compound (Young 1961).

Lydia E. Pinkham's Vegetable Compound

After the financial 'panic' of 1873, the 54-yearold Lydia Pinkham, an abolitionist and school teacher, saw a business opportunity. She added ingredients to an herbal formula that her husband had received as part of a settlement for a debt and made it into a proprietary medicine, which she brewed and bottled in her cellar in Lynn, Massachusetts. Two years later, upon the advice of her son, she began marketing her product as Lydia E. Pinkham's Vegetable Compound for 'women's weaknesses,' including menstrual cramps. Lydia's motto was 'Only a woman understands women's ills' (Pinkus 2002). The compound had a pungent odour and a sharp aftertaste, and is thought to have contained black cohosh (roots and stems of a perennial herb), fenugreek seed, and at least 18 per cent alcohol (as a preservative, because Pinkham was a temperance supporter).

Pinkham was a pioneer in DTCA. After placing an elaborate first page newspaper ad in the *Boston*

Herald in 1876, sales of the product rose significantly, and Pinkham became convinced of the value of advertising. In 1879, her son suggested that she place a likeness of herself on the label, replete with her grandmotherly features. Sales of her product increased dramatically and her picture became one of the most well known female images in print at the time (Simmons 2002). She encouraged women to write to her in confidence for counsel, and answered their letters, a service which continued even after her death in 1883. These letters offered sterling testimonials of the product's efficacy.

Over the years, more maladies were added to the advertisements. For example, an 1887 ad in the *New York Times* proclaimed:

> LYDIA E. PINKHAM'S VEGETABLE COMPOUND Offers the SUREST REMEDY for the PAINFUL ILLS AND DISORDERS SUFFERED BY WOMEN EVERYWHERE. It relieves pain, promotes regular and healthy reoccurrence of periods and is a great help to young girls and women past maturity. It strengthens the back and the pelvic organs, bringing relief and comfort to tired women who stand all day in home, shop and factory. Leucorrhea, Inflammation, Ulceration and Displacements of the Uterus have been cured by it, as women everywhere gratefully testify. Regular physicians often prescribe it. Sold by all Druggists $1.00 (cited in Applegate 1998: 80).

Lydia Pinkham's advertising to consumers was innovative and ubiquitous. Her Vegetable Compound was everywhere; her face was on labels, in newspaper ads, on fences in rural America, on trading cards, and in drug store displays. Very few nostrums had such wide recognition. In 1912 sales exceeded $1 million. In 1914, in response to federal regulation, the company changed the formula to remove the alcohol so it would not be taxed as an alcoholic beverage and modified its claims about effectiveness (Applegate 1998). After 1925 or so, sales of the product declined. The patent medicine companies'

DTCA had been wildly successful for some companies but, increasingly, it was opposed by the medical profession and other articulate critics.

CAMPAIGNS AGAINST PATENT MEDICINES AND DTCA

In Paul Starr's (1982: 128) words, 'The nostrum makers were the nemesis of physicians'. They competed with physicians for medical business, offered supposedly safer but unproven 'cures', and undercut the authority of medicine. Patent medicines, with secret formulas and advertising to the public, posed a threat to physicians' still fledgling professional aspirations. Both patent medicines and physicians grew in popularity and use in the late 19th century. In fact, despite the competition, physicians also used patent medicines in their practices; by one count, in 1874 one per cent of physicians used patent medicines, increasing to over 20 per cent by 1902 (Starr 1982: 130). By another count, 90 per cent of doctors were prescribing proprietary medicines (Young 1961: 160).

The medical profession's concern about patent medicines manifested itself in a variety of campaigns against the industry. In 1900 the AMA started a campaign 'to make the "legitimate proprietary drugs" respond to the ethics of medicine', which included disclosing formulas and not advertising directly to the public (Starr 1982: 129). The AMA announced it would stop taking patent medicine advertisements around this time, then relaxed their standards for revenues' sake. As Young notes, 'In 1905, JAMA did not have as many bad ads as many medical journals, but that is only faint praise' (1961: 207). Medical journals and newspapers continued to rely on patent medicine advertising as a major source of revenue.

In 1906, the AMA set standards for both advertising and prescribing medications with the publication of *New and Nonofficial Remedies* (Starr 1982: 131). Drugs were not accepted if their manufacturers made false advertising claims, refused to disclose their drugs' composition, advertised directly to the public, or whose 'label, package or circular listed the diseases for which the drug was used' (Starr 1982: 132). Ethical drug companies had a 'gentleman's agreement' with physicians, under which physicians would legitimise the drugs with the 'ethical' label and the drug companies would acknowledge physicians' authority to diagnose illness and determine treatments. This agreement did not guarantee that drugs were safe, as ethical drugs might contain poisons such as arsenic. Rather, the term 'ethical' meant that the drug companies would be honest about the contents of their wares, would not knowingly make fraudulent claims about their efficacy, and would not bypass physicians' authority. The line was drawn. Companies could advertise to physicians only or they could not advertise to physicians at all. Despite losing revenues, newspapers began to cut back on DTCA for drugs that the AMA listed as fraudulent.

Muck-raking journalists were also on the case of exposing useless potions that were sold in the name of health. In 1903 the *Ladies Home Journal* published an exposé on the dangers of patent medicines. Samuel Hopkins Adams' in-depth investigative series, 'The Great American Fraud', published in *Colliers Weekly* in 1905, really made the public case against patent medicines. The articles named specific names and identified specific false promises and deceptions made in patent medicine advertising. The writers and editors of these magazines advocated for federal regulation on the promotion and sale of patent medicines (Applegate 1998).

Some states had already considered regulating patent medicines, but they were 'easily out-matched by the well funded lobby of the Proprietary Association of America' (Crossen 2004). The AMA distributed 150,000 copies of these articles from 1905 to 1910 (Starr 1982: 130). Adams' investigation, along with Upton Sinclair's *The Jungle*, a muckraking exposé of the meat packing industry, the AMA's campaign against nostrum marketing, and scientist and crusader Harvey W. Wiley's work with Congress, finally resulted in the Pure Food and Drug Act of 1906, the first federal legislation to control drugs and medications.

FEDERAL REGULATION AND DRUG ADVERTISING

The Act put constraints on advertising and marketing, stating that manufacturers had to print accurate ingredients on the label, they could not make false or exaggerated claims on the label, and that drugs had to meet certain standards of purity. As one indicator of the Act's impact, the 1897 Sears Roebuck catalogue had 17 out of 770 pages dedicated to the 'Drug Department'; the 1908 catalogue had fewer than two pages of 1200 on drugs (Isreal 1968 cited in Pinkus 2002). The federal law was amended in 1912 to include claims of effectiveness and in 1920 to cover newspaper advertising (Starr 1982: 132). By 1915, Lydia E. Pinkham's Vegetable Compound had to cease advertising specifically for women's disorders and instead made the innocuous claim, 'Recommended as a Vegetable Tonic in conditions for which the preparation has been adapted' (Starr 1982: 132).

Between 1906 and 1980, the FDA consolidated regulatory authority over prescription drugs and gained jurisdiction over all communication from the pharmaceutical industry. Likewise, in the first half of the 20th century, physicians continued to solidify their medical authority over diagnosis of illness and prescribing drugs as treatments (Starr 1982). Both the profession of medicine and the FDA operated to constrain the advertising of pharmaceuticals during most of the 20th century, thereby also constraining consumers' access to pharmaceuticals to treat their aches and troubles. This concurrent consolidation of medical and regulatory authority began to break down in the 1980s.

THE EMERGENCE OF DTCA OF PRESCRIPTION DRUGS: 1981–1996

Direct-to-consumer advertising for prescription medications has fuelled the medicalisation that analysts noted as increasing in Western societies in the 1980s (Conrad 1992). DTCA has become a major

source of expanding medical markets and public engagement with medical solutions for life's conditions and problems (Conrad and Leiter 2004).

In 1981, Boots Pharmaceutical (a British firm) issued the first DTC broadcast ad for an ibuprofen product called Rufen and Merck Sharp & Dohme advertised a pneumonia vaccine called Pneumovax (Pines 1999). According to Pines, who was at the FDA at the time, the FDA's first response was shock, and 'Physicians at the FDA generally felt that such advertising was inappropriate' (1999: 492). Yet the very next year, FDA Commissioner Arthur Hull Hayes, Jr. gave a speech before the Pharmaceutical Advertising Council, in which he stated that, 'In sum, my impression is that we may be on the brink of the exponential growth phase of direct-to-consumer promotion of prescription products' (U.S. House of Representatives 1984: 1).

In that speech, Hayes describes the changing dynamics between patients, physicians, and pharmaceutical companies:

> There was a time when prescription product advertising to consumers was limited to an occasional institutional ad. Physicians were your industry's sole target audience. Patients had an insignificant voice in choosing prescription products they were given. Generic drugs were not yet an issue. The demographics of consumer publications were such that a very high percentage of the exposures paid for by a prescription product advertiser would be to people who could not possibly use the product. And members of the advertising profession did not want to run the risk of offending physicians by appearing to circumvent them or undercut their freedom of judgment. It is no longer so. One result of the consumer movement has been increasing numbers of patients who demand a role in the selection of all their health care products. The *Physicians' Desk Reference*—as Charlie Baker would be pleased to tell you—is a best seller. It's difficult to remember the last time that the weekly book best seller lists didn't include several volumes about prescription

drugs and health care. Specialised health magazines have proliferated. And 90 per cent of prescriptions are now for drugs no one heard of only a generation ago (U.S. House of Representatives 1984: 23–24).

Hayes' speech describes a shift to more consumer-demanded healthcare, with lay persons playing a larger role in determining their own needs and treatments, opening the door to increased medicalisation by health 'consumers'.

In response to this speech, the FDA commissioned a study of physicians and pharmacists regarding patients and prescriptions, and the US House Subcommittee on Oversight and Investigations sent out letters to 37 pharmaceutical companies asking for their position on DTCA (U.S. House of Representatives 1984). Not surprisingly, almost all of the response letters said that the companies would engage in DTCA if their competitors did so. What is striking about the letters is that *they were almost unanimous in their negative responses to the potential of DTCA*. Wayne Davidson, president of the U.S. Pharmaceutical and Nutritional Division of the Bristol-Myers Company, wrote:

> It will be very difficult, if not impossible, for a federal agency (FDA or FTC) to distinguish between when self-diagnosis is possible and when it is not. Where the line is drawn will be the subject of much legal controversy. We are of the opinion it is much better not to attempt to draw the line, but to prohibit this type of advertising to the patient consumer. This type of advertising will also put the prescribing professionals on the defensive in the relationship with their patients, just the reverse of the most productive relationship . . . (U.S. House of Representatives 1984: 89).

Similarly, Thomas Collins, president of Smith Kline & French Laboratories, replied:

> We do not believe that PDAC [Prescription Drug Advertising to the Consumer] is a good idea. . . . We believe that the chances for damaging doctor-patient relations and for encouraging costly competitive battles are real, while the likelihood that meaningful patient education will occur is small. We certainly welcome, let me stress, the increased consumer participation in health decisions in recent years. It is well for patients to take part, to the extent they wish, in decisions affecting their care. It is however very important to differentiate the capabilities of advertising from those of educational programs. Advertising can inform, but it is not education; and PDAC should not be portrayed as part of the education process (U.S. House of Representatives 1984: 152–3).

Both of these letters voice concerns about consumers' ability to self-diagnose, essentially questioning consumers' medicalisation of their own problems and highlighting the important role that physicians play as gatekeepers in the medicalisation process. In September of 1982, at the beginning of these explorations, the FDA requested a formal, voluntary moratorium on DTCA (Feather 1998 cited in Pines 1999). In 1983, the FDA issued a policy statement calling for a 'period of cautious restraint on the part of would-be prescription drug advertisers' (50 Fed. Reg. 36677 (1985)). Then in 1985, the FDA withdrew its moratorium, concluding that 'for the time being, current regulations governing prescription drug advertising provide sufficient safeguards to protect consumers' (50 Fed. Reg. 36677 (1985)). According to Pines, the FDA's policy change was 'not intended to open the floodgates for DTC advertising. On the contrary, it was a reluctant recognition by the agency of a new trend, and was intended to ensure that FDA had jurisdiction and that the industry had a framework within which to consider DTC advertising' (1999: 493).

After the FDA withdrew the moratorium, companies increased their print advertising considerably, with companies spending $12 billion in DTCA in 1989 (Medical Advertising News 1999 cited in Pines 1999). However, the cumbersome 'fair balance' and 'brief summary' requirements indirectly kept companies from engaging in DTC broadcast advertising, constraining their outreach to consumers.

DTCA COMES TO TV: 1997 ONWARD

On 8th, August 1997, the FDA issued draft guidelines for DTCA of product-specific prescription drug broadcast advertisements (62 Fed. Reg. 43171), which described how television and radio ads might fulfill FDA requirements for 'adequate provision' of product information and a 'major statement' of the drug's major risks. Prior to this, these requirements made TV drug advertising all but impossible.

Under this new interpretation of the regulations, the FDA would allow DTC broadcast advertising if the advertising would provide consumers with the product's approved labelling information through one of four sources: a toll-free telephone number that consumers could call; a concurrent print advertisement containing a brief summary of risk information; a web page (URL) that included the package insert; or additional product information from pharmacists, physicians, or other healthcare providers (Food and Drug Administration 1999). The FDA also announced that it wanted the industry to conduct studies of the effects of DTCA and that it would evaluate the policy in two years (Pines 1999). On 6th, August 1999, the FDA issued its final guidance for DTCA of prescription drugs (64 Fed. Reg. 43197), making very few changes to its original guidelines.

Three types of prescription DTCA would be permitted: product claim advertisements, which included the product name and specific therapeutic claims; reminder advertisements, which gave the name of the drug but did not state its use; and so-called help-seeking advertisements, which told consumers about unspecified treatment possibilities for diseases or conditions (Goldman 2005). From our perspective, all three contribute to medicalisation, with the help-seeking ads the most likely to promote it.

This shift in policy was controversial. Those supporting the change suggested that there would be a public health benefit, depicting broadcast DTCA as 'an excellent way to meet the growing demand for medical information, empowering consumers by educating them about health conditions and possible treatments' (Holmer 1999 quoted in Hollon 2005). Critics voiced reservations, especially regarding how DTCA could lead to overprescribing, how it emphasised newer and more expensive medicines over cheaper existing ones, and regarding 'the medicalising of normal human experience' (Mintzes 2002, Frosch *et al.* 2007).

Broadcast DTCA has grown enormously in the past years, up from $55 million in 1991 to $4.2 billion in 2005 (USGAO 2006), with 330 per cent growth in DTCA from 1996 to 2005 (Donahue *et al.* 2007). The ads focus on chronic problems affecting relatively healthy people, with large potential treatment populations and long-term usage, including drugs for allergy, anxiety, obesity, arthritis, erectile dysfunction, and high cholesterol. About 20 prescription drugs make up 60 per cent of the pharmaceutical company spending on DTCA (Hollon 2005) and advertising for one specific drug can have ripple effects for all drugs that are touted for a particular condition. The US Government Accountability Office has estimated that 'each 10% increase in DTC spending within a drug class increases sales in that class by 1%' (2002: 15). DTC ads for drugs to treat erectile dysfunction have become common, especially on television.

DTCA AND ERECTILE DYSFUNCTION

The Viagra story is by now a familiar one. We need not repeat it in detail here (see Conrad and Leiter 2004, Loe 2004) but will review some points that are relevant to DTCA and medicalisation. In 1992 a consensus conference officially labelled what used to be called impotence as 'erectile dysfunction' and as a biogenic rather than psychogenic problem. In March 1998, the FDA approved

Viagra (sildenafil citrate) as a treatment for this condition. In the early days it was marketed primarily to older men with erectile problems and for erectile dysfunction associated with prostate cancer, diabetes, and other medical problems (Loe 2004). Estimates for prevalence ranged from 10 million to half of all American men (Laumann *et al.* 1999). The market potential was not lost on the drug companies, so within a short time Pfizer Pharmaceuticals began advertising Viagra more broadly. With an ageing population, a high prevalence of erectile dysfunction, and an even broader concern with sexual performance, the potential market was huge. DTCA expanded the market to include virtually *any* man who might consider himself as having erectile problems or just wanted a boost in performance (Conrad and Leiter 2004). Within a few years of Viagra's introduction, pharmaceutical competitors came on the scene.

Levitra was introduced in 2003 as a faster drug with fewer adverse effects than Viagra. Levitra ads focused more on recreational uses, targeting 'men who may have successful sexual relationships but simply want to improve the quality or duration of their erections' (Harris 2003). The most visible DTCA spokesman for Levitra was Mike Ditka, a former hardnosed football coach and Hall of Fame player. Levitra became an official sponsor of the National Football League (NFL) and in 2004 became the first pharmaceutical ad during the Super Bowl with its 'Levitra Challenge'. In the week after the Super Bowl, Levitra prescriptions grew by 15 per cent (GSK news release 2004). However, there may be limits to what kind of DTC ads are acceptable for television. The FDA asked Bayer Pharmaceuticals, maker of Levitra, to pull its 15-second spot of 'My Man' ads that promoted Levitra. The ads starred an attractive actress, Marie Silvia—hailed as 'Queen Levitra' by the *Wall Street Journal*—who said how the drug's 'strong and lasting effects' provide a 'quality experience' (Snowbeck 2005). Apparently the ad did not include enough safety information and made a misleading comparison with other drugs for the condition. While the short version of the Queen Levitra ad was pulled, the 45-second version continued to be aired (Snowbeck 2005).

DTCA has shaped and developed the erectile dysfunction drug market. In 2004, drug companies spent over $382 million in advertising these drugs in the US, with sales of $1.36 billion (Snowbeck 2005). The demand for these drugs may have stabilised; doctors wrote 10 per cent fewer new prescriptions in October 2005 than the year before (Berenson 2005). While erectile dysfunction has been firmly medicalised, there may be limits to the demand for medical solutions for sexual difficulties.

FROM QUEEN LYDIA TO QUEEN LEVITRA

Lydia Pinkham was the queen of patent medicine. Her product, cooked up in her cellar and composed of herbs and alcohol, epitomises the patent medicine industry in the late 19th and early 20th centuries, which was built largely upon proprietary recipes and grand promises printed on cheap, pulp paper. Patent medicines contributed to a cultural medicalisation of life problems. Advertisements told consumers that they could diagnose their own symptoms and use patent medicines to alleviate those symptoms, without having to resort to consulting physicians. These symptoms ranged from everyday aches and pains, such as being tired or nervous, to serious diseases such as tuberculosis. While over-the-counter medications have continued to fill this self-help niche, during most of the 20th century the profession of medicine and the FDA successfully constrained the advertising of pharmaceuticals to the public, making physicians key gatekeepers to prescription drugs.

More recently, 'Queen Levitra' was on television, touting Levitra's ability to produce 'strong and lasting effects' and a 'quality experience', alluding to the sexual ability that men may gain (to women's benefit) by taking Levitra. We have come a long way since the days of patent medicine 100 years ago. Yet DTCA hearkens back to those days, in that the pharmaceutical industry is once again reaching out to consumers directly when selling their products and creating wider avenues to the medicalisation of life problems. In this way, the advertising of pharmaceuticals is becoming more like the advertising of over-the-counter medications. In fact, the distinction between prescription drugs and these medications may be less clear now than in the mid-20th century, due to DTCA as well as some pharmaceuticals shifting from prescription to over-the-counter status. For example, Claritin, a well-known antihistamine that was advertised heavily on broadcast media early in the contemporary DTCA era, is now available over the counter.

Pharmaceutical companies' advertising activities have changed considerably, with important implications for medicalisation, as summarised in Table 23.1. Before 1906, drug manufacturers were split into two increasingly distinct camps: ethical drug manufacturers and patent drug manufacturers. Much of the distinction between these two types of manufacturers was based on the type of advertising that they used to sell their wares: ethical drug companies advertised to physicians only, while patent medicine companies advertised directly to consumers. This gentleman's agreement allowed physicians to legitimise ethical drugs and ethical drug companies to defer to physician's authority in diagnosis and prescribing. During this period, physicians, patent medicine manufacturers, and consumers contributed to expansion of medical definitions and treatments for life problems.

After Congress passed the Food and Drug Act of 1906, the AMA stepped up its efforts to police the boundaries between ethical and patent drug firms, working with the federal government to identify firms that violated the Act. Through this legislation, the government could disrupt the direct relationship between patent drug producers and consumers, protecting consumers in the name of public health. As a result of these efforts, advertising for prescription medications became restricted between 1906–1980 to physicians only and drug companies had a limited role in medicalisation. It is important to note that drug companies always had access to consumers for over-the-counter medications. They did not require a medical prescription and were advertised widely. These were typically cold remedies and headache medications, although they would occasionally also encourage medicalisation of new ills such as the 'halitosis' (bad breath) mentioned in Listerine mouthwash advertisements. However, physicians' control over access to pharmaceuticals limited medicalisation.

Around 1981 pharmaceutical companies began to test the gentleman's agreement concerning prescription advertising by initiating limited forays of DTCA. There were no laws against advertising drugs but firms were unsure of what was permissible. A 1985 FDA statement permitted the pharmaceutical industry sufficient latitude to allow a broader engagement with print ads for prescription drugs. The drug companies did not yet venture into broadcast ads due to the difficulty of fulfilling the FDA's requirements regarding the 'major statement' of risks and side effects of drugs.

TABLE 23.1 ■ Summary of Drug Advertising Activities and Implications for Medicalisation		
Time Periods	**Pharmaceutical Advertising Activities**	**Implications for Medicalisation**
Before 1906	Ethical: to physicians Patent: to consumers	Both consumers and physicians are agents of medicalisation
1906–1980	Advertising of prescription drugs to physicians only	Physicians dominate medicalisation
1981–1996	Advertising to physicians; growth in print ads to consumers	Consumers have more information to participate in medicalisation
1997–present	Advertising to physicians; widespread DTCA print and broadcast ads to consumers	Drug industry and consumers become more significant; physicians' centrality decreased

The reinterpretation of FDA advertising guidelines in 1997 had major implications for DTCA, especially on television. Now drug companies could market directly to consumers. Physicians became gatekeepers for drugs advertised direct to consumers rather than initiators of pharmaceutical treatments: 'Ask your doctor if [name of drug] is right for you'. The drug industry and consumers, facilitated by DTCA, have become major players in medicalisation with physicians relegated to somewhat less of a role (Conrad 2007). In fact, direct access to consumers has increased the pharmaceutical industry's incentive to medicalise human problems, encouraging consumers to self-diagnose and request drugs that they see on TV. Furthermore, the Internet has become another direct avenue from pharmaceutical companies to consumers, and one that is not limited to national boundaries. This electronic form of DTCA can already be considered as a factor in internationalising medicalisation. Some Internet sites bypass physicians altogether with a veneer of medical oversight.

The impacts of DTCA on medicalisation and health are complicated. DTCA can raise awareness about disease and risk, and provide some useful medical information for consumers, although most physicians believe that DTCA does not provide balanced information (Perri et al. 1999, Hollon 2005). DTCA has significant impact on patient demands, physicians prescribing, and by implication, medicalisation. DTC advertising leads to increased requests for advertised medicines and more prescriptions (Mintzes et al. 2003). A study by Kravitz et al. (2005) sent trained standardised patients to physicians. The 'patients' presented symptoms of either major depression or adjustment disorder and made DTC-related requests of a brand specific drug, a general class of drugs, or no request. 'Patients' who made brand-specific requests or general requests for drugs were much more likely than patients who made no requests for drugs to receive a prescription. Requesting medications increased the amount of prescribing, at least for these two disorders. What is disturbing here is that although there are no data to support the use of antidepressants for adjustment disorder, half of those who requested it, based on DTCA, received prescriptions. The authors conclude that DTCA 'may stimulate prescribing of more questionable than clear indications' (Kravitz et al. 2005: 2000).

The scrutiny and criticism of DTCA appears to be increasing from various quarters. U.S. Senate Majority Leader Bill Frist (a physician) expressed concerns that DTCA creates a wedge between physicians and patients (Henderson 2005). An article in *Advertising Age* questioned whether recent drug safety scares may shift the balance of power back to physicians (Thomaselli 2005) as consumers respond to cases such as Vioxx's well-advertised entry and quick removal from the market. In July 2005, the drug industry drafted guidelines that called for a period of notifying doctors about new drugs before advertising to consumers (Saul 2005a). These new voluntary guidelines would 'virtually eliminate 15-second spots' because they do not provide enough time to list risks, and require that all ads will be submitted to the FDA for review before they are used (Saul 2005b). While it is too early to judge the impact of these changes on medicalisation, it seems doubtful that these changes would significantly decrease the roles of DTC advertising and consumers on medicalisation.

CONCLUSION

While DTCA appears to be flourishing, even FDA personnel seem concerned about its effects on medicalisation. In a meeting about DTCA, Janet Woodcock, the director of the FDA's Center for Drug Evaluation and Research, highlighted two concerns: 'First, that many common and relatively minor complaints of daily life represent diseases. This has been called the medicalisation of life. And second, the perception that all life complaints can and perhaps should be treated with a pill' (Food and Drug Administration 2003: 22). Broadcast DTCA is now only permitted in the US and New Zealand and is prohibited in the United Kingdom and most developed countries. Should DTC advertising be introduced in Europe (Watson 2003), most of the same issues would exist (Metzl 2007).

One of the ironies of DTCA is that it expands the relationship of drug companies, physicians and consumers, returning it to a situation similar to Lydia Pinkham's day, when the drug manufacturers had a direct and independent relationship with consumers. It encourages self-diagnosis and requests for treatment. It allows pharmaceutical companies to create specific markets for their products and promote them to waiting customers. Of course, with stronger government regulation and a more powerful medical profession, the situation is also different from what it was a century ago. The extravagant claims of Lydia Pinkham's day are constrained by laws, but modern advertising is both more subtle and sophisticated than what was available to the patent medicine peddlers. It seems clear that the pharmaceutical industry and consumers are becoming increasingly important players in medicalisation and that DTCA facilitates this shift.

ACKNOWLEDGMENTS

An earlier version of this paper was presented at the Centennial Session 'One Hundred Years of Health Policy Research' at the meetings of the American Sociological Association, August 14, 2005. Thanks to Donald Light for the original impetus for this paper and to Phil Brown and anonymous reviewers for comments on this paper.

References

Anderson, A. (2000) *Snake Oil, Hustlers and Ham-bones: the American Medical Show.* Jefferson: McFarland and Company.

Applegate, E. (1998) *Personalities and Products: a Historical Perspective on Advertising in America.* Westport, CT: Greenwood Press.

Berenson, A. (2005) Sales of impotence drugs fall, defying expectations, *New York Times*, December 4, 1, (http://www.nytimes.com/2005/12/04/business/yourmoney/04impotence.html?ex=1178596800&en=9a037a1bdd97025e&ei=5070) (accessed May 5, 2007).

Conrad, P. (1992) Medicalization and Social Control, *Annual Review of Sociology*, 18, 209–32.

Conrad, P. (2005) The shifting engines of medicalisation, *Journal of Health and Social Behavior*, 46, 1, 3–14.

Conrad, P. (2007) *The Medicalisation of Society: On the Transformation of Human Conditions into Treatable Disorders.* Baltimore: Johns Hopkins University Press.

Conrad, P. and Leiter, V. (2004) Medicalisation, markets and consumers, *Journal of Health and Social Behavior*, 45, Extra Issue, 158–76.

Conrad, P. and Schneider, J.W. (1992) *Deviance and Medicalisation: From Badness to Sickness.* Philadelphia: Temple University Press.

Crossen, C. (2004) Fraudulent claims led U.S. to take on drug makers in 1900s, *Wall Street Journal*, Oct. 6, B1.

Donahue, J.M., Cevasco, M. and Rosenthal, M.B. (2007) A decade of direct-to-consumer advertising of prescription drugs, *New England Journal of Medicine*, 357, 673–81.

Feather, K.R. (1998) Presentation before the Institute for International Research, Washington, D.C., Sept. 14, 1998.

Food and Drug Administration. (1999) *Guidance for Industry: Consumer-Directed Broadcast Advertisements Questions and Answers.* (http://www.fda.gov/cder/guidance/1804q&a.htm) (accessed May 16, 2007).

Food and Drug Administration. (2003) *Direct-to-Consumer Promotion: Public Meeting, September 22 and 23, 2003.* (http://www.fda.gov/cder/ddmac/DTCmeeting2003.html) (accessed July 7, 2005).

Freidson, E. (1970) *The Profession of Medicine.* New York: Dodd, Mead.

Frosch, D.L., Krueger, P.M., Hornik, R.C., Cronholm, P.F. and Barg, F.K. (2007) Creating demand for prescription drugs: a content analysis of television direct-to-consumer advertising, *Annals of Family Medicine*, 5, 1, 6–13.

Goldman, M. (2005) Direct-to-consumer advertising: benefit to patients? Drug and Marketing Publications (http://www.drugandmarket.com/default.asp?section=feature&article=042205)

GSK news release. (2004) GlaxoSmithKline news release, (http://www.gsk.com/media/archive .htm#nolink) (accessed May 15, 2007).

Harris, G. (2003) Levitra, a rival with ribald ads, gains on Viagra, *New York Times*, September 18, C5.

Harrison-Barbet, A. (1994) *Thomas Holloway: Victorian Philanthropist: a Biographical Essay.* Egham: Royal Holloway, University of London.

Henderson, D. (2005) With advertising under siege, drug makers rethink their marketing message, *The Boston Globe*, July 31, E1.

Hollon, M.F. (2005) Direct-to-consumer advertising: a haphazard approach to health promotion, *Journal of the American Medical Association*, 293, 16, 2030–3.

Holmer, A.F. (1999) Direct-to-consumer prescription drug advertising builds bridges between patient and physician, *Journal of the American Medical Association*, 281, 4, 380–4.

Israel, F.L., (ed.) (1968) *1897 and 1908 Sears Roebuck Catalog.* New York: Chelsea House Publishers.

Kravitz, R.L., Epstein, R.M., Feldman, M.D., Franz, C.E., Azari, A., Wilkes, M.S., Hinton, L. and Franks, P. (2005) Influence of patients' requests for direct-to-consumer advertised antidepressants: A randomised controlled trial, *Journal of the American Medical Association*, 293, 16, 1995–2002.

Laumann, E.O., Paik, A. and Rosen, R.C. (1999) Sexual dysfunction in the United States: prevalence and predictors, *Journal of the American Medical Association*, 281, 6, 537–44.

Loe, M. (2004) *The Rise of Viagra.* New York: New York University Press.

Medical Advertising News. (1999) Chart, 20.

Metzl, J.M. (2007) If direct-to-consumer advertisements come to Europe: lessons from the USA. *Lancet* 369: 704–06.

Mintzes, B. (2002) Direct to consumer advertising is medicalising normal human experience, *British Medical Journal*, 324, 908–11.

Mintzes, B., Barer, M.L., Kravitz, R.L., Bassett, K., Lexchin, J., Kazanjian, A., Evans, R.G., Pan, R. and Marion, S.A. (2003) How does direct-to-consumer advertising (DTCA) affect prescribing? A survey in primary care environments with and without legal DTCA, *Canadian Medical Association Journal*, 169, 5, 405–12.

Perri, M., Shinde, S. and Banavali, R. (1999) The past, present and future of direct-to-consumer drug advertising, *Clinical Therapy*, 21, 10, 1798–811.

Pines, W.L. (1999) A history and perspective on direct-to-consumer promotion, *Food and Drug Law Journal*, 54, 489–518.

Pinkus, R.L. (2002) From Lydia Pinkham to Bob Dole: what the changing face of direct-to-consumer drug advertising reveals about the profession of medicine, *Kennedy Institute of Ethics Journal*, 12, 141–58.

Saul, S. (2005a) Drug industry proposes limits on advertising, *The New York Times*, July 22, C4.

Saul, S. (2005b) Drug makers to police consumer campaigns, *The New York Times*, August 3, C7.

Shorter, E. (1992) *From Paralysis to Fatigue: A History of Psychosomatic Illness in the Modern Era.* New York: Free Press.

Simmons, J.G. (2002) *Doctors and Discoveries: Lives That Created What Medicine is Today.* Boston: Houghton Mifflin.

Snowbeck, C. (2005) FDA tells Levitra to cool it with ad, *Pittsburgh Globe-Gazette*, April 19. (http://www.post-gazette.com/pg/05109/490334.stm) (accessed May 14, 2007).

Spillane, J.F. (2004) The road to the Harrison Narcotics Act: drugs and their control, 1875–1918. In Erlen, J. and Spillane, J.F., (eds) *Federal Drug Control: The Evolution of Policy and Practice*, New York: Pharmaceutical Products Press.

Starr, P. (1982) *The Transformation of American Medicine*, New York: Basic Books.

Thomaselli, R. (2005) PR seems to be the Rx to get around DTC rules: firms confirm pharma is seeking ways to live with (but not skirt) guidelines, *Advertising Age*, 26 September, 6.

U.S. Government Accountability Office. (2006) *Prescription Drugs: Improvements Needed in FDA's Oversight of Direct-to-Consumer Advertising.* Washington, D.C.: U.S. Government Accountability Office.

U.S. House of Representatives. (1984) *Prescription Drug Advertising to Consumers. Staff Report Prepared for the Use of the Subcommittee on Oversight and Investigations of the Committee on Energy and Commerce, House of Representatives*. Washington, D.C.: U.S. Government Printing Office.

Watson, R. (2003) EU health ministers reject proposal for limited direct to consumer advertising. *BMJ*, 326, 1284.

Wertz, R. and Wertz, D. (1989) *Lying In: a History of Childbirth in America*. New Haven: Yale University Press.

Young, J.H. (1961) *The Toadstool Millionaires: a History of Patent Medicines in America Before Federal Regulation*. Princeton, N.J.: Princeton University Press.

PRESCRIPTIONS AND PROSCRIPTIONS

Moralising Sleep Medicines

Jonathan Gabe,[1] Catherine M. Coveney,[2] and Simon J. Williams[3]

INTRODUCTION

Sleep is not just a personal or political matter but a moral one, including the very meanings we accord sleep and the ways we manage it in our everyday/ night lives. In this paper we take a closer look at these issues through the multiple meanings and moral dimensions of sleep medications in every day/ night life. Our paper, in this regard, is located at the intersection of newly emerging social scientific scholarship on sleep matters (Henry *et al.* 2013, Williams 2005, 2011, Williams *et al.* 2013, Williams and Wolf-Meyer 2013), wider sociological debates on the medicalisation and pharmaceuticalisation of life (Abraham 2010, Bell and Figert 2012, Gabe

et al. 2015, Williams *et al.* 2011), and other work in medical sociology (Lumme-Sandt and Virtanen 2002, Pound *et al.* 2005) and cognate fields such as science and technology studies (STS) (Coveney 2011, Oudshoorn 2008, Webster *et al.* 2009) on the meanings, cultural scripts and uses of pharmaceuticals and other socio-technological objects.

Redefining sleep as a medical problem requiring a pharmaceutical intervention is a contentious issue (cf. Anthierens et al. 2007, Kripke 2006, PCT 2011, Rogers et al. 2007). Sleep medications get a 'bad press' due to their potential for dependence and other side effects, including studies reporting increased mortality risks for long-term users (Kripke et al. 2012). Medically, the long term use of

Prescriptions and Proscriptions: Moralising Sleep Medicines, Jonathan Gabe, Catherine M. Coveney, and Simon J. Williams in *Sociology of Health & Illness,* 38(4), 2016, pp. 627–644.

hypnotics is not advised due to adverse side effects, including drowsiness, confusion and cognitive and psycho-motor impairment, effects which have been associated with fractures, falls and road-traffic accidents (Buysse 2013, Siriwardena et al. 2008,), in addition to problems of tolerance and dependence. In 2004, NICE (National Institute for Health and Clinical Excellence) in the UK issued guidance to physicians about these risks and advised against use for over 4 weeks, and only for severe insomnia. Previously similar advice had been issued by the Department of Health and Social Security in the 1980s about the dependence potential of benzodiazepines, including those marketed as sleeping tablets (Gabe and Bury 1988), yet in 2013, over 9.7 million hypnotics were still dispensed in the UK including 6.3 million 'z drugs', primarily zopiclone and 2.9 million benzodiazepines (HSCIC 2014). Approximately a quarter of these prescriptions were for four weeks or more, contrary to guidance from NICE (2004).

A small number of sociological studies have looked at patient experiences of taking sleeping pills. These studies found that both the prescription of benzodiazepine hypnotics in primary care and consumption of these medicines in daily life are highly moralised issues (Gabe and Lipshitz-Phillips 1982, 1984, Gabe and Thorogood 1986, North et al. 1995, Venn and Arber 2012). Ambivalence to using these medicines emerges as a common theme across different patient groups where the benefits or need to medicate sleep is juxtaposed with more negative feelings towards hypnotic medication (Gabe and Lipshitz-Phillips 1982, 1984, Gabe and Thorogood 1986). For instance a recent study looking at older people's experience of taking sleep medications found that hypnotic use was often viewed as being morally inappropriate—'an unnatural interference into a natural state'—and associated with loss of control and addiction (Venn and Arber 2012). Similarly, the women in earlier studies (Gabe and Lipshitz-Phillips 1982, 1984, Gabe and Thorogood 1986) expressed a strong dislike of taking drugs of any kind, and while accepting that the drug might do them some good also expressed fears of addiction and dependency.

Social scientific research on pharmaceuticals more generally has, amongst other things, drawn attention to how pharmaceuticals are understood and used in everyday life. Pharmaceutical technologies are socially embedded (Cohen et al. 2001) and their use shaped by cultural repertoires, social relationships, the medical condition being experienced and the identities of their consumers (Dew et al. 2015, Lumme-Sandt et al. 2000, Rose, 2007, Webster et al. 2009). They are thus imbued with not only technical meanings relating to their biomedical functions but also with strong social and cultural scripts for how they should be used (Hodgetts et al. 2011). Users are increasingly recognised as being knowledgeable and reflexive actors, assessing the risks and benefits and making informed choices about medicine use drawing on what Webster et al. (2009) call a 'lay pharmacology' about safety, efficacy and side effects. Such choices are sometimes made in consultation with professionals and sometimes not (Will and Weiner 2015).

Modifying medicine treatment regimens without prior discussions with medical professionals is common place. For example, in a review of qualitative studies Pound et al. (2005) reported that dosages were generally decreased by patients in their attempts to maintain control of medications and medicines were often supplemented or replaced with non-pharmacological treatments. Pharmaceutical drugs are thus but one part of a larger assortment of medical and non-medical technologies, devices, discourses and talking therapies aimed at modulating physical, behavioural, psychological and emotional states. Dew et al. (2014) argue that people 'hybridise these wellness practices', assimilating different forms of knowledge and expertise and recombining them in relation to their own understandings in the enactment of their daily routines and relationships. The availability of such non-medical technologies thus provides opportunities for de-pharmaceuticalisation at the lay or life world level.

In this way, we can think about hypnotic medicines as consumer goods that are personalised and reconfigured in the home. They are consumed within socio-technical networks that give meaning to their use and non-use. Through our interactions with medicines in daily life these bio-medical objects are translated into social objects that carry biographies, personal and shared meanings, thus becoming 'socio-pharmacological objects' (Hodgetts *et al.* 2011). Different meanings are given to medications in daily life and these meanings are important to understand the variations in how medicines are used. Hence, not only the practicality of taking one's medication, but the morality of medicine use, and associated ideas about 'good' and 'bad' behaviour, is an important consideration.

Lumme-Sandt *et al* (2000), in their study of the oldest old (aged 90 or over) in Finland found that their respondents called primarily on a moral repertoire when talking about medications (including sleeping pills). They presented themselves as moral and responsible drug users by explaining the 'objective reasons' for their use, playing down the extent of such use and comparing it favourably with assumed level of use by others. In a similar vein Dew *et al.* (2015), in their study of households in New Zealand, reported that respondents developed and articulated four distinct repertoires about the moral meaning of medications: a disordering society repertoire where pharmaceuticals evoked a society in an unnatural state which required active resistance; a disordering self-repertoire where drug use indicated a moral failing of the individual and a lack of control; a disordering substances repertoire involving a threat to a person's physical or mental state but where medicine use could be justified on the basis of a cost benefit assessment and the importance of acting responsibly; and finally a re-ordering substances repertoire where drug use was associated with a restoration of function in line with the advice of professionals.

This focus on moral judgments can be located in wider concerns to understand health and illness in terms of the accounts people give, the vocabularies they draw on and the contexts in which these accounts are constructed (Backett 1992, Radley and Billig 1996). This means that morality is not viewed as located in people's heads but instead is an aspect of the embodied interactional practices that people engage in as members of society (Sayer 2011, Turowetz and Maynard 2010). Such practices can

involve expressing approval or disapproval of others or presenting oneself as a moral being (Sayer 2011).

In this paper, as a further contribution to these moral matters concerning medicines in general and sleep medicines in particular, we aim to explore the ways in which the use/non-use of prescription hypnotics is understood and negotiated in daily life and how this is implicated in moral discourses about medicines. Drawing on focus group data we analyse collective views and experiences of hypnotic use across a range of social contexts, paying attention to the moral dimensions of respondents' talk and the repertoires they draw on to justify and legitimate hypnotic use/non-use in the management of sleep problems. By 'repertoire' we mean a relatively coherent system of meanings for 'characterizing and evaluating actions, events and other phenomena' (Potter and Wetherell 1987: 149). It is important to recognise that 'the same person may use different repertoires in different contexts and for different functions' (Lumme-Sandt *et al.* 2000: 1845). How users engage with hypnotics in their daily lives moreover, we argue, is an important yet under-researched dimension of understanding the dynamics of pharmaceuticalisation in an era where users of medicines, sleep related or otherwise, are increasingly active in the management of their own health and illness.

METHODS

Data were collected as part of a wider study looking at Medicated Sleep and Wakefulness in the UK since 2000, funded by the UK Economic and Social Research Council. Following ethics approval from the National Health Service in England we held 23 focus groups (99 participants), between 2012 and 2014, with people who might be expected to have particular views and experiences of sleep management. This included those currently taking hypnotics prescribed in a primary care setting, people who have been diagnosed with a sleep disorder (narcolepsy, sleep apnoea, insomnia), and general population groups including students, parents of young children, ambulance service staff (including technicians and paramedics), academics, lawyers and retired people living in sheltered housing. We purposively selected these groups in order to explore diversity in experiences of and attitudes towards sleeping pills rather than for representativeness.

Research participants were recruited in a number of ways. General practice patients were invited to participate by their GP, on the basis of having received a prescription for sleeping tablets. Those attending sleep apnoea clinics and narcolepsy clinics were invited to contact the researchers if they were interested in being part of the research by the clinician in charge of the clinic. Paramedics were recruited through advertisements in the local Trust newsletter and posters sent to ambulance stations, while students were invited through the local university student union, departmental student lists and personal contacts. Parents of young children were recruited through local parent and toddler groups. The focus groups made up of academics and lawyers were formed through personal contacts. Those who lived in a retirement complex were invited to participate via a gatekeeper who lived on site, following agreement from the manager and the residents' committee. To our knowledge none of those who accepted our offer to take part had been diagnosed as suffering from dementia, which would have had a significant impact on their sleep and their understanding of it.

The resulting 23 focus groups were quite diverse in terms of age, with approximately half the sample being 45 years of age or over. Around 60 per cent of participants were female and around 90 per cent identified as of white British or Irish ethnicity. Just over half the sample had, or had previously had before retirement, a higher managerial or professional job (See Table 24.1). Focus groups were moderated by two of the research team, with one leading and the other taking notes. In each focus group we asked participants to discuss how they managed sleep problems in their daily lives and what they thought the appropriate role of pharmaceuticals was in their management practices. Forty-one participants, across 21 of the focus groups, disclosed current or previous use of prescription hypnotic medications (see Table 24.1). Of these just over half

were members of the primary care or sheltered housing focus groups. Experience of use ranged from one short course of hypnotics to several years or in some cases, decades of use (up to 40 years). The medications used included benzodiazepines, Z drugs (e.g. Zopiclone) and other forms of sedative such as Melatonin, Sodium Oxybate (Xyrem) and sedative antidepressants.[4,5] The paper focuses particularly on those who said they were current or previous users of prescription sleep medicines and how they interacted with those (n = 58) who said they had never used these medicines.

Focus groups were used as the means of data collection in order to explore people's views about, and experiences of using hypnotics and issues around the use of sleeping pills in daily life. Focus groups were audio recorded and transcribed. Analysis of the transcripts was facilitated using the qualitative data analysis software package NVivo 10 (QSR International, Brisbane). We took an inductive approach to data analysis which involved reading and re-reading the transcripts, grouping data extracts together based on their main themes and developing a coding frame based on these emergent themes to identify major topics and issues. Codes and themes relating to major issues were discussed between the authors for purposes of reliability and validity. These were used to develop an interpretative analysis of the meaning of hypnotic use and draw out the implications for the research questions outlined above.

Subsequently each focus group member was given an identifying code, indicating the type of focus group they had participated in, the number of the group and the gender of the participant, and the sequence in which they first spoke in the focus group (for example PCFG1F1 indicates primary care focus group 1, Female 1). Focus groups can be distinguished from one-to-one interviews as during a focus group participants are encouraged to engage with one another and this interaction between participants is included as research data (Kitzinger 1994). This methodology generates data not only about what people think about a certain issue, but also draws out the moral dimensions of how they think about it and why they think as they do. Using focus groups as a research tool, therefore, enabled us

TABLE 24.1 ■ Medicated Sleep: Participant Demographics

Focus Groups	Number of Participants	Gender (M/F)	Age Range	Ethnicity	SES	Number Taken Hypnotics
Academics 2 groups (AFG1–2)	8	5M 3F	25–54	7 WB/Irish 1 mixed (White & Asian)	Higher managerial & professionals	2
Ambulance service staff 3 groups (ASFG1–3)	9	5M 4F	25–54	9 WB/Irish	Higher managerial & professionals	3
Lawyers 1 group (LFG1)	3	2F 1M	35–44	2 WB/Irish 1 White (other)	Higher managerial & professionals	2
Narcolepsy patients 2 groups (NFG1–2)	13	7F 6M	18–74	12 WB/Irish 1 BB (African)	5 Intermediate 4 Technical & craft 1 Not disclosed 1 Unemployed 1 Student 1 Higher managerial & professionals	3
Parents of young children 2 groups (PFG1–2)	10	6F 4M	25–44	8 WB/Irish 1 Asian or AB (Pakistani) 1 White (other)	6 Higher managerial & professionals 3 Intermediate 1 Technical & craft	1

Group	N	Gender	Age	Ethnicity	Occupation	N
Primary care patients 3 groups (PCFG1–3)	12	6F 6M	45–85+	12 WB/Irish	6 Higher managerial & professionals 1 Intermediate 3 Technical & craft 2 Not disclosed	12
Retirement complex 3 groups (RFG1–3)	15	14F 1M	65–85+	15 WB/Irish	9 Higher managerial & professionals 3 Intermediate 3 Technical & craft	10
Sleep apnoea patients 3 groups (SAFG1–3)	13	8M 5F	45–74	13 WB/Irish	10 Higher managerial & professionals 1 Intermediate 2 Technical & craft	4
Students 4 groups (SFG1–4)	16	11F 5M	18–44	10 WB/Irish 2 White (other) 1 Mixed (other) 1 Asian 2 Chinese	Students	4
Totals	99	41M 58F	18–24 (15) 25–34 (18) 35–44 (15) 45–54 (14) 55–64 (10) 65–74 (11) 75–84 (12) 85+ (3) Not disclosed (1)	88 WB/Irish 4 White (Other) 2 Chinese 1 Black British 2 Asian/Asian British 2 Mixed	52 Higher managerial & professionals 14 Intermediate occupations 12 Technical & craft 17 Students 1 Unemployed 3 Not disclosed	41

to: explore how people talk about sleep and the management of their sleep problems together; assess how ideas are formed and decisions are made regarding the 'appropriate' role of sleep medications in such management strategies and how they evaluate their own relationships with sleeping pills.

Below we consider six distinct repertoires about hypnotic use. These are constructed drawing on the cross-cutting themes of addiction and control, ambivalence and reflexivity. These crosscutting themes are considered in the discussion.

MORAL REPERTOIRES: THEMES AND TENSIONS

In focus group discussions participants drew on a range of moral repertoires which allowed them to present themselves and their relationships with hypnotics in different ways. We can identify six repertoires about hypnotic use in this regard—the 'deserving' patient, the 'responsible' user, the 'compliant' patient, the 'addict', the 'sinful' user and the 'noble' non-user. These are discussed in turn below.

The 'Deserving' Patient

Participants were asked if they had ever been to see a doctor about their sleep problems or if they had ever taken any prescribed medication for sleep. The answers to these questions tended to be given in the form of a series of short monologues, where each member of the group took turns to share their story, allowing each of them to explain and justify why they were taking sleeping pills or had taken this type of medication in the past. Typically, the other members of the group would listen to each story and wait for their turn, occasionally expressing their empathy by offering reassuring statements, agreeing with and backing up the experiences described by others. These accounts were very rarely questioned or challenged.

For example, the following brief accounts were provided in turn by four members of a primary care focus group, (two male and two female, aged 55–85+):

PCFG1M2: The reason I had [sleeping pills] was because I had a bad accident, several years ago and the particular hospital I was in said 'something to help you sleep and when you come out just go along and see your doctor for a prescription and continue' [. . .] Simple as that.

PCFG1M1: Well, when I approached my doctor about depression, brought on with my wife going to hospital for a major operation, as far as I was concerned, lack of sleep was driving me into depression. Of course I was worried about my wife, extremely, but if there was one factor that could help me through it all was the sleep.

PCFG1F2: And the lack of sleep means you can't actually cope, doesn't it, with what you need to cope with, I think.

PCFG1M1: That's right. [. . .].

PCFGIF1: With me it was I didn't sleep at the time my husband died. He died suddenly and I just struggled along for a number of years but various problems that I had, not really coping all that well at the time. Doctor gave me [. . .] a prescription for three. He said 'take one of these every second day and see how you go on'. Well, it was lovely, absolutely lovely but I was back within three days - 'can I have some more?' So, it's gone on from then, really.

Every one of the participants who had taken prescription medication to help them sleep acted to present themselves as deserving of a pharmaceutical solution for their sleep problem. Therefore, the deserving patient repertoire was found across all of our focus groups. A typical way of doing this was to present themselves as in need of sleeping pills, using this as moral justification for their medication use.

As shown in the next extract, many of the respondents described complex, enduring and severe health and social problems that contributed towards poor sleep. These ranged from cancer, pain, anxiety, depression and stress to social and relational problems such as bereavement, social isolation, redundancy, financial problems, relationship breakdowns, and caring for ill family members. Some clearly attributed these as causal factors in the development of their sleep problems. Others described their problems with sleep as existing alongside and often exacerbating or being exacerbated by other health conditions and social issues they had faced in their lives. Through discussion of their health, life circumstances and interactions with medical professionals, the participants depicted themselves as deserving patients who had had their sleep problems medically recognised and pharmaceuticals prescribed as a necessary medical treatment, which in turn acted to validate them as deserving patients who were justified in taking sleeping pills:

> SAFG2F1: Not sleeping? Well, all the doctors said it was because of the stressful life I had, and I had as I say a very sick child and my husband was away a lot, and a very, very stressful job, and so I went to a doctor and I just said, you know *I need something* [emphasis added] to get me to sleep' so they gave me some tablets. (Sleep Apnoea Focus Group Two, female, aged 55–64)

It was common for participants to talk about other medications that they took alongside (or instead of) sleeping pills. These included antidepressants and pain killers that have a sedative effect and non-sedative medications they took for a range of other conditions such as hypertension and diabetes. Thus they presented themselves as in need of a range of medical treatments and their use of sleeping pills as just one part of their medicated self.

These illness narratives allowed participants to present themselves as in distress and in need of help, to justify why they had sought medical advice and legitimate why they were taking, or had taken medications for sleep.

The 'Responsible' User

In addition to presenting themselves as deserving of and in need of medication, the respondents typically presented themselves as vigilant in self-monitoring their use of sleeping pills. It was common for participants to construct an image of themselves as being responsible users who used their medication appropriately. The 'responsible user' repertoire was drawn on by academics, ambulance service staff, primary care patients, retired persons, sleep apnoea patients and students. The responsible user is one who is knowledgeable about their medication and its effects and is reflexive about their use. They are actively concerned about becoming dependent on or addicted to sleeping pills and describe taking steps to minimise this. They were ambivalent about their use of hypnotics, indicated they knew about the medication they took and its effects on them, questioned medical expertise and advice and made choices which they felt were in their best interest, drawing on their own ideas about appropriate uses of medication in daily life. For instance, these participants told stories about asking their doctor for their dosage to be reduced if they felt they were becoming reliant on the medication and altering their pharmaceutical regimens outside of medical authority to safeguard against dependency or addiction. They did this in various ways, for example, by using medication intermittently or as a last resort when they were extremely fatigued and 'could not go on' without sleeping, reducing the dose by cutting pills in half or into quarters, and substituting their medicine for a herbal remedy. Typically, medicated sleep was classed as inferior to 'natural sleep'—or sleep without medication, with the latter idealised.

In the following exchange we see an example of such self-surveillance and self-governance. The participants present themselves as being responsible for their own drug use, carefully monitoring their levels of consumption and acting to minimise their use of the sleeping pills, of their own volition:

> RFG3F3: What frightens me, I had a hip operation and I have to take some medication to get me to sleep at night because of the

pain. The trouble is, after a few nights, you're beginning to rely on it. And that's frightening. And so you have to be, as [RFG3M1] said, self-controlling, and try to control the drug, and gradually lessen it.

RFG3F2: That's why you cut it down if you can.

RFG3F3: If you can. (Residential Focus Group, two female participants, aged 75–84)

In cases where there was only one person in the focus group who had taken sleeping pills in the past, the participant could find their need to use sleep medication being challenged by other members of the group, pushing them to justify and explain further why they had turned to sleeping pills, to demonstrate that they were not only deserving of sleeping pills but also responsible in their use of them.

The 'Compliant' Patient

When asked further questions about how they took their medication a small number of participants went on to present themselves as not only a deserving patient, but also a compliant one—someone who deferred to medical expertise, followed medical advice to the letter and respected medical authority. Talk of this kind was found across the three primary care patient groups and also in the focus groups held with retired persons and ambulance service staff. These participants described taking their medication in line with the dose and frequency recommended by their doctor. Presenting an image of being a compliant patient meant that in some cases they accepted that their use of this medication was 'for life'; in other cases, they explained how they were trying to cut down or stop using hypnotic medication because their doctor had told them to do so:

PCFG1M1: I was with Dr [name] at the time and she told me when she prescribed them 'you realise that you are on these for life?' I said 'yes, if they do what they say on the packet' and it does. I just take the recommended dose and that's it. (Primary care focus group 1, Male participant, aged 55–64)

Compliance with medical advice was also a frequent theme in focus group discussions amongst those who had never taken sleeping pills or seen a doctor about sleep problems. In such cases, it was common for participants to assert that they would take this type of medication, if it was prescribed to them and its use advised by their doctor.

Although presenting their use of sleeping pills as complying with medical advice, participants were also at times somewhat critical of this and expressed a high level of ambivalence about their use of these medicines. They acknowledged that sleeping pills helped them to get some sleep but at the same time talked about their unpleasant side effects, occasions when they did not work, and in some cases, feelings of guilt and embarrassment for their continued use. Despite presenting themselves as compliant patients, when asked directly about altering treatment regimens it was common for these patients to admit that they had increased the dosage of their medication at some point, but they stressed that it was a one-off, it was not worth it, or that it did not do anything for them:

Moderator: You take them every day?

PCFG2M2: I take them every night, yeah, about nine o'clock at night, 8.30 at night. I see them as placebo.

Moderator: Why do you still take them, then?

PCFG2M2: It's like I'm clutching at straws, I suppose, yeah.

PCFG2M1: Safety blanket.

PCFG2M2: Yeah, I suppose it's like, it serves its need.

Moderator: So, do you set them up in advance and take them as part of your routine?

PCFG2M2: I do, yeah [. . .] they go out before . . . antidepressant for the morning time. So, I went from being I thought I was physically fit, all of a sudden I went up to four prescriptions, four tablets a day, medication, I don't know what happened to myself.

Moderator: Do you actually vary the number you take?

PCFG2M2: No, it's only one. I have tried more than one just to see if it helps but no [. . .] I've done it on a few occasions. I limit myself when I go to sleep, I take two tablets but it's not much effect.

Moderator: Doesn't make that much difference?

PCFG2M2: No. They only give you a month's supply now so they do. They know, they keep track on how many you use, so they know, so you couldn't take them willy nilly. (Primary care focus group 2, two male participants, aged 45–64)

The stigma surrounding use of sleeping pills was apparent throughout the data. We asked participants if they had ever taken any medication for sleep, both on a short demographic questionnaire and during the focus group discussion. On occasion, when participants had said they had not taken sleeping pills on the questionnaire, it came out later in the discussion that in fact they had previously taken this type of medication.

In these cases, adopting the sick role and the identity of a compliant patient functioned to allow them to legitimate their previous use of sleeping pills as following doctor's orders. They had a medical need which was addressed by a medically prescribed treatment, which they took as advised by their doctor.

The 'Addict'

Typically, participants did not orientate themselves towards being an addict and were critical of being mis-represented as one. The addict repertoire

was drawn upon by participants across all focus groups with the exception of narcolepsy patients, who are on medication for life, regarding this in terms of medical necessity rather than through an addiction frame, and parents of young children, who were more concerned with short term effects of medication on their daily functioning rather than possible effects of long term use. Addiction was associated with escalating use and a loss of control over ones use of medication and oneself. Long term users of hypnotics in particular strove to distance themselves from being seen as an addict, by depicting themselves as deserving, responsible or compliant, as discussed above. There was a general reluctance to disclose any information that might suggest they were addicted to sleeping pills. However, acknowledging long term use of these pills and/or a need to take them in order to sleep could lead to feelings of ambivalence about being seen as an addict and, as seen in the next extract, to participants questioning whether they could be classified as an addict or not:

PCFG3M1: I remember vaguely I think talking about sort of getting addicted, and I think he [GP] said you know, you want to make sure you're not taking them too often. But I'm almost of the philosophy that if he doesn't say anything, then it's okay. And I find it very comforting that I've got them there for when I need them. But I do very much try and watch it myself.

Moderator: Is addiction an issue in your mind?

PCFG3M1: No, I mean, it's an issue in the fact that I don't want to become addicted, but I honestly don't think I am addicted. There's the occasion I've forgotten about them and absolutely got worried, but it hasn't been a disaster. If I was addicted to them, it really would cause problems.

PCFG3F1: I don't perceive myself as having an addictive personality. I think I could have been addicted in situations that have been offered to me in the past, I could have got myself addicted [. . .] So I don't perceive myself as being an addict. However, I don't sleep without them, so does that make me an addict? (Primary care focus group 3, one male and one female participant, aged 55–64)

The occasions on which individuals acknowledged their vulnerability towards addiction, dependency and tolerance tended to be when talking about previous rather than current medication use. In these cases, as discussed in the above sections, participants told stories about how they recognised that their use was getting out of control and how this acted as a trigger for them to attempt to reduce their reliance on medication or stop taking the medication altogether.

In some cases, the participant's doctor had spoken to them about reducing or withdrawing the medication, or told them outright that the medication they were prescribing should not be used long term, citing risks of the addictive potential of the drugs. Doctors telling their patients that they should not be taking these tablets long term whilst at the same time continuing to issue them a prescription can appear conflicting. On the one hand, it conveys the moral impression to patients that their prolonged use of these substances is 'wrong' and the people who use them long term could become 'addicts' rather than legitimate patients. On the other hand, they are still having their problem medically validated and pharmaceuticalised by being issued a prescription for sleeping pills. This can result in divided emotions amongst patients, where feelings of guilt and embarrassment about their continued use of this medication coexist with their belief that they still have a legitimate need for it:

PCFG1F2: I was told only the other day, you become addicted to this, you must try and stop taking them. I said, I've been trying to stop taking them for a very long time, but I don't sleep if I don't take them.

PCFG1M1: Do you feel guilty about taking the sleeping tablets?

PCFG1F3: It isn't guilt, really, it's just that I suppose I was told at the beginning 'you shouldn't take them for long, it will help you over this spell' and then 'it will help you over this' and it's because I'm told they are addictive and, yes, I feel I shouldn't be taking pills. Other people manage to sleep every night and get through a night without pills.

PCFG1F2: But they're not ill are they?

PCFG1M2: I think the word addictive is one of these words that you don't really want in your . . . You are eating the forbidden fruit.

PCFG1F3: But I don't particularly want to be taking pills.

PCFG1M3: I feel guilty to ask for them. (Primary care focus group 1, 3 male participants and 2 female participants, aged 55–85+)

In such cases, it was all the more evident how respondents strove to portray themselves as deserving patients and their use of sleeping pills as appropriate. They attempted to distance themselves from the idea that they might be an addict by emphasising how they did not want to take pills but their continued use was necessary for them to get some sleep, which they needed in order to function in daily life. As discussed previously, it was typical for participants to describe the strategies of self-surveillance and self-governance they adopted precisely for this very reason: to protect themselves from becoming an addict.

The 'Sinful' User

When discussing modifications they made to their treatment regimens participants also discussed a variety of medically unsanctioned practices that they had been 'guilty of'. These included increasing their dose of medication, stockpiling medicines, using medications prescribed for other reasons or to other people to help them sleep, and circumventing medical authority in order to obtain sleeping pills that they could not get on prescription, either because their doctor refused to prescribe or because the medication (such as melatonin supplements) was not readily available in the UK. Talk of this kind was found in the focus groups held with primary care patients, sleep apnoea patients, retired persons, students and lawyers. These activities were referred to by some of the participants as 'wrong', 'being naughty' or 'sinning'. In 'confessing' these practices participants acknowledged that they were going against medical advice, but were able to 'forgive' themselves due to being in additional need or finding themselves in exceptional circumstances, such as when experiencing 'a bad night' or finding themselves in unfamiliar surroundings. At the same time they were still careful to present themselves as deserving and responsible, reflexive users who remained in control of their use of sleeping pills. Consider for example, the following exchange between three members of a primary care focus group:

PCFG1M3: I have sinned occasionally. And done that when there has been a big day, a long travelling day or doing something and I haven't felt any side effects. I've been quite happy.

PCFG1M2: I must admit, the most I've ever had is two of these things in a night, but I haven't had any side effects, perhaps that's unusual . . .

PCFG1M1: Some nights it's a real bad night [. . .] and I know I should only have one tablet but - it might happen about once every two or three months [. . .] I might end up having 1.5 or two tablets, almost, but I've thought 'well, I've got to get some sleep some time'.

PCFG1F1: I think we all know the dangers of being over-sedated, and the dangers that there are of falling over the cat or something and breaking your leg or something. There is that danger, of course there is that danger,

but occasionally if you have an extra one, if you've got something coming up you've just got to forgive yourself and get on with your life. (Primary care focus group 1, 2 male participants and one female, aged 55-64)

In the next extract, participants from a residential focus group discuss how they shared tablets when not able to get them from the doctor:

Moderator: Because it's so difficult to get sleeping tablets, have you ever shared them with each other?

RFG1F4: When we run out.

RFG1F2: Be careful what you say [RFG1F4].

Moderator: Don't worry!

RFG1F2: She is inclined to slide me a few Temazepam.

RFG1F4: If she was running out, I'd say 'have some of mine'.

RFG1F7: See you shouldn't do that.

RFG1F4: But you were running out of your prescription.

Moderator: Anyone else share tablets?

RFG1F2: We don't share any tablets now; it was just if we were running out.

RFG1F4: Only because we couldn't get them.

RFG1F2: Because we couldn't get them. (Residential focus group 1, 3 female participants, aged 75–84).

It is clear that they were usually secretive about this and knew that it was not considered an appropriate way to obtain medication.

The 'Noble' (or 'Virtuous') Non-User

A prevalent theme in our data, found predominately in discussions of medicating sleep amongst non-users and previous users of hypnotics (ambulance service staff, academics, lawyers, parents of young children, retired persons, sleep apnoea patients, students), was the rejection of pharmaceuticalisation of sleep. This was tied in with the belief that it was a sign of moral strength not to rely on artificial props—a form of pharmaceutical Calvinism (Klerman 1972). The data we draw on here comes from participants who disclosed sleep problems or difficulties but were opposed to a pharmaceutical solution for them. Different reasons were given for the rejection or resistance to such pharmaceuticalisation. Some saw their sleep problems as not severe enough or not deserving of a medical solution. Difficulties sleeping were positioned as something people *should* be able to deal with themselves. In such discussions, respondents typically took an anti-medication stance and saw the use of hypnotics as 'giving in' to strong medication, 'taking the easy route' or a 'lazy' way to deal with one's problems, with a view of medicated sleep being 'unnatural'.

Others did not want to take sleeping pills, even in times of legitimate medical need (e.g. they had been prescribed sleeping pills but decided not to take them). In some cases this was due to past experiences of taking sleeping pills and experiencing negative side effects from the drugs. In others, it was because they worried about the effects the drug might have on them, including addiction, loss of control over their situation or impairing their ability to function.

For example, in the extract below from a Residential focus group, a male participant (RFG3M1) expresses his resistance to pharmaceuticalisation of sleep. The discussion in this particular group was moralistic and anti-medication, although several of participants had taken sleeping pills in the past. Although initially presenting himself as a non-user, later in the focus group this participant disclosed previous use of sleeping pills over a short period of time. He presented himself as a deserving patient at the time, but did not like the effect the medicine had had on him and rejected it subsequently, defying medical advice. Others in the group echoed his concerns about loss of control, and the side effects of medication and mentioned their own attempts to reduce the amount they took or their success in stopping taking the medication altogether.

RFG3M1: 50 years ago I had a serious illness, which lasted about 3 years. And I was admitted to hospital initially. And one of the things, I was in a lot of pain and I wasn't sleeping. So I was prescribed sleeping pills, which I took for two nights and woke up with a hangover the following morning. I was asked by the consultant why I wasn't taking my medication, because I thought I'm going to refuse to take it. He agreed because I was adamant that I didn't want the hangover in the morning. And I've never ever had any aid to sleeping in the form of a sleeping tablet since that one occasion [. . .] Unnatural sleep is hypnotic sleep. I think that induces adverse side effects very often.

RFG3F2: The side effects are terrible.

RFG3F1: Years ago, I had patches of not sleeping very well, and used to take a half a phenobarbitone, half a one just gave me a good night's sleep. Then I went for a long time and didn't need anything. Then I think I came here and I had a patch of sleeplessness, went to the doctor and he prescribed some tablets, which—he said he couldn't give phenobarbitone, they weren't allowed to prescribe them so I don't know what it was he gave me—but it gave me such an awful . . . it used to knock me out for two hours. And then I'd wake up wide awake, so I don't take them anymore. (Residential focus group 3, 1 male and two female participants, aged 75–85+)

Many of our focus group participants had not sought medical advice despite describing severe sleep problems because they did not want to be prescribed sleeping tablets and thought that this is what their doctor would offer. For these participants sleep problems were caused by lifestyle factors and although sleeping pills might be a remedy they were thought of as treating the symptom rather than the root cause of the problem. There was a general dislike of sleep medication, linked to the possibility of becoming addicted, the idea of sleeping pills being 'unnatural' and concerns that medicated sleep 'won't feel like real sleep'. Echoes of this narrative can be seen in the exchange below between two paramedics. Both had had sleep problems in the past.

> Moderator: What have you used to help to sleep or keep awake?
>
> ASFG2F3: Nothing.
>
> Moderator: Why not?
>
> ASFG2F3: Well, it's only because I'm quite a natural. I like the natural complementary side of . . . I don't particularly like the allopathic way of treating your body. So I like things more natural and so that's why I definitely would never go to the doctor and say 'Can I have some Zopiclone please.' and I would never think about taking anything orally to make me either stay awake or go to sleep.
>
> ASFG2M1: Not even any of the herbal type products?
>
> ASFG2F3: No. (Ambulance Staff Focus group 2, 1 female and 1 male participant, aged 25–54)

Instead of taking hypnotics those drawing on this repertoire described their efforts to manage their sleep through non-pharmacological means, including varying use of over-the-counter remedies, exercise, mediation, prayer, alcohol and other 'personalised strategies', similar to female respondents in a study by Hislop and Arber (2003). They criticised

doctors for handing out sleeping pills too freely and, through their talk, depicted a moral image of themselves as exhibiting strength of character and 'doing the right thing' by resisting the medication. Although not seeing themselves as deserving patients who were in need of sleeping pills, they did see a role for pills in special circumstances. However, they expressed concerns about negative side effects of taking this type of medication and saw medicated sleep as being different from and inferior to natural sleep.

DISCUSSION

Through their talk, participants in our study depicted themselves and their relationships with hypnotics in a range of ways, drawing on different moral repertoires. Six repertoires as we have seen are evident—the 'deserving' patient, the 'responsible' user, the 'compliant' patient, the 'addict', the 'sinful' user and the 'noble' or virtuous non-user. These repertoires clearly have much in common with the moral repertoires identified in other studies of medications use. Thus Lumme-Sandt et al. (2000), in their study of the oldest old (aged 90 or over) in Finland, found that their respondents presented themselves as moral and responsible drug users by explaining the 'objective reasons' for their use, playing down the extent of such use and comparing it favourably with the assumed level of use by others. Similarly Dew et al. (2015), in their study of households in New Zealand, reported that respondents developed and articulated four distinct moral repertoires: a disordering society repertoire; a disordering self repertoire; a disordering substances repertoire and finally a re-ordering substances repertoire. Our study has identified a broader variety of repertoires which have drawn on those described above but have honed them to legitimise the use or non-use of hypnotic medications. In our study addiction, sin and virtue were more to the fore than in Lumme-Sandt et al.'s (2000) study, while in comparison with Dew et al. (2015) we found a greater variety of repertoires relating to the 'restoration of function' (deserving user, compliant user). However, like Dew et al., we too found evidence of resistance to a disordered society (the virtuous non user), the disordering self (the addict) and the disordering substance (the responsible user). These differences may in part relate to the fact that we have focused on repertoires relating to a specific drug type—hypnotics.

While we have identified a range of distinctive moral repertoires in the data, in practice we found that participants orientated towards multiple repertoires which were often layered one on top of another. Use of these repertoires shifted over time and in response to what others revealed about their own pharmaceutical regimens and the moral discourse that was articulated around hypnotic use in the focus group. For example, the same person who initially presented themselves as a deserving patient claimed to be a responsible user and also a sinful user during subsequent discussion.

Each of the repertoires we have identified, we suggest, draws on the following crosscutting themes: addiction and control, ambivalence and reflexivity. Taking these in turn, it was common for our participants to attempt to distance themselves from sleeping pills by drawing on moralising talk, in recognition of the stigma around addiction and the associated imagery of illicit drug use. Concerns about addiction have long been reported in studies of benzodiazepine use (Gabe and Lipshitz-Phillips 1984, North *et al.* 1995). Typically, participants were concerned about being (mis)represented as being an 'addict' and attempted to distance themselves from this image, describing strategies of self-surveillance and self-governance they had adopted in order to protect themselves from becoming addicted to sleeping pills. Addiction was in turn related to the issue of control; claiming to be in control challenged the idea that they were addicted. Hence participants emphasised how they were in control over whether they chose to take their medication or not, how many pills they took, how often they took them and their ability to stop taking such medications.

A second key theme was that of ambivalence, a response to medicine and medications which is said to be ever more common in late modern society where traditional authority and expertise are increasingly

questioned (Nettleton 2006). Ambivalence towards sleeping pills was a prevailing theme across all the focus groups. For instance, participants articulating a compliant patient repertoire also acknowledged side effects and expressed doubts about the efficacy of their medication, regarding hypnotics as a 'necessary evil' (Gabe and Lipshitz-Phillips 1982). At the same time those expressing strong anti-medication sentiments could also see a role for sleeping pills in some circumstances. Some of this ambivalence may stem from the UK medical community's own ambivalent moral and political stance towards the pharmaceuticalisation of sleep problems. Although hypnotic medications are licensed for insomnia in the UK and doctors may see a role for them as a short term solution, they are viewed as far from perfect, being associated with various negative side effects. Furthermore, efforts have been made for some time to reduce hypnotic prescribing in UK primary care, measures which some of our participants at least, had experienced. These participants said their GP had advised about the risks of dependence and warned them that the drug should only be taken for a limited period. And yet it is clear from our respondents that it is still possible to obtain a prescription from some GPs and in some circumstances. Our data thus shed some further light on the ways in which processes of pharmaceuticalisation/ depharmaceuticalisation (Abraham 2011, Williams *et al.* 2011) work to shape the cognitive, cultural and affective framing of sleep problems. While long term hypnotic use continues to be commonplace in the UK it is now rarely embraced unquestioningly. Instead, it is reviewed in a critical and reflexive way, even by those who have been using this medication for a considerable period of time.

The final cross-cutting theme was that of reflexivity. This was clearly demonstrated in the way that many of our focus group participants rejected the image of the passive consumer of medications. They preferred to engage reflexively with the different normative frameworks and discourses around medicine use to justify their own medication taking practices. They often seemed to act as 'lay pharmacologists' assessing the safety, efficacy and side effects of the drug' (Webster *et al.* 2009). Like other studies

(Dew *et al.* 2014), the participants in our study also drew on advice from various quarters, including medical advice, as and when they deemed it necessary, in developing personal medication practices. This reflects the social lives and meanings of medications, as medication taking practices become entangled in domestic routines and meanings within the therapeutic environment of the home and the competing forms of knowledge that co-exist there. In domestic spaces these competing forms of knowledge can get mixed up or 'hybridised' (Dew *et al.* 2014). Consequently, forms of medical knowledge and clinical advice are reworked and reformed through the relationships people have with medications in daily life. As our analysis shows, responses to illness and wellbeing involve pragmatic decision-making based not only on what works for people with sleep problems, but also on what they deem to be appropriate and acceptable in the context of their daily lives, rather than simply adhering to the rules set by medical experts. Thus some of our focus group members reported taking 'drug holidays' while others reduced the dose to see what the effect would be. In both cases this was done without consultation with a doctor. Amongst those invoking the repertoire of the virtuous non-user, using alternative therapies to deal with sleep problems was often mentioned. All of these practices illustrate the desire of people to be reflexive about their medicines and reflect the nature of the late modern age where medical authority is no longer unquestionably accepted and lay experience if not expertise carries increasing weight (Williams and Calnan 1996).

At a broader level, our data therefore support conceptualisations of pharmaceuticalisation as being a dynamic bidirectional process, including various forms of expert patient/consumer resistance to pharmaceuticalisation. On the one hand, people may reject pharmaceuticals in the management of sleep problems and selectively alter therapeutic regimens in the home where pharmaceuticals may be used alongside or replaced by non-pharmacological means of therapy. On the other hand, they may also present various challenges to GPs' attempts (in line with current mandates) to reduce or restrict resorting to prescription hypnotics in primary care, through continuing to present themselves as deserving and in need of pharmaceuticals, questioning medical authority and knowledge and, on occasion, seeking prescription drugs outside the medical encounter, through practices such as sharing with friends, buying sleeping pills on the Internet and stockpiling medications for use at a later date.

Although documented cases of depharmaceuticalisation are rare, in the case of hypnotics to treat sleep problems at least, the process is best seen as being in a state of flux, particularly in the context of developments for more cognitive behavioural based forms of intervention, although doctors do not necessarily see Cognitive Behaviour Therapy for Insomnia (CBTi) as an alternative to medication. The degree to which sleep problems are subject to (de)pharmaceuticalisation in the future therefore remains uncertain and open to challenge.

ACKNOWLEDGMENTS

This study was funded by the UK Economic and Social Research Council (ES/H028870/1). We would like to thank the reviewers of this paper for their helpful comments and the research participants who took part in the focus groups.

Notes

1. Centre for Criminology & Sociology, Royal Holloway, University of London
2. Centre for Global Health Policy, University of Sussex
3. Department of Sociology, University of Warwick
4. It was common for those who had been using hypnotics for several years to have

used many different types and brands of medication. Of those who were taking prescription hypnotics at the time of the study (18), the majority (13) were taking Zopiclone or Zolpidem.

5. Xyrem has been included as it is prescribed to narcolepsy patients for the purpose of sedation and to help these patients consolidate their sleep at night. It also helps to reduce cataplexy during daytime.

References

Abraham, J. (2010) Pharmaceuticalization of society in context: theoretical, empirical and health dimensions, Sociology, 44, 4, 603–22.

Anthierens, S., Habraken, H., Petrovic, M. and Christiaens, T. (2007) The lesser evil? Initiating a benzodiazepine prescription in general practice, *Scandinavian Journal of Primary Health Care*, 25, 4, 214–9.

Backett, K. (1992) Taboos and excesses: lay health moralities in middle class families, *Sociology of Health and Illness*, 14, 2, 255–74.

Bell, S. and Figert, A. (2012) Medicalization and pharmaceuticalization at the intersections: looking backward, sideways and forward, *Social Science and Medicine*, 75, 5, 775–83.

Buysse, D. J. (2013) Insomnia, *Journal of the American Medical Association*, 309, 7, 706–16.

Cohen, D., McCubbin, M., Collin, J. and Perodeau, G. (2001) Medications as social phenomena, *Health*, 5, 4, 441–69.

Coveney, C.M. (2011) Cognitive enhancement? Exploring Modafinil use in social context. In Pickersgill, M. and Van Keulen, 1. (eds) *Sociological Reflections on the Neurosciences (Advances in Medical Sociology, Volume 13)*, pp 203–28. Bingley: Emerald.

Dew, K., Chamberlain, K., Hodgetts, D., Norris, P., *et al.* (2014) Home as a hybrid centre of medication practice, *Sociology of Health & Illness*, 36, 1, 28–43.

Dew, K., Norris, P., Gabe, J., Chamberlain, K., *et al.* (2015) Moral discourses and pharmaceuticalised governance in households, *Social Science and Medicine*, 131, 272–9.

Gabe, J. and Bury, M. (1988) Tranquillisers as a social problem? *Sociological Review*, 36, 2, 320–52.

Gabe, J. and Lipshitz-Phillips, S. (1982) Evil necessity? The meaning of benzodiazepine use for women patients from one general practice, *Sociology of Health & Illness*, 4, 2, 201–9.

Gabe, J. and Lipshitz-Phillips, S. (1984) Tranquillisers as social control? *Sociological Review*, 32, 3, 524–46.

Gabe, J. and Thorogood, N. (1986) Prescribed drug use and the management of everyday life: the experiences of black and white working class women, *Sociological Review*, 34, 4, 737–72.

Gabe, J., Williams, S., Martin, P. and Coveney, C. (2015) Pharmaceuticals and society; Power, promises and prospects, *Social Science and Medicine*, 131, 193–8.

Henry, D., Knutson, K. L. and Orzech, K. M. (2013) Sleep, culture and health: reflections on the other third of life, *Social Science and Medicine*, 79, 1–6.

Hislop, J. and Arber, S. (2003) Understanding women's sleep management; beyond medicalization-healthicization? *Sociology of Health & Illness*, 25, 7, 815–37.

Hodgetts, D., Chamberlain, K., Gabe, J., Dew, K., *et al.* (2011) Emplacement and everyday use of medications in domestic dwellings, *Health and Place*, 17, 1, 353–60,

HSCIC (2014) Prescription Cost Analysis England 2013 April. Available at http://www.hscic.gov.uk/catalogue/PUB13887/pres-cosi-anal-eng-2013-rep.pdf (accessed 4 April 2014).

Kitzinger, J. (1994) The methodology of focus groups: the importance of interaction between research participants, *Sociology of Health & Illness*, 16, 1. 103–21.

Klerman, G.L. (1972) Psychotropic hedonism vs. pharmacological Calvinism, *Hastings Center Report*, 2, 4, 1–3.

Kripke, D.F. (2006) Risks of chronic hypnotic use, In Lader, M., Cardinali, D.P. and Pandi-Perumal, S. R. (eds) *Sleep and Sleep Disorders*, pp 141–5. New York: Springer.

Kripke, D.F., Langer, R.D. and Kine, L.E. (2012) Hypnotics' association with mortality or cancer: a matched cohort study, *British Medical Journal Open*, 2, 1, e000850.

Lumme-Sandt, K. and Virtanen, P. (2002) Older people in the field of medication, *Sociology of Health & Illness*, 24, 3, 285–304.

Lumme-Sandt. K., Hervonen, A. and Jylha, M. (2000) Interpretative repertoires of medication among the oldest-old. *Social Science and Medicine*, 50, 12, 1843–50.

Nettleton, S. (2006) 'I just want permission to be ill': towards a sociology of medically unexplained symptoms, *Social Science and Medicine*, 62, 5, 1167–78.

NICE (2004) Guidance on the use of zaleplon, Zolpidem and zopicione for the short-term management of insomnia, Technology appraisal 77. April, http://www.nice.org.uk/nicemedia/pdt7TA077fullguidance.pdf (accessed 20 May 2015).

North, D., Davis, P. and Powell, A. (1995) Patient responses to benzodiazepine medicine: a typology of adaptive repertoires developed by long term users, *Sociology of Health & Illness*, 17, 5, 632–50.

Oudshoorn, N. (2008) Diagnosis at a distance: the invisible work of patients and healthcare professionals in cardiac telemonitoring technology, Sociology of Health & Illness, 30, 2, 272–88.

PCT (2011) PCT board prescribing report. Hypnotics—prescribing guidance and discussion points. www.nhsbsa.nhs.uk/Documents/PPDPCTReports/pctreport_20103.pdf (accessed 20 May 2015).

Potter, J. and Wetherell, M. (1987) Discourse and Social Psychology—Beyond Attitudes and Behaviour. London: Sage.

Pound, P., Britten, N., Morgan, M., Yardley, L., et al. (2005) Resisting medicines: a synthesis of qualitative studies of medicine taking, Social Science and Medicine, 61, 1, 133–55.

Radley, A. and Billig, M. (1996) Accounts of health and illness: dilemmas and representations, Sociology of Health & Illness, 18, 2, 220–40.

Rogers, A., Pilgrim, D., Brennan, S., Sulaiman, I., et al. (2007) Prescribing benzodiazepines in general practice: a new view of an old problem, Health, 11, 2, 181–98.

Rose, N. (2007) The Politics of Life Itself. Princeton: Princeton University Press.

Sayer, A. (2011) Why Things Matter to People. Social Science, Values and Ethical Life. Cambridge: Cambridge University Press.

Siriwardena, A.N., Qureshi, M.Z., Dyas, J.V., Middleton, H., et al. (2008) Magic bullets for insomnia? Patients' use and experiences of newer (Z drugs) versus older (benzodiazepine) hypnotics for sleep problems in primary care, British Journal of General Practice, 58, 551, 417–22.

Turowetz, J.J. and Maynard, D.W. (2010) Morality in the social interactional and discursive world of everyday life. In Hitlin, S. and Vaisey, S. (eds) Handbook of the Sociology of Morality. New York: Springer.

Venn, S. and Arber, S. (2012) Understanding older peoples' decisions about the use of sleeping medication: issues of control and autonomy, Sociology of Health & Illness, 34, 8, 1215–29.

Webster, A., Douglas, C. and Lewis, G. (2009) Making sense of medicines: 'lay pharmacology' and narratives of safety and efficacy, Science as Culture, 18, 2, 233–47.

Will, C. and Weiner, K. (2015) The drugs don't sell: DIY heart health and the over-the-counter statin experience, Social Science and Medicine, 131, 280–8.

Williams, S.J. (2005) Sleep and Society: Sociological Explorations and Agendas. London: Routledge.

Williams, S.J. (2011) The Politics of Sleep: Governing (Un)Consciousness in the Late Modern Age. Basingstoke: Palgrave Macmillan.

Williams, S.J. and Calnan, M. (1996) The 'limits' of medicalization? Modern medicine and the lay populace in 'late' modernity, Social Science and Medicine, 42, 12, 1609–20.

Williams, S.J and Wolf-Meyer, M (2013) Longing for sleep: Assessing the place of sleep in the 21st Century, Somatosphere, http://somatosphere. net/author/matthew-wolf-meyer (accessed 26 May 2015).

Williams, S.J., Coveney, C.M. and Gabe, J. (2013) Medicalisation or customisation? Sleep, enterprise and enhancement in the 24/7 society, Social Science and Medicine, 79, 40–7.

Williams, S.J., Martin, P. and Gabe, J. (2011) The pharmaceuticalisation of society? A framework for analysis, Sociology of Health & Illness, 33, 5, 710–25.

FINANCING MEDICAL CARE

Medical care is big business in the United States. Billions of dollars are spent each year on medical services, with nearly half of each dollar coming from public funds. Medical costs, a significant factor in the economy's inflationary spiral, were until quite recently practically unregulated. Most of the money spent on medical care in the United States is spent via *third-party payments*.[1] Unlike *direct* (or *out-of-pocket*) payments, third-party payments are those made through some form of insurance or charitable organization for someone's medical care. Third-party payments have increased steadily over the past forty years. In 1950, a total of 32 percent of personal health care expenditures were made via third-party payments; in 1965, that figure was up to 48 percent; and by 1974, the ratio of third-party payments had increased to 65 percent (*Medical Care Chart Book* 1976, 117). By 2013, only 12 percent of health care expenditures were out of pocket, with 33 percent paid by private health insurance and 47 percent paid by public funds (Chapter 25). Third-party insurers are thus central to the financing of medical care services in this country. This section examines the role of insurance in financing medical care and the insurance industry's influence on the present-day organization of medical services.

The original method of paying for medical services directly or individually, in money or in kind, has today largely been replaced by payment via insurance. Essentially, insurance is a form of "mass financing" ensuring that medical care providers will be paid and people will be able to obtain and pay for the medical care they need. Insurance involves the regular collection of small amounts of money (premiums) from a large number of people. That money is put into a pool, and when the insured people get sick, that pool (the insurance company) pays for their medical services either directly or indirectly by sending the money to the provider or patient.

The United States has both private and public insurance plans. Public insurance programs, including Medicare and Medicaid, are funded primarily by monies collected by federal, state, or local governments in the form of taxes. The nation has two types of private insurance organizations: *nonprofit* tax-exempt Blue Cross and Blue Shield plans and for-profit *commercial* insurance companies.

Blue Cross and Blue Shield emerged out of the Great Depression of the 1930s as mechanisms to ensure the payment of medical bills to hospitals (Blue Cross) and physicians (Blue Shield). The Blues (Blue Cross and Blue Shield) were developed as community plans through which people made small "prepayments" on a regular basis, generally monthly. If they became sick, their hospital bills were paid directly by the insurance plan.

Although commercial insurance companies existed as early as the nineteenth century, only after World War II did they really expand in this country. Blue Cross and Blue Shield originally set the price of insurance premiums by what was called "community rating," giving everybody within a community the chance to purchase insurance at the same price. Commercial insurers, on the other hand, employed "experience rating," which bases the price of insurance premiums on the statistical likelihood of the insured needing medical care. People less likely to need medical care are charged less for premiums than are people more likely to need it. By offering younger, healthier workers lower rates than could the Blues, commercials captured a large segment of the labor union insurance market in the 1950s and 1960s. In order to compete, Blue Cross and Blue Shield eventually abandoned community rating and began using experience rating as well. One unfortunate result of the spread of experience rating has been that those who most needed insurance coverage—the elderly and the sick—often had difficulty affording or obtaining it.

Congress created Medicare and Medicaid in 1965 as amendments to the Social Security Act. Medicare pays for the medical care of people over sixty-five years of age and other qualified recipients of Social Security. Medicaid pays for the care of those who qualify as too poor to pay their own medical costs. However, commercial and nonprofit insurance companies act as intermediaries in these government programs. Providers of medical care are not paid directly by public funds; instead, these funds are channeled through the private insurance industry. The Blues also act as intermediaries in many Medicaid programs, which are state-controlled. Public funding via private insurance companies has resulted in enormous increases in the costs of both of these public insurance programs; high profits for the insurance intermediaries and their beneficiaries, physicians, and hospitals; and the near exhaustion of available public funds for the continuation of Medicare and Medicaid. Before 1965, the federal government paid about 10 percent of all medical expenditures. By 1995, it paid for nearly 38 percent of health care costs. As noted previously, its contribution is now up to 47 percent of costs. The federal contribution to Medicare alone had risen from a couple of billion dollars in 1965 to $679 billion in 2016 (Centers for Medicare and Medicaid Services 2017a), and is still rising.

The Medicare/Medicaid response had a number of consequences. Medicare has provided basic medical insurance coverage for 99 percent of Americans over sixty-five. While the elderly still face significant out-of-pocket expenses, this widespread coverage is a stark contrast to their lack of coverage before 1965 (Davis 1975). Medicaid is much less comprehensive. Because it is a federal–state matching program, coverage varies from state to state, leaving many people without coverage. Utilization of services has increased under Medicaid because people who are poor are generally sicker than those who are not poor. The major impact of Medicaid has been on maternal and child health.

Although federal programs surely helped some sick people and reduced inequality and inaccessibility of medical services, their effect was limited. The Republican administrations in the 1980s cut back a number of these programs. But even before these cutbacks, Medicare covered less than half of the elderly's health expenses, and Medicaid

covered only a third of those of the poor (Starr 1982, 374).

The intent of Medicare and Medicaid is certainly worthy, even if the results are limited. But these programs also created new problems. They put billions of new dollars into the health system with no cost controls, and by the 1970s, Medicare and Medicaid were clearly fueling escalating health costs. Total U.S. health care costs now comprise 17.8 percent of the gross domestic product (Centers for Medicare and Medicaid Services 2017b). Some people were reaping enormous profits from the system, especially owners of shoddy nursing homes and so-called Medicaid mills. Tightening restrictions eliminated the worst offenders, but medical costs continued to soar.

In the early 1970s, the federal government began to mandate a series of programs aimed at reducing spiraling costs, especially with Medicare. In 1972, utilization review boards and hospital-based committees were instituted to review the appropriateness of medical utilization. These were followed by professional standard review organizations that were set up to monitor both quality and cost of care. There were even attempts to put a "cap" (ceiling) on the total amount that could be allocated to a program. Some cost-control programs had limited effects in specific situations, but the federal attempt to control costs has so far been generally a failure.

Diagnostically related groups were another federal attempt to control costs. Mandated in 1984 for Medicare, this program replaced the fee-for-service system with a form of "prospective reimbursement" whereby the government will pay only a specific amount for a specified medical problem. The prices of hundreds of diagnoses are established in advance. Medicare will pay no more, no less. If a hospital spends less than the set amount, it gets to pocket the difference. The idea is to give hospitals the incentive to be efficient and save money. The concern is that patients will get poorer treatment. The rise of managed care as a method for delivering health care is largely a response to rising costs. Managed care requires preapprovals for many forms of medical treatment and sets limits on some types of care in an effort to control medical expenditures. This has given third-party payers more leverage and constrained both the care given by providers and the care received by patients (subscribers).

This section investigates the origins and consequences of financing medical care in the particular way the U.S. medical system has evolved. One of the most obvious and vexing issues is why the United States is the only Western industrialized country without a national health insurance plan. This lack of universal health care leaves 9% of the U.S. population without health insurance (National Center for Health Statistics 2017). One reason is that the rise of employer-based private health insurance (e.g., Blue Cross) covered much of the middle class, and thus they never became an important force favoring government health reform (Rothman 1993).

Thomas Bodenheimer and Kevin Grumbach discuss the historical process of health care financing in an updated piece on "Paying for Health Care," illustrating the impact of shifts in payment mechanisms. Using vignettes, they show how each solution for financing health care created a new set of problems. In particular, they examine the emergence of four modes of payment for patients or consumers: out of pocket, individual private health insurance, employment-based group private insurance, and government financing. While private insurance certainly has helped many sick people, it has not been provided in a fair and equitable manner. The shift from community-rated to experience-rated insurance was a regressive policy change and had a negative effect on those who were old, sick, poor, or at risk. In other words, while experience rating gave the commercial insurers a competitive edge (Starr 1982), it undermined insurance as a principle of mutual aid and eroded the basis of distributive justice in insurance (Stone 1993).

President Clinton's attempts at national health reform in the early 1990s failed (see Starr 1995), but the health care system continued to change through the "market-based reform" of managed care. While managed care is changing and retreating from some of its original strictures, 160 million people are covered by some kind of managed care plan (National Conference of State Legislatures 2016). Managed care is an attempt to deliver medical care while reducing or controlling health costs. Health maintenance organizations (HMOs) are the key to managed care, linking hospitals, doctors, and specialists with the goal of delivering more effective care at lower costs and eliminating "unnecessary" or "inappropriate" care (see Wholey and Burns 2000). While this can create more coordinated care, it also puts restrictions on access to physicians and available treatments. In an effort to make health care more accountable, patients are treated as "cost units." Managed care has eroded physician autonomy (Chapter 19), endangered trust between doctors and patients (Mechanic 1996), and encouraged new systems for rationing services. The monetary incentives built into managed care can turn doctors into business people, resulting in higher potential incomes but poorer quality care (Stone 1997). While the old ideal about clinical care without regard to cost or profit is now unrealistic, the commercial nature of managed care encourages doctors to emphasize profits over patient care.

The Patient Protection and Affordable Care Act (ACA), signed into law by President Obama in 2010, attempted to encourage the free market while making coverage more accessible and affordable for individuals. Nicknamed "Obamacare," it accomplished a major expansion in health insurance coverage, requiring insurance to cover young adults under their parents' plans until the age of 26, preventing insurers from discriminating against people with preexisting conditions, requiring insurers to cover basic preventative care (such as vaccinations recommended by the Centers for Disease Control and Prevention), and expanding federal eligibility for Medicaid to all U.S. citizens and legal residents with income up to 133% of the federally defined poverty threshold. Critics of the ACA have stressed how the law limits individual freedoms by requiring that all residents have documented insurance coverage or pay a financial penalty, and intrudes on state prerogatives by regulating private health insurance markets (Blumenthal, Abrams, and Nuzum 2015).

In "The Origins of the Patient Protection and Affordable Care Act," Jill Quadagno examines the roots of the ACA. The ACA's key provisions borrow from the Clinton administration's attempted health insurance policy, particularly in its expansion of Medicaid and regulation of the insurance industry. Yet it also borrows ideas and principles from Republican health policy initiatives, especially the employer and individual mandates. Since President Obama signed it in 2010, the ACA has been credited with reducing the number of uninsured people from over 48 million in 2010 to 24.5 million in 2016 (National Center for Health Statistics 2017). However, at this writing, the ACA is under attack as Congress and the White House attempt to dismantle it.

In the third selection in this section, "The Debate Over Health Care Rationing: Déjà Vu All Over Again?" Alan Cohen examines the policy literature on medical care rationing over the past 25 years, examining the evolution of debates. Medical care rationing is implicit in the United States based on the ability to pay (through third-party insurance or out of pocket), whereas national health systems sometimes employ explicit rationing of medical care. Recent discussions about "death panels" of bureaucrats making health care decisions promoted fear among individuals, stymying cost containment efforts to curb the steady increases in health care spending in the United States. Cohen explores how rationing might be addressed in the future, increasing transparency and equity in access to health care resources.

Note

1. Third-party payments for services are a central feature of the economic organization of medicine in U.S. society. Since medical providers are paid a fee for every service they provide, many critics argue that this system creates a financial incentive to deliver unnecessary services, making medical care more profitable and costly.

References

Blumenthal, David, Melinda Abrams, and Rachel Nuzum. 2015. "The Affordable Care Act at 5 Years." *New England Journal of Medicine* 373: 2451–58.

Centers for Medicare and Medicaid Services. 2017a. *National Health Expenditures 2015 Highlights.* Accessed November 10, 2017. https://www.cms.gov/Research-Statistics-Data-and-Systems/Statistics-Trends-and-Reports/ReportsTrustFunds/index.html.

Centers for Medicare and Medicaid Services. 2017b. *Trustees Report & Trust Funds.* Accessed November 10, 2017. https://www.cms.gov/Research-Statistics-Data-and-Systems/Statistics-Trends-and-Reports/ReportsTrustFunds/index.html.

Davis, Karen. 1975. "Equal Treatment and Unequal Benefits: The Medicare Program." *Milbank Memorial Fund Quarterly* 53: 449–88.

Mechanic, David. 1996. "Changing Medical Organization and the Erosion of Trust." *Milbank Quarterly* 74: 174–89.

Medical Care Chart Book, 6th edition. 1976. School of Public Health, Department of Medical Care Organization, University of Michigan. Data on third-party payments computed from Chart D-15:117.

National Center for Health Statistics. 2017. *Early Release of Selected Estimates Based on Data From the 2016 National Health Interview Survey.* Accessed November 10, 2017. https://www.cdc.gov/nchs/data/nhis/earlyrelease/earlyrelease201705.pdf.

National Conference of State Legislatures. 2016. *Managed Care, Market Reports and the States.* Accessed November 10, 2017. http://www.ncsl.org/research/health/managed-care-and-the-states.aspx.

Rothman, David J. 1993. "A Century of Failure: Health Care Reform in America." *Journal of Health Politics, Policy & Law* 18 (2): 271–86.

Starr, Paul. 1982. *The Social Transformation of American Medicine*. New York: Basic Books.

Starr, Paul. 1995. "What Happened to Health Care Reform?" *American Prospect* (Winter): 20–31.

Stone, Deborah A. 1993. "The Struggle for the Soul of Health Insurance." *Journal of Health Politics, Policy and Law* 18: 287–317.

Stone, Deborah A. 1997. "The Doctor as Businessman: Changing Politics of a Cultural Icon." *Journal of Health Politics, Policy and Law* 22: 533–56.

Wholey, Douglas R., and Lawton R. Burns. 2000. "Tides of Change: The Evolution of Managed Care in the United States." In *Handbook of Medical Sociology*, 5th edition, edited by Chloe Bird, Peter Conrad, and Allen M. Fremont, 217–37. Upper Saddle River, NJ: Prentice Hall.

PAYING FOR HEALTH CARE

Thomas Bodenheimer and Kevin Grumbach

ealth care is not free. Someone must pay. But
how? Does each person pay when receiving
care? Do people contribute regular amounts in
advance so that their care will be paid for when
they need it? When a person contributes in
advance, might the contribution be used for care
given to someone else? If so, who should pay how
much?

Health care financing in the United States evolved
to its current state through a series of social interventions. Each intervention solved a problem but
in turn created its own problems requiring further
intervention. This chapter will discuss the historical
process of the evolution of health care financing.
The enactment in 2010 of the Patient Protection and
Affordable Care Act, commonly referred to as the
Affordable Care Act, ACA, or "Obamacare," created
major changes in the financing of health care in the
United States.

MODES OF PAYING FOR HEALTH CARE

The four basic modes of paying for health care are
out-of-pocket payment, individual private insurance, employment-based group private insurance,
and government financing (Table 25.1). These four
modes can be viewed both as a historical progression and as a categorization of current health care
financing.

Out-of-Pocket Payments

Fred Farmer broke his leg in 1913. His son
ran 4 miles to get the doctor, who came to the
farm to splint the leg. Fred gave the doctor
a couple of chickens to pay for the visit. His
great-grandson, Ted, who is uninsured, broke

his leg in 2013. He was driven to the emergency room, where the physician ordered an x-ray and called in an orthopedist who placed a cast on the leg. The cost was $2,800.

One hundred years ago, people like Fred Farmer paid physicians and other health care practitioners in cash or through barter. In the first half of the twentieth century, out-of-pocket cash payment was the most common method of payment. This is the simplest mode of financing—direct purchase by the consumer of goods and services (Fig. 25.1).

People in the United States purchase most consumer items and services, from gourmet restaurant dinners to haircuts, through direct out-of-pocket payments. This is not the case with health care (Arrow, 1963; Evans, 1984), and one may ask why health care is not considered a typical consumer item.

Need Versus Luxury

Whereas a gourmet dinner is a luxury, health care is regarded as a basic human need by most people.

For 2 weeks, Marina Perez has had vaginal bleeding and has felt dizzy. She has no insurance and is terrified that medical care

TABLE 25.1　■　Health Care Financing in 2013[a]	
Type of Payment	**Percentage of National Health Expenditures, 2013**
Out-of-pocket payment	12%
Individual private insurance	3%
Employment-based private insurance	30%[b]
Government financing	47%
Other	8%
Total	100%
Principle Source of Coverage	**Percentage of Population, 2013**
Uninsured	13%
Individual private insurance	7%
Employment-based private Insurance	47%
Government financing	33%
Total	100%

Note: These figures precede implementation of most of the Affordable Care Act.

[a]Because private insurance tends to cover healthier people, the percentage of expenditures is far less than the percentage of population ´covered. Public expenditures are far higher per population because the elderly and disabled are concentrated in the public Medicare and Medicaid programs.

[b]This includes private insurance obtained by federal, state, and local employees which is in part purchased by tax funds.

Source: Data extracted from Hartman M et al. National health spending in 2013; growth slows, remains in step with the overall economy. *Health Aff* 2015;34:150–160; US Census Bureau: Health Insurance Coverage in the United States, 2013. September, 2014.

might eat up her $500 in savings. She scrapes together $100 to see her doctor, who finds that her blood pressure falls to 90/50 mm Hg upon standing and that her hematocrit is 26%. The doctor calls Marina's sister Juanita to drive her to the hospital. Marina gets into the car and tells Juanita to take her home.

If health care is a basic human right, then people who are unable to afford health care must have a payment mechanism available that is not reliant on out-of-pocket payments.

Unpredictability of Need and Cost

Whereas the purchase of a gourmet meal is a matter of choice and the price is shown to the buyer, the need for and cost of health care services are unpredictable. Most people do not know if or when they may become severely ill or injured or what the cost of care will be.

Jake has a headache and visits the doctor, but he does not know whether the headache will

cost $100 for a physician visit plus the price of a bottle of ibuprofen, $1,200 for an MR1, or $200,000 for surgery and irradiation for brain cancer.

The unpredictability of many health care needs makes it difficult to plan for these expenses. The medical costs associated with serious illness or injury usually exceed a middle-class family's savings.

Patients Need to Rely on Physician Recommendations

Unlike the purchaser of a gourmet meal, a person in need of health care may have little knowledge of what he or she is buying at the time when care is needed.

Jenny develops acute abdominal pain and goes to the hospital to purchase a remedy for her pain. The physician tells her that she has acute cholecystitis or a perforated ulcer and recommends hospitalization, an abdominal CT scan, and upper endoscopic studies. Will

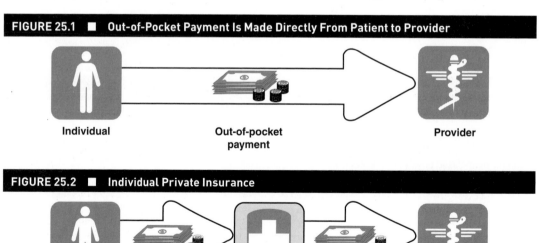

FIGURE 25.1 ■ Out-of-Pocket Payment Is Made Directly From Patient to Provider

Individual   Out-of-pocket payment   Provider

FIGURE 25.2 ■ Individual Private Insurance

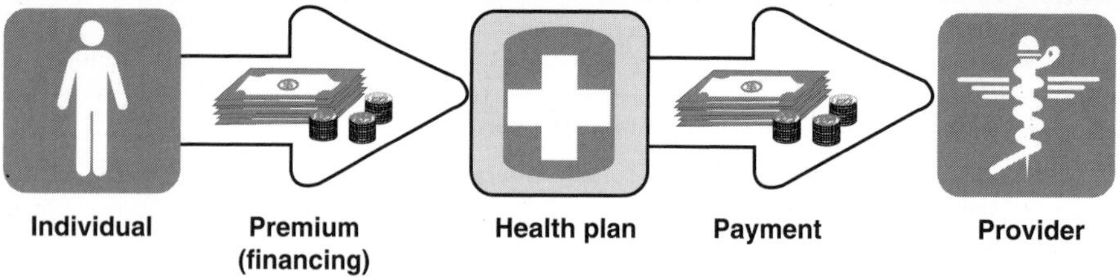

Individual   Premium (financing)   Health plan   Payment   Provider

Note: A third party, the insurance plan (health plan), is added, dividing payment into a financing component and a payment component. The ACA added an individual coverage mandate for those not otherwise insured and federal subsidy to help individuals pay the insurance premium.

Jenny, lying on a gurney in the emergency room and clutching her abdomen with one hand, use her other hand to leaf through a textbook of internal medicine to determine whether she really needs these services, and should she have brought along a copy of Consumer Reports to learn where to purchase them at the cheapest price?

Health care is the foremost example of asymmetry of information between providers and consumers (Evans, 1984). A patient with abdominal pain is in a poor position to question a physician who is ordering laboratory tests, x-rays, or surgery. When health care is elective, patients can weigh the pros and cons of different treatment options, but even so, recommendations may be filtered through the biases of the physician providing the information. Compared with the voluntary demand for gourmet meals, the demand for health services is partially involuntary and is often physician- rather than consumer-driven.

For these reasons among others, out-of-pocket payments are flawed as a dominant method of paying for health care services. Because the direct purchase of health services became increasingly difficult for consumers and was not meeting the needs of hospitals and physicians to be reliably paid, health insurance came into being.

Individual Private Insurance

In 2012, Bud Carpenter was self-employed. To pay the $500 monthly premium for his individual health Insurance policy, he had to work extra jobs on weekends, and the $5,000 deductible meant he would still have to pay quite a bit of his family's medical costs out of pocket. Mr. Carpenter preferred to pay these costs rather than take the risk of spending the money saved for his children's college education on a major illness. When he became ill with leukemia and the hospital bill reached $80,000, Mr. Carpenter appreciated the value of health insurance. Nonetheless he had to feel disgruntled when

he read a newspaper story listing his insurance company among those that paid out on average less than 60 cents for health services for every dollar collected in premiums.

With private health insurance, a third party, the insurer is added to the patient and the health care provider, who are the two basic parties of the health care transaction. While the out-of-pocket mode of payment is limited to a single financial transaction, private insurance requires two transactions—a premium payment from the individual to an insurance plan (also called a health plan), and a payment from the insurance plan to the provider (Fig. 25.2). In nineteenth-century Europe, voluntary benefit funds were set up by guilds, industries, and mutual societies. In return for paying a monthly sum, people received assistance in case of illness. This early form of private health insurance was slow to develop in the United States. In the early twentieth century, European immigrants set up some small benevolent societies in US cities to provide sickness benefits for their members. During the same period, two commercial insurance companies, Metropolitan Life and Prudential, collected 10 to 25 cents per week from workers for life insurance policies that also paid for funerals and the expenses of a final illness. The policies were paid for by individuals on a weekly basis, so large numbers of insurance agents had to visit their clients to collect the premiums as soon after payday as possible. Because of the huge administrative costs, individual health insurance never became a dominant method of paying for health care (Starr, 1982). In 2013, prior to the implementation of the individual insurance mandate of the ACA, individual policies provided health insurance for 7% of the US population (Table 25.1).

In 2014, Bud Carpenter signed up for individual insurance for his family of 4 through Covered California, the state exchange set up under the ACA. Because his family income was 200% of the federal poverty level, he received a subsidy of $1,373 per month, meaning that his premium would be $252 per month (down from his previous monthly premium of $500) for a silver plan with Kaiser Permanente. His deductible was $2,000 (down from $5,000). Insurance companies were no longer allowed to deny coverage for his pre-existing leukemia.

The ACA has many provisions, described in detail in the Kaiser Family Foundation (2013a) Summary of the Affordable Care Act. . . . One of the main provisions is a requirement (called the "individual mandate") that most US citizens and legal residents who do not have governmental or private health insurance purchase a private health insurance policy through a federal or state health insurance exchange, with federal subsidies for individual and families with incomes between 100% and 400% of the federal poverty level ($24,250 to $97,000 for a family of four). Details of the individual mandate are provided in Table 25.2.

Employment-Based Private Insurance

Betty Lerner and her schoolteacher colleagues each paid $6 per year to Prepaid Hospital in 1929. Ms. Lerner suffered a heart attack and was hospitalized at no cost. The following year Prepaid Hospital built a new wing and raised the teachers' prepayment to $12.

Rose Riveter retired in 1961. Her health insurance premium for hospital and physician care, formerly paid by her employer, had been $25 per month. When she called the insurance company to obtain individual coverage, she was told that premiums at age 65 cost $70 per month. She could not afford the insurance and wondered what would happen if she became ill.

The development of private health insurance in the United States was impelled by the increasing effectiveness and rising costs of hospital care. Hospitals became places not only in which to die, but also

in which to get well. However, many patients were unable to pay for hospital care, and this meant that hospitals were unable to attract "customers."

In 1929, Baylor University Hospital agreed to provide up to 21 days of hospital care to 1,500 Dallas school-teachers such as Betty Lerner if they paid the hospital $6 per person per year. As the Great Depression deepened and private hospital occupancy in 1931 fell to 62%, similar hospital-centered private insurance plans spread. These plans (anticipating health maintenance organizations [HMOs]) restricted care to a particular hospital. The American Hospital Association built on this prepayment movement and established statewide Blue Cross hospital insurance plans allowing free choice of hospital. By 1940, 39 Blue Cross plans controlled by the private hospital industry had enrolled over 6 million people. The Great Depression reduced the amount patients could pay physicians out of pocket, and in 1939, the California Medical Association set up the first Blue Shield plan to cover physician services. These plans, controlled by state medical societies, followed Blue Cross in spreading across the nation (Starr, 1982; Fein, 1986).

In contrast to the consumer-driven development of health insurance in European nations, coverage in the United States was initiated by health care providers seeking a steady source of income. Hospital and physician control over the "Blues," a major sector of the health insurance industry, guaranteed that payment would be generous and that cost control would remain on the back burner (Law, 1974; Starr, 1982).

The rapid growth of employment-based private insurance was spurred by an accident of history. During World War II, wage and price controls prevented companies from granting wage increases, but allowed the growth of fringe benefits. With a labor shortage, companies competing for workers began to offer health insurance to employees such as Rose Riveter as a fringe benefit. After the war, unions picked up on this trend and negotiated for health benefits. The results were dramatic: Enrollment in group hospital insurance plans grew from 12 million in 1940 to 142 million in 1988.

TABLE 25.2 ■ Summary of the Individual Mandate Provisions of the Affordable Care Act (ACA), 2015
U.S. citizens and legal residents are required to have health coverage with exemptions available for such issues as financial hardship. Those who choose to go without coverage pay a tax penalty of $325 or 2% of taxable Income in 2015, which gradually increases over the years. People with employer based and governmental health Insurance are not required to purchase the insurance required under the Individual mandate.
Tax credits to help pay health insurance premiums increase in size as family incomes rise from 100% to 400% of the Federal Poverty Level. In addition subsidies reduce the amount of out-of-pocket costs individuals and families must pay; the amount of the subsidy varies by income.
Under the individual mandate, health Insurance is purchased though insurance marketplaces called health insurance exchanges. Seventeen states have elected to set up their own exchanges, the remainder of states are covered by the federal exchange, Healthcare.gov.
Insurance companies marketing their plans through the exchange offer benefit categories: Bronze plans represent minimum coverage, with the insurer paying for 60% of a person's health care costs, with high out-of-pocket costs but low premiums Silver plans cover 70% of health care costs, with fewer out-of-pocket costs and higher premiums Gold plans cover 80% of costs, with low out-of-pocket costs and high premiums Platinum plans cover 90% of costs, with very low out-of-pocket costs and very high premiums
Most people who have obtained Insurance through the exchange have picked Bronze or Silver plans, and 87% have received a subsidy. A family of four with income at 150% of the federal poverty level receives an average subsidy of $11,000. At 300% of the federal poverty level the subsidy is about $6,000.

Source: Kaiser Family Foundation. Summary of the Affordable Care Act, 2013. http://kfforg/health-reform/fact-sheet/summary-of-the-affordable-care-act. Accessed March 12, 2015.

FIGURE 25.3 ■ Employment-Based Private Insurance

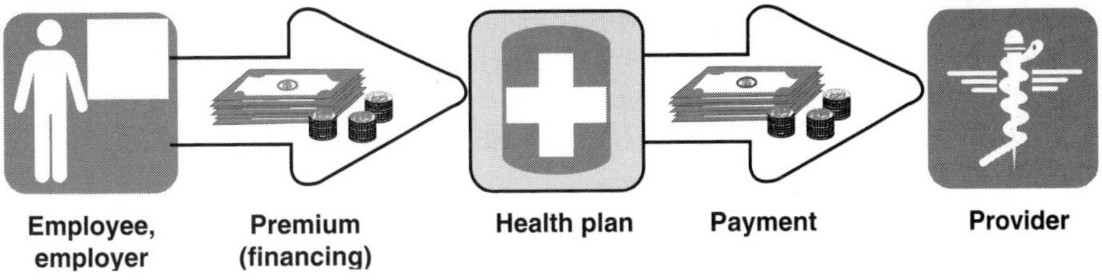

Employee, employer — Premium (financing) — Health plan — Payment — Provider

Note: In addition to the direct employer subsidy, indirect government subsidies occur through the tax-free status of employer contributions for health insurance benefits.

With employment-based health insurance, employers usually pay much of the premium that purchases health insurance for their employees (Fig. 25.3). However, this flow of money is not as simple as it looks. The federal government views employer premium payments as a tax-deductible business expense. The government does not treat the health insurance fringe benefit as taxable income to the employee, even though the payment of premiums could be interpreted as a form of employee income. Because each premium dollar of employer-sponsored health insurance results in a reduction in taxes collected, the government is in essence subsidizing employer-sponsored health insurance. This subsidy is enormous, estimated at $250 billion per year (Ray et al., 2014).

The ACA made a change in employer-based health insurance, requiring employers with 50 or more full-time employees to offer coverage or pay a fee to the government; the fee is meant to discourage employers from dropping employee health insurance, which they might be tempted to do since their employees could buy individual insurance through the health insurance exchanges (Kaiser Family Foundation, 2013b).

The growth of employment-based health insurance attracted commercial insurance companies to the health care field to compete with the Blues for customers. The commercial insurers changed the entire dynamic of health insurance. The new dynamic was called experience rating. (The following discussion of experience rating can be applied to individual as well as employment-based private insurance.)

> Healthy Insurance Company insures three groups of people—a young healthy group of bank managers, an older healthy group of truck drivers, and an older group of coal miners with a high rate of chronic illness. Under experience rating, Healthy sets its premiums according to the experience of each group in using health services. Because the bank managers rarely use health care, each pays a premium of $300 per month. Because the truck drivers are older, their risk of illness is higher, and their premium is $500 per month. The miners, who have high rates of black lung disease, are charged a premium of $700 per month. The average premium income to Healthy is $500 per member per month.
>
> Blue Cross insures the same three groups and needs the same $500 per member per month to cover health care plus administrative costs for these groups. Blue Cross sets its premiums by the principle of community rating. For a given health insurance policy,

> all subscribers in a community pay the same premium. The bank managers, truck drivers, and mine workers all pay $500 per month.

Health insurance provides a mechanism to distribute health care more in accordance with human need rather than exclusively on the basis of ability to pay. To achieve this goal, funds are redistributed from the healthy to the sick, a subsidy that helps pay the costs of those unable to purchase services on their own.

Community rating achieves this redistribution in two ways:

1. Within each group (bank managers, truck drivers, and mine workers), people who become ill receive benefits in excess of the premiums they pay, while people who remain healthy pay premiums while receiving few or no health benefits.

2. Among the three groups, the bank managers, who use less health care than their premiums are worth, help pay for the miners, who use more health care than their premiums could buy.

Experience rating is less redistributive than community rating. Within each group, those who become ill are subsidized by those who remain well, but among the different groups, healthier groups (bank managers) do not subsidize high-risk groups (mine workers). Thus the principle of health insurance, which is to distribute health care more in accordance with human need rather than exclusively on the ability to pay, is weakened by experience rating (Light, 1992).

In the early years, Blue Cross plans set insurance premiums by the principle of community rating, whereas commercial insurers used experience rating as a "weapon" to compete with the Blues (Fein, 1986). Commercial insurers such as Healthy Insurance Company could offer cheaper premiums to low-risk groups such as bank managers, who would naturally choose a Healthy commercial plan at $300 over a Blue Cross plan at $500. Experience rating helped commercial insurers overtake the Blues in the private health insurance market. While in 1945 commercial insurers had only 10 million enrollees, compared with 19 million for the Blues, by 1955 the score was commercials 54 million and the Blues 51 million.

Many commercial insurers would not market policies to such high-risk groups as mine workers, leaving Blue Cross with high-risk patients who were paying relatively low premiums. To survive the competition from the commercial insurers, Blue Cross had no choice but to seek younger, healthier groups by abandoning community rating and reducing the premiums for those groups. In this way, many Blue Cross and Blue Shield plans switched to experience rating. Without community rating, older and sicker groups became less and less able to afford health insurance.

From the perspective of the elderly and those with chronic illness, experience rating is discriminatory. Healthy persons, however, might have another viewpoint and might ask why they should voluntarily transfer their wealth to sicker people through the insurance subsidy. The answer lies in the unpredictability of health care needs. When purchasing health insurance, an individual does not know if he or she will suddenly change from a state of good health to one of illness. Thus, *within a group*, people are willing to risk paying for health insurance, even though they may not use it. *Among different groups*, however, healthy people have no economic incentive to voluntarily pay for community rating and subsidize another group of sicker people. This is why community rating cannot survive in a market-driven competitive private insurance system (Aaron, 1991).

In a major reform contained within the ACA, insurers are severely limited in using experience rating to set premiums; they can only vary premiums based on family size, geographic location, age, and smoking status. The ACA also limits how much premiums can differ between older and younger individuals (Kaiser Family Foundation, 2013b).

The most positive aspect of health insurance—that it assists people with serious illness to pay for their care—has also become one of its main drawbacks—the difficulty in controlling costs in an insurance environment. With direct purchase, the "invisible hand" of each individual's ability to pay holds down the price and quantity of health care. However, if a patient is well insured and the cost of care causes no immediate fiscal pain, the patient will use more services than someone who must pay for care out of pocket. In addition, particularly before the advent of fee schedules, health care providers could increase fees more easily if a third party was available to foot the bill.

Thus health insurance was originally an attempt by society to solve the problem of unaffordable health care under an out-of-pocket payment system, but its very capacity to make health care more affordable created a new problem. If people no longer had to pay out of their own pockets for health care, they would use more health care; and if health care providers could charge insurers rather than patients, they could more easily raise prices, especially during the era when the major insurers (the Blues) were controlled by hospitals and physicians. The solution of insurance fueled the problem of rising costs. As private insurance became largely experience rated and employment based, persons who had low incomes, who were chronically ill, or who were elderly found it increasingly difficult to afford private insurance.

Government Financing

In 1984 at age 74 Rose Riveter developed colon cancer. She was now covered by Medicare, which had been enacted in 1965. Even so, her Medicare premium, hospital deductible expenses, physician copayments, short nursing home stay, and uncovered prescriptions cost her $2,700 the year she became ill with cancer.

Employment-based private health insurance grew rapidly in the 1950s, helping working people and their families to afford health care. But two groups in the population received little or no benefit: the poor and the elderly. The poor were usually unemployed or employed in jobs without the fringe benefit of health insurance; they could not afford insurance premiums. The elderly, who needed health care the most and whose premiums had been partially subsidized by community rating, were hard hit by the trend toward experience raring. In the late 1950s, less than 15% of the elderly had any health insurance (Harris, 1966). Only one program could provide affordable care for the poor and the elderly: tax-financed government health insurance.

Government entered the health care financing arena long before the 1960s through such public programs as municipal hospitals and dispensaries to care for the poor and through state-operated mental hospitals. But only with the 1965 enactment of Medicare (for the elderly) and Medicaid (for the poor) did public insurance payments for privately operated health services become a major feature of health care in the United States. Medicare Part A (Table 25.3) is a hospital insurance plan for the elderly financed largely through social security taxes from employers and employees. Medicare Part B (Table 25.4) insures the elderly for physician services and is paid for by federal taxes and monthly premiums from the beneficiaries. Medicare Part D, enacted in 2003, offers prescription drug coverage and is paid for by federal taxes and monthly premiums from beneficiaries. Medicaid (Table 25.5) is a program run by the states that is funded by federal and state taxes, which pays for the care of millions of low-income people. In 2013, Medicare and Medicaid expenditures totaled $586 and $450 billion, respectively (Hartman et al., 2015).

With its large deductibles, copayments, and gaps in coverage, Medicare paid for only 58% of the average beneficiary's health care expenses in 2012. Ninety percent of the 50 million Medicare beneficiaries in 2012 had supplemental coverage: Thirty-three percent of beneficiaries had additional coverage from their previous employment, 19% purchased supplemental private insurance (called "Medigap" plans), 24% were enrolled in the Medicare Advantage program, and 14% were enrolled in both Medicare and Medicaid (Kaiser Family Foundation, 2015a).

The Medicare Modernization Act (MMA) of 2003 made two major changes in the Medicare program: the expansion of the role of private health plans (the Medicare Advantage program, Part C) and the establishment of a prescription drug benefit (Part D). Under the Medicare Advantage program, a beneficiary can elect to enroll in a private health plan contracting with Medicare, with Medicare subsidizing the premium for that private health plan rather than paying hospitals, physicians, and other providers directly as under Medicare Parts A and B. Beneficiaries joining a Medicare Advantage plan sacrifice some freedom of choice of physician and hospital in return for lower out-of-pocket payments and are only allowed to receive care from health care providers who are connected with that plan. Two-thirds of beneficiaries with Medicare Advantage plans are in health maintenance organizations (HMOs) . . . ; the remainder are in private fee-for-service plans. In order to channel more patients into Medicare Advantage plans, the MMA provided generous payments to those plans, with the result that they initially cost the federal government 14% more than the government paid for health care services for similar Medicare beneficiaries in the traditional Part A and Part B programs. The ACA reduced payments to Medicare Advantage plans with the goal of saving the Medicare program $136 billion over the following 10 years. In 2012, HMO Medicare Advantage plans on average cost the federal government 7% less than traditional Medicare while fee-for-service plans cost 12% to 18% more than traditional Medicare (Biles et al., 2015).

Medicare Part D provides partial coverage for prescription drugs. In 2013, 73% of Part D was financed through tax revenues, and 75% of Medicare beneficiaries had enrolled in the voluntary Medicare Part D program. Part D has been criticized because (1) there are major gaps in coverage, (2) coverage has been farmed out to private insurance companies rather than administered by the federal Medicare program, and (3) the government is not allowed to negotiate with pharmaceutical companies for lower drug prices. These three features of the program have caused confusion for beneficiaries, physicians, and pharmacists and a high cost for the program. Two-thirds of beneficiaries on Medicare Part D are enrolled in one of the 1,001 stand-alone private prescription drug plans and one-third receives their

TABLE 25.3 ■ Summary of Medicare Part A, 2015

Who is eligible?

Upon reaching the age of 65 years, people who are eligible for Social Security are automatically enrolled in Medicare Part A whether or not they are retired.

A person who has paid into the Social Security system for 10 years and that person's spouse are eligible for Social Security. People who are not eligible for Social Security can enroll in Medicare Part A by paying a monthly premium.

People under the age of 65 years who are totally and permanently disabled may enroll in Medicare Part A after they have been receiving Social Security disability benefits for 24 months. People with amyotrophic lateral sclerosis (ALS) or end-stage renal disease requiring dialysis or a transplant are also eligible for Medicare Part A without a 2-year waiting period.

How is it financed?

Financing is through the Social Security system. Employers and employees each pay to Medicare: 1.45% of wages and salaries. Self-employed people pay 2.9%.

The 2010 Affordable Care Act Increases the employee care for higher-income taxpayers (incomes greater than $200,000 for individuals or $250,000 for couples) from 1.45% to 2.35% starting in 2013.

What services are covered?[a]

Services	Benefit	Medicare Pays
Hospitalization	First 60 days[b]	All but a $1,260 deductible per benefit period
	61st to 90th day[b]	All but $315/day
	91st to 150th	All but $630/day
	Beyond 90 days if lifetime reserve days are used up	Nothing
Skilled nursing facility	first 20 days	All
	21st to 100th day	All but $157.50/day
	Beyond 100 days	Nothing
Home health care	Medically necessary care for homebound people	100% for skilled care as defined by Medicare regulations
Hospice care	As long as doctor certifies person suffers from a terminal illness	100% for most services, copays for outpatient drugs and coinsurance for inpatient respite care
Unskilled nursing home care	Care that is mainly custodial is not covered	Nothing

[a]For patients in Medicare Advantage plans, covered services and patient responsibility for payment changes based on the specifics of each Medicare Advantage plan.

[b]Part A benefits are provided by each benefit period rather than for each year. A benefit period begins when a beneficiary enters a hospital and ends 60 days after discharge from the hospital or from a skilled nursing facility.

[c]Beyond 90 days. Medicare pays for 60 additional days only once in a lifetime ("lifetime reserve days").

Part D coverage through a Medicare Advantage plan. Sixty-three percent are enrolled in one of five large companies. Different plans cover different medications and require different premiums, deductibles, and coinsurance payments. The standard benefit in 2015 has a $320 deductible and 25% coinsurance up to $2,960 in total drug costs, followed by a coverage gap. During the gap, enrollees are responsible for a larger share of their total drug costs until their total out-of-pocket spending reaches $4,700. Thereafter, enrollees pay only a small percentage of drug costs. The coverage gap, called the "donut hole," is a major problem for patients with chronic illness needing several medications. The ACA gradually reduces the amounts beneficiaries must pay in the donut hole (Kaiser Family Foundation, 2015b).

In 2009, the trustees of the Medicare program estimated that the Part A trust fund would be depleted by 2017. The ACA, by raising social security payments and reducing expenditures, extended Medicare's solvency through 2030.

The Medicaid program is jointly administered by the federal and state governments, with the federal government contributing at least 50% of the

---

TABLE 25.4 ■ Summary of Medicare Part B, 2015

Who is eligible?
People who are eligible for Medicare Part A who elect to pay the Medicare Part B premium of $104.90 per month. Some low-income persons can receive financial assistance with the premium. Higher income beneficiaries (over $85,000 for individual, $170,000 for couple) have higher premiums related to income.

How is it financed?
Financing is in part by general federal revenues (personal income and other federal taxes) and in part by Part B monthly premiums.

What services are covered?[a]

Services	Benefit	Medicare Pays
Medical expenses Physician services Physical, occupational, and speech therapy Medical equipment Diagnostic tests (no coinsurance for laboratory services)	All medically necessary services	80% of approved amount after a $147 annual deductible
Preventive care	Pap smears; mammograms; colorectal/ prostate cancer, cardiovascular and diabetes screening; pneumococcal and influenza vaccinations; yearly physical examinations	Included in medical expenses, and for some services the deductible and copayment are waived
Outpatient medications	Partially covered under Medicare Part D	All except for premium, deductible, coinsurance, and "donut hole," which vary by Part D plan
Eye retractions, hearing aids, dental services	Not covered	Nothing

[a]For patients in Medicare Advantage plans, covered services and patient responsibility for payment changes based on the specifics of each Medicare Advantage plan.

TABLE 25.5 ■ Summary of Medicaid Under the Affordable Care Act (ACA), 2015
Medicaid is a federal program administered by the states.
Eligibility
From 1965 through 2014, Medicaid while designed for low-income Americans, did not cover all poor people. In addition to being poor, Medicaid had required that people also meet "categorical" eligibility criteria such as being a young child, parent, pregnant, elderly or disabled, leaving out nonpregnant adults with dependent children. Income eligibility for Medicaid varied by state, typically children were covered up to 100%, adults to 61% and the elderly or disabled to 74% of the Federal Poverty Level. The federal government paid between 50% and 76% of total Medicaid costs; the federal contribution being greater for states with lower per capita incomes.
In 2015, Medicaid under the ACA varies widely between states participating in the Medicaid expansion and those not participating; for the latter states, the provisions summarized for the 1965 to 2014 period still apply. Participating states must make all individuals with incomes up to 138% of the federal poverty level eligible for coverage, with no categorical eligibility criteria. To finance Medicaid expansion for the participating states, the federal government pays 100% of the costs of the newly eligible from 2014 to 2016, decreasing to 90% in 2020 and beyond. Undocumented immigrants are not eligible for Medicaid.
State waivers
States can be granted waivers by the federal government to make changes in which services they provide to Medicaid recipients and whether recipients are required to receive the services through managed care plans.

funding to match state expenses for operating Medicaid programs. Although designed for low-income Americans, not all poor people have traditionally been eligible for Medicaid. In addition to being poor, until enactment of the ACA Medicaid required that people also meet "categorical" eligibility criteria such as being a young child, pregnant, elderly, or disabled.

The ACA (Table 25.5) eliminated the categorical eligibility criteria and required that beginning in 2014, states offer the program to all citizens and legal residents with family income at or below 138% of the Federal Poverty Line—about $16,000 in 2015. The ACA did not change Medicaid policies that continue to exclude undocumented immigrants from eligibility for federal funding, The ACA intended that it be mandatory for states to expand Medicaid eligibility, and provided states an incentive for expansion by having the federal government pay almost all the cost of the increased Medicaid enrollment (100% of the cost of expanded enrollment in 2014 to 2016, phased down to 90% in 2020 and thereafter). However, in June 2012, the Supreme Court ruled that the ACA's Medicaid expansion was optional for states. In February 2015, only 28

states plus the District of Columbia had expanded Medicaid (Obamacare Facts, 2015). Medicaid now covers one in six people in the United States, making it the single largest health program in the nation. Enrollment grew dramatically in recent years even before implementation of the ACA in 2014, with enrollment increasing from 32 million to 60 million people between 2000 and 2013 (9 million of whom were "dual eligibles" receiving both Medicare and Medicaid). By the end of 2014, an additional 6 million people had enrolled in states participating in ACA Medicaid expansion—falling short of the goal of 16 million new enrollees, if all states had participated in the expansion (Rosenbaum, 2014).

From 2000 to 2013, Medicaid expenditures rose from $200 billion to $450 billion. To slow down this expenditure growth, the federal government ceded to states enhanced control over Medicaid programs through Medicaid waivers, which allow states to make alterations in the scope of covered services, require Medicaid recipients to pay part of their costs, and obligate Medicaid recipients to enroll in managed care plans. . . . In 2014, more than half of Medicaid recipients were enrolled in managed care plans. Because Medicaid pays primary care physicians an average of 58% of Medicare fees, the majority of adult primary care physicians limit the number of Medicaid patients they will see.

In 1997, the federal government created the State Children's Health Insurance Program (SCHIP), a companion program to Medicaid. SCHIP covers children in families with incomes at or below 200% of the federal poverty level, but above the Medicaid income eligibility level. States legislating an SCHIP program receive generous federal matching funds. In 2012, 8 million children were enrolled in the program, some of whom are transitioning to Medicaid under the expanded eligibility criteria enacted in the ACA.

Government health insurance for the poor and the elderly added a new factor to the health care financing equation: the taxpayer (Fig. 25.4). With government-financed health plans, the taxpayer can interact with the health care consumer in two distinct ways:

1. The social insurance model, exemplified by Medicare, allows only those who have paid a certain amount of social security taxes to be eligible for Part A and only those who pay a monthly premium to receive benefits from Part B. As with private insurance, social insurance requires people to make a contribution in order to receive benefits.

2. The contrasting model is the Medicaid public assistance model, in which those who contribute (taxpayers) may not be eligible for benefits (Bodenheimer & Grumbach, 1992).

It must be remembered that private insurance contains a subsidy: redistribution of funds from the healthy to the sick. Tax-funded insurance has the same subsidy and usually adds another: redistribution of funds from upper- to lower-income groups.

FIGURE 25.4 ■ Government-Financed Insurance

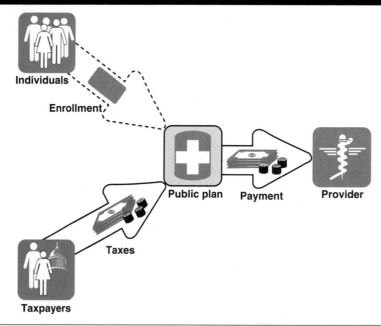

Note: Under the social insurance model (e.g., Medicare Part A), only individuals paying taxes into the public plan are eligible for benefits. In other models (e.g., Medicaid), an individual's eligibility for benefits may not be directly linked to payment of taxes into the plan.

Under this double subsidy, exemplified by Medicare and Medicaid, healthy middle-income employees generally pay more in social security payments and other taxes than they receive in health services, whereas unemployed, disabled, and lower-income elderly persons tend to receive more in health services than they contribute in taxes.

The advent of government financing improved financial access to care for some people, but, in turn, aggravated the problem of rising costs. The federal government and state governments have responded by attempting to limit Medicare and Medicaid payments to physicians, hospitals, and managed care plans.

THE BURDEN OF FINANCING HEALTH CARE

Different methods of financing health care place different burdens on the various income levels of society. Payments are classified as progressive if they take a rising percentage of income as income increases, regressive if they take a falling percentage of income as income increases, and proportional if the ratio of payment to income is the same for all income classes (Pechman, 1985).

What principle should underlie the choice of revenue source for health care? A central purpose of the health care system is to maintain and improve the health of the nation's population. . . . Rates of mortality and disability are far higher for low-income people than for the wealthy. Burdening low-income families with high levels of payments for health care (i.e., regressive payments) reduces their disposable income, amplifies the ill effects of poverty, and thereby worsens their health. It makes little sense to finance a health care system—whose purpose is to improve health—with payments that worsen health. Thus, regressive payments could be considered "unhealthy."

Rita Blue earns $10,000 per year for her family of 4. She develops pneumonia, and her out-of-pocket health costs come to $1,000, 10% of her family income.

Cathy White earns $100,000 per year for her family of 4. She develops pneumonia, and her out-of-pocket health costs come to $1,000, 1% of her family income.

Out-of-pocket payments are a regressive mode of financing. According to the 1987 National Medical Care Expenditure Survey, out-of-pocket payments took 12% of the income of families in the nation's lowest-income quintile, compared with 1.2% for families in the wealthiest 5% of the population (Bodenheimer & Sullivan, 1997). This pattern is confirmed by the 2000 Medical Expenditure Panel Survey (MEPS, 2003). Many economists and health policy experts would consider this regressive burden of payment as unfair. Aggravating the regressivity of out-of-pocket payments is the fact that lower-income people tend to be sicker and thus have more out-of-pocket payments than the wealthier and healthier.

Jim Hale is a young, healthy, self-employed accountant whose monthly income is $6,000, with a health insurance premium of $200, or 3% of his income.

Jack Hurt is a disabled mine worker with black lung disease. His income is $1,800 per month, of which $400 (22%) goes for his health insurance.

Experience-rated private health insurance is a regressive method of financing health care because increased risk of illness tends to correlate with reduced income. If Jim Hale and Jack Hurt were enrolled in a community-rated plan, each with a premium of $300, they would respectively pay 5% and 17% of their incomes for health insurance. With community rating, the burden of payment is regressive, but less so than with experience rating. Most private insurance is not individually purchased but rather obtained through employment. How is the burden of employment-linked health insurance premiums distributed?

Jill is an assistant hospital administrator. To attract her to the job, the hospital offered her a package of salary plus health insurance of $6,500 per month. She chose to take $6,200 in salary, leaving the hospital to pay $300 for her health insurance.

Bill is a nurse's aide, whose union negotiated with the hospital for a total package of $2,800 per month; of this amount $2,500 is salary and $300 pays his health insurance premium.

Do Jill and Bill pay nothing for their health insurance? Not exactly. Employers generally agree on a total package of wages and fringe benefits; if Jill and Bill did not receive health insurance, their pay would probably go up by nearly $300 per month. That is why employer-paid health insurance premiums are generally considered deductions from wages or salary, and thus paid by the employee (Blumberg et al., 2007). For Jill, health insurance amounts to only 5% of her income, but for Bill it is 12%. The MEPS corroborates the regressivity of employment-based health insurance; in 2001 to 2003, premiums took an average of 10.9% of the income of families in between 100% and 200% of the Federal Poverty Line compared with 2.3% for those above 500% of poverty (Blumberg et al., 2007). In 2012, employer-sponsored health insurance premiums represented 58% of family income for the bottom 40% of American families compared with 4% for the top 5% (Blumenthal & Squires, 2014).

Larry Lowe earns $10,000 and pays $410 in federal and state income taxes, or 4.1% of his income.

Harold High earns $100,000 and pays $12,900 in income taxes, or 12.9% of his income.

The progressive income tax is the largest tax providing money for government-financed health care. Most other taxes are regressive (e.g., sales and property taxes), and the combined burden of all taxes that finance health care is roughly proportional (Pechman, 1985).

In 2009, 46% of health care expenditures were financed through out-of-pocket payments and premiums, which are regressive, while 47% was funded through government revenues (Martin et al., 2011), which are proportional. The sum total of health care financing is regressive. In 1999, the poorest quintile of households spent 18% of income on health care, while the highest-income quintile spent only 3% (Cowan et al, 2002). Overall, the US health care system is financed in a manner that is unhealthy.

CONCLUSION

Neither Fred Farmer nor his great-grandson Ted had health insurance, but the modern-day Mr. Farmer's predicament differs drastically from that of his ancestor. Third-party financing of health care has fueled an expansive health care system that offers treatments unimaginable a century ago, but at tremendous expense.

Each of the four modes of financing health care developed historically as a solution to the inadequacy of the previous modes. Private insurance provided protection to patients against the unpredictable costs of medical care, as well as protection to providers of care against the unpredictable ability of patients to pay. But the private insurance solution created three new, interrelated problems:

1. The opportunity for health care providers to increase fees to insurers caused health services to become increasingly unaffordable for those with inadequate insurance or no insurance.

2. The employment-based nature of group insurance placed people who were unemployed, retired, or working part-time at a disadvantage for the purchase of insurance, and partially masked the true costs of insurance for employees who did receive health benefits at the workplace.

3. Competition inherent in a deregulated private insurance market gave rise to the practice of experience rating, which made insurance premiums unaffordable for many

elderly people and other medically needy groups.

To solve these problems, government financing was required, but government financing fueled an even greater inflation in health care costs.

As each "solution" was introduced, health care financing improved for a time. But rising costs have jeopardized private and public coverage for many people and made services unaffordable for those without a source of third-party payment. The problems of each financing mode, and the problems created by each successive solution, have accumulated into a complex crisis characterized by inadequate access for some and high costs for everyone.

References

Aaron HI. *Serious and Unstable Condition: Financing America's Health Care*. Washington, DC: Brookings Institution; 1991.

Arrow KJ. Uncertainty and the welfare economics of medical care. *Am Econ Rev*. 1963;53:941.

Biles B et al. Variations in county-level costs between traditional Medicare and Medicare Advantage have implications for premium support. *Health Aff (Millbank)*. 2015; 34:56–63.

Blumberg LJ et al. Setting a standard of affordability for health insurance coverage. *Health Aff (Millwood)*. 2007;26: w463-w473.

Blumenthal D, Squires D. Do health care costs fuel economic inequality in the United States? The Commonwealth Fund Blog, www.commonwealthfund.org/publications/blog/2014/sep/do-health-costs-fuel-inequality. Published September 9, 2014. Accessed February 15, 2015.

Bodenheimer T, Grumbach K. Financing universal health insurance: taxes, premiums, and the lessons of social insurance. *J Health Polit Policy Law*. 1992:17:439–462.

Bodenheimer T, Sullivan K. The logic of tax-based financing for health care. *Int. J Health Serv*. 1997; 27:409–425.

Cowan CA et al. Burden of health care costs: businesses, households, and governments, 1987-2000. *Health Care Financ Rev*. 2002; 23:131–159.

Evans RG. *Strained Mercy*. Toronto, Ontario, Canada: Butterworths; 1984.

Fein R. *Medical Care, Medical Costs*. Cambridge, MA: Harvard University Press; 1986.

Harris R. *A Sacred Trust*. New York, NY: New American Library; 1966.

Hartman M et al. National health spending in 2013: growth slows, remains in step with the overall economy. *Health Aff (Millwood)*. 2015;34:150–160.

Kaiser Family Foundation. Summary of the Affordable Care Act 2013a. http://kff.org/health-reform/fact-sheet/summary-of-the-affordable-care-act. Accessed March 12, 2015.

Kaiser Family Foundation. Health insurance market reforms: rate restrictions, 2013b. https://kaiserfamilyfoundation, fileswordpress .com/2013/01/8328.pdf. Accessed March 12, 2015.

Kaiser Family Foundation. Medicare publications, 2015a. http://kff.org/medicare. Accessed February 15, 2015.

Kaiser Family Foundation. The Medicare Part D prescription drug benefit. 2015b. http://files.kff.org/attachment/medicare-prescription-drug-benefit-fact-sheet. Accessed February 15, 2015.

Law SA. *Blue Cross: What Went Wrong?* New Haven, CT: Yale University Press; 1974.

Light DW. The practice and ethics of risk-rated health insurance. *JAMA*. 1992;267:2503–2508.

Martin A et al. Recession contributes to slowest annual rate of increase in health spending in five decades. *Health Affairs*. 2011;30;11.

Medical Expenditure Panel Survey. Health insurance coverage of the civilian non-institutionalized population, first half of 2002. Agency for Healthcare Research and Quality, June 2003. www.meps.ahrq.gov. Accessed November 11, 2011.

Obamacare Facts, February 2015. http://obamacarefacts.com/obamacares-medicaid-expansion

Pechman JA. *Who Paid the Taxes, 1966–1985*. Washington, DC: Brookings Institution; 1985.

Ray M et al. Tax subsidies for private health insurance. Kaiser Family Foundation, 2014. http://files.kff.org/attachment/tax-subsidies-for-private-health-insurance-issue-brief. Accessed February 15.2015.

Rosenbaum S. Medicaid payments and access to care. *N Engl J. Med*. 2014;371:2345–2347.

Starr P. *The Social Transformation of American Medicine*. New York, NY: Basic Books; 1982.

26

THE ORIGINS OF THE PATIENT PROTECTION AND AFFORDABLE CARE ACT

Jill Quadagno

On March 23, 2010, President Barack Obama signed into law the Patient Protection and Affordable Care Act (ACA). For the first time in more than a century, the federal government made a commitment to provide universal coverage through a complex mix of private incentives and public support. Its main features include state insurance exchanges, stringent regulations on insurance companies, fines on employers who do not offer coverage, a mandate that individuals purchase health insurance, subsidies to help low-income people with the costs, and a substantial expansion of Medicaid. To liberal supporters of a single-payer plan, the ACA represented a disappointing concession to private insurance companies, a scheme that would never achieve universal coverage. As Physicians for a National Health Program (PNHP 2010) reported, the legislation was like "seeing aspirin dispensed for

the treatment of cancer." For conservatives, however, Obamacare was a first step on the road to socialism (Grogan 2011). According to former House Speaker Newt Gingrich, a Republican presidential candidate in 2012, "The new law [is] a back door to socialized medicine that puts America at the edge of a possible catastrophic failure" (McDermott 2010).

Despite criticisms from both the Left and the Right, most analysts agree that the ACA represented a victory for the Democratic Party over Republican visions of limited government intervention. For Anne Beaussier (2012), the victory resulted from congressional Democrats' success in transcending institutional constraints. Hacker (2010) emphasizes the composition of the Democratic majority in Congress. As he explains, "The approach (of the ACA) was feasible only because so much intraparty agreement already existed about the proper direction forward. The three leading Democratic candidates in the presidential race endorsed not similar reform plans but essentially the same reform plan" (Hacker 2011: 440). Similarly, Lawrence Brown (2011: 421,425) claims that "Congress' accomplishment was not merely but entirely a triumph for the Democratic Party. . . . The ACA is a virtually pure Democratic product."

These claims are correct in the narrow sense of votes in Congress. The ACA passed without a single Republican vote in either the House or the Senate. Yet they are also inaccurate in other respects. First, despite howls from the Right that the ACA signified the victory of socialized medicine, its provisions were nearly identical to the Health Equity and Access Reform Today Act of 1993 (HEART), a Republican plan that was promoted as an alternative to President Bill Clinton's American Health Security Act of 1993. The HEART was consistent with a free-market approach and contained provisions, notably the employer mandate and the individual mandate, that had widespread Republican support in the two decades before the ACA was enacted. Second, contrary to conventional wisdom that President Clinton's health care reform was an utter failure, a road to nowhere (Hacker 1997), policies his administration pursued were critical for the ACA's eventual success. These include federal regulation of the private insurance industry through the Health Insurance Portability and Accountability Act of 1996 (HIPAA) and incentives for states to expand Medicaid coverage beyond the very poor, to near-poor and working-class families. How was the ACA transformed from a conservative Republican plan to protect the private insurance industry into an ambitious proposal for universal coverage favored by liberal Democrats? This article draws on archival research, congressional records, and secondary documents to elucidate the complex policy legacies that became the Patient Protection and Affordable Care Act.

THE ORIGINS OF THE INDIVIDUAL MANDATE

Policy learning effects come from political actors' experiences with past initiatives in which "the setting of a new agenda and the design of alternative responses may build on . . . past successes or may reflect lessons learned from past mistakes" (Pierson 1994: 4). For example, Hugh Heclo (2011), in his study of social policy in Britain and Sweden, emphasized an incremental policy-learning process in which past policies provided models for policy makers. What is initially puzzling about the ACA is that its policy legacy reflected neither conservatives' favored proposal for expanding health savings accounts nor liberals' proposal to extend Medicare to all (Quadagno and McKelvey 2010; Schlesinger and Hacker 2007). Rather, the ACA's core provisions were a legacy inherited from other health insurance proposals over nearly half a century following the enactment of Medicare and Medicaid in 1965.

The success of Medicare emboldened supporters of national health insurance regarding the prospects for universal coverage. As Dr. John Hogness, president of the Institute of Medicine, declared in 1973, "The feeling among experts is that it will take three to five years" (Hodgson 1973: 2). During the 1970s numerous bills were introduced in Congress, ranging from Senator Russell Long's (D-LA) plan to subsidize basic private health plans with federal payment for catastrophic costs to Senator Ted Kennedy's (D-MA) Health Security, which would fold all public and private health plans into a single federal program. When it appeared that Congress would enact some program, President Richard Nixon unveiled his own national health plan in 1974. Nixon's plan consisted of two parts: the Comprehensive Health Insurance Plan, which included an employer mandate administered by private insurance companies, and the Assisted Health Insurance Plan, where states would contract with private insurers to cover low-income and high-risk individuals (Quadagno 2005). The employer mandate won the endorsement of the Washington Business Group on Health, an organization of two hundred corporation members whose mission was to help firms design benefit packages that reduced costs. Another business group, the National Leadership Coalition, composed of executives from large companies, also supported the employer mandate. Although Nixon's impeachment ended Republican support for health insurance legislation, President Jimmy Carter included an employer mandate in his health insurance plan, which gained no traction in Congress because of a stalled economy (Quadagno 2005). Thus, the employer mandate originated with Republicans but was not anathema to Democrats.

In the 1980s, rising costs and increasing numbers of uninsured revived interest in health care reform. Most proposals for universal health care, except the liberal single-payer model, were based on an employer mandate. Yet some conservatives warned that an employer mandate contained perverse incentives, which could lead to job lock and create inflation as employers passed costs onto consumers. Looking for an approach that would not interfere with a free market, conservatives began to evaluate an alternative approach, an individual mandate. The virtues of an individual mandate were that it would avoid job lock and discourage free riders. As Stuart Butler (1989: 6) of the conservative Heritage Foundation explained the rationale for the individual mandate:

> Many states now require passengers in automobiles to wear seatbelts for their own protection. Many others require anybody driving a car to have liability insurance. But neither the federal government nor any state requires all households to protect themselves from the potentially catastrophic costs of a serious accident or illness. Under the Heritage plan, there would be such a requirement. This mandate is based on two important principles. First, that health care protection is a responsibility of individuals, not businesses. . . . Second, it assumes that there is an implicit contract between households and society, based on the notion that health insurance is not like other forms of insurance protection. If a young man wrecks his Porsche and has not had the foresight to obtain insurance, we may commiserate but society feels no obligation to repair his car. But health care is different. If a man is struck down by a heart attack in the street, Americans will care for him whether or not

he has insurance. . . . A mandate on individuals recognizes this implicit contract. Society does feel a moral obligation to insure that its citizens do not suffer from the unavailability of health care. But, on the other hand, each household has the obligation, to the extent it is able, to avoid placing demands on society by protecting itself.

In 1991 a group of conservative economists charged with developing a health insurance plan for President George H. W. Bush laid these principles out in greater detail (Roy 2012). Their plan endorsed an individual mandate as a counterpoint to either the employer mandate or the single-payer system favored by Democrats:

> The allocation of resources to health care should rest on individuals' choice of insurance in light of their different needs and desires. This will drive a competitive market and improve the efficiency of the health care system. . . . All citizens should be required to obtain a basic level of health insurance. . . . Permitting individuals to remain uninsured results in inefficient use of medical care, inequity in the incidence of costs of uncompensated care, and tax-related distortions. . . . [The individual mandate] avoids interfering with labor markets and employment contracts; it facilitates portability of coverage, employment mobility and a competitive market. (Pauly et al. 1991: 8)

Thus in its original formulation the individual mandate was consistent with conservative American values that favored a free market and limited state authority (Lipset 1996). It was incorporated into President Bush's plan, the Comprehensive Health Reform Act of 1992, which mandated that each individual purchase a basic benefit coupled with tax credits and deductions to help cover the costs. The Bush plan also would have created health insurance networks (HINs) that would arrange for the purchase of health insurance and negotiate payment rates and selective contracts with providers

(US Congress 1993: 25). Republicans tabled the plan, however, when it appeared they could not get enough Democratic support. Then Bush lost the 1992 election, and momentum shifted to the Democrats.

THE POLICY LEGACY OF THE CLINTON ADMINISTRATION

American Health Security Act

During the 1992 presidential election, Bill Clinton campaigned on a promise to enact legislation to guarantee universal coverage. Following his victory, he created an outside task force to draft a plan, ignoring ongoing work in congressional committees. The Clinton proposal, the American Health Security Act of 1993 (H.R. 3600,103d Cong. 1st Sess. [1993]), was released seven months later. Its central feature involved the purchase of cooperatives called "health alliances." Echoing aspects of Bush's HINs, the alliances would hold down costs by bargaining directly with health care providers. Further, Health Security would create an independent agency that would certify private insurance plans and set guidelines for a standard benefit package that all insurers would have to offer (Hacker 1997). Health Security also included federal regulations on insurance companies operating in the small-group and individual insurance market. These regulations would prohibit insurance companies from refusing coverage on the basis of age or health status (guaranteed issue) or terminating benefits for any reason. Firms with more than five thousand employees could self-insure but would have to pay a new payroll tax to expand the public program for the uninsured.

Purchasing cooperatives, standard benefit packages, and insurance company regulation were at the forefront of Health Security and received the bulk of the critical attention. Health Security also included a little-noticed provision, however, mandating that individuals purchase health coverage. Section 1002 of the Health Security Act specified that "each eligible individual (1) must enroll in an applicable health plan for the individual and (2) must pay any premium consistent with the Act, with respect to such enrollment." Eligible individuals according to Section 1001 included citizens, nationals, permanent alien residents, and long-term nonimmigrants. Thus virtually all Americans and people residing in the United States would be required to enroll in a health insurance plan.

The story of how a coalition of insurers, corporations, and small business groups mobilized against Health Security has been described in great detail elsewhere (Jacobs and Skocpol 2010; Quadagno 2011). Overall, the Center for Public Integrity estimated that 650 organizations spent at least $100 million to defeat the Clinton plan (Quadagno 2005; Skocpol 1997). Health Security never even came up for a vote. What is less well known is that Republican opponents of the Clinton plan adopted an alternative proposal that included a stringent employer mandate and a harsh individual mandate.

HEART

The Republican alternative, the Health Equity and Access Reform Today Act, was introduced in November 1993 by Senator John Chafee (R-RI). Chafee was the leader of a Republican task force that had met almost weekly for three years to develop a health care plan. When Chafee introduced his bill, Senator Robert Packwood (R-OR) called it "a culmination of these efforts [that] represents a cautious and sensible approach to reforming our health care system" (Cong. Rec. S16925 [November 22, 1993] ["Health Care Reform"]). The HEART would "guarantee every individual access to affordable and secure health coverage through substantial health insurance market reforms." Insurance plans would have to meet strict requirements, including guaranteed eligibility, no preexisting condition exclusions, guaranteed renewal, and a standard benefit package. Further, large employers would be required to offer coverage to all employees, and small employers (one hundred or fewer employees) would have to offer but not pay for a benefit package. Individuals would be required to purchase coverage or pay a substantial penalty "equal to the average yearly premium of the local area plus 20 percent" (Cong. Rec. E3078 [November 24, 1993] [Hon. William M. Thomas,

"Introduction of the Health Equity and Access Reform Today"]). However, vouchers would be provided to make insurance affordable for low-income individuals.

The HEART alternative was supported by half of the GOP Senate, including such knowledgeable members as Senate minority leader Bob Dole (R-KS), Robert Bennett (R-UT), John Danforth (R-MO), Pete Domenici (R-NM), David Durenberger (R-MN), and Richard Lugar (R-IN). It also had the support of key House Republicans, including Representative Newt Gingrich (R-GA), who declared on *Meet the Press* in 1993, "I am for people, individuals—exactly like automobile insurance—individuals having health insurance and being required to have health insurance. And I am prepared to vote for a voucher system which will give individuals, on a sliding scale, a government subsidy so we insure that everyone as individuals have health insurance" (Gingrich 1993), Yet when Chafee attempted to move his bill forward, conservatives within his own party declared that mandates were out of the question. As Senator Trent Lott (R-MS) said, "Republicans have to make clear we are not signed on to any of this government control and mandate stuff" (Johnson and Broder 1996: 364). The HEART was never debated in the Senate, and it disappeared from the national policy agenda for the remainder of the 1990s.

Insurance Company Regulation

It is accepted wisdom that Health Security was a failed policy initiative that led to a Republican takeover of the House and Senate in 1994 and undermined support for the Democratic Party for more than a decade (Skocpol 1997). Lost in this interpretation are the Clinton administration's policy legacies that paved the way for the ACA. One legacy was federal regulation of insurance companies. Ever since the McCarran-Ferguson Act of 1945 affirmed insurance regulation as a primary state responsibility, health insurance plans had been regulated by the states. In most states, legislatures enacted the laws under which insurance companies operated and state insurance departments enforced

those laws. Under Clinton that power shifted to the federal government.

During the early 1990s, the states responded to growing concerns about the disintegration of the insurance market for individuals and small groups by enacting numerous reforms (Hall 2000; Kail, Quadagno, and Dixon 2009). Many states enacted consumer protection policies that were designed to control the underwriting practices of insurance companies (Stream 1999). Rating restrictions compressed the range of prices insurers could charge to policyholders. Although insurers were allowed to vary premiums according to an individual's or group's risk profile, they could only do so to a defined extent within set "rating bands" (Hall 2000). Affordability and disclosure regulations required insurers to offer similarly priced plans with uniform benefits (Stream 1999). Guaranteed issue regulations required insurers to offer coverage to any individual or group, regardless of health.

States also attempted to restrict insurers' risk selection practices through accessibility reforms (Stream 1999). Guaranteed renewal laws require insurers to continue to cover previously insured groups, even if the members of the group suffered a change in health. Preexisting condition limitations set a maximum period for which an individual could be excluded from a group plan because of a prior health condition. Finally, portability rules guaranteed that a person who changed jobs or changed insurers within the same workplace could retain coverage without being subject to a new exclusion period (Barrilleaux and Brace 2007; Hall 2000).

For the most part, these reforms did little to reduce the number of uninsured, and in some cases they had the opposite effect (Kail, Quadagno, and Dixon 2009). For example, the guaranteed issue requirement for all small-group products prompted insurers to drop plans they were unwilling to sell under these conditions. Rating restrictions appear to have had a similar effect (Hall 2000). The failure of regulation may also reflect the fact that in many states insurers control the state insurance commissioner's offices. These offices have become a revolving door, with insurance industry executives often serving as commissioners and then returning to the industry (Bodenheimer 1990). As a result, at the state level insurers could influence legislation and insert loopholes to ensure that regulations were ineffective (Hall 2000; Light 1992).

Although states' efforts to regulate insurance practices largely failed, they set the stage for greater federal control. In 1995 Senators Ted Kennedy (D-MA) and Nancy Kassebaum (R-KS) drafted rigorous federal regulations including guaranteed renewal, guaranteed issue, prohibitions on experience rating, and tightening of preexisting condition exclusions. Following a barrage of opposition from the insurance industry, however, the proposal was watered down considerably. The bill that President Clinton signed into law, the Health Insurance Portability and Accountability Act of 1996 (HIPAA), limited the ability of private health plans to impose preexisting condition coverage exclusions on plan participants (Medill 1998), allowed employees who lost group coverage because of a change in personal circumstances to convert to individual coverage, prohibited insurers from charging different premiums for individuals within groups, and required insurers to guarantee renewal to any group. HIPAA did not include any price restrictions, however, and this made continuing coverage unaffordable for many individuals (Quadagno 2005). Nor did HIPAA guarantee that people shopping for coverage would not be rejected because of health. Further, HIPAA had many loopholes and applied only to small groups (Hall 2000). Despite these limitations, HIPAA set an important precedent for federal regulation of the insurance industry.

Medicaid Expansion

A less publicized achievement of the Clinton administration was the expansion of Medicaid beyond the very poor to near-poor and working-class families. This expansion was made possible by Section 1115 of the 1965 amendments to the Social Security Act, which allows states to apply for waivers to conduct research and demonstration projects within their Medicaid programs, thus bypassing strict federal rules and regulations. Throughout the 1970s and 1980s there were many approved demonstrations, but they were small in scope and driven mainly by state rather than federal interests. Most expansions targeted pregnant women and children, groups generally viewed as morally deserving (Grogan 2008; Grogan and Patashnik 2003). In 1993 the Clinton administration began actively promoting states' use of Section 1115 waivers to expand coverage beyond the very poor and issuing new guidelines that streamlined the process. States responded rapidly, raising income and asset limits and incorporating groups not categorically eligible (Schneider 1997). For example, Oregon extended Medicaid eligibility to *all* state residents with income below the federal poverty level (Gold et al. 2001). Tennessee's TennCare program made Medicaid available to families with income up to 400 percent of the poverty level (Ku and Garrett 2000).

The expansion of Medicaid to new beneficiary groups and to the near poor and working class helped to transform public perceptions of the program. During the 1995–96 budget showdown between President Clinton and Republicans, Clinton sought to rally support against the GOP budget by arguing that it would involve huge cuts in popular entitlement programs, not only Social Security and Medicare but also Medicaid. No longer was Medicaid merely a "welfare" benefit. This definition of Medicaid as an entitlement was incorporated into the 1996 Democratic Party platform, which promised to protect the program from "devastating cuts" (Grogan and Patashnik 2003: 845).

Medicaid was further entrenched as a popular entitlement when Congress enacted the State Children's Health Insurance Program (SCHIP) of 1997. This new program increased the federal match to the states from 50 percent to 65 percent and covered children in families with income up to 200 percent of poverty level. In response, some states created quite generous SCHIP programs (Blewett, Davern, and Rodin 2004; Cunningham 2003). Others, as allowed by law, implemented separate non-Medicaid programs for low-income children with more restrictive benefit packages, a strategy that reduced costs and also avoided any stigma associated with Medicaid. Between 1998 and 2001 Medicaid and SCHIP enrollment grew on average by 30 percent (Grogan and Patashnik 2003). Further, SCHIP rules were subsequently amended to allow states to cover uninsured parents as well as their children (Cunningham 2003; Kaiser Commission on Medicaid and the Uninsured 2005). As Grogan (forthcoming) notes, "By the end of the Clinton administration, [Medicaid] looked like a broad entitlement more than a welfare program."

Although the 1990s transformed Medicaid, both in regard to coverage expansions and in ideological terms, these changes also highlighted the limitations of state responsibility. TennCare provides an example of some of the challenges the states faced. Originally TennCare expanded subsidized coverage to all uninsured residents and allowed those ineligible for the subsidy to buy into what was essentially a public option. In its first year of operation, TennCare enrollment quickly grew close to the federal cap of 1.5 million people, meaning the federal government would not share in the cost of the number above that. In 1995, however, the fiscal strain caused by the growth in enrollment forced Tennessee to close eligibility to uninsured adults. Another budget crisis in 2005 resulted in the removal from TennCare of more than 160,000 people who were not Medicaid eligible, and the program's benefits were trimmed (Kaiser Commission on Medicaid and the Uninsured 2005). Thus the waiver experiments demonstrated the limits on what can be achieved at the state level and pointed to the need for a federal solution.

The Massachusetts Health Care Plan

One of the state experiments with coverage expansion was a rousing success. In 2006, after a six-month debate and a series of compromises between Democrats and Republicans, the Massachusetts legislature adopted the Massachusetts Health Care Reform Plan, with only four nay votes out of two hundred House and Senate members. On board was Senator Ted Kennedy, the single-payer advocate who became convinced that this approach could achieve his lifelong goal of universal coverage (Cooper 2012). Designed in large part with the assistance of the Heritage Foundation, the plan was "a hybrid approach that incorporated ideas from across the political spectrum" (Hyman 2007). The law included a state insurance exchange, which Governor Mitt Romney

touted as "a single consumer-driven marketplace for health insurance for small businesses, their employees and individuals" (quoted in Owcharenko and Moffit 2006: 1). It also contained an employer mandate requiring that all employers with more than eleven full-time employees make a "fair and reasonable" contribution toward their workers' health plans or face penalties. And for the first time, health insurance legislation included an individual mandate. In signing the bill, Romney (2006) explained its virtues: "No longer can individuals free ride [sic] by seeking healthcare and expecting society to bear the cost." To ensure that all residents could afford the premiums, health insurance was fully subsidized for adults earning up to 150 percent of the federal poverty level and for children of parents earning up to 300 percent of that level. Thus these provisions borrowed many features in HEART but also incorporated the Medicaid expansions that the Clinton administration had made possible.

Some observers believed that the Massachusetts plan would be as futile as other state-level reforms and, more worrisome, likely to detract from efforts for federal reform (Jacobson and Braun 2006–7). Yet such dire predictions proved unfounded. Before the law took effect in 2006, about 94 percent of state residents were insured. By 2010 more than 98 percent were insured, including 99.8 percent of all children, making Massachusetts's rate of uninsured the lowest in the United States (Kahn 2011). Thus Massachusetts provided the blueprint and the evidence that the individual mandate was a workable solution that could be achieved with bipartisan support.

HEALTHY AMERICANS ACT

The success of the Massachusetts plan encouraged members of Congress to consider moving toward universal coverage through an individual mandate, an option was gathering support among Democrats as well as Republicans. In 2004 Senator Ron Wyden (D-OR) began developing a proposal around the individual mandate, testing it out on both Democrats and Republicans. "Between 2004 and 2008, I saw over eighty members of the Senate, and there were very few who objected" (quoted in Klein 2012).

In December 2006, he unveiled the Healthy Americans Act (S. 334, 110th Cong. [2007]), and in May 2007, Robert Bennett (R-UT), who had been a sponsor of the 1993 Chafee bill, joined him. Two related House bills, H.R. 3163 and H.R. 6444, were introduced simultaneously.

The Healthy Americans Act was designed to transition away from employer-provided health insurance to employer-subsidized health insurance. It would do this by eliminating entirely the tax break for employer health insurance. This was a highly controversial feature because it meant abandoning the employer-based system, which had been the mainstay of health coverage since the 1940s. The Healthy Americans Act would also require those who did not have insurance coverage to enroll in Healthy American Private Insurance Plans (HAPIs). Individuals would choose their health care plan from state-approved private insurers. Endorsed by seventeen co-sponsors, including nine Republicans and seven Democrats, the bill won more bipartisan support than any universal health care proposal in the history of the Senate but died in the Senate Finance Committee.

Despite the failure of the Healthy Americans Act, a bipartisan consensus on the individual mandate seemed to be emerging. Not only did congressional members of both parties support the concept, but in the 2008 presidential election campaign, two Democratic candidates, Senators John Edwards (D-NC) and Hillary Clinton (D-NY), highlighted the individual mandate in their health care plans (Jacobs and Skocpol 2010). The holdout was Senator Barack Obama. Thus what began as a conservative, free-market approach to health care reform was beginning to morph into the liberal blueprint for change.

THE PATIENT PROTECTION AND AFFORDABLE CARE ACT OF 2010

Immediately after his victory in the 2008 election, President Obama urged committees in Congress to assemble the legislative specifics and the votes

to pass a bill. In contrast to President Clinton, who involved a task force of outsiders to draft his plan and delayed release for seven months, Obama did not attempt to reinvent the wheel but turned to policy options already on the agenda. Initially, it seemed that the Healthy Americans Act would provide the solution. Immediately after Obama became president-elect, Wyden and Bennett wrote a letter on November 20, 2008, recommending legislative goals reflected in the Healthy Americans Act. They reintroduced their bill on February 5, 2009, with fourteen co-sponsors—nine Democrats and five Republicans (S. 391). A companion bill (H.R. 1321) was introduced in the House with ten co-sponsors. Wyden-Bennett was also endorsed by Republican presidential aspirant Mitt Romney (2009a), who in a June 2009 interview on *Meet the Press* called it a plan "that a number of Republicans think is a very good health-care plan—one that we support." Yet in an interview on July 2009, President Obama said that although he agreed with many of the principles in Wyden-Bennett, he felt that the plan, like the plan promoted by single-payer advocates, was too radical. In theory, he said, those plans work, but "the problem is, we have evolved partly by accident into an employer-based system." Not only would a "radical restructuring" meet with "significant political resistance"; in addition, "families who are currently relatively satisfied with their insurance but are worried about rising costs . . . would get real nervous about a wholesale change" (Lane 2009).

Another obstacle was that a key Democratic constituency, organized labor, was opposed to the Healthy Americans Act. The trade unions were concerned about whether employment-based coverage could be sustained over the long run, but they were unwilling to support legislation that would undo it completely. In 2009 three large unions—the American Federation of State, County and Municipal Employees; the United Food and Commercial Workers; and the National Education Association—ran ads against the Healthy Americans Act, charging that it would unfairly tax health benefits (Robertson 2009).

A key constituency was the private insurance industry. Insurers were willing to accept stricter regulations, including price controls and guaranteed-issue without preexisting condition exclusions, as long as these regulations were accompanied by an individual mandate (Hacker 2011). An individual mandate would bring young, healthy people into the system to help pay the costs of older, sicker people. Insurers also supported Medicaid expansion. Indeed, a decade earlier the Health Insurance Association of America had endorsed a proposal that would use Medicaid as the cornerstone to expand coverage. Under this plan Medicaid would cover all individuals with income below 133 percent of the poverty level (Grogan and Patashnik 2003). What was unacceptable to insurers, however, was the public option, which would have offered an alternative to private insurance. Fearing that a new public program could out-compete private insurance on price and quality, insurers launched a campaign against it (Harwood 2009).

Physician organizations were less influential in 2010 than in previous health care reform debates (Quadagno 2005). The reason was that physicians were divided into multiple organizations and did not speak with a single voice. The liberal PNHP wanted to eliminate the private insurance industry entirely and opposed any solution other than a single-payer system. In contrast, the AMA favored expanding tax advantages for health savings accounts. Physicians' opposition was reduced by a concession that abrogated a 1997 provision that would have cut Medicare reimbursement rates by the end of the year (Beaussier 2012).

On July 14, 2009, three House committees reported out the House Tri-Committee America's Affordable Health Care Act (HB 3200). The following day the Senate Health, Education, Labor and Pension Committee, of which Obama had been a member when he was a senator, passed its own version, the Affordable Health Choices Act (S 1679). The legislation that emerged was much more comprehensive than the Healthy Americans Act and less committed to eliminating employer-based coverage. A key provision was the individual mandate, which the president now supported: "I was opposed to this idea because my general attitude was the reason people don't have health insurance is not because

they don't want it. It's because they can't afford it. I am now in favor of some sort of individual mandate" (quoted in Klein 2012). His change of heart was a pragmatic choice. Given the extensive bipartisan support won by previous health care reform plans based on an individual mandate, the president had reason to believe that he might receive a favorable response from Republicans. Romney, in fact, heralded the individual mandate's merits: "Our experience also demonstrates that getting every citizen insured doesn't have to break the bank. First, we established incentives for those who were uninsured to buy insurance. Using tax penalties, as we did, . . . encourages free riders to take responsibility for themselves rather than pass their medical costs to others" (Romney 2009b). This optimism proved unfounded, however, for the final bill that made it through the House and Senate on March 21, 2010, had no Republican support. Republicans united against it, hoping for the complete victory they had achieved against the Clinton plan (Hacker 2010).

Yet the ACA's main provisions were nearly identical to the Republican-supported HEART plan. As Table 26.1 shows, both the HEART plan and the ACA included an individual mandate, an employer mandate, a standard benefit package, state-based purchasing exchanges, subsidies for low-income people, efforts to improve efficiency, controls on Medicare spending growth, and controls on high-cost plans. Both measures also included stringent regulations on insurance companies, including a ban on denying coverage because of preexisting conditions, and prohibited insurers from canceling coverage because of health.

The HEART plan and the ACA also differed on a few provisions that, to a large degree, reflected changes that had occurred in the health insurance system during the Clinton administration. One difference was that the ACA but not HEART prohibited insurers from setting lifetime limits on health benefits. In 1996 Representative Anna Eshoo (D-CA) had first introduced a bill, the Christopher Reeve Health Insurance Reform Act (H.R. 3030), banning lifetime caps, which had been set at $1 million in the 1970s but had failed to keep pace with inflation. Her bill failed to win support

TABLE 26.1 ■ Provisions of the ACA (2010) and HEART (1993)

Major Provisions	ACA 2010	HEART Bill 1993
Individual mandate	Yes	Yes
Fines on employers	Yes	Yes
Standard benefits package	Yes	Yes
Bans on denying medical coverage for preexisting conditions	Yes	Yes
Establishes state-based exchanges/purchasing groups	Yes	Yes
Offers subsidies for low-income people to buy insurance	Yes	Yes
Improves efficiency of health care system	Yes	Yes
Equalizes tax treatment for insurance of self-employed	Yes	Yes
Reduces growth in Medicare spending	Yes	Yes
Controls high-cost health plans	Yes (taxes plans over $8,500 for single coverage, $23,000 for family plan)	Yes (caps tax exemption for employer-sponsored plans)
Prohibits insurance company from canceling coverage	Yes	Yes
Prohibits insurers from setting lifetime spending caps	Yes	No
Expands Medicaid	Yes	No
Extends coverage to dependents	Yes (up to age 26)	No

Source: Adapted from Henry J. Kaiser Family Foundation 2010

in the Republican-controlled House, and it died in committee. By 2007 more than half of all health insurance plans had a lifetime cap, often buried in the fine print (Henry J. Kaiser Family Foundation 2007). With Democrats in control of the House in 2008, Representative Eshoo reintroduced the bill (H.R. 6228), while Senator Byron Dorgan introduced a similar bill in the Senate. That provision was included in the ACA.

Another difference was that the ACA but not HEART extended coverage on private plans to dependents up to age twenty-six. This age group stood out because young adults had the lowest rate of insurance coverage and, unlike children under age eighteen, were ineligible for SCHIP benefits (Sommers et al. 2013). Allowing young adults to remain on their parents' plans would immediately reduce the number of uninsured.

Both HEART and the ACA included an employer mandate, but whereas it was stringent under HEART, it was watered down under the ACA to a fine of $750 for each full-time employee. The individual mandate was also more modest. Under HEART individuals who failed to purchase coverage would pay a penalty equal to the average yearly premium in the area plus 20 percent. Under the ACA the penalty for those who failed to purchase coverage was $95 in 2014, rising to $750 in 2016 and indexed thereafter. Another difference was that HEART would have equalized the tax treatment of premium costs for the self-employed with workers who received benefits through their jobs, a provision not included in the ACA.

The ACA also expanded Medicaid by universalizing a process that had escalated in the states throughout the 1990s, thus eliminating the need for waivers. Specifically, the ACA extended Medicaid to all children, parents, and childless adults with family incomes up to 133 percent of federal poverty level. As an incentive to participation, the federal government would pay for 100 percent of the expansion for three years and 90 percent thereafter, plus a 23 percent increase in the SCHIP federal match.

Although many Republicans had previously supported the core provisions of the ACA, once it was enacted, they launched an assault against it. Republican governors in several states refused to set up insurance exchanges and said that they would refuse to expand their Medicaid programs (Cohen 2012). The individual mandate, in particular, came under the heaviest fire, as polls showed that this was the most unpopular element of the law (Klein 2012). On the day that President Obama signed the ACA into law, fourteen Republican state attorneys general filed suit against it on the grounds that it was unconstitutional. Heritage's Butler (2012) also repudiated his previous support for the individual mandate:

> I headed Heritage's health work for 30 years. And make no mistake; Heritage and I actively oppose the individual mandate. Nevertheless, the myth persists. . . . The confusion arises from the fact that 20 years ago, I held the view that as a technical matter, some form of requirement to purchase insurance was needed in a near-universal insurance market to avoid massive instability through

"adverse selection." At that time, President Clinton was proposing a universal health care plan, and Heritage and I devised a viable alternative. . . . But the version of the health insurance mandate Heritage and I supported in the 1990s had three critical features. First, it was not intended to push people to obtain protection for their own good but to protect others. . . . Second, we sought to induce people to buy coverage through the carrot of a generous health credit or voucher. . . . And third, in the legislation we helped craft that ultimately became the preferred alternative to ClintonCare, the mandate was actually the loss of certain tax breaks for those not choosing to buy coverage, not a legal requirement. . . . Heritage-funded research . . . caused me to conclude that we had made a mistake in the 1990s. . . . Changing one's mind about the best policy to pursue—but not one's principles—is part of being a researcher at a major think tank.

On June 28, 2012, the Supreme Court upheld the constitutionality of the ACA but gave the states the right to opt out of the Medicaid expansion. As of February 2013, eleven states with Republican governors had announced they would not participate. However, some Republican governors, responding to pressures from Latino voters and the potential loss of billions in federal matching funds and health care jobs, did decide to expand their Medicaid programs. A prime example is Arizona, historically a welfare laggard, which did not participate in Medicaid at all until 1982. Yet in January 2013 Governor Jan Brewer, an outspoken critic of Obamacare, nonetheless announced that Arizona would expand its Medicaid program. In 2014, the first full year of expansion, Arizona would gain $1.6 billion in federal matching funds. It is likely that such fiscal concerns, coupled with hard lobbying by the health care industry, will eventually result in universal participation (Burton, Dooren, and Lippman 2012). Thus what began as a program of welfare medicine will probably play a major role in the move toward universal coverage. As Grogan (forthcoming) explains,

"The ACA . . . puts Medicaid on par with Medicare and Social Security—our sacrosanct middle-class entitlements."

CONCLUSION

When Bill Clinton was elected president, he set the ambitious but ultimately unsuccessful goal of providing health insurance for all. His Health Security proposal is usually viewed as a total failure, a presidential initiative that foundered "quickly and completely" (Hacker 1997: xi). What is often not recognized is that the Clinton administration left a policy legacy that made possible the success of an equally ambitious plan for health care reform nearly two decades later. Specifically, Clinton encouraged states to apply for waivers to extend their Medicaid programs to new groups and enacted SCHIP, which expanded coverage for children and some adults. He also signed into law the HIPAA, which incorporated into federal law many of the state regulations on insurance companies that had been enacted in the early 1990s. This legacy of insurance company regulation and Medicaid expansion paved the way for core provisions of the ACA.

Yet the policy legacy of the ACA extends beyond the Clinton plan to Republican proposals from the 1970s to the 1990s, notably the employer mandate and the individual mandate developed in opposition.

The employer mandate was initially introduced during the Nixon administration and remained favored by Republicans under the Bush administration and in HEART. The individual mandate first made a formal appearance in the Bush plan, was revived under the Republican-sponsored HEART in 1993, then reappeared under the bipartisan Healthy Americans Act of 2006. It appeared to have bipartisan support until 2009, when Republicans turned against it. Instead, it became the favored option of Democrats.

The ACA represents a curious stew of provisions that simmered for nearly four decades. Those who claim it represents a liberal takeover of the health care system, a major step on the road to socialism, ignore the fact that the employer mandate and the individual mandate were both devised by conservatives who claimed these provisions were consistent with free-market principles and conservative ideals. At the same time, liberal supporters of a single-payer plan who view the ACA as a right-wing victory should take comfort in the Medicaid expansion, low-income subsidies, and opportunity for states to introduce a public option down the road. The ACA does adhere to the objectives of those who believe that the health care system should encourage market competition. Yet the subsidies will make coverage more affordable for low-income individuals and families, and the insurance company regulations will make coverage more accessible and reliable.

References

Barrilleaux, Charles, and Paul Brace. 2007. "Notes from the Laboratories of Democracy: State Government Enactments of Market- and State-Based Health Insurance Reforms in the 1990s." *Journal of Health Politics, Policy and Law* 32: 655.

Beaussier, Anne L, 2012. "The Patient Protection and Affordable Care Act: The Victory of Unorthodox Lawmaking." *Journal of Health Politics, Policy and Law* 37, no. 5: 741-78.

Blewett, Lynn, Michale Davern, and Holly Rodin. 2004. "Covering Kids: Variation in Health Insurance Coverage Trends by State, 1996–2002." *Health Affairs* 23, no. 6: 170–80.

Bodenheimer, Thomas. 1990. "Should We Abolish the Private Health Insurance Industry?" *International Journal of Health Services* 20, no. 2: 199–220.

Brown, Lawrence D. 2011. "The Elements of Surprise: How Health Reform Happened." *Journal of Health Politics, Policy and Law* 36, no. 3: 419–27.

Burton, Thomas, Jennifer Dooren, and Daniel Lippman. 2012. "Hospitals Urge Medicaid Expansion." *Wall Street Journal,* June 29. online.wsj.com/article/SB100014240527023048307045774 97123131684982.html.

Butler, Stuart M, 1989. "Assuring Affordable Health Care for All Americans." Heritage Lectures, 218. Washington, DC: Heritage Foundation.

Butler, Stuart M. 2012. "Don't Blame Heritage for ObamaCareMandate."USAToday.com,February6. usatoday30.usatoday.com/news/opinion/forum/story/2012-02-03/health-individual-mandate-reform-heritage/52951140/1.

Cohen, Tom. 2012. "House Republicans Vote, Again, to Repeal Health Care Law." CNN.com, July 11. www.cnn.com/2012/07/ll/politics.

Cooper, Michael. 2012. "Conservatives Sowed Idea of Health Care Mandate, Only to Spurn It Later." *New York Times,* February 14. www.nytimes.com/2012/02/15/health/policy/health-care-mandate-was-first-backed-by-conserva tives.html?_r=0.

Cunningham, P. J. 2003. "SCHIP Making Progress: Increased Take-Up Contributes to Coverage Gains." *Health Affairs* 22, no. 4: 163–72.

Gingrich, Newt. 1993. *Meet the Press* transcript. October 3. www.mediaite.com/tv/newt-gingrich-releases-video-opposing-individual-mandate-he-defended-yesterday/.

Gold, M., J. Mittler, A. Aizer, B. Lyons, and C. Schoen. 2001. "Health Insurance Expansion through States in a Pluralistic System." *Journal of Health Politics, Policy and Law* 26, no. 3: 581–616.

Grogan, Colleen. 2008. "Medicaid: Health Care for You and Me?" In *Health Politics and Policy,* 4th ed., edited by James Morone, Theodor Litman, and Leonard Robins, 329–54. New York: Delmar.

Grogan, Colleen. 2011. "You Call It Public, I Call It Private, Let's Call the Whole Thing Off." *Journal of Health Politics, Policy and Law* 36, no. 3: 401–12.

Grogan, Colleen. Forthcoming. "Medicaid: Designed to Grow." In *Health Politics and Policy,* 5th ed., edited by James Morone, Theodor Litman, and Leonard Robins. New York: Delmar.

Grogan, Colleen, and Eric Patashnik. 2003. "Between Welfare Medicine and Mainstream Entitlement: Medicaid at the Political Crossroads." *Journal of Health Politics, Policy and Law* 28, no. 5: 821–58.

Hacker, Jacob. 1997. *The Road to Nowhere.* Princeton, NJ: Princeton University Press.

Hacker, Jacob. 2010. "The Road to Somewhere: Why Health Reform Happened." *Perspectives on Politics* 8, no. 3: 861–76.

Hacker, Jacob. 2011. "Why Reform Happened." *Journal of Health Politics, Policy and Law* 36, no. 3: 437–41.

Hall, M. A. 2000. "The Impact of Health Insurance Market Reforms on Market Competition." *American Journal of Managed Care* 6: 57–67.

Harwood, John. 2009. "The Lobbying Web." *New York Times,* August 1. nytimes.com/2009/08/02/weekinreview/02harwood.html?page wanted=all&_r=0.

Heclo, Hugh. 2011. *Modern Social Policies in Britain and Sweden.* 2nd ed. ECPR Press Classics Series. Colchester, UK: European Consortium for Political Research Press.

Henry J. Kaiser Family Foundation. 2007. *Employer Health Benefits 2007 Annual Survey.* www.kff.org/insurance/7672/index.cfm.

Henry J. Kaiser Family Foundation. 2010. "Summary of a 1993 Republican Health Reform Plan." *Kaiser Health News,* February 23. kaiserhealth-news.org/stories/2010/february/23/gop-1993-health-reform-bill.aspx.

Hodgson, Godfrey. 1973. "The Politics of American Health Care: What Is It Costing You?" *Atlantic Monthly,* October, www.theatlantic.com/past/politics/healthca/hodgson.htm.

Hyman, David. 2007. "The Massachusetts Health Plan: The Good, the Bad and the Ugly." *University of Kansas Law Review* 55, no. 5: 1103–18.

Jacobs, Lawrence, and Theda Skocpol. 2010. *Health Care Reform and American Politics: What Everyone Needs to Know.* New York: Oxford University Press.

Jacobson, Peter, and Rebecca Braun. 2007. "Let 1000 Flowers Wilt: The Futility of State Health Care Reform." *University of Kansas Law Review* 55, no. 5: 1173–1202.

Johnson, Haynes, and David Broder. 1996. *The System: The American Way of Politics to the Breaking Point.* Boston: Little, Brown.

Kahn, Huma. 2011. "Has Mitt Romney's Massachusetts Health Care Law Worked?" *The Note* (blog), May 12. abcnews.go.com/blogs/politics/2011/05/has-mitt-romneys-massachusetts-health-care-law-worked.

Kail, Ben, Jill Quadagno, and Marc Dixon. 2009. "Can States Lead the Way to Universal Coverage? The Effect of Health Care Reform on the Uninsured." *Social Science Quarterly* 90, no. 5: 1–20.

Kaiser Commission on Medicaid and the Uninsured. 2005. *Medicaid Section 1115 Waivers: Current Issues.* Key Facts, January 2005. Washington, DC: Kaiser Family Foundation.

Klein, Ezra. 2012. "Unpopular Mandate: Why Do Politicians Reverse Their Positions?" *New Yorker,* June 25. www.newyorker.com/reporting/2012/06/25/120625fa_fact_klein#ixzz2K-K6q961t.

Ku, Leighton, and Bowen Garrett. 2000. "How Welfare Reform and Economic Factors Affected Medicaid Participation: 1984–1996." Urban Institute Discussion Paper. Washington, DC: Urban Institute.

Lane, Dee. 2009. "Obama Calls Wyden Health Plan Radical." *Oregonian,* July 9. www.oregonlive.com/politics/index.ssf/2009/07/obama_calls_wyden_health__plan.html.

Light, Donald. 1992. "The Practice and Ethics of Risk-Related Health Insurance." *Journal of the American Medical Association* 267, no. 18: 2503–4.

Lipset, Seymour M. 1996. *American Exceptionalism: A Double-Edged Sword.* New York: Norton.

McDermott, Karyn. 2010. "Gingrich Says Obamacare 'Socialized Medicine.'" *Richmond Republican Examiner,* May 15. www.examiner.com/republican-in-richmond/gingrich-says-obamacare-socialized-medicine.

Medill, Colleen. 1998. "HIPAA and Its Related Legislation: A New Role for ERISA in the Regulation of Private Health Plans?" *Tennessee Law Review* 65, no. 2: 485–510.

Owcharenko, Nina, and Robert Moffit. 2006. "The Massachusetts Health Plan: Lessons for the States." *Backgrounder No. 1953* (Heritage Foundation), July 18. heritage.org/research/reports/2006/07/the-massachusetts-health-plan-lessons-for-the-states? ac=l.

Pauly, Mark, Patricia Damon, Paul Feldstein, and John Hoff. 1991. "A Plan for Responsible National Health Insurance." *Health Affairs* 10, no. 1: 5–25.

Pierson, Paul. 1994. *Dismantling the Welfare State.* New York: Cambridge University Press.

PNHP (Physicians for a National Health Program). 2010. "Pro-Single-Payer Doctors: Health Bill Leaves 23 Million Uninsured." News release, March 22. www.pnhp.org/news/2010/march/pro-single-payer-doctors-health-bill-leaves-23-million-uninsured.

Quadagno, Jill. 2005. *One Nation, Uninsured: Why the US Has No National Health Insurance.* New York: Oxford University Press.

Quadagno, Jill. 2011. "Interest Group Influence on the Patient Protection and Affordability Act of 2010: Winners and Losers in the Health Care Reform Debate." *Journal of Health Politics, Policy and Law* 36, no. 3: 449–54.

Quadagno, Jill, and J. Brandon McKelvey. 2010. "The Consumer-Directed Health Care Movement." In *Social Movements and the Transformation of American Health,* edited by Mayer Zald, Sandra R. Levitsky, and Jane Banaszak-Holl, 50–63. New York: Oxford University Press.

Robertson, Lori. 2009. "Half the Story on Health Care." FactCheck.org, May 21. www.factcheck.org/2009/05/half-the-story-on-health-care/.

Romney, Mitt. 2006. Letter to the Honorable Senate and House of Representatives, April 12. www.ncsl.org/Portals/l/documents/health/veto.

Romney, Mitt. 2009a. *Meet the Press* transcript. June 28. www.nbcnews.com/id/31584983/ns/meet_the_press/t/meet-press-transcript-june/.

Romney, Mitt. 2009b. "Mr. President, What's the Rush?" *USA Today,* July 7. usatoday30.usatoday.com/printedition/news/20090730/column30_st.art.htm.

Roy, Avit. 2012. "The Tortuous History of Conservatives and the Individual Mandate." *Forbes,* February 7. www.forbes.com/sites/aroy/2012/02/07/the-tortuous-conservative-history-of-the-individual-mandate/.

Schlesinger, Mark, and Jacob Hacker. 2007. "Secret Weapon: The 'New' Medicare as a Route to Health Security." *Journal of Health Politics, Policy and Law* 32, no. 2: 247–91.

Schneider, S. K. 1997. "Medicaid Section 1115 Waivers: Shifting Health Care Reform to the States." *Publius* 27, no. 2: 89–109.

Skocpol, Theda. 1997. *Boomerang: Health Care Reform and the Turn against Government* New York: Norton.

Sommers, Benjamin D., Thomas Buchmueller, Sandra L. Decker, Colleen Carey, and Richard Kronick. 2013. "The Affordable Care Act Has Led to Significant Gains in Health Insurance and Access to Care for Young Adults." *Health Affairs* 32, no. 1: 165–74.

Stream, Christopher. 1999. "Health Reform in the States: A Model of State Small Group Insurance Market Reforms." *Political Research Quarterly* 52, no. 3: 499–525.

US Congress. 1993. *Coverage of Preventive Services: Provisions of Selected Current Health Care Reform Proposals.* September 1993. Office of Technology Assessment. OTA-BP-H-110, NTIS Order No. PB94-126976. Washington, DC: Library of Congress.

27

THE DEBATE OVER HEALTH CARE RATIONING

Déjà Vu All Over Again?

Alan B. Cohen

It has been almost three decades since Henry Aaron's and William Schwartz's 1984 book, *The Painful Prescription: Rationing Hospital Care*, touched off a policy debate over the need to employ stern measures to bring rising health care costs under control. Since then, the debate over health care rationing has been confined mostly to the pages of academic journals. In 2009, however, it erupted violently in newspaper headlines across America when Sarah Palin and others charged that proposed end-of-life counseling for Medicare beneficiaries constituted "death panels" that would ration care and decide the fate of elderly Americans (Saltonstall 2009; Rutenberg and Calmes 2009). Although these false claims were quickly challenged (Allen 2009; Blumenauer 2009; Bookman 2009; Diaz 2009; Farley 2009; Parker 2009), such counter measures often fail (Nyhan and Reifler 2010), and in this case,

the myth of death panels persisted and became so pervasive (Holan 2009) that it instilled fear about health care reform and triggered an unfortunate retreat from advanced care planning (Tinetti 2012). Hyperbolic claims of "rationing" and "death panels" subsequently were used as weapons at different times (and with varying effect) to: oppose the appointment of Donald Berwick as administrator of the Centers for Medicare and Medicaid Services; disparage the Food and Drug Administration's decision to withdraw the breast cancer drug Avastin from the market; and bludgeon the Independent Payment Advisory Board (IPAB), whose mission under the health reform law is to rein in Medicare spending that exceeds pre-set limits *Arkansas Democrat-Gazette* 2011; Cohn 2011; Ferrer 2011; *New York Times* 2012; Nocera 2011; Ornstein 2011; *USA Today* 2011).

The Debate Over Health Care Rationing: Déjà Vu All Over Again, Alan B. Cohen in *Inquiry, 49* (Summer 2012), 90–100. Copyright © 2012 Excellus Health Plan, Inc. With permission from SAGE Publications, Inc.

What is it about rationing of care that evokes such heated, visceral reaction? Perhaps it strikes a nerve in individuals who legitimately fear that rationing schemes will limit their access to health care. More likely, the concept of "rationing" bewilders many people, leading to the mistaken belief that it exists only in other countries. Whatever their source of discomfort, Americans respond negatively to the slightest mention of the word. Capitalizing on these misconceptions and fears, reform opponents routinely invoke the specter of rationing to discredit various provisions of the Patient Protection and Affordable Care Act (ACA) and to distract the public from the law's true aims. Ironically, the Medicare budget plan proposed by Rep. Paul Ryan and supported by many ACA critics has been cited by the Congressional Budget Office as likely to produce the very kind of rationing that reform foes claim to detest (Rovner 2011).

Twenty-five years ago, the late Jeff Merrill and I wrote a guest editorial in *Inquiry* that tried to dispel myths about rationing in U.S. health care (Merrill and Cohen 1987). We argued that our health care system always had rationed care based on price and ability to pay and that these mechanisms, together with the indirect effects of several cost containment policies (e.g., certificate-of-need regulation and chronically low Medicaid payment rates to providers), had conspired to limit access to care for vulnerable segments of the population. However, because these forms of rationing were less publicly visible than the methods employed in other countries (e.g., wait lists in Great Britain and Canada), rationing became a straw man in the debate over ways to control health care costs. Several scholars (Aaron and Schwartz 1984; Evans 1983a; Evans 1983b; Fuchs 1984; Thurow 1984; Callahan 1987) predicted that explicit rationing would soon become the policy tool of choice for constraining health care spending. We, on the other hand, held out hope that American cultural values would instead join with economic imperatives to assure a minimum level of care for all Americans without requiring unpalatable forms of rationing.

Neither scenario unfolded as envisioned, with policymakers generally shunning explicit rationing schemes and the nation failing to achieve universal coverage. Today, the financial condition of the U.S. health care system is more precarious than it was a quarter century ago and we have yet to come to terms with rationing of care. Thanks to the Affordable Care Act, however, the nation stands on the threshold of defining essential health benefits for all Americans and significantly reducing the number of uninsured citizens. But the fate of health reform is also precarious, awaiting a momentous Supreme Court ruling on the law's constitutionality and the November 2012 national elections. Whatever the outcomes of those events, the nation ultimately must face the arduous challenge of implementing effective cost containment measures to slow health care spending growth. Therefore, it is necessary once again to engage in serious dialogue about rationing and its role in U.S. health care. Like so many aspects of U.S. health care plagued by years of ceaseless argument and policy inaction, the rationing debate has a sense of "déjà vu all over again."[1]

A RETROSPECTIVE LOOK AT THE LITERATURE ON RATIONING

The literature on rationing since 1987 may be divided into three somewhat overlapping areas of inquiry that:

- Define (or redefine) rationing and resource allocation, with an emphasis on understanding these terms and the methods for accomplishing them (Mariner 1995; Mechanic 1997; Aaron 2005; Reinhardt 2009; Meltzer and Detsky 2010);

- Build the case for rationing as a cost containment tool to stem rising health care costs (Schwartz and Mendelson 1992; Aaron and Schwartz 2005; Aaron 2005; Callahan 2009a; 2009b; Singer 2009); or

- Promote rationing as an ethical policy to assure equitable allocation of resources (Callahan 1987; Young 1994; Callahan 2009b; Singer 2009; Brody 2012).

These complementary lines of scholarship have shaped the debate in academia, but have had little impact in policy circles—at least not until the advent of the Obama reforms.

Defining (or Redefining) Rationing

In a free market economy, resources are allocated efficiently to consumers based on price, and consumers' decisions to purchase goods and services reflect their preferences, willingness to pay, and personal wealth (Mariner 1995; Meltzer and Detsky 2010). When resources are extremely scarce and valued by all market participants, their allocation through the price mechanism confronts important issues of fairness and ability to pay. As a result, explicit rationing may be used as an alternative approach to market allocation. Rationing, in simple terms, is the allocation of scarce resources among individuals in society according to a fixed allotment scheme (Mariner 1995). Rationing implies that the allocation of goods and services is "disconnected" from prices and based instead on criteria other than consumers' preferences and characteristics (Meltzer and Detsky 2010). For these reasons, Americans generally harbor the belief that rationing is always a government-controlled alternative to the free market. Reinhardt (2009), however, asserts that prices also ration scarce resources, such that free markets are *not* an alternative to rationing but rather a particular form of rationing. Health care rationing by price poses serious barriers for those unable to pay for care, causing them to "self-ration" care when they are sick, with attendant costs for the health care system as a whole (Davidson 2011). Because of these perverse effects, discussions about health care rationing often gravitate toward finding methods that will distribute resources equitably as well as efficiently (Mariner 1995).

Older Americans may recall World War II rationing of sugar, canned foods, aluminum pots, and gasoline as an apportionment of scarce goods. Rationing was described as "a little less for some of us, but a fair share for all" in a radio program from that era (Fein 2012). It was understood that a fair share might not necessarily be an equal share, but

rather an *equitable* share in accordance with one's need. Americans of that generation saw rationing as a means through which all citizens were summoned to sacrifice individually to achieve a common purpose. In contrast, many Americans today fail to see a need for shared sacrifice both in terms of the "common good" and in controlling health care spending despite strong evidence that spending growth threatens U.S. economic security. Instead, a widespread sentiment seems to be: "Why should I be forced to pay for the health care of others who are 'undeserving' either because of their indolence or their ineligibility for such benefits (e.g., undocumented immigrants)?" For some, this viewpoint gives rise to an unwillingness to join with others in a health insurance pool, waiting instead to purchase insurance only when serious illness or injury generates substantial medical expense. Unfortunately, the perceived lack of a common bond in health care is fueled by ideological and political forces that oppose many elements of ACA reform, especially the individual mandate to purchase insurance. Rationing, in this context, is often portrayed as "soulless" government bureaucrats (or, in the case of IPAB, as "unaccountable" expert panels) wielding a harsh, punitive instrument that severely limits access to needed health care (Singer 2009; Cohen 2012).

Although there is universal agreement among scholars today that rationing pervades U.S. health care, definitions and classification schemes still vary. For example, we (Merrill and Cohen 1987) had defined *explicit* rationing as conscious policy decisions to limit access to certain services (e.g., the use of wait lists in the British health care system) and *implicit* rationing as global constraints that limit the availability of resources for providing care, such as certificate-of-need limitations on imaging technologies that can indirectly ration care for population segments depending on where they live. In contrast, others have defined explicit rationing as "decisions made by an administrative authority" regarding the levels and mix of resources to be made available to eligible populations, with specific rules for allocation, and implicit rationing as "discretionary decisions made by managers, professionals, and other health care personnel" operating within a fixed budget (Mechanic 1997). Thus, while some consider rationing in the British National Health Service (NHS) to be explicit in nature, others see the NHS as relying on implicit rationing methods (Mechanic 1997). Likewise, scholars have had different views of the Oregon Health Plan's (OHP) pioneering use of statewide Medicaid funding priorities for health care, with some citing it as a prime example of explicit rationing (Young 1994; Mechanic 1997), others contending that it never operated in that manner (Oberlander, Marmor, and Jacobs 2001), and still others questioning whether it involves more politics than science (Klein 1991). Differences in interpretation aside, both forms of rationing have been assailed over time. In particular, implicit rationing decisions by insurers and health plans to deny coverage for certain conditions or procedures were bitterly attacked by consumers during the managed care backlash of the 1990s (Friedman 1997; Mechanic 2001).

The dichotomous labels of explicit versus implicit rationing have limited value. An alternative classification scheme proposed by Mariner (1995) distinguishes among three types of allocation decisions:

- Macroallocation decisions by policymakers that determine how much money is allocated to health care in a country;

- Microallocation decisions by individual firms (that affect their employees' access to and use of health care) and by insurance companies and health plans (that are made on behalf of firms and their employees); and

- Physicians' decisions to recommend specific treatments for individual patients.

Rationing may occur in all three types of decisions, but the specific criteria and methods employed to make such decisions will vary. Ubel and Goold (1997), for example, highlighted the key role that physicians play in "bedside rationing" of care. Overall, the most commonly used methods tend to limit utilization of health care. Meltzer and Detsky (2010) point out that, to limit service use,

decisions must be made about the circumstances under which insurance will cover specific services, and that coverage policies represent "rationing from a practical perspective just as much as rationing systems that are more explicit in preventing consumers from acting on their preferences." Mariner (1995) argues, though, that the only way to limit the use of resources is by "limiting the supply of those resources."

When one considers the type of service to be limited, *first-dollar* versus *last-dollar* rationing remains a more useful dichotomy (Merrill and Cohen 1987). First-dollar rationing has been the dominant form of rationing in this country, with both public and private payers limiting access to basic services and primary care—either by denying coverage or by imposing high deductibles and coinsurance—even as they pay for more expensive tertiary care, often at the end of life (Merrill and Cohen 1987). In most other industrialized nations, last-dollar rationing has been the norm, with consumption of high-cost services limited via wait lists and constrained supply of costly technology, while universal coverage assures access to basic primary and secondary care. The ACA aims to reduce first-dollar rationing by promoting access to primary care and preventive services.

Rationing as a Cost Containment Tool

In a 1992 commentary, Schwartz and Mendelson posited that managed care would not be able to constrain rising health care costs without employing some form of rationing. Citing three chief factors responsible for cost growth—demographic changes, rising costs of labor and supplies, and new medical technology—they argued that the first two factors were beyond the control of managed care (or any public policy initiative) but that the introduction and diffusion of new technology could be controlled, *only if* managed care providers were willing to limit the availability of expensive new services (Schwartz and Mendelson 1992). To do this, they recommended that cost-effectiveness analysis be used to guide decision making. But they also recognized that, as cost pressures mounted, providers might become more likely to engage in price rationing that would raise "difficult social and medical issues" in the future (Schwartz and Mendelson 1992).

Aaron and Schwartz (2005) later argued that rationing in the form of health care spending priorities would become increasingly necessary as spending continued to rise, and that a framework for evaluating the worth of improvements in diagnosis and treatment would be critical to setting those priorities. To construct such a framework, an infrastructure supporting both clinical and health services research would be essential (Aaron and Schwartz 2005). Two decades earlier, Bulger (1992) had anticipated a research framework in which academic health centers would play a leading role. In addition to advancing the use of rationing as a cost containment tool, Aaron (2005) argued for the adoption of universal coverage in U.S. health care on the grounds that it not only would be fair and just, but also would be a "precondition for effective and equitable cost control."

In his 1987 book *Setting Limits,* Daniel Callahan proposed a rationing plan that would limit particular diagnostic or therapeutic interventions using age-based rules. Arguing that individuals above a certain age threshold should not receive aggressive care (e.g., tests, treatments) at public expense, he advocated placing age limits on resource use (Callahan 1987). More recently, he reiterated this theme in the context of controlling costs associated with the use of expensive medical technology (Callahan 2009a, 2009b). By reducing excessive use of medical technology, particularly when it may be of marginal value to individuals in their 70s, he believes that overall health care spending may be controlled and considers an age-based approach to be the most equitable means of rationing health care (Callahan 2009b). Constraining the adoption and use of medical technology, in his view, would free up resources that could be applied by government to other sectors of the economy for social needs, such as housing and education (Callahan 2009b). Kane and Orszag (2003) have shown that as Medicaid spending climbs, states rob higher education to pay for Medicaid during economic downturns and that public universities consequently suffer declines

in quality. Thus, slowing the growth of health care costs may pay dividends in reversing this trend and helping future generations to attend high-quality public colleges (Orszag 2010).

Callahan's views have been challenged for failing to account for differences among individuals in physiological (rather than chronological) age, for neglecting the importance of private sector activity in resource allocation, and for ignoring the role of "properly incentivized" consumers as decision makers in their own health care (Kapp 2009). Regardless, his point that we need to address intergenerational trade-offs in resource allocation cannot be easily ignored.

Rationing as an Ethical Policy for Equitable Resource Allocation

Bioethicists have long approached the allocation of scarce resources from the standpoint of distributive justice, arguing that: finite resources must be distributed in an equitable way, and avoidance of explicit rationing will force us to resort to implicit (and likely unfair) rationing methods (Brody 2012). In the Clinton health reform era, Young (1994) lauded the Oregon Health Plan for having "squarely faced up" to these challenges by recognizing that Medicaid beneficiaries could not have all the medical services that they wanted, but rather could have only what the state could afford under a fixed Medicaid budget. Noting that Americans generally fail to distinguish needs from wants, he challenged the wisdom of "single-tier" health reform based on universal access to the same basic package of benefits for all (Young 1994). Instead, he recommended a three-tiered system of services consisting of: 1) universal access to basic services, with emphasis on primary care, prevention, and health promotion; 2) access to a limited array of medical, surgical, and psychiatric services for those with exceptional or catastrophic needs caused by genetic and social circumstances; and 3) supplemental services not included in either of the first two tiers that could be purchased through insurance by those able to pay for such services. Only under a system of this kind, he argued, could people be treated fairly according to need (Young 1994).

But any system that purportedly allocates resources fairly must have a set of guiding principles to set spending priorities. Borrowing from the Swedish health care system, Caplan (1995) espoused three core principles that should be embodied in any priority-setting system: "that all human beings are equally valuable; that society must pay special attention to the needs of the weakest and most vulnerable; and that, other things being equal, cost-efficiency and gaining the greatest return for the amount of money spent must prevail." These principles are a blend of egalitarian and utilitarian values intrinsic to Swedish culture, but may be considerably more difficult to adopt in an American context, given our historical emphasis on free markets and a tendency toward libertarian views. Nevertheless, Caplan (1995) noted that the Swedes injected ethics into the debate about rationing priorities "not because there is consensus about what is right when it comes to rationing, but because there must be consensus about what is wrong."

In a provocative *New York Times* article, Singer (2009) argued in favor of rationing on both ethical and economic grounds, insisting that unbalanced media coverage had corrupted the reform debate and that rationing in some form not only is inescapable but desirable. The only question in his mind was how best to ration care, and he recommended keeping decisions about the allocation of health care resources separate from judgments about the moral character or social value of individuals (Singer 2009). In his view, a reformed U.S. health care system that explicitly accepts rationing as legitimate policy, with quality-adjusted life-years (QALYs) as a measure for comparing the benefits of different therapies, would be the most socially desirable way to make resource allocation decisions. While acknowledging that the QALY is an imperfect measure, Singer maintained that it is superior to alternative methods and may be modified to suit specific needs, such as giving greater weight to benefits that accrue to those who generally are worse off than others, assuming that there is a social consensus that priority be given to such individuals.

Other prominent bioethicists recently have joined with economists to reframe the rationing debate as one embracing "waste avoidance" (Brody 2012) and "frugality" (Bloche 2012). Brody (2012), for example, offers two ethical arguments for avoiding waste—that patients should not be deprived of useful medical services so long as money is being wasted on useless interventions, and that useless tests and treatments cause harm through false-positive results and complications. Thus, wasteful, non-beneficial medicine imposes opportunity costs for patients in need and also conflicts with the medical maxim of "First, do no harm." Berwick and Hackbarth (2012) estimate that spending on non-beneficial interventions may consume 30% of all health care dollars in the U.S., and call for actions to reduce waste in six areas: overtreatment; failures of care coordination; failures in execution of care processes; administrative complexity; pricing failures; and fraud and abuse.

IS IT REALLY DÉJÀ VU ALL OVER AGAIN?

How, then, does the present situation compare with that in 1987? Four similarities are particularly striking. First, although the recent financial crisis and recession have been much deeper and of longer duration than the recession of the early 1980s, economic pressures in both eras were sparked by rising government spending on health care, mounting federal budget deficits, and an expanding share of the gross domestic product (GDP) attributable to health care. Second, system-wide problems in health care pertaining to cost, quality, access, efficiency and equity have been in continuous crisis since 1987, becoming arguably more severe and complex over time. Third, Americans persist in their worship of technology (Callahan 2009b), believing that the most advanced (and, often, most expensive) medical treatments should be made available in life-threatening circumstances regardless of age, prognosis, or cost. Not only have we fostered a cultural view that "death should be avoided at all cost," but we seem to have cultivated a growing sense of entitlement to technological advances as they diffuse into medical practice. Finally, because so many Americans still fail to realize that we ration care through price barriers, the powerful anti-rationing rhetoric of today effectively twists an "inconvenient truth" into a convenient lie for political and/or financial gain.

Even though these economic, social, and technological forces have not changed appreciably over time, there are a few notable differences between the two eras. First, the clear shift in policy thinking and managerial focus toward obtaining "value" for our health care investment in 2012 signals that we no longer are preoccupied with cost containment just for the sake of cost containment (Singer 2009). Rather, we have acquired a greater appreciation for employing evidence-based medicine, comparative effectiveness studies, cost-effectiveness analysis, and other tools to distinguish between services and therapies that confer high value versus those that offer marginal or no benefit. Second, the Medicare program in 1987 did not cover outpatient prescription drugs, forcing many chronically ill seniors who could not afford either Medigap coverage or out-of-pocket payments for their medications to "self-ration." However, since the introduction of the Part D prescription drug benefit in 2006, barriers to such drugs for many senior citizens have been effectively lowered or, in some cases, eliminated altogether. Third, the ACA seeks to reduce *socially undesirable* rationing of care by eliminating insurance limitations on preexisting conditions, by mandating coverage of annual physical exams and other preventive services, and by defining essential health benefits that will set a "floor" rather than a "ceiling" on care. And, last, even though the ACA establishes entities that some critics claim will ration care, such as IPAB and the Patient-Centered Outcomes Research Institute (PCORI), IPAB is explicitly prohibited from engaging in rationing decisions (Aaron 2011) and PCORI's mission is to produce information regarding the comparative effectiveness of medical therapies and procedures that will assist decision making by patients, clinicians, purchasers, and policymakers (Selby, Beal, and Frank 2012). When fully implemented, both entities hold promise to achieve more rational and equitable allocation and consumption of health care resources.

On balance, it would appear that we have come full circle in 25 years, but it is not exactly déjà vu all over again. Recent developments, most notably those emanating from the ACA, offer hope that the current climate may be "warming" to the concept of rationing. Nonetheless, persuading critics and elected officials that the time has come to confront this challenge straightforwardly will not be easy.

TOWARD MORE RATIONAL WAYS OF RATIONING CARE

Health care now consumes nearly 18% of our gross domestic product and few would dispute that we do not obtain good value for our health care investment. Despite health care's role as a vital economic engine generating jobs in many communities at a time of high unemployment, the current rate of spending growth is unsustainable without trading off spending in other sectors of the economy or across generations (Orszag 2010; Baicker and Chernew 2011; Glaeser 2012; Callahan 1987). Thus, the search for effective cost containment continues, but there are limits to what can plausibly be accomplished under the ACA. As Baicker and Chernew (2011) point out, the economics of financing Medicare is complex. Without even a modest tax increase, it will be difficult to finance the program in the long run, and the bitter Congressional clash over Medicare payment cuts to providers seems inherently myopic. Any short-term savings wrung from Medicare or Medicaid with such blunt instruments is likely to come at the expense of both quality and access to care. And no one knows for certain whether the payment and delivery system reforms of the ACA will ultimately be successful.

Given these uncertainties, rationing based on factors *other than* price and ability to pay will be required to curtail future spending. Are we, as a nation, willing to adopt such rationing schemes? Thurow (1984) long ago argued that our nation's capitalist heritage dictated that we not deny treatment to anyone who could afford to pay for it, but also that our egalitarian ethos compelled us to make treatment available to all. Yet, before the advent of the ACA, guaranteed access to care extended only to emergency care[2] and we silently tolerated annual growth in the number of uninsured, suggesting that our egalitarianism has been eroding over time. Even if we now accept the premise that health care rationing is both ethically sound and economically exigent, we will need to muster the requisite political will to ration care based on criteria and methods that emphasize equity.

Rationing criteria and priorities based on need and clinical effectiveness should be the goal. First-dollar rationing makes little sense if we want to obtain the highest value for our long-term investment in health care. Instead, *first-dollar coverage* of primary care and evidence-based preventive services should be the norm, as the ACA strives to attain. Rationing, then, should apply to services that are wasteful or non-beneficial, and in this respect, last-dollar rationing makes more sense because of diminishing marginal returns on expensive tertiary care, especially in end-of-life situations.

But can we learn to accept death as a part of life? Getting people to alter long-held beliefs, cultural values, and attitudes toward death is a daunting challenge. At the same time, it will be important to differentiate between non-beneficial consumption of care and above-average consumption by those with clear medical need. Research has shown that a disproportionately large share of health care expenditures is concentrated in a relatively small proportion of the population (Berk and Monheit 2001; Monheit 2003). Data from the 2009 Medical Expenditure Panel Survey indicate that the sickest 10% of patients account for 65% of all health care expenses (Blumenthal 2012). In a reformed health care system, it will be critical to design rationing schemes that take these factors into account. For rationing to gain broader acceptance in American society, the methods must be definitive, fair, and transparent.

There are encouraging signs that we may be able to accomplish this. Equity in health care is an explicit aim of the ACA, and the proposed Health Equity and Accountability Act of 2012 (S. 2474) would further strengthen ACA efforts to eliminate health and health care disparities (NHeLP

2012). There also may be opportunities to capitalize on lessons from the experience of the Oregon Health Plan, whose multi-tiered, prioritized list of health care services under-girds an essential benefits package that contains higher cost-sharing for lower-priority services (Saha, Coffman, and Smits 2010). The package includes first-dollar coverage for "value-based" services—low-cost, evidence-based services, such as routine childhood and adult vaccinations, prenatal care, chronic disease management, and smoking cessation treatment, all of which are intended to minimize downstream costs and adverse outcomes (Saha, Coffman, and Smits 2010). States now have responsibility for defining essential benefits for health insurance exchanges under the ACA (Health Policy Brief 2012), and the Oregon approach offers a model for designing tiered priority-setting systems that employ best-available clinical evidence, take into account public values, and foster prudent spending.

In the end, we must learn to accept equitable rationing as a fair and just way to distribute scarce resources. Thorny implementation issues remain, though. Foremost is the question: *Who* should make policy decisions involving health care rationing? As Meltzer and Detsky (2010) observe, it is a matter of whom to entrust with these decisions—private enterprises (driven by profit motives), government officials (likely influenced by political motives), or independent experts (presumably apolitical and uninfluenced by financial or other factors). The political battle over IPAB is one such example (Aaron 2011; Cohen 2012). To obtain better value for our health care investment, we need to move toward more rational ways of rationing while striking a balance among efficacy, efficiency, and equity goals. This will require increased use of analytic tools, such as evidence-based medicine, comparative effectiveness research (Selby, Beal, and Frank 2012), and cost-effectiveness analysis (CEA), as well as novel ways to ensure fairness, such as lotteries for distributing resources in some cases (Aaron 2005; Baicker and Finkelstein 2011). Even so, there will be formidable obstacles to overcome, including the ACA's prohibition against the use of QALYs by PCORI (Neumann and Weinstein 2010) and the controversies that often result from unpopular analyses and their recommendations, as was the case with screening mammography and with the prostate-specific antigen test (Truog 2009). Fuchs (2010) cautions against a policy that cuts off new interventions prematurely because some may not be cost-effective at first but, with time, may prove to be so. In addition, because people may place greater importance on equity than is reflected by CEA, basing health care priorities on CEA may require that explicit considerations of equity be incorporated into these analyses or the policy process used to develop the priorities (Ubel et al. 1996).

In conclusion, the way forward with health care rationing will require a paradigm shift in our present thinking. We consider ourselves a generous and caring people who are among the first to respond with humanitarian aid in times of global crisis or disaster (e.g., the 2009 Haitian earthquake and the 2011 Japanese tsunami). But we also possess a curious blind spot that makes us neglect our own—be they inhabitants of New Orleans and the Gulf coast following Hurricane Katrina or the millions of uninsured citizens in our midst. A chilling reminder of this reality was evident during a Republican presidential candidate debate when Wolf Blitzer of CNN asked whether an uninsured person should be left to die and audience members responded with cheers of approval (Kaiser Health News 2011). As Starr (2011) wonders in his book on U.S. health reform, will Americans ever be able to "summon the elemental decency toward the sick that characterizes other democracies"? This fundamental question is clouded by a mix of ideology, politics, and complexity that hampers efforts to find common ground among patients, physicians, hospitals, insurers, pharmaceutical firms, medical device manufacturers, advocacy groups, and policymakers. However, the need to confront our fears about rationing, engage in open and honest dialogue about potential options, and reach consensus on a solution is undeniable and urgent.

Notes

1. After witnessing Roger Maris and Mickey Mantle repeatedly hit back-to-back home runs in the early 1960s, Yogi Berra is reported to have said, "It's déjà vu all over again."

2. Through the Emergency Medical Treatment and Active Labor Act of 1986.

References

Aaron, H. J. 2005. Health Care Rationing: What It Means. Washington, D.C.: Brookings Institution.

_____. 2011. The Independent Payment Advisory Board—Congress's "Good Deed." *New England Journal of Medicine* 364(25):2377–2379.

Aaron, H. J., and W. B. Schwartz. 1984. *The Painful Prescription: Rationing Hospital Care.* Washington, D.C.: The Brookings institution.

_____. 2005. *Can We Say No? The Challenge of Rationing Care.* Washington, D.C.: The Brookings Institution.

Allen, D. 2009. Health Reform's Hearing Problem; Both Sides Are Deaf to the Real Debate about Consequences. *Washington Post* August 11: A13.

Arkansas Democrat-Gazette. 2011. Editorial: They're . . . BACK! Return of the Death Panels. *Arkansas Democrat-Gazette* January 2:80.

Baicker, K., and M. E. Chernew. 2011. The Economics of Financing Medicare. *New England Journal of Medicine* 365(4): e7.

Baicker, K., and A. Finkelstein. 2011. The Effects of Medicaid Coverage—Learning from the Oregon Experiment. *New England Journal of Medicine* 365(8):683–685.

Berk, M. L., and A. C. Monheit. 2001. The Concentration of Health Care Expenditures, Revisited. *Health Affairs* 20(2):9–18.

Berwick, D. M., and A. D. Hackbarth. 2012. Eliminating Waste in U.S. Health Care. *Journal of the American Medical Association* 307:1513–1516.

Bloche, M. G. 2012. Beyond the "R Word"? Medicine's New Frugality. *New England Journal of Medicine* 366(21): 1951–1953.

Blumenauer, E. 2009. My Near Death Panel Experience. *New York Times* November 15:12.

Blumenthal, D. 2012. Performance Improvement in Health Care—Seizing the Moment. *New England Journal of Medicine* 366(21): 1953–1955.

Bookman, J. 2009. Even Reasonable Get Steamed in Health Debate. *Atlanta Journal-Constitution* August 14:18A.

Brody, H. 2012. From the Ethics of Rationing to an Ethics of Waste Avoidance. *New England Journal of Medicine* 366(21): 1949–1951.

Bulger, R. J. 1992. The "R" Word. "Rationing" of Health Care and the Role of Academic Health Centers. *Western Journal of Medicine* 157(2):186–187.

Callahan, D. 1987. *Setting Limits: Medical Goals in an Aging Society.* New York: Simon & Schuster.

_____. 2009a. Cost Control—Time to Get Serious. *New England Journal of Medicine* 361(7): e10.

_____. 2009b. *Taming the Beloved Beast: How Medical Technology Costs Are Destroying Our Health Care System.* Princeton, N.J.: Princeton University Press.

Caplan. A. L. 1995. Straight Talk about Rationing. *Annals of Internal Medicine* 122(10):795–796.

Cohen, A. B. 2012. Sunday Dialogue: Equitable Health Care. *New York Times* March 25: SR2.

Cohn, J. 2011. The Avastin Decision: A Rational Decision or Rationing? *The New Republic* January 4:1–3.

Davidson, S. M. 2011. The Self-Rationing of Medical Care. *New York Times* May 22. http://www.nytimes.com/2011/05/23/opinion/123health.html

Diaz, J. 2009. When Lies Get in the Way of Reform. *San Francisco Chronicle* August 16: E2.

Evans, R. W. 1983a. Health Care Technology and the Inevitability of Resource Allocation and Rationing Decisions: Part I. *Journal of the American Medical Association* 249(15):2047–2052.

_____. 1983b. Health Care Technology and the Inevitability of Resource Allocation and Rationing Decisions: Part II. *Journal of the American Medical Association* 249(16):2208–2219.

Farley, R. 2009. Health Care "Rationing" Sounds Scarier Than It Is. *St. Petersburg Times* August 31:1A.

Fein, R. 2012. Personal communication.

Ferrer, R. 2011. "Death Panel" Rhetoric Mutes Elderly. *San Antonio Express-News* January 14:6B.

Friedman, E. 1997. Managed Care, Rationing, and Quality: A Tangled Relationship. *Health Affairs* 16(3):174–182.

Fuchs, V. R. 1984. The "Rationing" of Medical Care. *New England Journal of Medicine* 311: 1572–1573.

_____. 2010. How to Think about Future Health Care Spending. *New England Journal of Medicine* 362(11):965–967.

Glaeser, E. L. 2012. Health Care: Schools vs. End-of-Life? *Boston Globe* May 17: A15.

Health Policy Brief. 2012. Essential Health Benefits. *Health Affairs* April 25.

Holan, A. D. 2009. Lie of the Year. *St. Petersburg Times* December 20:1 A.

Kaiser Health News. 2011. Transcript: GOP Candidates Squabble over Health Care during Tampa Debate. *Kaiser Health News* September 13:1–8.

Kane, T. J., and P. R. Orszag. 2003. *Higher Education Spending: The Role of Medicaid and the Business Cycle.* Washington, D.C.: The Brookings Institution.

Kapp, M. B. 2009. Health Care Technology, Health Care Rationing, and Older Americans: Enough Already? http://ssrn.com/abstract= 1561924.

Klein, R. 1991. On the Oregon Trail: Rationing Health Care. More Politics than Science. *British Medical Journal* 302:1–2.

Mariner, W. K. 1995. Rationing Health Care and the Need for Credible Scarcity: Why Americans Can't Say No. *American Journal of Public Health* 85(10):1439–1445.

Mechanic, D. 1997. Muddling Through Elegantly: Finding the Proper Balance in Rationing. *Health Affairs* 16(5):83–92.

———. 2001. The Managed Care Backlash: Perceptions and Rhetoric in Health Care Policy and the Potential for Health Care Reform. *Milbank Quarterly* 79(l):35–54.

Meltzer, D. O., and A. S. Detsky. 2010. The Real Meaning of Rationing. *Journal of the American Medical Association* 304(20):2292–2293.

Merrill, J. C., and A. B. Cohen. 1987. The Emperor's New Clothes: Unraveling the Myths about Rationing. *Inquiry* 24:105–109.

Monheit, A. C. 2003. Persistence in Health Expenditures in the Short Run: Prevalence and Consequences. *Medical Care* 41(7 Suppl): III-53–III-64.

New York Times. 2012. Editorial: We Thought They Were Worried About Costs. *New York Times* March 9: A30.

National Health Law Program (NHeLP). 2012. NHeLP Welcomes Introduction of the Health Equity and Accountability Act of 2012. www .healthlaw.org. Accessed April 27.

Neumann, P. J., and M. C. Weinstein. 2010. Legislating against Use of Cost-Effectiveness Information. *New England Journal of Medicine* 363(16): 1495–1497.

Nocera, J. 2011. Why Doesn't No Mean No? *New York Times* November 21:1–3.

Nyhan, B., and J. Reifler. 2010. When Corrections Fail: The Persistence of Political Misperceptions. *Political Behavior* 32:303–330.

Oberlander, J., T. Marmor, and L. Jacobs. 2001. Rationing Medical Care: Rhetoric and Reality in the Oregon Health Plan. *Canadian Medical Association Journal* 164(11):1583–1587.

Ornstein, N. J. 2011. The Real Death Panels. *Washington Post* January 1: A17.

Orszag, P. 2010. A Health Care Plan for Colleges. *New York Times* September 18. http://www .nytimes.com/2010/09/19/opinion/19orszag .html.

Parker, K. 2009. Easing the "Death Panel" Fear. *Washington Post* August 12: A21.

Reinhardt, U. E. 2009. "Rationing" Health Care: What Does It Mean? *New York Times* July 3:1–3.

Rovner, J. 2011. Budget Office: GOP Medicare Plan Could Lead to Rationing. *NPR Blog* April 6. http:// www.npr.org/blogs/health/2011/04/08/1351 87359/budget-office-gop-medicare-plan-could-lead-to-rationing.

Rutenberg, J., and J. Calmes. 2009. Getting to the Source of the "Death Panel" Rumor. *New York Times* August 14: A1.

Saha, S., D. D. Coffman, and A. K. Smits. 2010. Giving Teeth to Comparative-Effectiveness Research— The Oregon Experience. *New England Journal of Medicine* 362(7): el8.

Saltonstall, D. 2009. We're Not Gonna "Pull the Plug on Grandma." Obama Nixes Rumors of

"Death Panel" Health Care. *New York Daily News* August 12:9.

Schwartz, W. B., and D. N. Mendelson. 1992. Why Managed Care Cannot Contain Hospital Costs Without Rationing. *Health Affairs* 11(2): 100–107.

Selby, J. V., A. C. Beal, and L. Frank. 2012. The Patient-Centered Outcomes Research Institute (PCORI) National Priorities for Research and Initial Research Agenda. *Journal of the American Medical Association* 307(15): 1583–1584.

Singer, P. 2009. Why We Must Ration Health Care. *New York Times* July 19:1–10.

Starr, P. 2011. *Remedy and Reaction: The Peculiar American Struggle over Health Care Reform.* New Haven, Conn.: Yale University Press.

Thurow, L. C. 1984. Learning to Say "No." *New England Journal of Medicine* 311:1569–1572.

Tinetti, M. E. 2012. The Retreat from Advanced Care Planning. *Journal of the American Medical Association* 307(9):915–916.

Truog, R. D. 2009. Screening Mammography and the "R" Word. *New England Journal of Medicine* 361(26):2501–2503.

Ubel, P. A., M. L. DeKay, J. Baron, and D. A. Asch. 1996. Cost-Effectiveness Analysis in a Setting of Budget Constraints—Is It Equitable? *New England Journal of Medicine* 334(18): 1174–1177.

Ubel, P. A., and S. Goold. 1997. Recognizing Bedside Rationing: Clear Cases and Tough Calls. *Annals of Internal Medicine* 126(1):74–80.

USA Today. 2011. Editorial: Nonsense about "Death Panels" Springs Back to Life. *USA Today* January 7:8A.

Young, E. W. D. 1994. Rationing—Missing Ingredient in Health Care Reform. *Western Journal of Medicine* 161:74–77.

MEDICINE IN PRACTICE

The social organization of medicine is manifested on the interactional as well as the structural levels of society. There is an established and rich tradition of studying medical work firsthand in medical settings, through participant observation, interviewing, or both. Researchers go "where the action is"—in this case, among doctors and patients—to see just how social life (i.e., medical care) happens. Such studies are time consuming and difficult (Charmaz and Olesen 1997), but they are the only way to penetrate the structure of medical care and reveal the sociological texture of medical practice. For it is here that the structure of medicine shapes the type of care that is delivered.

There are at least four traditional, general foci for these qualitative studies. Some studies focus on the organization of the institution itself, such as a mental hospital (Goffman 1961), a nursing home (Gubrium 1975), or an intensive care unit (Zussman 1992). Others examine the delivery of services or practitioner–patient interaction ranging from childbirth (Davis-Floyd 1992) to dying (Timmermans 1999). A third general focus is on collegial relations among professionals (e.g., Anspach 1993; Mesman 2008). A fourth focus for research examines the impact of specific health policies on medical work and care (Kellogg 2011). All of these studies give us a window on the backstage world of medical organization. No matter what the focus, they bring to life the processes through which organizations operate and how participants manage in their situations. It is worth noting also that most of these close-up studies end up with the researchers taking a critical stance toward the organization and practice of medicine. Because of some ethical and bureaucratic research constraints, it has become increasingly difficult to do such firsthand research in medical settings (Anspach and Mizrachi 2006). Government regulations that limit some forms of observational research and protect the privacy of

medical records have prevented some kinds of firsthand research in medical institutions.

The four selections in this section reveal different aspects of medicine in practice. The readings represent a range of medical settings and situations: outpatient encounters, intercultural communication, an emergency department, and families negotiating care at an elite hospital. As well as illuminating the texture of medical practice, the selections individually and together raise a number of significant sociological issues.

In "The Struggle Between the Voice of Medicine and the Voice of the Lifeworld," Elliot G. Mishler offers a detailed analysis of the structure of doctor–patient interviews. His analysis allows us to see two distinct voices in the interview discourse. In this framework, the "voice of medicine" dominates the interviews and allows physicians to control the interview. When "the voice of the lifeworld"—patients talking "about problems in their lives that were related to or resulted from their symptoms or illness" (Mishler 1984, 91)—disrupts the voice of medicine, it is often interrupted, silenced, or ignored. This perspective shows how physician dominance is recreated in doctor–patient encounters, and it gives some clues to why patients may say their doctors don't understand them.

Ming-Cheng Miriam Lo's article "Cultural Brokerage: Creating Linkages Between Voices of Lifeworld and Medicine in Cross-Cultural Clinical Settings" takes Mishler's concept of voice of the lifeworld and examines how it manifests itself in different cultural settings. There have been frequent calls for "culturally competent health care," where the health care provider understands enough about a patient's culture to modify his or her interaction in order to be sensitive to cultural differences. But it is often difficult for a physician to adapt the voice of medicine to a patient's cultural understandings. In this article, Lo explores how doctors perform this "cultural brokerage" on the job. This calls for a mutual inclusion of different frameworks that people use to organize their assumptions and understandings. In her firsthand research, Lo identifies four different but related forms of cultural brokerage that can facilitate understanding and health care. As our society becomes more multicultural, cultural brokerage becomes an increasingly important skill in medical care. It is equally interesting that the need for cultural brokerage can work in two directions; the editors of this volume have had students in class who, as children, became translators and cultural brokers for their immigrant parents or grandparents who could not speak English well enough to communicate with doctors. In this case, these children would often need to translate sensitive personal information from their sick relatives or technical medical information back to their relatives. Adequate cultural brokerage could have made these interactions much easier and smoother for all parties.

In the third selection, "Social Death as Self-Fulfilling Prophecy," Stefan Timmermans demonstrates how staff evaluations of patients' "social worth" affects whether and how the staff will attempt to resuscitate them. Sociologists have frequently shown that medical staff make moral judgments of patients' worthiness based on their evaluations of the patients' social attributes. Timmermans (1999) observed the use of cardiopulmonary resuscitation (CPR) in two emergency departments and compared his findings with a benchmark study conducted

30 years earlier (Sudnow 1967). Despite great changes in the health care system and a refinement of CPR techniques, Timmermans found a persistence of social rationing of medical interventions. The allocation of medical care based on perceived social worth not only reflects existing inequalities in society but also creates new ones as well.

In the final selection, "'I Want You to Save My Kid!': Illness Management Strategies, Access, and Inequality at an Elite University Research Hospital," Amanda M. Gengler interviewed and observed eighteen families whose children were diagnosed with life-threatening illnesses. Since highly specialized and technologically advanced care was necessary in such cases, and not all families had the same resources to access such care, Gengler shows how "cultural health capital" becomes an important explanation for understanding how such advanced medical care may be distributed. Thus, the different family illness management strategies rather than medical need encourage the reproduction of inequalities in the types and levels of care rendered to these sick children.

All four selections highlight the structure of medical practice. Each illustrates how the social organization of medicine constrains and shapes the physician's work. Firsthand qualitative studies like these place sociological researchers right in the midst of the action and can highlight how dilemmas and solutions are manifested and negotiated as part of ongoing medical work.

References

Anspach, Renée. 1993. *Deciding Who Lives.* Berkeley: University of California Press.

Anspach, Renée, and Nissim Mizrachi. 2006. "The Field Worker's Fields: Ethics, Ethnography and Medical Sociology." *Sociology of Health and Illness* 6: 713–31.

Charmaz, Kathy, and Virginia Olesen. 1997. "Ethnographic Research in Medical Sociology: Its Foci and Distinctive Contributions." *Sociological Methods and Research* 25: 252–94.

Davis-Floyd, Robbie. 1992. *Birth as an American Rite of Passage.* Berkeley: University of California Press.

Goffman, Erving. 1961. *Asylums.* New York: Doubleday.

Gubrium, Jabar. 1975. *Living and Dying at Murray Manor.* New York: St. Martin's Press.

Kellogg, Katherine A. 2011. *Challenging Operations: Medical Reform and the Resistance in Surgery.* Chicago: University of Chicago Press.

Mesman, Jessica. 2008. *Uncertainty in Medical Interventions: Experienced Pioneers in Neonatal Care.* London: Palgrave.

Mishler, Eliot G. 1984. *The Discourse of Medicine: Dialectics of Medical Interviews.* Norwood, NJ: Ablex.

Sudnow, David. 1967. *Passing On: The Social Organization of Dying.* Englewood Cliffs, NJ: Prentice Hall.

Timmermans, Stefan. 1999. *Sudden Death and the Myth of CPR.* Philadelphia: Temple University Press.

Zussman, Robert. 1992. *Intensive Care.* Chicago: University of Chicago Press.

THE STRUGGLE BETWEEN THE VOICE OF MEDICINE AND THE VOICE OF THE LIFEWORLD

Elliot G. Mishler

INTRODUCTION

The work reported here assumes that the discourse of patients with physicians is central to clinical practice and, therefore, warrants systematic study. . . . Principal features of the approach and the general plan of the study will be outlined briefly in this introductory section.

The inquiry begins with a description and analysis of "unremarkable interviews." This term is applied to stretches of talk between patients and physicians that appear intuitively to be normal and nonproblematic. The interviews are drawn from the large sample collected by Waitzkin and Stoeckle[1] in their study of the informative process in medical care (Waitzkin & Stoeckle, 1976; Waitzkin et al. 1978). In these interviews patients and physicians talk to each other in ways that we, as members of the same culture, recognize as contextually appropriate. Our sense of appropriateness depends on shared and tacit understandings; on commonly held and often implicit assumptions of how to talk and of what to talk about in this situation.

Our intuitive sense of the unremarkable nature of these interviews merely locates the phenomenon for study. The central task of this chapter is to develop and apply concepts and methods that allow us to go through and beyond our ordinary, implicit, and shared understanding of the "normality" and "unremarkableness" of these interviews. The aim is to make explicit features of the talk that produce and warrant our sense as investigators and, by implication, the sense made by physicians and patients that the talk is unremarkable, and that the interview is going as it "should" go. The investigation proceeds through four analytically distinct but intertwined phases discussed in the review of alternative approaches to the study of discourse: description, analysis, interpretation, and interruption.

An adequate description is a prerequisite to further study. As noted earlier, a transcription of speech is neither a neutral or "objective" description. Transcription rules incorporate models of language in that they specify which features of speech are to be recorded and which are to go unremarked. Thus, they define what is relevant and significant. The typescript notation system used here is a modification and simplification of one developed by Gail Jefferson (1978) and used by many conversation analysts; . . . The general aim is to retain details of the talk believed to be significant for clarifying and understanding the structure and meaning of patient-physician discourse. The relevance of particular details will be demonstrated in the analyses.

In reviewing various approaches to the analysis of discourse, I noted a number of problems in the use of standardized coding systems. A particularly serious limitation is its neglect of the structure and organization of naturally occurring talk between speakers. For this reason alone, this method would be inappropriate to the study of medical interviews which, like other forms of human discourse, is both structured and meaningful. Speaking turns are connected both through the forms of utterances, as in question and answer pairs, and by content. The analyses undertaken here are directed to determining the organization of medical interviews with respect to both form and content.

A structural unit of discourse is proposed that appears to be typical and pervasive in such interviews. It consists of a sequential set of three utterances: Physician Question-Patient Response-Physician Assessment/Next Question. The specific features and functions of this unit will be examined. Problems that arise during the interview are discussed in terms of the disruption and repair of this unit. Finally, the ways in which meaning is developed and organized over the course of the interview are documented and shown to be related to this basic structure.

The effort to make theoretical sense of analytical findings is the work of interpretation, referred to here as the third stage of an investigation. This is usually considered the last stage, but I have adopted a distinction made by Silverman and Torode (1980) between interpretation and interruption. The latter will be discussed below. Interpretations, as would be expected, may take many forms, reflecting different theories of language and of social action. All of them, nonetheless, focus primarily on the questions of "what" is done in and through the talk, and "how" it is done. Thus, in their sociolinguistic analysis of a therapeutic interview, Labov and Fanshel (1977) state their interest as the discovery of "what is being done." They conclude that much of the talk of therapy consists of "requests" and "responses to requests." The framework for the analysis of discourse that they develop and apply is, in large part, a set of definitions, rules, and methods for describing, locating, and interpreting the interactional functions of different types of requests and responses.

The analytic question for ethnomethodologists and conversation analysts shifts toward the "how." For any particular instance of a "request," for example, conversation analysts wish to determine how speakers "do the work" of requesting. That is, how do speakers convey to each other their mutual recognition that what their talk is about is "requesting." But more is involved than a shift from "what" to "how." For conversation analysts, forms of requests and general rules of use cannot be specified and listed in a coding manual, as Labov and Fanshel attempt. The contextual embeddedness of speech would make any such manual a poor guide for conversationalists, and for investigators as well. The "how" of discourse for ethnomethodologists concerns the speaker practices through which "requesting" is routinely done, or "accomplished," to use the ethnomethodologists' term, in any context, despite the problem that a formal rule cannot take into account the specific features of particular contexts.[2]

Much of the work of conversation analysts, like that of sociolinguists, is directed to the study of how general tasks of conversation are accomplished, how conversations are initiated and terminated, how turns are taken, how topics are switched, and how mistakes are repaired. All these conversational tasks are "done" in medical interviews, as in all other types of discourse. One aim of the present study is to determine if there are systematic and typical ways in which patients and physicians accomplish these general tasks of a conversation. For example, there are a number of ways in which speakers may ask and answer questions. How is questioning and answering done by patients and physicians?

Linked to this approach is another level of interpretation that represents a more central topic in our inquiry, namely, the nature of clinical work. Our speakers are physicians and patients, and in how they begin their discourse, take their turns, and take leave of each other they are also doing the work of doctoring and patienting. Interpretation of findings on conversational practices is directed to an understanding of how the work of doctoring and patienting is done. For example, the strong tendency for physicians to ask closed- rather than open-ended questions is interpreted as serving the function of maintaining control over the content of the interview. In turn, this assures the dominance of the biomedical model as the perspective within which patients' statements are interpreted and allows doctors to accomplish the "medical" tasks of diagnosis and prescription. At the same time, the fact that their utterances are almost exclusively in the form of questions gives doctors control of the turn-taking system and, consequently, of the structure and organization of the interview. The interpretation of particular discourse practices developed here will refer to both form and content.

Finally, borrowing from Silverman and Torode, I have referred to a second mode, or line of theorizing, as interruption. Of particular relevance to our purpose is Silverman and Torode's notion of "voices." As I understand it, a voice represents a particular assumption about the relationship between appearance, reality, and language, or, more generally, a "voice" represents a specific normative order. Some discourses are closed and continually reaffirm a single normative order; others are open and include different voices, one of which may interrupt another, thus leading to the possibility of a new "order." There are occasions in medical interviews where the normal and routine practice of clinical work appears to be disrupted. In order to understand both the routine, fluent course of the interview as well as its occasional disruption, a

distinction will be introduced between the "voices" representing two different normative orders: the "voice of medicine" and the "voice of the lifeworld." Disruptions of the discourse during interviews appear to mark instances where the "voice of the lifeworld" interrupts the dominant "voice of medicine." How this happens, and whether the discourse is then "opened" or remains "closed" will be of major interest in succeeding analyses.

In sum, the principal aim of this chapter is to develop methods for the study of discourse that are informed by considerations of the research tasks of description, analysis, interpretation, and interruption. The methods are applied to a set of unremarkable interviews to bring out more clearly those features that are associated with our intuitive recognition of the interviews as instances of routine, normal, and ordinary clinical practice. After a close look at how these interviews work to produce a sense of normality and appropriateness, stretches of talk between patients and physicians that depart in some way from the normal and typical pattern will be examined. The departures suggest that something has become problematic. The analysis of problematic interviews is undertaken in the context of the findings from analyses of nonproblematic or unremarkable interviews. This will provide an initial set of contrasting features and their functions for use in further analyses that compare the "voice of medicine" with the "voice of the lifeworld."

UNREMARKABLE MEDICAL INTERVIEWS

Diagnostic Examination (W:02.014)[3]

The excerpt presented as Transcript 28.1 is taken from the beginning of an interview. Through this opening series of exchanges the patient (P) responds to the physician's (D) questions with a report of her symptoms. After each response, the physician asks for further details or other symptoms with the apparent aim of determining the specific nature of the problem and arriving at a diagnosis. On its surface, their talk proceeds as we would expect in a routine medical interview; it is unremarkable.

The physician initiates the interview with a question that Labov and Fanshel (1977, pp. 88–91) would code as a request for information: "What's the problem." Although its syntactic form is that of an open-ended Wh-question, the physician's voice does not carry question intonation. For that reason, the transcript does not show a question mark. The utterance is a request in the imperative mode, a paraphrase of a statement such as, "Tell me what the problem is." The phrasing of a request for action or information as an imperative is not unusual, and Labov and Fanshel argue that "the imperative is the unmarked form of a request for action" and "the central element in the construction of requests" (pp. 77–78).

In his first turn, the physician has set the general topic of discussion, namely, the patient's "problem." Or, more precisely, the physician's request is mutually understood to be germane and to express their joint recognition of the reason for the patient's presence in this setting: she is here because she has, or believes she has, a medically relevant problem. We, as investigators, knowing that this is a medical interview, are able to "read" the physician's utterance in the same way as the patient does. More than simply expressing a mutual understanding of the situation, his request confirms it and by confirming it contributes to the definition of the situation as a medical interview. It is in this sense that the "fact" that a medical interview is taking place is constructed through discourse. Such a definition of the situation excludes others. It is not a social occasion, a casual conversation, or an exchange of gossip, and we do not find initial greetings, an exchange of names, or other courtesies with which such conversations commonly begin. (Their absence must be treated with caution since it may reflect when the tape recorder was turned on).

The patient responds to the physician's request for information; she begins to report her symptoms, when they began, and the change from a sore throat that began a week ago, "which turned into a cold," "and then a cough." As she gives her account, the physician indicates that he is attending to her, understands, and wants her to continue by a go-ahead signal, "hm hm."

TRANSCRIPT 28.1

```
   W:02.014
       001 D   What's the problem.
  I ⌐                        (Chair noise)
    |                                    [
    |  002 P                          (...) had since . last
    |  003      Monday evening so it's a week of sore throat
    |  004 D                                        hm hm
    |  005 P    which turned into a cold .......... uh:m ..........
    |  006      and then a cough.
    |  007 D                   A cold you mean what? Stuffy nose?
    |  008 P    uh Stuffy nose yeah not a chest ........ cold. ..........
    |                                        [
    |  009 D                              hm hm
    |  010 P    uhm
    |           [
    |  011 D    And a cough.
    |  012 P                  And a cough .. which is the most irritating
    |  013      aspect.
    └           [
     ⌐014 D   Okay. (hh) uh Any fever?
  II |015 P                      ...... Not that I know of.
    |016      .... I took it a couple of times in the beginning
    |017      but . haven't felt like-
    └          [
     ⌐018 D      hm                 How bout your ears?
```

```
III ⎡019 P                                              ........
    |020 P   (hh) uhm .... Before anything happened .... I thought
    |021     that my ears ...... might have felt a little bit
    ⎣022     funny but (....) I haven't got any problem(s).
     023 D                                        Okay.
IV  ⎡024     .........(hh) Now this uh cough what are you producing
IV' |025     anything or is it a dry cough?
    |026 P                             Mostly dry although
    |027     ....... a few days . ago it was more mucusy ....
    |028     cause there was more (cold). Now (there's) mostly cough.
IV" |                [                                      [
     029 D           hm hm                              What
V   ⎡030     about the nasal discharge? Any?
    |031 P                                ....A little.
    |032 D                                       What
    |033     color is it?
    |034 P           ...... uh:m ........ I don't really know
    |035     .... uhm I suppose a whitish- (....)
    |                          [
    |036 D                     hm hm What?
    |037 P                                 There's been
    |038     nothing on the hankerchief.
    |                  [
    ⎣039 D             hm hm    Okay. .... (hh) Do you have
VI  ⎡040     any pressure around your eyes?
    ⎣041 P                          No.
                                       Okay. How do you feel?
     042 D   .......... uh:m ........ Tired. heh I couldn-(h)
VII ⎡043 P   I couldn't(h) sleep last night(h) uhm
    |044                  [
    |                     Because of the . cough.
    |045 D                              [
    |                                   Otherwise-
    |046 P   Yup. Otherwise I feel fine.
    |047                       Alright. Now . have you .
     048 D   had good health before (generally).
VIII⎡049                               Yeah . fine.
    ⎣050 P              (1'25")
```

As the patient responds to his opening question, the physician requests further clarification and specification: "A cold you mean what? Stuffy nose?" A little later he asks for confirmation of what he heard her say earlier, "And a cough." Through his questions the physician indicates that although he has asked her to talk about the nature of her "problem," the topic remains under his control. That is, his questions define the relevance of particular features in her account. Further, when the patient mentions a cold, sore throat, and cough as her symptoms, the physician suggests additional dimensions and distinctions that may be of medical relevance that the patient has neglected to report. Thus, a "cold" is not a sufficient description for his purpose; he must know what is "meant" by a cold and what kind of cold it is, "Stuffy nose?" The patient recognizes that there are at least two kinds, nose colds and chest colds, and introduces this contrast pair in order to specify her own: "uh stuffy nose yeah not a chest . . . cold."

The physician acknowledges her distinction, "hm hm," and adds to it the other symptom she has mentioned, "And a cough." The patient reconfirms his addition and goes on to give this symptom particular emphasis: "And a cough . . . which is the most irritating aspect." The physician's "Okay," inserted to overlap with the end of the patient's utterance, terminates the first cycle of the interview. He acknowledges the adequacy of the patient's response to his opening question, "What's the problem," and his "Okay" serves to close this section of the interview; no more is to be said about the problem in general and he will now proceed with more specific questions.

The first cycle is marked on the transcript by a bracket enclosing utterances 001–014 under Roman Numeral I. Its basic structure may be outlined as consisting of: a request/question from the physician, a response from the patient, and a post-response assessment/acknowledgment by the physician, to which is added a new request/question to begin the next cycle. The remainder of the excerpt is made up of seven additional cycles with structures identical to the first one. The first six cycles focus on the "cold" symptoms, the last two open with more general questions.

There are two variants within the basic structure. In the first type, the basic structure is expanded internally by requests from the physician for clarification or elaboration of the patient's response; this occurs in the first, fifth, and seventh cycles. In the second variant, the physician's assessments are implicit. Although his post-response assessments are usually explicit (an "Okay" or "Alright" comment), there are occasions when they are implicitly conveyed by the physician proceeding immediately to a next question. Alternatively, his assessment may occur before the patient's completion of her utterance through an overlapping "hm hm"; this occurs in the linkage between cycles IV and V.

This three-part utterance sequence is a regular and routine occurrence in the talk between patients and physicians. For that reason, I will refer to it as the basic structural unit of discourse in medical interviews. We recognize and accept interviews with these structures as normal, standard, and appropriate—as unremarkable. The medical interview tends to be constituted, overwhelmingly, by a connected series of such structural units. They are linked together through the physician's post-response assessment utterance that serves the dual function of closing the previous cycle and initiating a new one through his next question.

I do not mean to imply that this structure is unique to medical interviews, although it is one of their distinctive features. The same general type of structure appears in other settings of interaction where the aim is assessment, diagnosis, or selection, that is, when one person has the task of eliciting information from another. Thus, the same three-utterance sequence initiated by questions is found in classroom exchanges between teachers and pupils, although these are not interviews and teachers may direct successive questions to different pupils.[4] We might also expect to find it in psychological test situations and personnel interviews. Further work would be needed to determine how these discourses with similar general structures differed in their particular features.

Since I am proposing that this discourse structure is the basic unit of the medical interview and that its pervasive presence in a linked series is what makes this interview unremarkable, it is important to look more closely at how it is constructed and how it functions. The first and most obvious impression is of the physician's strong and consistent control over the content and development of the interview. . . . Here, I am trying to show how physicians exercise control through the structure of their exchanges with patients in the course of an interview.

There are a number of ways in which the physician uses his position as a speaker in this structure to control the interview: he opens each cycle of discourse with his response/question; he assesses the adequacy of the patient's response; he closes each cycle by using his assessment as a terminating marker; he opens the next cycle by another request/question. Through this pattern of opening and terminating cycles the physician controls the turn-taking process; he decides when the patient should take her turn. He also controls the content of what is to be discussed by selectively attending and responding to certain parts of the patient's statements and by initiating each new topic.

The physician's control of content through the initiation of new topics is particularly evident. After the first cycle in which the patient introduces her problem, there are seven new topics, each introduced by the physician through a question that opens a new cycle. In sequence, the physician asks the patient about: presence of fever, ear problems, type of cough, presence and type of nasal discharge, pressure around her eyes, how she feels, and her general state of health. The list is hardly worth noticing; these are the questions we might expect a physician to ask if a patient reports having a sore throat and a cold. The fit between our expectations and the interview is very close, which is why I have referred to it as an unremarkable interview.

We may learn more, however, about the significance and functions of the physician's control if we examine how his questions not only focus on certain topics, but are selectively inattentive to others. Through the questions he asks the physician constructs and specifies a domain of relevance; in Paolo Freire's phrase, he is "naming the world," the world of relevant matters for him and the patient (Freire, 1968).[5] The topics that the patient introduces, all of which are explicit, but not attended to by the physician, are: the history and course of her symptoms, and the effects they have had on her life that the cough is the most irritating aspect, that she's tired and has had a sleepless night. Both of these latter topics, opened up by the patient but not pursued by the physician, bear on a question that remains unasked but whose potential "relevance" is close to the surface: why she has come to see the physician at this point even though the problem began a week before.

In summary, this analysis shows that the physician controls the content of the interview, both through his initiation of new topics and through what he attends to and ignores in the patient's reports. Further, there is a systematic bias to his focus of attention; the patient's reports of how the problem developed and how it affects the "life contexts" of her symptoms are systematically ignored. The physician directs his attention solely to physical-medical signs that might be associated with her primary symptoms, such as ear or eye problems, or

to the further physical specification of a symptom, such as type of cough or color of nasal discharge. . . .

. . . We may now move beyond this level of interpretation to the stage referred to earlier as "interruption." The particular patterning of form and content shown in the analysis documents and defines the interview as "unremarkable," a characterization that was made on intuitive grounds. The clear pattern suggests that the discourse expresses a particular "voice," to use Silverman and Torode's (1980) term. Since the interview is dominated by the physician, I will refer to this as the "voice of medicine."

The topic introduced by the patient in VII, her tiredness and difficulty sleeping, is in another voice; I will call it the "voice of the lifeworld." It is an interruption, or an attempted interruption, of the ongoing discourse being carried on in the "voice of medicine." It is of some interest that the patient's introduction of another voice occurs in response to the open-ended question: "How do you feel?" Except for his initial question, this is the only open-ended question asked by the physician in this excerpt. In this instance, the second voice is suppressed; it does not lead to an opening of the discourse into a fuller and more mutual dialogue between the two voices. Rather, the physician reasserts the dominance of the voice of medicine through his response: "Because of the cough." Interruptions of the discourse and their effects will receive further attention in the following analyses.

It is instructive to examine in some detail the patterns of pauses and hesitations in the respective utterances of physician and patient. The findings of this analysis that pauses are not randomly distributed, but located systematically at certain points, particularly in the transitions between speakers, reinforces the argument made earlier about the importance of including such details of speech in transcripts. If we look at the cycle transition points (that is, from I–II, II–III, etc., that the physician controls through his utterance with a dual function terminating the previous cycle with a post-response assessment and initiating the new cycle with a question), we find a relatively consistent pattern. The physician either breaks into the patient's statement before she has completed it, thus terminating her statement with his own comment an "Okay" or "hm hm" as in I–II, II–III, IV–V, and V–VI, or he takes his next turn without pause as soon as the patient finishes, as in III–IV, VI–VII, and VII–VIII. Often, the assessment-terminating part of his utterance is followed by a pause, filled or unfilled, before the question that begins the next cycle, as in the utterances marking the beginnings of cycles II, III, IV, and VI.

. . . Findings from this analysis of one "unremarkable" interview will be summarized at this point. They provide a characterization, albeit tentative and preliminary, of normal and routine clinical practice, and can be used as a framework for comparing and contrasting analyses of other interviews.

First, the basic structural unit of a medical interview is a linked set of three utterances: a physician's opening question, a patient's response, and the physician's response to the patient which usually, but not always, begins with an assessment followed by a second question. The second utterance of the physician serves the dual function of terminating the first unit, or cycle, and initiating the next. In this way, the separate units are connected together to form the continuous discourse of the interview.

The primary discourse function of the basic structure is that it permits the physician to control the development of the interview. His control is assured by his position as both first and last speaker in each cycle, which allows him to control the turn-taking system and the sequential organization of the interview. This structure of dominance is reinforced by the content of the physician's assessments and questions that he asks, which selectively attend to or ignore particulars of the patient's responses. The physician's dominance is expressed at still another level through the syntactic structure of his questions. These tend to be restrictive closed-end questions, which limit the range of relevance for patient responses. At all these levels, the focus of relevance, that is, of appropriate meaning, is on medically relevant material, as is defined by the physician.

Within utterances, two patterns of pauses were identified that are consistent with the overall structure and its functions. Typically, in physician utterances there is a pause between the assessment and the next question. This serves to mark the termination of the prior unit and the initiation of the next one. The length of initial pauses in patient responses appears to depend on the location of a cycle within a sequence of cycles. Patient utterances in the first cycle of a series are preceded by a short pause, in the second cycle by a long pause, and in the third cycle by no pause. This seems to be related to the degree of disjunction between successive physician questions and whether or not he "helps" the patient prepare for a response by making his next question relevant to her prior response.

Finally, all the features and functions of this unit of discourse have been brought together under a general analytic category referred to as the "voice of medicine." The physician's control of the interview through the structure of turn-taking and through the form and content of his questions expresses the normative order of medicine. The dominance of this voice produces our intuitive impression of the interview as an instance of normal clinical practice, that is, as unremarkable. Patients may attempt to interrupt the dominant voice by speaking in the "voice of the lifeworld." This alternative voice may be suppressed, as it was in this interview, or may open up the interview to a fuller dialogue between voices. Relationships between the two voices will be explored further. . . .

THE INTERRUPTION OF CLINICAL DISCOURSE

The structure of clinical discourse has been explicated through analyses of two unremarkable interviews. The basic three-part unit of such discourse and the ways in which these units are linked together has been described, as well as the functions served by this structure the physician's control of organization and meaning. I referred to this patterned relationship between structure and function as the "voice of medicine," and suggested that it expressed the normative order of medicine and clinical practice. This voice provides a baseline against which to compare other medical interviews that depart in some way from normal and routine practice.

Some preliminary comparisons have already been made. In each of these unremarkable interviews the patient interrupted the flow of the discourse by introducing the "voice of the lifeworld." In both instances, the new voice was quickly silenced and the physician reasserted his dominance and the singularity of the clinical perspective. In the following interview, the patient makes more of an effort to sustain an alternative voice. Examining how the patient does this and how the physician responds will extend our understanding of the specific features and functions of medical interviews and will also alert us to problems that develop when there are departures from normal and routine clinical work. This discussion will also bring forward an issue that will be central to later analyses; the struggle between the voices of medicine and of the lifeworld.

Symptom and Lifeworld Context: Negotiation of Meaning (W:13.121/01)

The patient is a 26-year-old woman with stomach pains, which she describes as a sour stomach beginning several weeks prior to this medical visit. The excerpt (Transcript 28.2) begins about 3½ minutes into the interview, preceded by a review of her history of peptic ulcers in childhood and the time and circumstances of the present complaint.

In the excerpt, the first four cycles and the beginning of the fifth are similar in structure to the interviews analyzed earlier. Each one begins with the physician's question about the symptom. This is followed by a response from the patient, sometimes preceded by a pause, and is terminated by the physician's next question. His question is sometimes preceded by an assessment, which then initiates the next cycle.

Two other features of the first four cycles may be noted. Although there are occasional pauses prior to the patient's responses and some false starts as she appears to search for an appropriate answer, there are few within-utterance pauses and those that occur are of short duration. For the physician, the pattern found earlier of a pause between assessment and question is occasionally present, but there are no false starts or pauses between the patient's responses and the physician's next questions. Again, there is a high degree of fluency in his speech.

TRANSCRIPT 28.2

```
W:13.121/01
        ┌001 D   Hm hm .... Now what do you mean by a sour stomach?
   I    │ 002 P   .................. What's a sour stomach? A heartburn
        │ 003     like a heartburn or something.
        │                                        [
        └004 D                                   Does it burn over here?
  II    ┌005 P                                                      Yea:h.
        │ 006     It li- I think- I think it like- If you take a needle
        │ 007     and stick ya right .... there's a pain right here ..
        │               [           [                        [
        │ 008 D         Hm hm Hm hm                          Hm hm
        └009 P   and  and then it goes from here on this side to this side.
         010 D   Hm Hm Does it go into the back?
 III   ┌                              [
       │ 011 P                        It's a:ll up here. No. It's all right
       │ 012     up here in the front.
       │              [
       └013 D   Yeah               And when do you get that?
  IV   ┌014 P                                                   ........
       │ 015     ........... Wel:l when I eat something wrong.
        016 D                                         How- How
```

(Continued)

TRANSCRIPT 28.2   ■   (Continued)

V	017	soon after you eat it?
V′	018 P	............................Wel:l
	019	.... probably an hour .... maybe less.
		[
V″	020 D	About an hour?
	021 P	Maybe less .... I've cheated and I've been
	022	drinking which I shouldn't have done.
	023 D	....
	024	Does drinking making it worse?
VI		[
	025 P	(...) Ho ho uh ooh Yes. ....
	026	.... Especially the carbonation and the alcohol.
VII	027 D	.... Hm hm .... How much do you drink?
VII′	028 P	......
	029	.... I don't know. .. Enough to make me
	030	go to sleep at night .... and that's quite a bit.
VII″	031 D	One or two drinks a day?
	032 P	O:h no no no humph it's (more
	033	like) ten. ...... at night.
		[
	034 D	How many drinks- a night.
	035 P	At night.
	036 D	.....
	037	..... Whaddya ta- What type of drinks .... I (...)-
VIII		[
	038 P	Oh vodka
	039	.. yeah vodka and ginger ale.
	040 D	....
IX	041	...... How long have you been drinking that heavily?
IX′	042 P	.... Since I've been married.
	043 D	......
IX″	044	.. How long is that?
	045 P	(giggle..) Four years. (giggle)
	046	huh Well I started out with before then I was drinkin
	047	beer but u:m I had a job and I was .... ya know ......
	048	had more things on my mind and ya know I like- but
	049	since I got married I been in and out of jobs and
	050	everything so .... I- I have ta have something to
	051	go to sleep.
	052 D	...... Hm:m.
	053 P	.... I mean I'm not
	054	gonna- ...... It's either gonna be pills or it's
	055	gonna be .. alcohol .... and uh alcohol seems
	056	to satisfy me moren than pills do .... They don't
	057	seem to get strong enough .... pills that I have
	058	got I had- I do have Valium .... but they're two
	059	milligrams .... and that's supposed to
	060	quiet me down during the day but it doesn't.
	061 D	......
X	062	How often do you take them?
		(1′47″)

The routine breaks down in cycle V. The patient's response to the physician's question with its false start includes a signal of trouble: "How–How soon after you eat it?" The patient's response is preceded by her longest pre-utterance pause (one of 2.50), and contains two relatively long intra-utterance pauses. A major change comes in her next response, after restating her previous answer, "Maybe less," in response to his clarification question: "About an hour?" This physician question is treated as an internal expansion within V, although it might also be considered as beginning a new cycle, V9. Her answer, "Maybe less," is followed by a moderately long intra-utterance pause of 1.20, after which she introduces a new topic, her drinking.

This new topic comes in the form of a "tag" comment added to her answer to the physician's question and it has some features that mark it as different from what has previously been said. ". . . I've cheated and I've been drinking which I shouldn't have done," has a quality of intonation that is unusual when compared with her earlier responses. Those who have heard the tape recording easily recognize the difference and describe her speech as "teasing," "flirtatious," or "childish."

The physician's next question, which terminates V and initiates VI, is preceded by his first long pre-question hesitation: ". . . Does drinking make it worse?" This is the first break in the fluency of his pattern of questioning. Further, he talks over the patient's attempt to say something more. His uncertainty, indicated by his pause, reflects two changes in the nature of the interview. The patient's comment introduces her drinking and, since this new topic is not in response to a direct question from the physician, it also shifts the control of the interview from physician to patient. I pointed out in earlier analyses that the basic structure of the medical interview, physician question-patient response-physician (assessment) question, permits the physician to control the form and content of the interview. As the "questioner," the physician controls the turn-taking structure and through the focus of his assessments and questions controls the development of meaning; he defines what is and what is not relevant. By her tag comment, the patient has taken control both of form and meaning; she has introduced another voice.

With this tentative hypothesis that the normal structure of the medical interview has been interrupted and that as a result, the normal pattern of control has also been disrupted, we might expect to find evidence of: (a) other indicators of disruption and breakdown in the continuing exchange, and (b) efforts on the part of the physician to repair the disruption, to restore the normal structure, and to reassert the dominant voice of medicine.

The physician's pre-question hesitation after the patient introduces the new topic has already been noted as a sign of disruption, a change from his usual response timing: ". . . Does drinking make it worse?" Similar and frequently longer pauses appear before all of his succeeding questions initiating new cycles at VII, VIII, IX, and X. The regularity of these pauses is quite striking, particularly when it is contrasted with the equally striking occurrence of no pauses preceding questions in cycles with a normal structure (I–IV).

Throughout the second half of this excerpt, from cycles VI–X, there is a continuing struggle between physician and patient to take control of the interview. The patient tries to maintain her control by restatements of the problem of drinking in her life situation exemplifying the voice of the lifeworld. The physician, on the other, persistently tries to reformulate the problem in narrower, more medically relevant terms. For example, to his question, "How much do you drink?" (the transition between cycles VI and VII), she replies, after a long pause of 2.2, "I don't know . . . Enough to make me go to sleep at night . . . and that's quite a bit." He persists with two further questions, within cycle VII, requesting the specific number of drinks. In this manner, the physician attempts to recapture control of the meaning of her account; he is excluding her meaning of the function of drinking in her life and focusing on "objective" measures of quantity.

The physician persists in this effort. To his question about how long she has been drinking heavily (IX), she responds, "Since I've been married," again preceding her response with a long pause. But this is not considered an adequate or relevant answer from the physician's point of view and he asks for an actual, objective time, "How long is that?" Finally, in a relatively extended account in cycle IX, the patient talks about her drinking, of problems since her marriage, and her preference for alcohol over pills. There is much surplus information in her story to which the physician might respond. He chooses to attend selectively to that part of her account which is of clear medical relevance, the taking of pills, and asks again for a precise, objective, and quantitative answer. "How often do you take them?"

Another way to indicate that a significant change has taken place in the structure of the interview during the fifth cycle is to take note of the difficulty encountered in attempting to describe this interview in terms of the structural units found in the analyses of the first two interviews. Although I have marked the cycles of the interview in the same way, distinguishing such successive series of physician question-patient response-physician (assessment) question exchanges, there are problems in using this unit here. This structural unit assumes that an exchange is initiated by the physician's question and that the three-part exchange cycle is then terminated by the physician as he initiates the next cycle.

The problem may be seen in cycle V, at the point of the patient's comment about her drinking. This statement is not in response to a direct question; rather it is a statement introducing a new topic. The physician's next question refers to this new topic and he thus remains "in role." The reader will note that all of the physician's statements, except for his "Hm" assessments, are questions. The implicit

function of questions remains which is to control the form and content of the interview; however, in this instance there is a break in the continuity of the physician's control. As an alternative structure to the one presented, we could ask whether a new cycle should begin with the patient's tag comment. If that were done, the physician's next question would be treated as a "response" to her statement, even though it is framed as a question. I'm not proposing an answer to the problem of structural analysis at this preliminary stage. However, I am suggesting that the change in the interview resulting from the patient's comment introduces problems for analysis. These problems provide another line of evidence for the assertion that there has been a breakdown in the normal structure of the clinical interview. . . .

. . . In this discussion, I have been using the occurrence of a noticeable change in the structure and flow of an interview to raise questions about how to analyze and understand the workings of medical interviews. The introduction of a new topic by the patient altered the routine pattern of the interview found in earlier "unremarkable" interviews. The features of physician and patient utterances varied in specific ways from those found earlier. These changes raised questions about which speaker was controlling the development of the interview, and hence controlling the development of meaning. The idea of "voices," and the distinction between the "voice of medicine" and the "voice of the lifeworld," was introduced to characterize alternative orders of meaning and the struggle between them. . . .

Notes

1. Waitzkin and Stoeckle's original corpus of nearly 500 interviews included a stratified random sample of physicians in private and clinic sessions in Boston and Oakland. For the present study, a small series of about twenty-five tapes was selected initially from the larger sample. Male and female patients were equally represented in the series, and both single and multiple interviews of a patient with the same

physician were included. The original tapes were sequentially ordered by code numbers assigned to physicians and each of their successive patients. The selection procedure was to choose the "next" code number in the sequence where the interview met the criteria noted earlier until the cells were filled. Although this was not a random sampling procedure it ensured heterogeneity among the interviews and there was no reason to believe that the series was biased in a systematic way with reference to the original sample. The analyses presented here are based on a small number of interviews drawn from this series. Further, analyses are restricted to brief excerpts from the full interviews which exemplify issues of primary theoretical interest. This description of the procedure is intended to clarify the grounds on which the claim is made that the interviews examined in this study are "typical" medical interviews. This claim does not rely on statistical criteria or rules for selecting a "representative" sample. Rather, it rests on a shared understanding and recognition of these interviews as "representative," that is, as displays of normatively appropriate talk between patients and physicians.

2. Examples of these studies may be found in Schenkein (1978); and in Psathas (1979). A perceptive discussion of the way that ethnomethodology approaches the study of talk, and some of its unresolved problems, is found in Wooton (1975).

3. The typescript numbers used here are the codes on the tapes assigned by Waitzkin and Stoeckle; the number is preceded by a "W" to indicate the source.

4. In earlier studies of classroom interaction, I referred to the set of three utterances initiated by a question as an Interrogative Unit. Connections between units through the dual function of the second question were called Chaining (see Mishler 1975a, 1975b, 1978).

5. Another example of the ways in which a physician's selectivity of attention and inattention, through his pattern of questioning, shapes the development of meaning in a medical interview may be found in Paget (1983).

References

Freire, Paulo. 1968. *Pedagogy of the Oppressed.* New York: Seabury Press.

Jefferson, Gail. 1978. "Sequential aspects of storytelling in conversation." Pp. 219–248 in *Studies in the organization of conversational interaction*, edited by Schenkein. New York: Academic Press.

Labov, William, and David Fanshel. 1977. *Therapeutic Discourse: Psychotherapy as Conversation.* New York: Academic Press.

Mishler, Elliot. 1975a. "Studies in Dialogue and Discourse: I. An Exponential Law of Successive Questioning." *Language in Society* 4:31–51.

_____. 1975b. "Studies in Dialogue and Discourse: II. Types of Discourse Initiated by and Sustained Through Questioning." *Journal of Psycholinguistic Research* 4(2):99–121.

_____. 1978. "Studies in Dialogue and Discourse: III. Utterance Structure and Utterance Function in Interrogative Sequences." *Journal of Psycholinguistic Research* 7(4): 279–305.

Paget, Marianne. 1983. "Experience and Knowledge." *Human Studies* 6(1):67–90.

Psathas, George. 1979. "Organizational features of direction maps." Pp. 203–26 in *In Everyday Language: Studies in Ethnomethodology,* edited by George Psathas. New York: Irvington.

Schenkein, Jim (editor). 1978. *Studies in the Organization of Conversational Interaction.* New York: Academic.

Silverman, David, and Brian Torode. 1980. *The Material Word: Some Theories of Language and Its Limits.* Boston: Routledge and Kegan Paul.

Waitzkin, Howard, and John Stoeckle. 1976. "Information Control and the Micropolitics of Health Care: Summary of an Ongoing Project." *Social Science and Medicine* 10:263–276.

Waitzkin, Howard, John D. Stoeckle, Eric Beller, and Carl Mons. 1978. "The Informative Process in Medical Care: A Preliminary Report with Implications for Instructional Communication." *Instructional Science* 7(4):385–419.

Wooton, Anthony. 1975. *Dilemmas of Discourse: Controversies About the Sociological Interpretation of Language.* London: George Allen & Unwin Ltd.

29

CULTURAL BROKERAGE

Creating Linkages Between Voices of Lifeworld and Medicine in Cross-Cultural Clinical Settings

Ming-Cheng Miriam Lo

CULTURALLY COMPETENT HEALTHCARE IN THE UNITED STATES

In the USA, it is well established among public health scholars and practitioners that certain racial and ethnic groups receive poorer care, experience lower life expectancy, and have higher rates of mortality and morbidity relative to whites. On the basis of this shared recognition, healthcare professionals and social scientists of medicine wrestle with the puzzle of how these disparities are reproduced and whether policy changes can effectively address inequalities. In this context, the notion of 'culturally competent healthcare' emerges as an umbrella concept that captures the sensitivity to racial and ethnic cultures in healthcare delivery (Betancourt et al., 2005). Broadly defined as 'a set of congruent behaviors, attitudes, and policies that come together in a system, agency, or among professionals that enables effective work in cross-cultural situations' (Office of Minority Health, 2001: 4), the movement for cultural competency began more than 20 years ago and gained initial traction in the fields of mental health and nursing (Brach and Fraserirector, 2000; Good et al., 2002). Renewed interest in the topic emerged in response to the Institute of Medicine's report *Unequal Treatment* (Smedley et al., 2003), which documents the scope of disparities even after controlling for income, education, and insurance status. Examples of cultural competency

Cultural Brokerage: Creating Linkages Between Voices of Lifeworld and Medicine in Cross-Cultural Clinical Settings, Ming-Cheng Miriam Lo in *Health*, *14*(5), 484–504. First Published August 27, 2010. Reprinted with permission from SAGE Publications, Inc.

efforts include sensitivity training of physicians and other healthcare providers, both in medical school and on the job; patient support services, such as translators; and ethnicity-specific preventive health campaigns (see Lo and Stacey, 2008 for a comprehensive review).

While our understanding of cultural competency in healthcare is largely in the formative stage (Paez et al., 2008; Perloff et al., 2006), existing research suggests that patient-centeredness is an important component of culturally competent healthcare. Empirical studies have shown that attempts at culturally competent healthcare that fail to incorporate patient-centeredness can lead to inappropriate stereotyping, despite doctors' best intentions (Hunt and De Voogd, 2005). Identifying the patients' values alone without giving patients adequate opportunities to voice their concerns does not enhance the quality of care (see also Kagawa-Singer and Blackhall, 2001).

At a theoretical level, a rigorous conceptualization of patient culture also implies that it is impossible to deliver culturally competent care without engaging in patient-centered communication. Building upon Lo and Stacey's (2008) Bourdieu-informed theorization of patient culture,[1] I conceptualize patient culture as a set of broad orientations or sense-making schemas, of which patients themselves may or may not be conscious. Such orientations or schemas are shaped by multiple, intersecting structural forces, including, for example, race or ethnicity, immigration, gender, poverty, or religion (see also Liamputtong, 2005). Furthermore, patients 'mix and match' their available schemas and sometimes pick up new ones, as they navigate through clinical encounters. Given that cultural schemas and orientations are multiple, hybridized, and adaptable, doctors cannot know *a priori* the patient's culture, but must learn it by orienting themselves toward careful communication (see also Connelly, 2005).

Thus, patient-centered communication is recognized as a central component of culturally competent healthcare. Yet to date, there exists little empirical research on doctors' on-the-ground work and specific strategies for achieving patient-centeredness in inter-ethnic, cross-cultural settings. Based on

qualitative analyses of 24 in-depth interviews with primary care physicians, the current study takes up this issue.

PATIENT-CENTERED CARE: GIVING VOICE TO THE LIFEWORLD

Long before the culturally competent healthcare campaign became popular, the notion of patient-centeredness was widely discussed among both healthcare practitioners and researchers. In an extensive review of the literature, Mead and Bower (2000) propose a five-dimension framework for conceptualizing patient-centeredness: biopsychological perspective, 'patient-as-person', sharing power and responsibility, therapeutic alliance, and 'doctor-as-person'. A broad, multifaceted concept, patient-centeredness generally highlights the importance of understanding, and negotiating with, the patient's thoughts, needs, preferences, and illness experiences, which are grounded in her life context. Mishler (1984), drawing upon Habermas's theory of communicative action, conceptualizes the patient's accounts of these personal, context-sensitive illness experiences as the voice of the 'lifeworld'.[2] Whereas the voice of medicine is technology-centered and goal-oriented, the voice of the lifeworld is oriented to meanings, understanding, and a sense of groundedness in everyday life. In the conventional doctor-centered models, the patient's lifeworld voice is largely fragmented during medical interviews. The doctor's biomedical framework reduces the lifeworld voice to a set of abstract symptom presentations, which are in turn treated as the scientific basis of diagnosis and treatment options (Good and Good, 2000; Hunter, 1991).

The suppression of the lifeworld voice by the voice of medicine is considered highly problematic, as it often leads to distorted communication, erratic diagnoses, or inappropriate treatment plans (Barry et al., 2001). Furthermore, a rich and diverse literature has elaborated on the healing power of narrative itself—patients need to be heard and understood, not just cured, for the completion of the healing process (Brody, 1994; Frank, 1995; Hunter, 1991, 1996; Kleinman, 1988; Mattingly, 1998a). The art of listening helps make the practice of modern medicine more humane and allows doctors to become more complete caretakers (Charon, 2001; Connelly, 2005). Some researchers also point out that while operating within a biomedical framework, doctors themselves rely on narrative reasoning in their sense-making process; doctors need to connect the dots (their data points) in meaningful ways and they do so by figuring out a most plausible story (Mattingly, 1998b; see also Good, 2004). If doctors rely on 'storytelling' in their clinical reasoning, it is crucial that the patients' lifeworld concerns and narratives are heard and incorporated in this process.

These characterizations of the struggle between medical and lifeworld voices reinforce the importance of patient-centeredness for culturally competent healthcare, while also revealing its challenges. If 'culture' often appears to be an abstract and illusive object for doctors to grasp, the patient's lifeworld narratives offer some concrete articulations of her culture. As the patient's narratives are informed and organized by her cultural orientations and sense-making schemas, the former is the concrete manifestation of the latter. For the very same reason, however, as patients from different cultural backgrounds resort to their own sense-making schemas to organize and tell their stories, it can be difficult for doctors to comprehend these narratives. These cultural barriers are further compounded, as Mishler's argument would suggest, by the institutionalized domination of the lifeworld by medicine. Cultural incommensurability and power inequalities can render the gaps between medical and lifeworld voices especially difficult to bridge in cross-cultural settings.

Clinicians and scholars have explored various models for eliciting the patient's lifeworld voice. Mishler (1984) himself suggests listening, using open-ended questions, and power-sharing during clinical encounters. Viewing clinical interactions as a process of negotiations between diverse 'explanatory models' for illness experiences, Kleinman's (1980, 1988) now classic research outlines a list of concrete questions that a provider could use to elicit a patient's 'explanatory model'. More recently, scholars have proposed more diverse lists of questions for eliciting patient input (Cooper et al., 2003; Hunt and De Voogd, 2005). For example, Kagawa-Singer and Blackhall (2001: 2999) expand the list to include sets of open-ended questions about 'patients' and families' attitudes, beliefs, context, decision-making [style], and environment (ABCDE)'. Conversely, focusing on how physician authority may serve to silence patients' lay voices, scholars explore how interactional styles (e.g. humor, friendliness, positive reassurance) can help cultivate trust and reach beyond patients' self-censorship (Beck et al., 2002; Hunter, 1991; Street et al., 2007).

Although the aforementioned proposals by Kleinman and others focus on unblocking lifeworld narratives while operating from within the world of medicine, it is unclear how doctors create linkages between these two sets of meaning systems when they appear drastically different, as in the case in cross-cultural clinical encounters. Addressing this issue, the analysis in this article will show how doctors' 'cultural brokerage' helps to create such linkages. Originally developed by anthropologists Eric Wolf and Clifford Geertz, the notion of cultural brokerage has generally been defined as bridging, linking, or mediating between groups or persons from different cultures. Scholars have applied this notion to the context of clinical interactions, especially for studying the roles of nurses and medical interpreters (Barbee, 1987; Hsieh, 2006; Jezewski, 1990; Tripp-Reimer and Brink, 1985). Informed by my earlier discussion of patient culture as multiple, flexible, and hybridized schemas and orientations, I further specify cultural brokerage as the mutual inclusion of seemingly incongruent sets of schemas or orientations with which people organize their meanings and information (see also Gershon, 2006). This mutual inclusion provides the foundational work that makes the sharing of meanings and information possible.

I document and explain four aspects of this cultural work next. As my empirical examples suggest, in cross-cultural clinical encounters, doctors often find their patients operating with different conceptual schemas and cultural orientations than their own for understanding and acting upon illness experiences, clinical procedures, the role of institutionalized medicine itself, or the process of handling new knowledge and information. To enable, at least to some extent, the mutual inclusion of theirs and their patients' conceptual schemas, doctors often engage in practices of cultural translation between the two sets of sense-making frameworks. This is illustrated in the discussion of aspects 1 and 2 of cultural brokerage ('Translating between Health Systems' and 'Bridging Divergent Images of Medicine'). Aspect 3 of cultural brokerage, 'Establishing Long-Term Relationships', discusses how doctors rely on cultivating long-term relationships with their patients in order to create a relational context in which they might gradually comprehend their patients' subtler, less easily observable cultural orientations. The fourth aspect of cultural brokerage, 'Working with Patients' Relational Networks', addresses how doctors approximate or approach patients' own communal networks to create an environment that feels familiar to the patients and is conducive to their open discussion of new medical concepts and practices. With these cultural brokerage efforts, doctors begin to depart from the model of 'standard practice plus patient voice', moving, instead, toward an attempt to embed and transform the voice of medicine in the patient's life context. This cultural work must be understood as concrete 'cultural labor', which involves specific tasks and requires time and resources. By the same token, this analysis suggests that without recognizing cultural brokerage as concrete cultural labor, scholars and policy makers may fail to comprehend key limitations of the current cultural competency campaign.

Finally, it might be useful to offer one brief qualifying note before moving on to my data, method, and empirical findings. Given the widely documented gaps between the cultures of medicine and lifeworld, one can argue that cultural brokering is required, potentially, in any doctor–patient interaction, and not just in cross-cultural settings. Indeed, existing models of sensitive and open-ended questioning can be conceptualized as one form of cultural brokerage. Even so, not all patients are equally distanced,

culturally speaking, from their providers (Malat and Hamilton, 2006). In cases in which patients come from marginalized class, educational, or ethnic backgrounds, the lifeworld–medicine gap may be further widened and complicated, thus additional cultural brokerage work is needed. What cultural brokerage in clinical encounters consists of, beyond sensitive and open-ended questions, has largely been under-studied and is the empirical focus of the current study. But it is more intellectually fruitful to place cultural brokerage along with other models of patient-centered communication on the same conceptual continuum than to treat them as mutually exclusive categories.

DATA AND METHOD

This study is part of a larger project that examines the understandings and experiences of cultural barriers in healthcare from the perspectives of policy makers, healthcare professionals, and immigrant patients. The current article draws upon 24 open-ended, in-depth interviews with primary care physicians (in family practice, internal medicine, or pediatrics) in Northern California during 2005–2006. Through purposeful sampling, I recruited physicians who self-identified as having worked extensively with LEP (limited English proficiency) patients and who expressed interest in promoting culturally competent healthcare. The current study is therefore not intended to be representative of the general views of medical doctors; instead, it focuses on the experiences of those doctors who have attempted cultural brokerage work. In other words, the dominance of the biomedical framework in American medicine notwithstanding, there are variations among how the agents of the profession respond to its critiques, with some now consciously aspiring to understand the patient's lifeworld—raising questions about how and whether they do so.

The interviewees were evenly divided by gender. Nine of the interviewees worked at a teaching hospital and 15 were from a community clinic or county hospital. Fifteen of the interviews self-identified as belonging to an immigrant or minority group. The interviews typically took place at the physician's office or home or, on occasion, at my office. On average, each interview lasted 90 minutes. All interviews were audio-taped and then transcribed. To preserve confidentiality, all interviewees are identified by pseudonyms.

A flexible interview schedule allowed respondents to talk freely about their understanding and experiences of cultural competency, including how they defined the term, the cultural competency training they had received, and their perceived barriers and preferred changes at individual, organizational, and societal levels. Doctors were then asked to offer and elaborate on concrete examples of their attempts at cultural competency, and then to describe how they thought these efforts impacted the quality of care they provided.

Interview transcripts and corresponding field notes were first read in their entirety to gain a holistic understanding of the providers' views and experiences. After that, systematic inductive coding was conducted, using the software program NVivo7. Doctors' own accounts of cultural competency efforts were first coded into two broad categories: successful versus failed. Four facilitating mechanisms emerged from the 'successful' category. The absence of several facilitating mechanisms corresponded with the 'failed' category, along with two 'institutional constraints'. Certainly, doctors' discussions of their cultural competency efforts are not to be conflated with patient satisfaction or experience; what these accounts do tell us is what it takes for doctors to perform this cultural work on the job.

ASPECTS OF CULTURAL BROKERAGE

Li-Chin, a Chinese-American pediatrician at a community clinic, shared an honest reflection on her failed cultural competency effort. The pediatrician recalled treating a female Muslim teenage patient who:

> has not been out of the house, has not completed her education, and an arranged marriage is about to happen. . . . So [this

patient] comes in and says, 'I have a stomachache'. I don't find anything medically that I can do for the stomachache. But what else could be causing the stomachache, or this headache? Lots of stuff, stuff that I don't understand enough.

As she told the story, Li-Chin expressed an urgent desire to engage this patient in an in-depth conversation about her life context, but conceded that she did not have the 'culturally meaningful' vocabulary to initiate an in-depth conversation about such matters:

> It's my not knowing which things were most important to her, and where she felt constraints. What were the bases for those constraints? I mean, I can't just say, you don't want to do this [arranged marriage], this isn't a good idea, you know?

Li-Chin viewed the patient as an 'experiencing subject' and wanted to understand her illness experience as shaped in part by social and psychological factors (Mead and Bower's dimensions 1–2). She was also eager to partner with the patient (Mead and Bower's dimensions 3–4) and quite capable of reflecting on her own limitations (Mead and Bower's dimension 5). But what was frustrating for Li-Chin—and debilitating for her ability to deliver patient-centered care—was the lack of cultural brokerage skills. As she put it, she lacked the 'culturally meaningful' vocabulary to bridge the gap with her Muslim patient.

Other interviewees shared similar frustrations. But they also offered more positive accounts that allowed us to discern mechanisms of successful cultural brokerage. The following discussion illustrates these mechanisms.

1. Translating Between Health Systems

Complicating the dichotomy between the voices of lifeworld and medicine, doctors in this study pointed out that the practice of medicine itself was pluralistic, organized in different systems in different countries and traditions. Immigrant patients often brought with them distinct health concepts, expectations of treatment procedures, or norms of clinical interactions. The medical community had certainly been aware that it needed to respect such differences, but what remained unclear was how to implement this principle. My interviewees' experiences suggested that one concrete strategy was to 'translate' for the patients what their familiar concepts and practices might look like in the US health system. The work of cultural translation aspired to the same goals as did general models of patient-centered care (e.g. sharing power and responsibility and building therapeutic alliance), but in cross-cultural settings, cultural translation was an important prerequisite.[3]

Maria, a Caucasian family doctor at a community clinic, shared her experience of interacting with a Cambodian woman who refused to take calcium but kept telling Maria, 'Oh, yes, doctor, oh, yes, I'll take the calcium.' Eventually, Maria found out that the patient refused calcium supplements because she was concerned about the hot/cold balance of her diet and medication. As Maria engaged the patient in a long conversation on the subject, the patient finally offered that she 'didn't want to tell me this, because she knew I wouldn't believe her. . . . So she never even mentioned to me why.' Having understood their different health concepts, Maria recruited her patient's help to translate the concern about hot/cold diet into Western food categories:

> So we talked about different foods. I don't think patients—their system doesn't necessarily correspond exactly to calcium. So when you understand the origin, you can go through, 'Well, is spinach hot or cold? Is cheese? Is milk? . . .' Oh, orange juice fortified with calcium is warm, so you can do that. . . . When you understand that this is what they believe, they're really not going to change, it forces you to come up with another plan.

Maria's example illustrated how the work of cultural translation between different health concepts provided the necessary basis for successful doctor–patient negotiation.

Health concepts, however, were not the only dimension of the broader health systems in which doctors and their immigrant patients were grounded, and which thus required cultural translation. Sometimes the work of cultural translation focused on other dimensions, such as different norms of clinical interaction. Daniel, a Caucasian family doctor at a community clinic, offered some thoughtful comments when discussing how some immigrant patients wanted to yield their decision-making power to him, which contradicted the concept of patient autonomy that Daniel practiced:

> So I've said, 'You could . . . , if you [do] A, B, C, or D', and they have no idea of what the benefits or risks of A, B, C, or D are. So, I would go through, 'Well, A has this benefit, but you're kind of old, and you might die from this. B, less risk of dying, but it won't cure you. You're still gonna have the problem, you're just going to feel better. C, might do nothing. If you do nothing, then you're probably going to die in about six months. Then they still might say, 'Well, what do you think I should do?'

Daniel translated the patient's preferred model of medical paternalism into, 'Okay, I'm going to tell you what I would advise for my own mother', and then he tried to show the patient that there was another perspective:

> But in America we don't make you do things. So now you have to adjust to the fact that we don't make you do things. . . . I want them to feel that it's a free choice, and they can change their mind if they want.

The work of cultural translation helped to restate the patient's request in more understandable and legitimate terms in the US health system. On the basis of being accepted, the patient was in turn asked to consider making adjustments in this new context.

In his own words, Daniel described this as a way of 'hybridizing' the American medical culture and the patients' model.[4] In the process of hybridizing, patients' norms and interaction styles were translated and respected, but at the same time their potential for learning new concepts and practices was also valued and encouraged:

> So I'm going to bend a little bit, but they have to bend a little bit, too, 'cause they're not in Cambodia or Vietnam; they're here. *So I think most people can understand they're here, and things work differently, but I have to give them enough information.*

Through hybridizing, the patient and doctor shared negotiated authority over clinical interaction.

Similarly, Daniel discussed how to work with different expectations of treatment procedures. Drawing from his experiences with Russian immigrant patients, Daniel noted that some of them were used to a much lengthier and more extensive form of physical therapy. These patients were often disappointed at the brevity of sessions here; they sometimes complained that the physical therapist did nothing for them except for ordering them to do all the work at home:

> If somebody says to me, they didn't do anything at physical therapy, I don't want to tell them, 'that's not true', or 'that's stupid'. 'Physical therapy in Russia didn't do anything, this is better.' What I want to say is, well, that's how we do it in the United States. Maybe it's not as good, but that's all we can afford. You know? And just *allow people to retain their respect for their own institutions, their own conceptions.*

Daniel did not judge the other models to be inferior to the American model; rather, he encouraged some pragmatic transitions, since the only available treatment for the patient was now from the American system. Again, Daniel helped the patient to translate her expectation of specific treatment (e.g. 'physical therapy sessions should be longer') into a motivation for working within the new system (e.g. 'maybe it's not as good, but that's all we can afford'). In short, the doctors who engaged in cultural translation

recognized the validity of health concepts, clinical interaction styles, or treatment procedures that were rooted in different health systems, and they worked to help patients restate these notions and sometimes hybridize them with the American model.

2. Bridging Divergent Images of Medicine

Another aspect of the doctors' cultural brokerage focused on negotiating appropriate roles for medical intervention that would make sense in the patient's lifeworld. These doctors found that culturally and socially marginalized groups had often developed conceptual frameworks that categorized medical institutions as agents of social authority, which aimed to punish deviance and were indifferent to their welfare. In these situations, sensitive questioning and skillful interactions alone, though helpful, often proved insufficient for bridging divergent understandings of the doctors' roles. Instead, the doctors needed to present the role of medicine in a framework that resonated with their patients. Similar to the translational work between different healthcare systems, establishing shared understandings of the role of medicine formed an important basis for building therapeutic alliances across ethnic and class divides.

Oftentimes, doctors did so by offering a picture of medicine that was less ambitious and more prone to mistakes. Such conceptualizations overlapped with the patients' understandings and experiences to some extent. On these shared grounds, doctors could then explain what medicine could potentially offer for the patient. For example, José, a Mexican-American internist at a teaching hospital, spoke of the experience of treating a diabetic African American patient who vehemently refused an eye exam that was long over-due. Upon his inquiry, the patient told a story of having been humiliated 'like a dog' by the staff at ophthalmology several years ago. José decided to 'take this corporate responsibility' and apologized to the patient:

> So I apologize to the patient. I say, 'You know, this may be coming very late, and it may not come from the person that needs to

apologize, but on behalf of Valley University Hospital [pseudonym], let me apologize to you, and let me say that this is not the way we want to practice medicine. And that we let you down once, and I don't want this to happen again, but we need to take care of your eyes.' There's a happy ending here in that, after encouraging her, she did go back to ophthalmology, saw a different provider, had an entirely different experience, and she was grateful at the end.

José's admission about the hospital staff's wrongdoings affirmed the validity of the patient's experience and feelings. This laid the ground for the doctor to introduce some redeeming features of the medical institution and to ask for a second chance. The clinical interaction reached a turning point.

Some patient groups were alienated from the medical profession through past experiences and, even if they believed medicine could be a caring institution, they were predisposed to thinking that this caring was mainly designed for other, more mainstream groups. Sudha, an internist of Indian descent, noted that in her experiences, African American patients appeared guarded and un-engaged during clinical encounters. To relate to these patients, Sudha used a framework to introduce medical intervention that was grounded in substantial understandings of, and identification with, the problems with the medical institution that the group had experienced. Sudha described it as the 'we thing', or a mutual inclusion:

> Remember I was saying before with the 'we thing'? I think there's an inclusion. . . . So, I educate myself about African American health. So I'll say, 'You know, African American women are among the bottom of the barrel when it comes to heart disease. I bet that you guys get served the absolute worst.' . . . [Then,] it's like—oh, you're paying attention to my people? . . . So your care is tailored to my thing, my health problems? I'd say, 'For unknown reasons, your population doesn't do well with AIDS inhibitors. We

don't know why, but you don't.' And when I make comments like that, there's a trust.

A similar example was offered by José about an African American patient who was in the hospital with a series of small heart attacks. The medical interviews indicated that the patient had refused all study or intervention, with full understanding of the risks of his course of action. When José assumed his care, he 'sat down and spoke to him at length':

> I said, 'It's interesting, because the literature tells us that often African Americans get these procedures less often.' So he said, 'Well, what are we talking about in terms of the procedure that I might have?' And so I explained to him what a bypass operation was, a revascularization procedure was, and after all of that, he said, 'Really? That's what we're talking about?' I said, 'Yes.' He said, 'So, let me get this straight, now. If I had this done, is it possible that I could live another year?' 'Sir, I mean, you might live *many* years, you know, if this were done.' And he looked at me quite seriously, 'You know, no one's ever taken the time to explain that to me'. . . . For this patient, I don't know . . . did he think it was experimental?

Like Sudha, José's knowledge of medicine's 'unequal treatment' for certain patient groups both acknowledged particular failings of the health-care system and conveyed a sense of identification with the patient's predicament. On this basis, the doctors found connections between understandings framed in 'medicine-as-it-should-be' (doctors' ideals) and 'medicine-as-it-is' (patients' experiences), with the hope of finding an acceptable role for medical intervention in their patients' life contexts.

3. Establishing Long-Term Relationships

Beyond the cultural translation between health systems or images of medicine, my interviewees had to decipher other puzzling modes of expression or sense-making schemas, which were informed less by health systems than by patients' life contexts. The distance between the culturally and socially marginalized patients and their doctors made this medicine–lifeworld gap wider than usual. To bridge this cultural gap, doctors emphasized that it was often through long-term interactions that they were able to piece together patients' life contexts that might have shaped their puzzling expressions or schemas. This aspect of cultural brokerage helped doctors pursue patient-centered goals such as better understandings of 'patient-as-person' and the social and psychological factors of their diseases.

My interviewees' discussions revealed three reasons why continuity of care was particularly important for their cultural brokerage work in inter-ethnic settings. First, patients were not always aware of their own cultural frameworks and therefore could not always explicitly convey them to their doctors. Instead, doctors needed to observe these lifeworld orientations over time. For example, Maria recalled being puzzled and overwhelmed by some patients' expressions of pain. It was only through long-term interactions that Maria realized that, in some cultures, '[patients] don't express emotional pain very comfortably, and so they do it in the context of physical pain'.

Second, doctors also observed that patients sometimes felt shame for their life conditions and were reluctant to discuss them. In these situations, long-term interactions provided an important context in which patients might gradually become comfortable with sharing relevant lifeworld concerns. Maria recalled having treated several Latino male patients for depression, who had left their entire family at home and crossed the border illegally in order to work wage-earning jobs and send remittances home. Her patients often interpreted these experiences as their failures and therefore refused to discuss them. Maria needed to establish continuity of care with them before they might be open to broaching these topics.

Furthermore, it is noteworthy that continuity of care surfaced as an important theme in doctors' discussions of how to avoid stereotyping. Most

interviewees considered general understandings of group cultures as useful guidelines for what to ask or observe during clinical interactions, but they also emphasized the importance of capturing individual variations. For some, this meant understanding how multiple structural forces came together to shape a patient's cultural orientation, for example, gender, class, education experience, and immigration history, in addition to ethnicity. Others did not explicate the connection between culture and multiple structures, but they too debunked the common assumption that ethnicity defines one's culture, favoring a more contextual and nuanced understanding of culture. In practice, either the former constructionist perspective or the latter 'thick description' approach might not completely resolve the tensions between group categories and individual traits; upon probing, most doctors conceded as much. They acknowledged that important details were inevitably left out during the 15-minute clinical consultations, however sensitive and interactive they attempted to be. Thus, they needed the 'second chances', only available in long-term relationships, in order to approach a more multifaceted understanding of their patients.

Operating with the understanding that a female Peruvian diabetic patient of hers might be predisposed to being overly agreeable for cultural reasons, Maria made extra efforts to confirm that 'the patient's yes really meant yes'. For a while, Maria was getting reassuring signs. The patient's self-recorded blood sugar levels showed great improvement. She was extremely happy that her diabetes was finally being controlled. But as it turned out, the patient was becoming hypoglycemic without telling Maria: 'She didn't want me to feel bad . . . she was even checking her sugar but she wouldn't write down the ones that were too low because she didn't want to worry me.'

Although Maria was sensitive to how female Peruvian patients generally 'had this upper respect of doctors', she could not have anticipated that this patient's cultural orientation would be manifested, in this particular context, in her deliberate alteration of 'disappointing' information in her written records. It was only in their long-term interactions that Maria could eventually learn of what she had missed:

> [The patient] ended up in the hospital, and then when I went to see her, I was like, 'Are you sick? Did something happen? Did you not eat?' 'No, I've been feeling dizzy for a while, and my daughter came to visit from Peru, and decided I should come to the hospital.

Had Maria seen the patient only on a short-term basis, she might not have had a chance to learn the complete story. Yet these forms of short-term care were often the only available healthcare services for many low-income immigrant patients, as the following example shows.

Perla, a Hispanic American medical student who volunteered at a Spanish-speaking community clinic, recalled how her brokerage work between medicine and lifeworld was sabotaged by the conditions that prevented long-term interactions. According to the medical records of an elderly Latina patient with diabetes, for two years she had repeatedly refused insulin, allegedly with full understanding of the risks of her course of action. When Perla engaged her in longer and less structured conversations, it eventually became clear that the patient was almost blind and thus fearful of injecting herself with the wrong dosage of insulin. She was poor, spoke only Spanish, and therefore could receive care only at Perla's clinic, which operated only on Saturdays and could not come to her aid if she were to overdose herself on other days of the week. The patient revealed that, in her mind, it was more important to avoid crises than to manage her chronic illness. As Perla understood her patient's sense-making schemas—how she evaluated short-term risks (e.g. wrong dosages of insulin) versus long-term health (e.g. controlling the diabetes), the provider realized that the patient had good reasons to be 'non-compliant'. The important understanding and trust that Perla established through her sensitive communication and relational styles, however, was short-lived. The community clinic was staffed almost exclusively by voluntary, Spanish-speaking medical students, and soon Perla's term of voluntary work there was

over and someone else took over her post. When asked whether the patient continued to discuss possible courses of action with her new doctor, Perla admitted, with regret, that she did not know.

4. Working With Patients' Relational Networks

For some doctors, time constraints, the unavailability of quality medical interpretation, and their own limited language ability or cultural familiarity all presented significant barriers for them to individually shoulder the burden of navigating between different health systems or brokering between medicine and a cross-cultural lifeworld. These doctors explored an alternative—working with a variety of community figures or networks. This model provided an avenue for doctors to achieve the same goal as directly engaging themselves in various dimensions of cultural brokerage, while keeping some boundaries around their responsibilities and workload.

Most often, however, working with community networks served a different purpose. Doctors viewed this as a way to retain or recreate part of the familiar milieu in which patients would feel comfortable with in-depth sharing and adopting new ideas and practices. This dimension of cultural brokerage focused on grounding clinical communication in the relational networks deemed most conducive to enacting patients' 'habitus' for sharing, learning, and accepting medical intervention. Thus, working with community networks pursued similar goals as the emphasis on 'patient-as-person' in general patient-centered care. But here doctors noted the limits of cultural brokerage that relied solely on bettering their own cultural knowledge and communication skills. Rather than incorporating information about life contexts into clinical communication, they viewed communication itself as context-bound.

The most common example of the effort to work with community networks took a semi-institutionalized form. Known as 'group visits' among the medical community, these settings turned peers into cultural brokers for each other. Typically, a clinic organized small (10–12 people) groups consisting of patients of the same ethnicity and/or the same medical condition, which would meet weekly to discuss their issues, progress, and questions. A physician or nurse practitioner usually coordinated the meeting, but informal discussion and interaction was actively encouraged.

Most interviewees were extremely positive about the effects of group visits. They observed that the setting turned medical encounters into more enjoyable social gatherings among peers. Thomas, a family physician of Japanese descent at a county hospital, noted that patients were much more forthcoming in sharing their life stories in these gatherings. Alice, a Jewish family doctor at a community clinic, felt that when patients heard solutions from each other instead of directly from her, they seemed to remember better. Sue, a Caucasian family doctor at a community clinic, thought that they were able to provide reassurance for each other as fellow travelers in ways that she could not imitate. For doctors who found it challenging to tap deeply into an individual patient's life context, group visits reproduced parts of these contexts at the clinic for them.

Some physicians worked with patients in the context of their relational networks, especially among patient groups that lived in tightly woven communities. Having worked extensively with Mien and Khmu immigrant groups, Thomas observed that written materials, institutionalized procedures, and the like, were foreign and ineffective problem-solving mechanisms for these groups, because 'that's not the training from their lives. That's not the experience [that they are used to]'. Instead, working with networks and community leaders was more accepted:

> It's, 'I'm going to ask my neighbor for this thing, for this farming implement, or help the harvest thing', or whatever it was. . . . So, if it's not right there within their community, it's hard to access, so if we could promote these relationships among them where they know, 'Oh, this is the go-to person who I could call in Mien, and not have to deal with any office or anything', it seems to help them better. *It's almost more dealing with their network than with them as an individual.*

Doctors like Thomas thought that the provider's recommendations, even culturally sensitive ones, could be ineffective with these groups, because learning new things from an office was 'not the practice'. Rather, his patients' 'practice' of adopting new messages or changed behaviors was channeled through their social networks. These examples illustrate a Bourdieu-informed understanding of clinical communications. They suggest that as much as clinical communication involves information exchange and sharing of meanings, it is also a social practice, whose form must be rendered familiar through patients' cultural schemas.

LIMITATIONS OF CULTURAL BROKERAGE

Taken as a whole, the doctors in this study strived for successful cultural brokerage through micro-level clinical interactions. While their efforts as individual providers were important, their experiences also revealed that the room for cultural brokerage was limited by macro cultural and structural forces of the healthcare system. Doctors could certainly fail in aspects of cultural brokerage, as Li-Chin's earlier confession testified, but it would be a misconception to expect that sharpened skills of cultural competency alone could overcome these institutional hurdles.

The Cultural Constraint

As they engaged in the work of cultural brokerage, the doctors often encountered a dilemma: their Western notion of personhood would at times be challenged, while satisfactory alternatives were not easily available. Patient autonomy defines one of the predominant ethical principles in American medicine: patients are regarded as autonomous, rational actors who, upon receiving adequate input from physicians, are ultimately in charge of making their own healthcare decisions. In clinical interactions, doctors are called to respect and carefully respond to patients' specific concerns. They also must respect the patient's ability and freedom to carry out their responsibilities. To encroach upon the patient's autonomy would be an act of disempowering paternalism.

This ideal of patient autonomy, however, may sometimes contradict the goal of cultural competency. Most interviewees noted that immigrant and minority patients were particularly disadvantaged, as they had little cultural resources to enact the role of the ideal 'autonomous patient'. At a deeper level, the individualistic assumption implied in patient autonomy sometimes clashed with other cultural heritages. Aaron's experience was illustrative. This Caucasian pediatrician, who once helped his Hmong patients' family sacrifice a pig at the hospital, was highly devoted to patient advocacy. But when interacting with patients or families who deviated from the norm of autonomous individuals, Aaron found himself at a loss:

> I have had Muslim families where the father makes the decision, and the mother, it's not her business. . . . If he says one thing, and then she later says that she feels something else, what do you do with that? . . . If I say to her, 'Well, why don't you say that when we're sitting all together?' she says, 'I can't say that, because he's there.' *It's these kinds of things that just become this quagmire.*

Pattie, a Caucasian family doctor at a county hospital, described it well. With some of her immigrant patients:

> I feel like whatever [the patient] is telling me or is being presented is sort of the family agreement. . . . I'm not really sure whether she's communicating what she wants to say, *or if there is such a thing as 'what she wants to say', versus what the family wants.*

Whereas the dominant model of medical ethics was limited by its narrow focus on patient autonomy, the newer practices of narrative ethics (e.g. Charon, 2001) were more attentive to grounding clinical experiences in the patient's lifeworld relationships. But this new model seemed under-developed in its

notion of privacy rights and, at times, would fail to adequately inform decision making in delicate situations. Maria, for example, struggled intensely with who to release her diagnosis to, when she found out that a patient, to whom she had been communicating through the patient's daughter, had terminal cancer. In some cases, the patient's family simply insisted on protecting her from this type of depressing information. Seen through their cultural frameworks, discussion of death with the patient was extremely ill-omened; the family would naturally assume agency for the patient in such conversations. While my interviewees were committed to adapting their care to their patients' relational personhood and family connectedness, they nevertheless felt that the notion of relational ethics or narrative medicine provided limited tools for them to 'evaluate' this connectedness when it directly compromised patient autonomy or doctor–patient confidentiality.

Thus, the 'culture' of American medicine is itself rooted in and structured by certain philosophical understandings of personhood, autonomy, and confidentiality. Discussions of illness experiences and narratives as well as multicultural clinical encounters have encouraged welcomed reflections upon these basic tenets of American medical ethics, but an alternative model is still in the making and leaves some challenging questions unanswered.

The Structural Constraint

The doctors' cultural brokerage work, as discussed earlier, sometimes required material conditions that could nurture deeper clinical interaction and continuity of care. But given the current political economy of the US healthcare system, there were few resources available to fund longer consultations, continuity of care, or regular group visits, especially at low-income clinics frequented by immigrant and minority patients. To be sure, the impact of limited resources on access to healthcare has been widely documented, but what I wish to point out here is that the issue of resources also has a serious impact on how well doctors' cultural skills can be performed.

Sheri, a Jewish family doctor, offered an interesting example from the teaching hospital where she worked. As an attempt to help their patients adjust to the relatively rigid regimen of Western medicine, staff at the hospital had developed a visual system for organizing medications at home:

> We have these cards that have a picture of the sun, the morning, and then in the afternoon, and then at night, and then the moon, so that you could . . . tape the pills in the order that the patient needs to take them. . . . If they need to take their pills twice a day, you'll tape one pill on the little sun rising, and then one where the sun's coming down.

Sensitive to a more relaxed notion of time among some patient groups, the doctors at Sheri's hospital designed this approach to help these patients learn to adopt a new practice—taking their medication regularly. While it was a good example of cultural translation, some things were inevitably lost in the process. Sheri recalled an encounter in which the doctor used this visual system to explain to the patient how to take her medication. When the patient came back a few weeks later, her blood pressure remained dangerously high. The patient became angry, because she had ventured out of her comfort zone to follow, in her mind, everything her doctor asked of her. But as it turned out, the patient had just taken the pills off of the card, using them for only one day—she did not understand that she needed to take them every day following the card as an example.

From the doctor's perspective, in an ideal world, she should try even harder to help the patient understand the new practice, but in the fast-paced everyday reality of the hospital, she could not afford to endlessly delay seeing her other patients. Similarly, Perla's earlier example showed how the lack of continuity of care prematurely ended her cultural brokerage work just as she was making a breakthrough.

My interviewees expressed frustration, despair, or even cynicism about their pursuits of cultural competency under these conditions. Most admitted to resorting to personal solutions to the structural problems. Working overtime was common, though so were feelings of burn-out. Several, like Sudha, reflected that their cultural brokerage efforts were inconsistent:

> Sometimes you just feel overwhelmed . . . you just want to be able to write that prescription, and 'Here [you] go.' . . . [You] don't try to get into the mind, because it takes so much time. You don't have enough time. . . . You mean well, but. . . . So, no, right now as it stands, *the sociopolitical pressures of the practice of medicine, no we don't have those resources.*

Aaron put it bluntly:

> [Policy makers] want people to become culturally competent . . . , but they don't want to pay for [longer talking time]. And the problem is, until people pay for it, it ain't gonna happen. . . . I think that actually a lot of the issues about improving communication and cultural competence are going to *go absolutely nowhere.*

CONCLUSION

A rich and diverse literature exists on how to achieve goals of cultural competency and patient-centeredness through lifeworld-oriented questions, sensitive communication skills, and power-sharing interaction styles. While these models focus on how to elicit patients' lifeworld voices, in cross-cultural settings, the gap between the culture of medicine and the patients' health concepts as well as lifeworld cultures can be so wide that it requires additional bridging work. Without this bridging work, a doctor lacks the cultural tool to incorporate her patient's assumptions (e.g. about food and nutrition or about the relationships between doctors and minority patients) and habitus (e.g. predispositions for feeling ashamed about own life conditions or feeling reluctant to learn new things from a medical office) into the voice of medicine, rendering it difficult to

TABLE 29.1 ■ Mechanisms of Cultural Brokerage		
	Rendering Patient Cultures Recognizable by Medicine	Rendering Medicine Recognizable by Patient Cultures
Cultural translation between incongruent frameworks	Translating between health systems	Bridging divergent images of medicine
Cultivating relational contexts that enable learning	Establishing long-term relationships	Working with patients' relational networks

(at least partially) expand and transform the latter from within.

This study explores how doctors perform this cultural work, conceptualized as cultural brokerage, on the job. Cultural brokerage entails the mutual inclusion of two sets of seemingly incommensurate sense-making schemas or orientations so that there is a basis for sharing meanings and narratives. Doctors perform this cultural work through translating conceptual categories between the two meaning systems and creating relational contexts that extend beyond the standard brief clinical visits. This cultural work aims to render patient cultures more recognizable by medicine and vice versa. Table 29.1 provides a brief summary of these empirical patterns of cultural brokerage.

The last aspect, working with patient's relational networks, merits a clarifying note. This mechanism stresses the importance of recreating or retaining the relational milieu in which the patient actually feels familiar, rather than relying on community organizations or leaders that claim representativeness for the group. The distinction registers the possibility that doctors might romanticize the community, overlooking distrust, in-fighting, and other nuanced group dynamics (see Wayland and Crowder, 2002). Healthcare professionals should be aware that their understanding of the community might differ from how patients actually negotiate their social ties.

The notion of cultural brokerage extends Lo and Stacey's (2008) Bourdieu-informed conceptualization of patient culture, which theorizes how patients 'mix and match' cultural schemas in the lifeworld. While Lo and Stacey (2008) acknowledge that the 'mixing and matching' process is likely to continue

through clinical interaction, they do not specify how. The mechanisms of cultural brokerage explicate the interaction and mutual inclusion between the techno-professional meaning system and the patient's hybridized, less than fully aware, cultural schemas. Healthcare professionals should be aware that they do not simply stand apart from and study patient culture; rather, they actively participate in its transformation through their successful, failed, or neglected cultural brokerage.

Cultural brokerage is concrete 'work'; the performance of this 'cultural labor' must be recognized as embedded in the organizational contexts of the clinic and, more broadly, the structure of American healthcare. While individual physicians' cultural skills are essential, their practice of cultural brokerage cannot be sustainable or consistent without the resources to fund in-depth consultations and continuity of care. Certainly, no one is naïve enough to assume that cultural competency will solve the problem of resources, but this study emphasizes that even to adequately handle cultural barriers, structural changes are essential. The pretense that a cultural solution can address structural problems is costly; as we have seen, it leads to despair and cynicism among providers.

Similarly, the dominant notion of patient autonomy in American medicine sometimes clashes with other cultural traditions. But as doctors explore more relational modes of interaction, they too face difficulties with properly protecting their patients' privacy and confidentiality. For future research, social scientists are challenged to strive for a richer understanding of doctor–patient partnership that may better integrate the principles of rationality and relationality.

Notes

1. Bourdieu (1977) conceptualizes 'habitus' as mental structures, or dispositions, orientations, and schemas, that develop from an individual's constant exposure to social conditions from her class position. Bourdieu emphasizes that social actors, for the most part, operate with their 'habitus' without much self-awareness. 'It is because subjects do not, strictly speaking, know what they are doing that what they do has more meaning than they know' (Bourdieu, 1977: 79). Drawing upon recent sociological theories of structure and agency, Lo and Stacey (2008) further develop the notion of 'hybrid habitus', which expands Bourdieu's habitus in a number of ways: (1) individuals' orientations and schemas are recognized as shaped by not only class structure but multiple social structures (see also Sewell, 1992); (2) these orientations and schemas are seen as functioning not only in a habitual manner, but sometimes with a great deal of the individual's awareness and creativity (see also Emirbayer and Mische, 1998).

2. The lifeworld can be briefly defined as the everyday social world where 'individuals interact with others to decide and organize their affairs in the private sphere of their own families or households or in the wider public sphere' (Greenhalgh et al., 2006: 1171). In this everyday world, according to Habermas, interaction and communication are largely grounded in life experiences and oriented toward the goal of mutual understanding. In contrast, the system, for Habermas, is comprised of the State and the market, whose agents operate with decontextualized rules and pursue goals that are defined in technical and instrumental terms. Habermas argues that the system constantly intrudes into the lifeworld in late modern societies, distorting communication and social interactions.

Viewing Western medicine as an aspect of the system, scholars have drawn upon Habermas's theory to study how the technocratic biomedical framework distorts patients' everyday experiences and narratives during clinical interactions. See Barry et al. (2001), Greenhalgh et al. (2006), Mishler (1984), and Porter (1998).

3. The term 'cultural translation' generally refers to the reproduction of the same statement or story across cultural divides. As meaning is relationally produced and context-specific, cultural translation necessarily entails the paradox of telling the same story in different terms, or creating 'the difference of the same' (Bhabha, 1994: 22). Taking this paradox as the point of departure, many scholars of multiculturalism investigate cultural translation in terms of a process in which dominant groups learn to recognize how their own cultural values and ideals are manifested in diverse, minority cultures (e.g. Alexander, 2001), thereby debunking the black/white, East/West, or more generally self/other dichotomy. Conversely, postcolonial scholars often focus on the transformative and disruptive nature of cultural translation, emphasizing that 'placed in a new discursive structure, deformation and displacement of the 'original' meaning are inevitable' (Sakamoto, 1996: 115; see also Bhabha, 1994). As will be illustrated below, doctors' cultural translation centers on deciphering the very paradox of how a core idea can be expressed differently. For example, how can a prescription for calcium pills be effectively

re-stated in the patient's system of health concepts? Alternatively, if an immigrant patient desires to work effectively with her physical therapist in the American context, what new habits and understandings might she need to develop?

4. It is interesting that Daniel chose the word 'hybridizing' to describe the 'mix and match' between the American doctor's and the immigrant patient's models. Theoretically minded readers will find his notion suggestive of some postcolonial scholars'

argument that cultural translation, itself an act of boundary-crossing, inevitably creates a hybrid identity that brings together elements from both cultures. Scholars have debated long and hard over the political implications of hybridity, with varying arguments about its potential for critical and creative thinking (e.g. Bhabha, 1994) or the limitations of such potential (e.g. Marotta, 2008; Sakamoto, 1996). But it is beyond the scope of this article to detail these discussions here.

References

Alexander JC (2001) Theorizing the 'Modes of Incorporation': Assimilation, Hyphenation, and Multiculturalism as Varieties of Civil Participation. *Sociological Theory* 19(3): 237–249.

Barbee E (1987) Tensions in the Brokerage Role: Nurses in Botswana. *Western Journal of Nursing Research* 9(2): 244–256.

Barry CA, Stevenson FA, Britten N, Barber N, and Bradley CP (2001) Giving Voice to the Lifeworld: More Humane, More Effective Medical Care? A Qualitative Study of Doctor–Patient Communication in General Practice. *Social Science & Medicine* 53(4): 487–505.

Beck RS, Daughtridge R, and Sloane PD (2002) Physician–Patient Communication in the Primary Care Office: A Systematic Review. *Journal of the American Board of Family Practice* 15(1): 25–38.

Betancourt JR, Green AR, Carrillo JM, and Park ER (2005) Cultural Competence and Health Care Disparities: Key Perspectives and Trends. *Health Affairs* 24(2): 499–505.

Bhabha H (1994) *The Location of Culture*. London: Routledge.

Bourdieu P (1977) *Outline of a Theory of Practice*. Cambridge: Cambridge University Press.

Brach C, Fraserirector I (2000) Can Cultural Competency Reduce Racial and Ethnic Health Disparities? A Review and Conceptual Model. *Medical Care Research and Review* 57(Suppl. 1): 181–217.

Brody H (1994) 'My Story Is Broken; Can You Help Me Fix It?' Medical Ethics and the Joint Construction of Narrative. *Literature and Medicine* 13(1): 79–92.

Charon R (2001) Narrative Medicine: A Model for Empathy, Reflection, Profession, and Trust. *Journal of the American Medical Association* 286(915): 1897–1902.

Connelly JE (2005) Narrative Possibilities: Using Mindfulness in Clinical Practice. *Perspectives in Biology and Medicine* 48(1): 84–94.

Cooper LA, Roter DL, and Johnson RL (2003) Patient-Centered Communication, Ratings of Care, and Concordance of Patient and Physician Race. *Annals of Internal Medicine* 139(11): 907–915.

Emirbayer M, Mische, A (1998) What Is Agency? *American Journal of Sociology* 103(4): 962–1023.

Frank A (1995) *The Wounded Storyteller: Body, Illness and Ethics.* Chicago, IL: University of Chicago Press.

Gershon I (2006) When Culture Is Not a System: Why Samoan Cultural Brokers Can Not Do Their Job. *Ethnos* 71(4): 533–558.

Good BJ, Good MJD (2000) 'Fiction' and 'Historicity' in Doctors' Stories: Social and Narrative Dimensions of Learning Medicine. In: Mattingly C, Garro LC (eds) *Narrative and the Cultural Construction of Illness and Healing.* Berkeley, CA: University of California Press, 50–69.

Good MJD (2004) Narrative Nuances on Good and Bad Deaths: Internists' Tales from High-Technology Work Places. *Social Science & Medicine* 58(5): 939–953.

Good MJD, James C, Good BJ, and Becker AE (2002) *The Culture of Medicine and Racial, Ethnic, and Class Disparities in Health.* Russell Sage Foundation Working Paper #199.

Greenhalgh T, Robb N, and Scambler G (2006) Communicative and Strategic Action in Interpreted Consultations in Primary Health Care: A Habermasian Perspective. *Social Science & Medicine* 63(5): 1170–1187.

Hsieh E (2006) Conflicts in How Interpreters Manage Their Roles in Provider–Patient Interactions. *Social Science & Medicine* 62(3): 721–730.

Hunt LM, De Voogd KB (2005) Clinical Myths of the Cultural 'Other': Implications for Latino Patient Care. *Academic Medicine* 80(10): 918–924.

Hunter KM (1991) *Doctors' Stories: The Narrative Structure of Medical Knowledge.* Princeton, NJ: Princeton University Press.

Hunter KM (1996) Narrative, Literature, and the Clinical Exercise of Practical Reason. *Journal of Medicine and Philosophy* 21(3): 321–340.

Jezewski MA (1990) Cultural Brokering in Migrant Farmworker Health Care. *Western Journal of Nursing Research* 12(4): 497–513.

Kagawa-Singer M, Blackhall LJ (2001) Negotiating Cross-Cultural Issues at the End of Life: 'You Got to Go Where He Lives'. *Journal of the American Medical Association* 286(23): 2993–3001.

Kleinman A (1980) *Patients and Healers in the Context of Culture: An Exploration of the Borderland between Anthropology, Medicine, and Psychiatry.* Berkeley, CA: University of California Press.

Kleinman A (1988) *The Illness Narratives: Suffering, Healing, and the Human Condition.* New York: Basic Books.

Liamputtong P (2005) Birth and Social Class: Northern Thai Women's Lived Experiences of Caesarean and Vaginal Birth. *Sociology of Health and Illness* 27(2): 243–270.

Lo MCM, Stacey CL (2008) Beyond Cultural Competency: Bourdieu, Patients and Clinical Encounters. *Sociology of Health & Illness* 30(5): 741–755.

Malat J, Hamilton MA (2006) Preference for Same-Race Health Care Providers and Perceptions of Interpersonal Discrimination in Health Care. *Journal of Health and Social Behavior* 47(2): 173–187.

Marotta VP (2008) The Hybrid Self and the Ambivalence of Boundaries. *Social Identities* 14(3): 295–312.

Mattingly C (1998a) *Healing Dramas and Clinical Plots: The Narrative Structure of Experience.* Chicago, IL: Cambridge University Press.

Mattingly C (1998b) 'In Search of the Good: Narrative Reasoning in Clinical Practice. *Medical Anthropology Quarterly* 12(3): 273–297.

Mead N, Bower P (2000) Patient-Centeredness: A Conceptual Framework and Review of the Empirical Literature. *Social Science & Medicine* 51(7): 1087–1110.

Mishler EG (1984) *The Discourse of Medicine: The Dialectics of Medical Interviews.* Norwood, NJ: Ablex.

Office of Minority Health (2001) *National Standards for Culturally and Linguistically Appropriate Services in Health Care: Final Report.* Washington, DC: US Dept of Health and Human Services, OPHS.

Paez KA, Allen JK, Carson KA, and Cooper LA (2008) Provider and Clinic Cultural Competence in a Primary Care Setting. *Social Science & Medicine* 66(5): 1204–1216.

Perloff RM, Bonder B, Ray GB, Ray EB, and Siminoff LA (2006) Doctor–Patient Communication, Cultural Competence, and Minority Health: Theoretical and Empirical Perspectives. *American Behavioral Scientist* 49(6): 835–852.

Porter S (1998) *Social Theory and Nursing Practice.* London: Macmillan.

Sakamoto R (1996) Japan, Hybridity and the Creation of Colonial Discourse. *Theory, Culture, and Society* 13(3): 113–128.

Sewell WH (1992) A Theory of Structure: Duality, Agency and Transformation. *America Journal of Sociology* 98(1): 1–29.

Smedley BD, Stith AY, and Nelson AR (eds) (2003) *Unequal Treatment: Confronting Racial and Ethnic Disparities in Health Care.* Committee on Understanding and Eliminating Racial and Ethnic Disparities in Health Care, Board on Health Sciences Policy, Institute of Medicine. Washington, DC: National Academy Press.

Street RL, Jr, Gordon H, and Haidet P (2007) Physicians' Communication and Perceptions of Patients: Is It How They Look, How They Talk, or Is It Just the Doctor? *Social Science & Medicine* 65(3): 586–598.

Tripp-Reimer T, Brink PJ (1985) Culture Brokerage. In: Bulechek GM, McCloskey JC (eds) *Nursing Interventions: Treatments for Nursing Diagnoses.* Philadelphia, PA: Saunders, 352–364.

Wayland C, Crowder J (2002) Disparate Views of Community in Primary Health Care: Understanding How Perceptions Influence Success. *Medical Anthropology Quarterly* 16(2): 230–247.

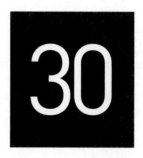

SOCIAL DEATH AS
SELF-FULFILLING PROPHECY

Stefan Timmermans

Although death is supposedly the great equalizer, social scientists have abundantly documented the social inequality of death via mortality statistics (see e.g., Feinstein 1993; Kitagawa and Hauser 1973; Waldron 1997). Recently researchers have paid less attention to possible social inequality in the dying process itself. One of the most powerful and detailed sociological formulations to account for social inequality in the process of dying is still David Sudnow's classical study *Passing On* (1967). Sudnow argued that the health care staff decided how to administer their care giving based on *the patient's social value:* patients with perceived low social worth were much less likely to be resuscitated aggressively than patients with a perceived high social value. Since Sudnow's study, the health care field has undergone dramatic change (Conrad 1997; Starr 1982). Especially with the advent and widespread use of resuscitation techniques, biomedical researchers have encapsulated medical knowledge

about lifesaving in sophisticated protocols, and legislators have instituted legal protections both to encourage resuscitative efforts and to secure patient's autonomy. The objective of this article is to evaluate the extent to which Sudnow's earlier claims about social inequality are still relevant in a transformed health care context that promotes a rational approach to medical practice and is influenced by extensive legal protections.

The purpose of resuscitative interventions is to reverse an ongoing dying process and preserve human lives. In most resuscitative efforts, however, the final result is a deceased patient (Eisenberg, Horwood, Cummins et al. 1990). When this result is the likely outcome of the resuscitative attempt, the staff's task is to avoid prolonged and unnecessary suffering and prepare for the patient's impending death. Saving lives requires an aggressive approach, whereas alleviating suffering demands that the staff intervenes minimally in the dying process and

Social Death as Self-Fulfilling Prophecy, Stefan Timmermans in *The Sociological Quarterly, 39*(3), 453–472, June 1998. With permission from Taylor & Francis.

focuses on relieving pain and assisting relatives and friends. An aggressive resuscitative effort for an irreversibly dying (or already biologically dead) patient is not only futile but robs the dying patient of dignity (Callahan 1993; Moller 1996). It becomes a violation of the patient, a caricature of medical acumen (Illich 1976). A low-key resuscitative effort without much conviction for a still viable patient is regarded as passive euthanasia (Siner 1989).

How does the staff—as gatekeepers between life and death (Pelligrino 1986)—decide in the relative short time span of a resuscitative trajectory (Glaser and Strauss 1968) to resuscitate aggressively or to let the patient go with minimal medical interference? In the early 1960s, social scientists demonstrated that those apparently moral questions rest upon deep social foundations (Fox 1976). In death and dying, the fervor of the staff's intervention depends mostly on the patient's perceived social worth (Glaser and Strauss 1964; Sudnow 1967). In one of the first studies of resuscitative efforts in hospitals, Sudnow provided appalling insights into the social rationing[1] of the dying process. He argued that depending on striking social characteristics—such as the patient's age, "moral character," and clinical teaching value—certain groups of people were more likely than others to be treated as "socially dead." According to Sudnow (1967, p. 74), social death is a situation in which "a patient is treated essentially as a corpse, though perhaps still 'clinically' and 'biologically' alive." The most disturbing aspect of Sudnow's analysis was his observation that social death becomes a predictor for biological death during resuscitative attempts. People who were regarded as socially dead by the staff were more likely to die a biological death sooner as well. Under the guise of lifesaving attempts, the staff perpetuated an insidious kind of social inequality.

Zygmunt Bauman has questioned whether Sudnow's observations are still relevant. Bauman (1992, p. 145) postulated that because resuscitative efforts have "lost much of their specularity and have ceased to impress, their discriminating power has all but dissipated."[2] Biomedical researchers and legislators appear to agree by omitting social rationing from a vast medical, legal, and ethical resuscitation literature.[3] The rationalization of medical knowledge

was supposed to turn the "art" of medical practice into a "science" (Berg 1997) and eliminate the social problems of a still experimental medical technology. After countless pilot and evaluation studies, national collaborations, and international conferences, medical researchers created uniform and universally employed resuscitation protocols supported by a resuscitation theory (CPR-ECC 1973; 1992). Biomedical researchers have interpreted clinical decision making in terms of formal probabilistic reasoning and algorithms that link clinical data inputs with therapeutic decision outputs (Schwartz and Griffin 1986; Dowie and Elstein 1988). Health care providers reach decisions during lifesaving efforts by simply following the resuscitation protocols until they run into an endpoint. The data taken into consideration consist solely of observable clinical parameters and biomedical test results. In lifesaving, social factors should be irrelevant and filtered out.

In addition, legislators instituted extensive legal protections against any form of discrimination, including social rationing. Legislators made it obligatory for health care providers to initiate cardiopulmonary resuscitation (CPR) in all instances in which it is medically indicated (CPR-ECC 1973). Paramedics and other health care providers have the legal duty to respond and apply all professional and regional standards of care, that is, they should follow the protocols to the end. Consent is implied for emergency care such as resuscitative efforts. To further legally encourage resuscitative measures, first-aid personnel are immune from prosecution for errors rendered in good faith emergency care under the Samaritan laws.[4] Failure to continue treatment, however, is referred to as abandonment that "is legally and ethically the most serious act an emergency medical technician can commit" (Heckman 1992, p. 21). Basically, once the emergency medical system is alerted, the health care providers have the legal and ethical duty to continue resuscitating until the protocols are exhausted.

At the same time, ethicists and legislators have tried to boost and protect patient autonomy. The Patient Self-Determination Act of 1991[5] mandated that patients be given notice of their rights to make medical treatment decisions and of the legal instruments available to give force to decisions made in advance. This attempt at demedicalizing (Conrad 1992) sudden death again is indirectly aimed at diminishing social rationing. When patients have decided that they do not want to be resuscitated, the staff should follow the written directives regardless of the patient's social value.

Did these scientific and medicolegal initiatives remove the social rationing in sudden death exposed by Sudnow, and Glaser and Strauss? I will show that biomedical protocols and legal initiatives did not weaken but reinforced inequality of death and dying. In the emergency department (ED), health care providers reappropriate biomedical theory and advance directives to justify and refine a moral categorization of patients. Furthermore, although the legal protections indeed result in prolonged resuscitative efforts, this does not necessarily serve the patient. The goal of lifesaving becomes subordinated to other objectives. The result is a more sophisticated, theoretically supported, and legally sanctioned configuration of social discrimination when sudden death strikes. The unwillingness of Western societies to accommodate certain marginalized groups and the medicalization of natural processes neutralize the equalizing potential of the rationalization of resuscitation techniques and legal protections.

METHODOLOGY

This article is based on 112 observations of resuscitative efforts over a fourteen-month period in the EDs of two midwestern hospitals: one was a level-1 and the other a level-2 trauma center.[6] I focused my observations on medical out-of-hospital resuscitative efforts. This research was approved by the institutional review board of the two hospitals and by the University of Illinois. I was paged with the other resuscitation team members whenever a resuscitative effort was needed in these EDs. I attended half of the resuscitative efforts that occurred in the two EDs during the observation period.

In addition to the observations, I interviewed forty-two health care providers who work in EDs and routinely participate in resuscitative efforts.

This group includes physicians, nurses, respiratory therapists, nurse supervisors, emergency room technicians, social workers, and chaplains. These health care providers came from three hospitals: the two hospitals in which I observed resuscitative efforts and one bigger level-1 trauma center and teaching hospital. All responses were voluntary and kept anonymous. The interviews consisted of fifteen open-ended, semistructured questions. The interview guide covered questions about professional choice, memorable resuscitative efforts, the definition of a "successful" reviving attempt, patient's family presence, teamwork, coping with death and dying, and advanced cardiac life support protocols.

SOCIAL VIABILITY

The ED staff's main task is to find a balance of care that fits the patient's situation (Timmermans and Berg 1997). Based on my observations, whether care providers will aggressively try to save lives still depends on the patient's position in a moral stratification. Certain patient characteristics add up to a patient's presumed social viability, and the staff rations their efforts based on the patient's position in this moral hierarchy (Sudnow 1967; Glaser and Strauss 1964). A significant number of identity aspects that signify a person's social status and overall social worth in the community (e.g., being a volunteer, good speaker, charismatic leader, or effective parent), are irrelevant or unknown during the resuscitation process. In contrast with Sudnow's conceptual preference, I opt for social viability to indicate the grounds of rationing because social worth is too broad to indicate the variations in reviving attempts.

During reviving efforts, *age* remains the most outstanding characteristic of a patient's social viability (Glaser and Strauss 1964; Iserson and Stocking 1993; Kastenbaum and Aisenberg 1972; Sudnow 1967; Roth 1972). The death of young people should be avoided with all means possible. Almost all respondents mentioned this belief explicitly in the interviews. One physician noted, "You are *naturally* more aggressive with younger people. If I had a forty-year-old who had a massive MI [myocardial infarction], was asystolic for twenty minutes, or something like that, I would be very aggressive with that person. I suppose for the same scenario in a ninety-year-old, I might not be." A colleague agreed, "When you have a younger patient, you try to give it a little bit more effort. You might want to go another half hour on a younger person because you have such a difficult time to let the person go." According to a nurse, dying children "go against the scheme of things. Parents are not supposed to bury their children; the children are supposed to bury their parents." Although respondents hesitated uncomfortably when I asked to give an age cutoff point, the resuscitation of young people triggered an aggressive lifesaving attempt.

A second group of patients for whom the staff was willing to exhaust the resuscitation protocols were patients *recognized* by one or more team members because of their position in the community. During the interview period in one hospital, a well-liked, well-known senior hospital employee was being resuscitated. All the respondents involved made extensive reference to this particular resuscitative effort. When I asked a respiratory therapist how this effort differed from the others, he replied, "I think the routines and procedures were the same, but I think the sense of urgency was a lot greater, the anxiety level was higher. We were more tense. It was very different from, say, a 98-year-old from a nursing home." A nurse explained how her behavior changed after she recognized the patient.

> The most recent one I worked on was one of my college professors. He happened to be one of my favorites and I didn't even realize it was him until we were into the code and somebody mentioned his name. Then I knew it was him. Then all of the sudden it becomes kind of personal, you seem to be really rooting for the person, while as before you were just doing your job . . . trying to do the best you could, but then it does get personal when you are talking to them and trying to . . . you know . . . whatever you can do to help them through.

When the British Princess Diana died in a car accident, physicians tried external and internal cardiac massage for two hours although her pulmonary vein—which carries half of the blood—was lacerated. Dr. Thomas Amoroso, trauma chief in emergency medicine department at Beth Israel Deaconess Medical Center, reflected, "As with all human endeavors there is emotion involved. You have a young, healthy, vibrant woman with obvious importance to the world at large. You're going to do everything you possibly can do to try and turn the matter around, but I rather suspect, in their hearts, even as her doctors were doing all their work, they knew it would not be successful" (Tye 1997). The interviewed doctors agreed that "most other patients would have been declared dead at the scene, or after arriving at the emergency department. But with a patient as famous as Diana, trauma specialists understandably want to try extraordinary measures" (Tye 1997).

Staff also responded aggressively to patients with whom they *identified*. A nurse reflected, "incidentally, anytime there is an association of a resuscitation with something that you have a close relationship with—your family, the age range, the situation . . . there is more emotional involvement." Another nurse explained how a resuscitative effort became more difficult after she had established a relationship with the patient by talking to her and going through the routine patient assessment procedures.

How do these positive categorizations affect the resuscitation process? Basically, when the perceived social viability of the patient is high, the staff will go all out to reverse the dying process. In the average resuscitative effort, four to eight staff members are involved. In the effort to revive a nine-month-old baby, however, I counted twenty-three health care providers in the room at one point. Specialists from different hospital services were summoned. One physician discussed the resuscitative effort of a patient she identified with: "I even called the cardiologist. I very seldom do call the cardiologist on the scene, and I called him and asked him, 'Is there anything else we can do?'" Often the physician will establish a central line in the patient's neck, and the respiratory therapists will check and recheck the tube to make sure the lungs are indeed inflated. These tasks are part of the protocol, but are not always performed as diligently in resuscitative attempts in which the patient's social viability is viewed as less.

The physician may even go beyond the protocol guidelines to save the patient. For example, at the time of my observations, the amount of sodium bicarbonate that could be administered was limited, and often the paramedics had already exhausted the quota en route to the hospital. The physician was supposed to order more sodium bicarbonate only after receiving lab test results of the patient's blood gases. In the frenzy of one resuscitative effort in which the patient was known to the whole staff, a physician boasted to his colleague, "So much for the guidelines. I gave more bicarb even before the blood gases were back." When the husband of a staff member was being resuscitated, nurses and physicians went out of their way to obtain a bed in intensive care.

How does a resuscitative effort of a highly valued patient end? In contrast with most other reviving attempts, I never saw a physician make a unilateral decision. The physician would go over all the drugs that were given, provide some medical history, mention the time that had elapsed since the patient collapsed, and then turn to the team and ask, "Does anybody have any suggestions?" or "I think we did everything we could. Dr. Martin also agrees—I think we can stop it."

At the bottom of the assumed moral hierarchy are patients for whom death is considered an appropriate "punishment" or a welcome "friend." Death is considered a "friend" or even a "blessing" for *seriously ill* and *older patients*. For those patients, the staff agrees that sudden death is not the worst possible end of life. These patients are the "living dead" (Kastenbaum and Aisenberg 1972). The majority of resuscitation attempts in the ED were performed for elderly patients (Becker, Ostrander, Barrett, and Kondos 1991)—often these patients resided in nursing homes and were confronted with a staff who relied on deeply entrenched ageism. For example, one nurse assumed that older people would want to die. "Maybe this eighty-year-old guy just fell over at home and maybe that is the way he wanted to go.

But no, somebody calls an ambulance and brings him to the ER where we work and work and work and get him to the intensive care unit. Where he is poked and prodded for a few days and then they finally decide to let him go." According to a different nurse, older people had nothing more to live for: "When people are in their seventies and eighties, they have lived their lives."

The staff considered death an "appropriate" retaliation for *alcohol-* and *drug-addicted people*. For example, I observed a resuscitative attempt for a patient who had overdosed on heroin. The team went through the resuscitation motions but without much vigor or sympathy. Instead, staff members wore double pairs of gloves, avoided touching the patient, joked about their difficulty inserting an intravenous line, and mentioned how they loathed to bring the bad news to the belligerent "girlfriend" of the patient. Drunks are also much more likely to be nasally intubated rather than administered the safer and less painful tracheal intubation.

These negative definitions affect the course and fervor of the resuscitative effort. For example, patients on the bottom of the social hierarchy were often declared dead in advance. In a typical situation, the physician would tell the team at 7:55 A.M. that the patient would be dead at 8:05 A.M. The physician would then leave to fill out paperwork or talk to the patient's relatives. Exactly at 8:05, the team stopped the effort, the nurse responsible for taking notes wrote down the time of death, and the team dispersed. In two other such resuscitative efforts, the staff called the coroner before the patient was officially pronounced dead.

Even an elderly or seriously ill patient might unexpectedly regain a pulse or start breathing during the lifesaving attempt. This development is often an unsettling discovery and poses a dilemma for the staff: are we going to try to "save" this patient, or will we let the patient die? In most resuscitative efforts of patients with assumed low social viability, these signs were *dismissed or explained away* (Timmermans 1999a). In the drug overdose case, an EKG monitor registered an irregular rhythm, but the physician in charge dismissed this observation with, "This machine has an imagination of its own."

Along the same lines, staff who noticed signs of life were considered "inexperienced," and I heard one physician admonish a nurse who noticed heart tones that "she shouldn't have listened." Noticeable signs that couldn't be dismissed easily were explained as insignificant "reflexes" that would disappear soon (Glaser and Strauss 1965). In all of these instances, social death not only preceded but also led to the official pronouncement of death.

Some patient characteristics, such as age and presumed medical history, become "master traits" (Hughes 1971) during the resuscitative effort. The impact of other identity signifiers—such as gender, race, religion, sexual orientation, and socioeconomic status—was more difficult to observe (see also Sudnow 1983, p. 280). The longest resuscitative effort I observed was for a person with presumably low social viability because of his socioeconomic status. He was a white homeless man who had fallen into a creek and was hypothermic.7 I also noted how the staff made many disturbingly insensitive jokes during the resuscitative effort of a person with a high socioeconomic status: a well-dressed and wealthy elderly white woman who collapsed during dinner in one of the fanciest restaurants in the city. During a particularly hectic day, the staff worked very hard and long to save a middle-aged black teacher who collapsed in front of her classroom, whereas two elderly white men who were also brought in in cardiac arrest were quickly pronounced dead.

Epidemiological studies, however, suggest that race, gender, and socioeconomic status play a statistically significant role in overall survival of patients in sudden cardiac arrest. The emergency medical system is much more likely to be alerted when men die at home than when women experience cardiac arrest; this suggests a selection bias in the system (Joslyn 1994). Women also have much lower survival rates than men. In a Minneapolis study, the survival rate one year after cardiac arrest was 3.5 percent for women and 13.1 percent for men (Tillinghast, Doliszny, Kottke, Gomez-Marin, Lilja, and Campion 1991). A similar relationship has been observed for racial differences. Not only was the incidence of cardiac arrest in Chicago during 1988 significantly higher among blacks in every age group

than among whites, but the survival rate of blacks after an out-of-hospital cardiac arrest was only a third of that among whites (1 versus 3 percent) (Becker et al. 1993). Daniel Brookoff and his colleagues (1994) showed that black victims of cardiac arrest receive CPR less frequently than white victims. Using tax assessment data, Alfred Hallstrom's research team (1993) demonstrated that people in lower socioeconomic strata are at greater risk for higher mortality. In addition, lower-class people were also less likely to survive an episode of out-of-hospital cardiac arrest: "An increase of $50,000 in the valuation per unit of the home address increased the patient's chance of survival by 60%" (Hallstrom et al. 1993, p. 247).

Even after twenty-five years of CPR practice, Sudnow's earlier observations still ring true. The social value of the patient affects the fervor with which the staff engages in a resuscitative effort, the length of the reviving attempt, and probably also the outcome. The staff rations their efforts based on a hierarchy of lives they consider worth living and others for which they believe death is the best solution, largely regardless of the patient's clinical viability. Children, young adults, and people who are able to establish some kind of personhood and overcome the anonymity of lifesaving have the best chance for a full, aggressive resuscitative effort. In the other cases, the staff might still "run the code" but "walk it slowly" to the point of uselessness (Muller 1992).

LEGAL PROTECTIONS?

One of the aspects of resuscitation that has changed since Sudnow's ethnography is the drop in the prevalence of DOA or "dead on arrival" cases. Sudnow (1967, p. 100–109) noted that DOA was the most common occurrence in "County" hospital's emergency ward. Ambulance drivers would use a special siren to let the staff know that they were approaching the hospital with a "possible," shorthand for possible DOA. At arrival, the patient was quickly wheeled out of sight to the far end of the hallway. The physician would casually walk into the room, examine the patient, and in most cases confirm the patient's death. Finally, a nurse would call the coroner. Twenty-five years later, I observed DOA only when an extraordinarily long transportation time occurred in which all the possible drugs were given and the patient remained unresponsive. For example,

> Dr. Hendrickson takes me aside before the patient arrives and says, "Stefan, I just want to tell you that the patient has been down for more than half an hour [before the paramedics arrived]. They had a long ride. I probably will declare the patient dead on arrival." When the patient arrives, the paramedic reports, "We had asystole for the last ten minutes. We think he was in V-fib for a while but it was en route. It could have been the movement of the ambulance." The physician replies, "I declare this patient dead."

The DOA scenario has now diminished in importance for legal reasons. When somebody calls 911, a resuscitative effort begins and is virtually unstoppable until the patient is viewed in the ED by a physician. After the call, an ambulance with EMTs or paramedics is dispatched. Unless the patient shows obvious signs of death,[8] the ambulance rescuers start the advanced cardiac treatment as prescribed by their standing orders and protocols. The patient is thus transported to the ED, where the physician with the resuscitation team takes over. Legally, the physician again cannot stop the lifesaving attempt, because the physician needs to make sure that the protocols are exhausted. Stopping sooner would qualify as negligence and be grounds for malpractice. These legal guidelines, more than any magical power inherent to technology, explain the apparent technological imperative and momentum of the resuscitation technology (Koenig 1988; Timmermans 1998).

Patients who in Sudnow's study would be pronounced biologically dead immediately are now much more likely to undergo an extensive resuscitative effort. These patients cluster together in a new group of already presumed low-value patients. They are referred to as *pulseless nonbreathers, goners,* or *flat-liners*. Most of these patients are elderly or

suffer from serious illnesses. Sudden infant death syndrome babies and some adults might fulfill the clinical criteria for pulseless nonbreathers, but because they are considered valuable and therefore viable, the staff does not include them in this group.

A respiratory therapist described her reaction to these patients, "If it comes over my beeper that there is a pulseless nonbreather, then I know they were at home, I know that they were down a long time . . . I go and do my thing, [but] it's over when they get here." Some respondents added that this group does not leave a lasting impression: "they all blend together as one gray blur."

Instead of prompting health care workers to provide more aggressive care, the legally extended resuscitative effort has created a situation in which the staff feels obligated to go through some useless motions and they spend the time for other purposes. I observed that while they were compressing the patient's chest and artificially ventilating him or her, the staff's conversation would drift off to other topics such as birthday parties, television shows, hunting events, sports, awful patients, staffing conflicts, and easy or difficult shifts. Besides socializing, the staff also practiced medical techniques on the socially but not yet officially dead patient. I did not observe resuscitative efforts in a teaching hospital but still noticed how occasionally paramedics in training would reintubate the patient for practice.[9]

In addition, instead of attempting to save lives with all means possible, the process of accurately following the protocols became a goal in itself. A resuscitative effort could be rewarding for the staff based on the process of following the different resuscitation steps, regardless of the outcome of the resuscitative effort. A physician confessed, "As bad as it sounds, there are many times when I feel satisfied when it was done very well, the entire resuscitative effort was done very well, very efficiently even though the patient didn't make it." In this bureaucratic mode of thinking, following the legal guidelines à la lettre officially absolved the physician of the blame for sudden death. The physician could face the relatives and sincerely tell them that the staff did everything possible within the current medical guidelines to save the life of their loved one.

Finally, the staff used the mandated resuscitation time to take care of the patient's relatives and friends instead of the patient. A physician explicitly admitted that the current resuscitation set-up was far from optimal for the patient or relatives. He saw it as his responsibility to help the family as best he could:

Even when I am with the patient for the sixty or ninety seconds, if that, I almost don't think about the patient. I prepare myself for the emotional resuscitation or the emotional guidance of the family in their grief. The patient was gone before they got there [in the ED]. In a better world, they wouldn't be there because there is nothing natural or sanctimonious about being declared dead in a resuscitation. It is far more natural to be declared dead with your own family in your own home. We have now taken that patient out of their environment, away from their family, brought that family to a very strange place that is very unnatural only to be served the news that their loved one has died.

A nurse also shared the preoccupation with the needs of the family:

My thoughts throughout the entire resuscitative effort, even prior to the arrival, are with the family. Who is going to be with that family? Who is going to support them? And that they are being notified throughout the resuscitative effort what is going on, to prepare them if it is going to be a long haul, or if things are not good and are not going to get better. I think they deserve that. So it is kind of a combined feeling throughout. But I can focus on the one without being bogged down with the emotion of what is going on over there.

The "resuscitation" of the relatives and friends of the patient became more important than the patient's resuscitation attempt. The staff used the resuscitation motions and prescriptions as a platform to achieve other values. They might turn the resuscitative effort into a "good death" ritual in which they prolong the lifesaving attempt to give relatives and friends the option to say goodbye to their dying loved one (Timmermans 1997).

The legal protections guaranteeing universal lifesaving care have not resulted in qualitatively enhanced lifesaving but instead have created a new set of criteria that need to be checked off before a patient can be pronounced dead. In Sudnow's study, social death often preceded and predicted irreversible biological death. The staff of "Cohen" and "County" hospitals did not stretch the lifesaving effort unnecessarily. Once patients of presumed low social value showed obvious signs of biological death, the staff would quickly pronounce them officially deceased. Currently, many patients of presumed low social value in resuscitative efforts are already biologically dead when they are wheeled into the ED. The time it takes to exhaust the resuscitation protocols has created a new temporal interval with *legal death* as the endpoint. Legal requirements form a new instance of what Barney Glaser and Anselm Strauss (1965) originally called the closed awareness and mutual pretense awareness context. The staff is fully aware that the patient was irreversibly dead at arrival in the ED but they go through the motions for legal reasons and to allow the family to come to grips with the suddenness of the situation. If the relatives and friends catch on and know that their loved one is dying, the setup of the reviving attempt encourages them to pretend this is not really happening. This management of sudden death does not reduce any social inequality. The same situational identity features that marginalized certain groups of patients still predict the intensity of lifesaving fervor. As in Glaser and Strauss's and Sudnow's studies, social death now also has become a self-fulfilling prophecy for legal death.

In the wake of the hospice and patient-right movements, ethicists and legislators have also developed legal means such as advance directives, living wills, durable powers of attorney, and do-not-resuscitate orders to empower people to influence their own deaths. These diverse initiatives culminated in the Patient Self-Determination Act of 1991, that mandated that patients be given notice of their rights to make medical treatment decisions and of the legal instruments available to give force to decisions made in advance. The act is intended to enhance patient autonomy, so that if a patient expressed her or his wish not to be resuscitated, a resuscitative effort should be avoided regardless of how the staff perceives the patient's social value. The actual effect, however, is the opposite.

I observed eight resuscitative efforts in which the patient had signed an advance directive. In only two of those eight situations did the advance directive result in a terminated lifesaving attempt. The main problem with the advance directive was that the health care providers who made the initial decision to resuscitate (paramedics) were not authorized to interpret the documents. A chaplain said, "We tell people who have a living will or have been given power of attorney and wish not to be kept alive, if you have a heart attack at home, don't call 911. Don't call the EMTs because they are automatically obligated to do everything they can." To complicate the situation, physicians often did not find out about the living will until well into the lifesaving attempt (Eisendrath and Jonsen 1983). The inefficiency of the advance directive to stop the resuscitative effort has been confirmed in other studies as well. Medical researchers concluded that "advance directives did not affect the rate of resuscitation being tried" (Teno et al. 1997, p. 505). A retrospective study of 694 resuscitative efforts found that 7 percent of all resuscitative efforts were unwanted, and 2 percent of those patients survived to hospital discharge (Dull, Graves, Larson, and Cummins 1994).

Even when the advance directive was present and known, the extent to which the staff followed the written wishes of the advance directive depended mostly on the assumed social viability of the patient. During resuscitative efforts for patients with presumed high social value, I never observed the staff mention the possibility that the patient might have an advance directive. In an interview, a nurse supervisor prided herself on going against the wishes of a patient and his relatives, even though the patient still thought after regaining consciousness that they should not have revived him. A survey of emergency physicians found that 42 percent did not

stop a resuscitative effort when an advance directive instructed them to do so (Iserson and Stocking 1993). Health care providers were only willing to accept a living will when the patient fulfilled their criteria for having one; this meant that the patients were seriously ill or old *and* the staff believed that the patient's quality of life suffered. One nurse explained.

> I think if a person has made very clear their wishes beforehand . . . especially in light of a terminal illness, a cancer, or an awful respiratory disease—they know that they don't have long to live and the quality of their life is not very good—then it is very appropriate for these people to make their statements when they have a free mind and are conscious that they don't wish to have resuscitations started.

According to the nurse, the staff should always evaluate whether it is appropriate that a patient had an advance directive.

In contrast, the staff blamed patients with presumed low social value (mostly seriously ill patients) for not signing an advance directive. During a resuscitative attempt, the physician entered the room after talking to relatives and asked the nurse, "Got rid of that pulse yet?" When he saw my surprised expression, he added, "She had all kinds of cancer. They were stupid enough not to ask for a red alert and now we have to go through this nonsense." Normally, an advance directive needed to be verified by the physician in charge, but even when no advance directive could be found in the patient's file, the physician still might stop the reviving effort. In the following observation, the team was not sure whether the patient actually had an advance directive or was going to talk to her physician about it.

> The chaplain enters and says, "The neighbor said that she has an aneurysm in her stomach area. She also said that she did not want to be operated. She was going to talk to her doctor tomorrow to discuss this." The physician asks, "Is she a no-code?" "According to the neighbor she is." "Why do we find

this out after we have been working on her?" The head nurse takes the patient's file, which the department administrator brought into the room. She looks through it once and looks through it a second time, but she cannot find an advance directive. The physician takes the file, and together they check it again. No advance directive, no official document. The doctor then decides to let the patient go anyway. He considers the patient hopeless unless she wants to have surgery.

Advance directives certainly do not empower the patient. Under the guise of increasing the patient's autonomy, the opposite result—medical paternalism—is obtained (Teaster 1995). Health care providers followed the wishes set forth in the advance directive when these guidelines matched their own assessment of the patient's social value and did not undermine their professional jurisdiction (Abbott 1988).10

In general, the legal drive to create a resuscitation-friendly environment and the laws to protect patient autonomy have not abolished the social inequality of sudden death. In certain instances, resuscitative efforts are lengthened or shortened, but these changes occur regardless of the legal intentions. The basic problem of administering resuscitative care based on the social viability of the patient remains uncorrected. The staff works around the legal guidelines to enforce their view of lives worth living and good deaths (Timmermans 1999b).

RESUSCITATION THEORY

Not only does the staff use legal guidelines to perpetuate existing views of social inequality, but health care providers also reappropriate the accumulated medical knowledge about resuscitations to justify withholding care of *new groups with presumed low social value.* For a technique that is not really proved to be effective with national survival rates, the field of resuscitation medicine has a surprisingly high level of agreement as to what constitutes the best chances for survival.[11] From physician to technician

to chaplain in the ED, almost all respondents provided a more or less complete reflection of the dominant theory. The basics of resuscitation theory are very simple: the quicker the steps of the "chain of survival" are carried out (Cummins, Ornato, Thies, and Pepe 1991), the better the chances for survival. A weakness in one step will reverberate throughout the entire system and impair optimal survival rates.

The chain of survival is intended as a simple, rational tool for educators, researchers, and policy makers to evaluate whether a community obtains optimal patient survival. In the ED, however, the same theoretical notions underlying the chain of survival serve as a rationalization for *no.* trying to resuscitate particular patient groups. The professional rescuers in the ED are acutely aware of their *location* in the chain of survival's temporal framework. The ED is the last link of the survival chain, and many elements need to have fallen in place before the patient reaches the hands of the team. Anything that deviates from the "ideal" resuscitative pattern and causes more time to elapse is a matter of concern for the staff. One technician estimated how important every step in the resuscitation process is for the final outcome:

One of the most important things would be the time between when the patient actually went down until the first people arrive. That is like, I'd say, 30 percent and then the time that a patient takes to get to the hospital takes another, probably, 30–40 percent. Sixty to 70 percent of it is prehospital time.

A nurse explains the importance of location and timing by contrasting resuscitation of somebody who collapsed inside the ED with somebody who collapsed outside the ED:

A lot has to do with EMS [Emergency Medical System] and family response and getting them there. If you would drop dead right here, your chances would be pretty good that we would be able to resuscitate you without any brain damage or anything else. If you're at home out on a farm, sixty miles away, and you have to call out for help and that takes fifteen minutes for them to get there and nobody in the house knows CPR, I think your chances are pretty slim.

According to the nurse, if the situation had not been optimal in the first steps, the ED staff could not be expected to rectify the situation. The consequence of this acute awareness about their location in the chain of survival is that the emergency medical hospital staff feels only limited control over the outcome of the resuscitative effort. A physician reiterated this: "for a lot of these people, their outcome is written in stone before I see them." A colleague added "there are certainly many, many instances of cardiac arrest where the end result is predestined, where the chance of resuscitation is very slim." Most respondents echoed the nurse supervisor who remarked, "I think there are always factors involved whether a resuscitation is successful or not. But I don't know if there is any personal or even physical control."

Because of this perceived lack of control, health care providers were less willing to aggressively resuscitate patients who deviate from the ideal scenario. Often such a consensus was reached even before the patient arrived in the ED. I observed how the nurse in charge sent a colleague back to the intensive care unit when paramedics radioed that a patient was found with an unknown downtime, saying, "We will not need you. She'll be dead." Sometimes only the name of the patient's town was sufficient for the staff to know that it probably would be "a short exercise." The town would give an indication of the transportation time and the available emergency care. Once a patient with such low perceived survival chances arrived in the ED, the staff would go through the resuscitation motions without much conviction. A technician noted how in many cases he "start[s] to feel defeated already. To the point now, where it is pretty much decided already, we are not going to get anywhere with this."

The staff interprets the official theory of reviving as a justification for only lukewarmly attempting to resuscitate patients who did not fit the ideal lifesaving scenario. This rationing rests not on biological but on social grounds. Underneath the staff's

reluctance to revive patients who deviate from the ideal resuscitative scenario lies the fear that the patient would be only partially resuscitated and suffer from brain damage. According to the dominant resuscitation theory (CPR-ECC 1973), irreversible brain damage occurs after less than five minutes of oxygen deprivation. The staff is concerned that if they revive a patient after this critical time period, the patient might be severely neurologically disabled or comatose. When a nurse got a patient's pulse back, she exclaimed, "Oh no, we can't do that to him. He must be braindead by now." A physician stated, "There have been situations where after a prolonged downtime we get a pulse back. My first feeling is, 'My God, what have I done?' It is a horrible feeling because you know that patient will be put in the unit and ultimately their chances of walking out of the hospital without any neurological deficits are almost zero."

A physician described one scenario to be avoided—a resuscitative effort in which an adult survived in a vegetative state:

I remember there was a man who was having just an MRI scan done, and while he was in the machine he had a cardiac arrest for who knows what reason. And they brought him to the ER, and we started to resuscitate him, and as we did, it looked obvious that he probably wasn't going to survive. And we gave him what we call high-dose epinephrine, and with that high dose he actually returned to a normal heart rhythm. Unfortunately, he had an inadequate blood supply to his brain so he ended up having not too much cognitive function . . . I guess I remember that because I thought he was going to die, and I gave him a little more medicine, and he didn't. And I have always wondered whether that was the right thing to do or not.

[Do you think you did the right thing?]

Well, in retrospect I don't think that I did. The man is alive, but his brain is not alive, so he really is not the same person he was before. I think that from the family's point of view, they probably would have had an easier time dealing with the fact that he was dead and sort of would have gone out of their system instead of in the state he is in right now.

Health care providers generally consider this the ultimate "nightmare scenario," an outcome that will haunt them for years to come.[12] The patient survived in a permanent vegetative state, continuously requiring emotional and financial resources of relatives and society in general.

With those "excesses" in mind, several respondents made thinly veiled arguments in favor of passive euthanasia. A nurse stated that she felt that in many cases attempting to resuscitate patients meant "prolonging their suffering." A technician asserted that "with an extensive medical history it is inhumane to try." Another technician reflected, "Sometimes you wonder if it is really for the benefit of the patient." A chaplain even made a case for suicide (or euthanasia, depending on who the "them" are in his sentence): "I feel a bit of relief knowing that if a person couldn't be resuscitated to a productive life, that it is probably just as well to have them have the right to end life." The principle that guides the rescuer's work is that a quick death is preferable over a lingering death with limited cognitive functioning in an intensive care unit. A nurse said this explicitly, "The child survived with maximum brain injury and has become now, instead of a child that they [the parents] can mourn and put in the ground, a child that they mourn for years."

Although health care providers again hesitated to define a criterion for a quality of life they would find unacceptable, I found implicit in both interviews and observations a view that such lives were not worth living. Drawing from the dominant resuscitation theory, the *prospect* of long-term physical and mental disabilities was reason enough to slow down the lifesaving attempt to the point of uselessness. In an age of disability rights, health care providers reflect and perpetuate the stereotypic assumptions that disability invokes (Fine and Asch 1988; Mairs 1996; Zola 1984). People with disabilities are associated with perpetual dependency and helplessness;

they are viewed as victims leading pitiful lives, "damaged creatures who should be put out of their misery" (Mairs 1996, p. 120). Disability symbolizes a lack of control over life, and health care providers fall back on the outcome over which they have the most control. The *possibility* of disability is considered worse than biological death. In a survey of 105 experienced emergency health care providers (doctors, nurses, and EMTs), 82 percent would prefer death for themselves over severe neurological disability (Hauswald and Tanberg 1993).

Along with the dominant resuscitation theory, health care providers support the view that people with disabilities should not be resuscitated. To be fair, the same theory is also invoked as a warning about giving up too soon. Several respondents mentioned that one can never be sure whether a report about downtime and transportation time is accurate. Even if there was a long transportation time, one cannot know for sure when the patient went into cardiac arrest. Exactly because there exists this margin of uncertainty, many respondents considered it worthwhile to at least attempt to resuscitate and follow the protocols. In most observed resuscitative efforts, however, it appeared that the expectations were clearly set and became self-fulfilling prophecies.

SOCIAL RATIONING AND THE MEDICALIZATION OF SUDDEN DEATH

In the conclusion to *Passing On,* David Sudnow discussed the ways in which dying became an institutional routine and a meaningful event for the hospital staff. He emphasized that the staff attempted to maintain an attitude of "appropriate impersonality" toward death and how the organization of the ward and the teaching hospital favored social death preceding biological death. In ethnomethodological fashion, Sudnow (1967, p. 169) underscored how "death" and "dying" emerged out of the interactions and practices of health care providers, "what has been developed is a 'procedural definition of dying,' a definition based upon the activities which that phenomenon can be said to *consist in*."[13]

My update of Sudnow's study indicates that with the widespread use of resuscitation technologies, health care providers now have to make sense of engaging in a practice with the small chance of saving lives and the potential to severely disable patients. They cope with this dilemma by deliberately not trying to revive certain groups of patients. These groups are not distinguished by their clinical potential but by their social viability. The staff reappropriates biomedical protocols and legal guidelines to further refine a system of implicit social rationing. The bulk of resuscitative efforts are still characterized by a detached attitude toward patients. In most reviving efforts, the staff feels defeated in advance and reviving becomes an empty ritual of going through mandated motions. It is only when patients transcend anonymity and gain a sense of personhood that the staff will aggressively try to revive them.

With regard to the broader institutional context, resuscitation is now, less than in Sudnow's study, marked by the health care provider's desire to "obtain 'experience,' avoid dirty work, and maximize the possibility that the intern will manage some sleep" (Sudnow 1967, p. 170) as well as by the requirements of defensive medicine and managed care. With the gradual erosion of physician autonomy because of peer review and utilization boards, the wave of cost-effectiveness in medicine, the proliferation of medical malpractice suits, and the patient rights movement, physicians' practices have become more externally regulated. As several respondents commented, a resuscitative effort is as much an attempt to avoid a lawsuit as an endeavor to save lives. Health care providers try to maneuver within the boundaries of the law, professional ethics, and biomedical knowledge to maintain lives worth living and proper deaths for their patients. Every resuscitative effort becomes a balancing act of figuring out when "enough is enough" based on the clinical situation and prognosis, legal and ethical guidelines, the wishes of the patient and relatives, and—most importantly—the preferences and emotions of the resuscitation team. The latter are in charge, so ultimately their definitions of the situation and their values will prevail.

After thirty years, Sudnow's main contribution to the sociological literature is his disclosure of how the ED staff rations death and dying based on the presumed social value of the patient. Most studies of social inequality in health care rely on showing statistical race, gender, and socioeconomic variations in the prevalence, incidence, morbidity, and mortality rates of particular conditions (e.g., Wilkinson 1996), however, Sudnow showed that social inequality is an intrinsic part of negotiating and managing death. Surprisingly, though, Sudnow did not question the implications of the rampant social inequality he exposed in *Passing On*. His interpretation of social rationing as a routine institutional coping mechanism for death and dying—not as an important social issue—remains unsatisfactory because the former interpretation implies a theoretical justification of social inequality.

From a contemporary point of view, Sudnow's position has become even more problematic because health care providers keep dismissing similar groups of marginalized patients in a very different health care structure. Policies that should have diminished social inequality have instead strengthened it. Instead of concluding that such rampant social inequality is an inevitable part of the interaction between the patient and the care provider, I suggest that the policy changes did not address the broader societal foundations of social inequality.

Unfortunately, the attitudes of the emergency staff reflect and perpetuate those of a society generally not equipped culturally or structurally to accept the elderly or people with disabilities as people whose lives are valued and valuable (Mulkay and Ernst 1991). As the need for and problems with an Americans with Disabilities Act show, the disabled and seriously ill are not socially dead only in the ED but also in the outside world; this is the original sense in which Erving Goffman first introduced social death (1961). The staff has internalized beliefs about the presumed low worth of elderly and disabled people to the extent that more than 80 percent would rather be dead than live with a severe neurological disability. As gatekeepers between life and death, they have the opportunity to execute explicitly the pervasive but more subtle moral code of the wider society. Just as schools, restaurants, and modes of transportation became the battlegrounds and symbols in the civil rights struggle, medical interventions such as genetic counseling, euthanasia, and resuscitative efforts represent the sites of contention in the disability and elderly rights movements (Fine and Asch 1988; Schneider 1993).

In addition to the fact that social rationing takes place under the guise of a resuscitative effort, the prolonged resuscitation of anyone—including irreversibly dead people—in our emergency systems perpetuates a far-reaching medicalization of the dying process (Conrad 1992). Deceased people are presented more as "not resuscitated" than as having died a sudden, natural death. The resuscitative motions render death literally invisible (Star 1991); the patient and staff are in the resuscitation room while relatives and friends wait in a counseling room. The irony of the resuscitative setup is that nobody seems to benefit from continuing to resuscitate patients who are irreversibly dead. As some staff members commented, the main benefit of the current configuration is that it takes a little of the abruptness of sudden death away for relatives and friends. I doubt, though, that the "front" of a resuscitative effort is the best way to prepare people for sudden death. By engaging and investing in resuscitative efforts, we as a society facilitate the idea that mortality can be deconstructed (Bauman 1992) and that crisis interventions will correct a lack of prevention and healthy life habits (Anspach 1993). The result of engaging in resuscitative efforts on obviously dead patients is structurally sanctioned denial, a paternalistic attitude in which staff members keep relatives and friends in a closed awareness context or engage them in the slippery dance of mutual pretense awareness (Glaser and Strauss 1965). For the sake of preserving hope and softening the blow of sudden death, the staff decides that it is better for relatives not to know that their loved one is dying. Relatives and friends are separated from the dying process and miss the opportunity to say goodbye when it could really matter to them, that is when there is still a chance that their loved one is listening.

Rationalizing medical practice or providing legal accountability only accentuated the medicalization of the dying process and social inequality. The biomedical protocols are part of the problem of the medicalization of death because they promote aggressive care instead of providing means to terminate a reviving attempt (Timmermans 1999a), and the staff relies upon those theories to justify not resuscitating people who might become disabled. Legal initiatives mostly stimulated the predominance of resuscitative efforts at the expense of other ways of dying and have been unable to protect marginalized groups.

In the liminal space between lives worth living and proper deaths, resuscitative efforts in the ED crystallize submerged subtle attitudes of the wider society. The ED staff enforces and perpetuates our refusal to let go of life and to accommodate certain groups. Exactly because health care providers implement our moral codes, they are the actors who might be able to initiate a change in attitudes. On a personal level, many health care providers seem to have made up their minds about the limitations of reviving. Medical researchers presented emergency health care providers with a common forty-eight-minute resuscitation scenario with a relatively good prognosis and a reasonable time course. Only 2.9 percent of the respondents would prefer to be resuscitated for the entire episode (Hauswald and Tanberg 1993). If those who are the most informed and have the most personal experience with resuscitative efforts are reluctant to undergo lifesaving attempts, there is a simple solution for the twin problems of social rationing and the medicalization of sudden death. Instead of increasing the access to these technologies, we might want to provide overall less resuscitative efforts. I see two ways that such a goal could be obtained.

The most important step to avoid a resuscitative effort is not to alert the emergency system. I don't believe that more regulations and legal protections will circumvent lifesaving attempts. Even with the best intentions, deciding to let people die in an ED is still too much a violation of core medical values (e.g., the Hippocratic Oath). Discussions about advance directives have an important sensitizing function, but people (and their relatives and caretakers) who choose not to be resuscitated need to realize that the first step of avoiding a resuscitative effort implies not dialing 911. We cannot expect medical restraint from professionals who are socialized and legally obligated to fight death and dying with all means possible.

In addition, relatives and friends should have the opportunity to play a more active role during a resuscitative effort. This occurs already in some midwestern hospitals, where relatives are given the option to attend the resuscitative effort and say goodbye during the last moments that their loved one hovers between life and death. The presence of grieving relatives and friends is a constant reminder for the staff that they are dealing with a person entrenched in a social network and not with a mere body (Timmermans 1997). Such a policy change also entails a more explicit recognition that resuscitative efforts are not only performed for patients but also for relatives and friends who need to make sense of sudden death (Ellis 1993; Rosaldo 1984). These initiatives should stimulate an understanding that "passing on" to the final transition is inevitable and should be the same for everyone, regardless of their presumed social value.

ACKNOWLEDGMENTS

I thank Sharon Hogan, Norm Denzin, Margie Towery, and the anonymous reviewers for their useful comments.

Notes

1. Social rationing means the withholding of potentially beneficial medical interventions based on social grounds (see Conrad and Brown 1993).

2. Bauman does not argue that resuscitative efforts are not decided upon patients' presumed social worth any longer, but that social discrimination has shifted from "primitive" technologies to more advanced medical technologies such as organ donation and "the electronic computerized gadgetry."

3. Sometimes medical critics will discuss the ethical implications of individualized resuscitation scenarios. Part of Sudnow's contribution, however, was to show that social rationing was not an isolated, individualized event, but a widespread, social practice.

4. Massachusetts General Law c.111C, Paragraph 14 states that "No emergency medical technician certified under the provisions of this chapter . . . who in the performance of his duties and in good faith renders emergency first aid or transportation to an injured person or to a person incapacitated by illness shall be personally in any way liable as a result of transporting such person to a hospital or other safe place . . ."

5. Omnibus Budget Reconciliation Act of 1990 (OBRA-90), Pub. L. 101–508, 4206, and 4751 (Medicare and Medicaid respectively), 42 U.S.C. 1395cc (a) (I) (Q), 1295mm (c) (8), 1395cc (f), 1396a (a) (58), and 1396a (w) (Supp. 1991).

6. Level 1 and level 2 refer to different staffing requirements and to differences in severity of cases. Level 1 hospitals are required to have a neuro, trauma, and cardiac surgeon always on call in the hospital, and these hospitals take more serious cases than level 2 hospitals (the differences are head injuries, gunshot wounds, multiple complex wounds, etc.). The distribution of level 1 and level 2 trauma centers per region is regulated by law.

7. The staff found this resuscitative effort interesting because it involved the first hypothermic person they attempted to revive in a year. They were a little lost about how to warm up the patient. Some patients gain status because they constitute medically challenging or interesting cases.

8. Death is obvious when rigor mortis has set in, decapitation has occurred, the body is consumed by fire, or there is a massive head injury with parts missing.

9. This practice is not as marginal as one would think. Major medical journals regularly publish articles about the ethical implications of practicing intubation and other techniques on the "newly dead" (see for example Burns et al. 1994).

10. There is also some evidence from other research that having an advance directive is in itself related to age, gender, race, socioeconomic status, education. Schonwetter et al. (1994), for example, found a strong relationship between socioeconomic status and the desire for CPR.

11. Partly this is due to the fact that US (and international) resuscitation medicine is dominated by a limited number of research groups who mostly seem to agree with each other. According to Niemann about 85% of all CPR related research articles in the United States come from a community of 10 research groups (Niemann 1993 p. 8).

12. The physician told me this story six years after it happened. My original question was "Can you give me an example of a resuscitative effort that left a big impression on you?"

13. Although I did not emphasize Sudnow's ethnomethodological legacy in this paper, the idea of life-saving, the technology, and saving lives in itself are jointly accomplished in practice (see Timmermans and Berg 1997). The ironic aspect of resuscitation technology is that resuscitation techniques and practice establish the value of saving lives at all costs while the actual numbers of saved lives remain very low. I discuss this seeming paradox at length in my book (Timmermans 1997). I thank Norm Denzin for drawing my attention to the ethnomethodological importance of Sudnow's study.

References

Abbott, Andrew. 1988. *The System of Professions: An Essay on the Division of Expert Labor.* Chicago: University of Chicago Press.

Anspach, Renée R. 1993. *Deciding Who Lives: Fateful Choices in the Intensive-Care Nursery.* Berkeley: University of California Press.

Bauman, Zygmunt. 1992. *Mortality, Immortality and Other Life Strategies.* Stanford, CA: Stanford University Press.

Becker, Lance B., Ben H. Han, Peter M. Meyer, Fred A. Wright, Karin V. Rhodes, David W. Smith, and John Barrett. 1993. "Racial Differences in the Incidence of Cardiac Arrest and Subsequent Survival." *New England Journal of Medicine* 329:600–606.

Becker, Lance, B. M. P. Ostrander, John Barrett, and G. T. Kondos. 1991. "Outcome of CPR in a Large Metropolitan Area: Where Are the Survivors?" *Annals of Emergency Medicine* 20:355–361.

Berg, Marc. 1997. *Rationalizing Medical Work: A Study of Decision Support Techniques and Medical Practices.* Cambridge, MA: MIT Press.

Brookoff, Daniel, Arthur L. Kellermann, Bela B. Hackman, Grant Somes, and Perry Dobyns. 1994. "Do Blacks Get Bystander Cardiopulmonary Resuscitation as Often as Whites?" *Annals of Emergency Medicine* 24:1147–1150.

Burns, J. P., F. E. Reardon, and R. D. Truogh. 1994. "Using Newly Deceased Patients to Practice Resuscitation Procedures." *New England Journal of Medicine* 319:439–441.

Callahan, Daniel. 1993. *The Troubled Dream of Life: Living with Mortality.* New York: Simon and Schuster.

Conrad, Peter. 1992. "Medicalization and Social Control." *Annual Review of Sociology* 18:209– 232.

_____, ed. 1997. *Sociology of Health and Illness: Critical Perspectives.* New York: St. Martin's Press.

Conrad, Peter, and Phil Brown. 1993. "Rationing Medical Care: A Sociological Reflection." *Research in the Sociology of Health Care* 10:3–22.

CPR-ECC. 1973. "Standards for Cardiopulmonary Resuscitation and Emergency Cardiac Care." *Journal of American Medical Association* 227:836–868.

_____. 1992. "Guidelines for Cardiopulmonary Resuscitation and Emergency Cardiac Care." *Journal of American Medical Association* 268:2171–2295.

Cummins, Richard, Joseph P. Ornato, William H. Thies, and Paul E. Pepe. 1991. "The 'Chain of Survival' Concept." *Circulation* 83:1832–1847.

Dowie, J., and A. Elstein. 1988. *Professional Judgment: A Reader in Clinical Decision Making.* Cambridge: Cambridge University Press.

Dull, Scott M., Judith R. Graves, Mary Pat Larsen, and Richard O. Cummins. 1994. "Expected Death and Unwanted Resuscitation in the Prehospital Setting." *Annals of Emergency Medicine* 23: 997–1001.

Eisenberg, Michael, Bruce T. Horwood, Richard O. Cummins, R. Reynolds-Haertle, and T. R. Hearne.

1990. "Cardiac Arrest and Resuscitation: A Tale of 29 Cities." *Annals of Emergency Medicine* 19: 179–186.

Eisendrath, S. J., and A. R. Jonsen. 1983. "The Living Will: Help or Hindrance?" *Journal of American Medical Association* 249: 2054–2058.

Ellis, Carolyn. 1993. "Telling a Story of Sudden Death." *The Sociological Quarterly* 34:711–731.

Feinstein, Jonathan S. 1993. "The Relationships between Socioeconomic Status and Health." *Milbank Quarterly* 71:279–322.

Fine, Michelle, and Adrienne Asch. 1988. "Disability beyond Stigma: Social Interaction, Discrimination, and Activism." *Journal of Social Issues* 44: 3–21.

Fox, Renée C. 1976. "Advanced Medical Technology: Social and Ethical Implications." *Annual Review of Sociology* 2:231–268.

Glaser, Barney G., and Anselm L. Strauss. 1964. "The Social Loss of Dying Patients." *American Journal of Nursing* 64:119–121.

_____, 1965. *Awareness of Dying.* Chicago: Aldine.

_____, 1968. *Time for Dying.* Chicago: Aldine.

Goffman, Erving. 1961. *Asylums: Essays on the Social Situation of Mental Patients and Other Inmates.* New York: Doubleday Anchor.

Hallstrom, Alfred, Paul Boutin, Leonard Cobb, and Elise Johnson. 1993. "Socioeconomic Status and Prediction of Ventricular Fibrillation Survival." *American Journal of Public Health* 83:245–248.

Hauswald, Mark, and Dan Tanberg. 1993. "Out-of-Hospital Resuscitation Preferences of Emergency Health Care Workers." *American Journal of Emergency Medicine* 11:221–224.

Heckman, James D., ed. 1992. *Emergency Care and Transportation of the Sick and Injured.* Dallas: American Academy of Orthopaedic Surgeons.

Hughes, Everett C. 1971. *The Sociological Eye.* Chicago: Aldine.

Illich, Yvan. 1976. *Medical Nemesis: The Expropriation of Health.* New York: Pantheon Books.

Iserson, Kenneth V., and Carol Stocking. 1993. "Standards and Limits: Emergency Physicians' Attitudes toward Prehospital Resuscitation." *American Journal of Emergency Medicine* 11:592–594.

Joslyn, Sue A. 1994. "Case Definition in Survival Studies of Out-of-Hospital Cardiac Arrest." *American Journal of Emergency Medicine* 12:299–301.

Kastenbaum, Robert, and R. Aisenberg. 1972. *The Psychology of Death.* New York: Springer.

Kitagawa, Evelyn M., and Philip M. Hauser. 1973. *Differential Mortality in the United States: A Study in Socioeconomic Epidemiology.* Cambridge, MA: Harvard University Press.

Koenig, Barbara A. 1988. "The Technological Imperative in Medical Practice: The Social Creation of a 'Routine' Treatment." Pp. 465–497 in *Biomedicine Examined,* edited by Margaret Lock and Deborah R. Gordon. Dordrecht: Kluwer Academic Publishers.

Mairs, Nancy. 1996. *Waist-High in the World: A Life Among the Nondisabled.* Boston: Beacon Press.

Moller, David Wendell. 1996. *Confronting Death: Values, Institutions, and Human Mortality.* New York: Oxford University Press.

Mulkay, Michael, and John Ernst. 1991. "The Changing Position of Social Death." *European Journal of Sociology* 32:172–196.

Muller, Jessica H. 1992. "Shades of Blue: The Negotiation of Limited Codes by Medical Residents." *Social Science and Medicine* 34:885–898.

Niemann, James T. 1993. "Study Design in Cardiac Arrest Research: Moving from the Laboratory to the Clinical Population." *Annals of Emergency Medicine* 22:8–9.

Pelligrino, Edmund D. 1986. "Rationing Health Care: The Ethics of Medical Gatekeeping." *Journal of Contemporary Health Law and Policy* 2:23–44.

Rosaldo, Renato. 1984. "Grief and a Headhunter's Rage: On the Cultural Force of Emotions." Pp. 178–199 in *Text, Play, and Story: The Construction and Reconstruction of Self and Society,* edited by Edward Bruner. Plainsfield, IL: Waveland Press.

Roth, Julius A. 1972. "Some Contingencies of the Moral Evaluation and Control of Clientele: The Case of the Hospital Emergency Service." *American Journal of Sociology* 77:839–855.

Schneider, Joseph P. 1993. *No Pity: People with Disabilities Forging a New Civil Rights Movement.* New York: Random House.

Schonwetter, Ronald S., Robert M. Walker, David R. Kramer, and Bruce E. Robinson. 1994. "Socioeconomic Status and Resuscitation Preferences in the Elderly." *Journal of Applied Gerontology* 13(2): 157–71.

Schwartz, S., and T. Griffin. 1986. *Medical Thinking: The Psychology of Medical Judgment and Decision Making.* Springer, New York.

Siner, D. A. 1989. "Advance Directives in Emergency Medicine: Medical, Legal, and Ethical Implications." *Annals of Emergency Medicine* 18: 1364–1369.

Star, S. Leigh. 1991. "The Sociology of the Invisible: The Primacy of Work in the Writings of Anselm Strauss." Pp. 265–285 in *Social Organization and Social Process: Essays in Honor of Anselm Strauss,* edited by David Maines. New York: Aldine de Gruyter.

Starr, Paul. 1982. *The Social Transformation of American Medicine.* New York: Basic Books.

Sudnow, David. 1967. *Passing On: The Social Organization of Dying.* Englewood Cliffs, NJ: Prentice-Hall.

_____, 1983. "D.O.A." Pp. 275–294 in *Where Medicine Fails*, edited by Anselm Strauss. Lovelorn, NJ: Transaction Books.

Teaster, Pamela B. 1995. "Resuscitation Policy Concerning Older Adults: Ethical Considerations of Paternalism versus Autonomy." *Journal of Applied Gerontology* 14:78–92.

Teno, Joan, Joanne Lynn, Neil Wenger, Russell S. Phillips, Donald P. Murphy, Alfred F. Connors, Norman Desbiens, William Fulkerson, Paul Bellamy, and William Knauss. 1997. "Advance Directives for Seriously Ill Hospitalized Patients: Effectiveness with the Patient Self-Determination Act and the SUPPORT Intervention." *Journal of the American Geriatrics Society* 45:500–507.

Tillinghast, Stanley J., Katherine M. Doliszny, Thomas E. Kottke, Orlando Gomez-Marin, G. Patrick Lilja, and Bian C. Campion. 1991. "Change in Survival from Out-of-Hospital Cardiac Arrest and its Effect on Coronary Heart Disease Mortality." *American Journal of Epidemiology* 134:851–861.

Timmermans, Stefan. 1997. "High Tech in High Touch: The Presence of Relatives and Friends during Resuscitative Efforts." *Scholarly Inquiry for Nursing Practice* 11:153–168.

_____, 1998. "Resuscitation Technology in the Emergency Department: Toward a Dignified Death." *Sociology of Health and Illness* 20:144–167.

_____, 1999a. "When Death Isn't Dead: Implicit Social Rationing During Resuscitative Efforts." *Sociological Inquiry* 24:213–214.

_____, 1999b. *The Paradox of Resuscitation Technologies.* Philadelphia: Temple University Press.

Timmermans, Stefan, and Marc Berg. 1997. "Standardization in Action: Achieving Local Universality through Medical Protocols." *Social Studies of Science* 27:273–305.

Tye, Larry. 1997. "Doctor Had Little Hope of Success." *Boston Globe,* September 1, p. A6.

Waldron, Ingrid. 1997. "What Do We Know about Causes of Sex Differences in Mortality?" Pp. 42–55 in *Sociology of Health and Illness:* Cultural Perspectives. New York: St. Martin's Press.

Wilkinson, Richard. 1996. *Unhealthy Societies: The Afflictions of Inequality.* London: Routledge.

Zola, Irving K. 1984. *Missing Pieces: A Chronicle of Living with a Disability.* Philadelphia: Temple University Press.

31

"I WANT YOU TO SAVE MY KID!"

Illness Management Strategies, Access, and Inequality at an Elite University Research Hospital

Amanda M. Gengler[1]

Within the steeply hierarchical U.S. healthcare system, access to high-quality medical care is not equally available to all. Medical sociologists have recently turned greater attention to the institutional and individual-level processes driving inequalities in access to high-quality care (Lutfey and Freese 2005; Shim 2010). Access to newly developed, "cutting-edge" treatments is especially uneven (Chang and Lauderdale 2009; Goldman and Lakdawalla 2005), and, as I will argue, even after one accesses the most advanced medical care available, inequities in illness and treatment experiences remain.

Here, I examine the "critical case" of children with life-threatening illnesses receiving care at Kelly-Reed,[2] an elite university research hospital ranked among the top 10 hospitals in the United States. For these children, who required scarcely available or newly developed treatments and highly specialized medical expertise, getting to Kelly-Reed often meant gaining access to a select group of doctors with extensive experience treating children with their particular rare disorder. If anything could be done for their children within the limits of current medical knowledge and technology, these families had some of the best opportunities to access it.

"I Want You to Save My Kid!": Illness Management Strategies, Access, and Inequality at an Elite University Research Hospital, Amanda M. Gengler in *Journal of Health and Social Behavior,* 55(3), 342–359, 2014. Reprinted with permission from the American Sociological Association.

Yet accessing and negotiating such care could require significant effort. Drawing on ethnographic data, repeated interviews, and medical observations with 18 families, I show how parents developed different approaches to obtaining care and managing their child's illness depending on their ability to mobilize what Shim (2010) has termed "cultural health capital" (CHC). Shim defines CHC as "the repertoire of cultural skills, verbal and nonverbal competencies, attitudes and behaviors, and interactional styles" (p. 1) that patients bring to interactions, which "can be leveraged in healthcare contexts to effectively engage with medical providers" (p. 3). These differences in both resources and approach to managing illness resulted in divergences in the pathways families followed to this elite institution and their ability to influence their child's treatment once there.

Families with significant CHC who became actively involved in directing their child's treatment accessed care at the top levels of the U.S. medical system quickly, obtaining swift treatment and greater peace of mind. Once there they continued to influence their children's care, sometimes obtaining what I call *microadvantages* in doing so. In contrast, families with little CHC rarely intervened in medical decision making, deferring instead to healthcare professionals. Some families accessed care at this elite institution despite having little CHC but were often shuffled around lower rungs of the healthcare system for some time before being appropriately referred. Such families wielded much less influence over the provision of care throughout the treatment process even when they attempted to do so. These case studies show how different illness management strategies, undergirded by differing degrees of CHC, can produce subtle and not-so-subtle inequalities even among families who ultimately obtained treatment at a prestigious and richly resourced medical institution.

BACKGROUND

Much research has investigated the social roots of enduring health disparities across groups (see Marmot 2004; Williams 2012). Link and Phelan's (1995)

fundamental cause theory points to inequality itself as an underlying cause of disease. Building on this perspective, other researchers have examined how factors such as neighborhood environment (Robert 1999; Sampson 2003), residential segregation (Williams and Collins 2001), discrimination (Grollman 2014; Krieger 2000), education (Mirowsky and Ross 2003; Schnittker 2004), psychosocial stressors (House 2002), social networks (Christakis and Fowler 2009; Kawachi 2010; Liu, King, and Bearman 2010), and raced, classed, and gendered patterns in diet, exercise, and tobacco use (Pampel, Kreuger, and Denney 2010) contribute to health disparities.

Phelan, Link, and Tehranifa (2010) have also highlighted the importance of what they call "flexible resources" for mitigating the consequences of disease and making it easier to obtain effective treatment. Research on healthcare delivery has illuminated a number of dynamics that can affect the diagnosis and treatment process—from poor patient health literacy (Schillinger et al. 2002) to providers' racial biases (Feldman et al. 1997; van Ryn and Fu 2003) and ineffective communication between patients and healthcare providers (Johnson et al. 2004; Maynard 2003). Lutfey and Freese's (2005) ethnographic study of two diabetes clinics is a particularly compelling example of inequality in care provision. The clinic serving primarily middle-class patients offered greater continuity of care, more patient education, and more complex (and effective) treatment regimens. The clinic serving primarily poor and working-class patients offered little continuity of care or patient education and tended to prescribe simpler (but less beneficial) treatments, presuming these patients were more likely to adhere to simpler regimens. Often, shift-based work schedules, transportation difficulties, and less help with childcare and other responsibilities would have made adherence to complex treatment regimens impractical for some of these patients, particularly those who faced other obstacles—such as poor prescription insurance coverage. These findings point to complex interactions between structures of care delivery and structural constraints faced by patients that combine to perpetuate health inequalities.

Within a medical context in which the "meaning of patienthood" has shifted, "requiring patients to be actively involved in their care and become knowledgeable about managing illness" (Boyer and Lutfey 2010: S88), it is important to examine how patients' resources and actions also shape disparities in access and treatment. Shim (2010) suggested that a focus on CHC reveals how such inequalities permeate healthcare encounters. Shim pointed to skills and resources including "knowledge of medical topics and vocabulary . . . knowledge of what information is relevant to healthcare personnel [and the ability to efficiently communicate it] . . . an enterprising disposition and proactive stance toward health . . . and the ability to communicate social privilege and resources that can act as cues of favorable social and economic status and consumer savvy" (p. 3) as especially advantageous. Building on Bourdieu's (1977) theories of cultural capital and habitus, Shim argued that although CHC may be strategically deployed, it is often reflexively "embodied" as part of one's habitus, making its "accumulation and use . . . tacit and pragmatic" (p. 3). Shim stressed both patient agency and "upstream" structural constraints in cultivating and mobilizing CHC. CHC becomes even more conceptually useful when orientations toward help-seeking (Greil et al. 2011; Pescosolido 1992), information-seeking, or information-avoidance behaviors (Clark 2005; Czaja, Manfredi, and Price 2003; Gage and Panagakis 2012) and material resources are considered as well.[3]

This research represents great strides forward, yet few have empirically examined CHC in action. In one such study, Dubbin, Chang, and Shim (2013) showed how CHC can facilitate or hinder healthcare providers' efforts to achieve "patient-centered care," a movement in healthcare that seeks to improve understanding between patients and providers. Patients who possessed CHC that doctors valued could "jointly achieve a shared understanding of the clinical situation" (p. 117) with their provider. Without this match, patient-centered care was not achieved, and healthcare interactions faltered. Anspach's (1993) and Heimer and Staffen's (1998) research in neonatal intensive care units (NICUs) pointed to similar dynamics; interactions between parents and providers in these studies were more or less contentious depending on how actors understood their own and others' responsibilities in care provision and medical decision making.

While previous research has begun to consider how CHC shapes individual healthcare encounters and relationships, here I examine how CHC is mobilized throughout the illness and treatment process, facilitating swift access to highly specialized physicians and difficult-to-obtain and experimental treatments for families whose children had serious, life-threatening, and often rare conditions. CHC could also help families obtain small but valuable microadvantages during care delivery. I propose the concept of microadvantages here as a conceptual counterpoint to everyday microaggressions. *Microaggressions* are the potentially subtle but frequent everyday indignities experienced by members of marginalized groups (Sue 2010)—for example, the click of locked car doors as a black man walks past or the assumption that a same-sex partner is a sibling or friend. Within the healthcare context, I argue that microadvantages, conversely, might smooth interactions with providers, reduce suffering or discomfort, or offer emotional reassurance. These microadvantages were especially meaningful in the critical cases examined here.

DATA AND METHODS

I began conducting fieldwork at the Kelly-Reed University Hospital Ronald McDonald House (RMH)[4] in the fall of 2011. The RMH provides housing to families of seriously ill children who travel to receive care at Kelly-Reed. As a guest services volunteer, I answered phones; recorded donations; wrote thank-you notes; gave house tours to new families; hunted down extra towels, shampoo, or pillows; and transported families to and from the hospital as needed. I generally worked three- to six-hour shifts once or twice per week. Occasionally, I took families to the airport, to the grocery store, or on other various errands.

Fieldwork at the RMH offered an opportunity to immerse myself in families' social worlds. As they spoke with me about the technologically innovative procedures many had traveled great distances to obtain, I became increasingly interested in how they mobilized social, emotional, and economic resources to access cutting-edge and elite care for their children. Fieldwork at the RMH also allowed me (a white woman in my early thirties) to get to know families, build trust, and strategically select cases before asking them to meet for a formal interview.

Strategic case selection is a qualitative research strategy in which the researcher deliberately selects cases that offer the greatest analytic leverage on the research questions (Small 2009). Negative cases (Becker 1998), or those that might shed further light on initial findings, are intentionally sought to deepen developing analyses. Because my aim was to uncover generic processes that are not particular to a specific type of disease, regional culture, or social position, I selected cases that reflected a variety of life-threatening childhood illnesses and novel medical technologies. I recruited families from across geographic, educational, racial, and class backgrounds. This strategy allowed me to examine variations in families' illness and treatment trajectories. During a year and a half of fieldwork at the RMH, 18 families were recruited to the study.

Of these families, seven were white, six were black, two were biracial, two were Latino/a, and one was South Asian. Three travelled to Kelly-Reed from outside the United States (Canada, Puerto Rico, and Argentina). Eleven were married or partnered with their child's other parent. In two families, parents were divorced but coparenting. Three parents were single mothers, and two were custodial grandmothers (one single, one married). Eight families came to Kelly-Reed so that their children ($N = 9$) could undergo bone marrow, peripheral blood, or umbilical cord blood–derived stem-cell transplantation. Four children received different novel medical technologies, including enzyme replacement therapies, a unique organ-tissue transplant (currently available nowhere else in the world for children with a particular rare chromosomal deletion syndrome), or cancer vaccine immunotherapy. Six children underwent surgery to correct congenital defects, had standard organ transplants or cancer treatments, or received primarily life-sustaining intensive care. Nine families had at least one parent with a college degree and at least one parent in a professional or

managerial job. Nine remaining families held hourly-wage working-class jobs; had quit working-class jobs to care for ill children; were retired from working-class jobs; or were already unemployed or receiving disability before the child's illness.

Initial interviews averaged two hours, ranging in length from 90 minutes to more than three hours. If one parent or guardian was present at Kelly-Reed with a child, initial interviews included only the available parent. If both parents were present, parents were interviewed together—allowing them to add details to one another's responses and share similar and differing perspectives on the experience. I was often able to interview a nonpresent parent later or informally during future observations. All interviews were recorded and transcribed verbatim.

After initial interviews, I asked to accompany families on hospital visits or medical appointments so that I could observe interactions with their child's healthcare providers. I observed interactions during follow-up clinic visits (at which children were usually seen by a nurse, nurse practitioner, and one or more doctors); occupational, physical, and speech therapy sessions; patient-education sessions prior to clinical trial entry; stem-cell transplantation, magnetic resonance imaging (MRI) procedures, and lumbar punctures; and life-supporting care in the pediatric intensive care unit (PICU). During these observations,[3] I was able to gather direct empirical data on what kinds of questions families asked, what types of information and (potentially contradicting) recommendations healthcare providers offered, and how parents made medical decisions in the moment. These data allowed me to compare families' *accounts* (Scott and Lyman 1968) of their interactions with their lived experiences, enhancing the validity of my data. "Thick" descriptions of these interactions were recorded in detailed field notes as soon as possible following each observation.

During observations I also conducted informal, but often recorded, follow-up interviews during which I asked about the outcome of a test or treatment or learned new details of a family's ongoing efforts to coordinate care and make difficult medical decisions. Ongoing fieldwork at the RMH offered regular opportunities to check in with families whose treatments were sustained over some time.

Whenever possible, I continued to follow families even after they returned home through home visits, during phone interviews, or when families returned to Kelly-Reed for follow-ups.

While others have shadowed healthcare professionals in hospitals (see, for instance, Anspach 1993; Cadge 2012; Heimer and Staffen 1998), this family-centered ethnographic approach (loosely following Lareau 2003) gave me a different vantage point from which to view families' healthcare interactions. I was in the room with families before and after they were seen by healthcare providers, not only during the 10 to 20 minutes the provider was present. I was able to ask families immediately after observed interactions with a provider how they felt about something the doctor did or said, about how today's advice conflicted with previous advice or the evaluation of a different provider, or how they felt about a suggested course of action. By observing many of these families during their interactions across a variety of providers and settings, I brought a broad understanding of that particular family's situation and treatment history to my interpretation of the interaction and could discern patterns that developed across these interactions.

Following a grounded theory approach (Charmaz 2006), transcripts and field notes were coded for emerging themes early in data collection so that developing analyses could inform follow-up interview questions and case selection. Coding continued throughout the project and was followed by early and regular memo writing on emerging themes in the data. These classic ethnographic methods facilitated the twin goals of developing new theory (Tavory and Timmermans 2009) and uncovering generic social processes (Prus 1987; Schwalbe et al. 2000). By examining particularly "critical cases . . . [which] activate more actors and basic mechanisms in the situation studied" (Flyvbjerg 2001:78), this study explored CHC, illness management strategies, and the reproduction of inequalities in a situation where the stakes were highest. Families' abilities to obtain the best possible medical care—often requiring highly specialized medical expertise and groundbreaking medical interventions—were essential in these circumstances.

RESULTS

Families with high CHC often adopted an illness management strategy I call "care-captaining." If we think of navigating a child's life-threatening illness as akin to the metaphorical experience of guiding a ship through stormy waters, these parents regularly took the helm, steering and directing their children's medical care and treatment throughout their child's illness. Care-captaining involved negotiating with healthcare providers; conducting sophisticated research on available doctors, hospitals, and treatments; and successfully intervening to influence the care their children received. These parents also mobilized medical social networks on behalf of their children, gathering recommendations and calling in favors. These parents kept vigilant watch over the provision of their child's medical care, demonstrated the ability to hold key actors accountable, and held those actors accountable when they deemed necessary.

Families with less CHC often took a different approach—one in which they stayed on the medical sidelines. This strategy, which I call "care-entrusting," involved turning the wheel over to healthcare professionals who families hoped would steer the most effective course. Parents who primarily care-entrusted followed doctors' orders, ferried children to each institution and provider they were referred to, and focused their own efforts on the provision of everyday loving care, leaving medical decision making to healthcare professionals. Although some parents blended these strategies or shifted strategies at different points in the illness process (as I explicate below), high-CHC parents who regularly care-captained and those with less CHC who primarily care-entrusted tended to follow different paths to this elite institution and had different illness and treatment experiences after their arrival.

Getting Access

Care-Captaining: Climbing the Rungs of the U.S. Healthcare System. Parents who regularly care-captained—and who were well equipped with the CHC required to do so effectively—often accessed Kelly-Reed through self-referral or collaborative referrals. These parents did extensive research on the facilities and experts best equipped to treat their child's illness, sought favors from trusted medical social network ties, and deployed a host of resources and negotiation tactics to gain swift access to the care they deemed best for their children.

Todd and Savannah Marin are a case in point. When their then 6-month-old son, Jacob, was diagnosed with Tay-Sachs—a rare, fatal, genetic, degenerative neurological disorder—Savannah, a white, 32-year-old, first-time mother with a bachelor's degree in nursing, and Todd, a white, 35-year-old contractor, were devastated to learn that the only option for Jacob in their West Coast home state was palliative hospice care. Todd recalled the diagnosing physician telling them, "Go look for clinical trials—'you go do your homework and I'll do mine.'" But at their next visit, Savannah reported, "He hadn't done anything. Like . . . he had printed out another sheet from his database . . . and told us, 'Oh, looks like he has 2–4 years to live.'" Unwilling to accept this outcome, the Marins "did their homework" and scoured FDA databases for clinical trials. They contacted the founder of a Tay-Sachs research foundation who told them about an experimental observational study: an umbilical cord blood–derived stem-cell transplant at Kelly-Reed, thousands of miles from their home. He put them in touch with a family whose now 10-year-old son had received the transplant, reassuring the Marins that their son might also be able to enjoy a reasonable quality of life for a longer period of time.

While they waited for test results to identify Jacob's particular variant of the disease, Savannah began requesting therapies that might strengthen Jacob neurologically before the disease took root. She explained:

> My brain goes to, okay, if he has a neurological disease, that's going to affect the neural connections. Let's make *more* neural connections. He's a *baby*. The more we do with him, the more connections he'll have. So then maybe he would have more places that the [metabolic] waste would have to build

up, so . . . I'm like, we should be getting him therapy! Let's make him as strong as possible right now, so he has even *further* to have to deteriorate. *Nobody* at that point was recommending any type of therapies. So I request it. Hey, can he get PT? And OT? And, [after learning of an infant swim therapy program] I'm like, whoa! Let's do water therapy! And PT, and OT! [emphasis hers]

Savannah also flew Jacob to another highly ranked East Coast research hospital to be seen by national Tay-Sachs experts. These doctors' positive assessment of Jacob's neurological state reassured the Marins that the transplant at Kelly-Reed might be successful and buy them time until a longer-term cure was discovered. Savannah negotiated with her insurance company to get the million-dollar treatment covered. After multiple phone calls, Savannah recalled the case manager exclaiming, "Savannah, you don't know what you're asking!" to which she replied, "I *do* know: *I want you to save my kid!*" Their insurance company and Kelly-Reed ultimately signed an agreement to approve the transplant. The Marins put their house up for sale, placed their belongings in storage, and traveled across the country, hoping to give their son a rare chance at survival.

The Marins' efforts to secure every possible health advantage for their son illustrate the power of a care-captaining approach when used by parents with abundant CHC. Savannah possessed an understanding of neural connections and how they develop, allowing her to hypothesize that having more of them might slow the progression of a disease that systematically destroys them. She felt comfortable requesting therapies that "nobody at that point was recommending" and had a general sense of how to make such requests and from whom. Savannah knew what clinical trials were and how to search for them, and she understood the medical language used in their descriptions. She possessed a basic understanding of the hierarchy of the U.S. healthcare system and understood that research hospitals might offer options not yet available in other places. Savannah was able to parlay the more general skills associated with cultural capital (in particular, comfort interacting and negotiating with institutions and authority figures; see also Lareau 2003) into coverage for an otherwise prohibitively expensive experimental medical treatment. These skills and resources equipped her with the ability to regularly influence Jacob's care over the course of his treatment, as illustrated ahead.

Simone Brady-Fischer, a white, 40-year-old Canadian mother of five who worked for a local foundation before taking a medical leave to care for her 11-year-old son, Max, also did "lots of hours of research" on her son's condition, declaring herself a "research junkie." Max struggled for several years with a congenital malformation that blocked the proper flow of cerebrospinal fluid around his brain. Unsatisfied with the treatment Max was receiving at home, Simone visited "every website that was reputable," and, she explained:

> I listened to hours and hours of doctoral lectures . . . and after I listened to Dr. J's lecture, I knew he was the right doctor, because Max's symptoms all fit what he specialized in, so I knew he was just the right one.

When I asked Simone how she identified "reputable websites" or distinguished good information from bad, she had a hard time articulating her process beyond telling me, "You have to definitely use your judgment." She explained, however, that when one of Max's home doctors had insinuated that her sources might be unreliable, she replied, irritated, "And would you consider the Mayo Clinic to be a reliable resource?" Simone's response reveals not how the impulse to conduct research is a somewhat intangible component of CHC; that knowing which sources of information are prestigious enough to be taken seriously, either by parents or by healthcare providers, is largely invisible to those who possess this knowledge. Simone cannot explain *how* she knew Max's doctor would respect the Mayo Clinic, she just "knew." In sociological terms, it is part of her "habitus" (Bourdieu 1977; Dubbin et al. 2013). This automatic understanding of the hierarchies of prestige and resources within the healthcare system was a key resource that high-CHC families used to obtain useful information about their child's condition, locate the most specialized care for that condition, and get providers to take their input seriously. Simone's confidence that her online research could be taken seriously by medical authorities allowed her to feel comfortable challenging those authorities. After contacting Dr. J and being impressed by his attentiveness during a lengthy weekend phone consultation, Simone and her husband, a white, 60-year-old, provincial government official, wired nearly $9,000 to Kelly-Reed[5] so that Max could be evaluated and treated by the physician she had painstakingly selected for him.

Other families leveraged medically rich social networks to speed their climb up the rungs of the U.S. health system and feel confident in the choices they made. When Nora Bialy's then 12-year-old son Benjamin began having severe headaches, dizziness, and vomiting, Nora, a white mother of four in her late thirties who had previously worked as a dietician, and her husband William—a child psychiatrist in his early forties—pushed for testing that ultimately discovered Benjamin's brain tumor. Nora told me:

> We actually pushed for the neurology consult before they were really ready to give us a neurology consult . . . because [William] knew that something else . . . we were hoping it was nothing more serious, but we knew there was a chance of it.

After the Bialys obtained a swift referral, Ben was seen by a neurologist the very next day:

> Because we were really pressing on the symptoms, we kept saying, you know, "These symptoms, [could be serious]." And my husband actually called someone I guess that he knew and asked if he could get us in.

After using William's medical network ties to get Ben seen immediately, Nora turned to her own trusted medical ties upon diagnosis. Once the neurologist identified the brain tumor, Nora had a neurosurgeon she had used for her own spinal surgery in the past on the phone within "like 10 minutes." That doctor referred her to a particular physician at an elite research hospital in a neighboring state who specialized in Ben's specific type of pediatric tumor. Nora took Ben to a local hospital and requested an immediate medical transport to the recommended hospital. Ben was placed into the care of the doctor her neurosurgeon recommended and was in surgery hours later.

By turning to trusted medical social networks, the Bialys felt that they had gotten Ben to the "best" care available—offering the microadvantage of some comfort and reassurance during a terrifying time. Other families also turned to social network ties with medical expertise, sometimes seeking out "weak ties" (Granovetter 1973)—for instance, a friend's husband's brother (a physician) in another state—to confirm that Kelly-Reed was the best place to seek care.

Care-Entrusting: Following Orders and Navigating Mazes in the U.S. Health System. While care-captains often actively sought access to Kelly-Reed, families with less CHC who adopted a care-entrusting approach generally arrived at Kelly-Reed because a local physician sent them up the ladder. These referrals were sometimes serendipitous—without them, these families may not have gained access to potentially lifesaving treatments not available at local and regional hospitals and, in some cases, available only at this particular hospital.

Anaya Rowland, for example, was born with a congenital heart defect and treated at a regional hospital several hours from Kelly-Reed. At a scheduled five-month check-up, her doctors became concerned. Anaya's mother, Chanise, a black mother of five in her late twenties who received disability, explained, "The tube they put in her when she was born . . . was closing up on her." A few days later the doctors told her, "The only option she had left is for them to airlift her to Kelly-Reed to keep her alive. So I told them [to] do what they got to do to save her."

Anaya was airlifted to Kelly-Reed and went into cardiac arrest just hours later. She stopped breathing, was resuscitated, and was immediately taken into emergency surgery. While it is impossible to know what would have happened had Anaya not made it to Kelly-Reed before "crashing," Chanise understood this as the crucial step that saved her daughter's life. Chanise recalled that a nurse at Kelly-Reed, who was comforting Chanise during her distress, told her, "We got her back alive! Think about it, if she was still at [the regional hospital] you wouldn't have a little girl tonight!" This was particularly alarming to Chanise, because initially Anaya was not going to be transported until the following week. She credited her daughter's arrival at Kelly-Reed that evening to one "really good doctor" who "stayed right up on her" and pushed to get her airlifted immediately, as opposed to the following Monday as initially planned. In a situation where parents who care-captained may have taken control of the situation and insisted on an immediate transfer, Chanise left this decision to the doctors, depending on them to determine the timing and destination of Anaya's transfer.

Not all families encountered doctors who sent them up the ladder so quickly. Connie and Nicholas Henderson, poor white parents of two in their mid-forties from a rural area in a neighboring state, told me that they knew something was wrong when their youngest son, 4-year-old Elijah, complained of constant stomach pain, ran a fever, and stopped passing bowels. But the Hendersons were ill equipped to advocate for him when doctors at their local rural hospital told them to give him Tylenol and Miralax and sent them home repeatedly. Despite Elijah's continuing pain, the Hendersons felt helpless during that period to do more to get him the care he needed. Connie told me despairingly:

> What can you do when you can't get nobody to listen to you? I mean, we've made six trips in three weeks . . . and wouldn't nobody do anything, until that one doctor said, "Well, I think it's his appendix, we need to have a CT scan done," . . . and they did a CT scan and that's when they found the tumor on his liver. But it took that long just to get somebody to listen to us, you know?

For the Hendersons, who had little CHC that might have allowed them to push for more specific testing or specialized referrals, the process of getting their child to treatment was haphazard and confusing. When I asked what the doctors told them when they turned them away, the Hendersons reported:

Nicholas: They'd say, "Well, if there was too much wrong, his belly would be real tight"—which it was extended—" and he would be running a real real high fever." But . . . they weren't considering I was giving him Tylenol and Motrin around the clock [as he recalled being instructed to]. But then when we got to [the regional hospital] one of the younger doctors jumped on us because we was giving him Tylenol and Motrin around the clock. And I told her, "We're just doing what our doctor told us to do." And they said, "Well, you ain't supposed to do that, that's bad for the liver," and I'm like, "Well, I'm just doing what I'm supposed to do."

Connie: Or what they *told* us to do. [emphasis hers]

With little CHC, the Hendersons may not have received sufficient clarification about how much or how often to give Tylenol and/or Motrin. A care-entrusting strategy made it unlikely that they would subsequently propose that this might have masked more serious symptoms on future visits (highlighting the importance of continuity of care) or that they would ask doctors to look deeper given those factors.

After Elijah's tumor was identified, he was referred for standard treatment at the nearest regional hospital. Once doctors there determined that a liver transplant was necessary, the Hendersons were sent to Kelly-Reed. Without significant CHC, the Hendersons depended on local doctors and hospitals to facilitate access to appropriate care for their son. Although this eventually occurred, their child's health was at greater risk and his suffering was prolonged while they waited for providers to point them in the right direction.

Other families with little CHC also followed referrals that ultimately led them to Kelly-Reed: some after similarly lengthy periods of frustration, and others serendipitously when they happened to encounter a local doctor familiar with their child's rare condition who channeled them quickly to doctors with that particular expertise. Although some families accessed highly specialized, cutting-edge care with little CHC, there are likely many others who did not. Without the constellation of skills and resources mobilized by families with significant CHC, these families may have slipped through the cracks, accepted a fatal diagnosis as such, or remained unaware of developing technologies that might have offered other options for their children.

Managing Care

Once at Kelly-Reed, care-captaining and care-entrusting continued to produce very different illness and treatment experiences. Parents who regularly care-captained influenced their children's care throughout the treatment process by (1) keeping vigilant surveillance over the provision of their child's medical care, (2) negotiating with physicians to alter their child's treatment or medication plans, and (3) signifying the potential to hold providers accountable and then when required.

"Hovering Like Hawks": Vigilant Surveillance and Medical Intervention. Todd and Savannah Marin stayed with Jacob every day throughout his six-month hospitalization, reviewing his daily laboratory reports, monitoring medication administration, and speaking with doctors during every daily round. If Jacob was transferred to the PICU, often for weeks at a time, the Marins stepped up their surveillance, trading off 12-hour shifts from 7 a.m. to 7 p.m., so that one of them would be with him, and awake, night and day. Savannah explained:

If there was something funky Todd would text me, or call me, and be like [gasp] "Oh what's this about," you know? . . . "This is what they want to change on his meds," . . .

and then we'd have a conversation about it so he could advocate for him even when I wasn't there. Because in the PICU, you have to. Like . . . they are constantly trying to change meds and change schedules on the platelet transfusions, and all kinds of stuff.

Being constantly present allowed the Marins to remain aware of every detail of Jacob's status and treatment and to influence the care he received. The Marins felt that by being present they could steer Jacob away from medical interventions that might be implemented by a provider who was not familiar with Jacob's specific needs and prior reactions. As Todd explained:

> They have certain things that they follow too, if they hear something, this is automatically what we do. [But] I already know that Jacob had a negative response to certain things. We had a respiratory therapist come in, for instance, and, "Oh, I heard him doing this, so I'm going to automatically do this." I'm like, "No, you're not going to do that, because if you do that, then we're going to have more of a complication. Because we've already been through this process before, we already know he doesn't have a good response to this." And if I hadn't done that, and I hadn't been there, it would've just been done. And then we could've had more of a negative thing.

By being constantly present and asserting knowledge of Jacob's response to a host of medications and treatments, the Marins steered providers away from treatments Jacob had not tolerated well in the past, potentially minimizing unnecessary stress and discomfort for their child—a small, but for them priceless, microadvantage. The Marins worked to influence Jacob's medication regimen as well, particularly when they wanted him off of damaging medications, like steroids, as quickly as possible. Savannah told me:

> I can't tell you how many times we've asked about a medication, and they've changed

it sooner than they would have, or later, or whatever. . . . If you don't ask, then they're just going to keep going on their schedule, and if [on our unit] there's five docs involved and everybody has their own opinion, one doc might have taken that medication off three days ago, the doc that's on right now might not have even seen it on the list, you know? . . . then the doc next week might be like, "Oh no, he needs to have twice as much!"

Given doctors' differences in opinion, the Marins pushed providers in the direction that they judged best:

> We wanted him off steroids as soon as possible because we know, "Oh that could have contributed to the bleed in his gut" . . . and of course it contributes to like fluid retention, and high blood pressure, and immune suppression, and all those other bad things. . . . But then they had to put him back on when he had other surgeries and stuff, so it's like, "Okay then, let's hurry up and get him back off again." [But] the last time we took it off . . . his body went out of whack and he had adrenal suppression, and adrenal insufficiency. So then all of a sudden his electrolytes went out of whack, his blood pressure dropped and like, got weird fast, so this time we were like, "Okay, well we do want to wean it again, but we're not in a hurry."

Savannah spoke about the consequences of Jacob's medication changes in ways that demonstrated her technical understanding of the specific biological chain of events that occurred when Jacob went on and off steroids. That Savannah was able to converse with doctors at this level likely helped them see her requests as informed ones, worth consideration—even if they didn't always lead to perfect outcomes. Without this display of knowledge, doctors may have been less willing to make these adjustments. I personally witnessed Savannah's influence over Jacob's medication regimen during a clinic visit in which she successfully lobbied the doctor to remove a costly prescription for vitamin K because of dietary changes she had initiated. From my field notes:

> Savannah asked about Jacob's vitamin K because, "Everybody's kind of wishy-washy about whether he needs vitamin K anymore." Dr. L said that he's doing well on vitamin K. Savannah reminded her that it's a $200 prescription every month, and that he might just "hang out low anyway" in his vitamin K levels. Dr. L agreed that he may be doing better since Savannah began adding blended foods to the breast milk administered through his feeding tube, and offered the option of not giving him vitamin K for now and checking his labs without it. Savannah said, "Yeah, that's what I was wondering."
>
> At the end of the appointment, Dr. L reiterated, "So we're decreasing the tacrolimus, hold the vitamin K, we'll check the coags next week." She warned that even if the numbers were okay, Dr. S [Jacob's primary doctor] might want to keep him on it, but Savannah quickly offered, "No that's great, we can just check it out."

By speaking knowledgably, comfortably, and confidently with medical lingo, the Marins gained doctors' trust and exerted significant influence over the provision of all aspects of their son's medical care.

Although Savannah's medical background allowed the Marins to care-captain especially effectively, more general cultural capital allowed other care-captaining parents to develop CHC and exert influence. Edward Rivera and Juliana Cruz, middle-class parents in their early thirties who had two children, traveled to Kelly-Reed from Puerto Rico to obtain a cord blood–derived stem-cell transplant for their infant son, Noah (for mucopolysaccharidosis—another usually fatal genetic degenerative neurological disease). They also kept vigilant watch over their son's care and actively negotiated with physicians even though English was their second language. When Noah caught a virus shortly after his transplant (before his new immune system had taken root) and was transferred to the PICU, both

Edward and Juliana remained by Noah's side from morning until night watching the monitors, checking his urine output, suctioning his airways, and questioning doctors about his dialysis titration rates and next steps and options. Edward and Juliana thus obtained detailed explanations from doctors every few hours about Noah's condition, providing opportunities for these parents to develop CHC and participate in Noah's care. For instance, during one of my visits, Edward raised the possibility of a white blood cell infusion and asked the doctors to retest for the virus that spurred Noah's decline. The doctors agreed to do so, even though they suggested the results "wouldn't really affect his treatment." For Edward, though, the test offered potentially reassuring information that might help to allay his growing fears for his son's recovery; this represented a rather small microadvantage, but nonetheless a resource with which Edward might feel more hopeful or better prepare for a bad outcome.

Simone Brady-Fischer also altered the course of her son's treatment. Although Max's neurosurgeon in Canada decided that surgery to correct the malformation should not be performed in Max's case, attributing his frequent violent seizures to other causes, Simone was dubious. After finding information that suggested to her that increased intracranial pressure (ultimately confirmed by a lumbar puncture at Kelly-Reed) might not have been visible on the MRI, Simone sought a second opinion from doctors at a different top-ranked U.S. research hospital (the only one she found that offered remote consults) at her own expense:

> We sent his MRI disc, I bought it, like, paid 200 bucks for it . . . and then sent $1500 to [an elite U.S. research hospital] and checked off all three options, like, I could only have one option, but I checked off all three . . . either they send you a report directly, they have a conversation with your [home] physician, or you can have a conference call between the three of you, and I checked off all three boxes, and then I wrote beside it, "Whichever will get treatment the fastest!" . . . I said, "I don't care what you do, whatever gets us results."

Eight days later, Max's Canadian neurosurgeon performed the surgery. Here, Simone leveraged her research skills and comfort in challenging authority to influence Max's treatment. That Simone felt empowered to check off three boxes and write marginal notes expressing her distress to convey a sense of urgency to those she sought help from was a significant display of cultural capital and ease in interacting with institutional authorities similar to that embodied by parents in Lareau's (2003) ethnography.

The Brady-Fischers also influenced Max's medication regimen, particularly the psychotropic medications prescribed to manage his pain. Simone's narrative reveals her understanding of her role in this process:

> He's tried him on like every psychotic pill *that we would let him try.* . . . There were a few *we said no to* because we did some research, and were like, "Uh, no." Like the side effects potentially could be pretty harmful. [emphasis mine]

Simone presented herself and her husband as the ultimate decision makers. Although Simone conceded that when Max's doctor is "adamant" that Max try a medication, she doesn't immediately refuse it, she understands the process as a negotiation. When Max arrived at Kelly-Reed he was taking a medication she "really wanted him off of," but because his Kelly-Reed neurologist (whose credentials and publications she admired) hesitated to make multiple changes at once, she acquiesced. Yet, she still framed this as a concession and planned to request the change again soon. In this way, Simone could feel a degree of control over Max's illness and treatment. At times, these interventions were instrumental, as when a lumbar puncture at Kelly-Reed confirmed the significantly elevated intracranial pressure she had suspected—a serious problem that would have continued untreated without her exceptionally persistent care-captaining efforts.

Nora Bialy also intervened to influence the medical interventions Benjamin received during his treatment. While undergoing radiation for his brain tumor, burning on the back of Ben's esophagus led him to have pain when swallowing and to eat less. Nora told me, "Being a registered dietician, I knew when Ben's nutritional status was [declining]." So Nora lobbied Ben's medical team:

> I pushed for the feeding tube to be put in quickly because I have an understanding of feeding tubes, and like, people get freaked out by that . . . but he did great with it. He actually was able to gain weight on it, and [then we] got him off of it. It wasn't a permanent thing, but it needed to be there.

Nora brought her professional knowledge to bear on Ben's illness, and doctors agreed to her request to place a gastric feeding tube (G-tube)—a small tube inserted surgically into the abdomen allowing nutrition to be delivered directly into the stomach. Nora reported that this quickly increased Ben's weight and strength, improving his quality of life and potentially his body's receptiveness to treatment during this difficult period.

"What You Think Is the Way I Want to Go": Staying on the Medical Sidelines. Parents who primarily care-entrusted did not wield the same influence over their child's medical care, nor did they aim to. Families with less CHC advocated for their children but focused primarily on issues of basic hygiene or comfort: wanting to provide kids "home cooked meals," asking nurses to tape down the cords on a child's accessed port so they wouldn't be tugged on (causing discomfort), and so on. But when it came to the provision of a child's medical care and medically important decisions, families with less CHC often deferred to doctors and other experts who would "know better" than they did.

Lakira Harris, a 32-year-old black single mother of four who had previously worked as a security guard, followed a referral when she made the difficult decision to travel with her oldest child, 8-year-old Jayden Lacoste, to Kelly-Reed for a cord blood–derived stem-cell transplant. Jayden, who was born with a severe case of sickle-cell disease, had already suffered several life-threatening vaso-occlusive crises requiring lengthy hospitalizations. Lakira explained:

> Dr. J called me one day and told me that there was an opening for Kelly-Reed, and that they had research money for stem cell research. And he asked me if I wanted to go, because he felt like it was best for Jayden, in his case, to go. And, um, I prayed about it, and I was like, "If that's what you think is best for my child, then I will do it." And that's how we got here. It was all the doctors rooting for me and my son.

Lakira relied on Jayden's doctors to point her toward the best treatment option, and although she "decided" to follow their advice—a decision she understood as important and that she prayed about—she ultimately felt best about doing what the doctors recommended. Unlike the care-captaining parents in the previous section, Lakira turned to prayer rather than medical journal articles or medical social networks to make this consequential decision.

Lakira, whose warmth and demonstrative affection for her son may have encouraged doctors to see her as someone who would make good use of a scarce resource, continued to interact deferentially with Jayden's physicians at Kelly-Reed, even when she felt uncertain about the course of Jayden's treatment. For instance, although Lakira voiced unwavering confidence to the nurse coordinator after the patient education session in which the cord blood protocol was explained, in a conversation with me after the meeting concluded Lakira hinted at lingering concerns and misunderstandings. These concerns came to a head on the day of Jayden's transplant (which I also observed). The transplant involved a series of infusions of donor cord blood over a period of about eight hours while Jayden colored, played games, or watched television. Lakira had been in contact with someone at a local sickle-cell foundation in her southeastern home state who called her in the middle of that day and asked her a series of questions—such as how many other families had participated in the study and what survival rates were. They suggested

to her that Jayden might be one of the first children to undergo this particular type of cord blood transplant and told her she should ask about survival rates. Lakira, realizing that she was not certain about the answers to these questions, was visibly alarmed. But she got out a small notebook and wrote down a few questions she wanted to ask Dr. R (Jayden's primary physician at Kelly-Reed and head of this particular study). An hour later, while Jayden was taking a walk in the hall with a physical therapist, Dr. R poked his head into the room. Lakira grabbed her notebook and tried to ask the questions she had written down, but she phrased them as questions that "the lady at the sickle cell foundation wants to know, and I told her I didn't know the answers." From my field notes:

> Dr. R told her that if the foundation wants information about the protocol, they should contact the doctors, not her, and that she should tell them to page him or email Dr. M, the director of the unit. Lakira said, "Okay" several times, and then told Dr. R that they were "kind of scaring her." Dr. R reiterated that if she is not comfortable with their questions she should tell them that "Jayden is doing fine" and to contact the doctors. Lakira said, "Alright, thank you Dr. R." Shortly after he left, I asked Lakira if she felt like Dr. R had answered her questions. She gave me an exasperated look, and said, "No! I feel like he kind of brushed me off."

Because Lakira framed her questions as coming from the foundation rather than herself, she did not successfully communicate to Dr. R her worries about the procedure and her desire for answers. The doctor responded only to his concern—one that I shared—that the foundation was asking her for information (including her signed trial enrollment papers) that would be more appropriately requested directly from the program itself. Yet, when he failed to provide these answers, Lakira did not ask Dr. R again or clarify that she wanted him to give *her* those answers, now. Rather, she demurely acknowledged his instructions and politely thanked him anyway.

Often, deferring to doctors and following orders (particularly once they had accessed specialized care) was a relatively successful strategy and could alternatively allow families to feel confident in their child's care. Mary Shaw, a white, 58-year-old, retired working-class custodial grandmother to her 7-year-old grandson, Aaron, expressed no doubt that Aaron's doctors would provide him with any care he needed and took pride in following their recommendations diligently. Because of weekly infusions of several enzyme replacement therapies provided through successive clinical trials at Kelly-Reed, Aaron had already survived two years longer than doctors predicted for a child with his rare, genetic glycogen and lysosomal storage disorder. Aaron was doing well and attending public school, although he wore braces on his legs, used assistive devices to walk significant distances, and struggled to speak clearly because of weak jaw and facial muscles. Mary told me that she had followed a series of referrals from local doctors who identified Aaron's condition shortly after he was born, which led to Dr. C, one of the Kelly-Reed researchers who oversaw the clinical trials that had extended Aaron's life. Mary continued to follow Dr. C's referrals to related specialists and to physical, occupational, and speech therapies. Mary assured me that she dutifully followed all of the doctor's directives: "She'll tell me, 'Well, he needs to see this [specialist],' and whatever she said I need to see, he's seen." When I asked Mary how she made decisions about medications or other treatment options, she told me, "I always leave it up [to them]. I say, 'What you think [we should do] is the way I want to go.' [That's] the way I leave it with them." From this perspective, Mary did not need to become more deeply involved in directing Aaron's medical care, because she turned that role over to those she deemed most competent to perform it, and she took comfort in doing so.

Pauline Donnoly, a white, working-class, retired custodial grandmother to biracial (white/Latina) 7-year-old Isabelle Santos, also told me that she had confidence in Isabelle's Kelly-Reed providers, but she simultaneously recognized the potentially unsettling limits of her expertise. When I asked Pauline how she chose Kelly-Reed for Isabelle's treatment for a rare type of kidney tumor, she explained that doctors at their coastal home hospital had sent them there when Isabelle's cancer recurred. She continued:

> I mean if you think about it, you don't really have the knowledge base. If I had had time to have sought out different hospitals, *I still wouldn't have known what I was looking for, or what would have been right.*

Because Pauline was not as familiar with healthcare hierarchies and hospital rankings, she could not take the same comfort in Kelly-Reed's elite status or its physicians' publication records as those with more CHC could. Instead, she told me, "You're hoping. You're hoping they're doing [a good job]. And I feel confident that they are." Without the knowledge or networks to technically assess their children's healthcare providers or treatment plans, Pauline, Mary, and Lakira stayed on the sidelines and hoped the experts in charge would steer the best course.

Holding Providers Accountable. Being constantly present and regularly negotiating about their child's care and treatment allowed care-captaining parents to signify to doctors and other care providers that they had the knowledge and ability to hold them accountable if needed. The Marins' constant presence at Jacob's side meant they were there to witness any problems or mistakes and could intervene when needed—a phenomenon that led nurses in the NICU Heimer and Staffen (1998) studied to label hovering parents "pains in the neck." Often the Marins' presence simply meant making sure that medications were given on time and that Jacob's schedule didn't get "off" (resulting in medications being administered at nonideal times). But on a few occasions, the Marins caught what they considered "true med errors" and either prevented the mistake from happening or held the responsible party accountable for the mistake. Here, Savannah's medical knowledge as an RN was particularly advantageous:

Savannah: The couple times that he got the wrong dose or was going to get the wrong order, like . . .

the wrong flush before a med or something, it's like, "Okay, *this* is unacceptable" . . . like, if you can cause a serious issue.

Todd: We had that happen once. And that one, I wasn't very happy about that. Actually went and talked to the nurse practitioner and did get them thrown off our team. It was just too serious for me to [handle] . . . but that was an instance like, if Savannah had not been standing there, that would not have gotten caught, and it was a really serious offense.

Although Vivian Patterson, a black middle-class mother in her early forties, did not have Savannah's medical training, she kept her own careful log of all the medications her 17-year-old son, Shawn, was given during his inpatient treatment for a primitive neuroectodermal tumor. Vivian also caught a medication error when a nurse brought in a dose of three pills and Vivian knew the dose should be four pills. While at first the nurse insisted that Vivian was mistaken, Vivian surmised that the nurse must have gone out and "spoken to someone [who informed him], 'she really is paying attention, she is on the game'" because he came back and "owned up" to making the mistake and administered the fourth pill. Here, care-captaining and vigilant surveillance even without technical medical knowledge allowed Vivian to successfully hold providers accountable and prevent a medication error.

Simone Brady-Fischer took comfort in her capacity to hold providers accountable more publicly. Doctors at Kelly-Reed suggested that Max get ongoing treatment at an elite children's hospital in Canada, outside of her home province. I asked Simone whether the state insurance plan in her home province would cover his care there. She told me that "they have to approve it or not" but assured me (and herself) that they would approve it, because:

If they don't, I'm going to make a big stink in the media about it . . . CBC in Canada is like the equivalent of CNN down here. They're

already all over his story on Facebook. They want to interview me, like, in the worst way. But I want to go up the ladder in the right way. Because in the end, these two negligent doctors . . . need to be called up by the college of physicians in Canada, and [told], "Hey!" Like, "Take this shit seriously, and now pay for his suffering that has happened."

Although Simone quashed her immediate desire to go to the press, calculating that first trying to "go up the ladder in the right way" might get her the best results, she felt that she could take steps to hold her province's health bureau publicly accountable if she did not get the results she wanted. Simone not only felt comfortable questioning and challenging the competency of prestigious professionals but also possessed a basic understanding of how to report them, to whom, and what consequences she might be able to create for them.

Families with less CHC, however, struggled to hold providers accountable. Tina Morgan, a white, 30-year-old, working-class mother of two, was outraged when her infant daughter, Kassidy, who was born with a congenital diaphragmatic hernia requiring surgery and months of life-supporting care in the NICU, fell out of a bouncy-seat and hit her head "on a nurse's watch." Tina never did successfully report the nurse, whom she viewed as negligent for not preventing the incident or swiftly informing her of it, although she had tried, explaining:

It was quite aggravating to try to file, to figure out who was over them. I went to the information desk in the front of the hospital, or on the fourth floor. They don't want to tell you. "Oh, they're gone. Oh, they're on vacation." It's like you get the run around.

Tina was routinely frustrated by her interactions with providers at Kelly-Reed, with whom she was frequently at odds. Tina attempted to care-captain, but she had little CHC that might have encouraged providers to take her efforts seriously. After the tumble, Tina requested an MRI but was told it was not needed and would expose Kassidy to unnecessary radiation. Tina was displeased. Later, when doctors required a swallowing test before Kassidy could be bottle-fed, Tina withheld permission because she Googled the test and surmised that the radiation "was like off the charts" and might cause leukemia. Although Tina wanted to participate more in Kassidy's daily care by feeding and bathing her daughter herself and was frustrated when nurses discouraged those efforts, she instead chose to forgo her desire to bottle-feed and refused the test. Such clashes led to further contention and miscommunication with Kelly-Reed providers and additional frustration for Tina.

Families with less CHC who care-entrusted also could not signify the potential to hold providers accountable in the ways care-captains could. Unlike the Marins and Rivera-Cruzes, who remained by their child's side all or almost all of the time they were in the intensive care unit, Lakira Harris could not bear to spend much time in the PICU when Jayden's body rejected the donor stem cells and his organs began failing. Lakira walked over to the hospital to visit Jayden each morning, but found it too difficult to "stay positive" if she watched him sedated and suffering for long. This meant she was not present to encourage nurses to keep perfect timing with medication schedules, to double-check laboratory work, to suggest possible tests or treatments, or to gather detailed information about Jayden's condition that might increase her CHC and comfort participating in his care. But to be constantly present, without feeling she could do much for him, was simply too hard on her. Lakira already worried that perhaps she "should've fought harder" when Jayden began having the severe pain that preceded his decline and doctors did not immediately identify a cause, but lacked the CHC with which she might have researched possibilities or sought second opinions as care-captaining parents often did. "How can you fight when they're doing what they're supposed to do and you're looking at the test yourself and you're like, 'Well, I don't see nothing either?'" she asked me. Once he was in the PICU, Lakira felt she could best fight for Jayden by "refus[ing] to think anything negative"—a task that was harder to accomplish when facing evidence of his poor condition. Lakira explained that it was good for her to be back at the RMH, because she needed "time

away from being up there and worrying." In order to avoid becoming emotionally overwhelmed, then, Lakira moved further towards the sidelines during the final weeks of Jayden's life.

DISCUSSION

These findings demonstrate how CHC can be mobilized over the course of illness trajectories and point to important advantages (big and small) that CHC can help secure. It is impossible to quantify disparities in long-term health outcomes between the families in this study (and for some, these outcomes are not yet determined)—in part because of the unknowable conditions involved. Benjamin Bialy's tumor, a medulloblastoma, has just under a 70% five-year survival rate for teens aged 10 to 19 (Smoll 2012). Yet, despite his parents' and physicians' exceptional efforts, Ben died four and a half years after his cancer was diagnosed. One could surmise from this single outcome measure that the Bialys did not gain much through their interventions. However, it is also possible that Ben's particular tumor was so aggressive that his life might have been cut even shorter, or his quality of life further reduced, without his parents' efforts to obtain speedy referrals and cutting-edge treatments across several elite research hospitals. Ultimately, the course his individual illness might have taken with a different set of treatments and circumstances is simply unknowable. Future, larger-scale research might usefully explore differences in long-term outcomes or survival rates between patients and families who use the illness management strategies I have explicated here with differing amounts of CHC at their disposal. Future research might also examine the use of these illness management strategies in other settings and at different levels of the U.S. healthcare system.

My aim here is to identify and explicate the processes through which families negotiated illness and accessed and influenced children's medical care. These cases also illuminate the smaller microadvantages that care-captaining can yield for some parents and children. That Nora Bialy encouraged doctors to place a G-tube as soon as Ben developed pain with swallowing likely minimized discomfort and improved his overall strength and nutrition—which in turn may have allowed him to better enjoy the time he had and to accomplish his educational and philanthropic goals (Ben was awarded two honorary degrees before he died and served as a spokesperson for several foundations raising funds for pediatric cancer research). Preventing a medication error, discouraging the administration of a nonessential treatment that had ill-effects in the past, obtaining supplemental therapies, or shortening lengthy periods of nontreatment due to slow diagnosis or delayed access to specialists are a few of the many small and not-so-small advantages that can be obtained with a combination of resources derived from CHC and an approach to illness management rooted in care-captaining. These efforts also offered important emotional advantages for parents, who could avoid the anguish of being shuttled around the lower rungs of the healthcare system indefinitely, being frustrated or disappointed by their interactions with providers, or worrying that they could have done more to save their child.

Yet, care-captaining was not without costs. Constant research and surveillance could exact a high toll on families, requiring massive investments of time and energy. Care-captaining could also become an obstacle to doctors' ability to perform potentially lifesaving interventions, as it did at one key juncture for Jacob Marin. When Jacob was admitted to the PICU during a period of posttransplant deterioration, PICU doctors wanted to intubate him for mechanical ventilation (or "put him on the vent"). The Marins were hesitant to proceed because they worried that "If he's put on a ventilator, he probably won't get off the ventilator." They also worried that problems during a previous intubation indicated that Jacob might have a "delicate airway." They continued gathering opinions and were surprised when PICU doctors told them, as Savannah recalled, "Well if you're gonna put him on the vent, do it. Like, it's starting to get more and more pressing." The Marins called Jacob's primary doctor (who was away) on his cell phone to solicit his opinion. Dr. S assured them that "his organ systems are good" so, "if he needs to go on the vent, ask them when it's time, when it's a 'no going back' . . . and then put him on the vent if he needs to be on the vent." The

Marins then posed this question to the PICU doctors, whom they recalled saying, "'Um, that [the point of no return] was a couple hours ago.' We were like, 'Shit! Intubate him now then!'" Although the intubation was successful and Jacob did recover, had they waited longer to grant permission, their care-captaining may have inadvertently prevented the administration of lifesaving care.

Conversely, care-entrusting placed fewer medical demands on parents and could facilitate less agonizing decision-making processes. Not all parents with sufficient levels of CHC always chose to care-captain, often because care-entrusting allowed them to feel less insecurity about a course of action and greater confidence in their child's providers (Gengler 2014). A blend of care-entrusting and care-captaining seemed to be particularly useful when used by parents who had enough CHC to engage in care-captaining when needed and to step back when they felt confident in their child's providers and the broad outlines of a treatment plan. Sometimes parents with little CHC, like Tina Morgan, made efforts to care-captain, but doing so could lead to contentious interactions with providers and greater feelings of inefficacy since these parents' efforts were less influential than those of parents with more CHC to bolster their efforts.

For those who had little CHC, care-entrusting could be the only viable strategy to use the majority of the time, even when lingering doubts and anxieties left parents feeling nervous and uninformed (as for Lakira Harris during Jayden's transplant) or left children and families coping with painful symptoms indefinitely before accessing needed care (as for Elijah Henderson and his parents). Although it is impossible to know with certainty, Chanise Rowland's inability to care-captain for Anaya might have had fatal consequences had her doctor not gotten Anaya transferred before her heart failed. On an everyday basis, parents who primarily care-entrusted may have simply missed out on some of the microadvantages care-captains could achieve, like the Marins' financial savings by cutting Jacob's vitamin K prescription. Jeanetta Moore, a black mother of three in her early forties who struggled to make ends meet on her husband's income as a maintenance worker, also mentioned to me the excessive cost of her 5-year-old daughter's vitamin K prescription. Jeanetta did not consider questioning its necessity even years after her daughter's successful organ tissue transplant because she entrusted her daughter's care entirely to the doctor who had cured her daughter's fatal immunodeficiency disorder.

Without his parents' sophisticated research, negotiations with their insurance company, and willingness and ability to travel cross-country, Jacob Marin would have received palliative care and declined neurologically until Tay-Sachs ended his life. Whether extending life under these circumstances is in fact a positive outcome for children or families is an ethical question far beyond the scope of this paper and one that may shift based on currently unknown clinical trial outcomes and the possibilities of future technologies. Although Jacob Marin has thus far not developed neurologically as his parents had hoped, he is still with his parents as of this writing. Noah, the infant son of Edward Rivera and Juliana Cruz, died as a result of complications from his cord blood–derived stem-cell transplant, but for their older daughter, the same treatment was a success. Sophie is producing the enzyme she needs to avoid neurological deterioration and is now a plucky, active, and curious 5-year-old.

Although substantial caution should be exercised in concluding that care-captaining is always the best approach to illness management, the core interactional dynamics outlined here represent important processes through which microadvantages may accrue in the day-to-day experiences of illness. Not all parents can "choose" to strategically care-captain as needed, even if doing so might benefit their children during lapses in care provision or at strategic junctures, because they lack the resources required to do so effectively.

Phelan and colleagues (2010) argue that advances in medical technologies, such as pap smears or the polio vaccine, can either increase or reduce health disparities (see also Goldman and Lakdawalla 2005). Yet, they caution that such specific mechanisms can be short-lived, will shift over time, and are eventually replaced by new ones. Phelan and colleagues do not dismiss the importance of identifying inequalities in access to new medical technologies—which policy interventions might effectively address—but they astutely observe that mediating factors like these will continue to emerge, fade, and rise again in new form as long as broader, structural inequalities result in some people having more resources to protect their health and obtain care for illnesses than others.

This research sheds light on some of these more pervasive and durable interactional processes. My findings suggest that explanations for inequalities in care delivery must go beyond examinations of inequality in access to well-resourced institutions (although this remains vitally important) and draws attention to the seemingly minute microadvantages—a shorter course of steroids, fewer medication errors, early access to therapies, or a frightened parent's ability to take comfort in the prestigious publication record of their child's physician—which may be missed in the larger aggregate studies more commonly used to document health inequalities. Broadening conceptualizations of healthcare advantages to consider differences not only in long-term health outcomes but also in access, influence, and daily life throughout the treatment process can inform a more complete understanding of the interactional dynamics through which care is accomplished and illnesses are lived.

Notes

1. Department of Sociology, Wake Forest University, Winston Salem, NC, USA
2. All names used are pseudonyms.
3. Differences in health insurance, job flexibility, and other material resources combined with CHC to construct the overall set of constraints and opportunities within which families operated. Limited space prohibits a full discussion of these economic dynamics,

although they are clearly evidenced in the cases discussed.

4. I was able to conduct medical observations with all but five families who were observed only at the RMH because their treatment was near completion when I began formal

interviewing. All families consented to ongoing communication after they returned home.

5. International patients must pay anticipated treatment costs up front prior to their arrival.

References

Anspach, Renee R. 1993. *Deciding Who Lives*. Berkeley: University of California Press.

Becker, Howard S. 1998. *Tricks of the Trade*. Chicago: University of Chicago Press.

Bourdieu, Pierre. 1977. *Outline of a Theory of Practice*. Cambridge, UK: Cambridge University Press.

Boyer, Carol A. and Karen E. Lutfey. 2010. "Examining Critical Health Policy Issues within and beyond the Clinical Encounter: Patient-provider Relationships and Help-seeking Behaviors." *Journal of Health and Social Behavior* 51(1): S80–93.

Cadge, Wendy. 2012. *Paging God*. Chicago: University of Chicago Press.

Chang, Virginia W. and Diane S. Lauderdale. 2009. "Fundamental Cause Theory, Technical Innovation, and Health Disparities: The Case of Cholesterol in the Era of Statins." *Journal of Health and Social Behavior* 50(3):245–60.

Charmaz, Kathy. 2006. *Constructing Grounded Theory*. Thousand Oaks, CA: Sage.

Christakis, Nicholas A. and James H. Fowler. 2009. *Connected*. New York: Little, Brown and Company.

Clark, Jacqueline. 2005. "Constructing Expertise: Inequality and the Consequences of Information-seeking by Breast Cancer Patients." *Illness, Crisis, and Loss* 13(2):169–85.

Czaja, Ronald, Clara Manfredi, and Jammie Price. 2003. "The Determinants and Conse-

quences of Information Seeking Among Cancer Patients." *Journal of Health Communication* 8(6):529–62.

Dubbin, Leslie A., Jami Suki Chang, and Janet K. Shim. 2013. "Cultural Health Capital and the Interactional Dynamics of Patient-centered Care." *Social Science & Medicine* 93:113–20.

Feldman, Henry A., John B. McKinlay, Deborah A. Potter, Karen M. Freund, Risa B. Burns, Mark A. Moskowitz, and Linda E. Kasten. 1997. "Nonmedical Influences on Medical Decision Making: An Experimental Technique Using Videotapes, Factorial Design, and Survey Sampling." *Health Services Research* 32(3):343–66.

Flyvbjerg, Bent. 2001. *Making Social Science Matter*. Cambridge, UK: Cambridge University Press.

Gage, Elizabeth A. and Christina Panagakis. 2012. "The Devil You Know: Parents Seeking Information Online for Paediatric Cancer." *Sociology of Health & Illness* 34(3):444–58.

Gengler, Amanda Marie. 2014. "Cultural Health Capital, Emotion Management, and the Reproduction of Inequality in the Case of Life-threatening Childhood Illness." PhD dissertation, Department of Sociology, Brandeis University, Waltham, MA.

Goldman, Dana P. and Darius Lakdawalla. 2005. "A Theory of Health Disparities and Medical Technology." *Contributions to Economic Analysis & Policy* 4(1):1–32.

Granovetter, Mark S. 1973. "The Strength of Weak Ties." *American Journal of Sociology* 78(6):1360–80.

Greil, Arthur L., Julia McQuillan, Karina M. Shreffler, Katherine M. Johnson, and Kathleen S. Slauson-Blevins. 2011. "Race-ethnicity and Medical Services for Infertility." *Journal of Health and Social Behavior* 52(4):493–509.

Grollman, Eric Anthony. 2014. "Multiple Disadvantaged Statuses and Health: The Role of Multiple Forms of Discrimination." *Journal of Health and Social Behavior* 55(1):3–19.

Heimer, Carol A. and Lisa R. Staffen. 1998. *For the Sake of the Children*. Chicago: University of Chicago Press.

House, James S. 2002. "Understanding of Social Factors and Inequalities in Health: 20th Century Progress and 21st Century Prospects." *Journal of Health and Social Behavior* 43(2):125–42.

Johnson, Rachel L., Debra Roter, Neil R. Powe, and Lisa A. Cooper. 2004. "Patient Race/Ethnicity and Quality of Patient-physician Communication During Medical Visits." *American Journal of Public Health* 94(12):2084–90.

Kawachi, Ichiro. 2010. "Social Capital and Health." Pp. 18–32 in *Handbook of Medical Sociology*, edited by C. E. Bird, P. Conrad, A. M. Fremont, and S. Timmermans. Nashville, TN: Vanderbilt University Press.

Krieger, Nancy. 2000. "Discrimination and Health." Pp. 36–75 in *Social Epidemiology*, edited by L. Berkman and I. Kawachi. New York: Oxford University Press.

Lareau, Annette. 2003. *Unequal Childhoods*. Berkeley: University of California Press.

Link, Bruce G. and Jo Phelan. 1995. "Social Conditions as Fundamental Causes of Disease." *Journal of Health and Social Behavior* 36(Extra Issue):80–94.

Liu, Ka-Yuet, Marissa King, and Peter S. Bearman. 2010. "Social Influences and the Autism Epidemic." *American Journal of Sociology* 115(5):1387–434.

Lutfey, Karen, and Jeremy Freese. 2005. "Toward Some Fundamentals of Fundamental Causality: Socioeconomic Status and Health in the Routine Clinic Visit for Diabetes." *American Journal of Sociology* 110(5):1326–72.

Marmot, Michael. 2004. *The Status Syndrome*. New York: Times Books.

Maynard, Douglas W. 2003. *Bad News, Good News*. Chicago: University of Chicago Press.

Mirowsky, John and Catherine E. Ross. 2003. *Education, Social Status, and Health*. New York: Aldine De Gruyter.

Pampel, Fred C., Patrick M. Krueger, and Justin T. Denney. 2010. "Socioeconomic Disparities in Health Behaviors." *Annual Review of Sociology* 36:349–70.

Pescosolido, Bernice A. 1992. "Beyond Rational Choice: The Social Dynamics of How People Seek Help." *American Journal of Sociology* 97(4):1096–138.

Phelan, Jo C., Bruce G. Link, and Parisa Tehranifa. 2010. "Social Conditions as Fundamental Causes of Health Inequalities." *Journal of Health and Social Behavior* 51(S): S28–40.

Prus, Robert. 1987. "Generic Social Processes." *Journal of Contemporary Ethnography* 16(3): 250–93.

Robert, Stephanie A. 1999. "Socioeconomic Position and Health: The Independent Contribution of Community Socioeconomic Context." *Annual Review of Sociology* 25:489–516.

Sampson, Robert J. 2003. "The Neighborhood Context of Well-being." *Perspectives in Biology and Medicine* 46(3): S53–64.

Schillinger, Dean, Kevin Grumbach, John Piette, Frances Wang, Dennis Osmond, Carolyn Daher, Jorge Palacios, Gabriel Diaz Sullivan, and Andrew B. Bindman. 2002. "Association of Health Literacy with Diabetes Outcomes."

Journal of the American Medical Association 288(4):475–82.

Schnittker, Jason. 2004. "Education and the Changing Shape of the Income Gradient in Health." *Journal of Health and Social Behavior* 45(3):286–305.

Schwalbe, Michael, Sandra Godwin, Daphne Holden, Douglas Schrock, Shealy Thompson, and Michele Wolkomir. 2000. "Generic Processes in the Reproduction of Inequality: An Interactionist Analysis." *Social Forces* 79(2):419–52.

Scott, Marvin B. and Stanford M. Lyman. 1968. "Accounts." *American Sociological Review* 33(1):46–62.

Shim, Janet K. 2010. "Cultural Health Capital: A Theoretical Approach to Understanding Health Care Interactions and the Dynamics of Unequal Treatment." *Journal of Health and Social Behavior* 51(1):1–15.

Small, Mario Luis. 2009. "'How Many Cases do I Need?' On Science and the Logic of Case Selection in Field-based Research." *Ethnography* 10(1):5–38.

Smoll, Nicolas. 2012. "Relative Survival of Childhood and Adult Medulloblastomas and Primitive Neuroectodermal Tumors (PNETs)." *Cancer* 118(5):1313–22.

Sue, Derald Wing. 2010. *Microaggressions and Marginality*. Hoboken, NJ: Wiley.

Tavory, Iddo and Stefan Timmermans. 2009. "Two Cases of Ethnography: Grounded Theory and the Extended Case Method." *Ethnography* 10(3):243–63.

van Ryn, Michelle and Steven S. Fu. 2003. "Paved with Good Intentions: Do Public Health and Human Service Providers Contribute to Racial/Ethnic Disparities in Health?" *American Journal of Public Health* 93(2):248–55.

Williams, David R., and Chiquita Collins. 2001. "Racial Residential Segregation: A Fundamental Cause of Racial Disparities in Health." *Public Health Reports* 116(5):404–16.

Williams, David R. 2012. "Miles to Go Before We Sleep." *Journal of Health and Social Behavior* 53(3):279–95.

DILEMMAS OF MEDICAL TECHNOLOGY

Medical technology exemplifies both the promise and the pitfalls of modern medicine. Medical history is replete with technological interventions that have reduced suffering or delayed death. Much of the success of modern medicine, from diagnostic tests to heroic lifesaving individual interventions, has its basis in medical technology. For example, new imaging techniques, including CT scans, magnetic resonance imaging machines, and ultrasound devices, allow physicians to "see" body interiors without piercing the skin; powerful antibiotics and protective vaccinations have reduced the devastation of formerly dreaded diseases; and developments in modern anesthesia, lasers, and technical life support have made previously unthinkable innovations in surgery possible. Technology has been one of the foundations of the advancement of medicine and the improvement of health and medical care (cf. Timmermans 2000).

But along with therapeutic and preventive successes, various medical technologies have created new problems and dilemmas. There are numerous recent examples. Respirators are integral to the modern medical armamentarium. They have aided medical treatment of respiratory, cardiac, and neurological conditions and extended anesthetic capabilities, which in turn have promoted more sophisticated surgical interventions. Yet they have also created a new situation where critically injured or terminally ill persons are "maintained" on machines long after the brain-controlled spontaneous ability to breathe has ceased. These extraordinary life-support measures have produced ethical, legal, political, and medical dilemmas that have only been partially resolved by new definitions of death (Zussman 1992). The technology around neonatal infant care has allowed premature babies less than 500 grams to survive but has created new problems: great financial burdens (often over $250,000) and the babies' ultimate outcome. While some such babies go on to live a healthy life, many die, and others survive with significant and costly disabilities (Guillemin and Holmstrom 1986). Parental and staff decisions regarding these tiny neonates are often difficult and painful (Anspach 1987). One tragic example of medical technology is DES (diethylstilbestrol), a synthetic estrogen prescribed to millions of pregnant women up until the 1970s to prevent miscarriages. DES turned out not only to be ineffective but also years later to cause cancer and other reproductive disorders in the daughters of the women who took the drug (Bell 1986, 2009; Dutton 1988).

These examples raise two particularly important issues (see also Timmermans 2002). The first concerns our great faith in technological expertise and the general medical belief in "doing whatever can be done" for the sick and dying, which has created a "can do, should do" ethic. That is, if we can provide some type of medical intervention—something that would keep an individual alive—we ought to do it no matter what the person's circumstances are or the consequences of that intervention. This results in increasing the amount of marginal or questionable care, inflating medical expenses, and creating dilemmas for patients and their kin. The second issue is cost. Medical technology is often expensive and is one of the main factors in our ever-rising health care costs. We may reach a point soon, if we have not already, that as a society we will not be able to afford all of the medical care that our technology is capable of providing. Thus, we need to seriously consider what we can afford to do and the most effective ways to spend our health care dollars. This raises the issue of "rationing" (or apportioning) medical care. Do we ration explicitly, on the basis of need or potential effectiveness, or implicitly, as we often already do, by the ability to pay? In the United Kingdom, with more limited resources devoted to medical care, rationing is built into the expectations of health policy (since it is virtually completely government funded). For example, for many years, no one over fifty-five was begun on dialysis; it simply was not considered a suitable treatment for kidney disorders after that age (Aaron and Schwartz 1984). (Patients under fifty-five receive treatment comparable to U.S. patients.) In recent years, dialysis is still rationed in the United Kingdom but not so strictly (Stanton 1999).

This leads us to perhaps the most interesting example of a recent technological intervention—the case of end-stage renal disease (ESRD), or chronic kidney failure. Before the development of dialysis and kidney transplantation, kidney failure was a death warrant. For sufferers of renal failure, these medical technologies are lifesaving, or at least life extending. The dialysis machine, for all of its limitations, was probably the most successful of the first generation of artificial organs. Dialysis was expensive, and the choice of who would receive this lifesaving intervention was so difficult that the federal government passed a special law in 1972 to include dialysis coverage under Medicare. The number of patients involved and the costs of dialysis have far exceeded what legislators expected: By the middle 1980s, over $2 billion a year was spent on treating a disease that affected 70,000 people (Plough 1986). As of 2009, 871 million people were under treatment for ESRD, at a cost of $42.5 billion in public and private spending (National Kidney & Urologic Diseases Information Clearinghouse 2016). Given the cost-containment initiatives that dominate health policy now, it is unlikely that any other disease will be funded this generously.

The issues raised by dialysis treatment are profound. Before federal funding was available, the issue of who should receive treatment was critical and difficult. How should limited resources be allocated? Who would decide, and on what grounds (social worth, ability to pay)? Despite the greater availability of funds, important questions remain. Is it reasonable economically to spend billions of dollars on such a relatively small number of patients? Is this an effective way to spend our health dollars? Can we, as a society with spiraling health costs, make this type of investment in every new medical technology? For example, if an artificial heart were ever perfected, would we make it available to all the 100,000 patients a year who might benefit

from such a device? With the heart perhaps costing (at $50,000 each) up to $500 billion a year, who would pay for it? Beyond the economic issues is the quality of extended life. Dialysis patients must go three times a week for six- to eight-hour treatments, which means relatively few patients can work a conventional schedule (Kutner 1987). Quality-of-life issues are paramount, with many patients suffering social and psychological problems; they are significantly more likely to commit suicide (Kurella et al. 2005). Finally, a large percentage of the dialysis treatment facilities in the United States are owned by profit-making businesses, thus raising the question of how much commercialization should exist in medical care and whether companies should make large profits from medical treatment (Relman and Rennie 1980; Plough 1986). (See Chapter 16 for an article about home dialysis users.)

Medical technology makes and fulfills substantial promises for patients. Yet technology can also bring substantial dilemmas into modern medical care, as these examples demonstrate. Our first selection in this section, "Medical Sociology and Technology: Critical Engagements" by Monica Casper and Daniel Morrison, discusses how medical technology has reshaped the practice of medicine, and how sociologists have examined critical connections in medical technology. They explain that there has been a shift from addressing the effects of medical technology on medical care to thinking about how medical technology has changed the way that we think about human bodies. For example, women may now find themselves to be "risky subjects" in a "predisease" status carrying genetic markers for breast cancer and act upon that status, sometimes going so far as to have preventative mastectomies. Casper and Morrison conclude their piece with policy implications, addressing health disparities and rationing, asking who reaps the benefits of medical technology.

Our second selection addresses genetics, now a powerful paradigm in medicine. The Human Genome Project commenced in 1990 to map the entire human genetic structure in fifteen years; a draft of the genome was completed in 2002. The prime goal has been to locate the causes of the thousands of genetically related diseases and ultimately to develop new treatments and interventions. Research has already discovered genes for cystic fibrosis, Huntington's disease, types of breast and colon cancer, and other disorders, although we are clearly in the early stages of genetic research. Beyond diseases, some scientists have applied the genetic paradigm to behavioral traits, presenting claims for genetic predispositions to alcoholism, homosexuality, obesity, and intelligence. Although genetic discoveries may eventually yield treatments and preventions of diseases, genetic testing as a medical technology raises serious social and ethical issues. Some analysts have warned of the dangers of biological reductionism, especially in terms of "genetic essentialism," as an increasingly pervasive explanation of human problems (Nelkin and Lindee 1995; see also Duster 1990). One critic has suggested that "Genetics is not just a science. . . . It is a way of thinking, an ideology. We're coming to see life through a 'prism of heritability,' a 'discourse of gene action,' a genetic frame. Genetics is the single best explanation, the most comprehensive theory since God" (Rothman 1998, 13).

An appearance and allure of specificity creates a privileged position for genetic explanations in the public discourse; on closer examination, the specificity may prove to be what Conrad (1999) describes as a mirage. While current conceptualizing about

genes has become more complex, focusing more on "epigenetics" (interaction of genes with genes and with environments), the public's perception of genetic contributions likely is still similar to what Conrad suggests (Lock and Nguyen 2010)—focused on genetic determinism and susceptibility.

Prenatal testing is one of the social locations where genetics have had the most impact on health care and individuals' lives. Screening for prenatal genetic conditions is now routine in the United States, and genetic counselors are a recently developed health profession whose job it is to help pregnant women and their partners understand complex genetic information about their fetuses. The second selection in this section, "'It Just Becomes Much More Complicated': Genetic Counselors' Views on Genetics and Prenatal Testing" by Susan Markens, addresses central bioethics concerns. Markens found that genetic counselors are enthusiastic about genetic medicine but have what she calls "reflexive ambivalence" in that they express skepticism and concern about the consequences of the use of genetic information in this context.

Medical technology continues to expand, bringing new "miracles" and new dilemmas. Most poignantly reflected in the issues of quality of life and costs, the social and economic consequences of medical technology will need to be addressed in the next decade.

References

Aaron, Henry J., and William B. Schwartz. 1984. *The Painful Prescription: Rationing Hospital Care.* Washington, DC: Brookings Institution.

Anspach, Renée. 1987. "Prognostic Conflict in Life and Death Decisions: The Organization as an Ecology of Knowledge." *Journal of Health and Social Behavior* 28: 215–31.

Bell, Susan. 1986. "A New Model of Medical Technology Development: A Case Study of DES." In *The Adoption and Social Consequences of Medical Technology (Research in the Sociology of Health Care,* Volume 4), edited by Julius A. Roth and Sheryl Burt Ruzek, 1–32. Greenwich, CT: JAI Press.

Bell, Susan. 2009. *DES Daughters, Embodied Knowledge, and the Transformation of Women's Health Politics in the Late Twentieth Century.* Philadelphia: Temple University Press.

Conrad, Peter. 1999. "A Mirage of Genes." *Sociology of Health & Illness* 21: 228–41.

Duster, Troy. 1990. *Backdoor to Eugenics*. New York: Routledge.

Dutton, Diana B. 1988. *Worse Than the Disease: Pitfalls of Medical Progress*. New York: Cambridge University Press.

Guillemin, Jeanne Harley, and Lynda Lytle Holmstrom. 1986. *Mixed Blessings: Intensive Care for Newborns*. New York: Oxford University Press.

Kurella, Manjula, Paul L. Kimmel, Belinda S. Young, and Glenn M. Chertow. 2005. "Suicide in the United States End-Stage Renal Disease Program." *Journal of the American Society of Nephrology* 16: 774–81.

Kutner, Nancy G. 1987. "Social Worlds and Identity in End-Stage Renal Disease (ESRD)." In *The Experience and Control of Chronic Illness (Research in the Sociology of Health Care, Volume 6)*, edited by Julius A. Roth and Peter Conrad, 107–46. Greenwich, CT: JAI Press.

Lock, Margaret, and Vin-Kim Nguyen. 2010. *The Anthropology of Biomedicine*. Oxford: Wiley-Blackwell.

National Kidney & Urologic Diseases Information Clearinghouse. 2016. *Kidney Diseases Statistics for the United States*. Accessed November 22, 2017. https://www.niddk.nih.gov/health-information/health-statistics/kidney-disease.

Nelkin, Dorothy, and M. Susan Lindee. 1995. *The DNA Mystique: The Gene as a Cultural Icon*. New York: Freeman.

Plough, Alonzo L. 1986. *Borrowed Time: Artificial Organs and the Politics of Extending Lives*. Philadelphia: Temple University Press.

Relman, Arnold S., and Drummond Rennie. 1980. "Treatment of End-Stage Renal Disease: Free but Not Equal." *New England Journal of Medicine* 303: 996–98.

Rothman, Barbara Katz. 1998. *Genetic Maps and Human Imaginations*. New York: Norton.

Stanton, J. 1999. "The Cost of Living: Kidney Dialysis Rationing and Health Economics in Britain, 1965–1996." *Social Science and Medicine* 49: 1169–82.

Timmermans, Stefan. 2000. "Technology and Medical Practice." In *Handbook of Medical Sociology*, 5th edition, edited by Chloe E. Bird, Peter Conrad, and Allen M. Fremont, 309–21. Upper Saddle River, NJ: Prentice Hall.

Timmermans, Stefan. 2002. "The Impact of Medical Technology." *Sociology of Health and Illness* 25: 97–114.

Zussman, Robert. 1992. *Intensive Care*. Chicago: University of Chicago Press.

MEDICAL SOCIOLOGY AND TECHNOLOGY

Critical Engagements

Monica J. Casper and Daniel R. Morrison

The Medical Sociology Section of the American Sociological Association was founded in 1959, at the turn of a decade that had witnessed tremendous advances in medical technology. Cardiopulmonary resuscitation was innovated, and the first pacemaker was developed. Penicillin was chemically synthesized in the 1940s, ushering in an era of mass production of antibiotics. Salk fashioned a polio vaccine in 1952, and by 1955 it was being distributed to American school children (Oshinsky 2005). The first kidney transplants were performed, and dialysis was innovated to treat kidney failure. Heart transplants followed. Scientists researched the birth control pill in a shifting context of sexual politics, successfully but under ethically dubious conditions (Briggs 2002). The price of hospital care doubled in

the 1950s, and national health expenditures grew to 4.5 percent of the gross national product (GNP) (Starr 1982). Health insurance companies began to spread across the United States, inaugurating employer-based benefits, and limited private coverage for people who could afford it (Murray 2007; Quadagno 2006).

In 2009, 50 years later, health care accounted for 16 percent of the gross domestic product (GDP), the highest ratio among industrialized nations (Robert Wood Johnson Foundation 2009). And according to the American Public Health Association, approximately 47 million Americans (many employed at least part-time) were uninsured. The new millennium brought expanded use of genetic technologies, growth in nanotechnology, diffusion of knowledge

Medical Sociology and Technology: Critical Engagements, Monica J. Casper and Daniel R. Morrison in *Journal of Health and Social Behavior, 51*, Extra Issue: What Do We Know? Key Findings From 50 Years of Medical Sociology (2010), pp. S120–S132. Reprinted with permission from the American Sociological Association.

produced by the Human Genome Project (HGP), a booming transnational pharmaceutical industry, new reproductive technologies, standardization of care, and escalating visualization and digitalization of medicine. The twenty-first century ushered in biomedicalization across sectors (Clarke et al. 2003, 2010), new health movements (e.g., Brown et al. 2004; Brown 2007; Epstein 1996, 2008; Klawiter 2004, 2008), and translational research (the practical application of scientific research) (Wainwright et al. 2006)—alongside ongoing contention about U.S. health care. The 2008 election of President Obama, whose campaign platform emphasized health reform, deepened public debates.

Across the half-century lifespan of the Medical Sociology Section, during which sweeping changes have impacted American society as a whole, technologies have changed dramatically, too, from large "machines at the bedside" to tiny pills and devices that enter into and transform human bodies, and information technologies that have altered if not restructured health care provision. These have been central to health care practices and financing (or lack thereof), politics of reform, health outcomes, and scholarship. Medical sociologists have investigated both the category of technology writ large and specific drugs, devices, digital innovations, and technical practices such as neonatal intensive care (e.g., Anspach 1993; Zetka 2003). Many scholars explore the essential "nature" of technology; contestation surrounds the term and its application to specific devices, techniques, and practices (Nye 2006).

The substantive and theoretical questions medical sociologists have pursued are as complex and capacious as the shifting technological landscape itself—far too extensive to fully document here. In offering a half-century "snapshot" of research on biomedical technology, we briefly profile three major foci: how technologies have reshaped medical practices; how technologies have reconfigured human bodies and our conceptions of them; and how technologies have been crucial to the emergence of new health social movements. While there has been major work on medical technologies, until the turn of this century sociologists did not attend thoroughly to technical aspects of medical practice.

Only within a theoretical paradigm in which technology was considered peripheral could we get an account of the social transformation of American medicine that little discusses the role of key technologies (much less science) in professionalization (Starr 1982).

THEORETICAL DEVELOPMENTS

Part of our charge for this issue of *JHSB*, and the ASA session from which it originated in 2009, was to articulate our key findings about technology. Yet *what* we know is inextricably bound up with *how* we know. Technologies have varied across 50 years; so, too, have theories, concepts, and methods for understanding them. Thus, we cannot discuss shifts in our knowledge about technologies without chronicling the myriad ways in which scholars have approached the topic. These epistemological developments have contributed to our collective knowledge about technology, advancing medical sociology while also broadening its connections to other scholarly areas. Concepts such as medicalization and biomedicalization and a range of perspectives (e.g., symbolic interactionist, feminist, constructionist, social movement approaches) have significantly reconfigured what "technology" means, under what conditions, and for whom.

In the mid-twentieth century and beyond, nascent sociologists of health and medicine were interested in the impact of particular technologies, as medical professionals used them "at the bedside" (Reiser and Anbar 1984). These technologies, often framed as external to meatier intellectual topics, were studied to understand the social order of medical work and the people who engaged in it as practitioners and patients. The focus was not on technology per se, but rather on the practices altered by introduction of new devices. Theoretically, the goal was to elucidate the contours of biomedicine itself, and not necessarily the tools of the trade or their unique, varied technical histories (e.g., Strauss et al. 1985).

Medical technologies have long been criticized as one form of medicalization (Zola 1972), a potentially dehumanizing process that restricts the autonomy of both experts and nonexperts as they confront pain, suffering, and death. Illich (1975) claimed that interventions intended to make sick people well in fact made sick people sicker, turning progress into pathogenesis. Technologies designed to alleviate symptoms of disease, according to this view, prolong suffering needlessly, and at exorbitant cost. Illich's concern with iatrogenic diseases, medicalization, and the high costs and profits of pharmaceuticals and medical devices remain with us, and they constitute a subtext of contemporary debates about health care. Other scholars of the political economy of health care extended these debates (McKinlay 1984; Navarro 1986). Medical machinery now monitors fetuses during delivery, while magnetic resonance imaging (MRI) maps our brains—each technology one step in the process of defining (or divining) the normal and the pathological (Canguilhem 1991; Foucault 1994, 2008).

Further developments, such as more complicated understandings of medicalization and stratification, were spurred by women's health movements of the 1970s (Lorber and Moore 2002). Feminist scholarship has both celebrated and critiqued the medical profession and its practices and technologies (Clarke and Olesen 1999; Ruzek, Olesen, and Clarke 1997). These studies underscored power relations embedded in medical technologies, and their differential impact on women relative to men. Indeed, research on women's health has long emphasized that health care is stratified (Ginsburg and Rapp 1995), as are medicalization experiences (Bell 1995, 2009; Riessman 1983). Some women (usually white, middle-class women) receive too much care and unnecessary interventions while many other women (especially poor women and women of color) receive too little. This chronic tension has provided diverse perspectives on, and varying levels of appreciation for, women's health care.

Symbolic interactionists, rooted in pragmatism and the Chicago School, created an early and vital home within the sociology of medicine. These contributions have focused, in part, on social interactions within medicine (e.g., hospitals, clinics, nursing homes) as forms of work (Strauss et al. 1985). This approach led to surprising findings about ways in which doctors, nurses, and other health professionals make the work of others easier, for example smoothing out ruffled emotions or preparing families for bad news (Star and Strauss 1999; Strauss 1988). Symbolic interactionists also analyzed medical practices in terms that highlight processes instead of outcomes. From Glaser and Strauss's (1965) early work on dying, to Charmaz's (1991) portrait of chronic illness, to Timmermans's (1999) study of cardiopulmonary resuscitation (CPR), symbolic interactionists have documented and theorized medical work, technologies, and care, refreshing such stalwart sociological concepts as trajectory.

Strauss and colleagues analyzed uses of machines for diagnosis and treatment, including laboratory tests, mobile x-ray machines, and heart rate monitors, as well as the growing army of technicians who do the "articulation work" between human patients and medical technologies (Strauss et al. 1985; Wiener et al. 1997). Chronic illness, they found, led to a growing reliance on medical technologies for monitoring and maintaining health. The major thrust of this research investigated the role of technology in changing practices. How, for example, did doctors, nurses, and patients respond to new technologies? How did technologies affect patients' illness experiences? What was the relationship between technologies and new systems of professional knowledge? How did technology impact conceptions of the patient and his or her illness? These questions continue to drive sociological research on health care technologies (Conrad and Gabe 1999; Franklin 2007).

Working at the intersection of medical sociology and science and technology studies, scholars developed other concepts (Clarke and Star 2007). For example, Star and Griesemer (1989) theorized boundary objects, or those objects (such as fetuses, genes, and brains) whose meanings are common and flexible enough to be intelligible across social arenas, but distinct and obdurate enough to carry specific localized meanings. Cultural and material characteristics of these objects, both within and across social arenas, makes shared understandings, collaboration, and work itself possible. For example, Williams et al. (2008) show how human embryos as boundary objects link the biomedical worlds of embryonic stem cells and pre-implantation genetic diagnosis. Similarly, Fujimura's (1988, 1996) notion of "bandwagons" in clinical research made possible new understandings of the theory and method packages that clinicians and scientists use in advancing their work. And Clarke and Fujimura's (1992) theoretical elaboration of "the right tools for the job" offered new material, symbolic, and institutional parameters for locating technologies in practice. This body of work allowed scholars to see how previously invisible technologies *work* in the practical accomplishment of science.

Scholars have also generated new ideas about classification as an organizing concept for scientific and biomedical practice, and they also have shown how classification systems are themselves technologies. By unpacking the processes by which classification systems are created and sustained, Bowker and Star (2000) demonstrate the social and political impulses that animate these. Their work also illustrates the ways in which messy, complex practices are conceptually narrowed in order to "fit" within existing knowledge systems. These classification systems as technologies are crucial for organizing knowledge and practice. For example, proposed revisions to the *Diagnostic and Statistical Manual of Mental Disorders* (DSM) would remove Asperger's Syndrome, placing it under the more general "autism spectrum disorders" (ASD). Such changes have real consequences for patients, who often define themselves as distinct from people with autism (Grinker 2010; Tanner 2010).

Timmermans and Berg (2003) critique evidence-based medicine as a type of technology that provides (or claims to provide) "gold standard" care. Similar classification practices occur for large-scale projects, such as the "International Classification of Diseases," "Nursing Interventions Classification" (Bowker and Star 2000), and the DSM (Horwitz 2002). Clarke and Casper (1996; see also Casper and Clarke 1998) focus on practices of reading and classifying pap smears. Simple diagnostic practices allow many tests to be analyzed per day, while at the same time rendering classification more difficult for lab technicians who meticulously examine specimens and slides. Classification schemes thus attempt to make sense of nebulous biological material (Keating and Cambrosio 2002, 2003).

Clarke and colleagues (2003, 2010) reformulated a central concept in medical sociology—medicalization—that was not routinely associated with technology, turning our attention toward contemporary, cutting-edge forms of "biomedicalization." This term encompasses both old and new practices, such as genome-wide association studies, nanoscale medicine that upends common sense distinctions between organic and inorganic matter, and devices made to alter electrical signals within the brain. To some degree, biomedicalization brings us full-circle to earlier notions of medicalization (Zola 1972; Conrad 2005, 2007), but the concept is updated and expanded theoretically for the twenty-first century. Biomedicalization is inflected with characteristic symbolic interactionist and science and technology studies attention to (1) processes and knowledge, (2) an interweaving of medicine with science, (3) recognition of vertical and horizontal integration of health care markets and biocapital, (4) introduction of nascent technologies and reinventions of the old, and (5) new organotechnical configurations of human bodies (Cooper 2008).

Finally, medical sociologists have taken up Foucauldian concepts, including biopolitics, to theorize individual health in relation to governmentality and governance (Armstrong 1995; Cooper 2008; Waldby 1996, 2000). Others have utilized Foucault's notion of biopower to underscore the productive capacities of human bodies (Hatch 2009; Waldby and Mitchell 2006). While Foucault's work has been highly influential, he did not address the specific role of technologies (e.g., tests, prosthetics, drugs) in and on biopolitical processes. Rather, he focused on knowledge as a kind of social apparatus or technology that shaped systems of governance and attempted control over life. He described other social technologies, such as the panopticon, a prison system designed such that one guard could survey all prisoners without himself being seen (Foucault 1995). This form of governance, with its imagined (or real) surveillance, ultimately affected notions of human health and well-being. More recent Foucauldian work considers twenty-first century technologies in relation to new discursive and institutional formations, and the consequences of these for human bodies and lives (Casper and Moore 2009; Lakoff 2005; Talley 2008).

In sum, in mid-twentieth century theoretical paradigms, technologies were often black-boxed. That is, the object of analysis was not technology per se, but rather practices surrounding the technology and people who both used it and on whom it was used. Political, economic, and early feminist perspectives recognized the intensely political valence of technologies, yet these perspectives saw technology as fairly static. Technologies were conceptualized as inert, ahistorical objects, uninteresting in and of themselves but with a dynamic capacity to reshape social practices and reorganize human bodies. Symbolic interactionist, feminist, and science and technology studies approaches, while highlighting practices, began to focus on technologies themselves. Previously black-boxed medical technologies were dissected and their historical, cultural, and political innards examined. In newer approaches, there is vivid and sustained recognition that technologies, health care practices, bodies, and identities are continually and mutually shaped, with innumerable consequences for human lives.

KEY FINDINGS

Impact of Technologies in and on Practice

Over the past 20 years, a major shift has occurred in the organization and goals of medicine, in which technical innovations have reshaped the contours of practice (Clarke et al. 2003, 2010). Medical sociologists have engaged with technology, using a "technology in practice" perspective, akin to the "science in practice" perspectives utilized by science and technology scholars (Pickering 1992). They have shown how professionals, patients, and others interact with and through medical technologies (and with each other via technologies) while also showing how new and old technologies influence health care

practices and other aspects of social life. Through these interactions, new meanings and categories—of patienthood, humanity, disease, risk, and health—are forged. These shifts mark a move from enhanced control over external nature to the harnessing and transformation of internal nature, often rebuilding life itself (Franklin 2000; Rose 2007), along with its fundamental properties.

Thompson (2005), for example, shows how women undergoing in vitro fertilization mobilize different forms of argument, reflection, and dialogue to account for success or failure. Instead of lacking agency, we see agency made operative through objectification. This "ontological choreography," as Thompson (2005) termed it, describes the development of actions and ideas that link persons with (and through) reproductive technologies in domains of practice. Dumit (2003), by contrast, shows how positron emission tomography (PET) brain imaging technologies are used to bolster professional accounts of "knowing" human types or persons, tracking the technology from development to implementation to cultural impact. These studies are exemplary in their descriptions and analyses of people and medical technologies interacting.

The history of ultrasound is also revealing. Ultrasound was developed for detecting icebergs after the sinking of the Titanic, expanded into naval warfare during World War I, and later used in manufacturing of metals (Yoxen 1987). Early twentieth-century practitioners believed ultrasound could destroy tumors, and subsequent use grew exponentially between the 1930s and 1950s. Visual mapping of the body was infinitely more appealing as the hazards of x-rays became known (Caufield 1989). In the 1970s, ultrasound was central to the emerging field of fetal medicine as clinicians attempted to locate the "unborn" patient, thus advancing the field and playing a key role in the evolution of fetal surgery (Blizzard 2007; Casper 1998). Critics debate benefits vis-à-vis measurable risks, yet ultrasound has become a normal, even highly anticipated part of prenatal care in the United States, offering pregnant women their first "baby" snapshots to hang on the refrigerator (Taylor 2000). Ultrasound has significantly transformed medical practice, creating new forms of work (e.g., increasing the need for sonographers) across the past half-century; making possible new cultural meanings of fetuses, pregnancy, personhood, life, and patienthood; and altering public and private perceptions of what "good" mothers should do (e.g., abstain from alcohol, certain recreational activities, and sex) (Burri and Dumit 2008; Casper 1998; Oakley 1984; Taylor 2008).

In the new millennium, other technologies have become part of medical practice, transforming routine procedures, shifting contexts of care, and generating new meanings of expertise. For example, health care systems have increasingly relied on the Internet to connect patients and doctors across long (and even short) distances. Hospitals of all sizes and resource levels use electronic medical records to store patient information and log medical records, prognoses, and outcomes. These records have multiple uses beyond simple recordkeeping. For example, genome-wide association studies integrate genetic information from patients with de-identified medical records in a search for correlations between certain genetic profiles and disease (Roden et al. 2008). Biobanking—the establishment of repositories of human biological material—is also changing medical practice, providing new forms of bio-data for clinical research and practice (Gottweis and Petersen 2008). Research on attitudes toward DNA biobanking found widespread support among a sample of patients (Pulley et al. 2008).

Such examples of technoscientific developments—from MRI (Joyce 2008) to personalized medicine (Hedgecoe 2004)—can be seen across health care delivery and research infrastructures. Of course, as with women's health care described above, these "advances" are stratified in their application: Elites everywhere receive "too much" boutique care, while impoverished people in both the global North and South lack even the most basic levels of nutrition and hygiene.

Reconfigurations of Human Bodies

Medicine in the early- to mid-twentieth century could be characterized by a mechanical notion of widespread application of technologies to human bodies and use of technical objects on bodies. Such technologies, many innovated in military contexts, unquestionably affected bodies, as they were designed to do, with the aim of improving human health. Serlin (2004), for example, nimbly traces the origins and impacts of an "engineering" model in postwar America that resulted in new cultural meanings of the prosthetic and collective recognition of our "replaceable" body parts. Yet a key shift in medical technology has been introduction of novel pills, devices, and other objects, both small and large, which remake bodies, often from the inside out. Clarke (1995) described this move from technologies of control to technologies of transformation, marking an epochal shift from the "modern" to the "postmodern" period. These technical practices have produced variations in bodies across time and space, alongside new epistemological frameworks.

In 1989, Nelkin and Tancredi (1989) documented, in vaguely alarmist prose, the rise of "dangerous diagnostics"—a set of technologies, such as genetic testing for possible future maladies and IQ tests, that increasingly pervaded the social sphere and threatened individual bodies and rights. They analyzed genetic technologies and biological information in social context, but they did not delve into the historical and cultural configurations of the technologies themselves, or their impacts on bodies. One such "dangerous diagnostic" is amniocentesis. As Rothman (1993) argued, use of this prenatal test spurred a new ontological embodied category, the "tentative pregnancy." She found that until a negative test result proved optimal health of a fetus, pregnant women could not fully accept their pregnancies. On the other hand, a positive diagnosis of genetic aberration created moral and bodily dilemmas; in the absence of prenatal treatment options and/or counseling, women with "defective" fetuses were confronted with the hollow "choice" of abortion. Rapp (2000) later explored these dynamics among a more ethnically and economically diverse group of women, finding a more intricate set of embodied politics.

Duster ([1990] 2003) presented a nuanced analysis of genetic technologies and risks posed to civil liberties and bodies by recycled explanations of science, heredity, and race. He suggested that genetic information reproduces structural inequalities, thus diluting any potential impact toward alleviation of human suffering. In Duster's story, the technologies have both histories and politics, as do the humans. In 2004, Hedgecoe offered an ethnographic account of genetics in practice, documenting the ascendance of personalized medicine and its impact on patients and practices. Wailoo and Pemberton (2006) then placed race, ethnicity, and racialized bodies front and center in their historical analysis of Tay-Sachs, cystic fibrosis, and sickle cell disease.

One of the most startling and instructive examples of old and very new technologies reshaping human bodies and lives is that of pharmaceuticals. A special issue of *Sociology of Health and Illness* (Williams, Gabe, and Davis 2008) explored multifaceted issues including direct-to-consumer advertising, sleep drugs, the human papillomavirus (HPV) vaccine, antiretroviral therapy, and stem cells. For example, Casper and Carpenter (2008) showed, with respect to the innovative and controversial HPV vaccine, that new technologies transform clinical practices: "the vaccine reveals gendered aspects of the doctor-patient relationship while creating new categories of patients and new pathways to medicalization of girls' bodies. . . . New drugs may reorder or forge new health-care practices and markets" (p. 890). These transnational dynamics are increasingly played out on the bodies of women in developing nations, often those women most desperately in need of new preventive and healing technologies (Carpenter and Casper 2009).

Similarly, in their landmark volume, anthropologists Petryna, Lakoff, and Kleinman (2006) describe the state of affairs:

> Major pharmaceutical breakthroughs occurred during and after World War II . . . After the war, the industry used sophisticated marketing methods to transform from a commodity chemicals business . . . to one heavily concentrated in several large firms and dependent on large investments in research and marketing. Global pharmaceutical spending reached almost $500 billion in 2003; approximately half of that was attributed to the United States and Canada. (p. 2)

As they also note, however, "behind these figures lies a morass of economic and moral paradoxes." (p. 2)

Biehl (2006) highlights such paradoxes in his investigation of the AIDS Program in Brazil, where state-supported production of antiretroviral medication has become a key strategy for controlling the epidemic. Drawing on ethnography geared toward making visible the "people missing in official data," he writes that "Brazil's policy of biotechnology for the people has dramatically reduced AIDS mortality and improved the quality of life for the patients covered" (p. 236).

Abundantly clear in the literature on pharmaceuticals is their profound impact on human bodies and experiences. Lakoff's (2005) compelling ethnography of mental illness showcases the transformative role of the multinational pharmaceutical industry in forging connections across psychiatric diagnostic categories in the United States and Argentina. In order for future pharmaceutical treatments to apply worldwide, the classification of bipolar disorder had to be standardized. The patients who populate the Buenos Aires clinic in Lakoff's study must negotiate the complex intersections of embodied personhood with "expert" medical knowledge, and of local experience with global formations. Lakoff's (2008) more recent work follows "pharmaceutical circuits" of regulation, technical standards, and struggles over inclusion and exclusion in finding the "right patients" for pharmaceutical clinical trials. Greene (2007) similarly argues that increasing reliance on measures such as blood pressure or cholesterol levels turns people without illnesses into those with "pre-disease" that doctors may feel obligated to treat.

One result of this over-reliance on tests is that drugs for the management of not-yet-illnesses are continuously used in human bodies, requiring ongoing monitoring and adjustment. Lovell (2006) states, "The history of buprenorphine, like that of psychotropics more generally, is a narrative of effects in search of an application" (p. 138). To state this more baldly, the pharmaceuticals often come first via the operations of global capitalism ("Big Pharma"), and diagnoses and patients follow as drug-makers seek new markets (and bodies) for their goods. Biehl (2006) notes, regarding the Brazilian program, "as the AIDS policy unfolded, Brazil attracted new investments, and novel public-private cooperation over access to medical technologies ensued" (p. 237). These arrangements resulted in expanded markets for pharmaceutical manufacturers and a marketing support infrastructure for the supply of "pharmaceutical intelligence" and forecasting (e.g., Piribo Limited 2010). New arrangements have also led to intensification of clinical research targeting human bodies conceptualized in terms of disease or pre-disease categories.

Use of cochlear implants provides a fascinating example of technical transformations of bodies and ensuing social consequences (Blume 2009). Advocates for Deaf culture have vigorously opposed the technological "solution" of cochlear implants on the grounds that deafness is not a difference in need of intervention, particularly in children (Hyde and Power 2006; Sparrow 2005). For these advocates, Deafness is a source of pride, an identity with a culture unified by its own unique language. Like medical sociologists, disability studies scholars have contested the biomedical model, arguing that "disability" is a socially constructed category (Shakespeare 1998). The biomedical model focuses on individual-level therapy and treatment, neglecting social conditions that lead to loss of mobility and social interaction that turns "impairment" into a disability. A constructionist stance towards disability has reframed bodily differences, such as deafness, to highlight abilities rather than deficits. Siebers (2006) has called for an embodied ontology as a theoretical ground for disability studies, echoing medical sociologists' call for attention to human bodies and embodiment.

In short, while we have learned much about how technologies remake human bodies, we need empirical and theoretical works on new bio-subjectivities—work that can track formation of technoscientific identities alongside reconfigurations of bodies (Clarke et al. 2003, 2010; Sulik 2009). The questions then become

bigger: In what ways, with what consequences, and by whom are these technoscientific identities constructed? In what ways and with what meanings and consequences do people take up such embodied identities? Sulik (2009), for example, found that women with breast cancer diagnoses formed one such identity as a result of their immersion in professional knowledge, placing themselves discursively within this technoscientific framework, receiving support in this identity from the medical system, and prioritizing official classification over their own suffering. Future work might investigate, for example, relations between humans and their brain implants (Morrison 2009), emergent pharmaceutical relations, new "biosocial" collective identities (Gibbon and Novas 2008; Rabinow 1992), and social movements associated with technologies (Kenny 2009).

Technologies and Embodied Health Movements

Since pioneering work by Epstein (1996), sociologists of medicine have theorized and examined connections among health, illness, and social movements—what Brown et al. (2004) call embodied health movements (EHMs). These are social movements organized around health-related issues such as disease categories, access to care, illness experiences, and inequities. Regarding HIV/AIDS activism (Epstein 1996), diethylstilbestrol (DES) daughters (Bell 2009), environmental contaminants (Brown 2007), and other product- and practice-oriented movements (Hess 2005), scholars have analyzed connections between health statuses and movement formation, development, and activism. Communities have emerged on the basis of biosocial categories, deploying technoscientific identities and knowledge (Bell 2009; Epstein 2008). Scholars have analyzed novel group formations and strategies using terms such as "biosociality," "biological citizenship," and others that are Foucauldian in their understandings of power and dominance (Petryna 2002; Rabinow and Rose 2006; Rose and Novas 2005).

Klawiter's (2008) work on breast cancer, for example, shows how the breast cancer movement transformed fundamental terms of debate about the condition; coalitions of women, researchers, and funding agencies reshaped the landscape of scientific inquiry and lived experiences. Breast cancer has been transformed from an embodied experience of passive patienthood to active identification and solidarity with others, from victim to survivor. This solidarity, in turn, helps individuals take control of their health care decisions, while it also attempts to direct research funding at the federal level. Yet contestation surrounds the prioritizing of research on breast cancer treatment (including pharmaceuticals) at the expense of prevention (Ehrenreich 2001; Ley 2009). Screening mammographies had long been recommended for even very young women, enlarging the population of women considered "at risk" but who had not yet been diagnosed with cancer. New guidelines issued in 2009 by the U.S. Preventive Services Task Force recommended limiting routine mammography to women over 50 (Mandelblatt et al. 2009), sparking a firestorm of controversy (Rabin 2009).

Central to Klawiter's analysis, and to other work on breast cancer (e.g., Fosket 2004), is the figure of the "risky subject"—the woman who may carry a genetic marker predisposing her to breast cancer. Kenny's (2009) work on the "previvor" movement is one example of breast cancer activism that emerged from groups of women with the BRCA1 and BRCA2 gene mutations seeking support based on the knowledge that they are at greater risk for breast cancer. Previvors are women with the BRCA 1 and 2 genes but without the disease; marked with the "pre-disease," these women may ultimately make significant treatment decisions in the absence of actual symptoms (Koenig et al. 1998). This group of women is one of many who are advocating for research on young girls, seeking environmental causes for genetic variations even before birth (Ley 2009; Thomson 2009).

POLICY IMPLICATIONS

What implications derive from this retrospective of a half-century of research on technology? Although policy has not been an explicit focus of the analyses discussed here, many of the works implicitly urge policy at local, national, and transnational levels.

We want to stress that medical sociologists should continue to engage in critical analysis of medical practices and health policy (Harrington and Estes 2007; Mechanic 2007). Often this work takes the form of health disparities or health services research (e.g., Barr 2008); yet other fields in the discipline have much to offer. Medical sociologists interested in the effects of medical technology might, for example, examine the ways in which technologies such as electronic medical records, disease classification systems, and other artifacts and processes create and obscure certain forms of professional and lay work.

While medical sociologists will, of course, continue to produce intellectually rigorous, critical, and creative accounts of historical and contemporary medical practices, we also envision more sophisticated interdisciplinary work in the future. In forging links with bioethics and neuroethics, for example, medical sociologists may highlight inequities in resource allocation, informed consent, and institutional structures that obscure or make invisible the ethical practices of those who engage in medical work. Some sociologists practice "empirical bioethics" (De Vries and Kim 2008; Fisher 2009) while wearing the hat of faculty members in interdisciplinary academic centers for bioethics. These connections will become more important as new technologies enter the biomedical landscape, forging shifts in practice, innovative embodied identities, and as-yet-unknown social movements. As technologies become ever tinier—for example, nanotechnologies—scholars will need to attend to a host of issues concerning bodily integrity and autonomy, civil liberties, and the inner and outer reaches of medicine.

Medical sociologists play a substantial role in analyzing power relations within medicine, including the scope of medical authority, biopolitics, and health policy. Experts on medical technology should engage here as well. Despite passage of the federal Patient Protection and Affordable Care Act in March 2010, vociferous debates over health care reform in the United States continue at the time of this writing. Medical sociologists are poised to make key contributions to these debates, with the expertise to highlight connections between health economics and finance and inequalities in provision of services. Yet health disparities are not merely economic, in terms of too much or too little care; they also embody questions of social justice in distributing social resources. In an era when Americans spend too much money for care that is not equitably distributed, sociologists may highlight moral and ethical dimensions of this unequal distribution. Fears of rationing contribute to both public panic and political posturing instead of meaningful comparative analysis. Sociologists can contribute through studies of public and political discourse around policy change, as well as through empirical studies comparing health care systems locally, regionally, and nationally.

Additional research should be conducted transnationally and in dialogue with human rights theory and praxis (Gruskin 2006; Turner 2006). In the context of global flows of capital, bodies, and other resources, how do medical technologies, and the expertise it takes to use them, become distributed throughout the world? Who does what kinds of work, for whom, and with what consequences? What kinds of inequalities are created when MRI scans, x-rays, and other tests and techniques are performed in one location and analyzed in another? Some researchers have already documented the "outsourcing" of clinical trials research to the "Third World" (Cooper 2008; Sunder Rajan 2006). What kind of medicine do we get when drugs are created in the United States, tested abroad, and then marketed, sold, and consumed in wealthy nations? What kinds of technology do we get? Who benefits? Such questions of technology will continue to be at the core of medical sociology.

References

Anspach, Renée R. 1993. *Deciding Who Lives: Fateful Choices in the Intensive-Care Nursery.* Berkeley: University of California Press.

Armstrong, David. 1995. "The Rise of Surveillance Medicine." *Sociology of Health and Illness* 17:393–404.

Barr, Michael S. 2008. "The Need to Test the Patient-Centered Medical Home." *Journal of the American Medical Association* 300:834–35.

Bell, Susan E. 1995. "Gendered Medical Science: Producing a Drug for Women." *Feminist Studies* 21:469–500.

_____. 2009. *DES Daughters: Embodied Knowledge and the Transformation of Women's Health Politics.* Philadelphia, PA: Temple University Press.

Biehl, João. 2006. "Pharmaceutical Governance." Pp. 206–39 in *Global Pharmaceuticals: Ethics, Markets, Practices,* edited by A. Petryna, A.

Lakoff, and A. Kleinman. Durham, NC: Duke University Press.

Blizzard, Deborah. 2007. *Looking within: A Sociocultural Examination of Fetoscopy.* Cambridge, MA: MIT Press.

Blume, Stuart. 2009. *The Artificial Ear: Cochlear Implants and the Culture of Deafness.* New Brunswick, NJ: Rutgers University Press.

Bowker, Geoffrey C. and Susan Leigh Star. 2000. *Sorting Things Out: Classification and its Consequences.* Cambridge, MA: MIT Press.

Briggs, Laura. 2002. *Reproducing Empire: Race, Sex, Science, and U.S. Imperialism in Puerto Rico.* Berkeley: University of California Press.

Brown, Phil. 2007. *Toxic Exposures: Contested Illness and the Environmental Health Movement.* New York: Columbia University Press.

Brown, Phil, Stephen Zavestoski, Sabrina McCormick, Brian Mayer, Rachel Morello-

Frosch, and Rebecca Gasior Altman. 2004. "Embodied Health Movements: New Approaches to Social Movements in Health." *Sociology of Health and Illness* 26:1–31.

Burri, Regula Valerie and Joseph Dumit. 2008. "Social Studies of Scientific Imaging and Visualization." Pp. 297–318 in *The Handbook of Science and Technology Studies*, edited by E. Hackett, O. Amsterdamska, M. Lynch, and J. Wajcman. Cambridge, MA: MIT Press.

Canguilhem, Georges. 1991. *The Normal and the Pathological*. New York: Zone Books.

Carpenter, Laura M. and Monica J. Casper. 2009. "Global Intimacies: Innovating the HPV Vaccine for Women's Health." *Women's Studies Quarterly* 37:80–100.

Casper, Monica J. 1998. *The Making of the Unborn Patient: A Social Anatomy of Fetal Surgery*. New Brunswick, NJ: Rutgers University Press.

Casper, Monica J. and Laura M. Carpenter. 2008. "Sex, Drugs, and Politics: The HPV Vaccine for Cervical Cancer," *Sociology of Health and Illness* 30:886–99.

Casper, Monica J. and Adele E. Clarke. 1998. "Making the Pap Smear into the Right Tool for the Job: Cervical Cancer Screening in the U.S., c1940–1995." *Social Studies of Science* 28:255–90.

Casper, Monica J. and Lisa Jean Moore. 2009. *Missing Bodies: The Politics of Visibility*. New York: New York University Press.

Caufield, Catherine. 1989. *Multiple Exposures: Chronicles of the Radiation Age*. Chicago, IL: University of Chicago Press.

Charmaz, Kathy C. 1991. *Good Days, Bad Days: The Self and Chronic Illness*. Piscataway, NJ: Rutgers University Press.

Clarke, Adele E. 1995. "Modernity, Postmodernity, and Reproductive Processes, ca 1890–1990: or, 'Mommy, Where do Cyborgs Come from Anyway?'" Pp. 139–56 in *The Cyborg Handbook*, edited by C. H. Gray, S. Mentor, and H. Figueroa-Sarriera. New York: Routledge.

Clarke, Adele E. and Monica Casper. 1996. "From Simple Technique to Complex System: Classification of Pap Smears, 1917–1990." *Medical Anthropology Quarterly* 10:601–23.

Clarke, Adele E. and Joan H. Fujimura. 1992. "What Tools? Which Jobs? Why Right?" Pp. 3–44 in *The Right Tools for the Job: At Work in Twentieth Century Life Sciences*, edited by A. E. Clarke and J. H. Fujimura. Princeton, NJ: Princeton University Press.

Clarke, Adele E. and Virginia L. Olesen. 1999. *Revisioning Women, Health, and Healing: Feminist, Cultural, and Technoscience Perspectives*. New York: Routledge.

Clarke, Adele E., Janet K. Shim, Laura Mamo, Jennifer Ruth Fosket, Jennifer R. Fishman. 2003. "Biomedicalization: Technoscientific Transformations of Health, Illness, and U.S. Biomedicine" *American Sociological Review* 68:161–94.

_____. 2010. *Biomedicalization: Technoscience and Transformations of Health and Illness in the U.S.* Durham, NC: Duke University Press.

Clarke, Adele E. and Susan Leigh Star. 2007. "The Social Worlds/Arenas Framework: A Theory-Methods Package." Pp. 113–37 in *The Handbook of Science and Technology Studies*, edited by E. Hackett, O. Amsterdamska, M. Lynch, and J. Wajcman. Cambridge, MA: MIT Press.

Conrad, Peter. 2005. "The Shifting Engines of Medicalization." *Journal of Health and Social Behavior* 46:3–14.

_____. 2007. *The Medicalization of Society: On the Transformation of Human Conditions into Treatable Disorders*. Baltimore, MD: Johns Hopkins University Press.

Conrad, Peter and Jonathan Gabe. 1999. *Sociological Perspectives on the New Genetics*. Oxford, England: Blackwell.

Cooper, Melinda. 2008. *Life as Surplus: Biotechnology and Capitalism in the Neoliberal Era*. Seattle: University of Washington Press.

De Vries, Raymond and Scott Kim. 2008. "Bioethics and the Sociology of Trust: Introduction to the Theme." *Medicine, Health Care and Philosophy* 11:377–79.

Dumit, Joseph. 2003. *Picturing Personhood: Brain Scans and Biomedical Identity*. Princeton, NJ: Princeton University Press.

Duster, Troy. [1990] 2003. *Backdoor to Eugenics*. 2nd ed. New York: Routledge.

Ehrenreich, Barbara. 2001. "Welcome to Cancerland: A Mammogram Leads to a Cult of Pink Kitsch." *Harper's Magazine*, November 2001, pp. 43–53.

Epstein, Steven. 1996. *Impure Science: AIDS, Activism, and the Politics of Knowledge*. Berkeley: University of California Press.

_____. 2008. "Patient Groups and Health Movements." Pp. 499–540 in *The Handbook of Science and Technology Studies*, edited by E. Hackett, O. Amsterdamska, M. Lynch, and J. Wajcman. Cambridge, MA: MIT Press.

Fisher, Jill A. 2009. *Medical Research for Hire: The Political Economy of Pharmaceutical Clinical Trials*. New Brunswick, NJ: Rutgers University Press.

Fosket, Jennifer R. 2004. "Constructing 'High Risk Women': The Development and Standardization of a Breast Cancer Risk Assessment Tool." *Science, Technology and Human Values* 29:291–313.

Foucault, Michel. 1994. *The Birth of the Clinic*. New York: Pantheon.

_____. 1995. *Discipline and Punish: The Birth of the Prison*. New York: Vintage.

_____. 2008. *The Birth of Biopolitics: Lectures at the College de France, 1978–1979*. New York: Palgrave Macmillan.

Franklin, Sarah. 2000. "Life Itself." Pp. 188–98 and 215–27 in *Global Nature/Global Culture*, edited by S. Franklin, C. Lurie, and J. Stacey. London, England: Sage.

_____. 2007. *Dolly Mixtures: The Remaking of Genealogy*. Durham, NC: Duke University Press.

Fujimura, Joan H. 1988. "The Molecular Biological Bandwagon in Cancer Research: Where Social Worlds Meet." *Social Problems* 35:261–83.

_____. 1996. *Crafting Science: A Sociohistory of the Quest for the Genetics of Cancer*. Cambridge, MA: Harvard University Press.

Gibbon, Sahra and Carlos Novas. 2008. *Biosocialities, Genetics, and the Social Sciences: Making Biologies and Identities*. London: Routledge.

Ginsburg, Faye D. and Rayna Rapp. 1995. *Conceiving the New World Order: The Global Politics of Reproduction*. Berkeley: University of California Press.

Glaser, Barney G. and Anselm Strauss. 1965. *Awareness of Dying*. Chicago, IL: Aldine.

Gottweis, Herbert and Alan Petersen. 2008. *Biobanks: Governance in Comparative Perspective*. New York: Routledge.

Greene, Jeremy A. 2007. *Prescribing by Numbers: Drugs and the Definition of Disease*. Baltimore, MD: Johns Hopkins University Press.

Grinker, Roy Richard. 2010. "Disorder out of Chaos." *New York Times*, February 9, P. A23. Retrieved March 2, 2010 (http://www.nytimes.com/2010/02/10/opinion/10grinker.html).

Gruskin, Sofia. 2006. "Rights-Based Approaches to Health: Something for Everyone." *Health and Human Rights* 9:5–9.

Harrington, Charlene and Carroll L. Estes. 2007. *Health Policy: Crisis and Reform in the U.S. Health Care Delivery System*. 5th ed. Sudbury, MA: Jones and Bartlett.

Hatch, Anthony R. 2009. "The Politics of Metabolism: The Metabolic Syndrome and the Reproduction of Race and Racism." PhD dissertation, Department of Sociology, University of Maryland, College Park, MD.

Hedgecoe, Adam. 2004. *The Politics of Personalised Medicine: Pharmacogenetics in the Clinic*. Cambridge, England: Cambridge University Press.

Hess, David J. 2005. "Technology- and Product-Oriented Movements: Approximating Social Movement Studies and Science and Technology Studies." *Science, Technology, and Human Values* 30:515–35.

Horwitz, Allan V. 2002. *Creating Mental Illness*. Chicago, IL: The University of Chicago Press.

Hyde, Merv and Des Power. 2006. "Some Ethical Dimensions of Cochlear Implantation for Deaf Children and Their Families." *Journal of Deaf Studies and Deaf Education* 11:102–11.

Illich, Ivan. 1975. *Medical Nemesis: The Expropriation of Health*. London, England: Calder & Boyars.

Joyce, Kelly A. 2008. *Magnetic Appeal: MRI and the Myth of Transparency*. Ithaca, NY: Cornell University Press.

Keating, Peter and Alberto Cambrosio. 2002. "From Screening to Clinical Research: The Cure of Leukemia and the Early Development of the Cooperative Oncology Groups, 1955–1966." *Bulletin of the History of Medicine* 76:299–334.

_____. 2003. *Biomedical Platforms: Realigning the Normal and the Pathological in Late-Twentieth Century Medicine*. Cambridge, MA: MIT Press.

Kenny, Katherine E. 2009. "Breast Cancer Activism and the 'Previvor' Movement: Embodiment, Citizenship, and the Genetically 'at Risk.'" Presented at the meeting of the Society for the Social Studies of Science, Washington, DC, October 31.

Klawiter, Maren. 2004. "Breast Cancer in Two Regimes: The Impact of Social Movements on Illness Experience." *Sociology of Health and Illness* 26:845–74.

_____. 2008. *The Biopolitics of Breast Cancer: Changing Cultures of Disease and Activism*. Minneapolis: University of Minnesota Press.

Koenig, Barbara A., Henry T. Greely, Laura M. McConnell, Heather L. Silverberg, Thomas A. Raffin, and the Members of the Breast Cancer Working Group of the Stanford Program in Genomics, Ethics, and Society. 1998. "Genetic Testing for BRCA1 and BRCA2: Recommendations of the Stanford Program in Genomics, Ethics, and Society." *Journal of Women's Health* 7:531–45.

Lakoff, Andrew. 2005. *Pharmaceutical Reason: Knowledge and Value in Global Psychiatry*. Cambridge, England: Cambridge University Press.

_____. 2008. "The Right Patient for the Drug: Pharmaceutical Circuits and the Codification of Illness." Pp. 741–60 in *The Social Construction of Technological Systems*, edited by W. E. Bijker, T. P. Hughes, and T. Pinch. Cambridge, MA: MIT Press.

Ley, Barbara L. 2009. *From Pink to Green: Disease Prevention and the Environmental Breast Cancer Movement*. New Brunswick, NJ: Rutgers University Press.

Lorber, Judith and Lisa Jean Moore. 2002. *Gender and the Social Construction of Illness*. 2nd ed. Walnut Creek, CA: Rowman Altamira.

Lovell, Anne M. 2006. "Addiction Markets: The Case of High-Dose Buprenorphine in France." Pp. 136–70 in *Global Pharmaceuticals: Ethics, Markets, Practices*, edited by A. Petryna, A. Lakoff, and A. Kleinman. Durham, NC: Duke University Press.

Mandelblatt, Jeanne, Kathleen A. Cronin, Stephanie Bailey, Donald A. Berry, Harry J. de Koning, Gerrit Draisma, Hui Huang, Sandra J. Lee,

Mark Munsell, Sylvia K. Pleveritis, Peter Ravdin, Clyde B. Schechter, Bronislava Sigal, Michael A. Stoto, Satasha K. Stout, Nicolien T. van Ravesteyn, John Venier, Marvin Zelen, Eric J. Feuer, and for the Breast Cancer Working Group of the Cancer Intervention and Surveillance Modeling Network (CISNET). 2009. "Effects of Mammography Screening Under Different Screening Schedules: Model Estimates of Potential Benefits and Harms." *Annals of Internal Medicine* 151:738–47.

McKinlay, John B. 1984. *Issues in the Political Economy of Health Care*. New York: Tavistock.

Mechanic, David. 2007. "Population Health: Challenges for Science and Society." *The Milbank Quarterly* 85:533–59.

Morrison, Daniel R. 2009. "Brain and Machine: Deep Brain Stimulation and the Self." Presented at the meeting of the Society for the Social Studies of Science, Washington, DC, October 31.

Murray, John E. 2007. *Origins of American Health Insurance: A History of Industrial Sickness Funds*. New Haven, CT: Yale University Press.

Navarro, Vicente. 1986. *Crisis, Health, and Medicine: A Social Critique*. New York: Tavistock.

Nelkin, Dorothy and Laurence Tancredi. 1989. *Dangerous Diagnostics: The Social Power of Biological Information*. New York: Basic Books.

Nye, David E. 2006. *Technology Matters: Questions to Live With*. Cambridge, MA: MIT Press.

Oakley, Ann. 1984. *The Captured Womb: A History of the Medical Care of Pregnant Women*. Oxford, England: Blackwell.

Oshinsky, David M. 2005. *Polio: An American Story*. New York: Oxford University Press.

Petryna, Adriana. 2002. *Life Exposed: Biological Citizens after Chernobyl*. Princeton, NJ: Princeton University Press.

Petryna, Adriana, Andrew Lakoff, and Arthur Kleinman. 2006. *Global Pharmaceuticals: Ethics, Markets, Practices*. Durham, NC: Duke University Press.

Pickering, Andrew. 1992. *Science as Practice and Culture*. Chicago, IL: The University of Chicago Press.

Piribo Limited. 2010. "About Piribo." Retrieved March 6, 2010 (http://www.piribo.com/about_us/index.html).

Pulley, Jill M., Margaret M. Brace, Gordon R. Bernard, and Dan R. Masys. 2008. "Attitudes and Perceptions of Patients towards Methods of Establishing a DNA Biobank." *Cell and Tissue Banking* 9:55–65.

Quadagno, Jill. 2006. *One Nation, Uninsured: Why the U.S. Has No National Health Insurance*. New York: Oxford University Press.

Rabin, Roni Caryn. 2009. "New Guidelines on Breast Cancer Draw Opposition." *New York Times*, November 16. Retrieved March 6, 2010 (http://www.nytimes.com/2009/11/17/health/17scre.html).

Rabinow, Paul. 1992. "Artificiality and Enlightenment: From Sociobiology to Biosociality." Pp. 234–52 in *Incorporations*, edited by J. Crary and S. Kwinter. New York: Zone.

Rabinow, Paul and Nikolas Rose. 2006. "Biopower Today." *Biosocieties* 1:195–217.

Rapp, Rayna. 2000. *Testing Women, Testing the Fetus: The Social Impact of Amniocentesis in America*. New York: Routledge.

Reiser, Stanley Joel and Michael Anbar. 1984. *The Machine at the Bedside: Strategies for Using Technology in Patient Care*. New York: Cambridge University Press.

Riessman, Catherine Kohler. 1983. "Women and Medicalization: A New Perspective." *Social Policy* 14:3–18.

Robert Wood Johnson Foundation. 2009. "Health Care Spending as Percentage of GDP." Talking About Quality Part 1: Health Care Today. Retrieved March 5, 2010 (http://www.rwjf.org/pr/product.jsp? id=45110).

Roden, Dan M., Jill Pulley, Melissa Basford, Gordon Bernard, Ellen Wright Clayton, Jeffrey Balser, and Dan Masys. 2008. "Development of a Large-Scale De-Identified DNA Biobank to Enable Personalized Medicine." *Clinical Pharmacology and Therapeutics* 84:362–69.

Rose, Nikolas S. 2007. *The Politics of Life Itself: Biomedicine, Power, and Subjectivity in the Twenty-First Century.* Princeton, NJ: Princeton University Press.

Rose, Nikolas S. and Carlos Novas. 2005. "Biological Citizenship." Pp. 439–64 in *Global Assemblages: Technology, Politics, and Ethics as Anthropological Problems*, edited by A. Ong and S. J. Collier. Malden, MA: Blackwell.

Rothman, Barbara Katz. 1993. *The Tentative Pregnancy: How Amniocentesis Changes the Experience of Motherhood.* New York: W.W. Norton & Co.

Ruzek, Sheryl Burt, Virginia L. Olesen, and Adele E. Clarke. 1997. *Women's Health: Complexities and Differences.* Columbus: The Ohio State University Press.

Serlin, David H. 2004. *Replaceable You: Engineering the Body in Postwar America.* Chicago, IL: University of Chicago Press.

Shakespeare, Tom, (ed.). 1998. *The Disability Reader: Social Science Perspectives.* London, England: Continuum.

Siebers, Tobin. 2006. "Disability in Theory: From Social Construction to the New Realism of the Body." Pp. 173–84 in *The Disability Studies Reader*, 2nd ed., edited by L. J. Davis. New York: Routledge.

Sparrow, Robert. 2005. "Defending Deaf Culture: The Case of Cochlear Implants." *The Journal of Political Philosophy* 13:135–52.

Star, Susan Leigh and James R. Griesemer. 1989. "Institutional Ecology, 'Translations' and Boundary Objects: Amateurs and Professionals in Berkeley's Museum of Vertebrate Zoology, 1907–39." *Social Studies of Science* 19:387–420.

Star, Susan Leigh and Anselm Strauss. 1999. "Layers of Silence, Arenas of Voice: The Ecology of Visible and Invisible Work." *Computer Supported Cooperative Work* 8:9–30.

Starr, Paul. 1982. *The Social Transformation of American Medicine: The Rise of a Sovereign Profession and the Making of a Vast Industry.* New York: Basic Books.

Strauss, Anselm. 1988. "The Articulation of Project Work." *The Sociological Quarterly* 29:163–78.

Strauss, Anselm L., Shizuko Fagerhaugh, Barbara Suczek, and Carolyn Wiener. 1985. *Social Organization of Medical Work.* Chicago, IL: University of Chicago Press.

Sulik, Gayle A. 2009. "Managing Biomedical Uncertainty: The Technoscientific Illness Identity." *Sociology of Health and Illness* 31:1059–76.

Sunder Rajan, Kaushik. 2006. *Biocapital: The Constitution of Postgenomic Life.* Durham, NC: Duke University Press.

Talley, Heather Laine. 2008. "Face Work: Cultural, Technical, and Surgical Interventions for Facial 'Disfigurement.'" PhD dissertation, Department of Sociology, Vanderbilt University, Nashville, TN.

Tanner, Lindsey. 2010. "Proposed Autism Diagnosis Changes Anger 'Aspies.'" Associated Press, February 10, 2010. Retrieved March 5, 2010 (http://www.apa.org/news/psycport/PsycPORTArticle.aspx? id=ap_2010_02_11_ap.online.all_D9DQ25C80_news_ap_org.anpa.xml).

Taylor, Janelle S. 2000. "Of Sonograms and Baby Prams: Prenatal Diagnosis, Pregnancy, and Consumption." *Feminist Studies* 26:391–418.

_____. 2008. *The Public Life of the Fetal Sonogram: Technology, Consumption, and the Politics of Reproduction.* New Brunswick, NJ: Rutgers University Press.

Thompson, Charis. 2005. Making *Parents: The Ontological Choreography of Reproductive Technologies*. Cambridge, MA: MIT Press.

Thomson, L. Katherine. 2009. "Transdisciplinary Knowledge Production of Endocrine Disruptors: 'Windows of Vulnerability' in Breast Cancer Risk." PhD dissertation, Department of Social and Behavioral Sciences, University of California, San Francisco, CA.

Timmermans, Stefan. 1999. *Sudden Death and the Myth of CPR*. Philadelphia, PA: Temple University Press.

Timmermans, Stefan and Marc Berg. 2003. *The Gold Standard: The Challenge of Evidence-Based Medicine and Standardization in Health Care*. Philadelphia, PA: Temple University Press.

Turner, Bryan S. 2006. *Vulnerability and Human Rights: Essays on Human Rights*. University Park, PA: The Pennsylvania State University Press.

Wailoo, Keith and Stephen Pemberton. 2006. *The Troubled Dream of Genetic Medicine: Ethnicity and Innovation in Tay-Sachs, Cystic Fibrosis, and Sickle Cell Disease*. Baltimore, MD: Johns Hopkins University Press.

Wainwright, Steven P., Clare Williams, Mike Michael, Bonnie Farsides, and Alan Cribb. 2006. "From Bench to Bedside? Biomedical Scientists' Expectations of Stem Cell Science as a Future Therapy for Diabetes." *Social Science and Medicine* 63:2052–64.

Waldby, Catherine. 1996. *AIDS and the Body Politic: Biomedicine and Sexual Difference*. New York: Routledge.

_____. 2000. *The Visible Human Project: Informatic Bodies and Posthuman Medicine*. New York: Routledge.

Waldby, Catherine and Robert Mitchell. 2006. Tissue Economies: Blood, Organs, and Cell Lines in Late Capitalism. Durham, NC: Duke University Press.

Wiener, Carolyn, Anselm Strauss, Shizuko Fagerhaugh, and Barbara Suczek. 1997. "Trajectories, Biographies, and the Evolving Medical Technology Scene." Pp. 229–50 in *Grounded Theory in Practice*, edited by A. Strauss and J. Corbin. Thousand Oaks, CA: Sage.

Williams, Clare, Steven P. Wainwright, Kathryn Ehrich, and Mike Michael. 2008. "Human Embryos as Boundary Objects: Some Reflections on the Biomedical Worlds of Embryonic Stem Cells and Pre-Implantation Genetic Diagnosis." *New Genetics and Society* 27:7–18.

Williams, Simon J., Jonathan Gabe, and Peter Davis. 2008. "The Sociology of Pharmaceuticals: Progress and Prospects." *Sociology of Health and Illness* 30:813–24.

Yoxen, Edward. 1987. "Seeing with Sound: A Study of the Development of Medical Images." Pp. 281–303 in *The Social Construction of Technological Systems*, edited by W. E. Bijker, T. P. Hughes, and T. Pinch. Cambridge, MA: MIT Press.

Zetka, James R. 2003. *Surgeons and the Scope*. Ithaca, NY: ILR Press/Cornell University Press.

Zola, Irving Kenneth. 1972. "Medicine as an Institution of Social Control." *Sociological Review* 20:487–504.

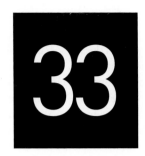

"IT JUST BECOMES MUCH MORE COMPLICATED"

Genetic Counselors' Views on Genetics and Prenatal Testing

Susan Markens

As scholarly and bioethical debates continue about the larger social significance of genetic medicine, research on genetic medicine often examines why patients accept or decline the tests that are offered to them, as well as their responses to genetic information they are provided (Rothman 1986; Browner and Press 1995; Press and Browner 1997; Hallowell 1999; Markens, Browner, and Press 1999; Rapp 1999; Taylor 2004; Featherstone et al. 2006; Kuppermann et al. 2006; Remennick 2006; Atkin et al. 2008; Garcia, Timmermans, and van Leeuwen 2008; Kelly 2009; Markens, Browner, and Preloran 2010; McAllister et al. 2011; Shostak, Zarhin, and Ottman 2011). This growing body of research has provided rich insight into the multi-layered implications of the increased availability of genetic testing and the proliferation of genetic information. For instance, studies have shown how prenatal testing has become simultaneously straightforward (i.e. normalized and routine) and complex (i.e. more options and information, and along with that more ambiguity). Meanwhile, research on attitudes towards genetics has found that opinions vary. On the one hand, people with more education and knowledge often express more favorable opinions about genetics than those with less knowledge; yet, research has also found that those with more knowledge or direct professional experience with medical genetics may have more doubts and concerns than the lay public (Michie et al. 1995; Jallinoja and Aro

It Just Becomes Much More Complicated: Genetic Counselors' Views on Genetics and Prenatal Testing, Susan Markens in *New Genetics and Society*, *32*(3), 302–321, 2013. Reprinted with permission from Taylor & Francis.

2000; Toiviainen et al. 2003; Morren et al. 2007; Singer et al. 2008).

Although understanding patients' perspectives and public opinion is important for understanding the impact of genetic medicine's recent acceleration, genetic counselors' perspectives are also important for social science research to focus on. As genomic knowledge and genetic technologies become more diffuse and complex, the specialized knowledge possessed by genetic counselors is more likely to be in demand throughout healthcare settings (e.g. see Pollack 2012). Indeed, genetic counselors constitute a key new profession situated between the ascendant complex genetic knowledge and the lay public, patients, and other medical professionals. In this sense, they occupy a space for "meso-level" analysis, as they traverse between the formal knowledge arena and the situational practice arena.

Today, genetic counselors in the USA who earn master's degrees to qualify for their profession can be the primary link between information on genetics and patients, including pregnant women seeking information about their fetus. Although medical workers other than master's-trained genetic counselors provide genetic counseling in the USA, there is a need to study this specific professional group because medical doctor (MD) clinical geneticists, a group of physicians that provide genetic counseling in the USA and elsewhere, account for only 0.18% of all physicians in the USA. Indeed, currently fewer physicians are board certified annually in clinical genetics than 30 years ago (Wicklund 2008; Korf, Irons, and Watson 2011). Meanwhile, with the rapid expansion and complexity of genetic knowledge, and the structure of clinical care in the twenty-first-century USA, most primary care and specialty physicians will likely have neither the expertise nor the time to provide adequate information to patients about genetic testing and the information it provides.[1] Thus, we can expect the non-MD, master's-trained genetic counselor to be in demand and to take on an increasingly integral role in the sphere of genetic knowledge and practice.

Yet, there is relatively little research focused on genetic counselors. As a result, a study focused on this particular genetic professional opens a relatively unexplored and important analytic window to investigate genetic medicine's cultural and social impact. Specifically, this study asks how these highly trained professionals think about the larger ethical debates and the uncertainties that patients face in the context of recent advances in genetic medicine and the work that they do, with a particular focus on prenatal testing. In doing so, this article builds on the rich scholarly literature that examines how (bio)medicalization processes affect how people think about and respond to health and illness, with a focus on interrogating the role that a specific group of providers may play in such processes, both in its institutionalization and in "resistance" to it (Conrad 2007; Clarke et al. 2010). Before presenting the study, the next section reviews the history of the master's-trained genetic counselor in the USA and the relevant literature in which this article is situated and builds on.

GENETIC MEDICINE, PRENATAL TESTING, AND THE GENETIC COUNSELING PROFESSION

Since the discovery of the DNA helix in the 1950s through the decoding of the human genome at the beginning of the twenty-first century, scholars of medicine have examined the "geneticization" of health and illness (Lippman 1991; Conrad 1999). Commentators of genetic medicine, and the increasingly prevalent "genetic worldview," have questioned its ethical and social impact from its effects on conceptions of health and illness and concerns about genetic reductionism and misunderstandings of risk to the dangers of genetic engineering and the drive for "designer babies" (Duster 1990; Lewontin 1993; Shakespeare 1995; Conrad 1999; Nelkin and Lindee 2004; Petersen 2006). Since prenatal testing is one of the main clinical sites in which genetic testing has been offered, and because some of the central bioethical concerns about genetic testing and knowledge are clearly salient when it comes to reproductive decision-making, social science research has often focused on prenatal genetic testing.

For instance, as prenatal genetic testing became normalized as a "routine part of prenatal care" (Browner and Press 1995) and institutionalized through state and medical policies, social scientists raised concerns about the causes and consequences of these developments. Some early concerns included: views of prenatal genetic diagnosis as a "backdoor to eugenics" in terms of the desire to eliminate certain traits from the population (Duster 1990); practices of prenatal testing as potentially expanding the medicalization of pregnancy, in turn causing women to experience a "tentative pregnancy" (Rothman 1986); and tensions around positioning women as "moral pioneers" if they are given responsibility for making decisions about under which conditions they would or would not terminate a pregnancy (Rapp 1999). Such critiques have continued in the twenty-first century, particularly regarding the impact on women as "decision-makers," the imposition of and responsibility for "risks," and the false and narrow sense of "choice" and "control" the availability of these tests provide (Samerski 2006, 2009; Roberts 2009). Meanwhile, much of this research on pregnant women's experiences with prenatal testing implicitly and explicitly positions genetic counselors as an unreflexive social actor implicated in the (bio)medicalization and geneticization of pregnancy in their role of providing information about testing options. In the USA, who are these genetic counselors?

The distinct *profession* of genetic counseling was born in the USA over 40 years ago when the first master's program was established at Sarah Lawrence College, New York, in 1969. In 1979, a professional organization, the National Society of Genetic Counselors (NSGC), was formed, and two years later a credentialing organization, the American Board of Genetic Counselors, which accredited graduate programs in genetic counseling and oversees a certification examination for those graduating from master's programs, was also established. Recently in 2013, the Accreditation Council for Genetic Counseling (ACGC) was formed as a separate accrediting body for training programs while ABGC continues

to certify individual counselors (American Board of Genetic Counselors 2013). The establishment of a master's-trained genetic counseling professional was thus created and institutionalized in the USA over a decade or two before separate training and certification programs emerged in other countries (Sahhar et al. 2005; Skirton, Arimori, and Aoki 2006; Barnes et al. 2012; Sagi and Uhlmann 2013; Skirton et al. 2013).[2] In the meantime, this specifically graduate-trained and credentialed genetic professional—both in the science of genetics and in the psychosocial aspects of counseling—has vastly expanded in the USA. The profession's growth to 32 accredited programs and over 3000 board-certified counselors in the USA by the end of the twenty-first century's first decade has been termed as a "quiet revolution" (Stern 2009; see also American Board of Genetic Counseling 2013).

Yet, with the exception of historical studies focused on the development of genetic counseling as a profession (Heimler 1997; Keenan 1997; Stern 2009, 2012), little research focuses solely on the professional genetic counselor described earlier. For instance, qualitative studies on "genetic counselors," as well as comparative survey and opinion research, usually investigates the work practices and views of health professionals other than the board-certified genetic counselor who is becoming increasingly prevalent in the USA (Wertz and Fletcher 1988a, 1988b, 1989; Bosk 1992; Michie et al. 1998; Williams Alderson, and Farsides, 2002a, 2002b; Hashiloni-Dolev 2006; Samerski 2006; Kerr, Cunningham-Burley, and Tutton 2007; Samerski 2009; Hashiloni-Dolev and Raz 2010; Arribas-Ayllon, Sarangis, and Clarke 2011; Schwennesen and Koch 2012). Another limit of previous research that examines genetic counselors is that much of the work on genetic counseling is centered on patients' understandings and experiences (Hallowell 1999; Featherstone et al. 2006, McAllister et al. 2011); thus, studies of prenatal genetic counseling, for instance, are usually part of a larger project in which the analytic focus is on the pregnant woman (Rothman 1986; Kolker and Burke 1994; Press and Browner 1997; Rapp 1999; Pilnick 2008; Samerski 2009).

So what has been learned and what do we still need to investigate from this scholarship on genetic counseling more broadly? Ethnographic studies on the genetic counseling process tend to focus on how genetic counselors actively negotiate and have difficulty living up to professional and ethical ideals, particularly the professional norm of nondirectiveness—to provide information and options, but not to "advise" (Karlberg 2000; Williams, Alderson, and Farsides 2002a; Pilnick 2002a, 2002b; Hashiloni-Dolev 2006; Schwennesen and Koch 2012). Yet, less attention is paid in this research to how genetic counselors view the impact of genetic knowledge and the availability of genetic testing at the personal as well as the population level. Likewise, while survey research has addressed personal value issues such as abortion, as well as the complexity and ambivalence that counselors feel about their work, including their views on professional norms (Wertz and Fletcher 1988a, 1989; Bartels et al. 1997; Pirzadeh et al. 2007), these attitudinal studies usually fail to interrogate counselors' broader perspectives about genetic medicine and the usefulness of genetic testing for real and potential patients. Research that has analyzed the broader views and "stories" of genetic professionals often focuses on elites, research scientists and "experts" (Kerr, Cunningham-Burley, and Amos 1997; Ettorre 1999; Rabino 2006). Missing still, are the perspectives of the very genetic professionals—genetic counselors[3]—whose work usually revolves around clinical interactions with patients (National Society of Genetic Counselors 2012). These gaps in the literature are compounded by the fact that much of the previous research on genetic counseling, especially survey research on attitudes, predates the current and continuing expansion of genetic information and technologies. We are left then with very little knowledge of how these genetic counseling professionals view the implications of the recent genetic revolution for the work they do and for the patients they see.

To address these lacunae, I interviewed genetic counselors about their perspectives on genetic medicine and prenatal testing. In doing so, this paper investigates whether this growing profession of front-line genetic workers is aware of and concerned about the ethical issues raised by social scientists and commentators. I ask: (1) are board certified/eligible genetic counselors unreflexive enthusiasts or thoughtful critics of genetic medicine more broadly? and (2) more specifically, how do genetic counselors view the impact of genetic decision-making for the patients they serve? Building on previous research that has recognized ambivalence and complexity among genetic workers, I find that this distinct genetic professional exhibits what I term "reflexive ambivalence." That is, in simultaneously occupying two worlds—the world of genetic science and the world of clinical care—genetic counselors vacillate between optimism and skepticism as they consider the promises and limits of science, as well as their ethical and professional obligations to patients.

As a result, while previous scholars have recognized that patients do not necessarily acquiesce to biomedicalization processes (Clarke et al. 2010), by placing genetic counselors at the center of analysis, the findings from this study extend such observations beyond patients to highlight how a medical actor—genetic counselors—whose work is necessarily implicated in (and is often blamed for) such processes not only express ambivalences themselves, but also may resist and negotiate them as well. At the same time, in my discussion, I discuss how the impact of genetic counselors' critiques and concerns may be muted due to conflicting professional norms and the larger social context that shape their personal and professional beliefs.

DATA AND METHODS

Data for this study consist of 26 semi-structured recorded interviews with master's-trained and board-certified (or eligible) genetic counselors. Participants were identified through lists of professional organizations and hospital directories publicly available on the web, as well as through snowball sampling. The interview length varied between 45 min and 2.5 h with the average length around 1 h and 25 min. The majority of interviews were conducted in their offices, but several were conducted in cafes, in a park, and one was conducted in a participant's home. All participants read and signed an Institutional Review Board approved consent form. No identifying information is provided in order to protect their anonymity.

The study participants were all recruited in one major US metropolitan area; however, they attended 10 different graduate programs located throughout the USA, and work at over 15 different clinical sites, significantly diversifying the intra-city sample. As with the profession as a whole, the majority of the counselors work or have previously worked in prenatal (n = 21), and all have experience in prenatal through their training programs. The median time at current job at the time of the interview was between 3.5 and 4 years (Table 33.1). The counselors interviewed range in age from 24 to 75 years with a median age of 30 years which is slightly younger than the profession as a whole. Thirty-one percent of the participants are non-white or mixed race, a much higher proportion than the profession as a whole. Yet, like the NSGC, most are white women under 40 years with less than 10 years on the job (National Society of Genetic Counselors 2012).

This study harnesses qualitative interview data to utilize a modified form of grounded theory (Glaser and Strauss 1967; Bryant and Charmaz 2010). The interview schedule covered four broad topics: (1) educational/professional background and views on the profession; (2) experiences with and goals of genetic counseling; (3) views of patients and institutional context; and (4) general views on genetics and genetic testing. The focus of this article's analysis is on responses given in Sections 1 and 4 of the interview guide, but includes relevant excerpts that occurred throughout interviews. Although I looked for particular topics in the transcripts (e.g. views on genetics), concepts and ideas emerged during the data collection process and as I read and coded the data. Upon identifying significant themes and patterns, I went back through the data to see if and where other examples appeared in the interview transcripts. While the methods used in this paper may limit the generalizability of its findings, qualitative methods, and grounded theory in particular, are viewed as especially suitable for understanding complex ethical and analytical issues in emergent

TABLE 33.1 ■ Characteristics of Study Participants		
	N = 26	**%**
Age		
20s	9	37
30s	13	50
>40	4	15
Race/ethnicity		
White	18	69
Asian/mixed	5	19
Hispanic/mixed	3	12
Years working as genetic counselor		
<5	16	62
5–15	6	23
>20	4	15

phenomena, such as those surrounding the work of genetic counselors (Brock 1995; Beeson 1997; Grubs and Piantanida 2010).

In the remainder of the paper, I first discuss genetic counselors' views on genetic medicine writ large; then, I analyze their assessment of and experience with prenatal testing more specifically. In each of the topics interrogated here, my analysis of the interviews revealed that most genetic counselors expressed variable sentiments. As a result, within each issue I juxtapose genetic counselors' enthusiasm and optimism with their simultaneous skepticism and awareness of disadvantages. In doing so, this study contributes unique data with its focus on a relatively understudied player in the genetic decision-making process, as well as important findings regarding the nuance expressed by these sometimes maligned genetic health care workers in the social science literature.

FINDINGS

Views Toward Decoding the Human Genome and the Future of Genetic Medicine: "There Are Benefits and Then There Are Very Scary Points as Well"

What are genetic counselors' thoughts about recent advances in genetic knowledge and medicine more broadly? Not surprisingly, given their scientific background and training, when asked about their views on the decoding of the human genome many of the counselors expressed much optimism. Some described the decoding of the human genome as a "positive thing" and "very exciting," and another counselor explained, "[I] think it's important." Examples of the import put on, and belief in, genetic medicine and the decoding of the human genome ranged from Counselor 4 who stated how it allows us to "understand how our body works better" to Counselor 7 who remarked, "[I] really believe everything is genetic." The counselors' positive reactions to and feelings about genetics' role in health care seem to reflect their overall optimism about and belief in science as both important and beneficial.

A main focus of their enthusiasm about genetic science was the potential impact new genetic knowledge would have for *personalized medicine*, a term mentioned spontaneously by several of the counselors, and an issue that has also been the focus of much optimism about and expectations for the applications of genetic science (Pollack 2008; Collins 2010; Hamburg and Collins 2010; Markoff 2012). This anticipated positive impact of decoding the human genome is illustrated in Counselor 2's prediction for the future of medicine and health care:

> I think where it [decoding the human genome] kind of leads to is more personalized genomics. . . . I think it is great that we can get to the point where we can understand more about common conditions like heart disease and diabetes and things like that. I think that is where it's really helpful . . . it's kind of where genetics is moving in the future and where a lot of genetic counseling services would be helpful.

Yet, despite expressing an overall hopeful outlook about genetic science for its promising impact on medical care, very few counselors were fully positive about the impact of decoding the human genome when they considered the potential consequences at the societal and patient levels. That is they exhibited *reflexive ambivalence:* the very things that excited them about what genetic science might offer also raised concerns for them. Indeed, the vast majority, without prompting, provided qualified responses, acknowledging the downsides to our increasing genetic knowledge, as well as skepticism regarding what genetic medicine may offer. More than one counselor, for instance, described the human genome project as a "slippery slope," while Counselor 5 was concerned about "abuse" and remarked that "perfect health" scares her. Counselor 12 mentioned it was "opening a can of worms" and "could be scary like Gattaca.[4]" An example of the simultaneous acknowledgment of the benefits and misuses of genetic knowledge is found in the following comment by Counselor 8:

Obviously we're understanding more about conditions and about how genes function and how they interact and perhaps providing better medical care because of that. And then, I think that there's the potential to take it back to that information either in a way that might not be most beneficial to the patient. . . . Taking it all the way to understanding what eye color, and people start making decisions that are not . . . medically necessary . . . so for eugenic things that seem more frivolous. . . .

Similarly expressing ambivalence, Counselor 17 explained that genetic information was useful if utilized for the "right purposes," which this counselor defined as for health but not for esthetic purposes. As she remarked, "[genetic medicine] can get out of control . . . with all this testing." Thus, genetic counselors' enthusiasm about the science of genetics in the abstract was dampened when considering how it may be misused in its implementation. In other words, while counselors are optimistic about the promise of genetic science they do express skepticism when considering how genetic information will be disseminated and the impact on patients.

A specific area that concerned counselors regarding the application of genetic medicine was the issue of direct to consumer (DTC) companies, a topic spontaneously mentioned by almost half the study participants.[5] Genetic counselors conveyed apprehension not just about the commercialization of health care DTCs represent, but the very poor understanding of risk that most people have which they feared would lead to problems with the information provided by DTCs. In particular, several counselors remarked about the lack of follow-up with DTC testing and not having results interpreted properly. For instance, Counselor 11 commented that, "Tricky new companies [were] giving out risks . . . [with] no follow-up," while Counselor 18 stated that the problem with DTCs was "not having the right people to interpret results." Expressing the unease about the information people receive from genetic testing, particularly those who use

DTC without any medical support, Counselor 28 remarked "most of us [people] are bad with numbers."

In addition to concerns about potential abuse and lack of understanding of risk, reflexive ambivalence was also expressed by many of the counselors interviewed who said they were troubled by the hype around the decoding of the human genome, particularly with regard to what they viewed as naïve expectations about its direct impact on disease prevention. Several, for instance, spoke of their belief that medical conditions are not strictly determined by genes, specifically mentioning that in the long-term we are going to learn much more about gene–environment interaction. Other counselors commented on how complicated the role of genes is in the expression of disease. Meanwhile, many of the counselors emphasized how much is still unknown, referring to the decoding of the genome as providing "too much" and "exaggerated" expectations. In this way, while their background and belief in science made them enthusiastic about the promise of genetic medicine, their scientific training also provided them with tempered expectations of how, and if, new genetic discoveries will matter for patient care.

Indeed, for some, the decoding of the human genome has revealed how much we do not know. As Counselor 3 remarked: "It has gotten really confusing . . . decoding hasn't made it obvious . . . [we] learn now about what we don't know." Similarly, Counselor 4 commented on the complexity of genetic knowledge despite recent advances: "Coding is all fine and good, [but we] still don't know what all the genes do . . . [it's] probably more intricate than we realize," Meanwhile Counselor 13 focused on the "hype," the complexity, and the lack of what can be done with new genetic discoveries:

On the one hand people will have more information than ever about their constitutional makeup. And yet at the same time, there's not a whole lot we can do with that information. . . . The hype of having this information at our fingers is enticing but I think we're overselling it . . . because we just don't know enough about these variances.

Genetic counselors, in their professional awareness of the limits of what genetic science can and will offer with regard to disease prevention and health promotion, were thus concerned about the unrealistic expectations about genetic medicine that the lay public and their patients may have. These sentiments about the exaggerated expectations and the long-term prospects for genetic medicine and personalized medicine, despite their professional hopes for and beliefs in genetic science, are summed up by Counselor 1 who described decoding the genome as learning "the alphabet" but not "the language":

> I think it was really important to do, but people don't, in general, understand that we basically . . . learned the alphabet, but we don't know the language at all . . . the implications are really in better understanding gene-gene interactions, gene-environment interactions, what is a gene . . . because, I think we misunderstood that all along. So, in the long term, yeah, maybe we can get towards more personalized medicine. . . . But in the long term. I don't think that's coming anytime soon, and I think the public has been misled on that.

It seems, then, that genetic counselors' investment in the world of science did produce excitement and enthusiasm about its promise in the abstract; yet, their involvement in the world of patients also made them ambivalent about real-world applications of genetic science.[6] In particular, they were concerned about abuse and misunderstandings. Additionally, although genetic counselors saw genetic medicine as possibly and positively leading toward personalized medicine, they were also skeptical of what this new form of medicine offered for health care delivery in the near future. Counselor 14 summed up this professional reflexive ambivalence regarding the promise and limits of genetic medicine when she remarked that we are "not there yet."

Perspectives on Prenatal Testing: "It's Kind of a Fine Line to Draw"

How did genetic counselors' nuanced views on genetics more broadly translate into their views on prenatal testing specifically? Perhaps because of their direct experience with prenatal counseling, as well as its established clinical history, counselors expressed more unbridled enthusiasm when asked about prenatal testing relative to their ambivalence about the impact of genetic medicine more broadly. As with genetic medicine in general, several mentioned the health care benefits of prenatal testing. As Counselor 3 commented, prenatal testing affects "medical management," making a difference for rare single-gene disorders, while Counselor 17 remarked that prenatal testing is "good for care" if a woman chooses not to abort. These perceived and specific benefits toward "obstetrical management" are described in the following remarks by Counselor 2:

> [Prenatal testing is] important in a situation where it can help with obstetrical management . . . if you know that baby is going to have something, you know the appropriate things that are going to happen post-natally. You know in certain situations . . . when you get a diagnosis of this then we know the baby might be susceptible to hypoglycemia . . . so you're going to keep a better eye on it.

In addition to their belief in the concrete benefit of medical management, most of the counselors perceived prenatal testing as providing useful information to pregnant women, reflecting once again that they generally view scientific knowledge as "good." For instance, when asked why they thought prenatal testing was important, counselors provided answers such as: "[Prenatal testing] provides information people want" (Counselor 6) and "knowledge is good" (Counselor 17).

The overwhelming reason why genetic counselors viewed genetic information and its availability as useful in the prenatal context was because of the choices they saw it as providing. As two of the study participants reasoned, it is "important for people to have options" (Counselor 19) and the "more options the better" (Counselor 11). Knowledge and choice, in turn, were seen as providing empowerment to pregnant women. This perceived link between "choice" and "empowerment," and the value given to both, is articulated by Counselor 1 when describing what she liked about her current job:

> . . . giving people the opportunity to make decisions about their futures and their lives. . . . I've always thought that the power of choice was very important. And when I took this job [in prenatal] I figured if I could empower patients to understand more about their decisions, that would be great.

These views about patient choice seem to reflect personal beliefs in and professional commitment to informed and autonomous patients that is central to the genetic counseling profession, as well as American medicine and society more generally.

Yet, while generally positive about how knowledge and choice can be empowering for patients, many counselors also acknowledged, when reflecting on actual clinical care, that empowerment varied by patient. In particular, they were attuned to whether or not all women wanted to have such genetic information as well as to the reasons why some women might not want testing. As Counselor 1 who, as we saw earlier, viewed her role as empowering patients put it, "[there are] disadvantages for knowing and not knowing and it really depends on the person." Counselor 2 explained when information available through prenatal testing may or may not be desired:

> . . . is getting an answer important to you? It can be important if you are going to make a decision. . . . I think for a lot of patients if it is something they can test the baby for afterwards, which obviously in every case you probably can, they say then let's just test the baby when the baby is born and we'll figure it out then. For some it's the anxiety, they just don't want to go through that, they don't want to think about it. Some people just don't want to face the test. . . .

Genetic counselors do reflect, then, about the emotional impact the availability of prenatal genetic information may have on patients.

In the end, despite enthusiasm about prenatal testing, most genetic counselors did qualify their positions on prenatal testing when directly asked if there were disadvantages. For these genetic counselors, their concerns about the anxiety prenatal testing can cause were often informed by their professional knowledge about the problems with the type of information prenatal diagnostic testing currently provides. As they explained, this is because there may be "ambiguous results" or it may just be "stressful to know little things." Representative of the many counselors who acknowledged the downsides to prenatal counseling is Counselor 3 who explained that the information provided by prenatal testing can be a "double-edged sword" as "test results aren't always so clear" and often provide "limited information." Genetic counselors' scientific knowledge and clinical experience with patients, once again, shapes a reflexive ambivalence toward the application and consequences of genetic testing and information.

An example of this ambivalence is Counselor 14 who recounted an example of how the results of genetic testing may provide patients with information they may have never needed or wanted. In a case in which she was recently involved, a pregnant woman's fetus was diagnosed with XYY sex chromosome after she had an amniocentesis to rule out other conditions. Since this rare male sex chromosomal abnormality is not associated with major health or developmental problems, the counselor explained that this woman, like most with this diagnosis, is "likely to continue the pregnancy if all the rest of the testing goes well." As a result, she told the woman:

> You don't have to tell anybody about this . . . because every time he falls over or doesn't say a word right, you're already going to think, 'Is this because he has an extra Y chromosome?' Do you want your parents thinking that too, or his siblings? . . . if you never had this test, you may never have known this because he may not have any of that stuff.

Therefore, on the one hand, genetic counselors as a group are committed to and believe in the increased options and information genetic testing can provide; on the other hand, they also express apprehension about the usefulness and impact of new genetic information for patients as they are increasingly confronted with unwanted genetic information that produces liminal social and medical identities (Timmermans and Buchbinder 2010).

Genetic counselors' reflexive concerns about ambiguous and complicated information provided by prenatal testing were sometimes focused on recent developments in genetic testing, in particular microarrays which test the whole genome of a DNA sample for deletions and duplications. In describing the problems of using these new techniques, Counselor 15 remarked, "Unfortunately . . . [it can] identify unknown things." The relationship between possible ambiguous results and the anxiety it can produce for patients was addressed by Counselor 2:

> How do you interpret . . . ambiguous results for a family? Or sometimes you get . . . if there's a certain deletion, or a duplication, you do your best to counsel a patient based on the literature that's out there but maybe there isn't much literature. So then they're left with, like ok there's nothing wrong so what do I do? . . . Our technology is getting better . . . we are able to pick up some minute things that sometimes you stop and you think well maybe you have this . . . and you pick up tons of things that are absolutely meaningless, so how do you differentiate what's meaningful and not? And where do you really increase anxiety with that? So, it's kind of a fine line to draw.

As a result, rather than empowering patients, genetic counselors do acknowledge the problems of too much and perhaps unwanted information generated by advances in genetic medicine, knowledge and testing—from microarrays to tests for late-onset diseases. Recent accelerations in genetic knowledge and technologies may particularly highlight the reflexive ambivalence that counselors experience in the traditional realm of prenatal counseling more broadly. As Counselor 8 explained:

> There are potentially things like microarrays which . . . [detect things that] might not be defined as either deleterious or not. . . . Or, predictive testing for conditions that may be late onset. It just becomes much more complicated. I think a lot of people come here knowing information they wished they didn't know but they've been told because of whatever screening or testing has been done.

In sum, as has been found with other medical professionals, genetic counselors in the USA are neither naïve about nor unaware of the downsides to prenatal testing. Drawing on their knowledge of genetic science, as well as on their clinical interactions with patients, genetic counselors view the availability of genetic testing and information as not only "empowering" but also as a mixed-bag. Their nuanced views are also evidenced by their observations that mirror bioethical issues raised by social science/feminist critics. For instance, returning to early critics of prenatal testing, when discussing the case of sex selection, one genetic counselor expressed concerns about "using information not clinically" that were similar in nature to Duster's (1990) themes of a "slippery slope" and a "backdoor to eugenics." Another counselor evoked Rapp's (1999) concept of "moral pioneers" when admitting that the results from prenatal testing in essence "forces you to have to decide." Likewise, findings here are also reminiscent of Rothman's (1986) concerns about the "tentative pregnancy" as counselors discuss how prenatal testing is "frequently anxiety provoking" and "overwhelming" taking "the fun out of pregnancy." As a result, genetic counselors express a reflexive ambivalence—they view the information available to their patients as part of "choices" which they value both professionally and personally, while at the same time they are aware of the personal and societal costs that are also produced with increasing genetic knowledge and "choices."

DISCUSSION

The rise of genetic medicine is emblematic and constitutive of broader trends in the biomedicalization of health and illness from the emphasis on personalized medicine, the increasing focus on risk and risk management and the increasing reliance on technology to a shifting view of patients as consumers who make "choices," the focus on interior bodies, and the molecularization of disease (Rose 2006; Clarke et al. 2010). Genetic testing, and in particular prenatal diagnosis, exemplifies these trends as well as ethical debates about a myriad of social consequences to which these transformations give rise.

The findings from this study confirm that master's-trained genetic counselors are aware of ethical concerns and critiques regarding genetic testing. For instance, although they see the potential for personalized medicine with more knowledge about the human genome, most are also skeptical about how much we really know and can do in the foreseeable future. Study participants additionally expressed concern about how biomedical notions of risk may be interpreted and how this in turn may impact people's sense of self and health.

With specific regard to prenatal testing, genetic counselors, unlike critics of genetic medicine, generally view its availability as providing choice and empowerment for patients. As such, genetic counselors do articulate a neo-liberal individualized discourse about genetic testing that focuses on maximizing health and minimizing risk via biomedical choices while less often acknowledging the social relations and institutions that shape the choices that are available and eventually made (Roberts 2009; Samerski 2009; Clarke et al. 2010). Additionally, they do tend to ignore their own role in these processes (Kerr, Cunningham-Burley, and Tutton 2007). Despite all of this, and perhaps contrary to critics of genetic professionals, they are also clearly aware of the disadvantages of prenatal genetic information and the uncertain and anxiety-laden decision-making it can induce.

Although I did not explore this theme in significant depth, I did detect a similar awareness of

ethical concerns when counselors discussed the costs and benefits of genetic testing for adult-onset diseases (see also Browner and Preloran 2010). Given genetic medicine's expansion into other clinical specialties in the last decade (especially cancer), further research on genetic counselors' views on the clinical growth of genetic technologies should also investigate the extent to which personal, professional, and institutional characteristics affect counselors' degree of optimism or skepticism with regard to the proliferation and increased availability of genetic information (Conrad and Markens 2001). Since this study focused solely on counselors in the USA, further research should also compare genetic counselors to other medical professionals who engage in genetic counseling (Kerr, Cunningham-Burley, and Tutton 2007) and examine how national/cultural context affects the views, training, and work of master's-trained genetic counselor (Hashiloni-Dolev 2006; Hashiloni-Dolev and Raz 2010), particularly as this specific genetic professional expands globally (Sahhar et al. 2005; Barnes et al. 2012; Sagi and Uhlmann 2013; Skirton et al. 2013).

Do the findings presented here mean that concerns about eugenics, abuse, and consequences raised by social scientists and critics of genetic technologies should be ignored? There is understandably much debate within social science research, as well as the genetic counseling profession itself, about the usefulness of nondirectiveness and genetic counselors' actual engagement with it (Brunger and Lippman 1995; Bartels et al. 1997; Williams, Alderson, and Farsides 2002a; Bennett et al. 2003; Resta 2006; Weil et al. 2006; Schwennesen and Koch 2012; Markens 2013). On the one hand, the fact that nondirectiveness is a guiding principle of the profession may facilitate that their specialized knowledge and professional positions are not used in authoritative and coercive ways. At the same time, and perhaps ironically, the nondirective ethos of genetic counseling may also impede counselors from engaging in more nuanced and critical discussions in clinical encounters. Indeed, other research has found that genetic counselors have difficulty in expressing their doubts and ambivalence in the workplace (Kerr, Cunningham-Burley, and Tutton 2007). From my reading of the interview data, I attribute this to a tension between their professionally informed concerns about genetic medicine and a personal, professional—and perhaps specifically American—commitment to autonomy and "choice." Paradoxically then, the very genetic professionals who are aware of the limits and problems of genetic diagnosis, through both their clinical experiences with patients and their knowledge about genetic science, often participate in the expansion of genetic medicine because of their simultaneous commitment to the ethics of disclosure, informed consent, "choice," and patient autonomy in decision-making. Further research should more closely examine these dynamics, tensions, and contradictions between genetic counselors' personal and professional views and knowledge and the work in which they engage. More research that both critically and empirically examines genetic counselors' views and experiences can provide a more informed analysis of how abstract ethics about genetic medicine may and can be enacted and negotiated in everyday clinical encounters.

In the end, although genetic counselors in the USA do exhibit some professional blinders (e.g. a narrow focus on individual "autonomous" choice), the findings from this study show clear acknowledgment, concern, and awareness of the disadvantages, limits, and abuses of genetic information and testing. As Thomas et al. (2005, 2142) write, health professionals "need to inform the public about the strengths, limitations, and costs of genomic tools." As a result, genetic counselors are situated to play an important role of patient and consumer advocate. In particular, the skepticism and concern elucidated in this article suggests that genetic counselors could provide necessary caution in clinical settings,[7] as well as in the policy arena, about the pursuit and use of genetic testing. In this way, genetic counselors, like other clinicians, may play an important and delicate role in a health care system characterized by increasing use of technology with sometimes questionable benefits. In other words, the reflexive ambivalence produced by genetic counselors' social location positions them as crucial social actors who can and may "resist" some of the biomedicalizing trends in the geneticization of health and illness.

Notes

1. This knowledge gap is mostly likely in clinical specialties that only recently have been impacted by genetic medicine, but it is also likely to increasingly occur even in a specialty such as obstetrics in which providers have a lengthier history and more familiarity with providing genetic counseling to their patients about what are now "routine" prenatal screenings in pregnancy care in the USA (e.g. ultrasounds and blood screens, as well as the offer of invasive testing for women of "advanced maternal age").

2. It should also be noted that unlike other countries, the master's-trained genetic counselor in the USA is not a medical professional such as nurse or sonographer that is then trained to conduct genetic counseling. Additionally, also unlike other countries, in the USA genetic nurses (with both BA and MS backgrounds) constitute both a very small and separately certified group of genetic counseling practitioners (Lea et al. 2006; Skirton, Arimori, and Aoki 2006).

3. For the remainder of the paper, the term "genetic counselors" refers specifically to the master's trained genetic counselors that are the focus of this study.

4. *Gatiaca* is a 1997 Hollywood science fiction film that depicts a world where genetic traits are chosen for future children to make sure

they possess the best health and behavioral dispositions in the belief that this will assure their future success and well-being.

5. The official journal of the National Society of Genetic Counselors, *Journal of Genetic Counseling*, published a special issue on DTC genetic testing in June 2012, demonstrating the professions' concern about and interest in this topic.

6. Of note, when asked what drew them to the profession of genetic counseling the vast majority of study participants responded

that they were attracted to the field because it involved both science and clinical care with patients, two things in which they were interested and invested.

7. Of course, the rise of DTC companies can leave genetic counselors out of the process which is a reason so many of them seem to be concerned about DTCs. Additionally, since the reflexivity expressed in this study may be a product of the interview setting itself, further research should explore how genetic counselors navigate real life quandaries.

References

American Board of Genetic Counseling. 2013. "Bylaws/History." Accessed July 18, 2013. http://www.abgc.net/About_ABGC/ABGCBylaws.asp

Arribas-Ayllon, M., S. Sarangis, and A. Clarke. 2011. *Genetic Testing: Accounts of Autonomy, Responsibility and Blame*. London: Routledge.

Atkin, K., S. Ahmed, J. Hewison, and J. M. Green. 2008. "Decision-Making and Ante-Natal Screening for Sickle Cell and Thalassaemia Disorders." *Current Sociology* 56 (1): 77–98.

Bartels, D. M., B. S. LeRoy, P. McCarthy, and A. L. Caplan. 1997. "Nondirectiveness in Genetic Counseling: A Survey of Practitioners." *American Journal of Medical Genetics* 72 (2): 172–179.

Beeson, D. 1997. "Nuance, Complexity and Context: Qualitative Methods in Genetic Counseling Research." *Journal of Genetic Counseling* 6 (1): 21–43.

Bennett, R. L., H. L. Hampel, J. B. Mandell, and J. H. Marks. 2003. "Genetic Counselors: Translating Genomic Science into Clinical Practice." *The Journal of Clinical Investigation* 112 (9): 1274–1279.

Bosk, C. 1992. *All God's Mistakes: Genetic Counseling in a Pediatric Hospital*. Chicago, IL: University of Chicago Press.

Brock, S. 1995. "Narrative and Medical Genetics: On Ethics and Therapeutics." *Qualitative Health Research* 5 (2): 150–168.

Browner, C. H., and H. M. Preloran. 2010. *Neurogenetic Diagnoses: The Power of Hope, and the Limits of Today's Medicine*. New York: Routledge.

Browner, C. H., and N. Press. 1995. "The Normalization of Prenatal Diagnostic Testing." In *Conceiving the New World Order: The Global Politics of Reproduction*, edited by F. Ginsburg and R. Rapp, 307–322. Berkeley: University of California Press.

Brunger, F., and A. Lippman. 1995. "Resistance and Adherence to the Norms of Genetic Counseling." *Journal of Genetic Counseling* 4 (3): 151–167.

Bryant, A., and K. Charmaz, eds. 2010. *Sage Handbook of Grounded Theory*. Thousand Oaks, CA: Sage Publications.

Clarke, A. E., J. K. Shim, L. Mamo, J. R. Fosket, and J. R. Fishman. 2010. "Biomedicalization: A Theoretical and Substantive Introduction." In *Biomedicalization: Technoscience, Health, and Illness in the U.S.*, edited by A. E. Clarke, L. Mamo, J. R. Fosket, J. R. Fishman and J. K. Shim, 1–44. Durham, NC: Duke University Press.

Collins, F. 2010. "Has the Revolution Arrived?" *Nature* 464 (7289): 674–675.

Conrad, P. 1999. "A Mirage of Genes." *Sociology of Health & Illness* 21 (2): 228–241.

Conrad, P. 2007. *The Medicalization of Society: On the Transformation of Human Conditions into Treatable Disorders*. Baltimore, MD: Johns Hopkins University Press.

Conrad, P., and S. Markens. 2001. "Constructing the 'Gay Gene' in the News: Optimism and Skepticism in the American and British Press." *Health: An Interdisciplinary Journal for the Social Study of Health, Illness and Medicine* 5 (3): 359–386.

Duster, T. 1990. *Backdoor to Eugenics*. New York: Routledge.

Ettorre, E. 1999. "Experts as 'Storytellers' in Reproductive Genetics: Exploring Key Issues." *Sociology of Health & Illness* 21 (5): 539–549.

Featherstone, K., P, Atkinson, A. Bhardawah, and A. Clarke. 2006. *Risky Relations: Family, Kinship and the New Genetics*. New York: Berg Publishers.

Garcia, E., D. R. M. Timmermans, and E. van Leeuwcn. 2008. "The Impact of Ethical Beliefs on Decisions about Prenatal Screening Tests: Searching for Justification." *Social Science & Medicine* 66 (3): 753–64.

Glaser, B. G., and A. Strauss. 1967. *The Discovery of Grounded Theory*. Chicago, IL: Aldine.

Grubs, R. E., and M. Piantanida. 2010. "Grounded Theory in Genetic Counseling Research: An Interpretive Perspective." *Journal of Genetic Counseling* 19 (2): 99–111.

Hallowell, N. 1999. "Doing the Right Thing: Genetic Risk and Responsibility." *Sociology of Health & Illness* 21 (5): 597–621.

Hamburg, M. A., and F. S. Collins. 2010. "The Path to Personalized Medicine." *New England Journal of Medicine* 363 (4): 301–304.

Hashiloni-Dolev, Y. 2006. "Genetic Counseling for Sex Chromosome Anomalies (SCA) in Israel and Germany: Assessing Medical Risks According to the Importance of Fertility in Two Cultures." *Medical Anthropology Quarterly* 20 (4): 469–486.

Hashiloni-Dolev, Y., and A. E. Raz. 2010. "Between Social Hypocrisy and Social Responsibility: Professional Views of Eugenics, Disability and Repro-Genetics in Germany and Israel." *New Genetics and Society 29* (1): 87–102.

Heimler, A. 1997. "An Oral History of the National Society of Genetic Counselors." *Journal of Genetic Counseling* 6 (3): 315–336.

Jallinoja, P., and A. R. Aro. 2000. "Does Knowledge Make a Difference? The Association Between Knowledge About Genes and Attitudes Towards Genetic Tests." *Journal of Health Communication* 5 (1): 29–39.

Karlberg, K. 2000. "The Work of Genetic Care Providers: Managing Uncertainty and Ambiguity," *Research in the Sociology of Health Care* 17: 81–97.

Keenan, R. 1997. "Opportunities and Impediments for a Consolidating and Expanding Profession: Genetic Counseling in the United States." *Social Science & Medicine* 45 (9): 1377–1386.

Kelly, S. E. 2009. "Choosing Not to Choose: Reproductive Responses of Parents of Children with Genetic Conditions or Impairments." *Sociology of Health & Illness* 31 (1): 91–97.

Kerr, A., S. Cunningham-Burley, and A. Amos. 1997. "The New Genetics: Professionals'

Discursive Boundaries." *The Sociological Review* 45 (2): 279–303.

Kerr, A., S. Cunningham-Burley, and R. Tutton. 2007. "Exploring Ambivalence About Genetic Research and Its Social Context." *Social Theory & Health* 5 (1): 53–69.

Kolker, A., and B. M. Burke. 1994. *Prenatal Testing: A Sociological Perspective.* Westport, CT: Bergin & Garver.

Korf, B. R., M. Irons, and M. S. Watson. 2011. "Competencies for the Physician Medical Geneticist in the 21st Century." *Genetics in Medicine* 13 (11): 911–12.

Kuppermann, M., L. A. Learman, E. Gates, S. E. Gregorich, R. F. Nease, J. Lewis, and A. E. Washington. 2006. "Beyond Race or Ethnicity and Socioeconomic Status: Predictors of Prenatal Testing for Down Syndrome." *Obstetrics & Gynecology* 107 (5): 1087–1097.

Lea, D. H., J. K. Williams, J. A. Cooksey, P. A. Flanagan, G. Forte, and M. G. Blitzer. 2006. "US Genetic Nurses in Advanced Practice." *Journal of Nursing Scholarship* 38 (3): 213–218.

Lewontin, R. C. 1993. *Biology as Ideology: The Doctrine of DNA.* New York: Harper Perennial.

Lippman, A. 1991. "Prenatal Genetic Testing and Screening: Constructing Needs and Reinforcing Inequities." *American Journal of Law and Medicine* 17: 15–50.

Markens, S. 2013. "'Is this Something you Want?': Genetic Counselors' Accounts of Their Role in Prenatal Decision-Making." *Sociological Forum* 28 (3): 431–451.

Markens, S., C. H. Browner, and H. M. Preloran. 2010. "Interrogating the Dynamics Between Power, Knowledge and Pregnant Bodies in Amniocentesis Decision-Making." *Sociology' of Health & Illness* 32 (1): 37–56.

Markens, S., C. H. Browner, and N. Press. 1999. "'Because of the Risks': How US Pregnant Women

Account for Refusing Prenatal Screening." *Social Science & Medicine* 49 (3): 359–469.

Markoff, J. 2012. "Breaking a Gene Barrier." *New York Times*, March 8, B1.

McAllister, M., A. M. Wood, G. Dunn, S. Shiloh, and C. Todd. 2011. "The Genetic Counseling Outcome Scale: A New Patient-Reported Outcome Measure for Clinical Genetics Services." *Clinical Genetics* 79 (5): 413–424.

Michie, S., A. Allanson, D. Armstrong, J. Weinman, M. Bobrow, and T. M. Marteau. 1998. "Objectives of Genetic Counselling: Differing Views of Purchasers, Providers and Users." *Journal of Public Health Medicine* 20 (4): 404–408.

Michie, S., H. Drake, T. Marteau, and M. Bobrow. 1995. "A Comparison of Public and Professionals' Attitudes Towards Genetic Developments." *Public Understanding of Science* 4 (3): 243–253.

Morren, M., M. Rijken, A. N. Baanders, and J. Bensing. 2007. "Perceived Genetic Knowledge, Attitudes Towards Genetic Testing, and the Relationship Between These Among Patients with Chronic Diseases." *Patient Education and Counseling* 65 (2); 197–204.

National Society of Genetic Counselors. 2012. *2012 Professional Status Survey: Professional Satisfaction.* May 1.

Nelkin, D., and M. S. Lindee. 2004. *The DNA Mystique: The Gene as a Cultural Icon.* Ann Arbor: University of Michigan Press.

Petersen, A. 2006. "The Genetic Conception of Health: Is it as Radical as Claimed?" *Health: An Interdisciplinary Journal for the Social Study of Health, Illness and Medicine* 10 (4): 481–500.

Pilnick, A, 2002a. "'There are "No Rights and Wrongs in the Situations': Identifying Interactional Difficulties in Genetic Counseling." *Sociology of Health & Illness* 24 (1): 66–88.

Pilnick, A. 2002b. "What 'Most People' Do: Exploring the Ethical Implications of Genetic Counselling." *New Genetics and Society* 21 (3): 339–350.

Pilnick, A. 2008. "'It's Something for you Both to Think About': Choice and Decision Making in Nuchal Translucency Screening for Down's Syndrome." *Sociology of Health & Illness* 30 (4): 511–530.

Pirzadeh, S. M., P. M. Veach, D. M. Barrels, J. Kao, and B. S. LeRoy. 2007. "A National Survey of Genetic Counselors' Personal Values." *Journal of Genetic Counseling* 16 (6): 763–773.

Pollack, A. 2008, "Patients DNA may be Signal to Tailor Drugs." *New York Times*, December 20, A1.

Pollack, A. 2012. "The Ethics of Advice." *New York Times*, July 14, B1.

Press, N., and C. H. Browner. 1997. "Why Women say Yes to Prenatal Screening." *Social Science & Medicine* 45 (7): 979–989.

Rabino, I. 2006. "Research Scientists Surveyed on Ethical Issues in Genetic Medicine: A Comparison of Attitudes of US and European Researchers." *New Genetics and Society* 25 (3): 325–342.

Rapp, R. 1999. *Testing the Woman, Testing the Fetus*, New York: Routledge.

Remennick, L. 2006. "The Quest for the Perfect Baby: Why do Israeli Women Seek Prenatal Genetic Testing?" *Sociology of Health & Illness* 28 (1): 21–53.

Resta, R, 2006. "Defining and Redefining the Scope and Goals of Genetic Counseling." *American Journal of Medical Genetics* 142C (4): 269–275.

Roberts, D. 2009. "Race, Gender, and Genetic Technologies: A New Reproductive Dystopia?" *Signs: Journal of Women in Culture and Society* 34 (4): 783–804.

Rose, N. 2006. *The Politics of Life Itself Biomedicine, Power, and Subjectivity in the Twenty-First Century*. Princeton, NJ: Princeton University Press.

Rothman, B. K. 1986. *The Tentative Pregnancy: Prenatal Diagnosis and the Future of Motherhood*. New York: Viking Penguin.

Sagi, M., and W. R. Uhlmann. 2013. "Genetic Counseling Services and Training of Genetic Counselors in Israel: An Overview." *Journal of Genetic Counseling*, Published Online 24 February. Accessed March 8, 2013. http://link.springer.com/article/10.1007/s10897-013-9576-4

Sahhar, M. A., M. A. Young, L. J. Sheffield, and M. A. Aitken. 2005. "Educating Genetic Counselors in Australia: Developing an International Perspective." *Journal of Genetic Counseling* 14 (4): 283–93.

Samerski, S. 2006. "The Unleashing of Genetic Terminology: How Genetic Counseling Mobilizes for Risk Management." *New Genetics and Society* 25 (2): 97–208.

Samerski, S. 2009, "Genetic Counseling and the Fiction of Choice: Taught Self-Determination as a New Technique of Social Engineering." *Signs: Journal of Women in Culture and Society* 34 (4): 735–761.

Schwennesen, N., and L. Koch. 2012. "Representing and Intervening: 'Doing' Good Care in First Trimester." *Sociology of Health & Illness* 34 (2): 283–298.

Shakespeare, T. 1995. "Back to the Future? New Genetics and Disabled People." *Critical Social Policy* 15 (44–45): 22–35.

Shostak, S., D. Zarhin, and R. Ottman. 2011. "What's at Stake? Genetic Information from the Perspective of People with Epilepsy and their Family Members." *Social Science & Medicine* 73 (5): 645–654.

Singer, E., M. P. Couper, T. E. Raghunathan, J. Van Hoewyk, and T. C. Antonucci. 2008. "Trends in U.S. Attitudes Toward Genetic Testing, 1990–2004." *Public Opinion Quarterly* 72 (3): 446–458.

Skirton, H., N. Arimori, and M. Aoki. 2006. "A Historical Comparison of the Development of Specialist Genetic Nursing in the United Kingdom and Japan." *Nursing and Health Sciences* 8 (4): 231–236.

Skirton, H., L. Kerzin-Storrar, C. Barnes, G. Hall, M. Longmuir, C. Patch, G. Scott, and J. Walford-Moore. 2013. "Building the Genetic Counsellor Profession in the United Kingdom: Two Decades of Growth and Development." *Journal of Genetic Counseling*, Published Online 22 January. Accessed March 8, 2013. http://link.springer.com/article/10.1007/sl0897-012-9560-4#page-1

Stern, A. M. 2009. "A Quiet Revolution: The Birth of the Genetic Counselor at Sarah Lawrence College, 1969." *Journal of Genetic Counseling* 18 (1): 1–11.

Stern, A. M. 2012. *Telling Genes: The Story of Genetic Counseling in America.* Baltimore, MD: Johns Hopkins University Press.

Taylor, S. D. 2004. "Predictive Genetic Test Decisions for Huntington's Disease: Context, Appraisal, and New Moral Imperatives." *Social Science & Medicine* 58 (1): 137–149.

Thomas, J. C., D. E. Irwin, E. S. Zuiker, and R. C. Millikan. 2005. "Genomics and the Public Health Code of Ethics." *American Journal of Public Health* 95 (12): 2139–2143.

Timmermans, S., and M. Buchbinder. 2010. "Patients-in-Waiting." *Journal of Health and Social Behavior* 51 (4): 408–423.

Toiviainen, H., P. Jallinoja, A. R. Aro, and E. Hemminki. 2003. "Medical and Lay Attitudes Towards Genetic Screening and Testing in Finland." *European Journal of Human Genetics* 11 (8): 565–572.

Weil, J., K, Ormand, J. Peters, K. Peters, B. B. Biesecker, and B. LeRoy. 2006. "The Relationship of Nondirectiveness to Genetic Counseling: Report of a Workshop at the 2003 NSGC Annual Education Conference." *Journal of Genetic Counseling* 15 (2): 89–93.

Wertz, D. C., and J. C. Fletcher. 1988a. "Attitudes of Genetic Counselors: A Multinational Survey." *American Journal of Human Genetics* 42 (4): 592–600.

Wertz, D. C. and J. C. Fletcher. 1988b. "Ethics and Medical Genetics in the United States: A National Survey." *American Journal of Medical Genetics* 29 (4): 815–27.

Wertz, D. C., and J. C. Fletcher. 1989. "Moral Reasoning among Medical Geneticists in Eighteen Nations." *Theoretical Medicine* 10 (2): 123–38.

Wicklund, C. 2008. "Genetics Education Pipeline and Workforce." July 28. Accessed March 6, 2013. http://www.iom.edu/~/media/Files/Activity%20Files/Research/GenomicBasedResearch/Wicklund.pdf

Williams, C., P. Alderson, and B. Farsides. 2002a. "Is Nondirectiveness Possible within the Context of Antenatal Screening and Testing?" *Social Science & Medicine* 54 (3): 339–347.

Williams, C., P Alderson, and B. Farsides. 2002b. "Too Many Choices? Hospitals and Community Staff Reflect on the Future of Prenatal Testing." *Social Science & Medicine* 55 (5): 743–53.

CONTEMPORARY CRITICAL DEBATES

Up until this point, we have presented our analysis of health and medical care as if all critical analysts were more or less in agreement. But in health care, as in any social and intellectual enterprise, controversies rage over the sources of problems and over appropriate solutions. In Part 3, we present two central controversies on the relevance of risk and the medicalization of American society.

THE RELEVANCE OF RISK

For most of modern history, medicine has been concerned with the causes and treatment of *diseases*. In recent years, medicine has become much more concerned with the reduction and prevention of *risks*. The forefront of public health medicine and research in the United States attempts to identify *risk factors* associated with various diseases.

Risk factors are usually statistically based associations derived from epidemiological research. As mentioned in an earlier section, epidemiology is "the study of the distributions and determinants of states of health in human populations" (Susser 1973, 3). Risk is derived from a multidimensional assessment of factors and related to the probability of an event or illness occurring. For example, researchers have found a strong association between cigarette smoking and rates of lung cancer and heart disease; thus, we can say cigarette smoking is a risk factor for cancer and heart disease. In a different arena, obesity increases the risk for diabetes. To take another kind of example, women with the BRCA1 or BRCA2 genetic mutation are at higher risk for the development of breast cancer.

There are several types of health risks: biological, environmental, and behavioral. Biological risks reside in the body, such as genes or genetic markers that have been shown to be associated with particular diseases. Environmental risks stem from environmental conditions that research has found to be related to disease, such as pollutants increasing the risk for asthma (see "The Health Politics of Asthma: Environmental Justice and Collective Illness Experience in the United States," Chapter 9). Behavioral risks are essentially lifestyle factors that have been shown to be associated with an increased incidence of particular diseases: cigarette smoking, alcoholism, obesity, sedentariness, not using seat belts, and so forth. A major distinction among risks is whether or not they are modifiable. For example, with heart disease, risks present in family history (have there been heart attacks under age 50 in your family?) or genetic structure are not modifiable. On the other hand, risks like smoking, stress,

hypertension, high cholesterol, and lack of exercise are all modifiable and can be targeted as risk factors that can be changed to reduce the likelihood of heart disease. Public health has traditionally focused on changing modifiable risks as a major initiative toward disease prevention and health promotion.

The news media reports new findings about health risks regularly, but these reports can be confusing or even contradictory. One year we read that butter is bad for us (too much cholesterol and fat) and margarine is healthier; another year we read that margarine is bad for us (it has trans fat and too many artificial additives) and butter is less unhealthy. Alcohol overuse is a health risk, but a glass or two of red wine a day may reduce the risk of heart disease. There are many more such examples about how the air we breathe, food we eat, sex we enjoy, transportation we use, and land we live on all contain health risks. One might even conclude that living is a risk to our health.

While one could debate about the validity of each putative risk factor, or about how ubiquitous risk is in modern society (Beck 1992), these are not the issues at hand here. This debate is more concerned about the meaning and the relevance of risk in medical discourse and intervention. The first selection in Part 3 critiques the contemporary framing of risk and responsibility. Deborah Lupton, in "Risk as Moral Danger: The Social and Political Functions of Risk Discourse in Public Health," raises questions about the whole risk-factor approach to public health. She suggests that risk is not a simple measure but is a complex sociocultural concept that often is used in a rhetorical way in public health discourses. Lupton sees the concept of "risk" as ideologically loaded; in the health discourse, it only has negative meanings and suggests danger. She is particularly critical about the uses of "lifestyle risk," where risk is moralized (it is often seen as the fault of the person at risk) and there is a certain amount of "victim blaming." The notion of identifying a risk suggests that an individual should do something to modify it. The question becomes who has the power to define risk? How do we know a risk when we see it? Who is deemed at risk? Who is seen as responsible for creating the risk? Who is encouraged or required to do what about the risk, and under what circumstances? Lupton makes it clear that *risk* is not a neutral term in health and its use has political implications. While scientists have been good at showing us our health risks, they have been less clear about the social meaning of these risks. We should seek modification of health risks that make sense, but be sensitive to the anxiety, guilt, and blame that the risk discourse can produce and the ways in which social, physical, and policy environments constrain the ability of individuals to change their behaviors.

Our second selection, "The Pursuit of Preventive Care for Chronic Illness: Turning Healthy People

Into Chronic Patients" by Meta J. Kreiner and Linda M. Hunt, highlights how risk reduction is embedded in preventative medicine. Evidence-based clinical guidelines are based on rigid test thresholds that are based on population norms. These norms are then applied to individuals, and one result is that at-risk states are equated with illness and medical interventions framed as "treatment" rather than prevention. Risk and disease are conflated, and aggressive treatments are used to reduce the risk of anticipated future health problems. The authors question the degree to which population-based health thresholds actually benefit individual patients, and call attention to the potential for adverse events associated with treatments for anticipated conditions that have not yet occurred.

References

Beck, Ulrich. 1992. *Risk Society.* London: Sage.

Susser, Mervyn. 1973. *Causal Thinking in the Health Sciences: Concepts and Strategies in Epidemiology.* New York: Oxford University Press.

34

RISK AS MORAL DANGER

The Social and Political Functions of Risk Discourse in Public Health

Deborah Lupton

We live in a society that has become more and more aware of risks, especially those caused by technology and "lifestyle" habits. According to Douglas and Wildavsky, modern individuals are afraid of "Nothing much . . . except the food they eat, the water they drink, the air they breathe, the land they live on, and the energy they use" (1, p. 10). Health risks seem to loom around every corner, posing a constant threat to the public (2). They constantly make headlines in the news media and are increasingly the subject of public communication campaigns. Risk assessment and risk communication have become growth industries. In short, the word "risk" itself has acquired a new prominence in Western society, becoming a central cultural construct (3, p. 2).

Risk is a concept with different meanings, according to who is using the term. The proliferation of usages of the term in both vernacular and professional applications means that its meanings are both complex and confusing. In its original usage, "risk" is neutral, referring to probability, or the mathematical likelihood of an event occurring. The risk of an event occurring could therefore relate to either a positive or negative outcome, as in the risk of winning the lottery. Used in the more mathematical areas of the growing field of risk analysis, this strict sense of the term is adhered to. Thus, risk analysts speak of the statistical likelihood that an event may occur, and use the mathematical model produced to assist in decision-making in such areas as economics and management. The risk, or likelihood, of an event happening can be calculated to numerical odds—one in fifty chance, one in a hundred, one in a million—as can the magnitude of the outcome should it happen (4, 5).

Risk as Moral Danger: The Social and Political Functions of Risk, Deborah Lupton in *International Journal of Health Services, 23*(3), 425–435, 1993. Baywood Publishing Company, Inc. Reprinted with permission from SAGE Publications, Inc.

Most industries devoted to the quantification of risk place a great deal of importance in measuring risk assessment, risk perception, and risk evaluation on the part of individuals in the general population. In the past two decades the field of risk assessment of technologies has grown in prominence in concert with the interest of the public in environmental hazards. Risk assessment applied in this field deals with the complex process of evaluating the hazards of technologies, as well as the communication of information about potential risks and developing appropriate controls (5–8). Risk in this content has been defined as "the probability that a potential harm or undesirable consequence will be realized" (8, p. 321).

This definition points to the new meaning of risk. As Douglas (3) has suggested, the word "risk" has changed its meaning in contemporary Western society. No longer a neutral term, risk has come to mean danger; and "high risk means a lot of danger" (3, p. 3). Any risk is now negative; it is a contradiction in terms to speak of something as a "good risk." According to Douglas, the use of "risk" to mean danger is preferred in professional circles because "plain danger does not have the aura of science or afford the pretension of a possible precise calculation" (3, p. 4).

In public health the word "risk" as a synonym for danger is in constant use. A "discourse of risk" has evolved with particular application to health issues. Individuals or groups are labeled as being "at high risk," meaning that they are in danger of contracting or developing a disease or illness. Epidemiologists calculate measures of "relative risk" to compare the likelihood of illness developing in populations exposed to a "risk factor" with the likelihood for populations that have not been thus exposed. State-sponsored health education campaigns in the mass media are conducted to warn the public about health risks, based on the assumption that knowledge and awareness of the danger of certain activities will result in avoidance of these activities.

Risk discourse in public health can be separated loosely into two perspectives. The first views risk as a health danger to populations that is posed by environmental hazards such as pollution, nuclear waste, and toxic chemical residues. In this conceptualization

of risk, the health threat is regarded as a hazard that is external, over which the individual has little control. The common response to such risks on the part of the layperson is anger at government authorities, feelings of powerlessness and anxiety, and concern over the seemingly deliberate and unregulated contamination of the environment by industry (9, 10). Risk communication on the part of those in authority is then cynically directed toward defusing community reaction, building trust and credibility for the "risk creator," the "risk regulator," and the "risk analyst," and facilitating "risk acceptance" on the part of the public (11).

Methodologies used to assess health risk perception and acceptance on the part of the layperson are deemed to be objective, systematic, and scientific, able to discern "rational" means to make decisions about health hazards. The layperson's assessment of risk is viewed as a cognitive process that can be measured in the laboratory, divorced from social context. Psychologists in the field of decision analysis employ laboratory experiments, gaming situations, and survey techniques to understand risk perception, attempting to arrive at a quantitative determination of risk acceptance. Individuals are given the names of technologies, activities, or substances and asked to consider the risks each one presents and to rate them (12–14).

The second approach to health risk focuses upon risk as a consequence of the "lifestyle" choices made by individuals, and thus places the emphasis upon self-control. Individuals are exhorted by health promotion authorities to evaluate their risk of succumbing to disease and to change their behavior accordingly. Risk assessment related to lifestyle choices is formally undertaken by means of health risk appraisals and screening programs in which the individual participates and is given a rating. Such health risk appraisals (also termed health risk assessment or health hazard appraisal) are used to counsel individuals about prospective threats to their health that are associated with behaviors deemed to be modifiable. The object is to promote awareness of potential dangers courted by lifestyle choices, and then to motivate individuals to participate in health promotion and health education programs (15, 16).

Research into the layperson's acceptance of personal lifestyle risk again tends to use quantitative methods, usually based upon pen-and-paper questionnaires that incorporate questions such as "How much at risk (from the illness or disease in question) do you think you are personally?", with available responses ranging from "At great risk" to "Not at all at risk." Most questionnaires use only close-ended and pre-categorized items that provide very little opportunity for respondents to give unprompted opinions and to expand upon their answers. These kinds of research methods into risk perception fail to take into account respondents' belief systems relating to causes of disease and health behaviors. Too narrow a range of explanatory variables results in many research studies failing to expose the impact of differing cultural factors upon behavior (17, 18).

As a consequence, the literature on risk acceptance and risk perception in the health domain tends not to account for the influence of the sociocultural contexts within which risk perception takes place and the political uses to which risk discourse is put. Despite the wealth of literature on risk perception, analysis, and assessment, and the extremely common use of the concept of "risk" in public health literature, little critical examination of the meaning and rhetorical use of risk discourse has taken place by scholars within these fields.

In recent years a small number of qualitative sociologists, anthropologists, and philosophers have focused their attention upon other aspects of risk, viewing risk not as a neutral and easily measurable concept, but as a sociocultural concept laden with meaning. The remainder of this article explores this dimension of risk discourse, which has been largely ignored in the public health and risk analysis literature.

EXTERNAL RISK RHETORIC

Interpretive analyses of the meanings of risk discourse in public health argue that there is more to risk than the disclosure of technical information and the mathematical determination of probabilities,

and more to the individual's perception of risk than the assimilation and rational weighing up of impartial technical information (1; 3; 7, p. 96; 19; 20). For example, Douglas and Wildavsky (1) contend with respect to external threats that the selection of risks deemed to be hazardous to a population is a social process: the risks that are selected may have no relation to real danger but are culturally identified as important. People's fears about risks can be regarded as ways of maintaining social solidarity rather than as reflecting health or environmental concerns.

Nelkin argues that "definitions of risk are an expression of the tensions inherent in given social and cultural contexts, and that these tensions frequently come to focus on the issue of communication" (7, p. 96). Definitions of risk may serve to identify Self and the Other, to apportion blame upon stigmatized minorities, or as a political weapon. Risk therefore may have less to do with the nature of danger than the ideological purposes to which concerns about risk may be put (7). In history the scapegoating of ethnic minorities when an epidemic such as smallpox or the plague broke out is an example of how the concept of risk has been used for political purposes in public health discourse (21).

The notion of external risk thus serves to categorize individuals or groups into "those at risk" and "those posing a risk." Risk, in modern society, has come to replace the old-fashioned (and in modern secular society, now largely discredited) notion of sin, as a term that "runs across the gamut of social life to moralize and politicise dangers" (3, p. 4). Although risk is a much more "sanitized" concept, it signifies the same meanings, for, as Douglas comments, "the neutral vocabulary of risk is all we have for making a bridge between the known facts of existence and the construction of a moral community" (3, p. 5).

Douglas believes that "being at risk" is the reciprocal of sinning, for the emphasis is placed upon the danger of external forces upon the individual, rather than the dangers afforded the community by the individual: "To be 'at risk' is equivalent to being sinned against, being vulnerable to the events caused by others, whereas being 'in sin' means being the cause of harm" (3, p. 7). Her analysis of the concept of risk is closely tied to the term as it is used in politics, especially with reference to the risks placed by environmental hazards upon individuals who have little personal power to deal with them.

Douglas's distinction, however, while enlightening, is accurate only when applied to risk that is believed to be externally imposed. The theory is less apt when viewed in the light of health risks considered to be the responsibility of the individual to control. When risk is believed to be internally imposed because of lack of willpower, moral weakness, venality, or laziness on the part of the individual, the symbolic relationship of sin and risk is reversed. Those who are deemed "at risk" become the sinners, not the sinned against, because of their apparent voluntary courting of risk. The next section addresses the moral meanings ascribed to health risks deemed to be "voluntary."

HEALTH EDUCATION AND LIFESTYLE RISK DISCOURSE

Ironically, there has been an increasing emphasis upon apprising individuals of their own responsibility for engaging in risky behaviors at the same time as the control of individuals over the risks in their working and living environments has diminished. An important use of risk discourse in the public health arena is that employed in health education, which seeks to create public awareness of the health risks posed by "lifestyle" choices made by the individual.

Cultural theorists interested in risk as a sociocultural phenomenon have tended to focus their speculations upon the moral meanings and political function of external risk. However, I would argue that greater attention needs to be paid to the implicit meanings and functions of lifestyle risk discourse. Just as a moral distinction is drawn between "those at risk" and "those posing a risk," health education routinely draws a distinction between the harm caused by external causes out of the individual's control and that caused by oneself. Lifestyle risk discourse overturns the notion that health hazards

in postindustrial society are out of the individual's control. On the contrary, the dominant theme of lifestyle risk discourse is the responsibility of the individual to avoid health risks for the sake of his or her own health as well as the greater good of society. According to this discourse, if individuals choose to ignore health risks they are placing themselves in danger of illness, disability, and disease, which removes them from a useful role in society and incurs costs upon the public purse. Should individuals directly expose others to harm for example, by smoking in a public place, driving while drunk, or spreading an infectious disease there is even greater potential for placing the community at risk.

Why has lifestyle risk discourse gained such cultural resonance in late-capitalist society? There are historico-cultural roots to this discourse. Rosenberg links the public health discourse of risk with the ancient and powerful "desire to explain sickness and death in terms of volition of acts done or left undone" (22, p. 50). He suggests that the decrease in incidence of acute infectious disease in contemporary Western society has led to an increasing obsession with regimen, and the control of individuals' diet and exercise, to reduce real or sensed risks, to "redefine the mortal odds that face them" (22, p. 50). The other side of the coin, according to Rosenberg, is a tendency to explain the vulnerability of others to disease and illness in terms of their own acts or lifestyle choices; for example, overeating, alcoholism, or sexual promiscuity.

The modern concept of risk, like that of taboo, has a "forensic" property, for it works backwards in explaining ill-fortune, as well as forwards in predicting future retribution (3). Thus the experience of a heart attack, a positive HIV test result, or the discovery of a cancerous lesion are evidence that the ill person has failed to comply with directives to reduce health risks and therefore is to be blamed for his or her predicament (23–28). As Marantz has commented of health education: "Many within the profession now think that anyone who has a [heart attack] must have lived the life of gluttony and sloth. . . . We seem to view raising a cheeseburger to one's lips as the moral equivalent of holding a gun to one's head" (26, p. 1186).

The current irrational discrimination, fear, and prejudice leveled against people with AIDS is a prime example of the way in which being "at risk" becomes the equivalent of sinning. Research undertaken by the anthropologist McCombie (29) illustrates the moral meanings attributed to the state of being "at risk" in the context of AIDS. She studied the counseling given by health workers to individuals deemed either "high risk" or "low risk" after a test for HIV antibodies had been performed. McCombie noticed that high-risk individuals, whether HIV positive or negative, were treated differently from low-risk individuals: "the high risk person is chastised, admonished and warned, while the low risk person is consoled and reassured" (29, p. 455). She evaluated this behavior in the context of taboo violation, pollution, and punishment for sin. High-risk individuals were being punished for their deviant behavior and were held responsible for their own behavior if HIV positive. By contrast, individuals deemed at low risk were looked upon more as innocent victims. The blood test itself was a ritual, acting an anxiety-reducing measure for those who were concerned that the virus was getting out of control as well as implicitly acting as a tool for detecting social deviance (29).

DEFINING RISK AND THOSE "AT RISK": THE POLITICAL FUNCTION OF RISK DISCOURSE

The rhetoric of risk serves different functions, depending on how personally controllable the danger is perceived as being. Douglas has pointed out that "blaming the victim is a strategy that works in one kind of context, and blaming the outside enemy, a strategy that works in another" (30, p. 59). She believes that both types of attributions of risk serve to maintain the cohesiveness of a society; the first in protecting internal social control, and the second in bolstering loyalty.

The categorization of which risks are deemed to be external and which internal influences the moral judgments made about blame and responsibility for placing health in jeopardy. It is important to consider which institutions have the power to define these categories of risk. Sapolsky (31) suggests that the political system of industrialized countries is responsible for the current obsession with risk. Because members of the general public do not have access to sufficient information to assess environmental risks, they must rely upon intermediaries such as scientists, government officials, environmental campaigners, and the news media to inform them. These intermediaries have their own agenda, and therefore tend to exaggerate and distort the "facts" to further their own cause, making it difficult for the layperson to conceptualize risk in the face of conflicting perspectives (31, p. 90).

The news media, for example, have an integral role in disseminating information about health risks. The news media can have an important influence on shaping public policy and setting the agenda for the public discussion of risks. They are interested in attracting a large audience or readership, and tend to over-dramatize and simplify information about health risks accordingly. If they are relying upon the news media for information and advice, members of the lay audience can be left feeling panicked and confused (32–34). Politicians must react to new risks in a concerned manner, to avoid the backlash of seeming apathy in the face of a new health scare and to bolster their position: "careers are as much at risk in risk controversies as is the public's health" (31, p. 94). They have the power to gain the attention of the news media, and their opinions are therefore privileged over those of the ordinary person.

Personal health risk appraisals have been shown to have serious limitations in their predictive capabilities. These limitations include their use of epidemiological data produced from population research not designed to be applied to personal health risk, and problems with the available statistical methods for estimating risk as a quantitative score using disparate items of measurement (15, 16). Despite these problems, little research has been undertaken into the practical and ethical consequences of such risk appraisals, including their capacity to arouse anxiety in the well and their appropriate use in patient counseling. Some critics have expressed concern that by instituting such programs as health risk appraisals, drug and other screening, and fitness assessments into the workplace, large corporations are able to maintain control over the worker even when she or he is not at the workplace. Programs such as drug screening may be used as tools to identify the "desirable" employees; in other words, those whose lifestyles are deemed acceptable. They also enable employers to determine what workers are doing in their spare time, casting the net of corporate control ever wider (2, 35, 36).

The use of public information campaigns on the part of governments has increased in recent years. According to Wikler (37) there is danger in allowing governments the power to publicize health risks. Knowledge and risk factors may be misinterpreted; interventions may be ineffective or counterproductive. Health education can be coercive when it gives only one side of the argument, and if it attempts to persuade rather than simply give information to aid rational decision-making. Health education campaigns, in their efforts to persuade, have the potential to manipulate information deceptively and to psychologically manipulate by appealing to people's emotions, fears, anxieties, and guilt feelings (38).

Risk definitions may therefore be considered hegemonic conceptual tools that can serve to maintain the power structure of society. The voice of Everyman and Everywoman is rarely accorded equal hearing with that of big business and politicians. The two latter are in a position both to define health risks and to identify their solutions.

People working in the field of health risk communication tend to hold naive views about the ethics and point of such messages. Analysis of the moral and ethical implications of risk communication tends to implicitly accept that public communication of risk is desirable in most circumstances, with no further need to evaluate the ethical implications other than those posed by the involvement of journalists and public relations firms. Public knowledge, or "general edification," as bestowed by the state, is privileged as being in the public's "best interest" (39). The endeavor of risk communication sponsored by the state itself is rarely questioned in the risk communication literature as a political practice that can serve to maintain the interests of the powerful.

More insightful critics have argued that the use of the term "risk" is rarely neutral or devoid of political implications or moral questions. Risk communication, whether it is made by government, industry, or other bodies, can readily be regarded as a "'top-down' justification exercise in which experts attempt to educate an apparently misguided public into the real world of probability and hazard" (11, p. 514).

Government-sponsored arguments for public health education campaigns that employ lifestyle risk discourse include: (*a*) a basic responsibility to protect and promote the nation's health; (*b*) providing resources through collective action to help individuals improve their health; (*c*) containing costs; and (*d*) preventing individuals from harming others through their lifestyle choices (38, pp. 33–34). However, the arguments against government health education campaigns are also compelling. Should the minority be forced to bow to the wishes of the majority? Do health education campaigns constitute paternalism, by telling individuals what they should do with their lifestyle choices and reducing personal autonomy? Moral arguments can be brought to bear against the harm to others and cost-containment justifications (37). Implicated in these arguments is the use of health education campaigns as a cynical means of acting in response to a health problem while perpetuating the structural status quo that helps maintain the problem.

Foucault has remarked that "Every educational system is a political means of maintaining or modifying the appropriation of discourse with the knowledge and powers it carries with it" (40, p. 227). Health education emphasizing risks is a form of pedagogy, which, like other forms, serves to legitimize ideologies and social practices. Risk discourse in the public health sphere allows the state, as the owner of knowledge, to exert power over the bodies of its citizens. Risk discourse, therefore, especially when it emphasizes lifestyle risks, serves as an effective Foucaldian agent of surveillance and control that is difficult to challenge because of its manifest benevolent goal of maintaining standards of health. In doing so, it draws attention away from the structural causes of ill-health.

CONCLUSION

There are ethical questions in the use of risk discourse in public health that have been little questioned. Public health rhetoric has often posited that all individuals should have the right to information about risks. The implication of this assertion is that all individuals should have the right to be warned of the dangers of their behavior. What is left out of this equation is the corollary: that all individuals should have the right *not* to be continually informed of the risks they might be taking when engaging in certain actions, or that they should have the right not to act upon warnings if so preferred. The discourse of risk ostensibly gives people a choice, but the rhetoric in which the choice is couched leaves no room for maneuver. The public is given the statistics of danger, but not the safety margins. The discourse of risk is weighted toward disaster and anxiety rather than peace of mind. Rather than inform the public, for example, that the probability of not contracting HIV in a single sexual encounter is 999 out of 1000, the focus is placed upon the one in 1000 probability that infection will occur.

This emphasis upon a negative outcome, the inducement of anxiety and guilt in those who have received the message about the risks but do not change their behavior, might be said to be unethical. People tend to avoid anxiety by believing that they will not be the victims of a negative outcome. Is the constant assault upon the public's need to feel personally invulnerable ethical? Should employers be allowed to demand health risk appraisals in the name of ameliorating employees' health prospects? Should the discourse of risk give way to more positive statements? Are there ways to induce behavioral change amongst those really at risk other than inciting anxiety?

Risk discourse as it is currently used in public health draws upon the *fin de millennium* mood of the late 20th century, which targets the body as a site of toxicity, contamination, and catastrophe, subject to and needful of a high degree of surveillance and control (41). No longer is the body a temple to be worshipped as the house of God: it has become a commodified and regulated object that must be strictly monitored by its owner to prevent lapses into health-threatening behaviors as identified by risk discourse. For those with the socioeconomic resources to indulge in risk modification, this discourse may supply the advantages of a new religion; for others, risk discourse has the potential to create anxiety and guilt, to promote hopelessness and fear of the future.

There needs to be a move away from viewing risk perception as a rational cognitive process that can and should be influenced by the external efforts of health promotion, to more critical and theoretically informed investigations into the meaning of risk to individuals in contemporary society. Lifestyle risk discourse as it is used in public health should be examined for its ethical, political, and moral subtext. Recent developments in the sociology, anthropology, and philosophy of risk discourse have pointed the way for such investigations.

References

1. Douglas, M., and Wildavsky, A. *Risk and Culture*. Basil Blackwell, Oxford, 1982.
2. Stoeckle, J. D. On looking risk in the eye. *Am. J. Public Health* 80: 1170–1171, 1990.
3. Douglas, M. Risk as a forensic resource. *Daedalus*, Fall 1990, pp. 1–16.
4. Starr, C. Social benefit vs. technological risk. *Science* 165: 1232–1238, 1969.

5. Short, J. F. The social fabric at risk: Toward the social transformation of risk analysis. *Am. Soc. Rev.* 49: 711–725, 1984.
6. Fischoff, B., et al. *Acceptable Risk.* Cambridge University Press, New York, 1981.
7. Nelkin, D. Communicating technological risk: The social construction of risk perception. *Annu. Rev. Public Health* 10: 95–113, 1989.
8. National Research Council Committee on Risk Perception and Communication. *Improving Risk Communication.* National Academy Press, Washington, D.C., 1989.
9. Dandoy, S. Risk communication and public confidence in health departments. *Am. J. Public Health* 80: 1299–1300, 1990.
10. Kahn, E., et al. A crisis of community anxiety and mistrust: The Medfly Eradication Project in Santa Clara County, California, 1981–82. *Am. J. Public Health* 80: 1301–1304, 1990.
11. O'Riordan, T., et al. Themes and tasks of risk communication: Report of an international conference held at KFA Julich. *Risk Analysis* 9: 513–518, 1989.
12. Otway, H., and Wynne, B. Risk communication: Paradigm and paradox. *Risk Analysis* 9: 141–145, 1989.
13. Tversky, A., and Kahneman, D. Judgment under uncertainty: Heuristics and biases. *Science* 185: 1124–1131, 1974.
14. Slovic, P. Perception of risk. *Science* 230: 280–285, 1987.
15. De Friese, G. H., and Fielding, J. E. Health risk appraisal in the 1990s: Opportunities, challenges, and expectations. *Annu. Rev. Public Health* 11: 401–418, 1990.
16. Fielding, J. E. Appraising the health of health risk appraisal. *Am. J. Public Health* 72: 337–340, 1982.
17. Kaplan, H. B., et al. The sociological study of AIDS: A critical review of the literature and suggested research agenda. *J. Health Soc. Behav.* 28: 140–157, 1982.
18. Nickerson, C. A. E. The attitude/behavior discrepancy as a methodological artefact: Comment on "Sexually Active Adolescents and Condoms." *Am. J. Public Health* 80: 1174–1179, 1990.
19. Teuber, A. Justifying the risk. *Daedalus,* Fall 1990, pp. 235–254.
20. Douglas, M., and Calvez, M. The self as risk taker: A cultural theory of contagion in relation to AIDS. *Soc. Rev.* 38: 445–464, 1990.
21. Brandt, A. No Magic Bullet: A Social History of Venereal Disease in the United States since 1880. Oxford University Press, New York, 1985.
22. Rosenberg, C. E. Disease and social order in America: Perceptions and expectations. *Milbank Mem. Fund. Q.* 64(Suppl.): 34–55, 1986.
23. Sontag, S. Illness as Metaphor/AIDS and Its Metaphors. Anchor, New York, 1989.
24. Crawford, R. You are dangerous to your health: The ideology and politics of victim blaming. *Int. J. Health Serv.* 7: 663–680, 1977.
25. Becker, M. H. The tyranny of health promotion. *Public Health Rev.* 14: 15–25, 1986.
26. Marantz, P. R. Blaming the victim: The negative consequence of preventive medicine. *Am. J. Public Health* 80: 1186–1187, 1990.
27. Grace, V. M. The marketing of empowerment and the construction of the health consumer: A critique of health promotion. *Int. J. Health Serv.* 21: 329–343, 1991.
28. Kilwein, J. H. No pain, no gain: A puritan legacy. *Health Ed. Q.* 16: 9–12, 1989.
29. McCombie, S. The cultural impact of the "AIDS" test: The American experience. *Soc. Sci. Med.* 23: 455–459, 1986.
30. Douglas, M. Risk Acceptability According to the Social Sciences. Routledge & Kegan Paul, London, 1986.
31. Sapolsky, H. M. The politics of risk. *Daedalus,* Fall 1990, pp. 83–96.
32. Stallings, R. A. Media discourse and the social construction of risk. *Soc. Probl.* 37: 80–95, 1990.

33. Nelkin, D. Selling Science: How the Press Covers Science and Technology. W. H. Freeman, New York, 1987.

34. Klaidman, S. How well the media report health risk. *Daedalus,* Fall 1990, pp. 119–132.

35. Stone, D. A. At risk in the welfare state. *Soc. Res.* 56: 591–633, 1989.

36. Conrad, P., and Walsh, D. C. The new corporate health ethic: Lifestyle and the social control of work. *Int. J. Health Serv.* 22: 89–111, 1992.

37. Wikler, D. Who should be blamed for being sick? *Health Ed. Q.* 14: 11–25, 1987.

38. Faden, R. R. Ethical issues in government sponsored public health campaigns. *Health Ed. Q.* 14: 27–37, 1987.

39. Morgan, M. G., and Lave, L. Ethical considerations in risk communication practice and research. *Risk Analysis* 10: 355–358, 1990.

40. Foucault, M. The Archaeology of Knowledge and the Discourse on Language. Pantheon, New York, 1972.

41. Kroker, A., and Kroker, M. Panic sex in America. In *Body Invaders: Sexuality and the Postmodern Condition,* edited by A. Kroker and M. Kroker, pp. 1–18. Macmillan Education, London, 1988.

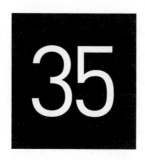

THE PURSUIT OF PREVENTIVE CARE FOR CHRONIC ILLNESS

Turning Healthy People Into Chronic Patients

Meta J. Kreiner and Linda M. Hunt

Clinical medicine in the US has been transformed in recent years to embrace an expanding emphasis on preventive care. Medicine's traditional focus on treating the signs and symptoms of existing disease is systematically being reframed in terms of risk assessment and control (Starfield *et al*. 2008). Preventive health care is now a prominent part of medical education and clinical guidelines in the US increasingly call for risk management interventions intended to avoid the future development of disease (Kelley *et al*. 2004).

Benign conditions that have been associated at a population level with a risk for developing serious illness—such as mildly elevated blood pressure, glucose or cholesterol—have received especially vigorous attention and their control has become a public health priority (Centers for Disease Control and Prevention 2010). Diagnostic and treatment criteria have been systematically expanded for these conditions and new categories of "borderline disease" or "pre-disease" have also been added. With these changes, risk factors for disease have been converted into disease entities themselves (Moynihan 2011, Yudkin *et al*. 2011) and now as many as 45 per cent of American adults have been diagnosed and are being treated for these conditions (Cory *et al*. 2010, Kaiser Family Foundation 2010).

Despite the pervasive enthusiasm for preventive medicine, critics point out some serious concerns with these practices. For example, they note that research linking marginal blood pressure, glucose or cholesterol levels to serious illness is inconclusive

The Pursuit of Preventive Care for Chronic Illness: Turning Healthy People Into Chronic Patients, Meta J. Kreiner and Linda M. Hunt in *Sociology of Health & Wellness, 36*(6), 870–884, July 2014. Reprinted with permission from John Wiley & Sons.

and that while most individual patients will experience no benefit from maintaining tight control of these levels, they are exposed to potentially serious harm from the medications (Aronowitz 2009, Brody and Light 2011, Greaves 2000, Light 2010, Moynihan 2011, Starfield *et al.* 2008, Yudkin *et al.* 2011).

Even so, these expanded diagnostic and treatment standards for chronic illness management are being rapidly institutionalised into clinical guidelines and medical practice, as they are incorporated into increasingly pervasive systems for monitoring clinical performance and quality of care. Equating quality health care with managing risk factors in healthy individuals may reduce the incidence of disease and healthcare costs for the total population but the value to each individual is uncertain. Rose (2001) has pointed out an inherent tension in such an approach, which he describes as the prevention paradox: "A preventive measure which brings much benefit to the population, but offers little to each participating individual" (p. 432). Such trade-offs are reasonable in terms of a public health agenda but their implications for the clinical agenda are less straightforward.

While clinical success is being redefined in terms of reducing the threat of possible future illness, little is known about the consequences of equating risk prevention with disease management for individual clinicians and their patients. Drawing on qualitative data from a study of chronic illness management in primary care, this article explores how this phenomenon is manifested in clinical care and considers some of the factors that promote and sustain this trend.

BLURRING OF PREVENTION AND DISEASE

The expansion of preventive medicine and its growing clinical dominance began with a number of theoretical and clinical innovations which developed synergistically in the 1950s in the US. Prior to this time, the diagnosis and treatment of chronic diseases such as diabetes and hypertension had been reserved for relatively rare cases where patients experienced symptoms of manifest pathology. Over time, many chronic conditions were reconfigured to be understood as occurring on a continuum, with non-pathological test levels redefined as clinically relevant, indicating an early stage of disease or the risk of the future development of a disease (Greene 2007).

Through the 1960s widespread screening arose as a strategy to reduce the population burden of chronic illness (Armstrong 2012) and new medications that were safer and more convenient than existing ones were rapidly entering the market. Clinicians were increasingly screening asymptomatic individuals for these conditions, in order to target them for preventive treatments (Greene 2007). With these innovations, conditions like marginally elevated blood pressure and cholesterol came to be understood as existing somewhere between being a risk factor for developing cardiovascular disease and a manifestation of the illness itself. At the same time, the definition of diabetes was expanded to include those who are only at risk for the disease, further blurring prevention and disease (Rosenberg 2009). This represents a fundamental alteration of the goals of clinical medicine, from identifying and managing illness towards the routine monitoring and management of risk in healthy people (Armstrong 1995. Fosket 2010).

RISK, POPULATION NORMS AND CLINICAL GUIDELINES

The idea of being at risk is a construction based on statistical observations of the distribution of health-related states and events in the general population. When identifying and managing risk becomes the focus of clinical medicine, population level trends provide the basis for definitions of normal and abnormal, shifting attention away from attending to the condition of the individual patient (Bluhm and Borgerson 2011). Canguilhem (1989) has criticised this approach for confusing statistical norms with biological norms, noting that while a certain range of test levels may be statistically defined as normal for a population, many individuals who fall outside that range will never experience any actual pathology. It may be of no benefit to a patient to bring their test levels into conformity with population norms if their particular variation presents no potential harm to them. Because population norms are a probabilistic concept, they apply to an aggregate of individuals and cannot be simply translated into a single, correct test value appropriate for all patients (Hunt *et al.* 2006, Lambert 2006, Rockhill 2001).

Nevertheless, population-level norms have become a cornerstone of how risk and illness are defined and understood in medicine, and clinical goals and evaluation criteria for many conditions are increasingly informed by such data. When professional organisations first began publishing diagnostic and treatment guidelines in the 1970s, these emphasised numeric definitions of risk status, elevating statistical norms to a central place in medical practice (see, for example, Davidson 2000, the Joint National Committee on Prevention, Detection, Evaluation and Treatment of High Blood Pressure [JNC] 1977). Throughout the next 40 years, in the name of improving disease prevention, the numeric thresholds defining diabetes, hypertension and high cholesterol have been repeatedly pushed downwards (Dumit 2012, Hunt *et al.* 2012), and definitions of pre-diabetes and pre-hypertension are now set at numbers approaching population averages (American Diabetes Association [ADA 2003], Chobanian *et al.* 2003, Davidson 2000).[1] With diagnostic cut-off points set at near population averages, by definition of an average, it follows that nearly half the population will be above the cut-off point and therefore now eligible for such diagnoses.

It is noteworthy that each downward revision of diagnostic and treatment criteria has expanded the percentage of people being treated not for pathology, but for the chance that they might develop pathology in the future. This represents a true transformation of the concept of disease, shifting clinical attention away from individual patients who are actually in decline from their disease, and instead to an as yet unaffected population (Aronowitz 2009, Starfield

et al. 2008). A key element of these evolving trends is the increasing reliance on the use of population based statistical modelling of risks and benefits to guide clinical decision-making, which gained momentum with the growth of evidence-based medicine.

While historically, evidence-based diagnostic and treatment guidelines had previously been followed by only a limited number of clinicians (Gallagher 2002), recent increases in the use of quality of care assessment has had a significant impact on adherence to guidelines. In the US most quality care assessment is carried out by one private, non-profit organisation—the National Committee for Quality Assurance (NCQA)—which ranks clinicians in part based on their adherence to professional practice guidelines, including a calculation of the percentage of their patients reaching target test levels (NCQA 2010, 2012). This approach was designed initially for the needs of large health insurance plans and corporate employers (Berman 1999), and the focus on population-level prevention is appropriate for such purposes. However, when such measurements are used to rank and reward individual clinicians, the provision of primary care may be redirected towards maintaining narrowly defined test threshold numbers, above other aspects of individual health status.

In order to better understand the ways the lens of preventive medicine may reconfigure the clinical agenda, we turn our attention to findings from an ethnographic study of chronic illness management in primary care clinics we have been conducting. We contrast clinician and patient perspectives, examining the way they understand and enact preventive strategies, their concepts of risk and disease and their criteria for evaluating treatment efficacy and defining clinical success.

THE STUDY

In 2009 we began conducting an ethnographic study in a midwestern US state of how primary care clinicians and their patients interpret and apply genetic and racial concepts of risk in their approaches to management of common chronic illnesses. As the project developed we were impressed with the intensity and uniformity with which clinicians responded to clinical indicators of disease risk. This began to make sense to us once we better understood the institutional context promoting clinicians' attention to those indicators.

Clinicians and patients were drawn from 44 primary care clinics, which included a wide variety of practices: suburban, urban and rural, private and public and large health system clinics, as well as small charitable clinics. We interviewed a purposive sample of 58 clinicians and 70 patients. We also observed 12 clinicians in over 100 of their clinical consultations with patients in treatment for diabetes or hypertension. The patients we interviewed were drawn from the consultations we had observed (see Tables 35.1 and 35.2).

TABLE 35.1 ■ Selected Characteristics for 58 Clinicians Interviewed, 2009–2010		
Characteristic	*n*	*Percent*
Sex		
Male	26	45
Female	32	55
Race/ethnicity		
Non-Hispanic White	37	63
African-American	10	17
Native American	2	3
Pacific Islander	2	3
Asian	5	9
Hispanic	2	3
Age (range: 27–77, median: 43)		
24–34	12	21
35–44	19	33
45–55	16	27
> 55	11	19

Degree		
Doctor of medicine	34	59
Doctor of osteopathic medicine	17	29
Physician assistant	2	3
Nurse practitioner	5	9
Graduation year		
< 1984	13	22
1985–1994	16	27
1995–2004	22	38
2005 +	7	12
Type of clinic		
University	3	3
Hospital/health system	21	36
Physician owned	21	36
Federally funded clinic	8	14
Other	5	9
Location of clinic		
Urban	40	69
Rural	7	12
Suburban	11	19

The interviews were open-ended and semi-structured, focusing on concepts of clinical risk and on strategies for managing diabetes and hypertension. They lasted about 1 hour and were recorded and transcribed. We also recorded careful notes of the clinical consultations we observed, capturing these interactions as fully as possible. All study participants gave their informed consent, following institutional review board-approved protocols. Names and personal details of the case material presented in this article have been changed to assure anonymity.

We developed quantitative and descriptive databases of patients' characteristics and open-coded variables, and used qualitative analysis software to

TABLE 35.2 ■ Selected Characteristics for 70 Patients Interviewed, 2009—2010		
Characteristic	*n*	*Percent*
Sex		
Male	38	54
Female	32	46
Race/ethnicity		
Non-Hispanic White	27	38
African-American	19	27
Native American	4	6
Pacific Islander	0	0
Asian	0	0
Hispanic	20	29
Age (range: 32–85, median: 58)		
24–34	2	3
35–44	9	13
45–54	17	24
55–65	20	29
> 65	22	31
Diagnosis		
Diabetes	15	21
Hypertension	14	20
Both	41	59
Interview language		
English	53	76
Spanish	17	24
Income level reported		
< $10,000	21	30
$11–20,000	16	23
$21–50,000	15	21
$51–70,000	4	6
$71–90,000	4	6
$90,000+	4	6
Unreported	6	9

code and analyse the interview transcripts. To minimise investigator bias the research team discussed and reviewed coding strategies and emerging findings throughout the project, reaching a consensus about coding procedures and honing analysis foci. Spot checks were also conducted to assure consistency in coding and classification procedures.

Risk as a Treatable Condition

In our study we were struck by how avidly and consistently the clinicians pursued narrowly defined test thresholds for their patients. They were well aware that guideline diagnostic criteria were subject to frequent revision but did not question these changes. They instead routinely incorporated the revised goals into their practices. The perspective of one physician who had been in practice throughout the various phases of these revisions is especially noteworthy. Dr Shields, who worked in a charity clinic in a large city, had practiced medicine for more than 40 years. In discussing current criteria for diabetes diagnosis and management, he remarked:

> Today standards are much more aggressive. The days are gone when we'd say to someone with pre-diabetes, "Okay, let's try behaviour modification for a few months." Now we just start them on metformin and other things, because the bulk of the damage is done early. So getting someone's blood sugar down after they've been diabetic 3 years is not enough . . . It makes sense. I mean, we know a lot more.

Dr Shields' certainty of the value of early, aggressive intervention reflects an important transformation in the way that preventive medicine is practiced. While when it first appeared in practice guidelines the diagnosis of pre-disease was presented as a wake-up call for individuals to pursue more healthy lifestyles, it has been converted into a treatable disease category. For example, in 2003 clinical guidelines did not recommend pharmaceuticals for pre-hypertension (Chobanian *et al.* 2003) but now the use of medications is promoted for such patients (Fuchs 2010, Julius *et al.* 2006). Similarly, the 2003 American Diabetes Association guidelines (ADA 2003) stated that pre-diabetes should be treated only with lifestyle modifications, not medications. However, the 2008 ADA guidelines recommend medications for pre-diabetic individuals who have other risk factors such as obesity, a family history or certain racial/ethnic identities (ADA 2008).

Most of the clinicians we interviewed agreed that marginally elevated test results require immediate action. For example, when asked about diabetes management, over half (60 per cent, 35/58) began their response by referring to pre-disease, and almost one-third (29 per cent, 17/58) said they begin hypertension treatment for patients in the pre-hypertensive range. Dr Morgan, a 56-year-old physician practicing in a private family medicine clinic in a suburban neighbourhood, described his approach for patients with pre-diabetes test results this way:

> They may not meet the definition of diabetes but we need to treat them like they are a diabetic and get more aggressive—starting on medications like metformin—And that may keep them from meeting the definition of diabetes for years.

Our study included a diverse group of clinicians—both recently trained and well-seasoned, both physicians and other healthcare professionals and both those in suburban private practices and in low-income clinics—yet they all cited nearly identical diagnostic criteria and detailed very similar treatment plans. Why would they respond so emphatically and uniformly to the ever-changing guideline criteria, above other indicators of patients' health status and needs?

MECHANISMS PROMOTING THE TREATMENT OF RISK

One factor behind this consistency seems to be the clinicians' heavy reliance on evidence-based electronic information sources in treating individual patients. Nearly three-quarters (71 per cent, 41/58) said they regularly use online subscription services as their primary source of information for making clinical decisions. Those we observed routinely turned to their computers in the course of clinical consultations—either a laptop during the consultation itself, or returning to their desktop computer briefly while the patient waited. Many (41 per cent, 24/58) remarked that such information sources helped them to keep up with the latest standards and treatment practices. It is also noteworthy that nearly three-quarters (74 per cent, 30/41) were using the same website—UpToDate (2013). This is an international evidence-based clinical decision support resource, to which wide-ranging healthcare institutions as well as private, independent clinicians subscribe. Heavy reliance on such information sources may contribute to the level of homogeneity we found in the clinicians' interpretation and response to even marginal test results.

Quality of care monitoring, which assesses clinician performance based on tight adherence to clinical guidelines, seems to further encourage clinicians to respond to risk as though it were pathology. The NCQA, the organisation currently responsible for setting most quality of care standards in the USA, defines specific numerical targets for diabetes and hypertension as the basis of clinician evaluation for management of these conditions. A clinician's score is calculated annually as a percentage, dividing the number of good control patients over the total number of patients diagnosed with that condition (NCQA 2010).

Our interviews and observations indicate that clinicians are particularly concerned with the very specific numbers set out in this ranking system. For example, in their discussions of diabetes care, all but one who named specific goal numbers (98 per cent, 47/48) said they strive to keep patients' test values below the current NCQA numeric threshold for "good control" (HbA1c below 7.0). Similarly, nearly all who named specific goal numbers for hypertension (95 per cent, 42/44) cited numbers consistent with current NCQA values (140/90 mmHg) (NCQA 2010).

To be clear, these clinicians did not express interest in pursuing these numbers in a cynical way but instead, viewed the threshold numbers as clinically meaningful goals. For example, regarding hypertension, Dr Shields said: "Every millimetre above 140/90 translates into a percentage risk for a stroke or heart attack." Similarly, Dr Jordan, a 58-year-old internal medicine physician made this observation about diabetes management:

> Anybody can get you down from a 12 to 9 [HbA1c], but we know that unless you are below 7, that the damage to the eyes, kidney, and heart continues. Getting you from 14 to 8.5 is no good. There's no merit in decreasing the numbers. Just getting close isn't good enough.

It is interesting, and concerning that in these examples the clinicians interpret the goal numbers as definitional of health for all patients, dismissing the value of lowering test levels for those with significantly elevated results, if they still remained outside the target range. In this way, quality monitoring systems may promote the conflation of risk and disease, encouraging clinicians to focus on at-risk patients who are diagnosed below the NCQA cut-off point and can readily remain on the controlled side of the equation. Ironically, to maximise their ranking, clinicians do well to prescribe medications to individuals with only marginal diagnoses and not focus on those who are more ill.

Because NCQA rankings are calculated annually they appear to be incentivising reaching goal numbers quickly and thereby encouraging clinicians to rely on medications to achieve a rapid response, rather than wait for the much slower effects of lifestyle modification. For example, 28 per cent (15/54)

of clinicians with whom we discussed treatment plans for hypertension made no mention of lifestyle modification at all. A clear majority of those who mentioned a time frame for diet and exercise to have an effect (86 per cent, 24/28) allowed their patients less than 3 months for this or started medications simultaneously. Consider, as an illustration, the remarks of Dr Jones, a doctor of medicine practicing in a private urban clinic, who explained her approach for patients who want to try diet and exercise rather than medications:

> I tell them, "I'll see you back in 1 month, and in that time you should have lost at least 6 to 8 pounds." ... If their test results have not improved, I tell them they have failed, and that I cannot allow them to walk around like that, and I put them on a low-dose, once-a-day pill.

What seems to be totally lost in this avid pursuit of lower test results is that, in all but the most extreme cases, these treatment efforts are not aimed at addressing a current disease but rather are preventive care, meant to reduce risk of developing disease sometime in the future (Saukko et al. 2012).

Thus far, we have considered how the distinction between risk reduction and disease treatment becomes blurred in the ways that clinicians understood and addressed these conditions. Next, we turn our attention to the patients we interviewed, to consider how they perceived and experienced this phenomenon.

THE URGENCY OF EARLY DIAGNOSIS

Researchers have reported that widespread screening, diagnosis and treatment of states of "risk" and "pre-disease" is creating a new category of patient experience, that of being a "partial patient"—one who is neither diseased nor well but exists in a liminal state between illness and health (Gillespie 2011,

Greaves 2000). This framing, however, does not fully capture what we found with the 70 patients we interviewed. Rather than perceiving themselves to be suspended between illness and health, they clearly understood themselves as ill—equally so for those diagnosed only in the borderline end of the continuum as for those with more elevated test results.

While a substantial number of those we interviewed had been diagnosed at borderline levels—33 per cent (18/55) with hypertension and 41 per cent (23/56) with diabetes—none, regardless of their test numbers, described their condition as "pre-diabetes" or "pre-hypertension." Rather than indicating they are at risk for developing diabetes or hypertension in the future, all described themselves as currently having a disease. Consider for example, the comments of Cindy, a retired schoolteacher in her early sixties, who has never had test results above the pre-diabetes range:

> When they discovered I was diabetic, I was in shock. I heard my doctor say "diabetic" and I could see his mouth moving, but I didn't hear another word he said that whole session. . . . It's not easy, I'm diabetic.

That the patients we interviewed so consistently equated being at risk with having a disease appears to be due, at least in part, to the way clinicians responded to their condition and how information was provided to them. Consider for example, the experiences of Stanley, a 59-year-old automobile engineering consultant. During his interview, he showed the researcher a lab printout he had received in the mail, which reported he had fasting plasma glucose of 103 mg/dL, which, while just over the pre-diabetes boundary of 100 mg/dL, was well below the current diagnostic boundary of 126 mg/dL. On the report, the glucose level was labelled "diabetes." Stanley said he had received a phone message from his primary care clinic telling him he had diabetes and needed to lose weight, watch his sugar intake and return to the clinic for a diabetes appointment.

Stanley's experience was by no means unique. Without exception, the pre-disease patients we observed were subject to the same clinical management strategies as were patients clearly above diagnostic thresholds. They received the same screening and diagnostic tests, the same patient hand-outs and pamphlets, the same clinical follow-up plans and home monitoring instructions and the same medications. At every juncture, the urgency of bringing test results below rigidly defined target levels was stressed.

The patients were deeply concerned about what they had been told could happen to them if they failed to get their test levels under control. All but two (97 per cent, 68/70) listed a set of very serious complications including death (54 per cent, 37/70), heart attack or stroke (67 per cent, 47/70) and, specifically for diabetes, blindness (46 per cent, 26/56) and amputations (38 per cent, 21/56). Patients in the pre-disease range expressed these same concerns and none mentioned the development of diabetes or hypertension as the outcome they were trying to prevent.

In some cases, this tendency to anticipate imminent danger from even marginally elevated metabolic levels clearly came from things clinicians told patients. For example, when we asked Marta, an elderly woman receiving care in a rural low-income clinic, what she thought could happen if she failed to keep her hypertension within the target range, she told us: "Well I could have a heart attack, or it could kill me. The doctor has told me that this is really bad."

We also found that patients may draw on the experiences of others they know to interpret their own at-risk state without distinguishing between preventive care and the management of advanced illness. This was especially true for diabetes, where almost half (48 per cent, 27/56) recounted such a story. For example, Jamie, a 58-year-old factory worker, told us:

> Years ago my doctor told me—these are his words. They used to call it "borderline," but now they say you are or you isn't. So I guess since I'm a little bit over the border, that I am.

Still, in Jamie's mind knowledge that his was a marginal diagnosis and that the diagnostic guidelines were subject to revision did not mitigate the weight of the diagnosis. He equated his own risk state with the condition of people he knew who had advanced disease. When asked what can happen when glucose levels are not controlled, he said:

> Man, you can go blind, a lot of stuff. . . . It's really like my uncle. He started off with one toe [amputated] . . . next thing you know they went to the ankle and then up to the knee. Then they started on the other leg. . . . Pretty soon he's 6 feet under. Diabetes took him right out of here.

Fear of the pain and suffering described in stories like this provides strong motivation for patients to follow treatment regimens. It was common in the consultations we observed for clinicians to encourage treatment compliance with remarks like this one, made by a physician to an elderly male patient: "Your diabetes is controlled right now but you need to keep on top of it, to avoid heart problems, stroke, and kidney problems." Equating the dangers of an at-risk state with imminent illness in this way promoted a sense of urgency for patients.

PREVENTIVE MEDICATION: IS TREATING RISK CAUSING HARM?

The urgency and intensity of the treatment efforts we observed for managing risk, even for marginal tests results, were impressive. Nearly all the patients interviewed (96 per cent, 67/70), including those with "pre-disease" diagnoses, had been prescribed medications for hypertension or diabetes and most (87 per cent, 61/70) had been given these prescriptions immediately upon diagnosis.

While heavy reliance on medications certainly can lower test results, it also may initiate a wide range of unintended health effects. Patients at the pre-disease end of the continuum are in particular danger of experiencing such effects. Because their metabolic

levels are only marginally elevated, medications may cause these levels to fall dangerously low (Dumit 2012, Hunt *et al.* 2012, Welch *et al.* 2011). Indeed, half the patients we interviewed (52 per cent, 36/70) reported suffering from symptoms of hypoglycaemia or hypotension, such as dizziness, headache, nausea, heart palpitations and blurred vision. In at least four cases, these were very serious episodes for which the patient had to be hospitalised. However, the patients rarely recognised that their medications might be the cause of these symptoms. In fact, most who had experienced episodes of hypoglycaemia or hypotension (68 per cent, 24/36) thought these were symptoms of the condition itself and did not consider them to be due to their medications.

Another concern with relying on medications to quickly achieve goal numbers is the rapid accumulation of prescriptions. This is especially true for diabetes because with this diagnosis, the guidelines set lower goal numbers for blood pressure and cholesterol. Once diagnosed with diabetes, patients are often prescribed new or additional medications to achieve goal levels for these other conditions. Most patients we interviewed (83 per cent, 57/69[2]) had some combination of diabetes, hypertension and high cholesterol and more than half (55 per cent, 38/69) had been diagnosed with all three. Nearly all (89 per cent, 62/70) were taking multiple drugs for these conditions. While these multiple diagnoses were routine for the clinicians, they were often overwhelming for patients.

For example, Marcos, a 34-year-old father of two, who was unemployed and uninsured, told us about his experience receiving marginally elevated test results when he went to a new doctor for a routine check-up. By the time he left he had been told he had diabetes, hypertension and high cholesterol and given prescriptions for each. He said, "Imagine what it's like to hear all of that in one day! When I came in I was perfectly fine and when I left, I had all of that."

Not surprisingly, as medications accumulate, associated adverse drug reactions often accumulate as well. Patients can quickly be drawn into a "Prescribing Cascade" (Rochon and Gurwitz 1997), taking more and more drugs to control the effects of drugs already prescribed. Indeed, this was often the case for patients in our study. For example, more than half of those taking medications for additional conditions (57 per cent, 24/42) had been prescribed drugs for respiratory or gastric symptoms, both well-known side-effects of the most common hypertension and diabetes medications.

The clinicians we interviewed were clearly aware of the potential harms of the medications they prescribe, resigned to managing these effects as a necessary step in managing these conditions. More than half (55 per cent, 32/58) noted specific drug side-effects they need to consider in prescribing medications but discussed these as the unfortunate but acceptable costs of attaining goal test results. For example, consider the remarks of two family practice physicians, referring to commonly used drugs for diabetes and for hypertension, respectively: "There's a lot of intolerance to metformin—gastro-intestinal side effects. It's unfortunate because it is a really good drug." And: "At higher doses the beta blockers cause bronco-spasm. That we treat with bronchodilator inhalers."

Like the clinicians, nearly all patients also viewed the use of medications as necessary for managing a life-threatening condition. Only two directly questioned the use of medications that cause adverse health effects. Cindy, the retired schoolteacher we introduced earlier, remarked:

> The side effects are worse than what you're trying to cure. I mean, the drugs might help you control it better, but what do you develop in the meantime from being on the stupid things?

And Eva, a 48-year old who is also a teacher commented:

> My concern is, you know, all these chemicals. . . . I'm afraid of these medicines. How is it that diabetics have all this kidney failure. Is it because of diabetes or is it because of all the medicine?

Still, these two, like almost everyone else in our study, patients and clinicians alike, saw attaining goal numbers as so important that they did not feel the adverse reactions to the drugs warranted stopping them. Throughout the consultations we observed we were struck by how much time and attention was devoted to adjusting medications, changing dosages or trying different combinations of medications, towards achieving goal numbers and managing negative drug effects, without questioning the urgency of pursuing preventive medicine in the first place.

DISCUSSION

When patients walk into the doctor's office, they might reasonably expect that the clinician will make diagnostic and treatment decisions by assessing their symptoms and medical history. In the primary care clinics where we conducted this study, it seems that the principles of preventive medicine have come to dominate the clinical agenda above more traditional clinical concerns. The clinicians in this study were largely focused on achieving rigidly defined treatment goals to manage risk as defined by clinical guidelines, evidence-based decision aids and quality of care assessment measures. At the same time, the patients accepted the treatments used to reach these goals and all the treatments' attendant burdens, believing they had a serious illness.

Despite the widespread belief that preventing illness is surely superior to treating it, it is not clear that the practice of allowing the logic of prevention to subsume the clinical agenda is necessarily in the best interest of individual patients. In recent years clinical goals have been steadily revised downwards for conditions like diabetes and hypertension and pre-disease has been elevated into a treatable condition based on population risk models. The clinicians received a consistent message that helping patients reach these numeric thresholds constitutes the best care they can provide.

Because both clinicians and patients equated at-risk states with actually being ill, they viewed the associated interventions not as prevention but as treatment. Such conflation redefines the notion of clinical success in a way that makes it difficult to evaluate benefit or harm. When prevention is equated with treatment, harms that might have been deemed unacceptable as a preventive strategy are transformed into the costs of a necessary, life-saving treatment. In assessing the value of intervention, clinicians and patients alike must navigate a complicated terrain where risk is equated with illness, the goal of treatment is reducing the threat of anticipated future illness, and treatments and any associated harms in the present appear to be necessary for protecting future health.

When prevention is the goal of treatment, criteria for assessing the treatment efficacy are recast as "positive deviation from a projected downhill trajectory" (Aronowitz 2009: 429). This places the diagnosis and treatment of at-risk and pre-disease conditions in an interesting light, wherein their accuracy can never be denied. Should the patient experience increasingly poor health, it is taken by both clinician and patient as confirmation that early or incipient disease had been identified. On the other hand, should the patient never develop illness, it is viewed not as diagnostic error but as a triumph of preventive medicine over disease.

Our analysis leads us to question the increasingly common practice of aggressively treating at-risk conditions as though failing to meet population norms presents real and immediate health threats to individual patients. This does more than create the illusion that healthy people are sick. It may in actuality be making them sick. There is growing evidence that tight control of blood glucose and blood pressure, especially at pre-disease levels, can have serious negative health consequences while providing little or no health benefit to the individual (see for example, Arguedas *et al.* 2009, Choe *et al.* 2010, Johnston *et al.* 2011, Montori and Fernandez-Balsells 2009, Montori *et al.* 2007). For example, in conducting a systematic review of studies of tight glycaemic control, Montori and Fernandez-Balsells (2009) observed that such efforts may expose many individuals to interventions "with still-uncertain benefits and certain harms" (p. 805).

In terms of a public health agenda, these may be viewed as acceptable costs for achieving societal gain: by managing risk factors in healthy individuals, the incidence of disease, disability and healthcare costs will be lower for the total population. Clinical guidelines and quality assessment criteria are increasingly defined by interests that lie outside clinical medicine, such as health insurers, public health agencies, large health system employers and the pharmaceutical industry (Conrad 2005, Dumit 2012). While for large institutions of this sort, lowering the disease burden across a population may be an appropriate goal, it is not equivalent to promoting quality of care for individual patients.

An individual walking into a doctor's office does not come there with the intention of improving the health profile of a population, but is there to pursue betterment of their own health. To enlist them unwittingly into the project of prevention, while exposing them to potential harm, in the absence of institutionally sanctioned mechanisms for tailoring clinical goals to individual patients, raises serious ethical concerns (Skrabanek 1990). While the expanding emphasis on preventive medicine may well improve the health profile of the total population, the implications of these innovations for the wellbeing of individual patients merits careful reconsideration.

ACKNOWLEDGMENTS

This research was supported by NIH grant #HG004710–03. We wish to thank the clinicians, clinical staff and patients who participated in this study, whose kind cooperation made this research possible. Amanda Abramson, Kristan Ewell, Linda Gordon, Heather Howard, Lynette King, Isabel Montemayor, Fredy Rodriguez, Kimberly Rovin and Nichole Truesdell provided invaluable assistance with a variety of data collection, analysis and literature review tasks. We also wish to thank two anonymous reviewers for their very helpful comments.

Notes

1. Since 2010 pre-diabetes has been defined as a fasting plasma glucose between 100–125 mg/dL or an Hb A1c between 5.7–6.4 per cent (ADA 2011). Pre-hypertension is defined as blood pressure between 120/80 and 140/90 (or 130/80 for someone diagnosed with diabetes) (Chobanian *et al.* 2003).

2. Information on the cholesterol status was missing for one patient, so *N* = 69 for these calculations.

References

American Diabetes Association (ADA) (2003) Standards of medical care for patients with diabetes mellitus, *Diabetes Care*, 26, Suppl 1, S33–50.

ADA (2008) Standards of medical care in diabetes—2008, *Diabetes Care*, 31, Suppl 1, S12–54.

ADA (2011) Standards of Medical Care in Diabetes—2011, *Diabetes Care*, 34, Suppl, S11–61.

Arguedas, J.A., Perez, M.I. and Wright, J.M. (2009) Treatment blood pressure targets for hypertension. *Cochrane Database of Systematic Reviews* 2010: CD004349.

Armstrong, D. (1995) The rise of surveillance medicine, *Sociology of Health & Illness*, 17, 3, 393–404.

Armstrong, D. (2012) Screening: mapping medicine's temporal spaces, *Sociology of Health & Illness*, 34, 2. 177–93.

Aronowitz, R.A. (2009) The converged experience of risk and disease, *Milbank Quarterly*, 87, 2, 417–42.

Berman, H.S. (1999) Performance measures: the destination or the journey?. *Effective Clinical Practice*. 2, 6, 284–6.

Bluhm, R. and Borgerson, K. (2011) Evidence-based medicine. In Gabbay, D.M., Gifford, F. Thagard, P. and Woods, J. (eds) *Philosophy of Medicine*. Philadelphia: Elsevier.

Brody, H. and Light, D.W. (2011) The inverse benefit law: how drug marketing undermines patient safety and public health, *American Journal of Public Health*, 101, 3, 399–404.

Canguilhem, G. (1989) *The Normal and the Pathological*. New York: Zone Books.

Centers for Disease Control and Prevention (2010) *Chronic Diseases and Health Promotion. Chronic Diseases and Health Promotion*. Atlanta: U.S. Department of Health and Human Services.

Chobanian, A.V., Bakris, G.L., Black, H.R., Cushman, W.C., *et al.* (2003) The seventh report of the Joint National Committee on prevention, detection, evaluation and treatment of high blood pressure: the JNC 7 Report, *Journal of the American Medical Association*, 289, 19, 2560–72.

Choe, H.M., Bernstein, S.J., Standiford, C.J. and Hayward, R.A. (2010) New diabetes HEDIS blood pressure quality measure: potential for overtreatment, *American Journal of Managed Care*, 16, 1, 19–24.

Conrad, P. (2005) The shifting engines of medicalization, *Journal of Health and Social Behavior*, 46, 1, 3–14.

Cory, S., Ussery-Hall, A., Griffin-Blake, S. and Easton, A. *et al.* (2010) Prevalence of selected risk behaviors and chronic diseases and conditions – steps communities, United States 2006–2007, *Morbidity and Mortality Weekly Report*, 59, SS08, 1–37.

Davidson, J.K. (2000) *Clinical Diabetes Mellitus A Problem-Oriented Approach*. New York: Thieme.

Dumit, J. (2012) *Drugs for Life: How Pharmaceutical Companies Define Our Health*. Durham: Duke University Press.

Fosket, J. (2010) Breast cancer risk as disease: biomedicalizing risk. In Clarke, E., Mamo, L., Fosket, J.R. and Fishman, J.R. *et al.* (eds) *Biomedicalization: Technoscience, Health and Illness in the U.S.A.* Durham: Duke University Press.

Fuchs, F.D. (2010) Prehypertension: the rationale for early drug therapy, *Cardiovascular Therapeutics*, 28, 6, 339–43.

Gallagher, E.J. (2002) How well do clinical practice guidelines guide clinical practice?, *Annals of Emergency Medicine*, 40, 4, 394–98.

Gillespie, C. (2011) The experience of risk as 'measured vulnerability': health screening and lay uses of numerical risk, *Sociology of Health & Illness*, 34, 2, 194–207.

Greaves, D. (2000) The creation of partial patients, *Cambridge Quarterly of Healthcare Ethics*, 9, 1, 23–37.

Greene. J.A. (2007) *Prescribing by Numbers: Drugs and the Definition of Disease*. Baltimore: Johns Hopkins University Press.

Hunt, L.M., Castaneda, H. and De Voogd, K. (2006) Do notions of risk inform patient choice? Lessons from a study of prenatal genetic counseling, *Medical Anthropology*, 25, 3, 193–219.

Hunt, L.M., Kreiner, M. and Brody, H. (2012) The changing face of chronic illness management in primary care: a qualitative study of underlying influences and unintended outcomes, *Annals of Family Medicine*, 10, 5, 452–60.

Joint National Committee on Detection, Evaluation and Treatment of High Blood Pressure (JNC) (1977) Report of the Joint National Committee on detection, evaluation and treatment of high blood pressure, *JAMA*, 237, 3, 255–61.

Johnston, S.S., Conner, C., Aagren, M., Smith, D.M., *et al.* (2011) Evidence linking hypoglycemic events to an increased risk of acute cardiovascular events in patients with type 2 diabetes, *Diabetes Care*, 34, 5, 1164–70.

Julius, S., Nesbitt, S.D., Egan, B.M., Weber, M.A., *et al.* (2006) Feasibility of treating prehypertension with an angiotensin-receptor blocker, *New England Journal of Medicine*, 354, 16, 1685–97.

Kaiser Family Foundation (2010) *Prescription drug trends*. Menlo Park: Kaiser Family Foundation.

Kelley, E., Moy, E., Kosiak, B., McNeill, D., *et al.* (2004) Prevention health care quality in America: findings from the First National Healthcare Quality and Disparities reports, *Preventing Chronic Disease*, 1, 3, A03.

Lambert. H. (2006) Accounting for EBM: notions of evidence in medicine, *Social Science & Medicine*, 62, 11, 2633–45.

Light, D.W. (2010) Bearing the risks of prescription drugs. In Light, D.W. (ed.) *The Risks of Prescription Drugs*. New York: Columbia University Press.

Montori, V.M. and Fernandez-Balsells, M. (2009) Glycemic control in type 2 diabetes: time for an evidence-based about-face? *Annals of Internal Medicine*, 150, 11, 803–8.

Montori, V.M., Isley, W.L. and Guyatt, G.H. (2007) Waking up from the DREAM of preventing diabetes with drugs, *BMJ*, 334, 882–4.

Moynihan, R. (2011) Surrogates under scrutiny: fallible correlations, fatal consequences, *BMJ*, 343. doi:http://dx.doi.org/10.1136/bmj.d5160.

National Committee for Quality Assurance (NCQA) (2010) *HEDIS 2010 Technical specifications for physician measurement*, national committee for quality assurance. Washington: NCQA.

NCQA (2012) Health insurance plan rankings 2012–2013. Available at: https://www.ncqa.org/tabid/1329/default.aspx (accessed 30 January 2013).

Rochon, P.A. and Gurwitz, J.H. (1997) Optimising drug treatment for elderly people: the prescribing cascade, *British Medical Journal*, 315, 7115, 1096–9.

Rockhill, B. (2001) The privatization of risk. *American Journal of Public Health*, 91, 3, 365–8.

Rose, G. (2001) Sick individuals and sick populations, *International Journal of Epidemiology*, 30, 3, 427–32, discussion 433–4.

Rosenberg. C. (2009) Managed fear. *Lancet*, 373, 9666, 802–3.

Saukko, P.M., Farrimond, H., Evans, P.H. and Qureshi, N. (2012) Beyond beliefs: risk assessment technologies shaping patients' experiences of heart disease prevention, *Sociology of Health & Illness*, 34, 4, 560–75.

Skrabanek, P. (1990) Why is preventive medicine exempted from ethical constraints? *Journal of Medical Ethics*, 16, 4, 187–90.

Starfield, B., Hyde. J., Gérvas, J. and Heath, J. (2008) The concept of prevention: a good idea gone astray? *Journal of Epidemiology and Community Health*, 62, 7, 580–3.

UpToDate (2013) Evidence-based clinical decision support resource. Available at: http://www.uptodate.com/home (accessed: 12 June 2013).

Welch, H.G., Schwartz, L.M. and Woloshin, S. (2011) *Overdiagnosed: Making People Sick in the Pursuit of Health*. Boston: Beacon Press.

Yudkin, J.S., Lipska, K.J. and Montori, V.M. (2011) The idolatry of the surrogate, *BMJ*, 343. doi.org/10.1136/bmj.d7995.

THE MEDICALIZATION OF AMERICAN SOCIETY

Only in the twentieth century did medicine become the dominant and prestigious profession we know today. The germ theory of disease, which proposed that microorganisms (germs) are the cause of many diseases and which achieved dominance after about 1870, provided medicine with a powerful explanatory tool and some of its greatest clinical achievements. It proved to be the key that unlocked the mystery of infectious disease, and it came to provide the major paradigm by which physicians viewed sickness. The claimed success of medicine in controlling infectious disease, coupled with the consolidation and monopolization of medical practice, enabled medicine to achieve a position of social and professional dominance. Medicine, both in direct and indirect ways, was called upon to repeat its "miracles" with other human problems. At the same time, some segments of the medical profession were intent on expanding medicine's jurisdiction over societal problems.

By the mid-twentieth century, the domain of medicine had enlarged considerably: childbirth, sexuality, death, as well as old age, anxiety, obesity, child development, alcoholism, addiction, and homosexuality, among other human experiences, were being defined and treated as medical problems. Sociologists began to examine the process and consequences of this *medicalization of society* (e.g., Freidson 1970; Zola 1972) and most especially the medicalization of deviance (Conrad and Schneider 1992; Conrad 1992). It was clear that the medical model focusing on individual organic pathology and positing physiological etiologies (causes) and biomedical interventions was being applied to a wide range of human phenomena.

Today, the medicalization of society as well as the debate over it continues. Human life, some critics observe, is increasingly seen as a sickness–wellness continuum, with significant (if not obvious) social consequences (Conrad 2007). One recent study found that 3.9% of our current health expenditures can be attributed to medicalization, which is about the same percentage that is spent on all of public health (Conrad, Mackie, and Mehrotra 2010). Other scholars, however, argue that although some expansion of medical jurisdiction has occurred, the medicalization problem is overstated (*Harvard Magazine* 2009).

Much of the debate over medicalization springs from a difference in how medicalization is defined. Conrad and Schneider (1992) suggested that medicalization occurs on three levels: (1) the conceptual level, at which a medical vocabulary is used to define a problem; (2) the institutional level, at which medical personnel (usually physicians) are supervisors of treatment organizations or gatekeepers to state benefits; and (3) the interactional level, at which physicians actually treat patients' difficulties as medical problems. This conceptualization reflects a broader view of medicalization than those that believe the medicalization of society has been overstated. In the last decade the debate has shifted, with some sociologists arguing for a still wider view of "biomedicalization," including the activities of most health-related institutions (Clarke et al. 2003), and others (e.g., Davis 2006) suggesting that medicalization should be limited to what doctors actually do (i.e., only physicians can medicalize problems). Thus, although it is by now accepted that there has been a significant increase in medicalization of human problems in the last four decades, there is still a debate about the boundaries and the origins of medicalization.

In "Medicine as an Institution of Social Control," Irving Kenneth Zola presents the medicalization thesis in terms of the expansion of medicine's social control functions. This classic sociological article was the first to call attention to the process of medicalization and to observe that the medical profession was challenging, and at times even replacing, religion, culture, and parts of the law as an institution of social control.

Peter Conrad, in "The Shifting Engines of Medicalization," argues that physicians and the medical profession are no longer the central forces in the increasing medicalization of society. He suggests that the new engines of medicalization are biotechnology (especially the pharmaceutical industry), consumers, and managed care. Doctors are still gatekeepers for medical care, but their role in the expansion of medicalization has become more subordinate. Medicalization is increasingly driven by commercial and market interests rather than medical professionals. New pharmacological treatments are especially important in the creation of new medical categories.

Nearly one-third of births in the United States are performed by cesarean section (C-section), and this medicalization of birthing has been increasing in the past fifty years. In "The Best Laid Plans?: Women's Choices, Expectations and Experiences in Childbirth," Claudia Malacrida and Tiffany Boulton examine the increase in the medicalization of childbirth in Western countries as evidenced by the rise of C-sections. A range of childbirth care providers have expressed concern about the impact of this increased medicalization while presenting differing views of the causes of the so-called C-section epidemic. The authors interviewed twenty-two women about their birth choices and their birth experiences. Finally, in a short analysis of the factors underlining the rise in C-sections, Theresa Morris interviewed fifty maternity clinicians and concluded it was external factors (e.g., hospital economic pressures, increased use of fetal monitor technology, clinicians' fear of malpractice suits) rather than individual childbirth circumstances or even clinical preferences that underlie this increased medicalization of childbirth. Both articles raise the question of the benefits and detriments of the increased medicalization of childbirth.

References

Clarke, Adele E., Janet K. Shim, Laura Mamo, Jennifer Ruth Fosket, and Jennifer R. Fishman. 2003. "Biomedicalization: Techno-scientific Transformations of Health, Illness, and U.S. Biomedicine." *American Sociological Review* 68: 161–94.

Conrad, Peter. 1992. "Medicalization and Social Control." *Annual Review of Sociology* 18: 209–32.

Conrad, Peter. 2007. *The Medicalization of Society: On the Transformation of Human Conditions Into Medical Disorders.* Baltimore: Johns Hopkins University Press.

Conrad, Peter, and Joseph W. Schneider. (1980) 1992. *Deviance and Medicalization: From Badness to Sickness* (expanded edition). Philadelphia: Temple University Press.

Conrad, Peter, Thomas Mackie, and Ateev Mehrotra. 2010. "Estimating the Costs of Medicalization." *Social Science and Medicine* 70: 1943–47.

Davis, Joseph E. 2006 "How Medicalization Lost Its Way." *Society* 43 (6): 51–56.

Freidson, Eliot. 1970. *Profession of Medicine.* New York: Dodd, Mead.

Harvard Magazine. 2009. "On the Medicalization of Our Culture." Accessed March 23, 2012. http://harvardmagazine.com/2009/04/medicalization-of-our-culture.

Zola, Irving Kenneth. 1972. "Medicine as an Institution of Social Control." *Sociological Review* 20 (November): 487–504.

36

MEDICINE AS AN INSTITUTION OF SOCIAL CONTROL

Irving Kenneth Zola

The theme of this essay is that medicine is becoming a major institution of social control, nudging aside, if not incorporating, the more traditional institutions of religion and law. It is becoming the new repository of truth, the place where absolute and often final judgments are made by supposedly morally neutral and objective experts. And these judgments are made, not in the name of virtue or legitimacy, but in the name of health. Moreover, this is not occurring through the political power physicians hold or can influence, but is largely an insidious and often undramatic phenomenon accomplished by "medicalizing" much of daily living, by making medicine and the labels "healthy" and "ill" relevant to an ever increasing part of human existence.

Although many have noted aspects of this process, by confining their concern to the field of psychiatry, these criticisms have been misplaced.[1]

For psychiatry has by no means distorted the mandate of medicine, but indeed, though perhaps at a pace faster than other medical specialties, is following instead some of the basic claims and directions of that profession. Nor is this extension into society the result of any professional "imperialism," for this leads us to think of the issue in terms of misguided human efforts or motives. If we search for the "why" of this phenomenon, we will see instead that it is rooted in our increasingly complex technological and bureaucratic system—a system which has led us down the path of the reluctant reliance on the expert.[2]

Quite frankly, what is presented in the following pages is not a definitive argument but rather a case in progress. As such it draws heavily on observations made in the United States, though similar murmurings have long been echoed elsewhere.[3]

Medicine as an Institution of Social Control, Irving Kenneth Zola in *The Sociological Review, 20*(4), 487–504, November 1, 1972. Reprinted with permission.

AN HISTORICAL PERSPECTIVE

The involvement of medicine in the management of society is not new. It did not appear full-blown one day in the mid-twentieth century. As Sigerist[4] has aptly claimed, medicine at base was always not only a social science but an occupation whose very practice was inextricably interwoven into society. This interdependence is perhaps best seen in two branches of medicine which have had a built-in social emphasis from the very start—psychiatry[5] and public health/preventive medicine.[6] Public health was always committed to changing social aspects of life—from sanitary to housing to working conditions—and often used the arm of the state (i.e. through laws and legal power) to gain its ends (e.g. quarantines, vaccinations). Psychiatry's involvement in society is a bit more difficult to trace, but taking the histories of psychiatry as data, then one notes the almost universal reference to one of the early pioneers, a physician named Johan Weyer. His, and thus psychiatry's involvement in social problems lay in the objection that witches ought not to be burned; for they were not possessed by the devil, but rather bedeviled by their problems—namely they were insane. From its early concern with the issue of insanity as a defense in criminal proceedings, psychiatry has grown to become the most dominant rehabilitative perspective in dealing with society's "legal" deviants. Psychiatry, like public health, has also used the legal powers of the state in the accomplishment of its goals (i.e. the cure of the patient through the legal proceedings of involuntary commitment and its concomitant removal of certain rights and privileges).

This is not to say, however, that the rest of medicine has been "socially" uninvolved. For a rereading of history makes it seem a matter of degree. Medicine has long had both a *de jure* and a *de facto* relation to institutions of social control. The *de jure* relationship is seen in the idea of reportable diseases, wherein, if certain phenomena occur in his practice, the physician is required to report them to the appropriate authorities. While this seems somewhat straightforward and even functional where certain highly contagious diseases are concerned, it is less clear where the possible spread of infection is not the primary issue (e.g. with gunshot wounds, attempted suicide, drug use and what is now called child abuse). The *de facto* relation to social control can be argued through a brief look at the disruptions of the last two or three American Medical Association Conventions. For there the American Medical Association members—and really all ancillary health professions—were accused of practicing social control (the term used by the accusers was genocide) in first, *whom* they have traditionally treated with *what*—giving *better* treatment to more favored clientele; and secondly, *what* they have treated—a more subtle form of discrimination in that, with limited resources, by focusing on some diseases others are neglected. Here the accusation was that medicine has focused on the diseases of the rich and the established—cancer, heart disease, stroke—and ignored the diseases of the poor, such as malnutrition and still high infant mortality.

THE MYTH OF ACCOUNTABILITY

Even if we acknowledge such a growing medical involvement, it is easy to regard it as primarily a "good" one—which involves the steady destigmatization of many human and social problems. Thus Barbara Wootton was able to conclude:

> Without question . . . in the contemporary attitude toward antisocial behaviour, psychiatry and humanitarianism have marched hand in hand. Just because it is so much in keeping with the mental atmosphere of a scientifically-minded age, the medical treatment of social deviants has been a most powerful, perhaps even the most powerful, reinforcement of humanitarian impulses; for today the prestige of humane proposals is immensely enhanced if these are expressed in the idiom of medical science.[7]

The assumption is thus readily made that such medical involvement in social problems leads to their removal from religious and legal scrutiny and thus from moral and punitive consequences. In turn the problems are placed under medical scientific scrutiny and thus in objective and therapeutic circumstances.

The fact that we cling to such a hope is at least partly due to two cultural-historical blindspots—one regarding our notion of punishment and the other our notion of moral responsibility. Regarding the first, if there is one insight into human behavior that the twentieth century should have firmly implanted, it is that punishment cannot be seen in merely physical terms, nor only from the perspective of the giver. Granted that capital offenses are on the decrease, that whipping and torture seem to be disappearing, as is the use of chains and other physical restraints, yet our ability if not willingness to inflict human anguish on one another does not seem similarly on the wane. The most effective forms of brain-washing deny any physical contact and the concept of relativism tells much about the psychological costs of even relative deprivation of tangible and intangible wants. Thus, when an individual because of his "disease" and its treatment is forbidden to have intercourse with fellow human beings, is confined until cured, is forced to undergo certain medical procedures for his own good, perhaps deprived forever of the right to have sexual relations and/or produce children, *then* it is difficult for the patient *not* to view what is happening to him as punishment. This does not mean that medicine is the latest form of twentieth century torture, but merely that pain and suffering take many forms, and that the removal of a despicable inhumane procedure by current standards does not necessarily mean that its replacement will be all that beneficial. In part, the satisfaction in seeing the chains cast off by Pinel may have allowed us for far too long to neglect examining with what they had been replaced.

It is the second issue, that of responsibility, which requires more elaboration, for it is argued here that the medical model has had its greatest impact in the lifting of moral condemnation from the individual. While some sceptics note that while the individual is no longer condemned his disease still *is,* they do not go far enough. Most analysts have tried to make a distinction between illness and crime on the issue of personal responsibility.[8] The criminal is thought to be responsible and therefore accountable (or punishable) for his act, while the sick person is not. While the distinction does exist, it seems to be more a quantitative one rather than a qualitative one, with moral judgments but a pinprick below the surface. For instance, while it is probably true that individuals are no longer directly condemned for being sick, it does seem that much of this condemnation is merely displaced. Though his immoral character is not demonstrated in his having a disease, it becomes evident in what he does about it. Without seeming ludicrous, if one listed the traits of people who break appointments, fail to follow treatment regimen, or even delay in seeking medical aid, one finds a long list of "personal flaws." Such people seem to be ever ignorant of the consequences of certain diseases, inaccurate as to symptomatology, unable to plan ahead or find time, burdened with shame, guilt, neurotic tendencies, haunted with traumatic medical experiences or members of some lower status minority group religious, ethnic, racial or socioeconomic. In short, they appear to be a sorely troubled if not disreputable group of people.

The argument need not rest at this level of analysis, for it is not clear that the issues of morality and individual responsibility have been fully banished from the etiological scene itself. At the same time as the label "illness" is being used to attribute "diminished responsibility" to a whole host of phenomena, the issue of "personal responsibility" seems to be re-emerging within medicine itself. Regardless of the truth and insights of the concepts of stress and the perspective of psychosomatics, whatever else they do, they bring man, *not* bacteria to the center of the stage and lead thereby to a re-examination of the individual's role in his own demise, disability and even recovery.

The case, however, need not be confined to professional concepts and their degree of acceptance, for we can look at the beliefs of the man in the street. As most surveys have reported, when an individual is asked what caused his diabetes, heart disease, upper respiratory infection, etc., we may be comforted by the scientific terminology if not the accuracy of his answers. Yet if we follow this questioning with the probe: "Why did you get X now?", or "Of all the people in your community, family, etc. who were exposed to X, why did you get . . .?", then the rational scientific veneer is pierced and the concern with personal and moral responsibility emerges quite strikingly. Indeed the issue "why me?" becomes of great concern and is generally expressed in quite moral terms of what they did wrong. It is possible to argue that here we are seeing a residue and that it will surely be different in the new generation. A recent experiment I conducted should cast some doubt on this. I asked a class of forty undergraduates, mostly aged seventeen, eighteen and nineteen, to recall the last time they were sick, disabled, or hurt and then to record how they did or would have communicated this experience to a child under the age of five. The purpose of the assignment had nothing to do with the issue of responsibility and it is worth noting that there was no difference in the nature of the response between those who had or had not actually encountered children during their "illness." The responses speak for themselves.

The opening words of the sick, injured person to the query of the child were:

"I feel bad"
"I feel bad all over"
"I have a bad leg"
"I have a bad eye"
"I have a bad stomach ache"
"I have a bad pain"
"I have a bad cold"

The reply of the child was inevitable:

"What did you do wrong?"

The "ill person" in no case corrected the child's perspective but rather joined it at that level.

On bacteria

"There are good germs and bad germs and sometimes the bad germs . . ."

On catching a cold

"Well you know sometimes when your mother says, 'Wrap up or be careful or you'll catch a cold,' well I . . ."

On an eye sore

"When you use certain kinds of things (mascara) near your eye you must be very careful and I was not. . . ."

On a leg injury

"You've always got to watch where you're going and I . . ."

Finally to the treatment phase:

On how drugs work

"You take this medicine and it attacks the bad parts. . . ."

On how wounds are healed

"Within our body there are good forces and bad ones and when there is an injury, all the good ones . . ."

On pus

"That's the way the body gets rid of all its bad things. . . ."

On general recovery

"If you are good and do all the things the doctor and your mother tell you, you will get better."

In short, on nearly every level, from getting sick to recovering, a moral battle raged. This seems more than the mere anthropomorphising of a phenomenon to communicate it more simply to children. Frankly it seems hard to believe that the English language is so poor that a *moral* rhetoric is needed to describe a supposedly amoral phenomenon—illness.

In short, despite hopes to the contrary, the rhetoric of illness by itself seems to provide no absolution from individual responsibility, accountability and moral judgment.

THE MEDICALIZING OF SOCIETY

Perhaps it is possible that medicine is not devoid of potential for moralizing and social control. The first question becomes: "what means are available to exercise it?" Freidson has stated a major aspect of the process most succinctly:

> The medical profession has first claim to jurisdiction over the label of illness and *anything* to which it may be attached, irrespective of its capacity to deal with it effectively.[9]

For illustrative purposes this "attaching" process may be categorized in four concrete ways: first, through the expansion of what in life is deemed relevant to the good practice of medicine; secondly, through the retention of absolute control over certain technical procedures; thirdly, through the retention of near absolute access to certain "taboo" areas; and finally, through the expansion of what in medicine is deemed relevant to the good practice of life.

1. The Expansion of What in Life Is Deemed Relevant to the Good Practice of Medicine

The change of medicine's commitment from a specific etiological model of disease to a multicausal one and the greater acceptance of the concepts of comprehensive medicine, psychosomatics, etc., have enormously expanded that which is or can be relevant to the understanding, treatment and even prevention of disease. Thus it is no longer necessary for the patient merely to divulge the symptoms of his body, but also the symptoms of daily living, his habits and his worries. Part of this is greatly facilitated

in the "age of the computer," for what might be too embarrassing, or take too long, or be inefficient in a face-to-face encounter can now be asked and analyzed impersonally by the machine, and moreover be done before the patient ever sees the physician. With the advent of the computer a certain guarantee of privacy is necessarily lost, for while many physicians might have probed similar issues, the only place where the data were stored was in the mind of the doctor, and only rarely in the medical record. The computer, on the other hand, has a retrievable, transmittable and almost inexhaustible memory.

It is not merely, however, the nature of the data needed to make more accurate diagnoses and treatments, but the perspective which accompanies it—a perspective which pushes the physician far beyond his office and the exercise of technical skills. To rehabilitate or at least alleviate many of the ravages of chronic disease, it has become increasingly necessary to intervene to change permanently the habits of a patient's lifetime—be it of working, sleeping, playing or eating. In prevention the "extension into life" becomes even deeper, since the very idea of primary prevention means getting there *before* the disease process starts. The physician must not only seek out his clientele but once found must often convince them that they must do something *now* and perhaps at a time when the potential patient feels well or not especially troubled. If this in itself does not get the prevention-oriented physician involved in the workings of society, then the nature of "effective" mechanisms for intervention surely does, as illustrated by the statement of a physician trying to deal with health problems in the ghetto.

> Any effort to improve the health of ghetto residents cannot be separated from equal and simultaneous efforts to remove the multiple social, political and economic restraints currently imposed on inner city residents.[10]

Certain forms of social intervention and control emerge even when medicine comes to grips with some of its more traditional problems like heart disease and cancer. An increasing number of physicians feel that a change in diet may be the most effective deterrent to a number of cardiovascular complications. They are, however, so perplexed as to how to get the general population to follow their recommendations that a leading article in a national magazine was titled "To Save the Heart: Diet by Decree?"[11] It is obvious that there is an increasing pressure for more explicit sanctions against the tobacco companies and against high users to force both to desist. And what will be the implications of even stronger evidence which links age at parity, frequency of sexual intercourse, or the lack of male circumcision to the incidence of cervical cancer, can be left to our imagination!

2. Through the Retention of Absolute Control Over Certain Technical Procedures

In particular this refers to skills which in certain jurisdictions are the very operational and legal definition of the practice of medicine—the right to do surgery and prescribe drugs. Both of these take medicine far beyond concern with ordinary organic disease.

In surgery this is seen in several different subspecialties. The plastic surgeon has at least participated in, if not helped perpetuate, certain aesthetic standards. What once was a practice confined to restoration has now expanded beyond the correction of certain traumatic or even congenital deformities to the creation of new physical properties, from size of nose to size of breast, as well as dealing with certain phenomena—wrinkles, sagging, etc.—formerly associated with the "natural" process of aging. Alterations in sexual and reproductive functioning have long been a medical concern. Yet today the frequency of hysterectomies seems not so highly correlated as one might think with the presence of organic disease. (What avenues the very possibility of sex change will open is anyone's guess.) Transplantations, despite their still relative infrequency, have had a tremendous effect on our very notions of death and dying. And at the other end of life's continuum, since abortion is still essentially a surgical procedure, it is to the physician-surgeon that society is turning (and the physician-surgeon accepting) for criteria and guidelines.

In the exclusive right to prescribe and thus pronounce on and regulate drugs, the power of the physician is even more awesome. Forgetting for the moment our obsession with youth's "illegal" use of drugs, any observer can see, judging by sales alone, that the greatest increase in drug use over the last ten years has not been in the realm of treating any organic disease but in treating a large number of psychosocial states. Thus we have drugs for nearly every mood:

to help us sleep or keep us awake

to enhance our appetite or decrease it

to tone down our energy level or to increase it

to relieve our depression or stimulate our interest.

Recently the newspapers and more popular magazines, including some medical and scientific ones, have carried articles about drugs which may be effective peace pills or anti-aggression tablets, enhance our memory, our perception, our intelligence and our vision (spiritually or otherwise). This led to the easy prediction:

We will see new drugs, more targeted, more specific and more potent than anything we have. . . . And many of these would be for people we would call healthy.[12]

This statement incidentally was made not by a visionary science fiction writer but by a former commissioner of the United States Food and Drug Administration.

3. Through the Retention of Near Absolute Access to Certain "Taboo" Areas

These "taboo" areas refer to medicine's almost exclusive license to examine and treat that most personal of individual possessions—the inner workings of our bodies and minds. My contention is that if anything can be shown in some way to affect the workings of the body and to a lesser extent the mind, then it can be labelled an "illness" itself or jurisdictionally "a medical problem." In a sheer statistical sense the import of this is especially great if we look at only four such problems—aging, drug addiction, alcoholism and pregnancy. The first and last were once regarded as normal natural processes and the middle two as human foibles and weaknesses. Now this has changed and to some extent medical specialties have emerged to meet these new needs. Numerically this expands medicine's involvement not only in a longer span of human existence, but it opens the possibility of medicine's services to millions if not billions of people. In the United States at least, the implication of declaring alcoholism a disease (the possible import of a pending Supreme Court decision as well as laws currently being introduced into several state legislatures) would reduce arrests in many jurisdictions by 10 to 50 percent and transfer such "offenders" when "discovered" directly to a medical facility. It is pregnancy, however, which produces the most illuminating illustration. For, again in the United States, it was barely seventy years ago that virtually all births and the concomitants of birth occurred outside the hospital as well as outside medical supervision. I do not frankly have a documentary history, but as this medical claim was solidified, so too was medicine's claim to a whole host of related processes: not only to birth but to prenatal, postnatal, and pediatric care; not only to conception but to infertility; not only to the process of reproduction but to the process and problems of sexual activity itself; not only when life begins (in the issue of abortion) but whether it should be allowed to begin at all (e.g. in genetic counselling).

Partly through this foothold in the "taboo" areas and partly through the simple reduction of other resources, the physician is increasingly becoming the choice for help for many with personal and social problems. Thus a recent British study reported that within a five year period there had been a notable increase (from 25 to 41 percent) in the proportion of the population willing to consult the physician with a personal problem.[13]

4. Through the Expansion of What in Medicine Is Deemed Relevant to the Good Practice of Life

Though in some ways this is the most powerful of all "the medicalizing of society" processes, the point can be made simply. Here we refer to the use of medical rhetoric and evidence in the arguments to advance any cause. For what Wootton attributed to psychiatry is no less true of medicine. To paraphrase her, today the prestige of *any* proposal is immensely enhanced, if not justified, when it is expressed in the idiom of medical science. To say that many who use such labels are not professionals only begs the issue, for the public is only taking its cues from professionals who increasingly have been extending their expertise into the social sphere or have called for such an extension.[14] In politics one hears of the healthy or unhealthy economy or state. More concretely, the physical and mental health of American presidential candidates has been an issue in the last four elections and a recent book claimed to link faulty political decisions with faulty health.[15] For years we knew that the environment was unattractive, polluted, noisy and in certain ways dying, but now we learn that its death may not be unrelated to our own demise. To end with a rather mundane if depressing example, there has always been a constant battle between school authorities and their charges on the basis of dress and such habits as smoking, but recently the issue was happily resolved for a local school administration when they declared that such restrictions were necessary for reasons of health.

THE POTENTIAL AND CONSEQUENCES OF MEDICAL CONTROL

The list of daily activities to which health can be related is ever growing and with the current operating perspective of medicine it seems infinitely expandable. The reasons are manifold. It is not merely that medicine has extended its jurisdiction to cover new problems,[16] or that doctors are professionally committed to finding disease,[17] nor even that society keeps creating disease.[18] For if none of these obtained today we would still find medicine exerting an enormous influence on society. The most powerful empirical stimulus for this is the realization of how much everyone has or believes he has something organically wrong with him, or put more positively, how much can be done to make one feel, look or function better.

The rates of "clinical entities" found on surveys or by periodic health examinations range upwards from 50 to 80 percent of the population studied.[19] The Peckham study found that only 9 percent of their study group were free from clinical disorder. Moreover, they were even wary of this figure and noted in a footnote that, first, some of these 9 percent had subsequently died of a heart attack, and, secondly, that the majority of those without disorder were under the age of five.[20] We used to rationalize that this high level of prevalence did not, however, translate itself into action since not only are rates of medical utilization not astonishingly high but they also have not gone up appreciably. Some recent studies, however, indicate that we may have been looking in the wrong place for this medical action. It has been noted in the United States and the United Kingdom that within a given twenty-four to thirty-six hour period, from 50 to 80 percent of the adult population have taken one or more "medical" drugs.[21]

The belief in the omnipresence of disorder is further enhanced by a reading of the scientific, pharmacological and medical literature, for there one finds a growing litany of indictments of "unhealthy" life activities. From sex to food, from aspirins to clothes, from driving your car to riding the surf, it seems that under certain conditions, or in combination with certain other substances or activities or if done too much or too little, virtually anything can lead to certain medical problems. In short, I at least have finally been convinced that living is injurious to health. This remark is not meant as facetiously as it may sound. But rather every aspect of our daily life has in it elements of risk to health.

These facts take on particular importance not only when health becomes a paramount value in society, but also a phenomenon whose diagnosis and treatment has been restricted to a certain group. For this means that that group, perhaps unwittingly, is in a position to exercise great control and influence about what we should and should not do to attain that "paramount value."

Freidson in his recent book *Profession of Medicine* has very cogently analyzed why the expert in general and the medical expert in particular should be granted a certain autonomy in his researches, his diagnosis and his recommended treatments.[22] On the other hand, when it comes to constraining or directing human behavior *because* of the data of his researches, diagnosis and treatment, a different situation obtains. For in these kinds of decisions it seems that too often the physician is guided not by his technical knowledge but by his values, or values latent in his very techniques.

Perhaps this issue of values can be clarified by reference to some not so randomly chosen medical problems: drug safety, genetic counselling and automated multiphasic testing.

The issue of drug safety should seem straightforward, but both words in that phrase apparently can have some interesting flexibility—namely what is a drug and what is safe. During Prohibition in the United States alcohol was medically regarded as a drug and was often prescribed as a medicine. Yet in recent years, when the issue of dangerous substances and drugs has come up for discussion in medical circles, alcohol has been officially excluded from the debate. As for safety, many have applauded the A.M.A.'s judicious position in declaring the need for much more extensive, longitudinal research on marihuana and their unwillingness to back legalization until much more data are in. This applause might be muted if the public read the 1970 Food and Drug Administration's "Blue Ribbon" Committee Report on the safety, quality and efficacy of *all* medical drugs commercially and legally on the market since 1938.[23] Though appalled at the lack and quality of evidence of any sort, few recommendations were made for the withdrawal of drugs from the market. Moreover there are no recorded cases of anyone dying from an overdose or of extensive adverse side effects from marihuana use, but the literature on the adverse effects of a whole host of "medical drugs" on the market today is legion.

It would seem that the value positions of those on both sides of the abortion issue needs little documenting, but let us pause briefly at a field where "harder" scientists are at work—genetics. The issue of genetic counselling, or whether life should be allowed to begin at all, can only be an ever increasing one. As we learn more and more about congenital, inherited disorders or predispositions, and as the population size for whatever reason becomes more limited, then, inevitably, there will follow an attempt to improve the quality of the population which shall be produced. At a conference on the more limited concern of what to do when there is a documented probability of the offspring of certain unions being damaged, a position was taken that it was not necessary to pass laws or bar marriages that might produce such offspring. Recognizing the power and influence of medicine and the doctor, one of those present argued:

> There is no reason why sensible people could not be dissuaded from marrying if they know that one out of four of their children is likely to inherit a disease.[24]

There are in this statement certain values on marriage and what it is or could be that, while they may be popular, are not necessarily shared by all. Thus, in addition to presenting the argument against marriage, it would seem that the doctor should—if he were to engage in the issue at all—present at the same time some of the other alternatives:

> Some "parents" could be willing to live with the risk that out of four children, three may turn out fine.
>
> Depending on the diagnostic procedures available they could take the risk and if indications were negative abort.
>
> If this risk were too great but the desire to bear children was there, and depending on

the type of problem, artificial insemination might be a possibility.

> Barring all these and not wanting to take any risk, they could adopt children.
>
> Finally, there is the option of being married without having any children.

It is perhaps appropriate to end with a seemingly innocuous and technical advance in medicine, automatic multiphasic testing. It has been a procedure hailed as a boon to aid the doctor if not replace him. While some have questioned the validity of all those test-results and still others fear that it will lead to second class medicine for already underprivileged populations, it is apparent that its major use to date and in the future may not be in promoting health or detecting disease but to prevent it. Thus three large institutions are now or are planning to make use of this method, not to treat people, but to "deselect" them. The armed services use it to weed out the physically and mentally unfit, insurance companies to reject "uninsurables" and large industrial firms to point out "high risks." At a recent conference representatives of these same institutions were asked what responsibility they did or would recognize to those whom they have just informed that they have been "rejected" because of some physical or mental anomaly. They calmly and universally stated: none—neither to provide them with any appropriate aid nor even to ensure that they get or be put in touch with any help.

CONCLUSION

C. S. Lewis warned us more than a quarter of a century ago that "man's power over Nature is really the power of some men over other men, with Nature as their instrument." The same could be said regarding man's power over health and illness, for the labels health and illness are remarkable "depoliticizers" of an issue. By locating the source and the treatment of problems in an individual, other levels of intervention are effectively closed. By the very acceptance of a specific behavior as an "illness" and the definition of illness as an undesirable state, the issue becomes not whether to deal with a particular problem, but *how* and *when*.[25] Thus the debate over homosexuality, drugs or abortion becomes focused on the degree of sickness attached to the phenomenon in question or the extent of the health risk involved. And the more principled, more perplexing, or even moral issue, of *what* freedom should an individual have over his or her own body is shunted aside.

As stated in the very beginning this "medicalizing of society" is as much a result of medicine's potential as it is of society's wish for medicine to use that potential. Why then has the focus been more on the medical potential than on the social-desire? In part it is a function of space, but also of political expediency. For the time rapidly may be approaching when recourse to the populace's wishes may be impossible. Let me illustrate this with the statements of two medical scientists who, if they read this essay, would probably dismiss all my fears as groundless. The first was commenting on the ethical, moral, and legal procedures of the sex change operation:

> Physicians generally consider it unethical to destroy or alter tissue except in the presence of disease or deformity. The interference with a person's natural procreative function entails definite moral tenets, by which not only physicians but also the general public are influenced. The administration of physical harm as treatment for mental or behavioral problems—as corporal punishment, lobotomy for unmanageable psychotics and sterilization of criminals—is abhorrent in our society.[26]

Here he states, as almost an absolute condition of human nature, something which is at best a recent phenomenon. He seems to forget that there were laws promulgating just such procedures through much of the twentieth century, that within the past few years at least one Californian jurist ordered the sterilization of an unwed mother as a condition of probation, and that such procedures were done by Nazi scientists and physicians as part of a series of medical experiments. More recently, there is the misguided patriotism of the cancer researchers under contract to the United States Department of Defense who allowed their dying patients to be exposed to massive doses of radiation to analyze the psychological and physical results of simulated nuclear fall-out. True, the experiments were stopped, but not until they had been going on for *eleven* years.

The second statement is by Francis Crick at a conference on the implications of certain genetic findings:

> Some of the wild genetic proposals will never be adopted because the people will simply not stand for them.[27]

Note where his emphasis is: on the people, not the scientist. In order, however, for the people to be concerned, to act and to protest, they must first be aware of what is going on. Yet in the very privatized nature of medical practice, plus the continued emphasis that certain expert judgments must be free from public scrutiny, there are certain processes which will prevent the public from ever knowing what has taken place and thus from doing something about it. Let me cite two examples.

> Recently, in a European country, I overheard the following conversation in a kidney dialysis unit. The chief was being questioned about whether or not there were self-help groups among his patients. "No," he almost shouted, "that is the last thing we want. Already the patients are sharing too much knowledge while they sit in the waiting room, thus making our task increasingly difficult. We are working now on a procedure to prevent them from even meeting with one another."

The second example removes certain information even further from public view.

> The issue of fluoridation in the U.S. has been for many years a hot political one. It was in the political arena because, in order to fluoridate local water supplies, the decision in many jurisdictions had to be put to a popular referendum. And when it was, it was often defeated. A solution was found and a series of state laws were passed to make fluoridation a public health decision and to be treated, as all other public health decisions, by the medical officers best qualified to decide questions of such a technical, scientific and medical nature.

Thus the issue at base here is the question of what factors are actually of a solely technical, scientific and medical nature.

To return to our opening caution, this paper is not an attack on medicine so much as on a situation in which we find ourselves in the latter part of the twentieth century; for the medical area is the arena or the example *par excellence* of today's identity crisis—what is or will become of man. It is the battleground, not because there are visible threats and oppressors, but because they are almost invisible; not because the perspective, tools and practitioners of medicine and the other helping professions are evil, but because they are not. It is so frightening because there are elements here of the banality of evil so uncomfortably written about by Hannah Arendt.[28] But here the danger is greater, for not only is the process masked as a technical, scientific, objective one, but one done for our own good. A few years ago a physician speculated on what, based on current knowledge, would be the composite picture of an individual with a low risk of developing atherosclerosis or coronary-artery disease. He would be:

> . . . an effeminate municipal worker or embalmer completely lacking in physical or mental alertness and without drive, ambition, or competitive spirit; who has never attempted to meet a deadline of any kind; a man with poor appetite, subsisting on fruits and vegetables laced with corn and whale oil, detesting tobacco, spurning ownership of radio, television, or motorcar, with full head of hair but scrawny and unathletic appearance, yet constantly straining his puny muscles by exercise. Low in income, blood pressure, blood sugar, uric acid and cholesterol, he has been taking nicotinic acid, pyridoxine, and long term anticoagulant therapy ever since his prophylactic castration.[29]

Thus I fear with Freidson:

> A profession and a society which are so concerned with physical and functional well-being as to sacrifice civil liberty and moral integrity must inevitably press for a "scientific" environment similar to that provided laying hens on progressive chicken farms—hens who produce eggs industriously and have no disease or other cares.[30]

Nor does it really matter that if, instead of the above depressing picture, we were guaranteed six more inches in height, thirty more years of life, or drugs to expand our potentialities and potencies; we should still be able to ask: what do six more inches matter, in what kind of environment will the thirty additional years be spent, or who will decide what potentialities and potencies will be expanded and what curbed.

I must confess that given the road down which so much expertise has taken us, I am willing to live with some of the frustrations and even mistakes that will follow when the authority for many decisions becomes shared with those whose lives and activities are involved. For I am convinced that patients have so much to teach to their doctors as do students their professors and children their parents.

Note

1. This paper was written while the author was a consultant in residence at the Netherlands Institute for Preventive Medicine, Leiden. For their general encouragement and the opportunity to pursue this topic I will always be grateful.

2. It was presented at the Medical Sociology Conference of the British Sociological Association at Weston-Super-Mare in November 1971. My special thanks for their extensive editorial and substantive comments go to Egon Bittner, Mara Sanadi, Alwyn Smith, and Bruce Wheaton.

References

1. T. Szasz: *The Myth of Mental Illness*, Harper and Row, New York, 1961; and R. Leifer: *In the Name of Mental Health*, Science House, New York, 1969.

2. E.g. A. Toffler: *Future Shock*, Random House, New York, 1970; and P. E. Slater: *The Pursuit of Loneliness*, Beacon Press, Boston, 1970.

3. Such as B. Wootton: *Social Science and Social Pathology*, Allen and Unwin, London, 1959.

4. H. Sigerist: *Civilization and Disease*, Cornell University Press, New York, 1943.

5. M. Foucault: *Madness and Civilization*, Pantheon, New York, 1965; and Szasz: *op. cit.*

6. G. Rosen: *A History of Public Health*, MD Publications, New York, 1955; and G. Rosen: "The Evolution of Social Medicine," in H. E. Freeman, S. Levine and L. G. Reeder (eds): *Handbook of Medical Sociology*, Prentice-Hall, Englewood Cliffs, N.J., 1963, pp. 17–61.

7. Wootton: *op. cit.*, p. 206.

8. Two excellent discussions are found in V. Aubert and S. Messinger. "The Criminal and the Sick," *Inquiry*, Vol. 1, 1958, pp. 137–160; and E. Freidson: *Profession of Medicine*, Dodd-Mead, New York, 1970, pp. 205–277.

9. Freidson: *op. cit.*, p. 251.

10. J. C. Norman: "Medicine in the Ghetto," *New Engl. J. Med.*, Vol. 281, 1969, p. 1271.

11. "To Save the Heart; Diet by Decree?" *Time Magazine*, 10th January, 1968, p. 42.

12. J. L. Goddard quoted in the *Boston Globe*, August 7th, 1966.

13. K. Dunnell and A. Cartwright: *Medicine Takers, Prescribers and Hoarders*, in press.

14. E.g. S. Alinsky: "The Poor and the Powerful," in *Poverty and Mental Health*, Psychiat. Res. Rep. No. 21 of the Amer. Psychiat. Ass., January 1967; and B. Wedge: "Psychiatry and International Affairs," *Science*, Vol. 157, 1961, pp. 281–285.

15. H. L'Etang: *The Pathology of Leadership*, Hawthorne Books, New York, 1970.

16. Szasz: *op. cit.*, and Leifer: *op. cit.*

17. Freidson: *op. cit.*; and T. Scheff: "Preferred Errors in Diagnoses," *Medical Care*, Vol. 2, 1964, pp. 166–172.

18. R. Dubos: *The Mirage of Health*, Doubleday, Garden City, N.Y., 1959; and R. Dubos: *Man Adapting*, Yale University Press, 1965.

19. E.g. the general summaries of J. W. Meigs: "Occupational Medicine," *New Eng. J. Med.*, Vol. 264, 1961, pp. 861–867; and G. S. Siegel: *Periodic Health Examinations Abstracts from the Literature*, Publ. Hlth. Serv. Publ. No. 1010, U.S. Government Printing Office, Washington, D.C., 1963.

20. I. H. Pearse and L. H. Crocker: *Biologists in Search of Material*, Faber and Faber, London, 1938; and I.

21. H. Pearse and L. H. Crocker: *The Peckham Experiment*, Allen and Unwin, London, 1949. Dunnell and Cartwright: *op. cit.*; and K. White, A. Andjelkovic, R. J. C. Pearson, J. H. Mabry, A. Ross and O. K. Sagan: "International Comparisons of Medical Care Utilization," *New Engl. J. of Med.*, Vol. 277, 167, pp. 516–522.

22. Freidson: *op. cit.*

23. *Drug Efficiency Study Final Report to the Commissioner of Food and Drugs*, Food and Drug Adm. Med. Nat. Res. Council, Nat. Acad. Sci., Washington, D.C., 1969.

24. Reported in L. Eisenberg: "Genetics and the Survival of the Unfit," *Harper's Magazine*, Vol. 232, 1966, p. 57.

25. This general case is argued more specifically in I. K. Zola: *Medicine, Morality, and Social Problems Some Implications of the Label Mental Illness*, Paper presented at the Amer. Ortho-Psychiat. Ass., March 20–23, 1968.

26. D. H. Russell: "The Sex Conversion Controversy", *New Engl. J. Med.*, Vol. 279, 1968, p. 536.

27. F. Crick reported in *Time Magazine*, April 19th, 1971.

28. H. Arendt: *Eichmann in Jerusalem A Report on the Banality of Evil*, Viking Press, New York, 1963.

29. G. S. Myers quoted in L. Losagna: *Life, Death and the Doctor*, Alfred Knopf, New York, 1968, pp. 215–216.

30. Freidson: *op. cit.*, p. 354.

THE SHIFTING ENGINES
OF MEDICALIZATION

Peter Conrad

Social scientists and other analysts have written about medicalization since at least the 1970s. While early critics of medicalization focused on psychiatry (Szasz 1970) or a more general notion of medical imperialism (Illich 1975), sociologists began to examine the processes of medicalization and the expanding realm of medicine (Freidson 1970; Zola 1972). As sociological studies on medicalization accumulated (see Conrad 1992, 2000) it became clear that medicalization went far beyond psychiatry and was not always the product of medical imperialism, but of more complex social forces. *The essence of medicalization became the definitional issue: defining a problem in medical terms, usually as an illness or disorder, or using a medical intervention to treat it.* While the medicalization process could be bidirectional and partial rather than complete, there is strong evidence for expansion rather than contraction of medical jurisdiction.

RISE OF MEDICALIZATION

Most of the early sociological studies took a social constructionist tack in investigating the rise of medicalization. The focus was on the creation (or construction) of new medical categories with the subsequent expansion of medical jurisdiction. Concepts such as moral entrepreneurs, professional dominance, and claims-making were central to the analytical discourse. Studies of the medicalization of hyperactivity, child abuse, menopause, post-traumatic stress disorder (PTSD), and alcoholism, among others, broadened our understanding of the range of medicalization and the attendant social processes (see Conrad 1992).

If one conducted a meta-analysis of the studies from the 1970s and 1980s several social factors would predominate. At the risk of oversimplification, I suggest that three factors underlie most of those analyses. First, there was the power and authority of the medical profession, whether in terms of professional dominance, physician entrepreneurs, or, in its extremes, medical colonization. Here, the cultural or professional influence of medical authority is critical. One way or another, the medical professional and the expansion of medical jurisdiction was a prime mover for medicalization. This was true for hyperactivity, menopause, child abuse, and childbirth, among others. Second, medicalization sometimes occurred through the activities of social movements and interest groups. In these cases, organized efforts were made to champion a medical definition for a problem or to promote the veracity of a medical diagnosis. The classic example here is alcoholism, with both Alcoholics Anonymous and the "alcoholism movement" central to medicalization (with physicians reluctant, resistant, or irresolute). But social movements were also critical in the medicalization of PTSD (Scott 1990) and Alzheimer's disease (Fox 1989). Some efforts were less successful, as in the case of multiple chemical sensitivity disorder (Kroll-Smith and Floyd 1997). In general, these were organized grassroots efforts that promoted medicalization. Third, there were directed organizational or inter or intra professional activities that promulgated medicalization, as was the case with obstetricians and the demise of midwives (Wertz and Wertz 1989) or the rise of behavioral pediatrics in the wake of medical control of childhood diseases (Pawluch 1983; Halpern 1990).

To be sure, there were other contributing factors that were implicated in the analyses. Pharmaceutical innovations and marketing played a role with Ritalin and hormone replacement therapy (HRT) in the medicalization of hyperactivity and menopause. Third-party payers were factors in the medicalization in terms of whether insurance would pay for surgery for "gender dysphoria," obesity, or detoxification and medical treatment for alcoholism. However, it is significant that in virtually all studies where they were considered, the corporate aspects of medicalization were deemed secondary to professionals, movements, or other claimsmakers. By and large, the pharmaceutical and insurance industries were not central to the analyses.

CHANGES IN MEDICINE

By the 1980s we began to see some profound changes in the organization of medicine that have had important consequences for health matters. There was an erosion of medical authority (Starr 1982), health policy shifted from concerns of access to cost control, and managed care became central. As Donald Light (1993) has pointed out, countervailing powers among buyers, providers, and payers changed the balance of influence among professions and other social institutions. Managed care, attempts at cost controls, and corporatized medicine changed the organization of medical care. The "golden age of doctoring" (McKinlay and Marceau 2002) ended and an increasingly buyer driven system was emerging. Physicians certainly maintained some aspects of their dominance and sovereignty, but other players were becoming important as well. Large numbers of patients began to act more like consumers, both in choosing health insurance policies and in seeking out medical services (Inlander 1998). Managed care organizations, the pharmaceutical industry, and some kinds of physicians (e.g., cosmetic surgeons) increasingly saw patients as consumers or potential markets.

In addition to these organizational changes, new or developed arenas of medical knowledge were becoming dominant. The long-influential pharmaceutical companies comprise America's most profitable industry and became more so with revolutionary new drugs that would expand their influence (Public Citizen 2003). By the 1990s the Human Genome project, the $3 billion venture to map the entire human genome, was launched, with a draft completed in 2000. Genetics has become a cutting edge of medical knowledge and has moved to the center of medical and public discourse about illness and health (Conrad 1999). The biotechnology industry has had starts and stops, but it promises a genomic, pharmaceutical, and technological future that may revolutionize health care (see Fukuyama 2002).

Some of these changes have already been manifested in medicine, perhaps most clearly in psychiatry where the cutting edge of knowledge has moved in three decades from psychotherapy and family interaction to psychopharmacology, neuroscience, and genomics. This is reinforced when third-party payers will pay for drug treatments but severely limit individual and group therapies. The choice available to many doctors and patient-consumers is not whether to have talking or pharmaceutical therapy but rather which brand of drug should be prescribed.

Thus, by the 1990s these enormous changes in the organization of health care, medical knowledge, and marketing had created a different world of medicine. How have these changes affected medicalization?

In a recent paper, Adele Clarke and her colleagues (2003) argue that medicalization is intensifying and being transformed. They suggest that around 1985 "dramatic changes in both the organization and practices of contemporary biomedicine, implemented largely through the integration of technoscientific innovations" (p. 161) coalesced as an expanded phenomenon they call biomedicalization. By biomedicalization they mean "the increasingly complex, multisited, multidirectional processes of medicalization that today are being reconstituted through the emergent social forms and practices of a highly and increasingly techno-scientific biomedicine" (Clarke et al. 2003:162). Clarke et al. paint with a very broad brush and create a concept that attempts to be so comprehensive and inclusive—incorporating virtually all of biotechnology, medical informatics and information technology, changes in health services, the production of technoscientific identities, to name just a few—that the focus on medicalization is lost. This new conception, in my judgment, loses focus on the definitional issues, which have always been a key to medicalization studies.[1]

Along with Clarke et al. (2003), I see some major changes in medicalization in the past two decades (cf. Gallagher and Sionean 2004). I see shifts, where they see transformations. I see medicalization as expanding and, to a degree, changing, but not morphing into a qualitatively different phenomenon. My task remains narrower and more focused on the medicalization process.

EMERGENT ENGINES OF MEDICALIZATION

In the remainder of this article, I want to examine how three major changes in medical knowledge and organization have engendered a shift in the engines that drive medicalization in Western societies: biotechnology, consumers, and managed care.

Biotechnology

Various forms of biotechnology have long been associated with medicalization. Whether it be technology such as forceps for childbirth (Wertz and Wertz 1989) or drugs for distractible children (Conrad 1975), technology has often facilitated medicalization. These drugs or technologies were not the driving force in the medicalization process; facilitating, yes, but not primary. But this is changing. The pharmaceutical and biotechnology industries are becoming major players in medicalization.

Pharmaceutical industry. The pharmaceutical industry has long been involved in promoting its products for various ills. In our 1980 book *Deviance and Medicalization* (Conrad and Schneider [1980] 1992) the examples of Ritalin, Methadone, and psychoactive medications were all a piece of the medicalization process. However, in each of these cases it was physicians and other professionals that were in the forefront. With Ritalin there were drug advertisements promoting the treatment of "hyperactivity" in children and no doubt "detailing" to doctors (e.g., drug company representative's sales visits to doctor's offices). But it was the physicians who were at the center of the issue.

This has changed. While physicians are still the gatekeepers for many drugs, the pharmaceutical companies have become a major player in medicalization. In the post-Prozac world, the pharmaceutical industry has been more aggressively promoting their wares to physicians and especially to the public. Some of this is not new. For most of the twentieth century the industry has been limited to promoting its wares to physicians through detailing, sponsoring medical events, and advertising in professional journals. However, since the passage of the Food and Drug Administration (FDA) Modernization Act of 1997 and subsequent directives, the situation has changed.

Revisions in FDA regulations allowed for a wider usage and promotion of off-label uses of drugs and facilitated direct-to-consumer advertising, especially on television. This has changed the game for the pharmaceutical industry; they can now advertise directly to the public and create markets for their products. Overall, pharmaceutical industry spending on television advertising increased six-fold between 1996 and 2000, to $2.5 billion (Rosenthal et al. 2002), and it has been rising steadily since. Drug companies now spend nearly as much on direct-to-consumer (DTC) advertising as in advertising to physicians in medical journals, especially for "blockbuster drugs that are prescribed for common complaints such as allergy, heart burn, arthritis, 'erectile dysfunction,' depression and anxiety" (Relman and Angell 2002:36). The brief examples of Paxil and Viagra can illustrate this, but there are many others (see Conrad and Leiter 2004).

Male impotence has been a medical problem for many years. In March 1998, the FDA approved Viagra (sildenafil citrate) as a treatment for erectile dysfunction (ED). When introduced, Viagra was intended primarily for the use of older men with erectile problems or ED associated with diabetes, prostate cancer, or other medical problems (Loe 2001). A demand for a drug for erectile problems surely existed before Pfizer began advertising Viagra. However, it was Pfizer who tapped into this potentially large market and shaped it by promoting sexual difficulties as a medical problem and Viagra as the solution. The initial Viagra promotion was modest (Carpiano 2001), but Pfizer soon marketed very aggressively to both physicians and the general public. At first it was with Bob Dole as a spokesman for elders, but soon it was with baseball star Rafael Palmeiro and the sponsorship of a Viagra car on the NASCAR circuit, expanding the audience and the market for the drug. Virtually any man might consider himself to have some type of erectile or sexual dysfunction. "Ask your doctor if Viagra is right for you," the advertisements suggest.

Viagra sales were sensational. In the first year alone, over three million men were treated with Viagra, translating into $1.5 billion in sales (Carpiano 2001). In 2000, Viagra was ranked sixth in terms of DTC spending and sales. By 2003 Viagra reached $1.7 billion in sales and was taken by six million men, which may not include all those who purchased it from Internet sites. By 2003, Levitra and Cialis were introduced as improvements and competitors for a share of this large market. The drug industry has expanded the notion of ED and has even subtly encouraged the use of Viagra-like drugs as an enhancement to sexual pleasure and relationships. Recent estimates suggest a potential market of more than 30 million men in the United States alone (Tuller 2004). The medicalization of ED and sexual performance has significantly increased in the past six years and shows no signs of abating.

When Prozac was introduced in 1987, it was the first wave of new antidepressants called selective serotonin reuptake inhibitors (SSRIs). SSRIs had the same or better efficacy than older antidepressants, with fewer disturbing adverse effects. These drugs caused a bit of a revolution in the pharmaceutical market (Healy 1998), and with $10.9 billion in sales in 2003 have become the third-best-selling class of drugs in the United States (IMS Health 2004). When Paxil (paroxetine HCl) was approved by the FDA in 1996 it joined a very crowded market for antidepressants. The manufacturer of Paxil, now called GlaxoSmithKline, sought FDA approval to promote their product for the "anxiety market," especially Social Anxiety Disorder (SAD) and Generalized Anxiety Disorder (GAD). SAD and GAD were rather obscure diagnoses in the *Diagnostic and Statistical Manual of Mental Disorders (DSM)*: SAD (or "Social Phobia") is a persistent and extreme "fear of social and performance situations where embarrassment may occur," and GAD involves chronic, excessive anxiety and worry (lasting at least six months), involving multiple symptoms (American Psychiatric Association 1994:411, 435–36).

Marketing diseases, and then selling drugs to treat those diseases, is now common in the "post-Prozac" era. Since the FDA approved the use of Paxil for SAD in 1999 and GAD in 2001, Glaxo-SmithKline has spent millions to raise the public visibility of SAD and GAD through sophisticated marketing campaigns. The advertisements mixed expert and patient voices, providing professional viability to the diagnoses and creating a perception that it could happen to anyone (Koerner 2002). The tag line was, "Imagine Being Allergic to People." A later series of advertisements featured the ability of Paxil to help SAD sufferers brave dinner parties and public speaking occasions (Koerner 2002). Paxil Internet sites offer consumers self-tests to assess the likelihood they have SAD and GAD (www.paxil.com). The campaign successfully defined these diagnostic categories as both common and abnormal, thus needing treatment. Prevalence estimates vary widely, from 3 to 13 percent of the population, large enough to be a very profitable pharmaceutical market. The marketing campaign for Paxil has been extremely successful. Paxil is one of the three most widely recognized drugs, after Viagra and Claritin (Marino 2002), and is currently ranked the number six prescription drug, with 2001 U.S. sales approximately $2.1 billion and global sales of $2.7 billion. How much Paxil was prescribed for GAD or SAD is impossible to discern, but by now both Paxil and SAD are everyday terms. While there have been some concerns raised about Paxil recently (Marshall 2004), it is clear that GlaxoSmithKline's campaign for Paxil increased the medicalization of anxiety, inferring that shyness and worrying may be medical problems, with Paxil as the proper treatment.

Children's problems constitute a growing market for psychotropic drugs. Ritalin for attention deficit hyperactivity disorder (ADHD) has a long history (Conrad 1975) but perhaps now can be seen as a pioneer drug for children's behavior problems. While the public may be ambivalent about using drugs for troubled children (McLeod et al. 2004), a wide array of psychotropic drugs are now prescribed for children, especially stimulants and antidepressants (Olfson et al. 2002). Whatever the benefits or risks, this has become big business for the drug industry. According to a recent survey, spending on behavior drugs for children and adolescents rose 77 percent from 2000 through 2003. These drugs are now the fastest growing type of medication taken by children, eclipsing antibiotics and asthma treatments (Freudenheim 2004).

At the other end of the life spectrum, it is likely that the $400 billion Medicare drug benefit, despite its limit, may increase pharmaceutical treatments for a range of elder problems as well. This policy shift in benefits is likely to encourage pharmaceutical companies to expand their markets by promoting more drug solutions for elders.

Genetics and enhancement. We are at the dawn of the age of genomic medicine. While there has been a great investment in the Human Genome Project and a celebration when the draft of the human genome was completed in 2000, most of genetic medicine remains on the level of potential rather than current practice. For example, we have known about the specific genes for cystic fibrosis and Huntington's disease for over a decade, but these have yet to translate into improvements in treatment. Thus far, genetics has made its impact mostly in terms of the ability to test for gene mutations, carriers, or genetic anomalies. Despite the publicity given to genetic studies (Conrad 1997), we have learned that only a few disorders and traits are linked to a single gene, and that genetic complexity (several genes operating together, gene-environment interactions) is the rule (Conrad 1999). But I have little doubt that genomics will become increasingly important in the future and impact medicalization.

Although the genetic impact on medicalization still lies in the realm of potential, one can imagine when some of the genetic contributors to problems such as obesity and baldness are identified, genetic tests and eventually treatments will soon follow. Obesity is an increasing problem in our society and has become more medicalized recently in a number of ways, from a spate of epidemiological studies showing the increase in obesity and body fat among Americans to the huge rise in intestinal bypass operations. Today physicians prescribe the Atkins or South Beach diet and exercise; it is possible in the future that there could be medical interventions in the genes (assuming they can be identified) that recognizes satiation. Gene therapy has not yet succeeded for many problems, but one could imagine the rush to genetic doctors if there were a way to manipulate genes to control one's weight. We know that baldness often has a genetic basis, and with Rogaine and hair transplants it has already begun to be medicalized. However, with some kind of medical genetic intervention that either stops baldness or regenerates hair, one could see baldness move directly into the medical sphere, perhaps as a genetic "hair growth disorder."

A large area for growth in genetics and medicalization will be what we call biomedical enhancement (Conrad and Potter 2004; Rothman and Rothman 2003; Elliott 2003). Again, this is still in the realm of potential, but the potential is real. There is a great demand for enhancements, be they for children, our bodies, or our mental and social abilities. Medical enhancements are a growing form of these. One could imagine the potential of genetic enhancements in body characteristics such as height, musculature, shape, or color; in abilities such as memory, eyesight, hearing, and strength; or in talents (e.g., perfect pitch for music) and performance. Enhancements could become a huge market in a society where individuals often seek an edge or a leg up. While many genetic improvements may remain in the realm of science fiction, there are sufficient monetary incentives for biotechnology companies to invest in pursuing genetic enhancements.

The potential market for genetic enhancements is enormous. To get a sense of the possible impact, I recently examined human growth hormone as an existing biomedical enhancement (Conrad and Potter 2004). Synthetic human growth hormone (hGH) became available in 1985, and it was approved for some very limited purposes, including growth hormone deficiency (a rare hormonal disorder). Shortness can be devalued and engender social problems for individuals. There is evidence that shorter people earn less money, get fewer promotions, can be stigmatized, and can have problems with such mundane tasks as finding proper fitting adult clothes (Conrad and Potter 2004; Rothman and Rothman 2003). Parents often have concerns that their children will be too short and now have the option of going to physicians for growth hormone treatments. Genentech, manufacturer of Protropin,

a brand of hGH, encouraged "off-label" uses of hGH for children who were extremely short but had no growth hormone deficiency. In a real sense these children with idiopathic short stature (ISS) can be called "normal" shorts; they are just short, from short parents or genetic makeup. Although hGH therapy can be very expensive ($20,000 a year for perhaps five years) and yield only moderate results (2–3 inches), in 1994 13,000 children with ISS were treated in the United States. These numbers are undoubtedly greater now, since the FDA recently approved an Eli Lilly growth hormone, Humatrope, for use for short statured children in the lowest 1.2 percent of the population. There are several lessons for biomedical enhancement here. First, a private market for enhancements for children, even involving significant expense, exists and can be tapped by biotechnology companies. Second, biotechnology companies, like pharmaceutical companies, will work to increase the size of their markets. Third, the promotion and use of biomedical enhancements will increase medicalization of human problems, in this case short stature. Imagine if genetic interventions to increase a child's height were available.

We do not yet have biotechnology companies promoting genetic enhancements, but we will. Biotech companies are already poised to use DTC advertising to promote genetic tests. They will employ many of the same marketing strategies as the pharmaceutical companies, which is no surprise, since many of them are the same or linked. The promotion of genetic tests may also contribute to medicalization. A positive finding on a genetic test—that one has a gene for a particular problem (cancer, alcoholism)— may create a new medicalized status, that of "potentially ill." This can have an impact on one's identity, social status, and insurability, and it may create new categories of pre-cancer, pre-alcoholism, or similar labels. This could expand medical surveillance (Armstrong 1995) and the medical gaze.

Consumers

In our changing medical systems, consumers of health care have become major players. As health care becomes more commodified and subject to market forces, medical care has become more like other products and services. We now are consumers in choosing health insurance plans, purchasing health care in the marketplace, and selecting institutions of care. Hospitals and health care institutions now compete for patients as consumers.

I will briefly cite several examples about how consumers have become a major factor in medicalization: cosmetic surgery, adult ADHD, hGH therapy, and the rise in pharmaceutical advertisements.

Cosmetic surgery is the exemplar of consumers in medicine (Sullivan 2001). Procedures from tummy tucks to liposuction to nose jobs to breast augmentation have become big medical business. The body has become a project, from "extreme makeover" to minor touch ups, and medicine has become the vehicle for improvement. In a sense, the whole body has become medicalized, piece by piece. To use just one example, from the 1960s through 1990 two million women received silicone breast implants, 80 percent for cosmetic purposes (Jacobson 2000; Zimmerman 1998). In the 1990s a swirling controversy concerning the safety of silicone implants became public when consumer groups maintained that manufacturers had mislead women about silicone implant safety, leading the FDA in 1992 to call for a voluntary moratorium on the distribution and implantation of the devices (Conrad and Jacobson 2003). The market for implants plummeted. In 1990 there were 120,000 implants performed; by 1992 there were 30,000. But with the introduction of apparently safer saline implants, breast augmentation increased by 92 percent from 1990 to 2000. According to the American Society for Aesthetic Plastic Surgery (2004), in 2003 there were 280,401 breast augmentations in the United States, making this procedure the second most popular cosmetic surgery following liposuction. While plastic surgeons do promote breast augmentation as a product (current cost around $3,000), the medicalization of breasts and bodies is driven largely by the consumer market. Overall, 8.3 million Americans had cosmetic medical procedures in 2003, a 20 percent rise from the previous year and a whopping 277 percent rise since 1997 (American Society for Aesthetic Plastic Surgery 2004). While the media and professional promotion fuel demand, virtually all of these procedures are paid for directly out of the consumer's pocket.

Since the early 1970s, Ritalin has been a common treatment for ADHD (formerly known as hyperactivity) in children. However, in the 1990s a new phenomenon emerged: adult ADHD. Researchers had shown for years that whatever ADHD was, it often persisted beyond childhood, but in the 1990s we began to see adults coming to physicians asking to be evaluated for ADHD and treated with medication. This was in part a result of several books, including one with the evocative title *Driven to Distraction* (Hallowell and Ratey 1994), along with a spate of popular articles that publicized the disorder. Adults would come to physicians and say, "My son is ADHD and I was just like him," "I can't get my life organized, I must have ADHD," or "I know I'm ADHD, I read it in a book." Since Ritalin for adult attention problems is an off-label use of the medication, the pharmaceutical companies cannot directly advertise either the disorder or its treatment, but there are other ways to publicize the disorder: There are any number of Internet Web sites describing adult ADHD and its treatment, and the advocacy group Children and Adults with Attention Deficit and Hyperactivity Disorder (CHAAD) has become a strong advocate for identifying and treating adult ADHD. It is well known that CHAAD gets most of its funding from the drug industry. Even so, CHAAD is a consumer-oriented group and, along with adults seeking ADHD treatment, has become a major force in what I have called elsewhere "the medicalization of underperformance" (Conrad and Potter 2000).

Adult ADHD is only one example of what Barsky and Boros (1995) have identified as the public's decreased tolerance for mild symptoms and benign problems. Individuals' self-medicalization is becoming increasingly common, with patients taking their troubles to physicians and often asking directly for a specific medical solution. A prominent example of this has been the increasing medicalization of unhappiness (Shaw and Woodward 2004) and expansive treatment with antidepressants.

Nonprofit consumer groups like CHAAD, National Alliance for the Mentally Ill (NAMI), and the Human Growth Foundation have become strong supporters for medical treatments for the human problems for which they advocate. These consumer advocacy groups are comprised of families, patients, and others concerned with the particular disorder. However, these consumer groups are often supported financially by pharmaceutical companies. CHAAD received support from Novartis, manufacturer of Ritalin; the Human Growth Foundation is at least in part funded by Genentech and Eli Lilly, makers of the hGH drugs; and NAMI receives over $6 million a year from pharmaceutical companies (Mindfreedom Online 2004). Spokespeople from such groups often take strong stances supporting pharmaceutical research and treatment, raising the question of where consumer advocates begin and pharmaceutical promotion ends. This reflects the power of corporations in shaping and sometimes co-opting advocacy groups.

The Internet has become an important consumer vehicle. On the one hand, all pharmaceutical companies and most advocacy groups have Web sites replete with consumer-oriented information. These often include self-administered screening tests to help individuals decide whether they may have a particular disorder or benefit from some medical treatment. In addition, there are thousands of bulletin boards, chat rooms, and Web pages where individuals can share information about illness, treatments, complaints, and services (Hardey 2001). This has for many individuals transformed illness from a privatized to a more public experience. On these Web sites people suffering from similar ailments can connect and share information in new ways, which, despite the pitfalls of misinformation, empower them as consumers of medical care. Both corporate and grassroots Web sites can generate an increased demand for services and disseminate medical perspectives far beyond professional or even national boundaries.

In our current medical age, consumers have become increasingly vocal and active in their desire and demand for services. Individuals as consumers rather than patients help shape the scope, and sometimes the demand for, medical treatments for human problems.[2]

Managed Care

Over the past two decades, managed care organizations have come to dominate health care delivery in the United States largely in response to rising health care costs. Managed care requires preapprovals for medical treatment and sets limits on some types of care. This has given third-party payers more leverage and often constrained both the care given by doctors and the care received by patients. To a degree, managed care has commercialized medicine and encouraged medical care organizations and doctors to emphasize profits over patient care. But this is complex, for in some instances managed care constrains medical care and in other cases provides incentives for more profitable care.

In terms of medicalization, managed care is both an incentive and a constraint. This is clearly seen in the psychiatric realm. Managed care has severely reduced the amount of insurance coverage for psychotherapy available to individuals with mental and emotional problems (Shore and Beigal 1996), but it has been much more liberal with paying for psychiatric medications. Thus managed care has become a factor in the increasing uses of psychotropic medications among adults and children (Goode 2002). It seems likely that physicians prescribe pharmaceutical treatment for psychiatric disorders knowing that these are the types of medical interventions covered under managed care plans, accelerating psychotropic treatments for human problems.

In the 1980s I would frequently say to my students that one of the limits on the medicalization of obesity is that Blue Cross/Blue Shield (then a dominant insurance/managed care company) would not pay for gastric bypass operations. This is no longer the case. Many managed care organizations have concluded that it is a better financial investment to cover gastric bypass surgery for a "morbidly obese" person than to pay for the treatment of all the potential medical sequelae including diabetes, stroke, heart conditions, and muscular skeletal problems. The number of gastric bypass and similar surgeries in the United States has risen from 20,000 in 1965 to 103,000 in 2003, with 144,000 projected for 2004 (Grady 2003). In the context of the so-called obesity epidemic (Abelson and Kennedy 2004), bypass operations are becoming an increasingly common way to treat the problem of extreme overweight, with the threshold for treatment decreasing and becoming more inclusive. The recent Medicare policy shift declaring obesity as a disease could further expand the number of medical claims for the procedure. As the *New York Times* recently reported, "the surgery has become big business and medical centers are scrambling to start programs" (Grady 2003: D1).

But managed care organizations affect medicalization by what they don't cover as well. When there is a demand for certain procedures and insurance coverage is not forthcoming, private markets for treatment emerge (Conrad and Leiter 2004). As noted earlier, prior to this year, hGH was only approved for the very few children with a growth hormone deficiency. The FDA approval of Humatrope expanded the number of children eligible for growth hormone treatment by 400,000. It will be interesting to see whether managed care organizations will cover the expensive hGH treatments for these children.

In effect, managed care is a selective double-edged sword for medicalization. Viagra and erectile dysfunction provides an interesting example; some managed care organizations' drug benefits cover (with co-pays) either four or six pills a month. While it is unclear how these insurance companies came up with these figures, it seems evident that managed care strictures both bolster and constrain the medicalization of male sexual dysfunction. Increasingly, though, managed care organizations are an arbiter of what is deemed medically appropriate or inappropriate treatment.

MEDICALIZATION IN THE NEW MILLENNIUM

The engines behind increasing medicalization are shifting from the medical profession, interprofessional or organizational contests, and social movements and interest groups to biotechnology,

consumers, and managed care organizations. Doctors are still gatekeepers for medical treatment, but their role has become more subordinate in the expansion or contraction of medicalization. In short, the engines of medicalization have proliferated and are now driven more by commercial and market interests than by professional claims-makers.

The definitional center of medicalization remains constant, but the availability and promotion of new pharmaceutical and potential genetic treatments are increasing drivers for new medical categories (cf. Horwitz 2002). While it is still true that medicalization is not technologically determined, commercial and corporate stakeholders play a major role in how the technology will or won't be framed. For example, if a new pharmaceutical treatment comes to market, the drug industry may well pursue the promotion of new or underused medical definitions to legitimate their product (e.g., Paxil and SAD/GAD), attempt to change the definitions of a disorder (e.g., hGH and idiopathic short stature), or expand the definitions and lower the treatment threshold of an existing medicalized problem (e.g., Viagra and erectile dysfunction). Thus drug companies are having an increasing impact on the boundaries of the normal and the pathological, becoming active agents of social control. This is worrisome for a number of reasons, but perhaps especially "because corporations are ultimately more responsible to their shareholders than to patients; shareholder desires are often at odds with patients' needs for rational drug prescribing" (Wilkes, Bell, and Kravitz 2000). It may well be to the shareholders' advantage for pharmaceutical companies to promote medications for an ever-increasing array of human problems, but this in no way insures that these constitute improvements in health and medical care. And what is the impact of the new engines of medicalization on the rising costs of health care?

In a culture of increasingly market-driven medicine, consumers, biotechnological corporations, and medical services interact in complex ways that affect social norms in changing definitions of behaviors and interventions. The relationship between normative changes and medicalization runs in both directions. For example, changing norms about breast augmentation are one cause of medicalization, while at the same time the processes of medicalization themselves lead to changes in the social norms surrounding breast enhancements. Similarly, advertisements for Viagra have destigmatized male erectile dysfunction, while a normalized notion of erectile dysfunction has increased the consumer demand for Viagra.

I would be remiss if I did not note the gendered nature of much corporatized medicalization. This should be no surprise, since women's bodies have long been objects of medical control (Riska 2003). We are now seeing the expansion of largely gendered markets for medicalization, such as Viagra and Ritalin for males and Prozac and cosmetic surgery for females (e.g., Blum and Stracuzzi 2004). And there may be more coming, with growing markets for andropause and baldness targeting men (Szymczak and Conrad 2006) and the pharmaceutical industry's ardent search for a female equivalent of Viagra (Hartley and Tiefer 2003). While corporate medicalizers might wish to include both men and women to increase their market potential, gender segmentation is a propitious strategy for defining problems and promoting medical solutions, both exploiting and reinforcing gender boundaries.

Medicalization is prevalent in the United States, but it is increasingly an international phenomenon. This is partly the result of the expanding hegemony of western biomedicine, but it is facilitated by multinational drug companies and the global reach of mass media and the Internet. As McKinlay and Marceau (2002) note, "Transnational corporations involved in the globalization of medicine (pharmaceuticals, services, medical insurance, and biotechnology) generate local demand for services . . ." (p. 399). The pharmaceutical companies' introduction and promotion of "mild depression" as an illness in Japan has resulted in a dramatic rise in SSRI treatment since 1999 (Schulz 2004). Furthermore, cyberspace knows no national boundaries, expediting the dissemination of medical knowledge, commercial promotion, and consumer desires. Perspectives that germinate in Boston today are available in Cairo or Moscow by the evening and in Calcutta and Yogyakarta, Indonesia, the next day. We have no idea yet what the Internet's impact is on the local and global nature of medical categories and treatments, but it is a safe assumption that medicalization will increase with globalization.

Professional and public concern about medicalization may be growing as well. The *British Medical Journal* (2002) devoted nearly an entire issue to medicalization topics, and we increasingly see the term medicalization used in the popular press. For years when I talked with people about medicalization I would always need to explain in detail what I meant. Now most people quickly understand what the term means. But despite the increased awareness and openness to the issue, we also need to develop our own understandings of medicalization in new and deeper ways.

I close with a challenge to sociologists. We need to shift our attention in medicalization research and study the emergent engines of medicalization. This means examining the impact of biotechnological discoveries, the influence of pharmaceutical industry marketing and promotion, the role of consumer demand, the facilitating and constraining aspects of managed care and health insurance, the impact of the Internet, the changing role of the medical profession and physicians, and the pockets of medical and popular resistance to medicalization. This means supplementing our social constructionist studies with political economic perspectives. Medicalization still doesn't occur without social actors doing something to make an entity medical, but the engines that are driving medicalization have changed and we need to refocus our sociological eye as the medicalization train moves into the twenty-first century.

ACKNOWLEDGMENTS

This is a revised version of the 2004 Leo G. Reeder Award lecture presented at the meetings of the American Sociological Association, August 16, 2004, in San Francisco, California. My thanks to Renee Anspach, Charles Bosk, Libby Bradshaw, Phil Brown, Stefan Timmermans, and the anonymous reviewers for comments on an earlier version of this article.

Notes

1. While this ambitious and analytically dense paper has many virtues, in my judgment, Clarke et al. (2003) lose sight of the process of medicalization itself. The authors are certainly correct in many of their contentions. It seems clear that the biotechnological and pharmaceutical industries—especially in the areas of scientific and commercial discoveries in genetics, neuroscience, and pharmacology—will have an increasing impact on the medicalization of human problems. The extension of "medical jurisdiction over health itself and the commodification of health" are seen as parts of medicalization, especially through risk factors and medical surveillance. They see the shift to biomedicalization as moving from medical control over external nature to controlling and transforming inner nature. These all seem to me to be astute observations. However, in the Clarke et al. conception one is hard-pressed to identify something related to biotechnology and medicine that is not part of biomedicalization.

   Further, the claim that the biomedicalization change represents a shift from modernity to postmodernity depends entirely on what one considers as postmodern. As Anspach (2003) points out, "Efforts to rationalize health care through data banks and practice guidelines may actually represent the new forms of bureaucratization, a quintessentially modern, rather than postmodern, phenomenon" (unpaged). Given its reliance on a scientific knowledge base and its bureaucratic organization, it is difficult to see biomedicine as predominantly a postmodern enterprise.

2. It is my contention that the consumer orientation toward medical care has expanded, subsuming or reorienting some of the social movements promoting medicalization. Moreover, there is an increasing amount of public and media promotion of health care products, procedures, and services that further spurs medicalization (including medications, surgical procedures, and other treatments). These are aimed at individuals, not as patients but as consumers.

References

Abelson, Phillip and Donald Kennedy. 2004. "The Obesity Epidemic." *Science* 304(June 4):1413.

American Psychiatric Association. 1994. *Diagnostic and Statistical Manual of Mental Disorders.* 4th ed. Washington, DC: American Psychiatric Association.

American Society for Aesthetic Plastic Surgery. 2004. Retrieved July 15, 2004 (http://www .surgery.org/press/news.release.php? iid5325).

Anspach, Renee. 2003. "Gender and Health Care." Department of Sociology, University of Michigan, Ann Arbor, MI. Unpublished manuscript.

Armstrong, David. 1995. "The Rise of Surveillance Medicine." *Sociology of Health and Illness* 17:393–404.

Barsky, Arthur J. and Jonathan F. Borus. 1995. "Somatization and Medicalization in the Era of Managed Care." *Journal of the American Medical Association* 274:1931–34.

Blum, Linda M. and Nena F. Stracuzzi. 2004. "Gender in the Prozac Nation: Popular Discourse and Productive Femininity." *Gender and Society* 18(3):269–86.

British Medical Journal. 2002. Special Issue on Medicalization. 234(7342):859–926.

Carpiano, Richard M. 2001. "Passive Medicalization: The Case of Viagra and Erectile Dysfunction." *Sociological Symposium* 21:441–50.

Clarke, Adele E., Janet K. Shim, Laura Mamo, Jennifer Ruth Fosket, and Jannifer R. Fishman. 2003. "Biomedicalization: Technoscientific Transformations of Health, Illness, and U.S. Biomedicine." *American Sociological Review* 68:161–94.

Conrad, Peter. 1975. "The Discovery of Hyperkinesis: Notes on the Medicalization of Deviant Behavior." *Social Problems* 32:12–21.

_____. 1992. "Medicalization and Social Control." *Annual Review of Sociology* 18:209–32.

_____. 1997. "Public Eyes and Private Genes: Historical Frames, News Constructions and Social Problems." *Social Problems* 44:139–54.

_____. 1999. "A Mirage of Genes." *Sociology of Health and Illness* 21:228–41.

_____. 2000. "Genetics, Medicalization and Human Problems." Pp. 322–33 in *The Handbook of Medical Sociology*, 5th ed., edited by Chloe Bird, Peter Conrad, and Alan Fremont. Upper Saddle River, NJ: Prentice Hall.

Conrad, Peter and Heather Jacobson. 2003. "Enhancing Biology? Cosmetic Surgery and Breast Augmentation." Pp. 223–34 in *Debating Biology: Sociological Reflections on Health, Medicine and Society*, edited by Simon J. Williams, Gilliam A. Bendelow, and Linda Berke. London: Routledge.

Conrad, Peter and Valerie Leiter. 2004. "Medicalization, Markets, and Consumers." *Journal of Health and Social Behavior* 45 (extra issue):158–76.

Conrad, Peter and Deborah Potter. 2000. "From Hyperactive Children to ADHD Adults: Observations on the Expansion of Medical Categories." *Social Problems* 47:59–82.

_____. 2004. "Human Growth Hormone and the Temptations of Biomedical Enhancement." *Sociology of Health and Illness* 26:184–215.

Conrad, Peter and Joseph W. Schneider. [1980] 1992. *Deviance and Medicalization: From Badness to Sickness.* Expanded ed. Philadelphia, PA: Temple University Press.

Elliott, Carl. 2003. *Better than Well: American Medicine Meets the American Dream.* New York: Norton.

Fox, Patrick. 1989. "From Senility to Alzheimer's Disease: The Rise of the Alzheimer's Disease Movement." *Milbank Quarterly* 67:57–101.

Freidson, Eliot. 1970. *Profession of Medicine.* New York: Dodd, Mead.

Freudenheim, Milt. 2004. "Behavior Drugs Lead in Sales for Children." *New York Times*, May 17, p. A9.

Fukuyama, Francis. 2002. *Our Posthuman Future: Consequences of the Biotechnology Revolution.* New York: Picador.

Gallagher, Eugene B. and C. Kristina Sionean. 2004. "Where Medicalization Boulevard Meets Commercialization Alley." *Journal of Policy Studies* 16:3–62.

Goode, Erica. 2002. "Psychotherapy Shows a Rise over Decade, but Time Falls." *New York Times*, November 6, p. A21.

Grady, Denise. 2003. "Operations for Obesity Leaves Some in Misery." *New York Times*, May 4, p. D1.

Hallowell, Edward M. and John J. Ratey. 1994. *Driven to Distraction.* New York: Pantheon.

Halpern, Sydney. 1990. "Medicalization as a Professional Process: Post War Trends in Pediatrics." *Journal of Health and Social Behavior* 31:28–42.

Hardey, Michael. 2001. "'E-Health': The Internet and the Transformation of Patients to Consumers and Producers of Health Knowledge." *Information, Communication and Society* 4:388–405.

Hartley, Heather and Leonore Tiefer. 2003. "Taking a Biological Turn: The Push for a 'Female

Viagra' and the Medicalization of Women's Sexual Problems." *Women's Studies Quarterly* 31(spring/summer):42–54.

Healy, David. 1998. *The Anti-depressant Era.* Cambridge, MA: Harvard University Press.

Horwitz, Allan V. 2002. *Creating Mental Illness.* Chicago, IL: University of Chicago Press.

Illich, Ivan. 1975. *Medical Nemesis.* New York: Pantheon.

IMS Health. 2004. "IMS Reports 11.5 Percent Dollar Growth in U.S. Prescription Sales." Retrieved July 15, 2004 (http://www.ims-health.com/ims/portal/front/articleC/0,2777,6599_3665_44771558,00. html).

Inlander, Charles B. 1998. "Consumer Health." *Social Policy* 28(3):40–42.

Jacobson, Nora. 2000. *Cleavage: Technology, Controversy, and the Ironies of the Man-Made Breast.* New Brunswick, NJ: Rutgers University Press.

Koerner, Brendan I. 2002. "Disorders, Made to Order." *Mother Jones* 27:58–63.

Kroll-Smith, Steve and H. Hugh Floyd. 1997. *Bodies in Protest: Environmental Illness and the Struggle over Medical Knowledge.* New York: New York University Press.

Light, Donald W. 1993. "Countervailing Power: The Changing Character of the Medical Profession in the United States." Pp. 69–80 in *The Changing Medical Profession: An International Perspective*, edited by F. W. Hafferty and J. B. McKinlay. New York: Oxford University Press.

Loe, Meika. 2001. "Fixing Broken Masculinity: Viagra Technology for the Production of Gender and Sexuality." *Sexuality and Culture* 5:97–125.

Marino, Vivian. 2002. "All Those Commercials Pay Off for Drug Makers." *New York Times*, February 24, sect. 3, p. 4.

Marshall, Eliot. 2004. "Antidepressants and Children: Buried Data Can be Hazardous to a Company's Health." *Science* 304(June 11):1576–77.

McKinlay, John B. and Lisa D. Marceau. 2000. "The End of the Golden Age of Doctoring." *International Journal of Health Services* 32(2):379–416.

McLeod, Jane D., Bernice A. Pescosolido, David T. Takeuchi, and Terry Falkenberg White. 2004. "Public Attitudes toward the Use of Psychiatric Medications for Children." *Journal of Health and Social Behavior* 45:53–67.

Mindfreedom Online. 2004. Retrieved July 15, 2004 (www.mindfreedom.org).

Olfson, Mark, S. C. Marcus, M. M. Weissman, and P. S. Jenson. 2002. "National Trends in the Use of Psychotropic Medications by Children." *Journal of the American Academy of Child and Adolescent Psychiatry* 41:514–21.

Pawluch, Dorothy. 1983. "Transitions in Pediatrics: A Segmental Analysis." *Social Problems* 30: 449–65.

Public Citizen. 2003. "2002 Drug Industry Profits: Hefty Pharmaceutical Company Margins Dwarf Other Industries." Retrieved July 15, 2004 (www.citizen.org/documents/Pharma_Report.pdf).

Relman, Arnold S. and Marcia Angell. 2002. "America's Other Drug Problem." *New Republic*, December 16, pp. 27–41.

Riska, Elianne. 2003. "Gendering the Medicalization Thesis." *Advances in Gender Research* 7:61–89.

Rosenthal, Meredith B., Ernst R. Berndt, Julie M. Donohue, Richard G. Frank, and Arnold M. Epstein. 2002. "Promotion of Prescription Drugs to Consumers." *New England Journal of Medicine* 346:498–505.

Rothman, Sheila M. and David J. Rothman. 2003. *The Pursuit of Perfection: The Promise and Perils of Medical Enhancement.* New York: Pantheon.

Schulz, Kathryn. 2004. "Did Antidepressants Depress Japan?" *New York Times Magazine*, August 22, pp. 38–41.

Scott, Wilbur J. 1990. "PTSD in DMS-III: A Case of the Politics of Diagnosis and Disease." *Social Problems* 37:294–310.

Shaw, Ian and Louise Woodward. 2004. "The Medicalization of Unhappiness? The Management of Mental Distress in Primary Care." In *Constructions of Health and Illness: European Perspectives*, edited by Ian Shaw and Kaisa Kauppinen. Aldershot, United Kingdom: Ashgate Press.

Shore, Miles F. and A. Beigal. 1996. "The Challenges Posed by Managed Behavioral Health Care." *New England Journal of Medicine* 334:116–18.

Starr, Paul. 1982. *The Social Transformation of American Medicine.* New York: Basic.

Sullivan, Deborah A. 2001. *Cosmetic Surgery: The Cutting Edge of Commercial Medicine in America.* New Brunswick, NJ: Rutgers University Press.

Szasz, Thomas. 1970. *Manufacture of Madness.* New York: Dell.

Szymczak, Julia E. and Peter Conrad. Forthcoming. "Medicalizing the Aging Male Body: Andropause and Baldness." In *Medicalized Masculinities*, edited by Dana Rosenfeld and Christopher Faircloth. Philadelphia, PA: Temple University Press.

Tuller, David. 2004. "Gentlemen, Start Your Engines." *New York Times*, June 21, p. F1.

Wertz, Richard and Dorothy Wertz. 1989. *Lying In: A History of Childbirth in America.* Expanded ed. New Haven, CT: Yale University Press.

Wilkes, Michael S., Robert A. Bell, Richard L. Kravitz. 2000. "Direct-to-Consumer Prescription Drug Advertising: Trends, Impact, and Implications." *Health Affairs* 19(2):110–28.

Zimmerman, Susan. 1998. *Silicone Survivors: Women's Experiences with Breast Implants.* Philadelphia, PA: Temple University Press.

Zola, Irving Kenneth. 1972. "Medicine as an Institution of Social Control." *Sociological Review* 20:487–504.

THE BEST LAID PLANS?

Women's Choices, Expectations and Experiences in Childbirth

Claudia Malacrida and Tiffany Boulton

INTRODUCTION

Over the past few decades, there has been an increase in the medicalization of childbirth, as evidenced by spikes in the rate of Caesarean sections (C-section) performed in many Western countries (Cherniak and Fisher, 2008; Lobel and DeLuca, 2007). In a rare moment of congruence, alternative health-care providers, feminist advocates for women's health and most recently, mainstream medical service providers have all expressed concerns about the rise in C-section rates (CSRs). However, this concern stems in each instance from divergent philosophical positions as well as differing assumptions about the causes for increasing CSRs (Lee and Kirkman, 2008). For natural (or alternative) birth advocates, rising CSRs reflect a medicalization of birth that limits women's control over their bodies, causing anxiety that in turn reduces women's natural capacity for birthing (Mansfield, 2008). Along similar lines, for feminists, the rise in CSRs reflects an increasing encroachment by technocratic and masculinist medicine over women's bodies in ways that disempower and alienate women while increasing medicine's power and reach (Beckett, 2005; Lee and Kirkman, 2008). Conversely, for those medical practitioners who have raised alarms about rising CSRs, the root of the problem is seen to lie in modern women's consumerist attitudes, where birth choices are moving too far into the hands of women who seek an easier birth on their terms without taking medical risks adequately into account (ACOG Committee, 2007; Klein, 2007; Minkoff et al., 2006; Robson et al., 2008). Embedded in each of these arguments, and despite their divergent imputed causal agents, there is an understanding that *someone*—either a doctor or a mother—is driving the CSR 'machine'. Furthermore, in these debates, there is a recurring assumption that women have, or should have, choices over the kinds of births they will experience and they can or should manage those choices by planning and preparing responsibly.

Drawing on elements of this debate, and particularly addressing the embedded arguments that modern birthing experiences are consumer driven because women have the capacity to plan for, make decisions about and choose a particular type of birth experience, we interviewed 22 recent mothers about their birthing choices, their expectations and their birth experiences. We did so in an attempt to understand how informed choice, consumer ideologies and medical influences interacted in the women's birth 'decisions' prior to and during birth. We asked women to tell us about their birth plans and experiences to examine tensions between women's choices and women's actual experiences of giving birth and to challenge assumptions about women's capacity to 'drive the machine' of birth, whether medicalized or natural.

Before we engage with the interview data, however, it is important to outline the contours of the C-section debates and to examine the implications of risk assessment and childbirth 'choices'. In the following, we articulate three contested positions concerning birth and intervention: medical perspectives, alternative and natural birth advocacy and feminist critiques (Lee and Kirkman, 2008). We recognize that the distinctions between these three perspectives are somewhat blurred, particularly in terms of feminist and natural birth perspectives. However, it is clear in the professional, lay and academic literature that contentions between these groups are persistent and form the contested backdrop against which women's birthing choices must be made.

Medical Perspectives on Birth

That birth has become increasingly medicalized in developed nations is clear, as is exemplified by increasing CSRs. In 1970, in Canada, the United States and Australia, the CSR was approximately 6 per cent (Cherniak and Fisher, 2008). In the intervening years, this rate has increased over fourfold: in Canada, in 2005, the CSR was 26.3 per cent (Canadian Institute for Health Information [CIHI], 2009); in the United States, in 2004, it was 29.1 per cent (Martin et al., 2006) and in 2007, in Australia, it was 28.5 per cent (Cherniak and Fisher, 2008).

The responses of medical practitioners to these shifts are varied. Many mainstream medical practitioners are supportive of medically managed birth, arguing that obstetricians rarely choose intervention needlessly and that medical intervention and C-sections, particularly when doctor driven, are life saving and risk reducing (Lee and Kirkman, 2008). However, from the perspective of some medical practitioners, these increases are alarming because of negative maternal and infant health outcomes attached to Caesarean delivery (Borgwardt et al., 2009; Dunn et al., 2009; Robson et al., 2008). Risks to the mother include pulmonary and circulatory problems, post-partum infections, evisceration and long-term risks associated with uterine scarring and weakening; risks to the child include surgical injuries and prematurity and poor lung development if fetal age calculations are inaccurate (Beil, 2008; Kotz, 2008). Medical practitioners also express concerns that women are not opting for medicalized birth to avoid real medical risks but are acting as consumers seeking an easier, controlled and pain-free experience (Lee and Kirkman, 2008). Indeed, recent issues of the *British Medical Journal* (*BMJ*) and *The Journal of Obstetrics and Gynaecology* were dedicated to the problem of increased CSRs, with most articles concluding that women were overstepping their patient role by pushing for inappropriate medicalization without a proper (i.e. doctor driven) assessment of the risks attached to C-section (Edwards and Davies, 2001; Irvine, 2001). A second *BMJ* special issue debated the connection between social class and elective C-sections, reflecting public discourse that characterizes many women who undergo C-sections as simply 'too posh to push' (Grant, 2004; Macfarlane, 2004). In these arguments, there is a clear sense that women, as medical consumers, are in a position to plan and execute the kind of birth experience they choose and that they are capable of and responsible for assessing and assuming the risks attendant with those choices.

Alternative or Natural Birth Advocacy Perspectives on Birth

While the use of technology in birth has become typical in Western cultures, it has also been critically linked by some to increasing medical control and authority over birth and the rise in CSRs (Davis-Floyd, 2004). Thus, natural or alternative birth advocates argue that the medical model focuses too heavily on the risks of birth, instilling fear in women and preventing them from fully embracing their natural ability to give birth (Mansfield, 2008). From this perspective, the increase in CSRs reflects the escalating medicalization of childbirth and how medical authority over birth takes away women's natural capacity (Lavender and Kingdon, 2006). In this view, the hospital setting is seen as, at the very least, contributing to rises in surgical interventions, because once a birthing woman enters a hospital, there is a seemingly natural 'transfer of power and responsibility for birth from a woman to her doctor' (Brubaker and Dillaway, 2009: 36).

In the early 1980s, Sally Inch (1982) and Sheila Kitzinger (1981) described a 'cascade of intervention', which begins with fetal heart monitoring and leads to progressively increasing intervention. Building on this idea, natural birth advocates (and feminists) have argued that the increasing rates of Caesarean births are not driven by maternal requests but are instead the outcome of the cascade of interventions that can occur in hospital births. Here, routine medical practices such as fetal monitoring, oxytocin induction and epidurals increase surveillance of the mother and, critically, can cause labour to stall, instigating the need for surgical interventions that might not have been necessary had the birth been allowed to proceed naturally (Diniz and Chacham, 2004; Irvine, 2001; Marx et al., 2001).

According to the natural birth perspective, a midwife-attended, intervention-free home birth is the 'gold standard', as it allows women to give birth in the way birth is 'meant' to be, and it is considered the safest option for the mother and for the baby (Beckett and Hoffman, 2005; Cheyney, 2008). Similar to the medical perspective, there is an embedded assumption that women can plan their birth process and manage the outcome by choosing a midwife or doula to attend hospital births, opting for home birthing or using methods such as hypnotherapy, water birthing, meditation or any number of birthing 'systems' such as Lamaze or the Bradley method. At the very least, women are encouraged to increase their likelihood of achieving a natural birth through constructing a *Birth Plan* (a detailed document outlining which procedures will be acceptable to the mother throughout labour and what limits the medical team should respect in terms of interventions at various stages in the process). These efforts in the natural/alternative discourse are seen as tools with which women can reduce the impositions of the medical model on the ideal, intervention-free birth, again reflecting an assumption that women have the capacity to plan and implement birth 'choices'.

Feminist Perspectives on Birth

Along similar lines to natural birth advocates, many feminists agree that medical dominance over all aspects of pregnancy and birth has served to undercut women's control and autonomy over their bodies and the birthing process (Kukla, 2005; Lane, 1996; Oakley, 1984). The medical model argument that women are using their consumer power to push for elective Caesarean sections—and that this is what is driving the rise in surgical births—is seen as problematic given the degree of medical authority over birth. Despite these critiques of the medical model, some feminists argue that the natural childbirth movement romanticizes 'natural' childbirth and thus has its own moral imperatives (Brubaker and Dillaway, 2009; Wolf, 2001); others have argued that the particulars of women's births are less important than that women should have real choice and control in making decisions about their birth experiences (Beckett, 2005; Bergeron, 2007). Indeed, critics argue that the strong promotion of a medication-free birth as the ideal is likely to be experienced by women as disciplining and controlling rather than empowering (Beckett, 2005; Brubaker and Dillaway, 2009; Crossley, 2007). In addition, the moral imperative to give birth naturally means that women who are unable to achieve this are likely to feel as though they have failed (Clift-Matthews, 2010). The feminist critique, with its understanding that birth 'choices' are clouded and that women's power and autonomy is compromised in both medical and natural births, is perhaps the least likely of the three perspectives to assume that women can and will be able to control their birth outcomes, although there remains a belief that women *should* have more choice and control. We take up this feminist, critical approach to inform our understanding of women's bodies, choices and risk management, drawing on the perspectives of women themselves.

Choice, Risk and Birth

Embedded in the debates about increasing CSRs are two key assumptions: first, at least some of these procedures are planned or unnecessary, and second, mothers are able to exercise considerable agency in choosing to have a natural, medical or self-directed style of birth (Anonymous, 2005; Edwards and Davies, 2001). Both of these assumptions are problematic. On a mundane level, figures on CSRs do not provide breakdowns between elective (itself a term without clear medical boundaries), emergency and planned C-sections, making it difficult to differentiate C-sections 'on request' from medically mandated procedures, let alone understand who or what drives those outcomes. More importantly, for the purposes of this article, the notion of an autonomous, fully informed, ideal medical consumer, who is not only capable of evaluating medical information but can also *implement* her informed choices, is a thorny one because women's choice has 'always been politically constrained . . . and shaped by hegemonic discursive orders and social practices that privilege the interests of one group of those over the individual' (McAra-Couper et al., 2011: 82).

In terms of risk and choice in the medical encounter, Michel Foucault's concept of governmentality is informative; he argued that individuals' actions, choices and self-concepts in relation to health and risk are informed, constrained and constructed through discourses emanating from medical, scientific, public and lay institutions and relationships (Foucault, 1991; Lupton, 2012). Ideas about what constitutes the ideal medical consumer, the imperative of the endlessly responsible mother, the authoritative position of medicine generally, the authority of the medical practitioner in the moment of the medical encounter and the idea of the innocent, precious and always vulnerable child are all discourses that weigh down upon and make complicated women's decisions (Crossley, 2007; Lupton, 2011, 2012; Malacrida and Boulton, 2012). Nevertheless, women are charged with—and themselves take up—the responsibility of making informed and conscientious birthing choices through engaging in 'reflexive modernity', characterized by collecting information about, understanding and evaluating risks and then working to minimize those risks (Lupton, 1999a; McCourt et al., 2007). This individualized model of risk assessment is particularly troubling given the contradictory feminist, natural and medical discourses about what constitutes the 'ideal birth' and what the benefits of natural versus medicalized birth are for women and, even more emphatically, their babies.

Women's attempts to evaluate and manage risk during childbirth, while framed as an individualized choice and responsibility, occur within a set of structural and social conditions. Among these is the reality that birth is an experience that is embedded in unequal power and knowledge relations between women and their medical caregivers, occurring within the organization of birth services that may privilege medicalized births or medical priorities and within an increasingly technocratic set of practices relating to childbirth more generally (Crossley, 2007; Lane, 1996; McAra-Couper et al., 2011). In this framing, women's knowledge of risk and their capacity to evaluate it are made within medical systems that are resistant to disclosures about medical practices or interests. The combination of an increasingly technocratic medical approach to birthing, an individualized and blaming model of patient/consumer risk evaluation and the contested discourses concerning the 'ideal' way of giving birth can make patient 'choice' and risk evaluation more difficult than usual. Finally, childbirth itself is not a predictable experience, and this can mean that consumer 'choices' can become irrelevant or come under tremendous pressures in the labour and delivery process.

These tensions concerning knowledge and responsibility about risk and choice led us to ask women about their reasons for preferring a particular type of birth, their intentions about their birth prior to labour and delivery, their expectations about birth and their actual experiences of birth and choice.

METHODOLOGY

We conducted qualitative, semi-structured, narrative interviews with 22 recent (during the previous 3 years) mothers, as part of a larger project examining the culture of birthing in Southern Alberta, Canada. Narrative interviews draw on feminist standpoint theories, which argue that it is crucial to understand the workings of discourse and power from the positions of those who are most oppressed by them. Because women are made responsible for birthing choices yet lack control over them, we anticipated that by asking women about their expectations, plans, choices and birth outcomes from their own perspectives, we would be best able to illuminate the tensions embedded in the expectations of women as birthing consumers/risk managers and their actual experiences in the medical encounter. As feminist narrative theorists have argued, by starting where women live and enquiring about social situations from women's perspectives, researchers are best able to understand how relations of power operate in women's lives (Smith, 1987; Sosulski, 2010). Additionally, narrative methods have the power to reclaim and refashion knowledge by offering individuals an opportunity to bear witness to their experience, to affirm personal perspectives, re-author experiences and challenge dominant discourses (Frank, 2002; Sakalys, 2000; Thomas, 2010). Thus, asking the women in this study to tell their stories of becoming and being mothers was a means of generating an emancipatory knowledge about choice, risk and responsibility in terms of birth choices and CSRs.

Participants were recruited in the city of Lethbridge and its surrounding communities, allowing for both urban and rural women to be included in this study. The Lethbridge Regional Hospital, where the majority of the women gave birth, has a CSR (27.4%) that is in keeping with national levels (CIHI, 2009). The women were recruited through support groups, email lists, public postings and snowball sampling. They ranged in age from 24 to 40 years, were predominantly middle classed and all identified as heterosexual; all but one were in committed relationships to their children's fathers. Their educations ranged from completing 10th grade to holding a medical degree, and their occupations ranged from living on disability pension to running a medical practice. Most of the women were born in Southern Alberta, all but one were Caucasian, and most identified as Christian or agnostic, so that there are significant racial, ethnic and cultural limitations to the sample.

Of the 22 women, only one indicated from the outset that she had arranged a planned Caesarean section. Because her perspectives on choice and planning sit so far outside the range of the rest of the women's insights, we have excluded her data from this article. The remaining 21 women all indicated a preference for as intervention-free a birth as possible, a topic we discuss more fully in the following. However, 11 of them experienced emergency Caesarean sections, and with the exception of two women who gave birth without any interventions, the remainder experienced medical treatments ranging from pain medication and epidurals to inductions and episiotomies.

Ethical Considerations

Prior to data collection, we obtained university ethics approval. All participants were fully informed about what their participation in the research would entail during our first contacts and in the interviews. Prior to each interview, we obtained informed consent, assuring participants of anonymity and confidentiality in data presentation and informing participants that they could withdraw from the research at any time without negative repercussions. Participants were offered the possibility of interview debriefing within a support group or counselling setting; none of the interviewees requested this service. Indeed, the women appeared to be generally positively affected by the opportunity to discuss their experiences.

Data Collection and Analysis

One of the research objectives of this study was to examine how circulating discourses about 'ideal' birth—whether 'natural' or medicalized—had influenced the women's expectations and plans concerning their own births. In addition, the interviews explored whether and how women engaged in planning for their births, what their birth expectations were prior to birth and how, if at all, women's expectations had changed subsequent to their children's births; sub-questions in the interview guide related to questions of risk, choice and decision-making. In the interviews, the women had the chance to respond to the interview questions at length and in their own words while exploring the specific issues outlined earlier. Interviewing women about their experiences and treating their insights as important sources of knowledge are rooted in feminist critiques of the traditional male-centred approach to research in the social sciences and the historical silencing of women's voices (Carter, 2010). Thus, engaging women in qualitative interviews is both individually and politically significant as it provides women with the rare opportunity to share their experiences from their own perspectives.

Data collection, transcription and analysis were completed through a team research approach, which can facilitate dialogue among multiple perspectives and result in a rich and nuanced analysis (Rogers-Dillon, 2005). Data were collected, coded and analysed reflectively, so that following initial interview transcription and coding, new questions and foci for enquiry and analysis were informed by emergent themes in the data; as the research project developed, we considered the data more deductively, adding depth and theoretical insight to our analysis (Fereday and Muir-Cochrane, 2005). Huberman and Miles (1998) argue that 'tighter designs' using a more theoretically informed analysis and offering a more explanatory approach are appropriate once the researcher has a grounded familiarity with the topic. Thus, we moved to a feminist theoretical framework to inform our analysis, taking women to be knowing subjects who offered meaningful and important insight into the workings of gender and knowledge in their lives. In the women's interviews, they were able to speak to questions of choice and their hopes and plans for specific kinds of birth and to compare those hopes to their actual birth outcomes. While findings for any qualitative research cannot be taken as generalizable, these accounts offer important insight into the tensions some women encountered between discourses of choice and responsibility and their actual childbirth experiences. We provide excerpts from this group in presenting our data in order to offer commentary from as many participants as possible, while also representing the core perceptions of the women we interviewed.

FINDINGS

As noted, in modern governmentality, it is assumed that women will be informed and active patients/consumers who are able to collect, evaluate and implement information and formulate informed birthing decisions. When we spoke with women about their birthing expectations, it was clear that they also ascribed to a model of patient/consumerism wherein they saw themselves as able to choose the kind of birth they would experience, and they understood themselves as responsible for planning and knowing about birth and its risks. Every woman we interviewed spoke about seeking information concerning birth from a very wide array of sources. All had attended prenatal classes and had received prenatal education books, both of which are free to mothers under publicly funded health care in Alberta. Additionally, they had all read popular books or magazines, viewed multiple on-line sources and spoken with family members and friends about what to expect in the birthing room. From the women's descriptions, it was clear that all the mothers spent considerable effort educating themselves and that most expected to make birthing choices based on that knowledge.

Efforts to Maximize 'Natural' Chances

As discussed elsewhere, prenatal education, both formal and informal, appeared to move most of the women towards choosing 'natural' birth (characterized as ranging from at-home, no pain medication or episiotomy to hospital based, with as little intervention as possible) (Malacrida and Boulton, 2012). Women spoke of 'natural birth' as 'less traumatic for the baby' (Shirley) or 'better for breastfeeding and bonding with the baby' (Carmen) or simply easier because 'you heal so much faster' (Stacy). Only four of the women described adopting a position of simply hoping things would turn out for the best, expressing faith in their physicians and in birth as a 'natural' process, but the remaining women had clear plans and expectations about how their birth would unfold. One of these women had arranged a planned elective C-section, but the remaining 18 'planners' described expectations firmly centred in the discourse of 'natural' birth as ideal. Although the primary hospital in the area of this study does not permit midwives to complete deliveries, two of the women chose midwives at another location and another six women chose to have a doula attend their births, expressing a belief that a doula or midwife would act as an advocate for them and hopefully increase their chances of having the kind of birth they hoped for. For example, Carmen said she 'researched, and researched and researched. And that's why I hired the doula. I was hoping for a natural birth, with no interventions—or the least amount possible'. Judith, reflecting this perspective, believed that the advocacy role of the doula was critical to reducing intervention because:

> I mean, you're at your most vulnerable then. You're not in a state of mind, you don't have. . . . Like, me sitting here right now, I would be able to say to a doctor, 'No, don't do that to me!' But in that position, you just can't. Like, maybe with a second birth, but not my first.

Judith's comments reflect an understanding that birth is something that can readily spin out of control and that doctors are to be defended against in the birthing process; in this interpretation, pain, worry about the baby and fatigue can all make resisting medical pressures difficult. Nevertheless, her choice of a doula reflects her understanding that it is her responsibility to ensure that safeguards are in place to avoid undesirable medical interventions.

Similar to Judith, many of the women assumed that their doulas' knowledge would provide a means of avoiding intervention. As Carmen noted, because of her presumed depth of experience, '[The doula] knew when to say 'Ok, time to go' so I wouldn't spend so much time in the hospital'. In her description, Carmen expressed an understanding that the longer she was in the hospital, the more likely would be her risk of having some sort of medical procedure; by waiting until the last moment to leave home, she hoped to ensure as natural a birth as possible.

In addition to hiring midwives and doulas, women adopted other strategies to maximize the potential for a natural birth. Three women chose to give birth in smaller local hospitals rather than the main city hospital in the region because they perceived these facilities to be less interventionist in orientation; none of the smaller centres have operating rooms in which to perform Caesarean sections so they transfer women to the larger hospital only when necessary. A further three women insisted on continuing seeing their general practitioners (GPs) throughout the term of their pregnancy rather than working with an obstetrician (which is typically recommended in Canadian hospitals) because they believed that seeing an obstetrician would invite more intervention than going with a family doctor. In each of these strategies—choosing a medical centre with limited facilities or opting for medical services from a less-qualified physician—we can see an ironic strategy. By choosing what to some might seem to be higher-risk medical services, these women were in actuality attempting to minimize their perceived risks of medical intervention.

A final means used by the women to manage their birth expectations came through the use of Birth Plans, a strategy that, as mentioned earlier, is firmly ascribed to by natural birthing advocates. In the region of this study, this tool is also strongly endorsed by mainstream birth educators; completing a Birth Plan is part of the standard prenatal course materials provided to mothers through government-subsidized health care in Alberta (Alberta Perinatal Health Program, 2007). In this effort, however, women's strategies reveal more ambiguity about their capacity to plan that one might expect. Despite that the prenatal classes encouraged all women to formulate a Birth Plan, several women described actively resisting such efforts. Stacy, for example, said,

> I didn't even bother with a Birth Plan because my girlfriend is a nurse, and she said, 'We don't follow your Birth Plan'. The prenatal classes just make it so ideal, like you can do what you want, whenever you want, but you can't. The nurses come in and they've done it a thousand times. They know.

For Stacy, the Birth Plan and its promise of control over the process are a chimera; from the outset, despite her wish for a natural birth and her assumption that the baby 'would just come out more or less naturally', there was already an acknowledgment that the outcome would be under medical knowledge and control. In contrast, Andrea decided against putting a Birth Plan in place so as to avoid not living up to expectations for a natural birth, saying, 'I don't want to set high expectations for myself and then feel like I didn't reach them'. For Andrea, although an intervention-free birth was what she held as ideal, reflecting the critique made by some feminists of hard-core natural birth advocacy, she also recognized the pressures of meeting that ideal as oppressive.

Most of the women did prepare Birth Plans, and these were described as a tool that would lay out their expectations of limiting medical intervention and help them to achieve the most 'natural' birth possible. While some women recognized that they might want medication for pain in their Birth Plans, only two included an agreement to consider epidurals, and several women specifically noted that they did not want Caesarean sections. In general, the tone of the women's Birth Plans was to limit interventions and increase women's control. Susan's description provides a sense of this:

> I really, really was opposed to being induced—I feel that that is the beginning of the end for natural childbirth . . . My hope was to call my doula, do most of my labour at my sister's house with the doula there, so she could help us spend the least amount of time in the hospital as possible. So that was the Birth Plan, without medication or interventions.

In this description, it is clear that the hospital is seen as a place of threat to natural birthing, and furthermore, interventions such as inducing birth are understood as the thin edge of the wedge when it comes to medical interventions, a topic we explore more fully later. Furthermore, it is clear that Susan saw her Birth Plan as a tool to help her resist intervention.

The women also adhered to natural birth ideology through specifying that they would use the hospital's birthing room, within an atmosphere they believed would facilitate natural labour. Andrea, who is described earlier as not having a Birth Plan, nevertheless had definite birth *plans*, noting,

> With the hypnobirthing thing, I've been trying to prepare. I have some music set already, a playlist on my iPod. We'll make the atmosphere very comfortable, we'll dim the lights, try to make it as quiet and as soothing as possible. . . . I've taken baths and tried to do the whole preparing of breathing and visualization in the bath.

Andrea's plans reflect the common theme that the women in this study hoped for a self-regulated birthing experience and saw themselves as patients/consumers, able to choose the kind of birth they would have and responsible for planning and knowing how to achieve that outcome.

'On a Train': Medical Interventions and Choice

While the majority of mothers assumed prior to birth that they could choose and plan for a specific type of birth, their birthing experiences often did not align with their expectations. As noted earlier, of 21 women who sought varying degrees of natural/intervention-free births, 11 ended with Caesarean sections, and all but two women experienced some form of medical intervention. The interviews reflect that, despite having planned for as natural a birth as possible, many of the women were unable to make meaningful decisions regarding medical interventions. In addition, the mothers explained that once they accepted one type of intervention, this inevitably led to a 'cascade of interventions', which further constrained their ability to control the birth process. Carmen, who had a Caesarean section despite wanting a non-medicalized birth, described how having one type of medical intervention such as an induction increases the likelihood of having other interventions:

> And what they call a 'cascade of interventions' seems to be absolutely true. If you get induced, your chance of a C-section goes up. If you get induced your chance of an epidural goes up, if you have an epidural, your chance of a C-section goes up again. Once that ball starts rolling, one thing tends to lead to another.

Later in the interview, Carmen elaborated on the lack of choice she felt following the induction, saying,

> And I didn't have any other choices presented to me. I was told nothing else would work. We can't do forceps, we can't do vacuum, this was it. . . . I realized that the C-section wasn't really a choice by then.

Similarly, Judith, who also planned a natural birth, explained that after she decided to have an epidural she was unable to intercede in further decisions concerning other interventions:

> It is true what they say about one type of intervention leading to another, and before you know it, you have all of them. That is absolutely true. At first, when I said yes to the epidural, then it was like, okay, the epidural.

Then suddenly it was like 'well, we'll put you on a drip'. So it was one thing after another.

As these comments reflect, once a decision was made to begin medical interventions, the idea that women are able to exercise free choice became increasingly problematic. Both Carmen and Judith stated that once they had the first medical intervention, it was no longer a matter of choosing further interventions but instead of accepting what the doctors and nurses recommended.

These themes were summarized by Shirley, who had a C-section despite planning a non-medicalized birth:

> You can't really just leave it once you started it [having an induction] and I didn't realize that. And he [the doctor] didn't really explain that to me. . . . I thought you could just try it . . . but I didn't get that option, because once I started it he came in and said, 'Ok we'll break your water next'. And I didn't feel qualified to question that. . . . But at that point I felt like I'm on a train and I have to keep going where it was going.

Shirley's initial acquiescence to her doctor's intervention was not adequately informed and left her feeling unqualified to question his expertise when it came to subsequent interventions. Shirley's comments reflect the imbalance of knowledge and power in the delivery room and the challenge this can pose for mothers who want to make informed and responsible birthing choices. It is revealing that Shirley uses the metaphor of being on a train to describe how she felt in the delivery room as it suggests that she felt out of control and swept away by the course of her birth.

Rita, who wanted a vaginal, intervention-free birth but underwent a Caesarean section, also employed the metaphor of being on a train to describe her experience:

> I think that [induction] started the, you know, heading towards the train wreck. That was the very first thing. I think that if they would

have allowed me more time even before they started Pitocin. If I had been allowed even to go home. . . . That makes a big difference because you are not in that unknown atmosphere. You can be at home and do what you need to do. Just more time. Things could have just been allotted a lot more time.

Rita's description highlights a further problem with the assumption that during labour, mothers are able to act as autonomous, rational patients/consumers. Women who are in labour are in pain, fatigued, worried about themselves and their babies, and unsure of what the 'right' decision might be (Carter, 2010). Given these factors, and the pressures and time constraints imposed on women in hospital delivery rooms, it is highly unlikely that women can take time to step back and dispassionately weigh the pros and cons before making a decision.

Susan's experience also reveals the difficulty women face when trying to make well-informed birthing choices. After many hours of labour, her doctor told her that labour had stalled and that she should consider a C-section. She described the experience as follows:

> When we were deciding to do the C-section, she didn't really give us much time to think about it, she was just standing there going, 'So what are you deciding?' And I didn't even think to ask, 'Can we think about it?'

Susan's experience challenges the assumption that women in labour have a range of options to evaluate and choose from or that mothers can assert informed choice or question the authority of medical professionals, especially when medical interventions are presented as being in the best interest of the child being born. Abby summarized this idea by stating, 'And I think women, you know, they trust their doctors, they don't want to hurt their babies . . . and so the doctor says we have to do this, then they do it'.

In many women's comments, it was clear that despite their initial expectations for as natural a birth as possible and despite their education about risk and birth, when it came to the moment of decision, they

were unable to clearly or rationally evaluate their options. In the moment, women did not—indeed, could not—know whether their pain would pass soon, whether the labour would progress quickly, whether the baby would arrive safely or whether the situation really was an emergency. Faced with this ambiguity, mothers often trusted experts' knowledge and acquiesced to medical pressure, hoping for the best.

Questions and Blame: Reconciling Birth Expectations With Experiences

Many of the women had hoped, even expected, that a birth plan would allow them some degree of certainty and control in the delivery room, and they engaged in the active, reflexive and responsible role of organizing and planning for an optimal outcome. As the earlier discussion reveals, however, the women's plans were rarely realized. Indeed, although the vast majority of these women 'chose' natural birthing as their hoped-for outcome, most ended with at least some sort of medical intervention. Rita's Birth Plan expressly stated that she wanted to have a vaginal birth and immediate skin-to-skin contact with her baby after delivery; however, because she had a Caesarean section, she says,

> I didn't get to hold my baby right away, I didn't get to look into her eyes undrugged for who knows how long. I did get to hear her cry for the first time, but still, it was kind of delusional with all the medication and everything else . . . I started crying and thinking, 'I really, really missed out' and the only thing that really consoled me was that my husband and daughter have a fantastic bond and it was good that he could be with her for those first few hours and experience some of those things that I didn't get to. . . . I just felt like my birth was taken away from me, really. . . . I think it's really just that I thought the whole experience was kind of taken.

The birth Rita had envisioned and planned differed significantly from her lived experience. Clearly, she feels she was robbed of a crucial mothering experience. While her bitter disappointment stems at least in part from the virulent discourse of bonding and natural birth as both optimal and critical to ideal birth and mothering, it also come from having a Birth Plan that promised her a false sense of control and certainty, yet failed to provide any real guarantees in the actual event.

Susan spoke directly to her belief that by preparing for childbirth and having a 'proper' Birth Plan in place, she would have had the capacity to achieve her ideal birth. Reflecting on her preparation for childbirth, Susan stated,

> And the worst thing is that I thought I was prepared. Like I really did. I had, you know, read up and read books, and taken the prenatal classes and surrounded myself with people that I hoped would help.

Susan planned to have a vaginal birth and 'immediate bonding' with her baby. Not surprisingly, when she had a C-section, she was left feeling as though she 'missed out'. Susan assumed that by acting as a responsible patient/consumer and risk manager in preparing for childbirth, she would safeguard herself against the unexpected. Thus, her experience further highlights how a Birth Plan can provide women with a heightened sense of individual responsibility in relation to childbirth, leaving women with a feeling of failed in their birth expectations and in their actual births.

The feeling of disappointment was common among the women. Katherine stated, 'As far as expectations versus disappointments. . . . My expectations were to go *au naturel* the way they have for years. [My] disappointments are that I went through pretty much every intervention you could possibly imagine'. Similarly, Tanya explained,

> It was exactly the opposite of what I'd hoped my birth would be. But I was also really happy that I was fine and my baby was fine. I thought, you know, it wasn't the birth I wanted but bottom line is I have a healthy baby and I was grateful to the doctor.

Tanya's comments are revealing. While she is upset and disappointed that her birth experience did not follow her plan, she also clearly expresses

a 'doctor knows best' attitude. Indeed, rather than assign responsibility for the birth outcome to her physician or the cascade of interventions attendant with modern, technocratic birthing, Tanya blames herself:

> I feel sort of like I failed in the birthing arena. . . . You hear these stories about women who went in there and they pushed four times and the baby just came out and you sort of compare yourself and think, you know, maybe if I'd have exercised more or maybe if I'd done something differently maybe I would have been one of those women who pushed. Because that's the ultimate standard. . . . I never expected that I'd be someone who had a C-section. Logically I know that it [the C-section] was necessary, but somehow I think, if I was slim and if I had walked every day and not eaten as much ice cream that would not have happened.

This excerpt reflects the feelings of guilt and inadequacy that many of the women felt when they did not have the birth that they had expected. In addition, Tanya's comments underline the assumption that women are responsible not only for the health of their children but also for ensuring that their Birth Plans are followed and that mothers should be in optimal physical and mental conditions to see that plan through. The implication is that mothers only have themselves to blame when their birth expectations are not met.

Looking back on their birth experiences, many of the mothers questioned what they could have done differently to fulfil their Birth Plans. Almost 3 years after the birth of her son, Shirley continues to wonder what she could have done to avoid a C-section:

> That's the only thing in the back of mind, is that if I wouldn't have said yes to the induction then maybe I wouldn't have had to have a C-section. But I mean that's 20-20 hindsight, right? Yeah that's looking back on it going, if I would have known that, that and that.

Similarly, when reflecting on her unplanned Caesarean section, Carmen stated,

> That's always the question, right? Would this have happened that way if I had been able to do this, this and this differently, right? Maybe if I hadn't had to lay in bed so much [due to fetal monitoring] and could have moved around. . . . Lots of questions like that.

Like others in the study, Shirley and Carmen are left with many questions when trying to reconcile the difference between their plans and their actual experiences. While Carmen considers how other factors might have impacted the birthing process—fetal monitoring, induction—both women clearly question what they could have done in order to alter the course of their births. Embedded within their words is the assumption, reflecting those expressed in both medical and natural birthing discourses, that they had the ability to make different choices and thus they are to blame for not having the births they expected.

CONCLUSION

The natural/alternative birth perspective assumes that women have the ability to plan and achieve their birth choices, encouraging women to employ various tools (including Birth Plans, employing a doula or midwife or using breathing and meditation techniques) in order to achieve a non-medicalized birth. The medical perspective on birth also assumes that women are medical consumers who can choose, plan and execute the birth experience they desire and that women are capable of assessing and managing risks attached to their choices. This assumption is evident in mainstream childbirth education's taking up and encouraging the use of a Birth Plan as part of a range of actions that responsible mothers must take. Despite their differences in orientation, both the medical perspective and the alternative perspective adhere to a discourse of a responsible, rational consumer/citizen who can choose, plan for and implement the type of birth she wants to have.

Rather than offering women an empowered capacity to choose, plan and control their births, however, birth planning discourse acts as a form of governmentality. The women's descriptions of the gaps between their plans and expectations and their actual birthing experiences illustrate for us that discourses about women's choice and capacity to plan and control their birth experiences, while operating superficially as a vehicle for women's empowerment, in practice are disciplining of women. By educating women that they have a 'choice' and positioning them to act responsibly as consumers and risk managers, both medical and natural birth discourses move the responsibility for birth outcomes to women as consumers, thus holding them culpable for the increasing technocratization of childbirth. From a medical perspective, this is evidenced overtly in the debates over 'who drives the machine' of increasing CSRs. From a natural birth perspective, this is evidenced by the unproblematized assertions that women not only should choose a natural, non-medicalized birth but that they also can implement such a birth, if they do the 'right' things.

Only a critical, feminist analysis provides us with a critique of the punitive discourses of risk and choice concerning childbirth and how they render women responsible for their health outcomes while failing to acknowledge the lack of power women have in the medical encounter. In line with the feminist critique on the medicalization of women's reproductive experiences, our research undermines medical and populist claims that women are 'driving the machine', that women have access to and the ability to control various birthing outcomes, that they can exercise agency in choosing their type of birth and that women's proclivities for a painless, controllable experience lead them to push for medicalized births. Similarly, the women's perspectives indicate the tremendous burden of blame and individualization that comes from natural birthing imperatives. The women's descriptions reveal that their birth outcomes were often the result of attempting to make well-informed choices and evaluate risk within a closed medical system and in relation to an individualized and blaming model of patient/consumerism. According to Deborah Lupton (1999b), the 'proliferation of risk discourse' in Western countries has rendered pregnancy a 'perilous journey' (p. 66). To navigate this journey, a pregnant woman is expected to act as a responsible patient, submit to medical scrutiny and engage in extensive self-surveillance in order to avoid risks and protect the health and well-being of her fetus (Lupton, 1999b). Women are thus made individually responsible for making fateful health-related decisions, for understanding the risks attached to these choices and they are held culpable for any negative outcomes that result from these decisions. In our study, the women we spoke with subscribed to this ethos as well; they made efforts to inform themselves and try to control their experiences in positive ways, but they also surrendered to medical knowledge and submitted to medical interventions in the interests of their children's well-being. The women we interviewed also internalized Lupton's notion of individualized responsibility by holding themselves responsible while simultaneously releasing medical professionals from blame for their undesired medicalized births.

While the assumption that women are 'driving the machine' of childbirth choices does not fit with the women's lived experiences, it aligns perfectly with the notion of the rational patient/consumer and the normative understanding that medical decisions are consumer driven. Here, not only is it assumed that women are responsible patients/consumers who can plan and choose, but, at least in the medical model, there is also a presumption that given such choices, women are increasingly opting for technocratic, predictable births in the form of planned Caesarean sections. However, the vast majority of women we interviewed ascribed to a natural birthing discourse and wanted a natural birth, and they planned to achieve this by employing various natural birth techniques and tools and by minimizing their exposure to the medical setting during childbirth. Thus, these women also subscribed to a belief in their capacities to assess, plan and control their own 'ideal birth', to manage the medical encounter and make meaningful birth-related decisions.

Although the women planned to have as natural a birth as possible, their lived experiences differed significantly from their birth plans. The majority of the women's accounts reveal that the decision to undergo medical interventions was not a free choice but a constrained decision made within the context of an unpredictable and disempowering event, where medical advice and intervention often led to escalating medicalization and undermined women's birthing efforts. The implications of these experiences have broader effects in terms of increasing the medicalization of birth and rising CSRs. In particular, for the 11 women who underwent 'emergency' Caesarean sections, their ability to 'choose' against having medical interventions in subsequent births was effectively foreclosed. Only one of the mothers experiencing a Caesarean in this group has gone on to experience a natural, vaginal birth, while a further six have experienced planned, 'chosen' Caesarean sections as a result of their histories, and another four reported that any subsequent births would almost certainly be accomplished through Caesarean because of their earlier 'choices'. Thus, not only were these women not able to make decisions along hoped-for lines in the births described in this study, but those decisions served to further limit women's 'choices' for subsequent births and further increased the likelihood of medicalized birth.

In the end, the women's descriptions provide little support for the current moral panic expressed in much medical and popular discourse that women control their medical choices and are simply 'too posh to push'. Rather, the women's experiences illuminate the difficulties of the medical encounter, the urgency and lack of clarity women feel when making birth decisions, and the responsibility and guilt women take on when their 'choices' go against plan. These findings lend support to the feminist critique of medicalized childbirth, where women's choices, while used to hold them responsible as effective and active consumers, are in reality profoundly limited in the labour and delivery room.

References

ACOG Committee (2007) Cesarean delivery on maternal request. *American College of Obstetricians and Gynecologists* 110(5): 1209–1212.

Alberta Perinatal Health Program (2007) *Alberta Prenatal Care Documentation: Guide and Resource for Prenatal Care Providers* (pp. 1–68) Edmonton, Alberta: Alberta Perinatal Health Program.

Anonymous (2005) C-sections: Becoming the popular choice. *Hospitals & Health Networks* 79: 1.

Beckett K (2005) Choosing caesarean: Feminism and the politics of childbirth in the United States. *Feminist Theory* 6(3): 251–275.

Beckett K and Hoffman B (2005) Challenging medicine: Law, resistance, and the cultural politics of birth. *Law & Society Review* 39(1): 125–170.

Beil L (2008) The case for keeping that bun in the oven. *Parenting* 22: 1.

Bergeron V (2007) The ethics of cesarean section on maternal request: A feminist critique of the American College of Obstetricians and Gynecologists' position on patient – Choice surgery. *Bioethics* 21(9): 478–487.

Borgwardt L, Bach D, Nickelsen C, et al. (2009) Elective caesarean section increases the risk of respiratory morbidity of the newborn. *Acta Paediatrica* 98(1): 187–189.

Brubaker SJ and Dillaway HE (2009) Medicalization, natural childbirth and birthing. *Sociology Compass* 3(1): 31–48.

Canadian Institute for Health Information (CIHI) (2009) CIHI health indicator reports. Available at: http://www.cihi.ca/hireports/SearchServlet.

Carter SK (2010) Beyond control: Body and self in women's childbearing narratives. *Sociology of Health & Illness* 32(7): 993–1009.

Cherniak D and Fisher J (2008) Explaining obstetric interventionism: Technical skills, common conceptualisations, or collective counter-transference? *Women's Studies International Forum* 31: 270–277.

Cheyney MJ (2008) Homebirth as systems-challenging praxis: Knowledge, power, and intimacy in the birthplace. *Qualitative Health Research* 18(2): 254–267.

Clift-Matthews V (2010) Vaginal birth as a rite of passage. *British Journal of Midwifery* 18(3): 140.

Crossley ML (2007) Childbirth, complications and the illusion of 'choice': A case study. *Feminism & Psychology* 17(4): 543–563.

Davis-Floyd RE (2004) Consuming childbirth: The qualified commodification of midwifery care. In: Taylor JS, Layne LL and Wozniak DF (eds) *Consuming Motherhood*. NJ: Rutgers University Press, pp. 211–248.

Diniz SG and Chacham AS (2004) 'The cut above' and 'the cut below': The abuse of caesareans and episiotomy in Sao Paulo Brazil. *Reproductive Health Matters* 12(23): 100–110.

Dunn C, Da Silva O, Schmidt G, et al. (2009) Outcomes of elective labour induction and elective caesarean section in low-risk pregnancies between 37 and 41 weeks' gestation. *Journal of Obstetrics and Gynaecology Canada* 31(12): 1124–1129.

Edwards GJ and Davies NJ (2001) Elective caesarean section – The patient's choice? *Journal of Obstetrics and Gynaecology* 21(2): 128–129.

Fereday J and Muir-Cochrane E (2005) Demonstrating rigor using thematic analysis:

A hybrid approach of inductive and deductive coding and theme development. *International Journal of Qualitative Methods* 5(1): 1–11.

Foucault M (1991) Governmentality. In: Burchell G, Gordon C and Miller P (eds) *The Foucault Effect: Studies in Governmentality: With Two Lectures by and an Interview with Michel Foucault*. Chicago, IL: The University of Chicago Press, pp. 87–104.

Frank AW (2002) Why study peoples' stories? The dialogical ethics of narrative analysis. *International Journal of Qualitative Methods* 1(1): 1–9.

Grant JM (2004) Social class and elective caesareans in the NHS. *British Medical Journal* 329(7460): 291.

Huberman AM and Miles MB (1998) Data management and analysis methods. In: Denzin NK and Lincoln YS (eds) *Collecting and Interpreting Qualitative Materials*. Thousand Oaks, CA: SAGE, pp. 179–210.

Inch S (1982) *Birthrights: What Every Parent Should Know about Childbirth in Hospitals*. New York: Pantheon.

Irvine ML (2001) Maternal request for caesarean section: Is it obstetrician driven? *Journal of Obstetrics and Gynaecology* 21(4): 373–374.

Kitzinger S (ed.) (1981) *Episiotomy: Physical and Emotional Aspects*. London: National Childbirth Trust.

Klein MC (2007) Women's views of elective primary caesarean section: Editorial. *Journal of Obstetrics and Gynaecology Canada* 29(3): 214.

Kotz D (2008) A risky rise in C-sections: Experts worry that the trend is bad for mom and baby. *U.S. News & World Report*, 7 April, 1.

Kukla R (2005) *Mass Hysteria: Medicine, Culture, and Mothers' Bodies*. Oxford: Rowman & Littlefield Publishers, Inc.

Lane K (1996) The medical model of the body as a site of risk: A case study of childbirth. In: Gabe J (ed.) *Medicine, Health and Risk: Sociological Approaches*. Oxford: Blackwell Publisher, pp. 53–72.

Lavender T and Kingdon C (2006) Caesarean delivery at maternal request: Why we should promote normal birth. *British Journal of Midwifery* 14(5): 2.

Lee ASM and Kirkman M (2008) Disciplinary discourses: Rates of cesarean section explained by medicine, midwifery, and feminism. *Health Care for Women International* 29: 448–467.

Lobel M and DeLuca RS (2007) Psychosocial sequelae of cesarean delivery: Review and analysis of their causes and implications. *Social Science & Medicine* 64: 2272–2284.

Lupton D (1999a) *Risk*. London and New York: Routledge.

Lupton D (1999b) Risk and the ontology of pregnant embodiment. In: Lupton D (ed.) *Risk and Sociocultural Theory*. Cambridge University Press, pp. 59–85.

Lupton D (2011) The best thing for the baby: Mothers' concepts and experiences related to promoting their infants' health and development. *Health Risk & Society* 13(7–8): 637–651.

Lupton D (2012) 'Precious Cargo': Foetal subjects, risk and reproductive citizenship. *Critical Public Health* 22(3): 329–340.

McAra-Couper J, Jones M and Smythe L (2011) Caesarean-section, my body, my choice: The construction of 'informed choice' in relation to intervention in childbirth. *Feminism & Psychology* 22(1): 81–97.

McCourt C, Weaver J, Statham H, et al. (2007) Elective caesarean section and decision making: A critical review of the literature. *Birth: Issues in Perinatal Care* 34(1): 65–79.

Macfarlane AJ (2004) Social class and elective caesareans in the NHS. *British Medical Journal* 329(7460): 291.

Malacrida C and Boulton T (2012) Women's perceptions of childbirth 'choices': Competing discourses of motherhood, sexuality, and selflessness. *Gender & Society* 26(5): 748–772.

Mansfield B (2008) The social nature of natural childbirth. *Social Science & Medicine* 66: 1084–1094.

Martin JA, Hamilton BE, Sutton PD, et al. (2006) *Births: Final Data for 2004 National Vital Statistics Report*, vol. 55. Hyattsville, MD: National Center for Health Statistics.

Marx H, Wiener J and Davies N (2001) A survey of the influence of patients' choice on the increase in the caesarean section rate. *Journal of Obstetrics and Gynaecology* 21(2): 124–127.

Minkoff H, Powderly KR, Chervenak F, et al. (2006) Ethical dimensions of elective primary cesarean delivery. *Journal of Obstetrics and Gynaecology* 103(2): 387–392.

Oakley A (1984) *The Captured Womb: A History of the Medical Care of Pregnant Women*. Oxford: Basil Blackwell.

Robson S, Carey A, Mishra R, et al. (2008) Elective caesarean delivery at maternal request: A preliminary study of motivations influencing women's decision-making. *Australian and New Zealand Journal of Obstetrics and Gynecology* 48(4): 415–420.

Rogers-Dillon RH (2005) Hierarchical qualitative research teams: Refining the methodology. *Qualitative Research* 5(4): 437–454.

Sakalys JA (2000) The political role of illness narratives. *Journal of Advanced Nursing* 31(6): 1469–1475.

Smith DE (1987) *The Everyday World as Problematic: A Feminist Sociology*. Toronto, ON, Canada: University of Toronto Press.

Sosulski MR (2010) Life history and narrative analysis: Feminist methodologies contextualizing Black women's experiences with severe mental illness. *Journal of Sociology and Social Welfare* 37(3): 29–57.

Thomas C (2010) Negotiating the contested terrain of narrative methods in illness contexts. *Sociology of Health & Illness* 32(4): 647–660.

Wolf N (2001) *Misconceptions: Truth, Lies, and the Unexpected on the Journey to Motherhood*. New York: Doubleday.

39

C-SECTION EPIDEMIC

Theresa Morris

The performance of cesarean section births has reached an epidemic level in the United States. In 2012, 32.8 percent of women who gave birth in the United States had c-sections. The World Health Organization warns that countries with a c-section rate over 15 percent put women's lives at risk, and a recent study finds that annual U.S. healthcare costs could be reduced by more than $5 billion if the C-section rate were reduced to 15 percent. In an attempt to understand the C-section trend, I interviewed 50 maternity clinicians—obstetricians, family physicians, certified nurse-midwives, and labor and delivery nurses—and 83 women who had given birth the day before. These sociological data illustrate the context of medical routines and practices that shape the decisions of pregnant women and their physicians and lead to a high rate of C-sections.

My research demonstrates that increased economic pressures on hospitals, as well as hospital administrators' and maternity clinicians' fear of lawsuits, are the main drivers of the C-section rate. Malpractice insurance cycles are a known phenomenon, and clinicians define malpractice crises in hard cycles, which are characterized by a shortage of malpractice insurance policies and high malpractice insurance premiums. Hard cycles have occurred in the American malpractice industry in 1975–1978, 1984–1987, and 2001–2004. Each of these periods coincides with a precipitous increase in the C-section rate, and the rate becomes institutionalized, continuing after the crisis subsides (see Figure 39.1). The C-section rate has increased by 34 percent since 2001, the beginning of the last defined crisis. Additionally, changes in Medicaid compensation mandated by Congress in 1982 spurred corporatization of hospitals and medical practices. As a result, physician autonomy has steadily declined, and hospitals face increased economic pressures. These structural changes, along with more intense attention to the economic threat of malpractice lawsuits, have led hospital administrators and maternity clinicians to search for an expedient mode of birth that will also protect them from lawsuits. The answer: C-sections.

C-Section Epidemic, Theresa Morris in *Contexts, 13*(1), 70–72, 2014. Reprinted with permission of SAGE Publications.

THE SPECTER OF MALPRACTICE SUITS

Many negative birth outcomes, like cerebral palsy, are unpredictable and, for the most part, unpreventable. Nevertheless, maternity clinicians are often held accountable, regardless of whether the care they provided *caused* the outcome. Obstetrics is a high-risk specialty in terms of malpractice allegations. Obstetricians have the third-highest lawsuit rate among physician specialties, third only to neurologists and neurosurgeons, and almost every obstetrician will be sued before age 65. Moreover, malpractice insurance premiums and average malpractice awards have been increasing. All of this heightens attention to liability in the obstetrics field; a concern that was prevalent among the maternity clinicians I interviewed.

Two types of C-sections are reflected in the epidemic rate—the increase in primary or first C-sections and the increase in repeat C-sections. In terms of primary C-sections, physicians are often intolerant of irregularities in fetal heart beat measurements and perform C-sections during the course of labor as a result. Yet, as a good example of Peter Berger's sociological insight that things are not always what they seem, there is no evidence that the increase in C-sections is due to better identification of problems with the baby during labor or that there has been any resultant improvement in outcomes.

Almost all hospital births in the United States include continuous monitoring of the fetal heartbeat. This is an increase from 44.6 percent in 1980. One might be surprised, then, to learn that these monitors *incorrectly* identify fetal distress 99.8 percent of the time, which means that 99.8 percent of babies identified to have "non-reassuring" heart rate patterns by continuous electronic monitoring will *not* be compromised at birth. Despite this lack of predictability, electronic fetal monitors are widely used continuously, and maternity clinicians intervene quickly when babies have "non-reassuring" fetal heart rate patterns, even though almost always the fetus is not compromised. Studies show that intermittently monitoring the fetal heart rate

produces outcomes that are just as good as continuous monitoring, but with a much lower c-section rate (see Alfirevic, Devane, and Gyte's 2013 review "Continuous cardiotocography [CTG] as a form of electronic fetal monitoring [EFM] for fetal assessment during labour" in the *Cochrane Database of Systematic Reviews*). Women's labors are monitored continuously not because fetal outcomes are improved, but because the strip of paper (or electronic record) produced from the monitor documents the fetal heart rate throughout the labor and can be used as evidence in court cases if there is a negative outcome.

Other practices, such as inducing women rather than allowing them to go into labor naturally, contribute to more C-sections, especially among first time mothers. Women whose labors are induced are twice as likely to have a C-section as women who go into labor spontaneously. Women are sometimes induced so that clinicians can avoid being sued if a bad outcome occurs in women who deliver past their due dates. Physicians also often induce or schedule C-sections for suspected "big" babies (defined as an estimated weight over 9 pounds 15 ounces), even though there is no scientific evidence of improved outcome over a vaginal delivery and professional guidelines discourage this practice. Further, women with twin pregnancies and women with babies in a breech position (bottom down) are routinely scheduled for C-sections. Maternity clinicians I interviewed reported that these C-sections are done to prevent blame for bad outcomes in vaginal deliveries, even though evidence suggests that vaginal birth leads to equally good outcomes as C-section in these situations.

The increase in repeat C-sections also contributes to the epidemic rates. For women who have had a C-section and become pregnant again, VBAC (vaginal birth after cesarean section) is an option in theory, if not always available in practice. Presently, 91 percent of women who give birth following a C-section have a repeat C-section, even though survey evidence suggests that nearly half would like to attempt a VBAC. VBACs are just as safe as first vaginal births and catastrophic outcomes are exceedingly rare, but because of the small risk of the

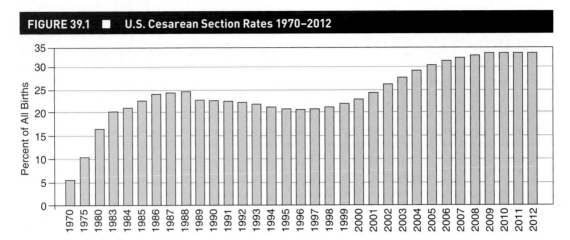

FIGURE 39.1 ■ U.S. Cesarean Section Rates 1970–2012

Source: Compiled from CDC; Taffel, Placek, and Liss (1987).

uterine scar rupturing during labor, many hospitals and physicians do not offer this option. Physicians know the risk of a catastrophic uterine rupture is slight, but fear they will be successfully sued if a uterine rupture occurs and the baby is injured or dies.

(MIS)LEADING ORGANIZATIONAL INFLUENCE

Organizational influence over individual decisions is particularly evident in the hesitation of physicians around VBACs. The professional organization of obstetricians in the United States, the American College of Obstetricians and Gynecologists (ACOG), officially recommends that obstetricians, anesthesiology staff, and operating rooms be immediately available in hospitals that offer women VBAC opportunities, even though there is no empirical evidence that such requirements improve outcomes and there are no similar recommendations that apply to other, more common, obstetric emergencies, such as hemorrhage.

Many hospitals face challenges in meeting these recommendations due to limited facilities and/

or staff. The only significant decrease in the past forty years in the c-section rate was between 1988 and 1998, when ACOG issued practice guidelines that encouraged VBACs and changed the language from its first VBAC practice guideline (issued in 1982) suggesting staff and resources be "immediately available" to a more flexible "readily available" requirement. The VBAC rate reached an all time high of 28.3 percent in 1996, and the C-section rate dropped to 20.7 percent. However, this ended in 1999 when ACOG issued a new VBAC practice guideline reverting back to the "immediately available" staff and resources guideline, which was reaffirmed in the most recent practice guideline issued in 2010. This ACOG stance stands out as one of its guidelines least tied to empirical evidence.

ACOG is not the only organization to bear responsibility for the low VBAC rate. Malpractice insurers may define VBACs as non-covered events, meaning that if an obstetrician oversees a VBAC attempt, the malpractice insurance company will not cover a malpractice suit resulting from that birth. In addition, reinsurance companies, which insure malpractice insurance companies against large claims, also may deny coverage for VBACs. In both cases medical care (including surgery) is not linked to medical science but, instead, is influenced by organizational recommendations or requirements outside the control of physicians and hospital administrators.

SOLUTIONS TO THE C-SECTION EPIDEMIC

Because maternity clinicians' fear of liability underlies much of the C-section epidemic, any effective solution must address this problem directly. For example, currently in most states, malpractice must be alleged for a family to seek compensation for an injured baby. The federal government should change the system of addressing malpractice to a no-fault system. In such a system, families of babies born with injuries would be compensated regardless of whether the injury was caused by medical negligence. Further, federal policy should prohibit malpractice and reinsurance companies from excluding established medical procedures, such as VBACs and vaginal twin and breech deliveries, from their range of coverage, and hospitals and obstetrical guidelines should refrain from banning these deliveries. In addition, the indiscriminate use of continuous electronic fetal monitoring on low-risk women should be abandoned. Finally, we all need to learn more about how economic and organizational pressures and guidelines may shape labor and birth practices in ways that contribute to patterns such as epidemic C-section rates.

EXPANDING HEALTH AND HEALTH CARE

In the past 20 years, there have been innumerable changes in health and health care, some of which we have discussed in the previous sections of this volume. The first part of the volume focused on the social production of disease and the meanings of illness. The second addressed how medical care is organized in the United States, and the third examined some contemporary critical debates about how we view health and illness. Here, we highlight three large areas of change: the impacts of the internet and hand-held personal device applications on health; social change through the politicization of health and through health social movements; and the globalization of our understandings of health in terms of comparative inequalities, the expansion of illnesses, and the migration of medical workers and diagnoses.

ILLNESS, MEDICINE, AND THE INTERNET

The Internet is one of the greatest social interventions of the past century. There are numerous ways it has impacted health and medicine, including vast amounts of easily accessible medical information, communication among people with illnesses, medical support for clinicians, and promotion of new and sometimes marginal or challenging medical theories and treatment. It is almost hard to believe, but this has all occurred in the past twenty-five years.

The invention of the web-browser-enabled Worldwide Web began in the 1990s. The Internet has grown enormously in the past two decades, as have the number of users. The number of Internet users keeps growing, with roughly 360 million users in 2000 and an estimated 3.7 billion users in 2017 (http://www.internetworldstats.com/stats.htm). The greatest penetration of usage is of course in the developed world, but China has pulled ahead of the United States as having the largest number of Internet users. According to recent statistics, North America has roughly 320 million Internet users. Sophisticated search engines like Google (founded in 1998) make accessing relevant information quick and simple. Virtually everything about the Internet is growing or increasing. The Internet revolution has affected health information and communication as well; nearly 150 million Americans access the Internet for health information regularly, with most focusing on specific diseases (see Conrad and Stults 2010). The Internet has become a global marketplace for health-related information.

One of the most interesting and widespread aspects concerning health on the Internet is the thousands of interactive or participatory websites, bulletin boards, discussion groups, social network groups, and other forums for virtually any illness or disorder one could imagine. These often become online communities, where many members participate regularly, some just visit occasionally, and others lurk by reading the posts without actively contributing. While the Internet has helped individuals become more active consumers, it has also transformed them into *producers* of knowledge. In this web 2.0 (more interactive) era, individuals now have the ability to construct their own websites, home pages, or develop blogs about their health issues, transforming them from consumers of health information to producers of health information and care (Hardey 1999). This has increased significantly with the growth of Facebook and other social media. The Internet is truly an interactive marketplace of communication about specific illnesses as well as discussions about health and treatments. Thus, the Internet has become a repository of lay knowledge as well as a medium for promoting alternative and challenging perspectives about particular problems and disorders. It has become a place where lay viewpoints exist alongside professional perspectives, at times supporting, questioning, or challenging medical knowledge.

There are now thousands of electronic support groups available online. Prior to the Internet, illness was a private affair for most people. Now, given the virtual online worlds, illness can be more of a shared and public experience. As Barker notes, "The process of understanding one's embodied distress has been transformed from an essentially private affair between doctor and patient to an increasingly public accomplishment among sufferers in cyberspace" (Barker 2008, 21). On occasion, these interactive Internet groups (or sets of web-based groups) develop distinctive and challenging perspectives to the dominant medical view.

In "Illness and the Internet: From Private to Public Experience," Peter Conrad, Julia Bandini, and Alexandria Vasquez describe how the experience of illness has transformed from a profoundly private experience to an increasingly public one. In pre-Internet time, a huge majority of people with a wide range of illnesses never spoke with any other individuals who had the same illness. As many sociologists had pointed out, for most patients illness was an extremely private affair. These days, when individuals experience symptoms, they may well go right to the Internet for a search for others who share the symptoms, or when diagnosed search for sites where contributors have the same diagnosis or treatment to find out what others have experienced or compare how others are treated with medical care. Increasingly, these discussions take place on social media like Facebook.

The Internet has begotten smartphones and hundreds of thousands of software applications, or "apps," affecting diagnosis and treatment. In "'It's Like Having a Physician in Your Pocket!' A Critical Analysis of Self-Diagnosis Smartphone Apps," Deborah Lupton and Annemarie Jutel explore the impact of self-diagnosis smartphone apps directed at lay people, sort of a digitized diagnosis via apps. The authors suggest that they inhabit a contested and ambiguous world of meaning and practice. Are they really valid medical information even if their developers provide disclaimers that they should not be taken as professional medical information and individuals should seek medical advice concerning the diagnosis? While we don't yet know the implications for health, privacy, and relations to medical care, these apps are used commonly and taken seriously by their users.

References

Barker, Kristin K. 2008. "Electronic Support Groups, Patient Consumers, and Medicalization." *Journal of Health and Social Behavior* 49 (1): 20–36.

Conrad, Peter, and Cheryl Stults. 2010. "The Internet and the Experience of Illness." In *Handbook of Medical Sociology*, 6th edition, edited by Chloe Bird, Peter Conrad, Allan Fremont, and Stefan Timmermans. Nashville, TN: Vanderbilt University Press.

Hardey, Michael. 1999. "Doctor in the House: Sources of Lay Knowledge and the Challenge to Expertise." *Sociology of Health and Illness* 21 (6): 20–36.

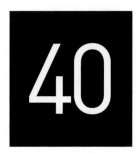

ILLNESS AND THE INTERNET

From Private to Public Experience

Peter Conrad, Julia Bandini,
and Alexandria Vasquez

Illness is a ubiquitous experience in all societies. Different cultures have different ways of responding to illness. Historically in Western cultures, illness is typically handled by self, kin, healers, or other specialized individuals. While the existence of illness may become a societal concern (e.g. various plagues, public health), the sufferers' experience and management of illness, while possibly culturally scripted, remain largely a private experience, until recently.

Sociologists have been studying the subjective experience of illness for nearly 50 years (Conrad and Stults, 2010). Until roughly the turn of this century, there were two consistent findings: (1) there were no illness subcultures, and (2) illness was a profoundly privatizing experience (with a few notable exceptions like the HIV/AIDS or breast cancer activist

and support groups). As the sociological theorist Talcott Parsons observed, "illness usually prevents the individual from attaching himself to a solitary subculture of similarly oriented deviants" (Parsons and Fox, 1952: 137). French sociologist Claudine Herzlich (2004) notes, "It is difficult to discern whether health and illness belong more in the private or public domain." The few studies available suggest that, even in institutions, illness experience remained individual and private, and even more so in the community (Conrad and Stults, 2010). As just one example, several decades ago, Schneider and Conrad (1983) interviewed 80 people with epilepsy and found that only 5 of the respondents had ever talked to anyone else who shared the same illness. For the overwhelming majority of people with chronic conditions, illness remained a private

Illness and the Internet: From Private to Public Experience, Peter Conrad, Julia Bandini, and Alexandria Vasquez in *Health*, *20*(1), 22–32, 2016. Reprinted with permission from SAGE Publications, Inc.

experience and shared only with family, medical personnel, and perhaps a few close friends. We are quite certain this would not be the case today. It would be an exaggeration to say that the Internet has changed everything, but it seems clear the Internet has revolutionized the interactive experience of illness, transforming illness experience for many people from a private to public experience. In this article, we will examine the role of the Internet in the facilitation of illness from a private to a public experience and the social consequences of the Internet in illness experience.[1]

The Internet, as we know it, with a browser for general use began in 1993 (e.g. Mosaic). Google, as an Internet search engine, appeared in 1998. This kind of potential access to online information and interconnectivity is the watershed event that made the Internet increasingly useful for obtaining information and connecting with others. There were about 360 million users in 2000, and by 2015, there are over 3 billion users worldwide (stastica.com). In the United States, 87 percent of US adults use the Internet, 72 percent of Internet users say they looked online for health information within the past year, 26 percent of Internet users have read or watched someone else's experience about health in the past year, and 18 percent of Internet users have gone online to find others who might have similar health concerns (Pew Internet Project, 2014). In short, there is a large and active number of people who use the Internet for health information and to interact with others about their illness or medical condition.

Based on their research, Ziebland and Wyke (2012) contend that there are seven health domains that drive the use of the Internet in peer-to-peer connections. The five major ones include finding information, feeling supported, maintaining relationships with others, affecting behavior, and experiencing health services. Not surprisingly, people with chronic illness and disability (or sometimes their caregivers) are among the largest users of health sites on the Internet.

As Ziebland and Wyke (2012) note, "the use of the Internet for peer-to-peer connection has been one of its most dramatic and transformational features" (p. 19). Whether people with illness go online

for information, support, advocacy, or comparative experiences, the Internet becomes a route to connections, often forming an illness subculture. In the first decade of online communities, there were a range of online mechanisms to make peer-to-peer connections including websites, blogs, bulletin boards, chat rooms, news groups, listservs, electronic support groups (ESGs), and forums. Some of these were asynchronous, in which individuals need not be online at the same time, while others were synchronous in which online users participated in real time.

Some of these websites required signing on to their accounts or joining, some had moderators, while many others were open to the public. While these Internet modes of connection differed in some ways, they all were available 24/7, many were anonymous or used screen names, most were globally available, and were "free" to anyone who had access to the Internet. Together, they created a vehicle that produced new connections, lay knowledge, and often vibrant online communities. It is difficult to know how many people these sites affected since only some participants actually posted material, while many more were observers, termed "lurkers," who would view the discussions, but did not post or actively participate. It is both the anonymity and lurking that make the actual participation difficult to measure. It is hard to estimate participation. The 1 percent rule states that 90 percent of online users do not actively contribute to Internet posts, while 9 percent somewhat contribute, and only 1 percent are responsible for generating new content. A recent study (Van Mierlo, 2014) found that this 1 percent rule was consistent across digital health social networks (DHSNs) as 1 percent of users actively contributed to content on these sites. This suggests that there are far more individuals silently participating in the various sites than are visible on screen. A study of 3000 respondents found that one in four Internet users living with a chronic condition reported going online to find others with similar health conditions (Fox, 2011). The utility of the Internet as a knowledge base and interactive venue for various diseases has transformed the nature of the experience of illness. Virtually any illness or medical condition has multiple sites online, openly accessible to anyone interested. Without question, illness in the 21st century has moved from a private to a public experience.

FROM WEB 1.0 TO WEB 2.0

In the past two decades, we have seen an enormous expansion of the Internet both in the number of users and in the amount of information and connections available. In terms of this article, one can see two kinds of Internet experiences, called in retrospect Web 1.0 and Web 2.0 (Cornode and Krishnamurthy, 2008). In Web 1.0, the vast majority of users are seeking already created content, which can be searched and retrieved from existing websites. Here, communication is largely in one direction, where information sought and retrieved has been already produced, often by professionally created websites (e.g. WebMD, the Mayo Clinic). In a sense, these websites are "passive": they can be accessed but not modified or contributed to by users.

In what is often called Web 2.0, the emphasis is on *user-generated* content and visibility. Here is where users can be interactive and collaborative with one another. The users create much of the content. In the past decade, Web 2.0 has expanded with a range of interactive websites (blogs, ESGs) and especially what is called "social media" (e.g. Facebook, Instagram, Twitter). With social media, the participants create, share, or exchange information, experiences, and even photos and videos in user-defined virtual communities and networks. The numerous kinds of Internet-based social media are built on the capabilities of Web 2.0 technologies and have significantly expanded the ways in which people with special interests (e.g. in our case an illness or condition) can connect with one another as "friends," network connections on Facebook, or through specifically created "Facebook pages." Together, these groups facilitate the interaction and exchange of user-generated content, often to a specific group of friends. One major difference from previous Internet interaction modes, social media does not emphasize online "anonymity," as did previous vehicles such as bulletin boards and

chat rooms. Yet, the Information Highway has been supplemented by the Interaction Highway.

WEB 2.0 AND THE PROLIFERATION OF PUBLIC ILLNESS EXPERIENCES

Interaction on the Internet became the norm after 2000 or so. There were thousands of websites, representing virtually any illness, both well-known and unknown. For example, Barker (2008) examined an ESG for the contested illness, fibromyalgia. This was one of numerous sites that provided support, information, and advocacy for the treatment of fibromyalgia. The wide reach of illness on the Internet can be exemplified by two unusual and controversial conditions that have spawned interactive websites that are at the same time supportive, informative, and involved in advocacy. Conrad and Rondini (2010) described support groups that are depicted as "proana" and "transabled." The proana websites claimed to provide support for anorexics, but in a particular way: claiming anorexia is a lifestyle and not a disease, providing advice on how to be a "better anorexic," and advocating for the demedicalization of anorexia. The second case Conrad and Rondini examined went under a number of names, including "amputees by choice" and "transabled." Subscribers who posted on these sites were individuals who believed that they were meant to be amputees (usually of some limb) and searched for others who shared the same orientation. They use a similar vocabulary as transgendered individuals: "I wasn't meant to be born with my 'left leg' or 'arm')." Because the phenomenon of transabled is very rare, it seems likely that without the Internet, this phenomena as a potential diagnosis would not exist, since each individual might believe only that he or she had these unusual desires. But with the Internet, there are a number of interactive websites that allow the transabled individuals to exchange information, engender support for their condition, and advocate that their condition become medicalized as Body Image Identity Disorder (BIID) in the American Psychiatric Association's *Diagnostic and Statistical*

Manual (DSM) with the hope that the medical profession will accept their disorder and thus provide the surgical amputation treatment they are seeking. (As of 2015, this condition is not a medically accepted diagnosis, nor are any surgeons willing to amputate healthy limbs.)

Most illnesses on the Internet are more common and have spawned many different websites, online support groups, and social networks. For example, if one googled "diabetes support group" in mid-2015, the results page tells us there are 13,300,000 hits. While it is likely the number is hugely exaggerated since there are probably hundreds of repeats, it gives an idea that there are at least "very many" diabetes support groups available on the Internet. To give another example, if one googled "celiac disease support group," one would see that there were 636,000 hits. As a comparison, "anorexia support groups" yielded about 1,490,000 hits and "transabled support groups" a mere 6130 hits. Such numbers indicate both a proliferation of opportunities to connect with similarly ill others and a redundancy from poorly filtered hits on the Internet search. It is unclear what these numbers mean except as comparative availability of potential "hits" of one illness relative to another.

We will use celiac disease, an autoimmune disorder in which the ingestion of gluten can cause damage in the small intestine, as our example for social media and health. It is treated by eliminating gluten from one's diet. Gluten-free diets and the diagnosis of celiac disease (and the more controversial claims to "gluten sensitivity") are issues that have come to the public forefront within the last two decades. Our choice of illness here lies partly on the currency of the publicity of gluten and celiac disease, with most of the Internet and social media interactions occurring in the past decade. Our focus is primarily on Facebook because it has the most users and overall activity of all social media platforms, it provides the most communication variation of all social media platforms (e.g. visual, textual, community pages), and because many social media users now have accounts on other social media platforms, such as Twitter, Instagram, Vine, Google+, to name a few, yet still consider Facebook to be their "homebase" platform (Duggan et al., 2015). This example will allow us to illustrate how individuals with celiac disease both create and interact using social media on the Internet.

SOCIAL MEDIA AND ILLNESS EXPERIENCE: CELIAC DISEASE

The advent of Web 2.0 and active media sites such as Facebook, Twitter, and Instagram is one avenue for exploring the experience of illness on the Internet. In particular, Facebook serves as a site in which people can both anonymously and visibly view a variety of Facebook pages devoted to particular diseases as well as engage in private or restricted Facebook groups. The case of celiac disease is a particularly interesting example for studying illness on the Internet because the treatment is a *lifestyle* change involving the gluten-free diet, rather than a medical regimen of prescription medications.

Viewers can anonymously view Facebook pages sponsored by national celiac disease or medical organizations, such as the Celiac Disease Foundation's Facebook page,[2] the National Foundation for Celiac Awareness,[3] Gluten Intolerance Group of North America,[4] and the University of Chicago Celiac Disease Center.[5] In addition to accessing basic information about celiac disease and recent medical updates, visitors to these public Facebook pages can view recent news articles about celiac disease, be alerted to product recalls for gluten-free products, watch videos for gluten-free recipes, and view photos of new gluten-free products and recipes. Public posts range from personal issues on how to talk to family members about screening for celiac disease to public announcements of upcoming gluten-free products by mainstream food companies. Regional support and advocacy groups for people with celiac disease have also created Facebook pages to facilitate local connectivity both online and offline through tips about new products and local gluten-free restaurants, as well as closed Facebook groups that are not accessible to the public enable individuals to connect on a more personal and private basis. Individuals also post questions and comments on many public pages, which can be viewed to outside anonymous visitors from all over the United States and globally, and other online users post responses to these questions. For example, on the National Foundation for Celiac Awareness public Facebook page under a post to a video on the diagnostic delay of women with celiac disease, one woman comments on her own experience of diagnosis:

> Years and years and years! That's how long! And then, after my primary doctor got a positive on the blood test, the gastro doc didn't want to take the time for the intestinal biopsy during my colonoscopy, telling me, "you're not celiac, you're only sensitive. You're numbers aren't high enough to actually be celiac," which was news to me because my primary had actually diagnosed me as celiac. So, I tell my primary doc and she tells my gastro doc to DO THE BIOPSY. After years of suffering, guess what! The biopsy was positive! Always be your own advocate. Be your best supporter and never take no for an answer but more importantly, don't ever be discredited or talked down to by a doctor.

Another online user agrees and comments,

> My GI doctor was the same way! Argued with me about performing the endoscopy . . . When he came into the recovery room (while I was still asleep but could hear everything he was saying) and said that everything was flattened and I needed to start a GF diet immediately. . . . All I wanted was to sit up and scream I told you so. Lol.

These posts are not anonymous and can be easily accessed by viewing the group's Facebook page, yet online users post personal information related to their diagnosis, family history, and symptoms on these Facebook pages, demonstrating a type of support community for individuals with celiac disease facilitated by social media. These open-access

Facebook pages exemplify the transformation of the experience of celiac disease from a private illness involving a change in diet to a public experience to which a community of online users contribute and provide suggestions and recommendations on the latest updates on the gluten-free diet. Unlike Web 1.0 and online support groups, the social media connectivity in these examples of celiac disease on Facebook represents the advance of Web 2.0 as they demonstrate the interactive and public nature of social media. They are indeed virtual communities creating an online subculture of celiac sufferers. Online posts about celiac disease also blur the boundary between medical treatment and food, as the medical regimen for celiac disease is a dietary change, and serve as an example of the transformation of the experience of illness from a private to public experience that is reinforced by an active community of online users.

IMPLICATIONS AND CONSEQUENCES OF ILLNESS AS A PUBLIC EXPERIENCE

In considering the implications of the Internet in the experience of illness, Conrad and Stults (2010) note that "the Internet has changed the experience of illness" (p. 180), particularly through illness subcultures and public notions around illness. The Internet has served as a catalyst in transforming the experience of illness from a private experience to a public one, particularly through its variety of its characteristics: (1) in serving as an information source for patients, (2) in becoming a repository of experiential knowledge, (3) in facilitating communication and support among individuals affected by a particular condition, (4) in shaping social movements (e.g. advocacy) around illnesses and collective illness identity, and (5) in playing a role in the changing nature of the doctor–patient relationship. We will comment briefly on all five aspects of social media and its impact on illness experience:

1. The Internet serves as a source of information for patients as well as for those who provide care to family members or others with an illness. Individuals can seek information online about their own condition and the recommended treatment rather than rely solely on the physician or standard medical sources as a resource of information about one's illness. This characteristic of the Internet is particularly notable for acute illnesses in which individuals may "self-diagnose" based upon symptoms described on the Internet. In addition, many aspects of Web 2.0 are interactive in that they bridge geographical spaces and time and allow illness peers to engage in online health communities (OHCs) and information seeking from their computers (or smart phones) 24/7. However, the notion of risk is an important consequence of seeking information related to health on the Internet and engaging in these OHCs, as patients may receive misinformation from other online users. Healthcare providers do not monitor online health forums and communities, and online users can post their own opinions and experiences around their condition and medical treatments they utilized, which is available to be read by all those who access the site. Advertisements to patients about specific medical treatments also appear online and may shape patients' ideas about their own health condition.

2. The Internet allows individuals to easily seek experiential knowledge. The Internet provides a different type of knowledge and empowerment to online users that they would otherwise not receive from a physician or other medical sources. For example, online users share knowledge around particular physicians to consult, preferences for medications, and issues around one's lifestyle that they can receive online without a visit to a clinician. In addition, non-ill others, including caretakers, can learn about the illness experience from these sites. Goffman (1963) might have called this the knowledge of the "wise," individuals who understand insider meanings of living with the illness. This availability of experiential knowledge represents more of the "soft" subjective side of an illness rather than the clinical or biomedical information one may receive in a clinic visit. In a fashion, this is like joining an Internet club where individuals with an illness can interact with similar others.

3. The Internet also facilitates communication among other patients and families, particularly caregivers, dealing with illness. This function of the Internet resonates more clearly with those with chronic rather than acute illnesses. Glenn's (2015) recent article of mothers of children with rare genetic disorders demonstrates the ways in which patients or caregivers can engage and connect with other individuals who are confronted with the same illness via the Internet, especially in cases in which the condition is rare and in which the individual has never met anyone with the illness in person. OHCs in particular serve as a source of emotional support for online patient seekers, as they allow individuals to learn about and engage in their illness experience without the potential stigma present in face-to-face interactions through the anonymity of the Internet (Broom, 2005), particularly in cases of psychiatric conditions (Berger et al., 2005). OHCs also enable patients to engage in various activities of activism around a particular cause for a disease. For example, "Glu,"[6] an online health community for Type 1 diabetes (T1D), allows participants to connect and emphasize the importance of research on T1D, as their mission statement reads: "Glu is an active and diverse type 1 diabetes online community designed to accelerate research and amplify the collective voice of those living with T1D."

Additionally, the weight-loss bloggers that Leggatt-Cook and Chamberlain (2012) study engaged in a more indirect method of activism through their comments on the meanings of being overweight in society and "offered critical commentary on fatness that went beyond individual struggles with weight" (p. 967). This article also points to the notion that blogs shift the private experience of weight loss to a public one, in which bloggers post their individual details, struggles, and experiences about their weight publicly.

4. The Internet has changed the notion of social movements and advocacy for various diseases and the collective identity around illness, as it facilitates the virtual connection of individuals through cyberspace. For example, the Internet has enabled connectivity and virtual interactions for parents of children with autism, aiding in the anti-vaccine movement as well as spawning the neurodiversity movement among some diagnosed with autism (Baker, 2006). Barker (2008) discusses such issues of collectivity in her piece on ESGs for patients with fibromyalgia, noting the ways in which ESGs provide the opportunity for patients to share information and become "experts" and advocates for their contested illness. Social movements surrounding certain diseases are possible with the Internet, as such a virtual place allows patients to collectively mobilize in cyberspace.

5. There is also a change in the doctor–patient relationship in which there is a resistance to the traditional hierarchy, as the patient becomes active in his or her disease management and lifestyle. Hardey's (1999) early notion when the Internet became more publicly available at the end of the 20th century that the Internet blurs the personal and professional aspects of illness remains true today, as patients are increasingly becoming active consumers of their own medical care

and knowledge around health. Conrad and Stults (2010) suggest that the Internet empowers patients and oftentimes "challenges physicians' expertise . . . which probably does erode physician authority to some degree, but to what extent and with what consequences are not yet understood" (p. 187).

Because the Internet is used among patients to seek information and learn about one's condition, it is important to recognize that there is no one term to describe the site of which online users gather to exchange information and share experiences. These terms are also followed by a certain acronym to shorten the phrase to describe these communities. Barker (2008) uses the term "electronic support groups," while others use the term "digital health social networks" (Van Mierlo, 2014) or "online health communities" (Glenn, 2015). The language of an OHC is a more neutral term to describe a location for the exchange of knowledge and information than solely a site for reasons of support. Similarly, it is important to consider the language we use to refer to these individuals who access the Internet for information and support around disease and illness. These individuals can be termed in different ways, including "patients," "visitors," "online users," and "online surfers," depending on their use of the Internet as a tool in illness experience. For example, the fact that the term to describe these individuals is unclear indicates that there are new ways of thinking about the experience of illness with advances in technology in our society and the ability to engage actively in one's own care.

CONCLUDING REMARKS

As this article has argued, the availability and use of Internet have transformed the experience of illness from a fundamentally private experience to an increasingly public one. This is a major transformation of the illness experience, one from which we believe there is no return. We expect that while there will of course always be private aspects of illness, the

Internet-facilitated public faces of illness will remain and probably grow. There are just too many benefits for ill or disabled people for the interactive sites to fade away. These sites are convenient, accessible from the comforts of home, via computer, tablet, and smart phone. Not only can these interactive sites now always be with us, they are 24/7 and globally accessible by our ever-present mobile phone. It is likely that as new dimensions of the Internet are created, experiential illness-oriented websites will adapt to new technologies and find ways to maintain or even expand their interactive capabilities. In this sense, there was a smooth transition from the early interactive Web 2.0 websites to the current social media connections (e.g. Facebook). Future technological advances in the Internet through new media avenues, mobile apps, or innovations that we cannot yet even imagine may change the shape of the interactive experience, but the existence of the public face of illness will adapt and remain vibrant.

There are a few characteristics of the Internet experience of illness that bear watching to see how they develop in future years. The potential of anonymity (e.g. screen names, lurking) has always been part of the attraction of the Internet and is already somewhat challenged by social media, where one of the main characteristics is individual identity (e.g. Facebook pages). Will social media or some future form of connectivity erode the anonymity that remains an attractive feature of the illness interaction sites? Related to this will many sites remain "open access" so that any interested party can join and participate? Will the Internet remain essentially "cost free" and globally available? The interactive illness websites have adapted as necessary for the past two decades, and one can only imagine that the demand is sufficient for continuing types of adaptation. The public face of illness, while recent in creation, is likely to remain a significant characteristic of illness well into the future.

Notes

1. While there is a multitude of Internet technologies that play a role in illness experience including websites, listservs, online chat rooms, social media sites, and mobile apps, we include all of these as Internet facilitators for the public experience of illness. For social media, we focus on Facebook, the largest and most popular Internet site.

2. https://www.facebook.com/CeliacDiseaseFoundation

3. https://www.facebook.com/NFCeliacAwareness

4. https://www.facebook.com/GlutenIntoleranceGroup

5. https://www.facebook.com/CureCeliac

6. https://myglu.org/?gclid=COf_k7S3psYCFREoaQodILcA0Q

References

Baker DL (2006) Neurodiversity, neurological disability and the public sector: Notes on the autism spectrum. *Disability and Society* 21(1): 15–29.

Barker KK (2008) Electronic support groups, patient-consumers, and medicalization: The case of contested illness. *Journal of Health and Social Behavior* 49(1): 20–36.

Berger M, Wagner TH and Baker LC (2005) Internet use and stigmatized illness. *Social Science & Medicine* 61(8): 1821–1827.

Broom A (2005) Virtually He@lthy: The impact of Internet use on disease experience and the doctor-patient relationship. *Qualitative Health Research* 15(3): 325–345.

Conrad P and Rondini A (2010) The internet and medicalization: Reshaping the global body and illness. In: Ettorre E (ed.) *Culture, Bodies and the Sociology of Health*. Farnham: Ashgate, pp. 107–120.

Conrad P and Stults C (2010) Internet and the experience of illness. In: Bird C, Conrad P, Fremont A, et al. (eds) *Handbook of Medical Sociology*. 6th ed. Nashville, TN: Vanderbilt University Press, pp. 179–191.

Cornode G and Krishnamurthy B (2008) Key differences between Web 1.0 and Web 2.0. *First Monday* 13: 6

Duggan M, Ellison NB, Lampe C, et al. (2015) *Social Media Update 2014*. Pew Research Center: Internet, Science & Tech. Available at: http://www.pewinternet.org/2015/01/09/social-media-update-2014/ (accessed 8 September 2015).

Fox S (2011) *The Social Life of Health Information, 2011*. Pew Research Center: Internet, Science & Tech. Available at: http://www.pewinternet.org/2011/05/12/the-social-life-of-health-information-2011/ (accessed 23 July 2015).

Glenn AD (2015) Using online health communication to manage chronic sorrow: Mothers of children with rare diseases speak. *Journal of Pediatric Nursing* 30(1): 17–24.

Goffman E (1963) *Stigma: Notes on the Management of Spoiled Identity*. Englewood Cliffs, NJ: Prentice Hall.

Hardey M (1999) Doctor in the house: The Internet as a source of lay health knowledge and the challenge to expertise. *Sociology of Health & Illness* 21(6): 820–835.

Herzlich C (2004) Health and illness at the Dawn of the 21st century: From private experience to public affair and back. *Michael* 1: 163–171.

Leggatt-Cook C and Chamberlain K (2012) Blogging for weight loss: Personal accountability, writing selves, and the weight-loss blogosphere. *Sociology of Health & Illness* 34(7): 963–977.

Parsons T and Fox R (1952) Illness, therapy and the modern urban American family. *Journal of Social Issues* 8(4): 31–44.

Pew Research Center: Internet, Science & Tech (2014) *Health Fact Sheet*. Available at: http://www.pewinternet.org/fact-sheets/health-fact-sheet/ (accessed 23 July 2015).

Schneider JW and Conrad P (1983) *Having Epilepsy: The Experience and Control of Illness*. Philadelphia, PA: Temple University Press.

Van Mierlo T (2014) The 1% rule in four digital health social networks: An observational study. *Journal of Medical Internet Research* 16(2): e33.

Ziebland S and Wyke S (2012) Health and illness in a connected world: How might sharing experiences on the internet affect people's health? *Milbank Quarterly* 90(2): 219–249.

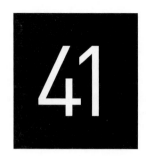

"IT'S LIKE HAVING A PHYSICIAN IN YOUR POCKET!"

A Critical Analysis of Self-Diagnosis Smartphone Apps

Deborah Lupton and Annemarie Jutel

INTRODUCTION

Mobile software applications ('apps') have become an important element of smartphone and tablet computer use since their emergence in 2008. Millions of apps designed for smartphones, tablet computers and other mobile devices have been developed since their first appearance. The two largest app stores by far, Google Play and the Apple App Store, both offered over a million apps each by mid-2014 (1.3 million for Google and 1.2 million for Apple) (Stastista, 2014). Medical and health apps constitute a major part of this market. (Both the Apple App Store and Google Play allow developers to categorise their apps in pre-determined categories

such as 'health and fitness' and 'medical', and it is the apps that are thus categorised to which we refer here.) Over 100,000 medical and health apps for mobile digital devices have now been listed in the Apple App Store and Google Play (Jahns, 2014).

Given the newness of the many digital health technologies that have recently emerged, including medical and health-related apps, little is known about how people are using these apps, whether the apparent benefits they promise are met and what their unintended consequences may be (Krieger, 2013; Lupton, 2014e, 2015b). However, some research suggests that they are becoming used by increasing numbers of lay people. One survey of adult smartphone users in the United States found

"It's Like Having a Physician in Your Pocket!" A Critical Analysis of Self-Diagnosis Smartphone Apps, Deborah Lupton and Annemarie Jutel in *Social Science & Medicine, 133*, 128–135, May 2015. Reprinted with permission from Elsevier.

that the average number of hours respondents spent per month on using apps exceeded 30 h, and that the respondents used an average of 26 apps each (Nielsen, 2014a). Other American research has found that one fifth of smartphone users have used their phone to download a medical or health-related app. The most popular of these apps were related to monitoring exercise, diet and weight (Fox and Duggan, 2012). A recent market research study found that almost one-third of American smartphone users (equivalent to 46 million people) had used apps from the health and fitness category in January 2014 (Nielsen, 2014b). Many medical practitioners and other healthcare workers are also beginning to use apps as part of their professional practice (Buijink et al., 2013).

Despite the prevalence and apparent popularity of medical and health apps, very little critical sociocultural analysis has been undertaken to investigate the ways in which app developers present their wares and to site apps within the broader landscape of digital health technologies. Studies of health and medical apps have predominantly appeared in the medical and public health literature, and have taken an instrumental approach, directed at such issues as their effectiveness for behaviour change, the medical accuracy of the content or legal and regulation issues. Yet from a sociological perspective, digital devices such as health and medical apps have significant implications for the ways in which the human body is understood, visualised and treated by medical practitioners and lay people alike, for the doctor–patient relationship and the practice of medicine (Jutel and Lupton, 2015: Krieger, 2013; Lupton, 2014e, 2015b).

The research reported in this article analyses apps that have been formulated for the purposes of self-diagnosis of medical conditions by lay people. Our study engages in a critical content analysis of these apps, seeking to provide a perspective that incorporates the sociology of diagnosis with a focus on the role played by digital technologies: that is, addressing the topic of digitised diagnosis. As such, the study fits the perspective adopted by one of us as part of a critical digital health studies that seeks to challenge a techno-utopian and solutionist approach to digital health (Lupton, 2014d, 2014b). We sought to examine the ways in which self-diagnosis apps were portrayed on the Apple App Store and Google Play websites; specifically how the developers sought to frame the apps as useful, important and authoritative to attract downloads, and the implications of the apps' content for medical authority, personal data, the doctor–patient relationship and power relations in the act of diagnosis.

Digitised Diagnosis

The sociology of diagnosis is concerned with diagnosis both as a process and as a category (Blaxter, 1978). It explores how these are socially framed, and in turn, frame the experience of health, illness, disease and medical care. A growing body of work has begun to focus on how diagnosis provides an important focal point for understanding the social and political elements of biomedicine. It offers a point of convergence and contestation for lay people and professionals; clinicians, administrators and politicians; corporations and scientists; and many others (Brown, 1990; Jutel, 2009, 2011; Jutel and Nettleton, 2011). Scholars addressing the sociology of diagnosis have contended that possessing the authority and legitimacy to make a diagnosis—to give a label to a collection of bodily signs and symptoms and thence to assert how illness and disease should be treated—is a source of power. This authority is a significant contributor to the status and dominance of the medical profession. The work of diagnosis legitimises the patient's complaint, organises the symptoms and gives sense to them, provides access to the sick role and distributes resources such as sick leave, benefits and therapies. It defines the lay–medical professional relationship, identifying the roles of the seeker and grantor of diagnosis, and creates sub-specialities with particular diagnosers responsible for specific diagnostic categories (Jutel, 2011).

In recent times, however, diagnosis as process and the authority of the medical profession to effect diagnoses have been confronted by changes in the practice of medicine and the doctor–patient relationship. The patient role in interpreting symptoms has entered a phase of liberalisation. Beginning with the emergence of the consumerist movement in healthcare emerging in the 1970s, patients have been encouraged to be 'empowered' and 'engaged' in their care, to view the medical encounter as a 'partnership' and to participate in self-management practices rather than passively accept medical advice (Andreassen and Trondsen, 2010; Bury and Taylor, 2008; Lupton, 1997b, 2013; Nettleton and Burrows, 2003).

Patient empowerment and engagement are related concepts and are often used interchangeably. Both terms tend to refer to lay people taking control over their healthcare and personal health promotion, behaving as self-responsible, knowledgeable actors who are able to make informed, autonomous decisions and position themselves as 'partners' with their healthcare professionals (Fox, Ward, and O'Rourke, 2005; Lupton, 1997a, 2013). The movement of medical information online has been viewed as contributing to patient empowerment and engagement (Nettleton and Burrows, 2003). The notion of the 'digitally engaged patient' brings digital technologies into these discourses of engagement and active participation on the part of lay people by championing the use of these technologies as part of learning more about one's health (Lupton, 2013).

This liberalisation of the patient role has changed the diagnostic process. A vast array of medical information is now available on websites and platforms, including patient support platforms and social media sites in which lay people are able to exchange their experiences of diagnosis and medical treatment (Kivits, 2013; Lupton, 2014a; Murthy, 2013). Given the panoply of online sources of information about illness and disease, the contemporary patient has much greater access to opportunities to self-diagnose. While the patient has always contributed to diagnosis—by instigating the medical consultation, presenting symptoms for consideration, and even negotiating the diagnosis offered by the doctor (Balint, 1964)—today a patient, with the help of technology, might seek out the doctor not for the purposes of deciding the diagnosis, but rather

for endorsing a diagnosis she or he brings to the consultation.

Contemporary diagnostic technologies include a growing array of self-diagnosis devices designed for the use of lay people. Home testing kits for such conditions as pregnancy and blood glucose levels and devices such as thermometers and blood pressure monitors pre-date the digital era. However new digital media and devices expand the range of technologies that are available to lay people to access information about illness and disease and perform self-diagnosis. There has been a trend towards self-diagnosis on the part of patients armed with the information they have been able to access online and the growing number of digital self-diagnosis instruments and direct-to-consumer kits that are now available on the internet (Goyder et at., 2010; Hynes, 2013). Such tools appear to be quite commonly used: one study (Fox and Duggan, 2013) found that one in three of the American adults surveyed had reported using online resources to self-diagnose or diagnose another individual.

The app offers one of the most recent digital tools by which self-diagnosis can take place. The mobility, ease of access and use of apps is a particular feature that differentiates them from earlier forms of digital diagnosis. Due to their simple format and location on mobile wireless devices, apps can be easily downloaded and carried around for constant reference or for updating information about, or comments from, the user and sharing these with others. A further important difference is the issues they raise for the security and privacy of the often very personal information that some of these apps generate about their users that are subsequently uploaded to the developers' archives and become their property. The data generated by apps and other software are now increasingly endowed with economic value, contributing to the 'big data' knowledge economy (Kitchin, 2014; Lesk, 2013). When people accept the terms and conditions of the developers when they install the app on their device, they typically are asked to give up their geolocation, unique phone identifier and details of their contact list even before they start using the app (McAllister, 2014). Once personal details are entered into an app, even more information is collected to which the developers have access. Many developers sell these data to third parties for profit (Dredge, 2013).

App and platform developers have not always taken appropriate steps to safe-guard the often very personal details that are collected, including data on sexual practices and partners and reproductive functions that are collected by some apps (Lupton, 2015b). Several reports recently published by privacy organisations have noted the lack of details offered by many medical and health app developers of what they do with users' personal data. These reports state that many developers failed to properly inform users how their personal data were being used or made excessive demands for personal data from users (see, for example, Ackerman, 2013).

No previous sociological research has been directed at exploring the place of such apps in the diagnostic process or about their role in changing the social dynamic around, as well the nature of, diagnosis. This is a lacuna that our analysis of self-diagnosis apps sought to address. Our analysis takes the approach that health and medical apps may be conceptualised as the products of the interplay between the human actors who make decisions about their form, content and use and the affordances offered by digital technologies which delimit the scope within which apps can be developed and used. They should be considered sociocultural artefacts that assume certain kinds of capacities, desires and embodiments and also construct and configure them. Importantly, apps can have material effects, with the possibility of changing human behaviours and bodies. Apps may further serve political purposes by championing or supporting vested interests and established forms of dominance and authority. They are therefore participants in networks of meaning and power relations (Jutel and Lupton, 2015; Lupton, 2014e, 2014c).

METHODS

The findings here reported draw from our larger study of medical diagnosis mobile apps directed at both health professionals and lay people. To identify relevant apps we undertook a search using the terms 'medical diagnosis' and 'symptom checker', that were available for download to smartphones in mid-April 2014 in the Apple App Store and Google Play. The descriptions of the apps that were listed under these terms were reviewed to determine whether they were directed at lay people for self-diagnosis or at medical professionals or medical students for use for differential diagnosis of patients or for education on carrying out diagnoses on patients. Only those apps that were in the English language were included. The apps that were assessed to be directed at a lay audience were singled out for separate analysis. Our analysis of the diagnosis apps for medical practitioners is described elsewhere (Jutel and Lupton, 2015).

A total of 35 apps claimed to assist lay people to engage in self-diagnosis for a range of conditions. Many more apps were directed at diagnosing specific illnesses or diseases, but they were excluded from the analysis because for our purposes here we wanted to focus on more comprehensive self-diagnosis apps that offered a diagnosis for a wide variety of conditions. The apps we examined typically adopt the approach of listing symptoms, asking a series of set questions based on the user's experiences of the symptoms and then producing a diagnosis based on the user's answers. Some then lead the user onto further information, including providing details of healthcare services.

Sixteen of the 35 self-diagnosis apps were available only in Google Play and 12 were offered only in the Apple App Store, while seven were offered in both stores. Details are provided in Table 41.1, including the name of each app, where it was offered, its price and number of times it had been downloaded where this was available (Google Play provides this information, but the Apple App Store does not).

Like other media representations of health and medicine, including other digital forms such as websites and platforms (Kivits, 2013; Seale, 2005), apps are communicative agents that employ carefully chosen images and discourses to represent their use and function. Examining the words used in the app titles and descriptions on the stores and the images used, including the logo and screenshots employed to illustrate what the app offers potential users, is a way of identifying the tacit assumptions that underpin them and their truth and authority claims. A critical content analysis of apps is directed at identifying these communicative aspects (Lupton, 2014e). In adopting this approach, we reviewed each of the apps for its content and iteratively identified common themes or assumptions across the apps. We investigated the discursive and visual features of the description and screen-shots provided for each app as it was presented in the app store websites. To accomplish this, for each app we reviewed the title, logo, app description text and screenshots provided. Where hyperlinks to the developer's website, terms and conditions and the privacy policy were provided, we clicked through to review these features, looking at how the developer described the intention of the app, where the content was derived from and how users' data were dealt with and used by the developers.

For all material examined we sought to identify the ways in which the categories of lay people and medical professionals and the authority to diagnose were portrayed. Following agreement about how the apps should be analysed, both authors conducted separate reviews and conferred about their findings. Any disagreements concerning interpretation of the apps content were reconciled by discussion between the authors. While such a content analysis cannot document how and why people may be using these apps, like analyses of other forms of media it can contribute insights into various aspects of the nature of apps, including the tacit assumptions and discourses on which they draw, trends and fashions in what kinds of medical and health conditions or problems are considered important to offer solutions, the portrayal of healthcare practitioners, patients and lay people or information about and the ways in which certain kinds of medical and health information are configured and reproduced (Lupton, 2014e, 2014c).

FINDINGS

Several of the self-diagnosis apps we examined appear to be popular. It is evident from the download figures provided for the Google Play apps that some have been downloaded by tens or hundreds of thousands, and in the case of WebMD and iTriage Health, millions of smartphone owners. The WebMD and iTriage apps also featured on the Apple App Store's list of popular health and fitness apps at the time of the study. While we cannot know whether these apps are in fact used following downloading, this information does suggest a high level of interest from the app-using public.

The app developers used various claims to entice users. Their app descriptions assert that they will save lay people's time and money (by potentially allowing them to avoid a visit to the doctor), allay their anxieties, improve their health by allowing them to diagnose a medical condition and then seek treatment, educate them by enhancing their medical knowledge and support patient empowerment by bestowing information about diagnoses. For instance the developers of the Best Android Symptom Checker represent the app as 'a symptom checker which helps you answer the question: "Do I need to see the doctor?". If you have any medical worries or symptoms she [the 'Virtual Nurse' avatar] will put your mind to rest and could save you an unnecessary visit to a physician. It's like having a physician in your pocket!'

The rhetoric and imagery employed in apps are a major element used by developers to attract potential users' attention and establish authority. It was notable that the titles of many of the apps alone represent them as possessing medical authority and credibility. While the terms 'symptom' and 'diagnosis' were most common in app titles, the titles of several apps suggest that they act as proxies for physicians ('Doctor Diagnose', 'WebMD', 'Doctor Online', 'Virtual Doctor', 'Dr Android MD Diagnosis' and 'Pocket Doctor'). Words such as 'medical', 'clinic' and 'triage' in app titles and medical symbols such as stethoscopes and red crosses and images of doctors or nurses in logos and artwork were commonly employed to further establish authority and credibility. The image provided for Doctor Diagnose Symptom Check, for example, features a cartoon-like drawing of a man with grey hair, wearing a white medical coat and a stethoscope around his neck, both potent and well-recognised symbols of the medical profession. Medicare's logo uses a stylised male head and shoulders, with a white coat and tie and with a red cross emblazoned on the coat. Screen-shot

TABLE 41.1 ■ Self-Diagnosis Smartphone Apps Available in the Apple App Store and Google Play, April 2014		
Google Play	Apple App Store	Both
WebMD	*Symptom MD*	*Isabel Symptom Checker*
Free, downloaded 5,000,000–10,000,000 times	$AU4.99	Free, downloaded 1,000–5,000 times on Google Play
Best Android Symptom Checker	*Dignity Health*	*iTriage Health*
Free, downloaded 100,000–500,000 times	Free	Free, downloaded 1,000,000–5,000,000 times on Google Play
Symptom Check by Symptomate	*CheckMySymptoms*	*Lenus*
Free, downloaded 10,000–50,000 times	Free	Free, downloaded 1,000–5,000 times on Google Play
MyClinic Symptom Checker	*iSymptom*	*Your Rapid Diagnosis*
AU$2.99, downloaded 1,000–5,000 times	$AU6.49	$AU5.49, downloaded 500–1,000 times on Google Play
Doctor Diagnose Symptoms Check	*Diagnoscope*	*Your Diagnosis*
Free, downloaded 10,000–50,000 times	$AU2.49	Free, downloaded 1,000–5,000 times on Google Play
Symptify—Symptoms Simplified	*Virtual Doctor*	*Pocket Doctor Lite*
Free, downloaded 1,000–5,000 times	$AU24.99	Free ($AU1.29 for the 'Pro' version with more features), downloaded 50,000–100,000 times on Google Play
Medical Handbook	*Medical Symptoms*	*Healthpedia*
Free, downloaded 100,000–500,000 times	$AU3.79	Free, downloaded 10,000–50,000 times on Google Play
The Common Symptom Guide	*Symptoms Checker*	
Free, downloaded 100,000–500,000 times	$AU6.49	
MediCare	*The Merck Manual Home Symptom Guide*	
Free, downloaded 5,000–10,000 times	$AU6.49	
Dr Moms Treatment Guide	*Child Symptom Checker*	
Free, downloaded 10,000–50,000 times	$3.79	

Doctor Online	Adult Symptom Checker	
Free, downloaded 10,000–50,000 times	$AU3.79	
Common Illnesses & Diagnosis	Medibank Symptom Checker	
Free, downloaded 5000–10,000 times	Free	
Quick Care		
Free, no download figures provided		
Doctor Android MD Diagnosis		
AU$1.06, no download figures provided		
Check My Symptoms		
Free, downloaded 10–50 times		
Diseases and Symptoms		
Free, downloaded 10,000–50,000 times		

images of the app's content use male and female avatars showed standing in a hospital room, with the male represented as an archetypal doctor dressed in a white coat and tie, and the female more ambiguously wearing blue scrubs (possibly a nurse or a doctor). Several apps also use full-colour anatomical drawings in the style of medical textbooks as part of the information provided on medical conditions.

Not only were medical symbols and terms used as a major claim for legitimacy of the information provided, but so too were those of computer science and data science. Technical computer terms such as 'algorithms', 'sensors', 'software engineers', 'deductive logic' and 'artificial intelligence' were often employed in the app descriptions to denote the aura of scientific objectivity and accuracy that supposedly can be established by computer software. This language was used to lend an additional layer of authority to that already maintained by medicine over the diagnostic domain. The Symptify app description, for example, claims: 'Created by top doctors and software engineers, Symptify is an online self-assessment tool that uses a patent-pending, algorithmic engine to help users educate themselves about the causes of their symptoms.' Your Diagnosis

also makes claims to authority based on 'medical algorithms' and 'a complex analysis of all information gathered about your symptoms and will produce a list of all possible and probable medical diagnoses'. Isabel Symptom Checker sells itself by claiming that it was an online tool originally developed for medical professionals but now 'for the first time' offered to lay people as an app. On the developer's website it is noted that: 'Using the latest searching technologies, the system can take a pattern of symptoms in everyday language and instantly compute from our vast database of 6,000 diseases.'

For the majority of apps we examined the discursive features that used reference to medical expertise was often not accompanied by details that were able to provide support for this expertise. Previous studies of medical apps have found that many do not nominate specific medical experts in contributing to the content, or are vague in their attribution of authorship, using such terms as 'doctors' or 'a medical team' (Hamilton and Brady, 2012; Rosser and Eccleston, 2011). Similar findings were evident in our study. It was difficult to ascertain from reading the app descriptions how accurate and authoritative was the information provided on the apps. Many apps made no statements at all about from where the information was sourced and provided no hyperlinks to the developer's website. Others gave only vague details. For example, both the app description and the developer's website for Best Android Symptom Checker make mention of the app content being contributed by the prestigious Harvard Medical School, but no further details are supplied to support this claim.

Sometimes clicking through to the developer's website does provide further information. No details are given about the credentials of information on the Your Diagnosis app description, for example, but the developer's website lists the names of Australian doctors who have contributed to the content. An examination of the other apps or online tools offered by the developers demonstrates a lack of persuasive medical focus or credentials. The developer of the Symptoms Checker app, for example, offers apps such as Mortgage Calculator, Shift Reminder and various games. Medical Symptom's developer has also produced Health Tips 1000, Buddha Quotes and Sex Secrets 1000, among others. The Common Illnesses & Diagnosis app is produced by a developer that has a range of other apps covering many topics, including some health-related apps but also apps focussing on logic puzzles, scary stories for kids and the history of Ancient Rome. This kind of developer offers little in the way of persuasive medical credentials.

Many of the apps employed the discourse of the engaged patient directly as part of their sales pitch. There were frequent references to these apps helping lay people to access medical information, assess their own symptoms and make decisions about whether or not to seek medical help. For instance the description for WebMD notes that it 'helps you with your decision-making and health improvement efforts'. It is claimed that the symptom checker part of the app allows users to '[s]elect the part of the body that is troubling you, choose your symptoms, & learn about potential conditions or issues'. The Rapid Diagnosis app description asserts that: '[the primary objective of this software is to encourage an active interest in health related problems, their diagnosis and treatment, and to empower patients

by providing them with accurate, up to date knowledge, so that they may understand and participate in their health care.' The Dr Moms—Treatment Guide app is explicit in its positioning of mothers as acting in an authoritative medical role for their family members, describing it as: '[a]n app dedicated to all you Doctor Moms out there who function as the "doctor of the family" whenever anybody gets sick.'

Despite such appeals to lay people to download the app in the pursuit of 'taking control' of their health, most of the apps also prevaricate in other parts of the app description or on the developer's website or terms of use page. Even while focused on self-diagnosis and clearly directed at lay users the wording in many of these apps expressed caution about suggesting that a lay person should use them as the only method of diagnosis. For example they prefaced the use of the word diagnosis in the app descriptions with adjectives such as 'possible', 'probable' and 'likely' in relation to the diagnoses to which these apps might lead.

Frequently direct warnings are made for users not to act on the information they access on the app and to seek medical help instead, often including a refutation that the app is indeed directed at self-diagnosis. The Symptify app description is vehement on this point: 'Symptify.com does not provide medical advice and it is NOT intended for medical diagnostic purposes' (emphasis in the original). It is commonly claimed that the apps are directed at developing lay people's awareness or assist them in better seeking healthcare rather than replacing a doctor's expertise. For instance it is noted on the app description for Doctor Diagnose Symptoms Check that: 'This application doesn't intend to replace a doctor but rather to inform the patients and make them more aware.' Several apps are tagged with the caution that they are for 'entertainment purposes only'.

Several of the apps that we examined were used for promotional purposes that were not always readily apparent at first sight Some apps, such as the Best Android Symptom Checker, provide contacts to actual physicians should users decide that their symptoms warrant further investigation. In this app, a list of doctors is provided for real-time contact, paid for by the minute. As such, the app acts as a conduit for promoting doctors' services in ways that are not readily apparent from first appraisal of the app's content and purpose. The Symptom Check by Symptomate invites users to fill in personal details such as their gender, age, height and weight. They are then offered a 'free online checkup report', which may include agreeing to receive a newsletter. Further investigation of the developer's website's terms and conditions page reveals that the app may lead to referral to one of the doctors listed by the app, advice to buy a health insurance policy or use an online pharmacy that is partnered with the company, and that 'Symptomate may receive financial compensation for such referrals and affiliate programs'.

As we noted earlier, many app developers collect personal information about users. Our analysis of the self-diagnosis apps found that information about users' data privacy was provided by only a minority of the app developers. The WebMD website notably provides a detailed privacy policy for users, outlining how their personal information may be used when they register on the website or apps (including the Symptom Checker app). It does advise that users' personal information may be shared with third parties such as vendors, advertisers or suppliers who provide products or services to the company and to provide users with 'more relevant content and advertisements'. The Privacy Policy for the Best Android Symptom Checker is brief, but notes that they do not share users' personal information with anyone else and that the data that they collect on users are used to develop and improve the product and the user experience. Location data and usage data are collected.

The terms of use of Symptom Check by Symptomate also assign to the developer the right to use the personal data uploaded by users for any purpose. The privacy policy notes that users must agree to the developer transferring their data to third parties with or without the users' consent, including physicians, insurers, pharmacies and other third party health-related businesses. The Privacy Policy for iTriage Health outlines that personal data may be used for marketing purposes (including direct marketing to users by advertisers) and that this may include geolocation details that may be provided to their marketing partners together with other information so that 'personalized content' may be delivered and the effectiveness of advertising campaigns assessed. Personal data about the user and their use habits, therefore, are used to deliver targeted advertising.

DISCUSSION

The very existence of self-diagnosis apps speaks to several important dimensions of contemporary patienthood and healthcare in the context of a rapidly developing ecosystem of digital health technologies. Self-diagnosis apps, like other technologies designed to give lay people the opportunity to monitor their bodies and their health states and engage with the discourses of healthism and control that pervade contemporary medicine (Crawford, 2006: Lupton, 2012, 2014e). They also participate in the quest for patient 'engagement' and 'empowerment' that is a hallmark of digital health rhetoric (Lupton, 2013). As the app description for Symptom Checker by Symptomate puts it, such apps are directed at those who are motivated to 'take care of your health'. Such technologies represent the vagaries of human embodiment as amenable to control if sufficient vigilance and self-responsibility are exercised on the part of lay people. The judicious gathering and use of information, including that provided on online forums and medical and health-related apps such as those examined here, is represented as the key to managing illness and disease.

The novel ways in which the digitisation of medical information is occurring are also dominant features of self-diagnosis apps. Many forms of digitised bodies can now be viewed using digital technologies, from YouTube videos of childbirth, surgical procedures, pro-anorexia, self-harming, body-building and fat activist websites to Facebook pages and blogs written about their illnesses by patients (Lupton, 2015a). Self-diagnosis apps are one such mode of digitised embodiment, which often rely on new digitised calculation technologies, as represented by the algorithms, large databases, artificial intelligence and so on that feature in apps' descriptions. As scholars writing about digital data practices have emphasised, the technical affordances of such software tends to represent computer codes and software as authoritative because they are positioned as independent of the frailties of human-decision making. Algorithms have played an increasingly dominant role in making decisions about people, predicting their behaviours and formulating solutions to problems. They offer a new form of logic (Totaro and Ninno, 2014), and a new form of expertise and power: that of 'algorithmic authority' (Cheney-Lippold, 2011).

In the context of self-diagnosis apps, these forms of calculation are portrayed as offering certainty and objectivity to the practice of self-diagnosis as part of participating as a digitally engaged patient. They overtly are positioned as neutral, objective technologies for effecting a diagnosis that differ from the traditional hands-on approach upon which medical practitioners rely. As we have found, however, the algorithmic authority offered by self-diagnosis apps and their appeals to healthism and patient empowerment are undermined by their disclaimers. Self-diagnosis apps inhabit an uneasy space between the engaged patient and the expert medical professional. While many of the apps seek to position lay people as empowered or engaged consumers of health information and healthcare, most shy away from suggesting that this empowerment go too far by challenging medical authority. Potential users of these apps are cautioned to use the information they derive from the apps judiciously by seeking further medical advice from the 'real' experts: qualified doctors.

While the cautions that are offered on the apps that they are for 'entertainment purposes only' and not designed to 'replace a diagnosis from a medical professional' may be added for legal reasons, they detract from the authority that the app may offer and indeed call into question why anyone should use it. In any diagnostic process, the lay person must initially engage in pre-diagnosis work before seeking medical attention (Balint, 1964; Jutel, 2011). However, the apps amplify the role of the lay person in this process. The symptom check list shapes the presentation of dysfunction and changes the locus of

authority (Ebeling, 2011). The app cannot be considered merely a simple tool for organising symptoms because of the pivotal ways in which discerning and interpreting symptoms shape diagnosis in general.

There also remains the issue of how healthcare practitioners may respond to patients who have attempted self-diagnosis using apps like these. For consumer and patient support groups, the ideal of the empowered patient is a means by which medical dominance may be challenged. For governments, this ideal is viewed as key to reducing healthcare costs in an age of austerity (De Vogli, 2011; Mort et al., 2013). Writers contributing to the medical literature demonstrate ambivalence, with some supporting the concepts of patient engagement and participatory medicine, but others articulating unease about the extent to which patients should 'take control' over their healthcare (Lupton, 2013; Prainsack, 2014). With respect specifically to diagnosis, the medical profession has been reluctant to surrender its professional authority to the lay person. While early recognition of symptoms is integral to many health promotion initiatives, with the exception of influenza (see Jutel and Bannister, 2013), we are unaware of any diagnoses where the diagnostic authority of the lay person is accepted formally by medical or public health organisations. A review of the medical literature on self-diagnosis highlighted that medical writers have argued for its utility in cases where early disease recognition is paramount for individual or public health protection, or where medical resources are scant (Jutel, 2010).

Lay people may struggle to know how to deal with the information they access from self-diagnosis apps. Users are placed in a position that many may find difficult: of evaluating the claims to authority and legitimacy of the content of each app and its developer. As we found in our research, determining how the content is created, who performs this content creation, how often it is updated, the commercial sponsors of the developers and the uses to which any personal data that are uploaded to the developers' data archives are put can involve thorough investigation, including time spent in following hyperlink trails. In many cases, such information is simply not provided.

The commercial interests underpinning self-diagnosis and other medical and health apps require further investigation. Many stakeholders now compete for lay people's attention in the world of digital health information, including members of the medical profession and allied health professionals, health insurance companies, pharmaceutical and medical technology companies, hospitals, patient support associations, government agencies and digital device and software developers (Lupton, 2014a: Rozenkranz et al., 2013). However, it is not always apparent where vested interests lie in the provision of medical information in digital formats either for lay people or members of the medical profession (Ebeling, 2011; Jutel and Lupton, 2015; Lupton. 2014a; Read, 2008).

Technologies designed for self-diagnosis are part of a lucrative commercial market, promoted in the interests of the manufacturers who sell these technologies or pharmaceutical companies whose products are recommended by the devices (Childerhose and MacDonald, 2013; Ebeling, 2011; Prainsack, 2014). Self-diagnosis apps are also part of a growing market aimed at promoting the digitally engaged patient. The emergence of self-diagnosis has been enabled by both technology and consumerism or, not unlike what Clarke et al. (2003, 167) refer to as 'Biomedical TechnoService Complex, Inc.' the 'corporatized and privatized (rather than state-funded) research, products and services made possible by technoscientific innovations that further biomedicalization'. At present there is no way of fully identifying the role that pharmaceutical companies or medical device developers may have played in contributing to the content of apps. Yet it is known that such companies are increasingly developing and distributing apps as part of their marketing efforts, raising issues of conflict of interest (Buijink et al., 2013; Ebeling, 2011).

One important difference between diagnosis apps and previous diagnostic technologies is the potential they hold for contravening the privacy of users. The value of big digital datasets for health and medical-related purposes is becoming increasingly recognised (Lupton, 2014a; Neff, 2013). In this context of the increasing collection, storage and monetisation of digital data, data security is a pressing concern for users of health and medical apps (McCarthy, 2013). For those apps which are designed for online use, in many cases users cannot be sure of how their data will be archived or on-sold to third parties because no details are given. Indeed in countries such as the United States, there are no legal requirements that app developers provide privacy policy statements on their information materials for users. A recent study of privacy policies on mobile health and fitness-related apps found that many lacked any kind of privacy policy, few took steps to encrypt the data they collect and many sent the data collected to a third party not disclosed by the developer on its website (Ackerman, 2013).

As our research demonstrated, the developers of medically-related apps, platforms and websites frequently sell the data that users contribute to third parties for commercial use (see also Lupton, 2014a). Furthermore, even though the majority of the apps we examined can be downloaded for free, they are often imbricated in a broader commodity culture by the app developers, several of whom are associated with private or public healthcare providers and health insurers. The commercial interests of app developers are not necessarily provided on the app description or the developer's website and thus may remain hidden to scrutiny. The different agendas that may lie behind these apps, therefore, are largely hidden from users' sight.

CONCLUSION

In this article we have adopted a perspective in our analysis of self-diagnosis apps that represent them as having potential sociocultural and material significance and effects. Our analysis of self-diagnosis apps suggests that they inhabit a contested and ambiguous site of meaning and practice. As sociologists of diagnosis emphasise, regardless of who undertakes the process of diagnosis, it is always contingent, an attempt to impose order upon a collection of bodily signs and symptoms. When medical practitioners undertake diagnosis their authority as doctors tends to obscure the contingency of their decision-making. When lay people undertake self-diagnosis using apps, by contrast, while the apps may promise a compelling combination of medical expertise and the algorithmic authority offered by their software, the uncertainty of their decision-making tends to be highlighted by virtue of their status as 'not medically qualified'. We would contend that despite the existence of devices such as self-diagnosis apps and other forms of digitised diagnosis, the diagnostic process is technically, administratively and legally still the preserve of medicine. This protected sphere is reproduced regularly by all the participants in the diagnostic process, including many of the self-diagnosis apps we examined. The app-generated diagnosis does not offer access to prescriptions, laboratory tests, sick leave or myriad other resources for which the doctor remains the gate-keeper even if diagnosis is the key.

Many questions have been raised by our study. While it is evident from download figures provided by Google Play that some self-diagnosis apps have been downloaded by tens of thousands or even millions of people, we do not know how the apps are used and how these diagnoses affect the doctor–patient encounter. What are lay users to make of the competing discourses of empowerment and acquiring medical knowledge and the insistence of the continuing authority of the medical profession to effect a 'proper' (expert) diagnosis that pervade many of these apps? What do they do with the diagnosis they extract from the app? How valid should they assume the diagnosis is? Do they seek further advice from medical professionals once a digitised diagnosis has been effected? How can lay people determine what commercial interests lie behind the apps' development and how their (often very personal) data may be used? How are medical practitioners responding to self-diagnoses effected by lay people and how do they negotiate these diagnoses with their patients? How are people in different geographical areas, with variable access to healthcare and of differing levels of education using these apps? All of these questions remain to be answered and require further critical sociological investigation.

References

Ackerman, L, 2013. *Mobile Health and Fitness Applications and Information Privacy*, Privacy Rights Clearing House, San Diego, CA.

Andreassen, H., Trondsen, M, 2010, The empowered patient and the sociologist, *Soc. Theory Health* 8 (3), 280–287.

Balint, M., 1964, *The Doctor, His Patient and the Illness*, second ed. Pitman Medical Kent, England.

Blaxter, M., 1978, Diagnosis as category and process: the case of alcoholism. *Soc. Sci. Med.* 12, 9–17.

Brown, P., 1990. The name game: toward a sociology of diagnosis, *J. Mind Behav.* 11 (3–4), 385–406.

Buijink, A.W.G., Visser, B.J., Marshall, L., 2013, Medical apps for smartphones: lack of evidence undermines quality and safety. *Evid. Based Med.* 18 (3), 90–92.

Bury, M., Taylor, D., 2008, Towards a theory of care transition: from medical dominance to managed consumerism. *Soc Theory Health* 6 (3), 201–219.

Cheney-Lippold, J., 2011, A new algorithmic identity: soft biopolitics and the modulation of control. *Theory Cult. Soc.* 28 (6), 164–181.

Childerhose, J., MacDonald, M., 2013, Health consumption as work: the home pregnancy test as a domesticated health tool. *Soc. Sci. Med.* 86 (1), 1–8.

Clarke, A.E., Shim, J.K. Mamo, L. Fosket, J.R., Fishman, J.R., 2003. Biomedicalization: technoscientific transformations of health, illness, and U.S. Biomedicine. *Am. Sociol. Rev.* 68 (2), 161–194.

Crawford. R., 2006, Health as a meaningful social practice, *Health* 10 (4), 401–420.

De Vogli, R., 2011, Neoliberal globalisation and health in a rime of economic crisis. *Soc. Theory Health* 9 (4), 311–325.

Dredge, S., 2013. Yes, Those Free Health Apps Are Sharing Your Data with Other Companies. *The Guardian.com*. http://www.theguardian.com/technology/appsblog/2013/sep/D3/fitness-health-apps-sharing-data-insurance (accessed April 9, 2013).

Ebeling, M., 2011, 'Get with the program!': pharmaceutical marketing, symptom checklists and self-diagnosis. *Soc. Sci. Med.* 73 (6), 825–832.

Fox, N.J., Ward. K.J., O'Rourke, A.J., 2005. The 'expert patient': empowerment or medical dominance? The case of weight loss, pharmaceutical drugs and the Internet. *Soc. Sci. Med.* 60 (6), 1299–1309.

Fox, S., Duggan, M., 2012. Mobile Health 2012. Pew Research Internet Project, http://www.pewinternet.org/Reports/2012/Mobile-Health.aspx (accessed December 21, 2012).

Fox, S., Duggan, M., 2013. Health Online. Pew Research Internet Project, http://www.pew-internet.org/2D13/0l/15/health-oniine-2Ol3/ (accessed December 12, 2013).

Goyder, C, McPherson, A. Glaszîou. P., 2010, Self diagnosis, *Br. Med. J.* 340 (7739), 204.

Hamilton, A., Brady, R., 2012, Medical professional involvement in smartphone 'apps' in dermatology, *Br. J. Dermatol.* 167 (1), 220–221.

Hynes, V., 2013, The trend toward self-diagnosis. *Can. Med. Assoc. J.* 185, E149–E150.

Jahns, R.-G., 2014, The 8 Drivers and Barriers That Will Shape the MHealth App Market in the Next 5 Years.*research2guidance*.http://mhealtheconomics.com/the-8-drivers-and-barriers-that-wiSl-shape-the-mhealth-app-market-in-the-next-5-years/ (accessed September 16, 2014).

Jutel, A, 2009. Sociology of diagnosis: a preliminary review, *Sociol. Health Illn.* 31 (2), 278–299.

Jutel. A., 2010. Self-diagnosis: a discursive systematic review of the medical literature. *J. Particip. Med.* 2, e8 (Sep. 15).

Jutel, A., 2011. *Putting a Name to It; Diagnosis in Contemporary Society*. Johns Hopkins University Press, Baltimore.

Jutel, A., Bannister, E., 2013, "I was pretty sure I had the flu": qualitative description of confirmed-influenza symptoms, *Soc. Sci. Med.* 99, 49–55.

Jutel, A, Lupton, D., 2015. Digitizing diagnosis: a review of mobile applications in the diagnostic process. *Diagnosis*, http://www.degruyter.eom/view/j/dx.ahead~of-print/dx-2014–0068/dx-2014–0068.xml.

Jutel, A., Nettleton, S., 2011. Towards a sociology of diagnosis: reflections and opportunities. *Soc. Sci. Med.* (Special Issue). 793–800.

Kitchin, R., 2014. *The Data Revolution: Big Data, Open Data, Data Infrastructures and Their Consequences*. Sage, London.

Kivits, J., 2013. E-health and renewed sociological approaches to health and illness. In: Orton-Johnson, K., Prior, N. (Eds.), *Digital Sociology: Critical Perspectives*. Palgrave Macmilian Houndmills. pp. 213–226.

Krieger, W., 2013, Medical apps: public and academic perspectives, *Perspect Biol. Med.* 56 (2), 259–273.

Lesk, M., 2013, Big data, big brother, big money, *IEEE Secur. Priv.* 11 (4), 85–89.

Lupton, D., 1997a, Foucault and the medicalisation critique. In: Petersen, A., Bunton, R. (Eds.). *Foucault, Health and Medicine*. Routledge, London, pp. 94–110.

Lupton, D., 1997b. Consumerism, reflexivity and the medical encounter, *Soc. Sci. Med.* 45 (3), 373–381.

Lupton, D., 2012. *Medicine as Culture: Illness, Disease and the Body*, third ed. Sage. London.

Lupton, D., 2013. The digitally engaged patient: self-monitoring and self-care in the digital health era. *Soc. Theory Health* (3), 256–270.

Lupton, D., 2014a. The commodification of patient opinion: the digital patient experience economy in the age of big data, *Sociol. Health Illn.* 36 (6), 856–869.

Lupton, D., 2014b. Beyond techno-utopia: critical approaches to digital health technologies. *Societies* 4 (4), 706–711.

Lupton, D., 2014c. Quantified sex: a critical analysis of sexual and reproductive self-tracking using apps. *Cult. Health Sex.* online first.

Lupton, D., 2014d, Critical perspectives on digital health technologies, *Sociol. Compass* 8 (12), 1344–1359.

Lupton, D., 2014e, Apps as artefacts: towards a critical perspective on mobile health and medical apps. *Societies* 4 (4), 606–622.

Lupton, D., 2015a, *Digital Sociology*, Routledge, London.

Lupton, D., 2015b, Quantified sex: a critical analysis of sexual and reproductive self-tracking using apps. *Cult. Health Sex.* 17 (4), 440–453.

McAllister. N., 2014. Free of Paid, Android or IOS. Your Apps Are Spying on YOU–Report *The Register*, http://www.theregister.co.uk/2014/02/21/appthority_app_privacy_study/ (accessed March 16, 2015.).

McCarthy, M., 2013, Experts warn on data security in health and fitness apps. *Br. Med. J.* (f5600) http://www.bmj.com/content/347/bmj.B600 (accessed February 27, 2014.).

Mort, M., Roberts, C., Callen, B., 2013, Ageing with telecare: care or coercion in austerity? *Sociol. Health Hin.* 35 (6), 799–812.

Murthy, D., 2013, *Twitter: Social Communication in the Twitter Age*, Wiley, Oxford.

Neff, G., 2013, Why big data won't cure us. *Big Data* 1 (3), 117–123.

Nettleton, S., Burrows, R., 2003, E-scaped medicine? Information, reflexivity and health, *Crit. Soc. Policy* 23 (2), 165–185.

Nielsen, C, 2014a. Smartphones: So Many Apps, So Much Time. *Nielsen Newswire*. http://www.nielsen.com/us/en/insights/news/2014/smartphones-so-many-apps-so-much-time.html (accessed October 20, 2014).

Nielsen, C, 2014b. Hacking Health: How Consumers Use Smartphones and Wearable Tech to Track Their Health, http://www.nielsen.com/us/en/newswire/2014/hacking-health-how-consumers-use-smartphones-and-wearable-tech-to-track-rheir-healrh.html (accessed May 10, 2014).

Prainsack, B., 2014. The powers of participatory medicine, *PLoS Biol.* (4) http:// www.plosbiology.org/article/infoX3Adoi%2F10.1371%2Fjournal.pbio.1001837 (accessed April 16, 2014).

Read, J., 2008, Schizophrenia, drug companies and the internet, *Soc. Sci. Med.* 66 (1), 99–109.

Rosser, B., Eccleston, C., 2011, Smartphone applications for pain management, *J. Telemecl. Telecare* 17 (6), 308–312.

Rozenkranz, N., Eckhardt, A., Kiihne, M., Rosenkranz, C., 2013. Health information on the internet: state of the art and analysis. *Bus. Inf. Syst. Eng.* 5 (4), 259–274.

Seale, C. 2005. New directions for critical internet health studies: representing cancer experience on the web. *Sociol. Health Illn.* 27 (4), 515–540.

Stastista, 2014. Number of Apps Available in Leading App Stories as of July 2014. http://www.sfatista.com/statistics/276623/number-of-apps-available-in-leariing-app-stores/ (accessed November 18, 2014).

Totaro, P., Nimio. D., 2014, The concept of algorithm as an interpretative key of modern rationality, *Theory Cult. Soc.* 31 (4), 29–49.

PREVENTION, MOVEMENTS, AND SOCIAL CHANGE

Prevention became a watchword for health in the 1980s and continues to resonate in society. A number of factors contributed to the renewed interest in prevention. While a few fresh concepts emerged (e.g., focus on lifestyle's effect on health) and a few new discoveries were made (e.g., relating hypertension to heart disease), the current attention paid to prevention has not been spurred by scientific breakthroughs. Rather, it is primarily a response to the situations described in this book: the dominant sick-care orientation of the medical profession; the increase in chronic illness; the continuing uncontrolled escalation of costs; and the influence of third-party payers. And prevention efforts are going beyond the medical profession. Insurance companies give rate reductions to individuals with healthy lifestyles (e.g., nonsmokers) and subsidize gym memberships, and numerous employers have introduced worksite wellness and health promotion programs. This new prevention orientation is occurring in a cultural environment that has become sensitized to various forms of health promotion including health foods, health clubs, jogging, and exercise.

If we are serious about reorienting our approach to health from cure to prevention of illness, medicine must become more of a social science. Illness and disease are socially as well as biophysiologically produced. For over a century, under the reign of the germ-theory medical model, medical research searched for specific etiologies (e.g., germs or viruses) of specific diseases. With the present predominance of chronic disease in American society, the limitations of this viewpoint are becoming apparent. If we push our etiological analysis far enough, as often as not we come to sociological factors as primary causes. We must investigate environments, lifestyles, and social structures in our search for etiological factors of disease with the same commitment and zeal with which we investigate bodily systems, and we must begin to conceptualize preventive measures

on the societal level as well as the biophysical. This is not to say that we should ignore or jettison established biomedical knowledge; rather, we need to focus on the production of disease in the interaction of social environments and human physiology. The current rise in obesity rates is a good example of a topic that requires social analysis.

The first surgeon general's report on disease prevention and health promotion, titled *Healthy People* (U.S. Department of Health, Education and Welfare 1979), took steps in this direction. The report recognized the "limitations of modern medicine" and highlighted the importance of behavioral and social factors for health. It deemphasized the role of physicians in controlling health activities and argued persuasively for the need to turn from "sick care" to prevention. Most significantly, the report officially legitimatized the centrality of social and behavioral factors in caring for our health. It argued that people must both take responsibility for changing disease-producing conditions and take positive steps toward good health. In some circles, *Healthy People* was deemed a revolutionary report, more significant even than the 1964 surgeon general's report on smoking. The fact, however, that many people have not yet heard about this 1979 report, much less are familiar with what it says, raises some questions about its potential impact on health behavior.

From a sociological perspective, the 1991 revision, *Healthy People 2000* (U.S. Department of Health and Human Services 1991), was something of a disappointment. While social and behavioral factors were depicted as central in causation and prevention of ill health, a close reading shows that most of those factors were little more than "healthy habits." The report exhorted people to adopt better diets, with more whole grains and less red meat, sugar, and salt; to stop smoking; to exercise regularly; to keep weight down; to seek proper prenatal and postnatal care; and so forth. Behavioral approaches focus on the individual and place the entire burden of change on the individual. From a strictly behavioral approach, individuals who do not or cannot change their unhealthy habits are not seen merely as "at risk." They are noncompliant patients, another form of the blame-the-victim response to health problems. In this interim phase, the *Healthy People* report hardly touched on significant social structural variables such as gender, race, and class, and was strangely silent about the corporate aspects of prevention (Conrad and Schlesinger 1980).

The most recent *Healthy People* report (U.S. Department of Health and Human Services 2011) represents a significant shift back toward the 1979 report, with an emphasis on creating changes in public health at the community level. Although individual behavior remains an issue, emphasis is placed first on broader political and social contexts. These contexts are then viewed as shaping people's hopes and expectations, their job and family demands, social problems (especially poverty), and public leadership around public health in powerful ways. In fact, the "social determinants of health" is included under topics and initiatives in the report for the very first time. Public health prevention at the national level once again recognizes that change needs to occur structurally, not simply at the individual level.

Today, we must conceptualize prevention more broadly and as involving at least three levels: medical, behavioral, and structural (see Table 1). Simply put, medical prevention is directed at the individual's body; behavioral prevention is directed at changing people's behavior; and structural prevention is directed at changing the society or environments in which people work and live. The Robert Wood Johnson Foundation is attempting to shift frameworks for health, moving toward greater equity, by addressing action areas that can improve population health, drivers that are systemic factors needed to improve health and measures to help track progress on these fronts. Focused primarily on community-based approaches to advancing public health, the foundation funds innovative approaches and awards a "Culture of Health" prize to communities that are striving to transform neighborhoods, schools, and other surroundings where people live, work, and play. These efforts address the structural levels that we discuss here.

The first selection in this section, "Politicizing Health Care" by John McKnight, describes a fascinating and innovative community effort to assess health needs and design local medical-care alternatives aimed at improving health in the community. In this project, people discovered a number of important things, including: (1) many "medical" problems had little to do with disease and could more accurately be termed *social problems*; (2) they could, as a community, take collective action to make real changes in their own health;

TABLE 1 ■ Conceptualization of Prevention			
Level of Prevention	**Type of Intervention**	**Place of Intervention**	**Examples of Intervention**
Medical	Biophysiological	Individual's body	Vaccinations; early diagnosis; medical intervention.
Behavioral	Psychological (and Social Psychological)	Individual's behavior and lifestyle	Change habits or behavior (e.g., eat better, stop smoking, exercise, wear seat belts); learn appropriate coping mechanisms (e.g., meditation).
Structural	Sociological (Social and Political)	Social structure, systems, environments	Legislate controls on nutritional values of food; change work environment; reduce pollution; fluoridate water supplies.

(3) they could build alternative organizations for meeting their health and social needs, and in the process include heretofore ignored groups (e.g., the elderly) as productive contributors to the community's health; and (4) they could develop new "tools" of production that would remain under their own control and serve their own particular needs. Despite these marvelous lessons, McKnight acknowledges the limitations of local efforts to change the basic maldistribution of resources and services, and notes the need for self-help efforts to come to grips with "external" authorities and structures.

In the second article, "Embodied Health Movements: Uncharted Territory in Social Movement Research," Phil Brown and his colleagues describe how health social movements can affect change in health and health care. This article focuses on a "new breed" of social movements, embodied health movements (EHMs), which address disease, disability, or illness experience and often challenge science and medicine on the etiology, diagnosis, treatment, and prevention. We frequently see EHMs with contested illnesses like fibromyalgia or Gulf War syndrome (e.g., see Moss and Teghtsoonian 2008). EHMs base their claims on the embodied experience of people with the illness and often involve collaboration with some scientists and health professionals. The goal and success of these movements is to change the definition and treatment of the illness. To achieve this goal, EHMs politicize the issues concerning an illness, functioning as important change agents in illness worlds.

References

Conrad, Peter, and Lynn Schlesinger. 1980. "Beyond Healthy Habits: Society and the Pursuit of Health." Unpublished manuscript.

Moss, Pamela, and Kathy Teghtsoonian, eds. 2008. *Contesting Illness*. Toronto: University of Toronto Press.

U.S. Department of Health, Education and Welfare. 1979. *Healthy People: The Surgeon General's Report on Health Promotion and Disease Prevention*. Washington, DC: U.S. Government Printing Office.

U.S. Department of Health and Human Services. 1991. *Healthy People 2000: National Health Promotion and Disease Prevention Objectives*. Washington, DC: Public Health Service.

U.S. Department of Health and Human Services. 2011. *Healthy People 2020: Improving the Health of Americans*. Accessed July 22, 2011. http://www.healthypeople.gov.

POLITICIZING HEALTH CARE

John McKnight

Is it possible that out of the contradictions of medicine one can develop the possibilities of politics? The example I want to describe is not going to create a new social order. It is, however, the beginning of an effort to free people from medical clienthood, so that they can perceive the possibility of being citizens engaged in political action.

The example involves a community of about 60,000 people on the west side of Chicago. The people are poor and Black, and the majority are dependent on welfare payments. They have a voluntary community organization which encompasses an area in which there are two hospitals.

The neighborhood was originally all white. During the 1960s it went through a racial transition and over a period of a few years, it became largely populated with Black people.

The two hospitals continued to serve the white people who had lived in the neighborhood before transition, leaving the Black people struggling to gain access to the hospitals' services.

This became a political struggle and the community organization finally "captured" the two hospitals. The boards of directors of the hospitals then accepted people from the neighborhood, employed Black people on their staffs, and treated members of the neighborhood rather than the previous white clients.

After several years, the community organization felt that it was time to stand back and look at the health status of their community. As a result of their analysis, they found that, although they had "captured" the hospitals, there was no significant evidence that the health of the people had changed since they had gained control of the medical services.

The organization then contacted the Center for Urban Affairs where I work. They asked us to assist in finding out why, if the people controlled the two hospitals, their health was not any better.

It was agreed that the Center would do a study of the hospitals' medical records to see why people were receiving medical care. We took a sample of the emergency room medical records to determine the frequency of the various problems that brought the people into the hospitals.

Politicizing Health Care, John McKnight in *Social Policy, 9*(3), 36–40, November–December 1978. Reprinted with permission from *Social Policy.*

We found that the seven most common reasons for hospitalization, in order of frequency, were:

1. Automobile accidents.

2. Interpersonal attacks.

3. Accidents (non-auto).

4. Bronchial ailments.

5. Alcoholism.

6. Drug-related problems (medically administered and nonmedically administered).

7. Dog bites.

The people from the organization were startled by these findings. The language of medicine is focused upon disease yet the problems we identified have very little to do with disease. The medicalization of health had led them to believe that "disease" was the problem which hospitals were addressing, but they discovered instead that the hospitals were dealing with many problems which were not disease. It was an important step in increasing consciousness to recognize that modern medical systems are usually dealing with maladies—social problems—rather than disease. Maladies and social problems are the domain of citizens and their community organizations.

A STRATEGY FOR HEALTH

Having seen the list of maladies, the people from the organization considered what they ought to do, or could do, about them. First of all, as good political strategists, they decided to tackle a problem which they felt they could win. They didn't want to start out and immediately lose. So they went down the list and picked dog bites, which caused about four percent of the emergency room visits at an average hospital cost of $185.

How could this problem best be approached? It interested me to see the people in the organization thinking about that problem. The city government has employees who are paid to be "dogcatchers," but the organization did not choose to contact the city. Instead, they said: "Let us see what we can do ourselves." They decided to take a small part of their money and use it for "dog bounties." Through their block clubs they let it be known that for a period of one month, in an area of about a square mile, they would pay a bounty of five dollars for every stray dog that was brought in to the organization or had its location identified so that they could go and capture it.

There were packs of wild dogs in the neighborhood that had frightened many people. The children of the neighborhood, on the other hand, thought that catching dogs was a wonderful idea so they helped to identify them. In one month, 160 of these dogs were captured and cases of dog bites brought to the hospitals decreased.

Two things happened as a result of this success. The people began to learn that their action, rather than the hospital, determines their health. They were also building their organization by involving the children as community activists.

The second course of action was to deal with something more difficult—automobile accidents. "How can we do anything if we don't understand where these accidents are taking place?" the people said. They asked us to try to get information which would help to deal with the accident problem, but we found it extremely difficult to find information regarding when, where, and how an accident took place.

We considered going back to the hospitals and looking at the medical records to determine the nature of the accident that brought each injured person to the hospital. If medicine was thought of as a system that was related to the possibilities of community action, it should have been possible. It was not. The medical record did not say, "This person has a malady because she was hit by an automobile at six o'clock in the evening on January 3rd at the corner of Madison and Kedzie." Sometimes the record did not even say that the cause was an automobile accident. Instead, the record simply tells you that the person has a "broken tibia." It is a record system that obscures the community nature of the problem, by focusing on the therapeutic to the exclusion of the primary cause.

We began, therefore, a search of the data systems of macroplanners. Finally we found one macroplanning group that had data regarding the nature of auto accidents in the city. It was data on a complex, computerized system, to be used in macroplanning to facilitate automobile traffic! We persuaded the planners to do a printout that could be used by the neighborhood people for their own action purposes. This had never occurred to them as a use for their information.

The printouts were so complex, however, that the organization could not comprehend them. So we took the numbers and transposed them onto a neighborhood map showing where the accidents took place. Where people were injured, we put a blue X. Where people were killed, we put a red X.

We did this for all accidents for a period of three months. There are 60,000 residents living in the neighborhood. In that area, in three months, there were more than 1,000 accidents. From the map the people could see, for example, that within three months six people had been injured, and one person killed, in an area 60 feet wide. They immediately identified this place as the entrance to a parking lot for a department store. They were then ready to act, rather than be treated, by dealing with the store owner because information had been "liberated" from its medical and macroplanning captivity.

The experience with the map had two consequences. One, it was an opportunity to invent several different ways to deal with a health problem that the community could understand. The community organization could negotiate with the department store owner and force a change in its entrance.

Two, it became very clear that there were accident problems that the community organization could not handle directly. For example, one of the main reasons for many of the accidents was the fact that higher authorities had decided to make several of the streets through the neighborhood major throughways for automobiles going from the heart of the city out to the affluent suburbs. Those who made this trip were a primary cause of injury to the local people. Dealing with this problem is not within the control of people at the neighborhood

level—but they understood the necessity of getting other community organizations involved in a similar process, so that together they could assemble enough power to force the authorities to change the policies that serve the interests of those who use the neighborhoods as their freeway.

The third community action activity developed when the people focused on "bronchial problems." They learned that good nutrition was a factor in these problems, and concluded that they did not have enough fresh fruit and vegetables for good nutrition. In the city, particularly in the winter, these foods were too expensive. So could they grow fresh fruit and vegetables themselves? They looked around, but it seemed difficult in the heart of the city. Then several people pointed out that most of their houses were two story apartments with flat roofs. "Supposing we could build a greenhouse on the roof, couldn't we grow our own fruit and vegetables?" So they built a greenhouse on one of the roofs as an experiment. Then, a fascinating thing began to happen.

Originally, the greenhouse was built to deal with a health problem—inadequate nutrition. The greenhouse was a tool, appropriate to the environment, that people could make and use to improve health. Quickly, however, people began to see that the greenhouse was also an economic development tool. It increased their income because they now produced a commodity to use and also to sell.

Then, another use for the greenhouse appeared. In the United States, energy costs are extremely high and a great burden for poor people. One of the main places where people lose (waste) energy is from the rooftops of their houses—so the greenhouse on top of the roof converted the energy loss into an asset. The energy that did escape from the house went into the greenhouse where heat was needed. The greenhouse, therefore, was an energy conservation tool.

Another use for the greenhouse developed by chance. The community organization owned a retirement home for elderly people, and one day one of the elderly people discovered the greenhouse. She went to work there, and told the other old people and they started coming to the greenhouse every day to help care for the plants. The administrator of the old people's home noticed that the attitude of the older people changed. They were excited. They had found a function. The greenhouse became a tool to empower older people—to allow discarded people to be productive.

MULTILITY VS. UNITILITY

The people began to see something about technology that they had not realized before. Here was a simple tool—a greenhouse. It could be built locally, used locally and among its "outputs" were health, economic development, energy conservation and enabling older people to be productive. A simple tool requiring a minimum "inputs" produced multiple "outputs" with few negative side effects. We called the greenhouse a "multility."

Most tools in a modernized consumer-oriented society are the reverse of the greenhouse. They are systems requiring a complex organization with multiple inputs that produce only a single output. Let me give you an example. If you get bauxite from Jamaica, copper from Chile, rubber from Indonesia, oil from Saudi Arabia, lumber from Canada, and labor from all these countries, and process these resources in an American corporation that uses American labor and professional skills to manufacture a commodity, you can produce an electric toothbrush. This tool is what we call a "unitility." It has multiple inputs and one output. However, if a tool is basically a labor-saving device, then the electric toothbrush is an anti-tool. If you added up all the labor put into producing it, its sum is infinitely more than the labor saved by its use.

The electric toothbrush and the systems for its production are the essence of the technological mistake. The greenhouse is the essence of the technological possibility. The toothbrush (unitility) is a tool that disables capacity and maximizes exploitation. The greenhouse (multility) is a tool that minimizes exploitation and enables community action.

Similarly, the greenhouse is a health tool that creates citizen action and improves health. The hospitalized focus on health disables community capacity by concentrating on therapeutic tools and techniques requiring tremendous inputs, with limited output in terms of standard health measures.

CONCLUSIONS

Let me draw several conclusions from the health work of the community organization.

First, out of all this activity, it is most important that the health action process has strengthened a community organization. Health is a political issue. To convert a medical problem into a political issue is central to health improvement. Therefore, as our action has developed the organization's vitality and power, we have begun the critical health development. Health action must lead away from dependence on professional tools and techniques, towards community building and citizen action. Effective health action must convert a professional-technical problem into a political, communal issue.

Second, effective health action identifies what you can do at the local level with local resources. It must also identify those external authorities and structures that control the limits of the community to act in the interest of its health.

Third, health action develops tools for the people's use, under their own control. To develop these tools may require us to diminish the resources consumed by the medical system. As the community organization's health activity becomes more effective, the swollen balloon of medicine should shrink. For example, after the dogs were captured, the hospital lost clients. Nonetheless, we cannot expect that this action will stop the medical balloon from growing. The medical system will make new claims for resources and power, but our action will intensify the contradictions of medicalized definitions of health. We can now see people saying: "Look, we may have saved $185 in hospital care for many of the 160 dogs that will not now bite people. That's a lot of money! But it still stays with that hospital. We want our $185! We want to begin to trade in an economy in which you don't exchange our action for more medical service. We need income, not therapy. If we are to act in our health interest, we will need the resources medicine claims for its therapeutic purposes in order to diminish our therapeutic need."

These three principles of community health action suggest that improved health is basically about moving away from being "medical consumers."

The experience I have described suggests that the sickness which we face is the captivity of tools, resources, power, and consciousness by medical "unitilities" that create consumers.

Health is a political question. It requires citizens and communities. The health action process can enable "another health development" by translating medically defined problems and resources into politically actionable community problems.

EMBODIED HEALTH MOVEMENTS

Uncharted Territory in Social Movement Research

Phil Brown, Stephen Zavestoski, Rachel Morello-Frosch,
Sabrina McCormick, Brian Mayer, Rebecca Gasior Altman,
Crystal Adams, Elizabeth Hoover, and Ruth Simpson

What we really need is a new women's health movement, one that's sharp and skeptical enough to ask all the hard questions: What are the environmental (and possibly lifestyle) causes of the breast cancer epidemic? Why are existing treatments, such as chemotherapy, so toxic and heavy-handed? And, if the old narrative of cancer's progression from "early" to "late" stages no longer holds, what is the course of this disease (or diseases)? What we don't need, no matter how pretty and pink, is a lady's auxiliary to the cancer-industrial complex.

—Ehrenreich 2009

INTRODUCTION: A NEW BREED OF SOCIAL MOVEMENT

When the U.S. Preventive Services Task Force recommended in late 2009 that regular screening mammography not start until age 50, it sparked uproar in the media, policy circles, and among women's health advocates. Although this new recommendation was based on a body of scientific studies demonstrating the limits of mammography in reducing breast cancer mortality rates among women under 50, it threatened to undermine dominant medical and public health messages regarding mammography as a reliable strategy for disease "prevention" or "early detection." Drawing from her personal experience with breast cancer, Barbara Ehrenreich boldly advocates for upstream approaches to preventing and treating breast cancer through a more politically and institutionally transformative women's health agenda. As a feminist and environmental breast cancer movement advocate, Ehrenreich's call epitomizes the unique characteristics that make embodied health movements (EHMs) such an important area of analysis for scholars of social movements, medical sociology, and environmental sociology.

Embodied health movements are a subset of a relatively recent and understudied type of social movement that we term "Health Social Movements" (HSMs). HSMs are social movements, centrally organized around health, that challenge medical policy and politics, belief systems, research, and practice. The United States has seen more than a century of social activism to improve health and health care, beginning in the Industrial Revolution with concerns about occupational health and continuing through to more recent fights for disability rights, mental health rights, women's health, and national health care. Some HSMs focus on improving access to health care services—these are "access health movements," including Physicians for a National Health Plan, local movements trying to prevent hospital closings, and movements seeking the legitimation of complementary and alternative medicine. Other HSMs target health inequalities. These "constituency health movements" focus on

a group membership, such as race, ethnicity, gender, class, disability, or sexuality. For example, the women's movement has advocated successfully for improved treatment of breast cancer and other illnesses, changed medical research practices, expanded funding and services in many areas important to women, and broadened reproductive rights (Ruzek 1978; Ruzek 1997; Morgen 2002). The HIV/AIDS movement expanded funding for AIDS research, fought the stigmatization of AIDS patients, gained medical recognition of alternative treatment approaches, and effected major shifts in how clinical trials are conducted (Epstein 1996). Indeed, constituency always matters, even if it is not the central orientation of an HSM or an HSM organization. That is because as individuals affected by disease affiliate with groups of people who experience a similar disease or condition, this can form the foundation for constituency-building through the development of a collective and politicized collective illness experience.

HSMs may emphasize one component (access, constituency, embodiment) over another for strategic and contextual reasons. Health access advocacy and constituency-building are important, but EHMs as a subset of HSMs tend to emphasize the embodied experience of illness. Indeed, EHMs, lift up the collective experience of health and illness as their core—a source of solidarity, motivation, and urgency. At the same time, EHMs link the personal experience of illness with collective illness experience and with the institutional and political economy structures that cause disease, as well as treat it.

Figure 43.1 demonstrates the diverse ways that HSMs interact with each other by emphasizing its different components. In Figure 43.1 the central component for the environmental breast cancer movement is embodiment. In the center of the field is the environmental breast cancer movement as an EHM, while it intersects with the access component of the mainstream breast cancer movement that seeks to alter research funding streams and with the women's health movement, which represents the health concerns of a broader constituency base. This frame highlights the new and emerging embodiment component that is central to the EBCM [Environmental Breast Cancer Movement].

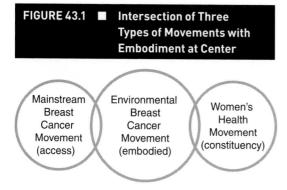

FIGURE 43.1 ■ Intersection of Three Types of Movements with Embodiment at Center

Mainstream Breast Cancer Movement (access)

Environmental Breast Cancer Movement (embodied)

Women's Health Movement (constituency)

Although we emphasize EHMs in this chapter, we are cognizant of the fact that there is much crossing-over from other types of HSMs. For example, constituency-based advocacy to improve working conditions for farmworkers in agricultural areas have historically taken up the embodied illness experiences of those affected by pesticide exposure and other occupational hazards (Pulido 1996). Like other social movements, HSMs include an array of formal and informal organizations, supporters, networks of cooperation, and media. Their influence extends beyond their stated objectives: as they pursue their health-related objectives, HSMs challenge political power, professional authority, and existing definitions of personal and collective identity.

In part, the emergence of HSMs is a response to the increase in industrial and technological risks in modern society (Beck 1992). Such risks are thought by many to have introduced new types of illness, and have raised concerns about possible connections between industrial hazards and disease, leading to the formation of health social movements committed to investigating and publicizing those links. The emergence of these industrial and technological risks both reflects and contributes to the "scientization" of society, where battles over policy-making are expected to involve experts, be scientific and "objective," and have the potential to discredit lay perspectives and the lived experience of illness. In this scientized world full of risk, these new health social movements use medical science and public health as important vehicles through which to marshal resources, conduct research, and produce their own scientific knowledge. These social movements

thus simultaneously embrace the principles of the science—the systematic use of theory, method, and evidence—and use it to challenge the unquestioned authority of scientific institutions in public debates about health.

Recently, various scholars have worked to synthesize this field of social movements in health. The past decade has seen several thematic conferences, special issues, and an increasing number of scholarly articles that focus attention on health social movements.[1] We see the study of HSMs in general, and EHMs in particular, as a new intellectual tradition that draws on multiple perspectives. Earlier studies of health-related activism typically did not adopt social movement perspectives, and social movement scholars have paid little attention to health-related movements. EHMs are the quintessential example of HSMs and have theoretical relevance for social movement theory, the sociology of medicine, environmental sociology, policy studies, and related fields. By studying EHMs, we hope to bridge the gap between the insights of individual experience with illness and healthcare and the implementation of effective policy for a community.

We begin with an in-depth description of embodied health movements, focusing on their unique features that are key to their theoretical relevance. We follow this by constructing a new type of theorizing that emerges from EHMs and helps us better understand them. Finally, we conclude by discussing the significance of EHMs for other HSMs, social movement theory, and for medical and environmental sociology.

EMBODIED HEALTH MOVEMENTS

Embodied Health Movements (EHMs) have as their primary motivating force the experience of a physical disease process within the biological bodies of individuals, and the related shared experience of treatment within and sometimes outside the healthcare system. EHMs address disease, disability, or illness experience by challenging science and medicine on etiology, diagnosis, treatment and prevention. EHMs often address "contested illnesses"—conditions whose causes are either unexplained by current medical knowledge or whose purported environmental explanations are in dispute—and organize to achieve medical recognition, treatment, and research. Not all EHMs necessarily center on contested illnesses. Some may primarily want improved medical care. Some established EHMs may include constituents that are not ill, but who perceive themselves as vulnerable to a disease. Many environmental breast cancer activists for example do not themselves suffer directly from breast cancer, but have joined the movement out of a collective sense of disease risk as women.

EHMs are defined by three characteristics. First, they introduce the biological body into social movements in central ways, particularly through the embodied experience of people who have the disease. Second, EHMs challenge how medical and scientific knowledge and practice define these experiences (such challenges also characterize the environmental movement, anti-nuclear movements, and other movements, though as we discuss later, EHMs are in an unusual position in their challenge to science). Third, EHMs involve activists collaborating with scientists and health professionals in pursuing treatment, prevention, research, and expanded funding. Though many other types of social movements have one or even two of these characteristics, EHMs are unique in possessing all three. We will begin with the defining quality of EHMs: the embodied experience of illness.

1) The Embodied Experience of Illness

In EHMs, the bodily experience of disease is a unifying and mobilizing force. The progression from aggrieved illness sufferer to a participant in collective action stems from an identity that emerges out of the biological disease process happening inside one's body and the ways that the disease is perceived and reacted upon by the outside world. This identity represents the intersection of social constructions of illness and the personal illness experience of a biological disease process. Our focus on embodied health movements meshes with recent social movements scholarship stressing the importance of

emotion and lived experience in the development of social movements and social movement activists (Goodwin et al. 2001; Morgen 2002). As Morgen writes, we cannot "understand the agency of political actors without recognizing that politics is lived, believed, felt, and acted all at once." (p. 230).

The body is often also implicated in other social movements, especially identity-based movements, but these are typically movements that emerge because a particular ascribed identity causes a group of people to experience their bodies through the lens of social stigma and discrimination. Such is the case with the women's and lesbian and gay rights movements, for example. With EHMs, on the other hand, the disease process happening within the body results in the development of a particular disease identity, which may or may not be stigmatized.

The significance of this embodied experience lies in how it constrains the options available to a movement once mobilized. Illness sufferers can work either within or against their target, in this case the system of the production and application of scientific and medical knowledge. They are less free, depending on the severity of their condition, to simply exit the system. Though some illness sufferers[2] seek alternative or complementary therapies, many others need or seek immediate care and are forced to pursue solutions within the system they perceive as failing their health needs. Most importantly, people who have the disease have the unique experience of living with the disease process, its personal illness experience, its interpersonal effects, and its social ramifications. Their friends and family, who may also engage in collective action, share some of the same experiences. These personal experiences give people with the disease or condition a lived perspective that is unavailable to others. It also lends moral credibility to the mobilized group in the public sphere and scientific world.

2) Challenges to Medical/Scientific Knowledge

Challenges to existing medical/scientific knowledge and practice are a second defining characteristic of EHMs, deriving directly from the embodied experience of illness. As science and technocratic decision-making have become increasingly dominant forces shaping social policy and regulation in the United States, social movements have begun encountering new sources of authority against which they must contend, and new types of resources that must be mobilized in order to undertake these challenges. The scientization of decision-making privileges those questions or decisions that can be asked of science and marginalizes those questions that may not be conducive to scientific analysis. Further, the framing of political and moral questions in exclusively scientific terms limits public participation in the decision-making process (Weinberg 1972) and can prevent outside scrutiny of the scientific process, which in turn can reduce the quality of the science produced. These outcomes of scientization have spurred existing social movements to challenge science's monopoly on the production of respected or legitimate knowledge and to develop new forms of scientific expertise.

EHM activists often judge science based on intimate, firsthand knowledge of their bodies and illness. EHMs often develop a strong critique of contemporary science, medicine, and policy by pointing out how ideological and political-economic factors shape medical research and treatment. Some EHMs work outside science altogether. In these embodied movements, adherents have a strong critique of the dominant science, but rather than working to produce alternate science (with or without professional allies), they reject scientific explanations. For example, some participants in the "psychiatric survivors" movement resist traditional psychiatry, eschew reform approaches, and oppose the very idea that they have, or have had, mental illness. Regardless of their relationship with science, however, these activists, like others in EHMs, frame their organizing efforts and critique of the system through their own personal awareness and understanding of their illness experience.

3) Activist Engagement With Science

EHMs' dependence on science leads us to a third characteristic—activist collaboration with scientists and health professionals in pursuing treatment, prevention, research, and expanded funding. Unlike

many other movements that confront science, and scientific knowledge and practice, EHMs must simultaneously challenge and collaborate with the scientific enterprise. Environmental groups, for example, quite often confront scientific justifications for risk-management strategies, global warming, or resource use by drawing on their own scientific evidence for alternative courses of action. However, some environmental groups can abandon scientific arguments by appealing instead, for example, to the public's desire to protect open spaces for psychological or spiritual reasons, or to preserve resources for enjoyment by future generations.

Such alternative organizing strategies are not available to EHMs, since treatment within the biomedical model requires scientific understanding of disease. While they may appeal to people's sense of justice or shared values, they nevertheless remain dependent to a large extent upon scientific understanding and continued innovation if they hope to receive effective treatment and eventually recover.[3] Disease groups are dependent on medical and scientific allies to help them press for increased funding for research, to raise money to enable them to run support groups, and to get insurance coverage. The more scientists can testify to those needs, the stronger patients' and advocates' claims are. Indeed, an EHM's success will likely be measured in part through any medical and scientific advances that may occur. Science is thus an inextricable part of EHMs, leading to a fundamentally different relationship with science than other social movements have.

Dependence on science is particularly apparent for EHMs involved with contested illnesses. When little was known about AIDS, activists had to engage the scientific enterprise in order to prod medicine and government to act quickly enough, and with adequate knowledge (Epstein 1996). However, even EHMs that focus on already understood and treatable diseases are dependent upon science. Although they may not have to push for more research, they typically must point to scientific evidence of causation in order to demand public policies for prevention.

What sets EHMs apart from other movements is less *that* they challenge science, and more *how* they go about doing it. EHMs often engage in *citizen-science alliances* (CSAs) in which activists collaborate with scientists and health professionals in pursuing treatment, prevention, research, and expanded funding. CSAs represent the willingness of citizens and scientists to go beyond a "we" vs. "them" paradigm in order to develop innovative organizational forms that can effectively address the social determinants of health. Citizens bring insights from their personal illness experience and scientists contribute their technical skills and knowledge. These alliances contribute to new knowledge, and they also challenge—and sometimes change—scientific norms by valuing the experience and knowledge of illness sufferers. CSAs may be citizen-initiated, professionally-initiated, or created through a joint-affinity model where lay and researcher interests are aligned.

There are numerous examples of CSAs in EHMs. AIDS activists have sought a place at the scientific table so that their personal illness experiences can help shape research design (Epstein 1996). Breast cancer activists have been involved in federal and state review panels, as well as informing foundation funding processes (Brown et al. 2006). Asthma activists have cooperated with scientists in projects linking air pollution to respiratory illnesses in urban neighborhoods that house bus depots and transit hubs (Shepard et al. 2002). CSAs have also been important in the environmental breast cancer, environmental justice, and environmental health movements, which are concerned with the role of chemical and industrial exposures in human health. Participants in these movements have become involved in a new form of activism that helps generate new evidence of the omnipresent chemical assault by petrochemicals, plastics, and other industrial sectors.

Community-based participatory research (CBPR) programs are the most far-reaching example of citizen-science alliances. In CBPR, members of an affected community engage in the research process alongside scientists, social scientists, medical professionals and other researchers. Drawing on their own experiences as members of the affected community, they participate in the definition of research questions and design, assist in carrying out the study,

help disseminate information back to the community, and actively help shape resulting policies. CBPR is thus inclusive of all affected parties and all potential end-users of the research, including community-based organizations, public health practitioners, and local health and social services agencies (Shepard et al. 2002; Israel et al. 1998; Minkler et al. 2003; Minkler et al. 2008). More comprehensive citizen involvement in research often occurs as the social problem becomes more public and the social movement gains strength and momentum. We will return to CBPR at the end of this chapter since it represents a central organizing frame for the methods we employ in studying EHMs.

At first glance, some HSMs may not appear to fit the three characteristics of EHMs. For example, the tobacco control movement may appear vastly different than the environmental breast cancer movement in terms of personal experience of illness, challenges to science, and collaboration with science. But a closer look at this movement shows that the movement started with intense health testimony from sufferers and their loved ones, and it is centered on the health concerns of smokers and their families and friends. It was also rooted in non-smokers' grievances about the health effects of second hand smoke. For example, a loosely organized group of organizations, GASP (Groups Against Smokers' Pollution), pushed for clean air policies at the state and national level (Wolfson 2001). Further, this movement challenged science for failing to adequately pursue its finding on primary tobacco use and for failing to take on secondary smoke hazards in a timely fashion. Even before the movement had a strong scientific foundation, the activists had made a logical extrapolation from primary to secondary exposure, and they knew they had to pressure researchers to examine this issue more closely. Indeed, one of the common features of EHMs is that they often initiate scientific directions in advance of medical science. The tobacco control movement also blurs several boundaries, as reflected in Wolfson's (2001) concept of state-movement interpenetration, in that it is comprised of single-issue groups, health voluntaries, state agencies, health care professionals, and health care organizations.

A NEW THEORY FOR A NEW BREED OF SOCIAL MOVEMENT

The emergence of social movements explicitly focused on health requires a new approach to analyzing and understanding those movements. Possibly because so much health activism has taken place within the framework and objectives of other forms of activism, there has been little effort to understand health social movements in their own right. Research has occurred across a range of disciplinary perspectives with no systematic attempt to organize a general conceptual framework around health social movements per se. Most of this research has not made use of social movement theory, and the social movement literature itself has paid little attention to health-related movements of all sorts, not just EHMs.

Drawing on social movement theory and the unique characteristics of embodied health movements, we develop a three-point theoretical approach. First, we use the concept of *politicized collective illness identity* to explain how individual disease sufferers become mobilized for action. Second we use the model of the *Dominant Epidemiological Paradigm* to describe the context in which embodied health movement organizations develop targets and identify the goals of their activism. Third, drawing on the concepts of "boundary work" and "boundary objects" from science studies, we conceptualize EHMs as *boundary movements* offering a new way to understand what constitutes movements and who their actors are, while also allowing us to observe the hybridity and fluidity of EHMs.

POLITICIZED COLLECTIVE ILLNESS IDENTITY

The centrality of the biological body in EHMs suggests a basic mechanism of mobilization: collective identity. We draw on the substantial body of work on collective identity (Poletta et al. 2001) and

oppositional consciousness (Groch 1994; Mansbridge et al. 2001) to arrive at what we term "politicized collective illness identity." Poletta and Jasper define collective identity as "an individual's cognitive, moral, and emotional connection with a broader community. It is a perception of a shared status or relation, which may be imagined rather than experienced directly, and it is distinct from personal identities, although it may form part of a personal identity" (Poletta et al. 2001). Illness identity, on the other hand, is the individual sense of oneself shaped by the physical constraints of illness and by others' social reactions to that illness (Charmaz 1991). When individuals, through the illness identity acquired as a result of their illness condition, develop a "cognitive, moral, and emotional connection" with other illness sufferers, a collective illness identity emerges. Collective illness identity, in other words, is the cognitive, moral, and emotional connection an individual has with a broader community of illness sufferers and their allies. A collective illness identity requires the perception of a shared status or relation, rooted in some aspect of the illness experience that is distinct from, though may form a part of, the personal illness identity.

A collective illness identity alone may be sufficient to form a support group or a self-help group. But for a *politicized* collective illness identity to form, the collective illness identity must be linked to a broader social critique that views structural inequalities and the uneven distribution of social power as responsible for the causes and/or triggers of the disease. The requirement for such a critique invokes another important concept. Oppositional consciousness (Groch 1994; Mansbridge et al. 2001) reflects a "state of mind" that binds members of a group against dominant ways of thinking (in this case, the dominant epidemiological paradigm) by attributing problems and grievance to structural factors. When the lived experience is subordinate to dominant groups and/or ideas, an oppositional consciousness often develops among lay persons who recognize that group-based inequalities are structural and unjust. These actors turn to collective action as a means to address perceived injustices (Mansbridge et al. 2001). The development of an

FIGURE 43.2 ■ The Dominant Epidemiological Paradigm's Process of Disease Discovery, Definition, Etiology, Treatment, and Outcomes

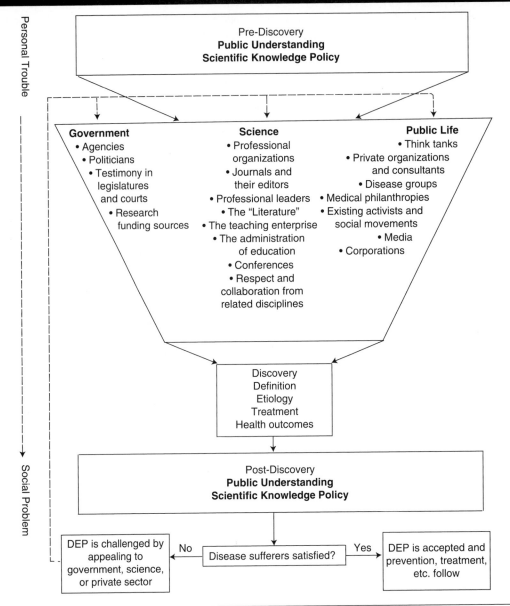

Note: Government, industry, academics, non-profit organizations, health voluntaries, the media, and other relevant actors draw on pre-existing public understanding, scientific knowledge, and policy frameworks to identify and define disease, as well as determine its etiology, proper treatment, and acceptable health outcomes which in turn influence the illness experience by shaping public understanding, scientific knowledge, and policy. The bottom of the figure illustrates how a disease sufferer may opt to challenge the DEP when dissatisfied with the resulting definition of the disease, beliefs about its etiology, norms for treatment, or accepted health outcomes. The left side of the figure captures what we see as a pattern in health social movement organizing: an organized challenge to the DEP's bias toward individualistic approaches to disease.

oppositional consciousness enables aggrieved people with an illness to politicize their collective illness identity.

The structural critique triggered by an oppositional consciousness and embedded in the politicized collective illness identity also places responsibility on social institutions, instead of individuals, for treating and preventing the disease (e.g., the potential impact of toxic substances, the failure of government to regulate industry and reduce population exposures to chemical pollutants). In short, a politicized collective illness identity begins the process of transforming a personal trouble into a social problem. At this stage, people with the disease no longer focus primarily on treatment access, support groups and expanded research, but on seeking structural explanations and the requisite structural changes. In this latter development, people without the disease can be part of the collective identity, either because they are friends or relatives of someone with the disease, or because they have reason to fear they will get the disease in the future. This latter stage clearly offers the potential of a larger critical mass of sufferers who will identify with and join EHMs.

Part of what causes individuals with illness to begin experiencing a politicized collective illness identity is their common experience within government, medical, and scientific institutions that create the dominant epidemiological paradigm, which we describe in the next section and illustrate in Figure 43.2. The pre-existing institutional beliefs and practices that shape the discovery and understanding of a disease also shape the illness experience for the affected population. As individuals experiencing illness enter into formal health care systems, these institutions shape their perceptions of the disease. When disease groups experience their conditions in ways that contradict scientific and medical explanations, and these contradictions are identified as a source of contention, a politicized collective illness identity may emerge.

In some cases, social movement spillover (Meyer et al. 1994) enables disease groups to make connections between their collective illness experience and some form of inequality. For example, environmental justice activists have influenced asthma activists

to view asthma as related to unequal racial exposure to air pollution and toxic substances. As Meyer and Whittier (1994: 281–282) explain, "taken together, one movement can influence subsequent movements both from outside and from within: by altering the political and cultural conditions it confronts in the external environment, and by changing the individuals, groups, and norms within the movement itself." Further, the notion of spillover captures the variety of outcomes movements can have, and moves beyond the notion that social movement successes are measured simply by impacts on the state. Such a conceptualization is ideally suited to EHMs, which are hybrid movements in which the collective identities, tactics, styles of leadership, and organizational structures of movements intersect with a disease's powerful effect on the body. Hybrid movements that benefit from social movement spillover transcend traditional conceptions of social movements and their attendant organizations. Observing the spillover that EHMs experience, and understanding these movements as hybrid movements that merge individuals, cultures, and strategies of various movements, invokes the notion of EHMs as boundary movements, which we discuss after elaborating on the concept of the dominant epidemiological paradigm.

EMBODIED HEALTH MOVEMENTS AS CHALLENGES TO THE DOMINANT EPIDEMIOLOGICAL PARADIGM

When challenging science, social movements confront a powerful set of institutions and belief structures, formed into a dominant epidemiological paradigm (DEP). The DEP is the codification of beliefs about disease and its causation by science, government, and the private sector. It includes established institutions entrusted with the diagnosis, treatment, and care of disease sufferers, as well as journals, media, universities, medical philanthropies, and government officials. There are many structures and institutions that contribute to a generally accepted view of disease, but people do not immediately see them. Actors can challenge the dominant epidemiological paradigm, attempt to reshape it at different locations, and take action on one or more of the components.

The creation, reinforcement, and influence of the dominant epidemiological paradigm comes from a complex set of interactions (Figure 43.2). Social actors such as government, industry, academics, non-profit organizations, health voluntaries, and the media draw on pre-existing public understanding, scientific knowledge, and policy frameworks to identify and define disease, as well as determine its etiology, proper treatment, and acceptable health outcomes. This process shapes future public understanding, scientific knowledge, and policies in ways that influence the illness experience of a disease sufferer.

A disease sufferer who is dissatisfied with the resulting definition of the disease, theories about its etiology, norms for treatment, or accepted health outcomes, may be motivated to challenge the DEP. A movement may mount an organized challenge to a DEP's individualistic approach to disease because the movement opposes the notion of holding individuals responsible for their health status. Embodied health movements point to population data that demonstrate the importance of social structural factors and environmental factors in determining health and disease in populations. They challenge the "lifestyle" approaches, implicit or explicit in the DEP, that single out apparent choices (such as smoking, diet, alcohol use). EHMs argue that this individualistic approach fails to see that personal behaviors are largely shaped by social structures, much as C. Wright Mills argued that we often miscast "social problems" as "personal troubles." In short, the process of challenging a DEP is often an attempt to move away from the idea that illness is a personal problem for which the individual is responsible and over which she or he has control, and move towards the idea that illness is a social problem that

must be dealt with systematically at higher levels of social organization.

Science and medicine have increasingly come under scrutiny by social movements, but differ from other institutions commonly targeted by social movements, making science and medicine open to a different set of strategies. Rapid changes in scientific innovation, investment in new areas of research, and the lack of a strongly held consensus on a scientific issue may create *windows of opportunity* for protest and action. Medicine and science are in a nearly constant state of flux as the growth and advancement of scientific knowledge progresses. In addition to creating new knowledge that may be contested by social movement actors, this process may also destabilize rules and relationships that govern institutions. When an organization receives a large influx of research dollars, or experiences rapid growth in membership or staffing, or when the expansion of the knowledge base triggers a paradigm shift, this may destabilize the organization, opening up opportunities for social movement actors to challenge the institutions. In such circumstances, the institution often lacks a unified center of gravity, and may be open to challenges by EHMs. As Moore (1999) notes, a scientific field undergoing rapid change presents "multiple locations of challenge and access for protesters and dissenting scientists (113)." Moore argues that social movement actors (including sympathetic scientists or the general lay public) can alter institutional practices when they capitalize on these windows of opportunity. For example, as breast cancer research funding expanded rapidly, it opened opportunities for different kinds of challenges, such as that related to improvement for detection devices and for better treatment (Casamayou 2001), and, for the environmental breast cancer movement, to very different types of demands about prevention (McCormick and Baralt 2006).

Second, the heterogeneous field of actors involved in creating and maintaining the DEP presents *multiple points of leverage* for social movement activists. Medical and scientific institutions are not completely unified around a single theory of disease causation or analytical approach to research. While the DEP is dominated by an emphasis on individual and behavioral risk factors for disease, over environmental or social factors, some elements of the DEP may be more accepting of environmental hypotheses (Zavestoski et al. 2004). With respect to breast cancer, for example, some scientific institutions have embraced the endocrine disrupter hypothesis (Krimsky 2000) and some institutes within the National Institutes of Health (especially the National Institute of Environmental Health Sciences, NIEHS) have funded extensive research on environmental causation of disease (McCormick et al. 2004). While environmental causation of breast cancer remains a controversial theory, and some segments of the DEP still de-emphasize the investigation of environmental causation in favor of individualized factors such as genes, diet, and health behaviors such as drinking or smoking, the existence of sympathetic elites in parts of the science policy arena creates opportunities for social movement actors to press their agenda. A lack of consensus among the scientific actors involved in creating or maintaining the DEP may make it possible for social movement actors to gain entry into an institution of authority. This example shows that the DEP may not necessarily be monolithic, and the presence of controversy and dissent among the actors create multiple possible points of entry for activists who are trying to influence the scientific agenda (Zavestoski et al. 2004).

Third, science policy is enacted at *multiple levels*, and activists can target local, statewide, or federal agencies. Activists may encounter medical and scientific institutions at multiple levels: locally, regionally, or nationally. Each scale adds a space for contestation. There may be locally-based research institutions that are responsive to local advocate interests. Silent Spring Institute is one such organization, founded by the Massachusetts Breast Cancer Coalition to conduct research on women's health and the environment with a strong component of citizen involvement. In addition, national-level research initiatives like those within NIEHS can respond to national organizations with sufficient credibility and membership. NIEHS has played a strong leadership role in federal initiatives to foster

academic-community collaborations that have a social justice component (Felix 2007). Medical institutions that attempt to resolve illnesses similarly operate on a multiplicity of scales. While local practitioners may see disease phenomena on a micro level that relate to community concerns, more macro-level health care foundations and philanthropic institutions get involved with movement leadership and elites that have transcended the concerns of one community. This has taken place with the panoply of breast cancer foundations like Komen for the Cure and the Breast Cancer Research Foundation that drive public attention (McCormick et al. 2006).

Finally, science policy presents *multiple targets* for the translation of scientific findings in regulations, presenting activists with multiple arenas for action. Many scientific and medical institutions are connected to the state through regulatory channels, which creates another potential target for social movement action. Scientific research is dependent on funding, and activists can mount challenges by questioning funding decisions or demanding additional government funding for certain projects. For example, forcing the passage of the Long Island Breast Cancer Study Project in 1993 was a part of breast cancer activists' establishment of a new agenda focused on elucidating environmental links to breast cancer and thus potential keys to disease prevention, rather than treatment and cure. This important milestone was preceded by activism around environmental links to breast cancer both in Long Island and across the country.

EMBODIED HEALTH MOVEMENTS AS BOUNDARY MOVEMENTS

Blurring the boundaries between social movements is just one example of how EHMs represent what we call *boundary movements*. In the sociology of science, the term "boundary work" describes the efforts of scientists and lay people to distinguish good science from bad science (Gieryn 1983), a process that occurs both within science, and also in its relationship to the public and the state. An attempt to secure authority and material resources, this demarcation effort is based not on a positivistic notion of truth, but on different kinds of proof and certainty that vary with the issue at hand. Star and Greisemer (1989) also focus on boundaries, examining how actors use them to leverage or create "boundary objects" that overlap different social worlds and are malleable enough to be used by different parties. For example, scientists can capitalize on the discovery of a DNA sequence that determines disease predisposition, by using it as a boundary object to justify funding for additional studies.

Because EHMs so often depend on challenging medical and scientific knowledge and practice, they constantly engage in boundary work and use boundary objects. Consequently, they can be thought of as boundary movements in four different ways. First, they attempt to reconstruct the lines that demarcate science from non-science, as well as lines demarcating good science from bad science. For example, environmental health activists have pointed to flaws and shortcomings in the science of chemical risk assessment for not adequately considering the health impacts of cumulative exposures, and have opposed the widespread notion that a detection technology (such as mammography) is a disease prevention strategy. By pushing science in new directions, or by participating in scientific processes as a means of bringing previously unaddressed issues and concerns to the clinical and bench scientists, EHMs are aimed at pushing the boundaries of science. EHMs can also use boundary objects in ways that blur the lines between science and non-science. For example, a particular scientific method may serve as a boundary object that an EHM can employ in order to produce scientific data to help scientists, but also to empower movement followers.

Second, EHMs also blur the boundary between experts and laypeople. Some EHM activists informally become experts by using the Internet and other resources to arm themselves with medical and scientific knowledge that can be employed in conflicts with their medical care providers. Others gain a more legitimate form of expertise by working with scientists and medical experts to gain a better level of understanding of the science underlying their disease. Through this process, boundary movements gain power and authority by obscuring the boundary between expert and layperson. In some cases, rather than just blur the boundary, activists redefine or even eliminate it, as with the National Breast Cancer Coalition's Project LEAD that helps activists become versed in the policy and scientific literature so that they can serve on peer review panels for the allocation of research funding (Dickersin et al. 2001). Some EHM organizations have evolved beyond "lay" organizations, since they deal so much with science and contend with the world of science. They become a hybrid through this process of breaking down long-existing boundaries.

Third, EHMs also cross boundaries with nonsocial movement institutions, as with the "interpenetration" in which tobacco control activists allied in varying combinations with health voluntary organizations and government units (Wolfson 2001). Hence, rather than distinct entities, EHMs are savvy social actors moving between social worlds. Additionally, this approach redefines who activists are, since scientists who have a fluid movement between lay and expert worlds of knowledge often play activist roles themselves in the role of "advocacy scientists" (Krimsky 2000).

Finally, EHMs take advantage of the malleability of boundary objects to acquire political resources to raise funds, recruit new members, or generate legitimacy for the social movement. For example, the Boston environmental justice organization, Alternatives for Community and Environment (ACE) pressured state and federal environmental agencies to install an air monitor on their roof. The monitor is a boundary object that crosses several social worlds: it is a symbol of ACE's political effectiveness; it is a teaching and community organizing device; and it is a scientific tool for research by ACE and public health researchers. Using the monitor, ACE was able to gather data to press for low-emissions buses.

For the environmental breast cancer movement, boundary objects include mammography machines, genetic testing for breast cancer, patents on the BRCA-1 and BRCA-2 sequences, pharmaceuticals, Breast Cancer Awareness Month, and Avon's "Breast Cancer Walk." The mammography machine is both a mainstay of hospitals and their breast cancer centers, but also a point of contention for activists who have critiqued its overuse and lack of attention to harmful consequences (radiation, false positives, unnecessary surgery), especially on younger women. This was highlighted in November 2009 when the US Prevention Services Task Force (USPSTF) issued new screening recommendations for women who are asymptomatic and who are not at elevated risk of breast cancer. The Task Force called for an end to routine mammography screening for women 40 to 49, and encouraged biannual (every two year) rather than annual mammograms for post-menopausal women. This has brought back to public light a major dispute that has long faced breast cancer activists, sufferers, clinicians, and policy makers—does the technology encourage false positives and hence more interventions than are useful, and does it expose people to more radiation, itself a cause of breast cancer? It is clear that the mammogram represents so much more than a mere imaging technology. Regarding another boundary object, the BRCA sequences are medical diagnostic tools to detect high levels of risk, yet also an example of the dangers of patenting gene sequences by private firms. Likewise, National Breast Cancer Awareness Month calls attention to breast cancer, but does so more from a treatment than a preventive approach. And, since the nonprofit healthcare foundation of pharmaceutical giant AstraZeneca holds the copyright over National Breast Cancer Awareness Month, this limits how breast cancer activists can be involved and the messages they can communicate to the broader public.

CONCLUSION

Health has emerged as a singularly powerful frame for many grievances, and numerous health movements have changed the political landscape of state and scientific institutions, and have played major roles in promoting social equality and change. The centrality of health as a human and social issue is clear in the way so many social movements not explicitly concerned with health have nonetheless come to champion health-related causes. Following Rachel Carson in the 1960s and Love Canal in the late 1970s, environmentalists pursued environmental health, expanding the environmental movement from its initial concerns with wildlife conservation and preservation, to consider how the environment affected human health. Civil rights activists cited the notorious Tuskegee syphilis experiment to demonstrate how the health care system itself promoted racism. Environmental justice activists expanded on this civil rights framework to make environmental health a social justice issue. Housing activists emphasized how poor housing conditions contributed to poor health, especially asthma. Repeatedly, social movements with disparate objectives often gravitate towards issues of health and healthcare.

Health social movements also feed off the growing public awareness of and involvement in health issues. Health consciousness has taken up struggles against targets that were previously seen as untouchable, such as tobacco, and in the U.S. there is growing sentiment that an expensive health care system, consuming sixteen percent of the country's gross domestic product fails to serve our needs adequately. A huge uninsured population, failures to treat new, mysterious chronic multi-system diseases, and dissatisfaction with the growing impersonal nature of managed care settings have led to a general distrust of the healthcare system and provided grounds for engaging in social movement activity, or at least for supporting others who do so.

Our emphasis on EHMs, and the theoretical insights they afford us, have implications for various fields, including social movement theory and the related fields of environmental sociology and medical sociology. For social movement theory, EHMs open new avenues of scholarship, as well as creative integration of existing social movement theories and approaches. For example, in social movement theory, the "political opportunity" approach argues that as political networks change, social movements may find allies among sympathetic political parties and government agencies where previously none existed, (Tilly 1978; McAdam 1982; McAdam et al. 2001). There are a number of cases where EHMs encountered and took advantage of such circumstances. For example, to a certain extent AIDS activism was feasible in light of more favorable opportunities for gay rights activism. Similarly, veterans struggled for years to get government acknowledgment that chemical and biological weapons had been present during the Gulf War. The eventual uncovering of evidence that thousands of soldiers had been exposed created opportunities for Gulf War veterans to appeal for increased funding for research and compensation for their health problems.

However, while EHMs demonstrate the importance of political opportunities for social movements, they also encourage us, as theorists, to temper the power and significance we attribute to those external opportunities. EHMs are strongly rooted in the illness experience and the exigency of health demands. The immediacy of healthcare needs means that illness sufferers cannot, and do not, wait for advantageous political opportunities before mobilizing. While they will likely be more successful when such opportunities exist, they often organize in the face of political constraints.

The example of EHMs also reminds us that social movements may contend with constraints from groups other than the state or formal political bodies, the most common focus in the political opportunity approach. Certainly, some EHMs are struggling against state action or inaction, but others focus on non-state targets such as scientific organizations and medical institutions, for example challenging the pharmaceutical firm AstraZeneca on promotion and direct advertising of the drug Tamoxifen for the prevention of breast cancer. EHMs also show us that a social movement can have a complex relationship with the state—both confrontational and strategically cooperative—allying with components of the state in their efforts to change the actions of the state as a whole. For example, some asthma activists have worked with the EPA to obtain stronger air quality regulation from the federal government.

Like many social movements, EHMs engage in "frame alignment," identifying problems, defining

solutions, motivating action and setting action agendas in ways that resonate with the personal experiences, values, and expectations of potential constituents (Snow et al. 1986; Benford et al. 2000). In EHMs this process centers on aligning the illness experience of potential constituents with the illness experience defined by the movement. Framing is vital in transforming an individual's illness experience from a personal trouble to a social problem that transcends the experience of the individual. Framing is also important to align both individual and collective illness experience with medicine, science, and government, since those sectors represent potentials for legitimation and resources.

EHMs also draw our attention to the continuing significance of social class in understanding health and access to healthcare. Class remains a salient feature of many, though not all, movements around health, and any approach that seeks to understand these movements must consider class and other social structures. For example, our research on asthma activism shows that poor, inner-city communities of color play a dominant role in organizing around asthma, and they integrate their asthma-centered organizing with efforts to address a host of class-based issues in housing, transportation access, and economic development (Brown et al. 2003).

We do not propose that our approach is necessarily a thoroughly new approach to *all* social movements. We do, however, think our approach represents a unique way of looking at *certain types* of movements, such as social movements concerned with scientific knowledge, whether they involve health concerns or not. Scholars who study social movements concerned with science issues that are not directly related to health might be examining social movements around natural resources, energy, genetically modified organisms, and hydroelectric dams. In all these cases, activists cross boundaries with scientists, are compelled to learn science in order to advance their movements, and eventually seek and even obtain seats at the table to make decisions based on science. David Hess (2002) addresses this in his notion of "technology-oriented social movements," including organic foods, nutritional therapeutics, renewable energy, recycling, and human-centered transportation. Kelly Moore (2008) does so in looking at challenges to military use of science, and Scott Frickel and Neil Gross (2005) do so in terms of "science and intellectual movements." As well, many identity-driven movements aim to remove the stigma of an identity by producing scientific knowledge that normalizes the identity.

For medical sociology, EHMs encourage us to pay attention to the intersection of health inequalities and environmental justice. Medical sociology has pioneered the area of health inequalities, but has not usually taken that interest to an applied or activist level, nor has the field grasped the connections with environmental justice. If we look at environmental justice scholars, some view health inequalities as central to environmental justice concerns. Still, even those who frame in terms of health inequalities rely more on justice frames than medical sociology approaches to make sense of EJ struggles.

Apart from medical sociology, environmental sociology is the field that most addresses health social movements. Environmental sociologists have addressed the problem of contaminated communities by explaining how conflicts emerge between ecological realities (e.g., contamination), and a community's attachment of symbolic meaning to the contamination (Kroll-Smith et al. 1991; Couch et al. 1994). Moving beyond a conflict between reality and symbolism, the framework we have laid out for understanding EHMs encourages us to view community contamination in terms of a more fundamental conflict between biological bodies and the social meaning of illness.

And, returning to our earlier discussion of community-based participatory research, we see how CBPR is so relevant to EHMs, because people in those movements need to be actively engaged in the science and policy work that involves their diseases. As affected members of a geographic community or a disease community, they draw on their own experiences to effectively participate in the definition of research questions and design, to work on the conduct of the study, to disseminate information back to the community, and to apply their work to affect social policy. Our approach to understanding EHMs synthesizes elements from a variety of social movement perspectives, and brings together material from multiple fields—social sciences, epidemiology, public health, environmental health science, and community-based participatory research. Our focus on the unique ways in which EHMs blur boundaries between lay and expert knowledge offers a new way of looking at health-related social movements.

Notes

1. This includes special streams at the 2001 and 2003 conferences of the Society for the Social Study of Science, a workshop at the American Sociological Association's Collective Behavior and Social Movements Section Conference in 2002, a Medical Social Movements symposium in Sweden in 2003 that led to a *Social Science & Medicine* special issue on Patient-based Social Movements in 2006, a special issue on "Health and the Environment" of *Annals of the American Academy of Political and Social Science* in 2002 (edited by Phil Brown), the *Sociology of Health and Illness* 2004 annual monograph on Health Social Movements (later a book edited by Phil Brown and Stephen Zavestoski), a 2005 conference at the University of Victoria on "Illness and the Contours of Contestation: Diagnosis, Experience, Policy," from which *Contesting Illness: Process and Practices* was published in 2007, a conference on Social Movements and Health Institutions at the University of Michigan 2007 from which a volume was published (Zald et al. 2009), and a workshop at the 2008 US-UK Medical Sociology conference.

2. Reflecting the contested nature of the illnesses that EHMs address, whatever term we choose is inevitably problematic from some perspective. Not all EHM actors identify as illness "sufferers" (antipsychiatry advocates, for example) and many prefer more empowered terms such as "survivor."
3. This claim should be qualified since, as previously acknowledged, some illness sufferers do choose to exit the system of Western medical care by seeking alternative and complementary therapies or abandoning treatment altogether. As this group of individuals represents a small minority of the ill who are seeking to restore their health, we choose to focus on the dependence on science that characterizes those who turn to mainstream medical care providers.

References

Beck, U. (1992). *Risk Society: Towards a New Modernity*. London, Sage.

Benford, R. D. and Snow, D. A. (2000). "Framing Processes and Social Movements: An Overview and Assessment." *Annual Review of Sociology* 26(1): 611.

Brown, P., Zavestoski, S., Luebke, T., Mandelbaum, J., McCormick, S. and Mayer, B. (2003). "The Health Politics of Asthma: Environmental Justice and Collective Illness Experience in the United States." *Social Science and Medicine* 57: 453–464.

Brown, P., Zavestoski, S., McCormick, S., Mayer, B., Morello-Frosch, R., Altman, R. G. and Senier, L. (2006). "'A Lab of Our Own': Environmental Causation of Breast Cancer and Challenges to the Dominant Epidemiological Paradigm." *Science, Technology, and Human Values* 31: 499–536.

Casamayou, M. H. (2001). *The Politics of Breast Cancer*. Washington, DC, Georgetown University Press.

Charmaz, K. (1991). *Good Days, Bad Days: The Self in Chronic Illness and Time*. New Brunswick, Rutgers University Press.

Couch, S. R. and Kroll-Smith, S. (1994). "Environmental Controversies, Interactional Resources, and Rural Communities: Siting Versus Exposure Disputes." *Rural Sociology* 59: 25–44.

Dickersin, K., Braun, L., Mead, M., Millikan, R., Wu, A. M., Pietenpol, J., Troyan, S., Anderson, B. and Visco, F. (2001). "Development and implementation of a science training course for breast cancer activists: Project LEAD (leadership, education and advocacy development)." *Health Expectations* 4(4): 213–220.

Ehrenreich, B. (2009) "We need a new women's health movement." Los Angeles Times. (2 December), URL (accessed 30 May 2012): http://articles.latimes.com/2009/dec/02/opinion/la-oe-ehrenreich2-2009 dec02.

Epstein, S. (1996). *Impure Science: AIDS, Activism, and the Politics of Knowledge*. Berkeley, University of California Press.

Felix, H. C. (2007). The Rise of the Community-Based Participatory Research Initiative at the National Institute for Environmental Health Sciences: An Historical Analysis Using the Policy Streams Model. *Progress in Community Health Partnerships: Research, Education, and Action*. 1: 31–39.

Frickel, S. and Gross, N. (2005). "A General Theory of Scientific/Intellectual Movements." *American Sociological Review* 70: 204–232.

Gieryn, T. F. (1983). "Boundary-work and the demarcation of science from non-science: Strains and interests in professional ideologies of scientists." *American Sociological Review* 48(6): 781–795.

Goodwin, J., Jasper, J. M. and Polletta, F., Eds. (2001). *Passionate Politics: Emotions and Social Movements*. Chicago, University of Chicago Press.

Groch, S. (1994). "Oppositional Consciousness: Its Manifestation and Development. The Case of People with Disabilities." *Sociological Inquiry* 64(369–395).

Hess, D. J. (2002). Technology-Oriented Social Movements and the Problem of Globalization. Unpublished paper.

Israel, B. A., Schulz, A., Parker, E. A. and Becker, A. B. (1998). "Review of Community-Based Research: Assessing Partnership Approaches to Improve Public Health." *Annual Review of Public Health* 19(1): 173–202.

Krimsky, S. (2000). *Hormonal Chaos: The Scientific and Social Origins of the Environmental Endocrine Hypothesis*. Baltimore, Johns Hopkins University Press.

Kroll-Smith, S. and Couch, S. (1991). "What Is a Disaster? An Ecological-Symbolic Approach to Resolving the Definitional Debate." *International Journal of Mass Emergencies and Disasters* 9: 355–366.

Mansbridge, J. and Morris, A. D. (2001). *Oppositional Consciousness: The Subjective Roots of Social Protest*. Chicago, University of Chicago Press.

McAdam, D. (1982). *Political Process and the Development of Black Insurgency, 1930–1970*. Chicago, University of Chicago Press.

McAdam, D., Tarrow, S. and Tilly, C. (2001). *Dynamics of Contention*. New York, Cambridge University Press.

McCormick, S. and Baralt, L. (2006). *The Breast Cancer Movement: Overlapping Success and Co-Optation*. Society for the Study of Social Problems Annual Meeting, Montreal, Quebec.

McCormick, S., Brody, J. G. and Brown, P. (2004). "Public involvement in breast cancer research: an analysis and model for future research." *International Journal of Health Services* 34: 625–646.

Meyer, D. S. and Whittier, N. (1994). "Social Movement Spillover." *Social Problems* 41: 277–298.

Minkler, M., Vasquez, V. B., Chang, C. and Miller, J. (2008). *Promoting Health Public Policy Through Community-Based Participatory Research: Ten Case Studies*. Oakland, PolicyLink.

Minkler, M. and Wallerstein, N., Eds. (2003). *Community-Based Participatory Research for Health*. San Francisco, Jossey-Bass.

Moore, K. (2008). *Disrupting Science: Social Movements, American Scientists, and the Politics of the Military, 1945–1975*. Princeton, Princeton University Press.

Moore, K. (1999). "Political Protest and Institutional Change: The Anti-Vietnam War Movement and American Science. *How Social Movements Matter*. M. Giugni, D. McAdam and C. Tilly. Minneapolis, University of Minnesota Press: 97–118.

Morgen, S. (2002). *Into Our Own Hands: The Women's Health Movement in the United States, 1969– 1990*. New Brunswick, Rutgers University Press.

Poletta, F. and Jasper, J. M. (2001). "Collective Identity and Social Movements." *Annual Review of Sociology* 27: 283–305.

Pulido, L. (1996). *Environmentalism and Economic Justice: Two Chicano Studies in the Southwest*. Tucson, University of Arizona Press.

Ruzek, S. B. (1978). *The Women's Health Movement: Feminist Alternatives to Medical Control.* New York, Praeger.

Ruzek, S. B., Virginia L. Olesen, Adele E. Clarke, Ed. (1997). *Women's Health: Complexities and Differences.* Columbus, Ohio State University Press.

Shepard, P. M., Northridge, M. E., Prakash, S. and Stover, G. (2002). "Preface: Advancing Environmental Justice Through Community-based Participatory Research." *Environmental Health Perspectives* 110(Supplement 2): 139–140.

Snow, D. A., Rochford, B., Worden, S. K. and Benford, R. D. (1986). "Frame Alignment Processes, Micromobilization, and Movement Participation." *American Sociological Review* 51: 464–481.

Star, S. L. and Greisemer, J. R. (1989). "Institutional Ecology, 'Translations,' and Boundary Objects: Amateurs and Professionals in Berkeley's Museum of Vertebrate Zoology, 1907–39." *Social Studies of Science* 19: 387–420.

Tilly, C. (1978). *From Mobilization to Revolution.* Reading, Addison-Wesley.

Weinberg, A. (1972). "Science and Transcience." *Minerva* 10(2): 209–222.

Wolfson, M. (2001). *The Fight Against Big Tobacco: The Movement, the State, and the Public's Health.* New York, Aldine de Gruyter.

Zavestoski, S., Morello-Frosch, R., Brown, P., Mayer, B., McCormick, S. and Altman, R. G. (2004). "Embodied Health Movements and Challenges to the Dominant Epidemiological Paradigm." *Research in Social Movements, Conflict and Change* 25: 253–278.

GLOBAL HEALTH ISSUES

While health and health care have long been seen as having international or comparative components, only in the past couple of decades have health and health care been depicted in a frame of global or globalization of health. The World Health Organization's (WHO's) "work on globalization and health focuses on assisting countries to assess and act on cross-border risks to public health security. Recognizing that domestic action alone will not be sufficient to ensure health locally," the WHO addresses health as a global public good (WHO 2001). Globalization has become a frame for seeing health-related problems in terms of worldwide issues as well as seeing global impacts of local health issues. In short, globalization analyses urge us to see health issues in the broadest possible framework and suggest we examine the global aspects of specific and local health problems. There are by now many books on global health (e.g., Lee 2003; Jacobsen 2015).

The three selections in this section reflect different global health issues. The first article, "Health Inequalities in Global Context" by Jason Beckfield, Sigrun Olafsdottir, and Elyas Bakhtiari, examines well-established findings about health inequalities in a global perspective. They reexamine the finding that social inequalities impact in a more comparative global frame, finding more variation in the "fundamental cause" explanation of health than might have been assumed. While this approach still finds education and income to have strong associations with self-rated health, a global perspective both reinforces these findings and makes potential interventions more complex.

The second article, Peter Conrad and Meredith Bergey's "The Impending Globalization of ADHD: Notes on the Expansion and Growth of a Medicalized Disorder," examines how attention-deficit/hyperactivity disorder (ADHD) went from being a mostly North American diagnosis through the 1990s to a global phenomenon today (see also Bergey et al. 2018). In a sense, they ask, how did ADHD migrate from the United States to a largely worldwide diagnosis and treatment today, and with what consequences? They examine five countries with different cultures and health care systems, and conclude there are at least five contributing factors in the globalization of ADHD, which essentially contribute to the globalization of medicalization as well.

The third article, Hannah Bradby's "International Medical Migration: Global Movements of Doctors and Nurses," looks at the explanations of the migration of trained health personnel from underserved countries to wealthier, more developed countries. This is often referred to as a *brain drain* from poorer countries to well-paying richer countries. This is clearly a global issue, leading to widespread shortages of doctors and other trained medical personnel in poorer countries. Bradby tries to reconsider this serious problem as a global issue and urges us to rethink it as an issue of global equity and quality of care.

References

Bergey, Meredith R., Angela M. Filipe, Peter Conrad, and Ilina Singh, eds. 2018. *Global Perspectives on ADHD*. Baltimore: Johns Hopkins University Press.

Jacobsen, Kathryn. 2015. *An Introduction to Global Health*, 2nd edition. New York: Barnes & Noble.

Lee, Kelley. 2003. *Globalization and Health: An Introduction*. London: Palgrave Macmillan.

World Health Organization. 2001. Special Theme—Globalization. *Bulletin of World Health Organization* 79 (9): 802.

HEALTH INEQUALITIES
IN GLOBAL CONTEXT

Jason Beckfield, Sigrun Olafsdottir, and Elyas Bakhtiari

The inverse relationship between social position and health—often referred to as the "health gradient"—is a central finding from decades of work on the social determinants of health (Cutler, Deaton, & Lleras-Muney, 2006; House, 2002; Kitagawa & Hauser, 1973; Mirowsky & Ross, 2003; Schnittker & McLeod, 2005; Williams, 1990; Williams & Collins, 1995). Indeed, low social standing has been theorized as a "fundamental cause" of disease that reproduces the health gradient through time and space (Link & Phelan, 1995; Phelan & Link, 2005). Although various types of inequality can represent a fundamental cause, the predominant research focus within this theoretical perspective has been on inequalities based on socioeconomic status. Research at the intersection of social inequality and health has tended to take two forms: On the one hand, researchers have examined individual-level inequalities in health within a single society, frequently the United Kingdom and the United States (Goesling, 2007; Lynch, 2006; Marmot, 2005; Schnittker, 2004; Warren, 2004; Yang, 2008), establishing social factors, such as income, education, gender, race/ethnicity, or immigration status, as predictors of various health outcomes. On the other hand, researchers have explored the relationship between aggregate indicators of income inequality and aggregate health outcomes across multiple, but usually advanced, industrialized nations (Babones, 2008; Beckfield, 2004; Wilkinson, 1996; Wilkinson & Pickett, 2006), finding mixed support for the relationship between income inequality and population-health indicators, such as life expectancy and infant mortality.

While research has focused on either inequalities *in* health within a single society or the relationship between inequality *and* health across societies, less is known about inequalities *in* health in comparative context (Beckfield, 2004; Beckfield & Krieger, 2009; Olafsdottir, 2007).

Health Inequalities in Global Context, Jason Beckfield, Sigrun Olafsdottir, and Elyas Bakhtiari in *American Behavioral Scientist, 57*(8), 1014–1039. Copyright © 2013 SAGE Publications. Reprinted with permission.

Cross-national comparison is essential because it can show how generalizable the relationship between inequality and health is at the individual level and can promote theoretical development and empirical testing of the broader social forces that shape health inequalities. For example, recent comparative work shows that generous family policies may have a positive impact on the health of parents in Iceland, while lack of such policies may negatively impact the health of parents in the United States (Olafsdottir, 2007). Our goal in this paper is to advance the comparative turn in research on health inequalities by conceptualizing and analyzing health inequality itself (as generated by markers of social position, such as education, income, sex, and migrant status) as a dependent variable. We illustrate the promise of this approach by developing cross-nationally comparable measures of health inequality and describing the global variability in health inequalities. The results suggest that the multidisciplinary debate over whether income inequality harms health (Beckfield, 2004; Jen, Jones, & Johnston, 2009; Kim, Kawachi, Vander Hoorn, & Ezzati 2008; Wilkinson & Pickett, 2006) can be extended in a new direction by investigating the determinants of inequalities in health.

Indeed, inequalities in health at the individual level are substantial, and income and education have been found to be key predictors of health outcomes. In general, those with lower levels of income and education experience worse health than those with higher levels (Mirowsky, Ross, & Reynolds, 2000; Robert & House, 2000; Schnittker & McLeod, 2005). Sex differences are more complex, with women typically disadvantaged relative to men on measures of morbidity and mental health but not mortality (Rieker, Bird, & Lang, 2010). U.S.-focused research shows that Blacks are disadvantaged relative to Whites across a range of health outcomes (Williams & Collins, 1995), and there are ongoing debates over the health effects of migration. Consequently, we focus on four indicators when creating our measures of cross-national variation in health inequalities: income, education, sex, and minority status (proxied by being foreign-born, a measure that generalizes outside the

United States). This is an important first step, since relatively little is known about how the strong associations observed in the United States and selected other countries translate into a diverse sample of developed and developing countries (see Eikemo, Huisman, Bambra, & Kunst, 2008; Kunst et al., 2004; Mackenbach et al., 2008; and Van Doorslaer & Koolman, 2004, for studies of health inequalities in Europe). We also know relatively little about the macrosocial factors that may differentially affect health inequalities based on social cleavages (Beckfield & Krieger, 2009; Putnam & Galea, 2008). After demonstrating the extensive cross-national variability of the health gradient, we then begin to explore the possible determinants of the health gradient. As noted, much of this research has focused on the impact of income inequality on health. While some researchers have enthusiastically supported the income inequality hypothesis (Wilkinson & Pickett, 2006), others have failed to find supportive evidence (Beckfield, 2004). Anticipating the following arguments and evidence, we argue for redirecting the debate on health and inequality by focusing on inequalities *in* health within and across countries rather than the relationship between inequality *and* health across countries (Olafsdottir & Beckfield, 2011).

In this paper, we use World Values Survey (WVS) data to address two overarching research questions: First, how much do health inequalities based on social position vary across 48 societies? Second, does income inequality at the societal level impact those health inequalities? Our paper proceeds in three steps. First, we review the literature on the relationship between inequality and health, focusing on inequalities *in* health across multiple nations and highlight recent work suggesting what factors may account for cross-national variation in health inequalities. Second, we provide figures that evaluate the health gradient in a cross-national perspective. We begin by using binary logistic regression models to evaluate the effects of income, education, gender, and migrant status on self-assessed health. We then create our new dependent variables and evaluate their relationships to income inequality. Third, in the concluding section, we discuss some of the implications (and the limitations) of our results and provide suggestions for further research.

SOCIAL INEQUALITIES GENERATE HEALTH GRADIENTS

The "fundamental-cause" perspective interprets the health gradient as a relationship between social position and health that reproduces itself through multiple mechanisms. Link and Phelan (1995) have directed health scholarship back to societal-level social inequality by arguing that social standing will always be linked to health because it represents a fundamental cause of disease, in that the impact of social standing on health cannot be eliminated by intervening on the mechanisms that link social standing to health disparities. The inverse relationship persists because access to resources (such as money, knowledge, power, and social networks) can be used to avoid health risks and to minimize the consequences of illness. This implies that mortality-reducing technologies and knowledge should steepen the health gradient, because the better off can take advantage of them faster (Cutler et al., 2006; Lutfey & Freese, 2005).

In this paper, we take the fundamental-cause approach as a point of departure for developing a comparative framework for theorizing health inequalities (see Olafsdottir, 2007, for an approach that focuses on social inequality and the welfare state and Beckfield and Krieger, 2009, for a review of the nascent empirical literature). We argue that societies establish systems for the distribution of resources, social hierarchies that generate relative social comparisons, and institutional mechanisms for translating social and individual resources into health. This opens up a new question: How much (and why) do health inequalities vary across societies? Following the logic of the fundamental-cause approach, one would expect to observe substantial cross-national variation in health inequalities, such that one finds steeper health gradients in richer,

healthier societies than in poorer, less-healthy societies, as people higher up the social hierarchy take disproportionate advantage of health-improving knowledge and technologies. Conversely, a case can be made that if social inequality translates into health inequality through mechanisms that vary in different social contexts, one would expect to observe constant health gradients across societies—especially if, as we do later for income and education, one measures social standing on *relative* scales. That is, in addition to reproducing itself over time, an extension of the fundamental-cause perspective might anticipate that the health gradient is a constant across a heterogeneous set of places. Existing evidence shows significant health gradients in the United States (Adler et al., 1994; Krieger et al., 2008; Mirowksy & Ross, 2003; Ross & Mirowsky, 1995; Ross & Wu, 1995, 1996; Schnitker, 2004; Williams, 1990; Williams & Collins, 1995) and most western European countries (Mackenbach et al., 2008), including the United Kingdom (Davey Smith, Bartley, & Blane, 1990; Macintyre, 1997; Townsend & Davidson, 1982) and Finland (Lahelma, Rahkonen, & Huuhka, 1997).

Health gradients are not unidimensional, reflecting the fact that there are multiple dimensions of social standing and multiple ways in which people can gain access to resources (Graham, 2007; House, Lantz, & Herd, 2005). Education, income, gender, and migrant status are all important cleavages in societies around the world. Education reflects social status in a broad manner and is related to both material and non-material resources (Lahelma, 2001). There are several advantages associated with using education as a source of stratification in health research. It is broadly stable across the life course, equally suitable for men and women, and more comparable across countries than occupation (Valkonen, 1989). However, educational structures change over time (Lahlema, 2001), and while perhaps more comparable than occupation, the meaning of education still varies across national contexts, especially, perhaps, between richer and poorer countries. Nevertheless, education is a crucial component of understanding why social class is related to health, since in addition to the material resources it may provide, it gives people knowledge that shapes their health behaviors that impact health and illness (Lahelma, 2001).

While education is associated with social status, health behaviors, health-related knowledge, and material resources (Kingston, Hubbard, Lapp, Schroeder, & Wilson, 2003; Mirowsky & Ross, 2003), it is important to isolate the role of material resources, most directly measured by income. Family income is, despite some problems associated with the measure, an indicator of the material resources individuals and families have at their disposal (Lahelma, 2001). Together, these two indicators provide insights into the material and non-material components of social standing that generate socioeconomic gradients in health. As Cutler and colleagues (2006, p. 114) point out, it is important to estimate the effects of income and education separately, both because different mechanisms are at work and because of the need to identify potential policy levers (see also Starfield, 2006). Indeed, estimating income-based and education-based health gradients separately and comparing them in a broad cross-section of societies can shed light on whether economic resources or social status matters more for health and how societal context itself might shape exactly how much resources and status matter for health.

While much of the cross-national work on health inequalities has focused on inequality based on socioeconomic status, it is important to consider other social cleavages that matter within and across societies. Research has shown that while women generally outlive men, they have worse health throughout the life course (Rieker et al., 2010). There may, of course, be some biological explanations for these differences, yet the largest part of the explanation can be found in the social roles assigned to men and women within societies. For example, research has indicated that women's lifestyle protects their health, compared to men, but that their vulnerable position in the workplace and within the home contributes to their worse health outcomes throughout their lives (Ross & Bird, 1994). Focusing on gender in a cross-national perspective, Bird and Rieker (2008) have developed the framework of constrained choice, highlighting how socially constructed social roles impact health behavior and health inequalities between men and women across

the globe. They particularly highlight the importance of social policies as a possible mechanism equalizing health across genders, a point that is supported by the impact of family policies on health of parents in Iceland (Olafsdottir, 2007).

Within the United States, much of the literature on health disparities focuses on racial and ethnic differences in health outcomes. As expected, minority groups often experience worse health than groups that hold a more advantageous position in society, and research consistently shows that African Americans experience some of the worst health outcomes in the United States, whereas Whites and Asian Americans generally have better health outcomes. Perhaps contradictorily, research has indicated that immigrants are often healthier than their native counterparts, but this difference decreases the longer a person resides in the United States. This has been explained both by positive impact of health selection and the negative impact of acculturation (Antecol & Bedard, 2006; Cho, Frisbie, Hummer, & Rogers, 2004; Kennedy, McDonald, & Biddle, 2006). As many of the countries that are included in the WVS do not have a similar history of multiple racial/ethnic groups living in the society, the survey does not have particularly good measures on race and ethnicity. Therefore, we rely on whether the respondent is an immigrant and look at whether that status results in better or worse health across our 48 countries.

Our first analytical step, then, is to examine the variation in the health inequalities based on social position in our sample of 48 countries. Drawing on the extensive literature that shows that those who have less education or less income have worse health outcomes, our *universal gradient* hypothesis (Hypothesis 1) predicts worse health for the relatively poor (vs. the relatively high income), the relatively less educated (vs. the relatively more educated), women (vs. men), and migrants (vs. the native-born) in all 48 nations.

Does Income Inequality Generate Health Inequalities?

The scholarship reviewed earlier has convincingly established that disadvantaged individuals in many affluent democracies have worse health than those in more advantageous positions. That is, there is consensus on the existence of social inequalities *in* health within many societies. Conversely, there is an ongoing, heated debate among comparative health researchers over whether the level of income inequality in a society is associated with aggregate, societal-level measures of population health, such as the infant mortality rate and life expectancy (Beckfield, 2004; Jen et al., 2009; Kim et al., 2008; Wilkinson & Pickett, 2006). That is, there is dissensus on the existence of a relationship between inequality *and* health. To take a recent characterization of the debate, Zimmerman (2008) colorfully notes that research on the association between inequality and health is now generating "far more heat than light, with two dug-in sides lobbing analyses back and forth with increasing sophistication and decreasing effect" (p. 1882). We argue that one way to generate some light is to examine whether and to what degree economic inequality in a society influences inequalities *in* health.

We anticipate that economic inequality within and among societies should be related to inequalities in health within societies. Researchers interested in comparative health care systems noted in the 1970s that inequality in capitalist societies creates and sustains health disparities (McKeown, 1979; Navarro, 1976), which gives reason to believe that some societies may have more health inequality than others, especially where market relations predominate. Moreover, there are dramatic differences between richer and poorer countries in aggregate measures of population health (Brady, Kaya, & Beckfield 2007; Goesling & Firebaugh, 2004), which is another reason to believe that social inequalities in the health of populations could differ dramatically across societies at very different levels of economic development. Following the logic of the fundamental-cause approach outlined earlier, we would expect steeper health gradients in richer societies. Comparative researchers have pointed out various societal factors, such as social inequality, that may impact health inequalities within and across countries (Beckfield & Krieger, 2009; Kunitz, 2007; Kunitz & Pesis-Katz, 2005; Olafsdottir & Beckfield, 2011; Wilkinson, 1996). However, this association has not

been systematically tested across multiple national contexts, nor has the focus been on the relationship between economic inequality and social inequalities in health.

We argue that economic inequality should be positively associated with the level of inequality in health in a society. Here, we can imagine that the effect of individual income on individual health is the same in two societies, but one has higher levels of income inequality, making the association between income and health stronger, mechanically, in the higher-income-inequality society. In addition, individuals with either educational or income advantage in a higher-income-inequality society may have even more resources that they can translate even more effectively into better health, and the poor would be even more deeply disadvantaged (Evans, Hout, & Mayer, 2004; Hout & Fischer, 2003). Furthermore, if income serves as a buffer against the strains of everyday life (Hall & Lamont, 2009), lower-income people in higher-inequality societies should be less healthy, generating a steeper gradient. Finally, if income inequality is an accurate index of the general level of social inequality in a society (in other words, if income inequality captures social stratification in a very general way), then income inequality should be positively associated with all four measures of health inequality. Thus, our *income inequality* hypothesis (Hypothesis 2) suggests that nations with higher levels of income inequality will have larger health inequalities.

DATA AND METHOD

Our analysis proceeds in two stages. In the first stage, we assess our first hypothesis—that health gradients exist across social contexts—by estimating health gradients based on education, income, gender, and immigration status in a heterogeneous set of societies. In the second stage, we assess our second hypothesis—that health gradients are steeper where income inequality is greater—by estimating the associations between our measures of inequality in health based on income, education, gender, and immigration status and our measures of income inequality at the societal level.

The WVS includes a wide range of societies, making it ideal for an exploration of cross-national variation in health inequalities (Hopcroft & Bradely, 2007). The original purpose of the WVS was to compare a wide array of societies in terms of general attitudes and values (Inglehart & Baker, 2000), but the data set also offers researchers interested in multiple topics, including health, a unique opportunity to examine cross-national differences. Each national sample is designed to be representative of the adult (ages 18 and over in most cases) non-institutionalized population. Sampling procedures vary slightly across the nations included but in general begin with geographically designated primary sampling units (e.g., ZIP codes in the United States). Respondents within these units are then randomly selected for in-person interviews. The "master survey" in English is translated into the predominant national language for non-English-speaking countries. Further details about the WVS can be found at worldvaluessurvey.org. We use data from the fifth (2005–2008) wave of the WVS. Again, the key advantage of the WVS data for our purposes is that they include a heterogeneous cross-section of societies that allows us to examine the generality of the health gradient and to explore one of its possible determinants. In detailing our data and methods discussed subsequently, we highlight our measurement and estimation efforts at ensuring cross-national comparability.

After deleting cases with missing data, we have 47,640 observations from 48 WVS countries, representing 74% of the world population, specifically the following: Australia (in the following figures, AUS), Burkina Faso (BFA), Bulgaria (BGR), Brazil (BRA), Canada (CAN), Chile (CHL), China (CHN), Columbia (COL), Cyprus (CYP), Ethiopia (ETH), Finland (FIN), France (FRA), Great Britain (GBR), Germany (GER), Ghana (GHA), Guatemala (GTM), Hong Kong (HKG), India (IND), Indonesia (IDN), Iran (IRN), Iraq (IRQ), Italy (ITA), Japan (JPN), Morocco (MAR), Moldova (MDA), Mexico (MEX), Mali (MLI), Malaysia (MYS), Netherlands (NLD), Poland (POL), Romania (ROM), Russia (RUS), Rwanda (RWA), Slovenia (SVN), South Africa (ZAF), South Korea (KOR), Spain (ESP), Sweden (SWE), Switzerland (CHE), Thailand (THA), Trinidad and Tobago (TTO), Turkey (TUR), Taiwan (TWN), Ukraine (UKR), Uruguay (URY), United States (USA), Vietnam (VNM), and Zambia (ZMB).

Self-Assessed Health

We use self-assessed health to create our new variables, health gradients based on education, income, gender, and immigration status. Survey respondents were asked, "All in all, how would you describe your state of health these days? Would you say it is . . ." and the response categories were *very good, good, fair, poor,* and *very poor*. We binarize this measure for analysis, coding *very good* and *good* as 1 and other responses as 0. This measure has been established as a valid indicator of health that predicts mortality and shows strong test-retest reliability (Davies & Ware, 1981; Idler & Benyamini, 1997; Idler, Hudson, & Levanthal, 1999; Lundberg & Manderbacka, 1996; Schnittker, 2004). Here, we follow a number of other comparative health researchers in employing this measure as an indicator of health status (Eikemo et al., 2007; Espelt et al., 2008; Kunst et al., 2004; Mackenbach et al., 2008; Mansyur, Amick, Harrist, & Franzini, 2008; Olafsdottir, 2007). In addition, this variable has been recommended as suitable for comparative research by the World Health Organization (de Bruin, Pichavet, & Nossikov, 1996). Self-assessed health is a partial but valid indicator of health status that has been validated as a predictor of mortality in a number of studies (Idler & Benyamini, 1997).

Education and Income

To create our four indicators of health inequalities, we first generate societal-level measures of health inequality using individual-level predictors of self-assessed health. The measures of gender and immigration status are created directly from a variable measuring whether the respondent is a woman or a migrant, but making comparable measures of education and income is more challenging. This is both a substantive and methodological issue. We address the comparability of measures in two ways:

First, rather than relying on absolute income or education, we transform our measures into relative measures that better capture what it means to have certain levels of education or income within societal context. Second, we use binary logistic regression to estimate measures of health inequalities that are margin-free in that they are unaffected by cross-national differences in the distributions of education and income.

Education is also measured with three relative categories to ensure cross-national comparability (Goesling, 2007); the original question from the English questionnaire asked, "What is the highest educational level that you have attained?" We construct the education measure as follows: Respondents in the top quartile of the national educational attainment distribution are coded as "relative high education," and respondents in the bottom quartile are coded as "relative low education," while others are coded as "relative middle education." The middle category is again the reference category in the regression models.

Income is measured for households, since it more accurately captures available resources than individual income (Lahelma, 2001). The original income measure in the WVS is a 10-category ordinal variable, but to enhance the cross-national comparability of income, we rely on relative indicators of affluence and poverty (Bolzendahl & Olafsdottir, 2008; Olafsdottir, 2007). Specifically, we create three dummy variables and classify respondents as "relative low income" if their income falls into the bottom quartile of the income distribution, as "relatively high income" if it falls into the top quartile of the distribution, and as "relative middle income" if it falls between those extremes. In the models, "relative middle income" serves as the reference category.

Female is an indicator variable, where 1 = female and 0 = male.

Immigration status is a binary variable where 1 = that the respondent has a parent who was not born in the country and 0 = both parents were born in the country. As this immigration indicator was available only in 37 countries, this variable is not included in the other models.

In addition, we use a limited number of essential control variables for basic demographic characteristics. Age is measured in years and is expected to have a negative association with the dependent variable. Employment status is an indicator variable, where 1 = full-time employment and 0 = else, and is expected to show a positive association with health. Because the focus of our paper is on social status health inequalities, we do not show the results for the controls in the figures and tables that follow. These results are as expected and are available from the authors.

Estimation of the Health Gradients

We use predicted probabilities, generated from binary logistic regression models, to measure health inequalities. For instance, we measure education-based health inequality by calculating the predicted probability of respondents with low relative education reporting good or very good health and subtracting that from the predicted probability of respondents with high relative education reporting good or very good health. This use of predicted probabilities is preferable to reporting differences in logistic regression coefficients because predicted probabilities do not require the assumption that the error variance is identical across countries.

Because income and education are significantly correlated, and because it has been argued that access to higher incomes accounts for part of the education-health association (Mirowsky & Ross, 2003), we enter income and education into the model separately (see Mackenbach et al., 2008, for another study that estimates the education and income associations with health separately). Gender inequality in health is also measured as a difference in predicted probability, specifically, the predicted probability that women report good or very good health minus the predicted probability that men report good or very good health. Unfortunately, the analysis of migrant status is limited to a smaller set of WVS countries, due to data availability. In the calculation of predicted probabilities, all covariates other than the focal covariate are held at their means.

Income Inequality and Health Inequalities

Once we have established the size of the health inequalities in each of the 48 nations, we examine the associations between our measures of health inequalities and a common measure of income inequality: the Gini coefficient. Data come from the UNU-WIDER database.

Given the relatively small number of countries in our sample, we show the data in a set of scatterplots. We estimate pairwise correlations between our contextual covariate and our measures of health inequalities based on income and education. We display scatterplots that show the data, the estimate of the linear fit between health inequality and income inequality, and the 95% confidence interval around the linear fit. Such descriptive analysis is appropriate in this case, since the structural correlates of health inequality have only begun to be assessed. Given the relatively small sample ($N = 48$) of countries in the WVS, we leave large-N assessments of these findings to future work. Our goal is to provide fresh evidence on the extent of variation in health inequality, and the relationship between health inequalities and income inequality, in as broad a cross-section of societies around the world as possible.

Analysis Plan

In sum, then, the plan for our analysis is as follows: (a) estimate binary logistic regressions of self-rated health on *relative income*, age, sex, and employment status; (b) estimate binary logistic regressions of self-rated health on *relative education*, age, sex, and employment status; (c) estimate binary logistic regressions of self-rated health on *sex*, age, and employment status; (d) estimate binary logistic regressions of self-rated health on *migrant status*, age, sex, and employment status; (e) calculate the difference in the predicted probability of good self-rated health for the higher-ranked social position versus the lower-ranked social position, using each of the four regression models (where each regression model is estimated separately for

each of our 48 societies); and (f) describe the associations between income-, education-, sex-, and migration-based inequalities in health and a general measure of income inequality, the Gini coefficient.

RESULTS

We begin our discussion of the results with our measures of cross-national differences in health inequalities, as estimated using individual-level data on our 48 societies. Then, we turn to our analysis of the relationship between societal-level health inequality and income inequality. We finish by showing our gradients based on gender and immigration status.

A Universal Gradient?

The first step of our analysis is to evaluate whether there is a universal health gradient across our sample of 48 societies. Figure 44.1 shows large cross-national differences in the extent to which the relatively affluent report better health than relatively poor people. The figure shows, for each country, the difference in the predicted probability of reporting good health for the relatively affluent versus the relatively poor, along with the 95% confidence interval calculated using the delta method (Xu & Long, 2005). Indeed, it shows that there are significant differences in health based on income in all of our countries except three (Hong Kong, Malaysia, and Switzerland). Overall, our results show that relative poverty harms health even in poor countries. Indeed, low income is associated with significantly worse self-reported health in nearly every country (45 out of 48 countries). Yet, importantly, there is substantial variation in the magnitude of the association. The effects of relative poverty or affluence appear to be sensitive to varying social conditions that do not merely reflect economic development, as the largest differences countries as diverse as Great Britain, Bulgaria, Ukraine, Rwanda, and Mexico. The universal gradient hypothesis is therefore largely supported regarding income.

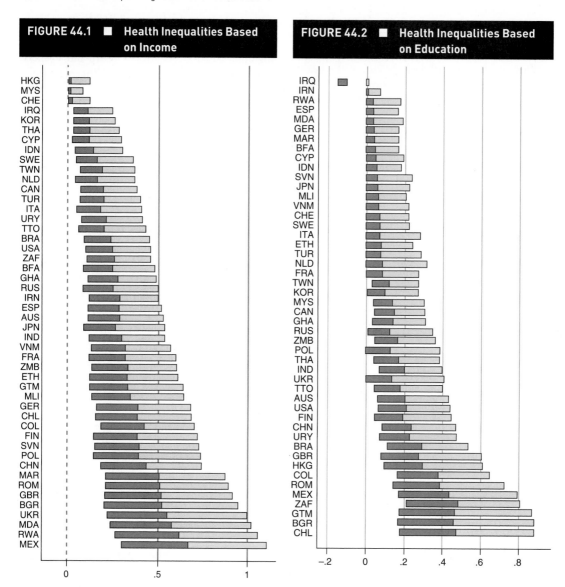

FIGURE 44.1 ■ Health Inequalities Based on Income

FIGURE 44.2 ■ Health Inequalities Based on Education

Figure 44.2 shows a similar relationship for the difference between those with high levels of education and those with low levels of education. In fact, the relationship is significant in all countries but Iraq, and the largest health inequalities based on education are in Chile, Bulgaria, Guatemala, and South Africa. Again, we find support for our universal gradient hypothesis.

Taken together, our results provide reasonably strong support for the universal gradient hypothesis. They show that those who are advantaged in terms of income or education have better health in more than half of our nations and conversely show that those who are disadvantaged in terms of income and education have worse health. Yet, and perhaps more importantly, the results show that there are important differences across the measures, underscoring the importance of looking at them separately.

Turning to health inequalities based on gender and immigration status, Figures 44.3 and 44.4 show a more complex picture. While it appears to be the case that those who are in a vulnerable socioeconomic

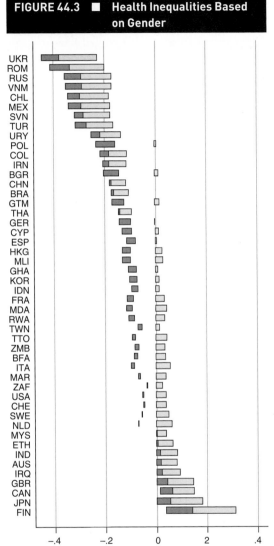

FIGURE 44.3 ■ **Health Inequalities Based on Gender**

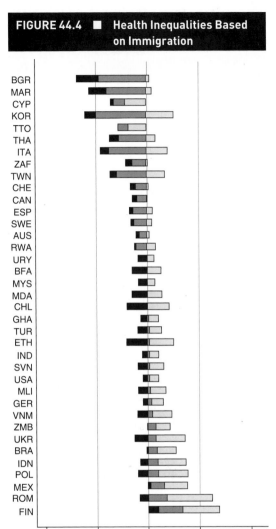

FIGURE 44.4 ■ **Health Inequalities Based on Immigration**

position across countries experience worse health, the way in which other forms of inequality, in our case, gender and immigration status, translate into health inequalities is more mixed. As an example, women experience significantly worse health than men in nine countries but significantly better health in nine countries. Similar patterns are observed for immigration status; immigrants have better health outcomes in some countries but worse in others. These mixed findings underscore the importance of considering what societal characteristics may be related to these types of health inequalities and what

it is about the social context that benefits women's health in some societies but harms it in others.

Income Inequality and the Health Gradient

The next step in our analysis is to explore how these variations are conditioned by income inequality in these 48 societies. Our second hypothesis, the income inequality hypothesis, suggests that health inequalities should respond to economic inequality, such that we observe steeper health gradients in societies with higher levels of income inequality. We

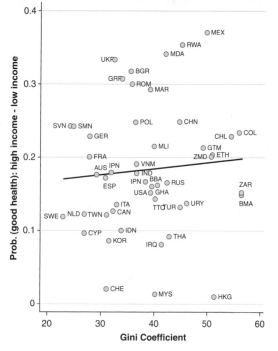

FIGURE 44.5 ■ The Relationship Between Income Inequality and Health Inequalities Based on Income

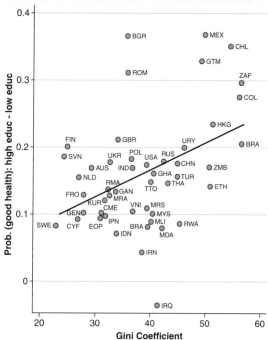

FIGURE 44.6 ■ The Relationship Between Income Inequality and Health Inequalities Based on Education

expect the level of income inequality at the societal level to be more strongly associated with the health inequalities based on income than health inequalities based on the other indicators. The results are displayed in Figures 44.5 through 44.8, which show scatterplots and linear regression fits. Figure 44.5 shows the results for our income inequality hypothesis: cross-national comparisons of *levels* of income inequality. Figure 44.5 shows that health inequalities based on income have a weak correlation with higher level of income inequality ($r = .09$). Conversely, Figure 44.6 shows that health inequalities based on education have somewhat of a stronger relationship with the level of income inequality ($r = .43$). Consequently, our income inequality hypothesis receives at best weak support.

Figures 44.7 and 44.8 show the relationship between income inequality and gender and migrant

status. Figure 44.7 shows that countries with higher levels of income inequality have a greater difference in health between men and women ($r = -.27$). Finally, Figure 44.8 indicates a very weak positive relationship between income inequality and migrant status ($r = .07$).

DISCUSSION

In this paper, we conceptualize and investigate inequality in health using a comparative framework. Building on the fundamental-cause perspective, we develop the hypothesis that inequalities in health should manifest in very heterogeneous social contexts. Building on the literature on income inequality and health, we develop the hypothesis that health inequalities should be sensitive to the

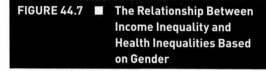

FIGURE 44.7 ■ The Relationship Between Income Inequality and Health Inequalities Based on Gender

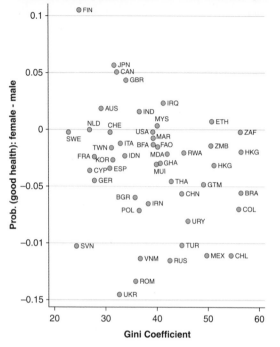

FIGURE 44.8 ■ The Relationship Between Income Inequality and Health Inequalities Based on Immigration Status

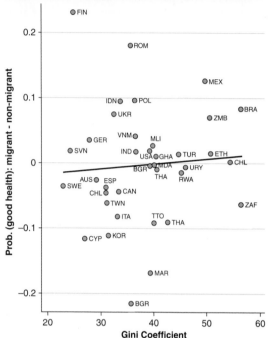

level of income inequality at the societal level. Both hypotheses are supported (although support for the second is weaker) by analysis of data from 48 heterogeneous societies represented in the WVS.

One of our central findings is that health inequality generalizes across a very broad range of societies but takes on diverse patterns in different social contexts. Most striking is the strong association between income inequality (measured at the societal level) and the education gradient in self-rated health. This implies that the fundamental-cause approach to the health gradient can be extended into a comparative framework to understand the variable "social conditions" that generates health gradients. Conceptualizing and measuring health inequality as a cross-national variable opens up a wide range of new research questions that invite new lines of inquiry. Much as the cross-national

(and historical) variability in income inequality has sparked critical new and multidisciplinary work on the institutional, demographic, and economic determinants of inequality (Alderson & Nielsen, 2002; Beckfield, 2006; Gottschalk & Smeeding, 1997; Guvenen & Kuruscu, 2007; Kenworthy, 2004; Korpi & Palme, 1998; Neckerman & Torche, 2007), we believe that research on the determinants of *health* inequality can generate important new theory- and policy-relevant questions and insights. In this paper, we have taken a step in this direction by showing how much the socioeconomic gradient in health shifts according to one social condition that varies widely among the countries in our sample: the level of income inequality. Our results imply that societal-level forces may matter significantly for health inequalities and suggest the promise of more work investigating the macro-sociological correlates of health inequalities (Hall & Lamont, 2009; Putnam & Galea, 2008).

Our findings also carry important implications for the debate over the association between income inequality and population health. Rather than focusing exclusively on aggregate measures of average population health, such as life expectancy and the infant mortality rate, we argue that progress can be made by investigating the social distribution of population health as a social fact that may respond to cross-national differences in, and historical changes in the structure of, social inequality. We have taken a step toward that larger goal by showing that education-based health inequalities are larger where income inequality is greater, but much work remains to be done. For instance, with finer-grained measures of health than we have access to here, quantile regression techniques can be used to model health at points across the health distribution other than the mean (see Martins & Pereira, 2004, for an application to wages). Also, trends in health inequalities within countries can be modeled using time-series techniques to estimate the impact of changes in income inequality within societies that have experienced particularly pronounced U-turns on income inequality, including the United States and the United Kingdom. Of course, the generality of the association between income inequality and health inequality should also be assessed using an even broader array of societies than we have assembled here.

As illustrated previously, our proposed global agenda has the potential to increase our understanding of some of the key debates within the health and inequality literature. Yet, variation in social conditions reflect more complicated patterns that inequalities across major fault lines in societies. Various macro-level factors have implications for health inequalities within and across nations. Clearly there are major differences between advanced, industrialized nations and developing nations, regarding both institutional arrangements and health profiles. While countries such as the United States have largely moved into a health trajectory of chronic illness, infectious diseases continue to be a major threat in many developing nations. More work is needed that places global health inequalities in the context of the broad global inequalities that characterize our world today. For instance, the highly uneven disease distribution across societies around the world could itself be related to social inequalities in health within societies, and a cross-nationally comparative analysis of cause-specific mortality could make progress on this question.

While it is important to acknowledge the very broad development differences across nations, we argue that more fine-grained comparisons across certain types of countries can shed further light on how health inequalities are created and sustained. We elected to focus on income inequality in this paper because there is an established cross-nationally comparative literature on income inequality and health, and because comparable measures of income inequality are available for the heterogeneous societies in our sample. With such a broad array of societies, it is possible to investigate other hypotheses as well. For instance, given the debate over the role of economic development in improving population health, it would be interesting to compare the association between development and aggregate health indicators (such as life expectancy and infant mortality) to the association between development and indicators of inequality in health like those we have used here. We would hypothesize that while development may be associated with average population health, it should be not be associated with health inequality, because development by itself does not distribute social goods. On the other hand, we would hypothesize that development combined with equitable social policy is positively associated with average population health and negatively associated with health inequality. These are examples of the sorts of questions that can be addressed only in a broad, cross-national, comparative framework.

Of course, there is also high utility in selecting theoretically relevant groups of societies for analysis. Within the set of advanced industrialized nations, the welfare state, as a political and cultural institution, represents a key institution determining the life chances of individuals. In previous work, we identified three mechanisms that link the welfare state to health inequalities (Olafsdottir & Beckfield, 2011). First, the level of decommodification (Esping-Andersen, 1990) shapes level of inequalities in general, which in turn shapes health inequalities. More specifically, it defines which social groups are excluded and included across a wide array of social policies that may have direct or indirect impact on health inequalities. Second, the way in which the welfare system is organized across the public/private domain of provision is likely to impact health inequalities within and across countries. Third, whether something is provided or not to individuals and groups is a dynamic process, and the kind of support one receives earlier matters for later outcomes. This highlights the importance of looking at health inequalities as a dynamic process, where cumulative advantages or disadvantages begin even before birth (Conley, Strully, & Bennett, 2003). Consequently, it is critical to link institutional arrangements and health inequalities; as such, inequalities are clearly embedded within specific political and cultural contexts.

Such work, in which we are currently engaged, can also help to overcome the limitations of this study, which should of course be noted. The WVS data we use here do not allow for an exploration of longitudinal change in health inequalities (see Krieger et al., 2008, for such an analysis using data from the United States). Nor do the data allow us to analyze potential biological mechanisms (see Avendano et al., 2005, for a study of stroke mortality). Also, self-rated health is but one of many measures that can be employed in research on health inequalities (see Kunst & Mackenbach, 1994, for alternatives). Moreover, because of the cross-sectional nature of our data, we cannot rule out health selection as a potential driver of income- and education-based health inequalities, although we believe it is as interesting to reveal cross-national differences in any health selection effect as it is to show cross-national differences

in social inequalities in health. We have as little evidence on the societal determinants of health selection (that is, what institutions and policies strengthen or weaken the health benefits that accrue to education and income?) as we do on the societal determinants of social causation. Finally, we note that there is controversy over whether questions about self-rated health mean the same thing across cultural groups (our method of comparing predicted probabilities avoids the assumption of equal error variances across societies, but there are most likely other differences that our method does not account for).

While country-specific studies of health inequalities have made great strides in documenting and explaining health inequalities, we think such research should be placed in a global context. A global context aids in the evaluation of health inequalities by providing a comparative scale for how much inequality is "large" or "small." A global context also identifies health inequalities as subject to social action—institutional variables that are not "natural" but instead systematically vary across societies.

ACKNOWLEDGMENTS

We thank Mauricio Avendano, Salvatore Babones, Lucy Barnes, Simon Cheng, Nitsan Chorev, Nathan Fosse, Jeremy Freese, Peter Hall, Ichiro Kawachi, Xander Koolman, Nancy Krieger, Peter Marsden, Bernice Pescosolido, Bo Rothstein, David Takeuchi, Rosemary Taylor, Chris Wildeman, Richard Wilkinson, and two anonymous reviewers for comments. We appreciate the research assistance of Maocan Guo. None of these kind scholars bears any responsibility for any errors.

Authors' Note

Previous versions of this paper were presented in the Robert Wood Johnson Health and Society Scholars Seminar at Harvard University, the Health of Nations Study Group at the Harvard University Center for European Studies, the Annual Meeting of the American Political Science Association, and the International Conference on Inequality, Health, and Society, convened at the University of Pittsburgh.

References

Adler, N. E., Boyce, T., Chesney, M. A., Cohen, S., Folkman, S., Kahn, R. L., & Syme, S. L. (1994). Socioeconomic status and health: The challenge of the gradient. *American Psychologist, 49,* 15–24.

Alderson, A. S., & Nielsen, F. (2002). Globalization and the great U-turn: Income inequality trends in 16 OECD countries. *American Journal of Sociology, 107,* 1244–1299.

Antecol, H., & Bedard, K. (2006). Unhealthy assimilation: Why do immigrants converge to American health status levels? *Demography, 43*(2), 337–360.

Avendano, M., Kunst, A. E., Van Lenthe, F., Bos, V., Costa, G., Valkonen, T., Mackenbach, J. B. (2005). Trends in socioeconomic disparities in stroke mortality in six European countries between 1981–1985 and 1991–1995. *American Journal of Epidemiology, 161,* 52–61.

Babones, S. (2008). Income inequality and population health: Correlation and causality. *Social Science and Medicine, 66,* 1614–1626.

Beckfield, J. (2004). Does income inequality harm health? New cross-national evidence. *Journal of Health and Social Behavior, 45,* 231–248.

Beckfield, J. (2006). European integration and income inequality. *American Sociological Review, 71,* 961–985.

Beckfield, J., & Krieger, N. (2009). Epi + demos + cracy: A critical review of empirical research linking political systems and priorities to the magnitude of health inequities. *Epidemiologic Reviews, 31,* 152–177.

Bird, C. E., & Rieker, P. P. (2008). *Gender and health: The effects of constrained choices and social policies.* Cambridge, MA: Cambridge University Press.

Bolzendahl, C., & Olafsdottir, S. (2008). Gender group interest or gender ideology? Comparing Americans' support of family policy within the liberal welfare regime. *Sociological Perspectives, 51,* 281–304.

Brady, D., Kaya, Y., & Beckfield, J. (2007). Reassessing the effect of economic growth on well-being in less developed countries, 1980–2003. *Studies in Comparative and International Development, 42,* 1–35.

Cho, Y., Frisbie, P. W., Hummer, R. A., & Rogers, R. G. (2004). Nativity, duration of residence, and the health of Hispanic adults in the United States. *International Migration Review, 38*(1), 184–211.

Conley, D., Strully, K. W., & Bennett, N. G. (2003). *The starting gate: Birth weight and life changes.* Berkeley: University of California Press.

Cutler, D., Deaton, A., & Lleras-Muney, A. (2006). The determinants of mortality. *Journal of Economic Perspectives, 20,* 97–120.

Davey Smith, G., Bartley, M., & Blane, D. (1990). The Black Report on socioeconomic inequalities in health 10 years on. *British Medical Journal, 301,* 373–377.

Davies, A. R., & Ware, J. E. (1981). *Measuring health perceptions in the health insurance experiment.* Santa Monica, CA: Rand Corporation.

de Bruin, A., Pichavet, H. S. J., & Nossikov, A. (1996). *Health interview surveys: Towards international harmonization of methods and instruments.* Copenhagen, Denmark: WHO Regional Publications.

Eikemo, T. A., Huisman, M., Bambra, C., & Kunst, A. E. (2008). Health inequalities according to educational level in different welfare regimes: A comparison of 23 European countries. *Sociology of Health and Illness, 30,* 565–582.

Espelt, A., Borrell, C., Rodriguez-Sanz, M., Muntaner, C., Pasarin, M. I., Benach, J., Navarro, V. (2008). Inequalities in health by social class dimensions in European countries of different political traditions. *International Journal of Epidemiology, 2008*, 1–11.

Esping-Andersen, G. (1990). *Three worlds of welfare capitalism.* Princeton, NJ: Princeton University Press.

Evans, W. N., Hout, M., & Mayer, S. E. (2004). Assessing the effect of economic inequality. In K. Neckerman (Ed.), *Social inequality* (pp. 933–968). New York, NY: Russell Sage.

Goesling, B. (2007). The rising significance of education for health? *Social Forces, 85*, 1621–1644.

Goesling, B., & Firebaugh, G. (2004). The trend in international health inequality. *Population and Development Review, 30*, 131–146.

Gottschalk, P., & Smeeding, T. M. (1997). Cross-national comparisons of earnings and income inequality. *Journal of Economic Literature, 35*, 633–687.

Graham, H. (2007). *Unequal lives: Health and socioeconomic inequalities.* New York, NY: Open University Press.

Guvenen, F., & Kuruscu, B. (2007). *A quantitative analysis of the evolution of the U.S. wage distribution: 1970–2000* (NBER Working Paper 13095). Cambridge, MA: National Bureau of Economic Research.

Hall, P. A., & Lamont, M. (Eds.). (2009). *Successful societies: How institutions and cultural frameworks affect health and capabilities.* New York, NY: Cambridge University Press.

Hopcroft, R. L., & Bradley, D. B. (2007). The sex difference in depression in 29 countries. *Social Forces, 85*, 1483–1508.

House, J. S. (2002). Understanding social factors and inequalities in health: 20th century progress and 21st century prospects. *Journal of Health and Social Behavior, 43*, 125–142.

House, J. S., Lantz, P. M., & Herd, P. (2005). Continuity and change in the social stratification of aging and health over the life course: Evidence from a nationally representative longitudinal study from 1986 to 2001/2002 (Americans' Changing Lives Study). *Journals of Gerontology Series B: Psychological Sciences and Social Sciences, 60*, S15–S26.

Hout, M., & Fischer, C. S. (2003). *Money and morale.* Working paper, University of California-Berkeley.

Idler, E. L., & Benyamini, Y. (1997). Self-rated health and mortality: A review of twenty-seven community studies. *Journal of Health and Social Behavior, 38*, 21–37.

Idler, E. L., Hudson, S. V., & Leventhal, H. (1999). The meanings of self-ratings of health: A qualitative and quantitative approach. *Research on Aging, 21*, 458–476.

Inglehart, R., & Baker, W. E. (2000). Modernization, cultural change, and the persistence of traditional values. *American Sociological Review, 65*, 19–52.

Jen, M. H., Jones, K., & Johnston, R. (2009). Global variations in health: Evaluating Wilkinson's income inequality hypothesis using the World Values Survey. *Social Science and Medicine, 68*, 643–653.

Kennedy, S., McDonald, J. T., & Biddle, N. (2006). *The healthy immigrant effect and immigrant selection: Evidence from four countries* (SEDAP Research Paper No. 164). McMaster University, Hamilton, Ontario, Canada.

Kenworthy, L. (2004). *Egalitarian capitalism: Jobs, incomes, and growth in affluent countries.* New York, NY: Russell Sage Foundation.

Kim, D., Kawachi, I., Vander Hoorn, S., & Ezzati, M. (2008). Is inequality at the heart of it? Cross-country associations of income inequality with cardiovascular diseases and risk factors. *Social Science and Medicine, 66*, 1719–1732.

Kingston, P. W., Hubbard, R., Lapp, B., Schroeder, P., & Wilson, J. (2003). Why education matters. *Sociology of Education, 76*, 53–70.

Kitagawa, E. M., & Hauser, P. M. (1973). *Differential mortality in the United States: A study of socioeconomic epidemiology.* Cambridge, MA: Harvard University Press.

Korpi, W., & Palme, J. (1998). The paradox of redistribution and strategies of equality: Welfare state institutions, inequality, and poverty in the western countries. *American Sociological Review, 63,* 661–687.

Krieger, N., Rehkopf, D. H., Chen, J. T., Waterman, P. D., Marcelli, E., & Kennedy, M. (2008). The fall and rise of US inequities in premature mortality: 1960–2002. *PLOS Medicine, 5,* 227–241.

Kunitz, S. J. (2007). *The health of populations: General theories and particular realities.* New York, NY: Oxford University Press.

Kunitz, S. J., & Pesis-Katz, I. (2005). Mortality of White Americans, African Americans, and Canadians: The causes and consequences for health of welfare state institutions and policies. *Milbank Quarterly, 83,* 5–39.

Kunst, A. E., & Mackenbach, J. P. (1994). *Measuring socioeconomic inequalities in health.* Copenhagen, Denmark: World Health Organization.

Kunst, A. E., Bos, V., Lahelma, E., Bartley, M., Lissau, I., Regidor, E., & Mackenbach, J. P. (2004). Trends in socioeconomic inequalities in self-assessed health in 10 European countries. *International Journal of Epidemiology, 34,* 295–305.

Lahelma, E. (2001). Health and social stratification. In W. C. Cockerham (Ed.), *The Blackwell companion to medical sociology* (pp. 64–93). Malden, MA: Blackwell.

Lahelma, E., Rahkonen, O., & Huuhka, M. (1997). Changes in the social patterning of health? The case of Finland 1986-1994. *Social Science and Medicine, 44,* 789–799.

Link, B. G., & Phelan, J. (1995). Social conditions as fundamental causes of disease. *Journal of Health and Social Behavior, 35,* 80–94.

Lundberg, O., & Manderbacka, K. (1996). Assessing reliability of a measure of self-rated health. *Scandinavian Journal of Social Medicine, 24,* 218–224.

Lutfey, K., & Freese, J. (2005). Toward some fundamentals of fundamental causality: Socioeconomic status and health in the routine clinic visit for diabetes. *American Journal of Sociology, 110,* 1326–1372.

Lynch, S. M. (2006). Explaining life course and cohort variation in the relationship between education and health: The role of income. *Journal of Health and Social Behavior, 47,* 324–338.

Macintyre, S. (1997). The Black Report and beyond: What are the issues? *Social Science and Medicine, 44,* 723–745.

Mackenbach, J. P., Stirbu, I., Roskam, A. J. R., Schaap, M. M., Menvielle, G., Leinsalu, M., & Kunst, A. E. (2008). Socioeconomic inequalities in health in 22 European countries. *New England Journal of Medicine, 358,* 2468–2481.

Mansyur, C., Amick, B. C., Harrist, R. B., & Franzini, L. (2008). Social capital, income inequality, and self-rated health in 45 countries. *Social Science and Medicine, 66,* 43–56.

Marmot, M. (2005). Social determinants of health inequalities. *Lancet, 365,* 1099–1104.

Martins, P. S., & Pereira, P. T. (2004). Does education reduce wage inequality? Quantile regression evidence from 16 countries. *Labour Economics, 11,* 355–371.

McKeown, T. (1979). *The role of medicine: Dream, mirage, or nemesis?* Princeton, NJ: Princeton University Press.

Mirowsky, J., & Ross, C. E. (2003). *Education, social status and health.* New York, NY: Aldine de Gruyter.

Mirowsky, J., Ross, C. E., & Reynolds, J. (2000). Links between social status and health. In C. E. Bird, P. Conrad, & A. M. Fremont (Eds.),

Handbook of medical sociology (5th ed., pp. 47–67). Upper Saddle River, NJ: Prentice Hall.

Navarro, V. (1976). *Medicine under capitalism.* New York, NY: Prodist.

Neckerman, K., & Torche, F. (2007). Inequality: Causes and consequences. *Annual Review of Sociology, 33*: 335–357.

Olafsdottir, S. (2007). Fundamental causes of health disparities: Stratification, the welfare state, and health in the United States and Iceland. *Journal of Health and Social Behavior, 48,* 239–253.

Olafsdottir, S., & Beckfield, J. (2011). Health and the social rights of citizenship: Integrating welfare state theory and medical sociology. In B. A. Pescosolido, J. K. Martin, J. D. McLeod, & A. Rogers (Eds.), *Handbook of sociology of health, illness, and healing* (pp. 101–115). New York, NY: Springer.

Phelan, J. C., & Link, B. G. (2005). Controlling disease and creating disparities: A fundamental cause perspective. *Journals of Gerontology Series B: Psychological Sciences and Social Sciences, 60,* S27–33.

Putnam, S., & Galea, S. (2008). Epidemiology and the macrosocial determinants of health. *Journal of Public Health Policy, 29,* 275–289.

Rieker, P. P., Bird, C. E., & Lang, M. E. (2010). Understanding gender and health: Old patterns, new trends, and future directions. In C. E. Bird, P. Conrad, & A. M. Fremont (Eds.), *Handbook of medical sociology* (5th ed., pp. 52–74). Upper Saddle River, NJ: Prentice Hall.

Robert, S. A., & House, J. S. (2000). "Socioeconomic inequalities in health: An enduring sociological problem. In C. E. Bird, P. Conrad, & A. M. Fremont (Eds.), *Handbook of medical sociology* (5th ed., pp. 79–97). Upper Saddle River, NJ: Prentice Hall.

Ross, C. E. and Bird, C. E. (1994). "Sex Stratification and Health Lifestyle: Consequences for Men's and Women's Perceived Health." *Journal of Health and Social Behavior* 35:161–78.

Ross, C. E., & Mirowsky, J. (1995). Does employment affect health? *Journal of Health and Social Behavior, 36,* 230–243.

Ross, C. E., & Wu, C. L. (1995). The links between education and health. *American Sociological Review, 60,* 719–745.

Ross, C. E., & Wu, C. L. (1996). Education, age, and the cumulative advantage in health. *Journal of Health and Social Behavior, 37,* 104–120.

Schnittker, J. (2004). Education and the changing shape of the income gradient in health. *Journal of Health and Social Behavior, 45,* 286–305.

Schnittker, J., & McLeod, J. D. (2005). The social psychology of health disparities. *Annual Review of Sociology, 31,* 75–103.

Starfield, B. (2006). State of the art in research on equity in health. *Journal of Health Politics, Policy and Law, 31,* 11–32.

Townsend, P., & Davidson, N. (1982). *Inequalities in health: The Black Report.* London, UK: Penguin.

Valkonen, T. (1989). Adult mortality and level of education: A comparison of six countries. In A. J. Fox (Ed.), *Health inequalities in European countries* (pp. 142–160). Aldershot, UK: Gower.

Van Doorslaer, E., & Koolman, X. (2004). Explaining the differences in income-related health inequalities across European countries. *Health Economics, 13,* 609–628.

Warren, J. R. (2004). Job characteristics as mediators in SES-health relationships. *Social Science and Medicine, 59,* 1367–1378.

Wilkinson, R. (1996). *Unhealthy societies: The afflictions of inequality.* London, UK: Routledge.

Wilkinson, R. G., & Pickett, K. E. (2006). Income inequality and population health: A review and explanation of the evidence. *Social Science and Medicine, 62,* 1768–1784.

Williams, D. R. (1990). Socioeconomic differentials in health: A review and redirection. *Social Psychology Quarterly, 53,* 81–99.

Williams, D. R., & Collins, C. (1995). US socioeconomic and racial differences in health: Patterns and explanations. *Annual Review of Sociology, 21,* 349–386.

Xu, J., & Long, J. S. (2005). Confidence intervals for predicted outcomes in regression models for categorical outcomes. *Stata Journal, 5,* 537–559.

Yang, Y. (2008). Trends in U.S. adult chronic disease mortality: Age, period, and cohort variations. *Demography, 45,* 387–416.

Zimmerman, F. J. (2008). A commentary on "Neo-Materialist Theory and the Temporal Relationship Between Income Inequality and Longevity Change." *Social Science and Medicine, 66,* 1882–1894.

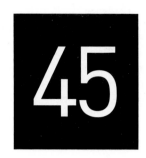

THE IMPENDING GLOBALIZATION OF ADHD

Notes on the Expansion and Growth of a Medicalized Disorder

Peter Conrad and Meredith R. Bergey

Attention Deficit Hyperactivity Disorder (ADHD) is a classic example in the study of medicalization. The first sociological study of the medicalization of deviance focused on hyperactive children (Conrad, 1975, 1976) and a key paper the rise of Adult ADHD is an exemplar of how diagnostic expansion contributes to the growth of medicalization (Conrad and Potter, 2000). While in recent years there have been important writings on the changes in medicalization (Clarke et al., 2003, 2010; Conrad, 2005; Conrad, 2007), these have mostly focused on the American context. But in the past two decades it has become apparent that medicalization is becoming an increasingly global phenomena and that this globalization is a significant change that needed sociological attention. Thus there is a gap in the sociological literature

on how a medicalized diagnosis is able to migrate from the U.S. to other countries. In line with previous studies we focus on ADHD as an exemplary case of medicalization, in this instance by examining the reception of ADHD in several countries, to provide fresh insights into impending globalized medicalization.

For the past forty years, ADHD has been among the most commonly diagnosed psychiatric conditions for children in the U.S. (Conrad, 1975; Kessler et al., 2006). With the rise of Adult ADHD the prevalence of ADHD continues to grow as it becomes seen as more of a lifespan condition than just a disorder for children. Recent studies suggest that up to 9% of U.S. children ages 4–17, and approximately 4.4% of U.S. adults have ADHD (Kessler et al.,

The Impending Globalization of ADHD: Notes on the Expansion and Growth of a Medicalized Disorder, Peter Conrad and Meredith R. Bergey in *Social Science & Medicine, 122*, 31–43, December 2014. Reprinted with permission from Elsevier.

2006). Until two decades ago, the ADHD diagnosis was primarily used in North America and a few other countries (e.g. Australia and Canada. (Mayes et al., 2009; Conrad, 2010). Growing evidence suggests that this is changing and that ADHD is now diagnosed in various countries across the globe (Polanczyk et al., 2007).

Analysts of medicalization see the forces behind medicalization as changing. Conrad (2005) has suggested that the engines of medicalization are shifting from the medical profession and social movements to biotechnology (e.g. the drug industry), consumers, and the insurance industry—with medical professionals increasingly taking more of a secondary role as gatekeepers. In a different frame, Clarke et al. (2003) suggest there is a greater impact of technoscience in what they call "biomedicalization." Both agree that medicalization is expanding and changing. Increased usage of pharmaceutical and drug interventions for various human issues, what Abraham (2010) and others refer to as the "pharmaceuticalization" of medicine, may also contribute to increased medicalization (Conrad, 2013).

One other important way medicalization is changing is that it is becoming more global. While most of the analysis of medicalization thus far has been limited to the U.S., there is a paucity of research examining how medicalization may be expanding in the international sphere. In this paper we explore how one example of a medicalized category, ADHD, has expanded beyond the U.S. More specifically, we examine how ADHD diagnosis and treatment have migrated from the U.S. to be used more globally. While this is not the same as the diagnostic expansion from children to adults (Conrad and Potter, 2000) and now to toddlers (Schwarz, 2014), it expands and extends the diagnostic application to different parts of the world. We first document the expansion of ADHD in a global context, present several specific examples, and then suggest vehicles by which this migration may be occurring. Finally, we discuss what this case of globalization of diagnosis and treatment reflects about the potential global medicalization of other conditions.

EVIDENCE FOR THE GLOBALIZATION OF ADHD

There is little evidence about ADHD diagnosis and treatment in countries other than the U.S. until roughly the 1990s. Indeed, some have suggested that ADHD might be a "culture bound syndrome" limited to the U.S. or English-speaking countries (Anderson, 1996; Canino and Alegria, 2008). What evidence does exist suggests lower diagnostic rates beyond the U.S. For example, research around the 1990s estimated that <1% of children in the U.K. and approximately 4% of children in Italy were diagnosed with ADHD, compared to an estimated 7–9% of children in regions in the U.S. (Camerini et al., 1996; Gallucci et al., 1993; Hinshaw, 1994; Prendergast et al., 1988). European perspectives on hyperactivity and ADHD differed significantly through the early 1990s, with lower prevalence associated with European perspectives (Sargeant and Steinhausen, 1992). There is also evidence that until the 1990s, the U.S. consumed about 90% of all the Ritalin (methylphenidate) produced, the signature psychoactive treatment for ADHD (Diller, 1997). As other countries adopted the treatment, this dropped to 75% by 2010 (Hinshaw and Scheffler, 2014: 126).

Several studies point to the spread of ADHD diagnosis and treatment beyond North America. Polanczyk et al. (2007) conducted a meta-analysis of 102 studies and calculated an estimated worldwide prevalence of 5.29%. While there is a wide range in the quality of the studies examined, and in the precision of the location-specific estimates underlying their analysis, Polanczyk et al.'s (2007) findings indicate that ADHD, and similar diagnoses, are being diagnosed in a large number of countries. Skounti et al. (2007) reviewed 39 studies1 conducted in various countries around the globe and described prevalence estimates ranging from 2.2 to 17.8%. Most of the studies indicated a prevalence of between 4 and 10%.

Drawing upon data from a cross-national workshop and survey, Hinshaw et al. (2011) describe diagnosis and treatment for ADHD in a number of countries for which ADHD research is increasingly available: Australia, Brazil, Canada, China, Germany, Israel, the Netherlands, Norway and the United Kingdom. The authors note that these countries have experienced large increases in ADHD medication usage and they describe social context factors that can shape service delivery. Timimi and Maitra (2009) discuss ADHD in global perspective—describing how diagnoses such as ADHD are being adopted into many Western and non-Western countries, and warning of problems associated with using a "uniform 'one-size-fits-all' approach to theory and practice."

Utilizing IMS Health data from 1993 to 2003, Scheffler et al. (2007) estimated the growth of ADHD worldwide by measuring changes in the global use of ADHD medications, a rough proxy for diagnosis. They found that the use of ADHD medications rose 3-fold concomitant with a 9-fold increase in global spending. While they found higher than predicted use for the U.S., Canada and Australia, increases in other parts of the world were also observed (e.g. the Netherlands, New Zealand, Mexico, and Turkey). The largest market remained the U.S., with an 83–90% share, but the number of countries using ADHD medications grew from 31 to 55 over the decade. The volume of ADHD medications also increased globally by 274%, averaging 13.2% per year, with Iceland now having the highest prescription rate of methylphenidate in the world (Einersdottir, 2008). As another indicator of increasing international interest in ADHD, we examined the locations of all 39 ADHD prevalence studies published in medical journals from 1992 to 2006 and found that while the U.S. dominated with 14, the other 25 studies were located in 20 countries throughout the world (see Table 45.1, constructed from Skounti et al., 2007).

Faraone et al. (2003) reviewed available international studies and contended that the difference in the prevalence of ADHD reflects variation in the definition of the condition as opposed to any real differences in behavior. They argue for the universal acceptance of the APA's (1994) *Diagnostic*

TABLE 45.1 ■ Location of ADHD Prevalence Studies in Medical Journals, 1992–2006[a]	
United States	14
Europe	11
Asia	4
Canada, Australia, New Zealand	3
Mideast	3
South America	3
Other	1

[a]All studies used DSM-IIIR or DSM-IV criteria.
Source: Skounti et al., 2007.

and Statistical Manual of Mental Disorders, 4th Edition, (DSM-IV) criteria for diagnosing ADHD and conclude that by using DSM criteria, the prevalence of ADHD is "at least as high in many non-U.S. children as in US-children" (Faraone et al., 2003: 104) "[with] no convincing difference between the prevalence of this disorder in the USA and most other countries or cultures" (111). They claim, for example, that ADHD rates of 1.4% in Russia and 1.3% in the U.K., considerably lower than U.S. rates, would range from 3.7% to 8.9% if the same method and criteria were used. Polanczyk et al. (2007) and others make similar arguments, suggesting that prevalence variation across geographic areas is due predominantly to variation in methodologies of prevalence studies. Such heterogeneity in practice, however, is precisely the sociological point; countries often do not use the same diagnostic criteria and that *is* a key difference. In a recent large European Union study, the authors' "best estimate" is that the European prevalence of ADHD among 6–17-year-olds is 5% (Wittchen et al., 2011).

While global data remain sparse, what data exist suggest a rising global prevalence of the diagnosis of ADHD and an increase in consumption of ADHD medications in a wide range of countries (See also Hinshaw et al., 2011). What is less evident, however, is how ADHD diagnosis and treatment are migrating to different regions of the globe. More specifically, what vehicles underlie the globalization of ADHD?

CASE EXAMPLES

In this section we present five brief sketches of countries where ADHD diagnosis and treatment have grown in roughly the past fifteen years. These countries include the United Kingdom, Germany, France, Italy and Brazil. We chose these countries because there was published research related to ADHD available for each, a review of that literature suggested that each of these countries experienced some change in ADHD diagnosis and treatment, and the cases present somewhat different experiences related to ADHD. For some countries we also supplemented this with key informants. While this is clearly an opportunity sample, together they can shed light on wider changes in ADHD diagnosis and treatment.

Overall ADHD diagnosis and treatment appear to be increasing in the countries we explored. We briefly describe the ADHD growth for each and identify specific differences among the selected cases. We then use these examples to point to vehicles for the globalization of ADHD. Owing to a paucity of systematic data on ADHD prevalence and migration in general and to a degree in our case countries as well, we are limited to using the best data available. Thus we rely on what data are available to reflect changes in the identification and treatment of ADHD: data on increases in diagnosis; on changes in prescription of medications; increases in prevalence, or some combination of these. We recognize that there are differences among these measures, but together they give use the best picture currently available on the changes in ADHD.

The United Kingdom

The case of ADHD in the U.K. points to the role different diagnostic criteria can play in shaping ADHD prevalence. The WHO's *International Classification of Mental and Behavioral Disorders* (ICD) was generally adopted in the U.K. after its release as the ICD-9 in 1979 and the ICD-10 in 1998. The ICD denotes a condition called hyperkinetic disorder (HKD), which provides a higher threshold to achieve a diagnosis than the DSM (see section comparing ICD and DSM diagnostic criteria for details). Mostly severe or extreme symptomology is classified as a disorder under the ICD (NICE, 2009), denoting a less prevalent and more severe condition than the DSM (Thapar et al., 1999). According to the National Institute for Health and Clinical Excellence (NICE, 2009), HKD thus refers to a "severe sub-group of the DSM-IV-TR combined subtype of ADHD." The prevailing use of the ICD criteria may account for the historically lower rates of ADHD in the U.K. than in the U.S. Research suggests that <1% of U.K. children were diagnosed with ADHD in the 1990s (Hinshaw, 1994; Prendergast et al., 1988; Taylor, 1994) and it was more difficult to receive an ADHD diagnosis in the U.K. than in the U.S. (Malacrida, 2003). Holowenko and Pashute (2000) suggest that use of ICD criteria likely under-represents the prevalence of ADHD in the U.K. population.

ADHD is now, however, the most prevalent behavioral disorder in the U.K. with an estimated 2–5% of school-aged children and young people having the condition (http://www.nhs.uk/conditions/attention-deficit-hyperactivity-disorder/Pages/Introduction.aspx). Stimulant-treatment for ADHD has also been on the rise since the 1990s (e.g. Bramble, 2003; Goldman et al., 1998; Orford, 1998; Robison et al., 1999), with an estimated increase from 183,000 prescriptions in 1991 to 1.58 million in 1995 (Parliamentary Office of Science and Technology, 1997). NICE (2009) notes a large rise in ADHD recognition and treatment, with approximately 0.5 per 1000 children diagnosed 30 years ago (Taylor, 1986), and 3 per 1000 receiving medication for ADHD in the late 1990s (NICE, 2006). The U.K. Department of Health estimates a 35-fold increase in Ritalin prescriptions between 1992 and 1997 and recent research suggests ADHD prescriptions approximately doubled from 2003 to 2008 for children, adolescents, and adults ages

45 years or older; results indicated an approximate 4-fold increase for adults 18–24 and 24–45 years old (McCarthy et al, 2012). Moreover, child psychiatrists in the early 2000s were twice as likely to use methylphenidate as a treatment option for ADHD, than in the mid-1990s (Bramble, 2003). A recent Care Quality Commission (2013) report suggests that methylphenidate prescriptions rose by 11% in primary care practices, and by 24% in private practices from 2011 to 2012, suggesting both increased ADHD diagnosis and treatment in the U.K.

Changes in diagnostic practice, with greater use of the DSM criteria, may contribute to these observed increases. Based on the ICD-10's narrower criteria, the prevalence of HKD is estimated to be between 1 and 2% of children and young people in the U.K. (Green et al., 2005; NICE, 2008). Using the broader DSM-IV criteria, ADHD prevalence in school-aged children and adolescents is estimated to be between 3 and 9% (NICE, 2008). NICE (2008) notes that the terminology in Europe has changed and 'ADHD' has become the diagnostic term most often used in clinical practice, even if more restrictive criteria are utilized. It is also important to note that, similar to the U.S., both specialists and general practitioners in the U.K. may prescribe and monitor treatment for ADHD (Frances et al., 2004). As discussed in more detail later, this is not the case for countries such as France and Italy, where specialists perform such tasks (Debroise, 2004; Panei et al., 2008).

Germany

When discussing ADHD in Germany the conversation often begins with the description of "Fidgety Phillip," an overactive "naughty boy" in the 1845 children's book by Heinrich Hoffman (Smith, 2010). In 1932 Franz Kramer and Hans Pollnow described behaviors in children that are similar to ADHD when they described Kramer-Pollnow Syndrome—a neurological disorder with hyperactivity and mental retardation. Their research did not, however, engender widespread diagnoses and treatment (Neumarker, 2005). There was some attention to the motor—as opposed to the attention—side of children's behavior problems in Germany, but there

is no evidence of any connection to Bradley's 1937 discovery about the 'paradoxical effect' of stimulants on children's behavior problems which so influenced ADHD research (Conrad, 1975). While there was some interest in the concept of 'minimal brain dysfunction' (a diagnostic precursor to ADHD) in Central Europe in the 1950s, it is unclear how widely used the diagnosis was (Fegert, personal communication, 2011).

The development of the ICD-9 criteria (1979–98) for "hyperkinetic disorder', generally adopted in Germany, presented European guidelines for diagnosing a hyperactive behavior disorder. In the 1980s, Ritalin was prescribed to many who were diagnosed with HKD in Germany, although insurance-covered behavioral training programs (e.g., "Ergotherapie," or Occupational Therapy) were also utilized. Some concern arose amongst parents and even some psychiatrists about the impact of 'labelling' children with a mental disorder, and there was a relatively critical public debate over the use of medications for these children (Fegert, personal communication, 2011).

Research suggests that an increase in diagnosis and prescription rates occurred in the 1990s (Ferber et al., 2001, 2003; Schubert et al., 2001). Drug reports suggest that from 1997, the volume of methylphenidate prescriptions increased approximately 10-fold; moreover, between 1999 and 2008, prescriptions for drugs to treat ADHD rose from 10 million defined daily doses to 53 million defined daily doses (Lohse et al., 2008; Lohse and Muller-Oerlinghausen, 2009). Up until the 1990s amphetamines played no role in Germany, as there were no approved formulations for children. Now, however, with federal drug agency (Das Bundesinstitut fur Arzneimittel und Medizinprodukte) approval, and the availability and promotion of slow release compounds, treatment numbers have continued to rise (Fegert, personal communication, 2011). Consistent with European guidelines, the German Society for Child and Adolescent Psychiatry and Psychotherapy recommends stimulant and behavioral interventions as part of a multimodal treatment approach (Dopfner et al., 2000; Overmeyer and Ebert, 1999; Taylor et al., 1998). ADHD prevalence also began to rise, in part responding to increased drug industry marketing and an increasing exchange of mental health experts between the U.S. and Europe. A study of one German state showed a 45% increase in the prevalence of ADHD between 2000 and 2007, although the percentage among individuals of ages 0–18 years was still only 2.21%; methylphenidate use was approximately 1% (Schubert et al., 2010). In another broader survey of German health (KiGGS), Huss et al. (2008) estimated the overall lifetime prevalence of ADHD diagnosis for children and adolescents to be 4.8% in Germany.

Several other factors may have led to an increase in ADHD diagnosis and treatment in Germany, and require further study. For example, Eli Lilly and other companies began sponsoring a speaker's bureau, meetings, parent's organizations, and other promotional efforts in Germany by the early 1990s (Fegert, personal communication, 2011). After a long debate between pediatricians and child psychiatrists, a consensus paper (see later discussion) emerged which allowed use of the DSM-IV criteria instead of the ICD-10, but apparently only for ADHD. ADHD research and talks at European scientific conferences also may have shaped practices around ADHD in Germany (http://www.adhdfederation.org/congress2013/congresshistory.html).

France

There is limited epidemiologic data regarding ADHD in France. Lecendreux et al. (2010) note that, prior to their own finding of 3.5–5.6%, ADHD prevalence in youth had not been examined in France. Research suggests that approximately 0.18% of French children take ADHD medications—versus 4–6%, for example, in the U.S. (Knellwolf et al., 2008; Robison et al., 2004; Winterstein et al., 2008) and 7.3% of French adults are diagnosed with ADHD (Fayyad et al., 2007). Recent studies also suggest an increase, albeit small, in the percentage (from 0.02% to 0.18%) of French children 6–18 years old who received pharmacologic treatment for ADHD between 1997 and 2005 (Frances et al., 2004; Debroise, 2004; Knellwolf et al., 2008).

ADHD's history in France appears to be shaped in large part by clinicians' preference for using the more restrictive *French Classification of Child and Adolescent Mental Disorders* (CFTMEA) or the ICD (Mises et al, 2002; Sechter, 1995) diagnostic approaches when examining symptoms related to hyperactivity (See Vallee, 2009, who first outlined some of this material, for more details.). Almost three decades ago Pichot et al. (1983) found that only 12% of French psychiatry professors utilized the DSM-III regularly in contrast to the more widely utilized ICD and French classification systems. Over a decade later, Sechter (1995) found that while >90% of French psychiatrists owned the DSM-IIIR, they used it irregularly, and predominantly for research purposes; 65% of French psychiatrists considered it unhelpful in the diagnostic process (Sechter, 1995). Mises et al., (2002) argue that the CFTMEA is the current "classification of reference for French child psychiatrists, who appear to be comfortable with it because it fits their diagnostic and therapeutic work."

A task force of the Federation Française de Psychiatrie developed the CFTMEA in 1983 in direct response to the release and growing influence of the DSM (then in its 3rd edition) (Mises et al., 2002). Drawing upon phenomenological and psychoanalytic perspectives, the CFTMEA was developed as an alternative nosography—one that was grounded in psychopathological and developmental approaches that aligned with French psychiatry (Squillante, 2014). The classification scheme's wide usage in France (Mises, 2012) is consistent with a psychopathological tradition, supporting broad assessments of disorders, and the establishment, when possible, of a structural diagnosis situated in psychodynamic psychopathology (Mises et al., 2002). French clinicians tend to perceive ADHD as a psycho-affective disorder, and favor psycho-social interventions—focusing less on the enumeration of symptoms and more on their meaning and their connection to a child's social context, and overall psychological functioning (Lafortune and Meilleur, 2014; Mises et al., 2002; Vallee, 2011). Psychostimulants are used as part of a comprehensive, multi-modal treatment when other approaches (e.g. educational and psychosocial) are insufficient alone (Agence Nationale de Securite du Medicament et des Produits de Sante, 2013; Bursztejn and Golse, 2006; Golse, 2004; Le Heuzey et al., 2006).

Regulatory policies regarding ADHD treatment have also shaped ADHD's history in France. Psychostimulants were approved over a decade after the U.S. (1975 vs. 1961), far fewer were approved (2 vs. 10), and strict controls were imposed (Knellwolf et al., 2008; Frances et al., 2004; Vallee, 2009). Only medical specialists could prescribe medication, from 3 authorized hospital pharmacies (all located in metropolitan areas) and only a week's supply could be granted (Debroise, 2004; Frances et al., 2004). Furthermore, in 1985, Ciba-Geigy allowed their license renewal to expire, essentially removing Ritalin from the French market (Debroise, 2004). Faced with strong public disapproval of Ritalin and low sales, Ciba-Geigy may have feared negative public relations associated with marketing the drug to children, and chose to distance itself from the product (Vallee, 2009).

The case of ADHD in France points in large part to diagnostic and treatment-related practices that are grounded in a strong psychopathological and psychoanalytic tradition. Many French clinicians prefer the more restrictive criteria presented in the CFTMEA or the ICD, and tend to choose psychosocial over pharmacologic interventions for ADHD. This dynamic may, however, be changing. For example, some medical specialists kept prescribing Ritalin after 1985—even encouraging parents to obtain medications for their children outside of France (Debroise, 2004; Vallee, 2009). Some specialists also urged Novartis (previously Ciba-Geigy) to reinstate Ritalin. It was later reapproved in 1995 and some of the controls relaxed (Chambry, 2006). For example, general practitioners may now provide 28-day prescriptions, and for up to a year at a time (Knellwolf et al., 2008; Vallee, 2009). In 2004, Concerta was also added to the French market (Knellwolf et al., 2008). Such changes may contribute toward the aforementioned small increase in the percentage of French children 6–18 years old who received pharmacologic treatment for ADHD between 1997 and 2005 (Frances et al., 2004; Debroise, 2004; Knellwolf et al., 2008).

Italy

Guareschi-Cazztullo and Mazzini-Tomazzolli (1971) are often credited with providing the first nosologic validity to something resembling an ADHD diagnosis in Italy when they described behavioral problems associated with hyperactivity as 'hyperkinetic syndrome.' Little other attention was given to ADHD, or "Disturbi di Attenzione/Iperattivia", in the Italian medical and epidemiologic literature until the 1990s (Bonati, 2005; Clavenna et al., 2007). The few existing studies estimate prevalence in school-aged children and adolescents to be <1–4% (Besoli and Venier, 2003; Camerini et al., 1996; Corbo et al., 2003; Gallucci et al., 1993; Marzocchi and Cornoldi, 2000; Swanson et al., 1998), with more recent estimates of 7% (Mugnaini et al., 2006) and 3% (Bianchini et al., 2013) among school-aged children.

The ADHD diagnosis has not been as widely adopted in Italy as it has been in countries such as the U.S. In the 1980s O'Leary et al. (1984, 1985) found differences in Italian and American psychologists' and psychiatrists' assessments of behaviors characteristic of ADHD. Italian professionals tended to diagnose 'learning disability' or 'personality disorder' where Americans denoted 'behavioral disorder' or 'hyperactivity' (Frazzetto et al., 2007). Until recently, many Italian clinicians had limited knowledge of ADHD as it is defined in the DSM and ICD—utilizing instead a predominantly psychodynamic–psychoanalytic approach and tending to use a fairly generic label of "problem child" or "developmental difficulties" (Bonati, 2005; Gallucci et al., 1993). In a 2001 study, approximately 60% of the primary care pediatricians were cognizant that ADHD existed but were unfamiliar with how to diagnose it; only 10% were following up ADHD cases directly (Bonati et al., 2001b; Marchini et al., 2000).

ADHD's history in Italy is intricately tied to that of Ritalin (methylphenidate). Ritalin first appeared on the Italian market in the late 1950s (similar to many other European countries). However, limited use of the ADHD diagnosis, preferences for less organic or drug-based psychiatry, and strict drug policies contributed to low clinical use of pharmacotherapy. Ritalin was restricted in 1989, due to increased illegal use among college students (Frazzetto et al., 2007) and Ciba-Geigy removed it from the market (Bonati, 2005; Panei et al., 2008). For well over a decade it was illegal to obtain.

This has since changed, due in large part to the efforts of patient and provider organizations (e.g. the Associazione Italiana Famiglie (AIFA) (www.aifaonlis.it) and the Italian Association of Paediatricians) that worked to raise awareness about ADHD and lobby for methylphenidate's reintroduction into the Italian market (Bonati et al., 2001a; Bonati, 2005; Frazzetto et al., 2007). Such efforts garnered further support in 2002 when the Societa' Italiana di Neuropsichiatria dell'Infanzia e dell' Adolescenza (SINPIA) published national guidelines for child and adolescent neuropsychiatry (see www.aifa.it/documenti/LGAdhdSINPIA02-doc), in an effort to synthesize and adapt existing ADHD research to the Italian context (Panei et al., 2008). The publication aligned with the American Academy of Pediatrics' international guidelines, introduced in 2000 and 2001, and was intended to facilitate systematic and rigorous diagnosis in Italy (Frazetto et al., 2007). A National Consensus Conference also formed, producing a statement that accepted and brought recognition to ADHD as a pathology of childhood, explained the diagnostic process, and justified pharmacotherapy as a possible treatment option (Maturo, 2012 personal communication; Zuddas and Bonati, 2003; Frazzetto et al., 2007).

In 2002, Italy's Drug Agency shifted methylphenidate to the less restrictive list of drugs (Bonati, 2005), and recognized it as a possible treatment option for children ≥6 years old. Ritalin and Strattera became available in 2007 (Panei et al., 2008)—the same year that a national drug registry was formed to collect and monitor diagnostic and management data on individuals receiving pharmacological treatment (Gazzetta Ufficiale, 2003; Bonati, 2005; Frazzetto et al., 2007). This registry determines the risk/benefit ratio of ADHD drugs and their safety in clinical practice (Germinario et al., 2013).

Pharmacologic treatment in Italy is not, however, the norm, and prescription rates for mental disorders

are relatively low (Clavenna et al., 2007). Research suggests that five times as many children receive psychotherapeutic interventions as pharmacologic interventions (Agency for Public Health, 2002) and 0.80% of individuals with ADHD are treated pharmacologically, compared to 57%, 11%, and 9% in the U.S., U.K., and France, respectively (Panei et al., 2008). Italy's lower rates have been attributed to the country's stricter treatment plans and the introduction of the National Register (Panei et al., 2008). The data also suggest a downward trend in psychotropic drug consumption in children from 2001 to 2006.

ADHD diagnosis and treatment therefore occur in Italy, though the country's history of ADHD points to a critical psychiatry legacy (Basaglia, 1982) coupled with a more psycho-dynamic orientation and a history of strong drug regulations. Several advocacy groups have also taken critical stances toward pharmacologic treatment for ADHD, such as the Associazione Italiana Disturbi di Attenzione/Iperattivita (AIDAI) (www.aidai.org) (Bonati, 2005).

Brazil

As in many South American countries, ADHD is called TDAH (Transtorno do deficit de attencao/hyperatividade) in Brazil. While published articles on ADHD in Brazil can be traced back as far as the early 1990s, acceptance of the notion of ADHD as a biomedical condition and the idea of medications as a primary treatment option has been slow (Hinshaw et al., 2011). Hinshaw et al. (2011) suggest that a strong clinical preference for psychoanalysis, and a dominant preference for "constructivism" in the education system, may contribute to a disinclination toward biomedical perspectives and medications in Brazil. Behavioral problems in Brazil tend not to be considered to be associated with clinical manifestations of disorders or syndromes (Hinshaw et al., 2011). Brazil's period as a military dictatorship also led to discourse regarding connections between medical treatment for behavioral problems and political depression, which may have contributed further toward a disinclination toward biomedical views and treatments related to ADHD (Hinshaw et al., 2011).

By the beginning of the 21st century, however, Brazil was home to several internationally-known ADHD researchers (e.g. Guilhermo Polanczyk and Luis Augusta Rohde). ADHD is now considered a highly prevalent disorder in Brazil and interest in the diagnosis has been growing dramatically in past decades (De Souza et al., 2008). Estimates of prevalence range from 0.9 to >6%, depending on the diagnostic criteria and the population studied. As one prominent researcher pointed out, there is a scarcity of studies using DSM-IV criteria (often considered the new diagnostic gold standard) in cultures from developing countries (Rohde, 2002). But there is no doubt there is "growing salience of DSM-IV derived categories" in Brazil (Behague, 2009, 461). This includes a 2004 study using DSM-IV criteria which found a prevalence of 4% in children (Goodman et al., 2005). ADHD is also increasingly seen as a lifelong disorder in Brazil; a recent household study of adults using a self-report screen reported a prevalence of 5.8% (Polanczyk et al., 2010).

As in developed countries, many children are identified in school by potential "sickness brokers for ADHD" (Phillips, 2006). A large scale Brazilian study showed that teacher suspicions of ADHD were important in identification (Ponde & Freire, 2007). A recent study revealed heterogeneous beliefs regarding ADHD among many Brazilian professionals including teachers—beliefs which were not based on scientific evidence; the authors noted that "it is urgent that these professional groups be trained and the information programs on ADHD be established for parents and schools" (Gomes et al., 2007). As in other countries, the first line of treatment for ADHD tends now to be stimulant medications (http://www.psiqweb.med.br/site/?area=NO/LerNoticia&idNoticia=277) though there has been some concern in Brazil around both under (Hinshaw et al., 2011) and overtreatment with such medications (Ortega et al., 2010).

There are a number of active groups promoting ADHD in Brazil, including a well-established information and advocacy website Associacio Brasil DTA (www.tdah.org.br), which is connected with kindred American groups. Ortega et al.

(2010) notes that the media, especially large circulation newspapers, has a significant impact on disseminating information about ADHD. There has, however, been some organized resistance to increased ADHD diagnosis and treatment. The first author (PC) was a featured speaker in November 2010 at "I Seminário Internacional—A Educação Medicalizada: Dislexia, TDAH e Outros Supostos Transtornos," a conference in San Paulo examining the medicalization and increased medication of children's behavior problems (especially dyslexia and ADHD). The event reflected some resistance to the bio-medicalization of psychiatry, especially by psychoanalysts and those identified with critical or anti-psychiatry, as others have noted (Behague, 2009). ADHD diagnosis may be somewhat slowed, however, because mental health practitioners are for the most part psychoanalytically oriented and are scarce beyond the main urban areas (Rohde, 2002); diagnoses of ADHD continue to increase nevertheless (Biatriz de Souza, personal communication 2010).

VEHICLES FOR ADHD'S GLOBAL MIGRATION

To the extent that there is a globalization of psychiatric diagnoses (Walters, 2010) such as ADHD, how do we understand the means of diagnostic migration? What is the potential impact of the globalization of ADHD? Hinshaw and Scheffler (2014) point to the rise of compulsory schooling and the pressures of global academic performance as the context for the rise of the identification and treatment of ADHD. We have identified five key vehicles that appear to contribute to the globalization of ADHD: 1) the transnational pharmaceutical industry, 2) the increasing influence of biologically-oriented American psychiatry as a standard, 3) the adoption of DSM-IV criteria for diagnosing ADHD, 4) the Internet, including the availability of specific and simple screening checklists, and 5) ADHD advocacy groups. We discuss each of these in more detail next.

The Transnational Pharmaceutical Industry

The pharmaceutical industry has long had an international presence. This is not news. What is relevant here is that ADHD and its medication have become a place for potential pharmaceutical market expansion. Private market research firms have documented the "growth potential for ADHD markets." One major report by Global Data, titled, "Attention Deficit Hyperactivity Disorder (ADHD) Therapeutics—Pipeline Assessment and Market Forecasts to 2018", states:

> Global Data estimates that the global ADHD therapeutics market was valued at $3855.6m in 2010, and is forecast to grow at a compound annual growth rate (CAGR) of 8.0% over the next eight years, to reach $7114.5m by 2018. . . . Between 2010 and 2018, the global ADHD market is expected to grow at a CAGR of 8%. The growth rate is similar across the US and European countries, but it is slightly high in Japan (18.4%). This difference across geographical markets exists because of the variation in the approval date for some of the drugs in the US, Europe and Japan. . . . During this forecast period, patents for various drugs such as Adderall XR, Daytrana, Concerta (methylphenidate), Strattera (atomoxetine) and Kapvay are set to expire. However, the losses due to expiry of these patents would be compensated by new drugs entering the market such as Vyvanse and Intuniv. Thus, the global ADHD market will show a steady growth from 2010 to 2018. (http://www.reportsnreports.com/reports/135322-attention-deficit-hyperactivity-disorder-adhd-therapeutics-pipeline-assessment-and-market-forecasts-to-2018.html)

The report proceeds to identify the following countries—the U.S., France, Germany, Italy, Spain, the U.K. and Japan—as key markets which have already been developing from 2005 to 2010. The lifting of severe legal restrictions on ADHD stimulants in countries like Italy and France make these markets more appealing and accessible to pharmaceutical companies.

Another market research firm, Global Industry Analysts issued a report which announced "Global ADHD Therapeutics Market Research to Reach $4.2 Billion by 2015" (http://www.strategyr.com/pressMCP-6195.asp). They suggest that the "global market for ADHD drugs is severely constrained by the lack of awareness of the disorder, even in developed countries such as the U.K., Germany and Japan" and they call for more marketing and advertising to physicians, and where possible, to potential consumers. Arguments are proposed for increased "education" about ADHD diagnosis and treatment.

The pharmaceutical industry has also expanded its marketing efforts to try to reach new groups. While efforts to target consumers (e.g. through direct-to-consumer advertising) and physicians (e.g. via physician-oriented lectures, meals and gifts, etc.) are not new, efforts to target non-medical professions such as teachers are more nascent. Teachers often play an integral role in ADHD diagnosis and treatment due to the extended periods of time they spend interacting with children throughout the school year. Teachers (as well as school nurses) also are often expected to participate in diagnostic assessments for ADHD and may be involved in administering ADHD medication. Phillips (2006) describes the teacher's role as one of "sickness and treatment broker", or "disease spotter" and notes how drug companies often attempt to influence teachers' views about ADHD:

> As teachers have some agency in diagnosing ADHD, and may in fact contest the diagnosis, the pharmaceutical industry has an interest in directing teachers toward medical treatment. Pharmaceutical companies have been able to exploit the Internet to access teachers and to influence their brokerage role. The approach to teachers tends to mirror strategies used to familiarize doctors with pharmaceuticals.

Pharmaceutical companies such as Pfizer and GlaxoSmithKline, as well as the Association of the

British Pharmaceutical Industry, have created a variety of "online science educational materials" for teachers (Phillips, 2006). While these sites might not explicitly promote their company's product, they may nonetheless "reinforce the place of the pharmaceutical industry as a benevolent and authoritative presence within the school, much as the provision of branded educational materials to doctors reinforces the position of the pharmaceutical industry within the clinic" (Phillips, 2006). The extent to which such Internet sites are used and/or shape educators' views and practices is unclear and requires empirical research. Such tactics may, however, play a role in the spread of ADHD diagnosis and treatment.

While the U.S. may be nearing saturation in ADHD diagnosis and treatment, much of the rest of the world represents attractive markets for the various ADHD medications. As the IMS Institute for Healthcare Informatics noted, "Rising incomes among consumers in emerging markets like China, India, and Brazil are poised to drive global growth in the pharmaceutical industry in the next five years" (Thomas, 2012). It is perhaps indicative of this goal to move beyond the increasingly saturated U.S. market that, similar to other reports, the Global Industry Report subdivides its publication in terms of the U.S. and the "Rest of the World."

Influence of Western Psychiatry

There is no question that U.S. psychiatry is increasingly dominated by modes of biological psychiatry (Watters, 2010; Carlat, 2010). Treatment of ADHD primarily with psychoactive medications (stimulants) has always been a biopsychiatric approach and may be viewed as a biological treatment harbinger for minor psychiatric disorders. While there are still countries where psychoanalytical approaches dominate (e.g. France, Italy), biological psychiatry appears to be extending its reach beyond the U.S.

There are a number of ways this may affect the globalization of ADHD diagnosis and treatment. Some recent observers have suggested that psychiatric training, foreign and U.S.-based, is becoming more similar (Zisook et al., 2007). Training opportunities in child psychiatry, are also often limited in

many countries. The WHO *Psychiatric Training Atlas* (WHO, 2005), which gathered information from >100 countries, reported that only 29 reported having child psychiatric training programs in their country. Twenty-eight of 74 countries had some agreement to send students to another country for specialized training. Gogineni et al. (2010) state that, "Historically, IMGs have played a critical role in filling positions in child psychiatry," in the U.S. though "the IMGs selected for training in child psychiatry decreased from 250 in 2006 to 226 in 2009." Thirty-five countries reported <500 psychiatrists were residing in the country while 11 countries reported that >30 psychiatrists had trained abroad (http://www.who.int/mental_health/evidence/Atlas_training_final.pdf).

International medical graduates (IMGs) come to the U.S. from 140 different countries and constitute 1/3 of the current residency positions (AMA, 2008). Some graduates remain in the U.S.; nearly 30% of practicing psychiatrists in the U.S. are IMGs (AMA, 2008). While it is unclear how many IMGs who are trained in psychiatry return to their original country, such psychiatric 'exchange' may influence whether psychiatric norms regarding diagnosis and treatment utilized in U.S. psychiatry migrate elsewhere.

In the past decade several jointly authored self-ascribed "international consensus statements" appeared in the psychiatric and medical literature. These statements may serve to supply professional support and promotion for the diagnosis. Most originated from North America with a global audience in mind. These documents recognized some controversies around ADHD and claimed some type of consensus in resolving them. The first one, released in 2002 as the "International Consensus Statement on ADHD" under the auspices of the prominent American ADHD researcher, Russell Barkley, expressed concern about the "periodic inaccurate portrayal of ADHD in media reports" and complained about the views of a "handful of non-expert doctors" who declare that "ADHD does not exist." The statement declares that the scientific evidence available overwhelmingly supports "ADHD as a valid disorder," a view which the report claims has been supported by half a dozen of psychiatry and psychology's most important professional organizations (Barkley et al., 2002). Elsewhere Barkley noted that the consensus statement has been "translated into several foreign languages" and "is being distributed internationally. . . ." (Barkley, 2002). It is interesting to note that while the report appears to reflect an international consensus, of the 86 cosigners of the statement 88% were from North America, barely an international representation.

In the next few years, several other purported consensus statements appeared in the psychiatric literature (e.g. Kutcher et al., 2004; Remschmidt et al., 2005; Kooij et al., 2010). These mostly attempted to justify and encourage ADHD diagnosis and treatment. For example, Remschmidt et al. (2005: 127) state, "This statement aims to re-affirm ADHD as a valid disorder that exists across different cultures, has a significant global impact, and should be diagnosed and treated where it occurs." Such statements have not gone unopposed. For example, Timimi and thirty-three co-endorsers (2004) challenged Barkley et al.'s (2002) assumption that ADHD identifies conclusively "a group of children who suffer from a common and specific neurobiological disorder." They contend that, "not only is it completely counter to the spirit and practice of science to cease questioning the validity of ADHD as proposed by the consensus statement, there is an ethical and moral responsibility to do so."

One point upon which the consensus statements did generally agree was the notion that the proper diagnosis of ADHD was based on the DSM-IV criteria. For example, as stated previously, an influential statement in Italy emanated from APA recommendations which were based upon DSM criteria. How much direct influence these specific statements had is difficult to say, but as the following section describes, the use of the DSM-based diagnostic criteria appears to have grown in global influence.

Moving From ICD to DSM

Related to the increasing influence of American Psychiatry is the growing usage of the DSM, as opposed to ICD criteria, for diagnosing attention and hyperactivity-related behaviors. Physicians throughout Europe have traditionally used the World Health Organization's ICD. A review of the global research literature, however, suggests that diagnostic criteria in the APA's DSM, now in its 5th edition, are increasingly being adopted to diagnose and treat ADHD. Table 45.2 illustrates several of the key differences between the two approaches. As stated previously, the ICD denotes a condition called hyperkinetic disorder (HKD), which in many ways is similar to ADHD, but provides a somewhat different and higher threshold for diagnosing ADHD-like symptoms.

For example, the ICD-10 diagnosis requires inattention, impulsivity and overactivity to be present

TABLE 45.2 ■ Criteria for ADHD and Hyperkinetic Syndrome	
DSM-IV	ICD-10
– ADHD	– Hyperkinetic Syndrome
– Symptoms in 2 dimensions*	– Symptoms in all 3 dimensions*
– Can do a diagnosis with symptoms in 1 dimension	– Requires all criteria in at least 2 situational contexts
– Requires some impairment in more than 1 setting	– Mood, anxiety, developmental disorders are exclusion diagnoses
– Comorbid conditions permissible	

*Inattention, overactivity, and impulsivity.

for HKD while the DSM-IV requires only two dimensions of these behaviors (Lee et al., 2008). The DSM-IV also counts a greater number of behaviors as indicators of overactivity/hyperactivity than does the ICD-10. Both criteria ascribe motor restlessness, excessive fidgeting, "off-task activity" and difficulty staying seated as part of their diagnosis (WHO 190; APA 79). The DSM-IV (79), however, also counts "blurting out answers," "talking excessively," "difficulty playing or engaging quietly," "difficulty awaiting one's turn" and "frequently interrupting or intruding on others". The two manuals also differ with respect to what qualifies as "inattentiveness." The DSM-IV stipulates more behaviors as indicators of inattention (e.g. carelessness, disobedience, forgetfulness, and trouble organizing activities). The ICD requires that diagnosable behaviors appear in ≥2 settings (e.g. home and school) while the DSM prefers symptoms in two settings, but allows a diagnosis in a single setting (e.g. school). In addition, the ICD-10 prohibits the diagnosis of HKD when the patient has certain comorbidities (e.g. anxiety disorders, mood disorders, pervasive developmental disorders or schizophrenia); the DSM-IV does not prohibit the diagnosis of ADHD in such cases. Considering the differences in diagnostic definitions described earlier, it is perhaps not surprising that Jensen (1999) reports far lower diagnostic rates for a disorder when the ICD-10 is used instead of the DSM-IV (~1% vs. 5%). When compared, it is easy to see why the DSM would yield higher rates of prevalence and treatment for disorder than the ICD (Moffitt and Melchior, 2007).

Sometimes the adoption of the DSM criteria is a stated option, as with NICE guidelines in the U.K. Other times it has become the preferred diagnosis, as with Brazil. As most of the research on ADHD was conducted using DSM diagnostic criteria, researchers have argued that it makes sense to align diagnostic practices with what may appear to be the standard approach (Fegert, personal communication, 2011). However, the DSM casts a bigger diagnostic net than the ICD and it appears to increasingly be the gold standard criteria. As noted previously, Hyperkinetic disorder (ICD-10) refers to a group that forms a severe subgroup of the DSM-IV

combined subtype of ADHD (NICE 2009). This can have important implications for increasing the prevalence of ADHD diagnosis and treatment. Only in rare cases (e.g. in France) do both diagnostic criteria appear to be predominantly replaced by a stricter diagnostic system.

The Internet

The advent of the Internet has had a significant effect on illness and medicine, by making health-related information more available (Akatsu and Kuffner, 1998; Fox, 2005), providing possibilities for health consultations (Ayers and Kronenfeld, 2007; Nettleton et al., 2005) and providing new opportunities for mutual support and self-help through numerous illness electronic support groups' newsgroups, list-serves, chat rooms, and bulletin boards (Eysenbach et al., 2004: Fox and Fallows, 2003; Barker, 2008; Conrad and Stults, 2010). Several studies show that health information is among the most frequently searched information on the Internet (Cohen and Sussman, 2010). Recent statistics estimate >2.2 billion Internet users, and the numbers continue to grow, with 500% growth since 2000 (http://www.internetworldstats.com/stats .htm). While there is undoubtedly global heterogeneity in terms of use (e.g. most users reside in North America, the fewest users reside in Africa), the Internet is essentially available globally.

While we have no way of easily measuring how often and in what ways the Internet is used for ADHD, much of our research into the global growth of ADHD points to its usage. The increase in parent support groups has altered the understanding, acceptance, and treatment of ADHD dramatically in various countries (Green and Chee, 1997: 202). The U.K.-based group "ADDers," for example, works "to promote awareness to Attention Deficit/Hyperactivity Disorder and to provide information and as much free practical help as we can to sufferers, both adults and children, and their families in the UK and around the World." Aforementioned groups from Italy also disseminate various ADHD-related information via the Internet. Such sites provide easy access to ADHD information and may well increase the number of individuals who consult a physician about a diagnosis. Many sites also describe ADHD in biomedical terms—providing lists of possible signs and symptoms, and noting the need to consult a physician for a diagnosis.

We have found ADHD Internet support groups in all five of the countries we examined, and in many others. Many of these interactive sites are connected to U.S. support groups like Children and Adults with Attention Deficit/Hyperactivity Disorder (CADD) or ADDers.org and thus are an important channel for sharing information. These support group sites appear in the native language of the country of origin, but with translation programs like "Google Translate" most information on the Internet is potentially accessible to people who speak different languages (see http://www.healthcentral.eom/adhd/c/1443/15863/adhd-world).

In addition to the online support groups, there are local medical websites, sometimes supported by professional associations. Major drug companies like Novartis and Shire have websites presenting ADHD information, screening devices (see checklists), and promotions for their drug products. These sites are typically in the language of the host country and sometimes provide translated pages as well. Google Scholar and other local journal search engines can also provide access to some professional and research articles and again, via online translation programs some kinds of rudimentary translations are possible.

The Internet knows no national boundaries and appears to be a major vehicle for ADHD diagnostic migration. Much of the ADHD information that emanates from the countries where the ADHD diagnosis is well-established (e.g. the U.S.) is almost equally available in countries where ADHD is as yet less frequently diagnosed. Most of these sites are open-access, available to anyone with access to the Internet who chooses to visit them.

Another Internet related vehicle for the migration of ADHD and other psychiatric disorders, is the wide availability of specific and simple "checklists" on the Internet, may facilitate pre and/or self-diagnosing, thus increasing the likelihood to seek or obtain a medical diagnosis and treatment (Ebeling, 2011). Online sites for ADHD (e.g. support groups, medical and pharmaceutical sites, etc.) often provide purportedly validated screening tools for identifying ADHD (e.g. Connor's Rating Scale, the Vanderbilt Scale). The ADDers group, for example, displays the Connor's Rating scale on its website (http://www.adders.org/info45.htm) as an example to parents of what they might encounter if they seek a diagnosis for their child.

These checklists typically emanate from the U.S. but are often modified into other languages to cater to people in other countries. AIFA, for example, provides a downloadable, Italian version of the Adult ADHD Self-Report Scale (ASRS-v1.1) Symptom Checklist on their website, titled "Scala di autovalutazione V1.1 (ASRS-V1.1) per l'ADHD nell'adulto da WHO Composite International Diagnostic Interview." The original checklist emerged from a collaboration between the Workgroup on Adult ADHD, which consisted of a team of three U.S. health professionals and the WHO.

Other online checklists are informal, abbreviated adaptations of scales, often consisting of a number of brief questions about behavior. One such checklist appears on the U.K.'s "netdoctor" site (http://www.netdoctor.co.uk/adhd/howdoiknowif ihaveadhd.htm), under the title "Questions to ask yourself." The site states that, "Not all people with ADHD have these symptoms. But if a lot of this sounds familiar, and you can recall these symptoms in childhood, it might help to speak to your family doctor about them." The preamble to another checklist suggests that their criteria may provide a point of departure for a formal medical diagnosis:

> When children have problems at school or with their behavior, it is often suggested that they have attention deficit hyperactivity disorder and that they should have further testing or evaluation. These evaluations often begin with parenting and teacher checklists to see if the child has enough symptoms of inattention, and/or hyperactivity and impulsivity to meet the criteria for having ADHD. While this form can't diagnose a child with ADHD, it can be helpful to guide you to see if your child does need additional testing.

When filling out this form, think about your child's behavior over at least the past six months.

At best, checklists are designed for screening or even self-screening; they can also become what Ebeling (2011) calls "a marketing of self-diagnosis." They do not, however, indicate a diagnosis per se. As Horwitz and Wakefield (2007) point out in a different context, checklists decontextualize behaviors, draining them of any meaning. Such screening devices sometimes get interpreted by parents, children, or even professionals as indicating the validity of a diagnosis. Without a proper understanding of the context in which the behavior occurs, however, it is sometimes difficult to discern its meaning.

In still other cases, sites provide information regarding how ADHD is diagnosed, providing a list of symptoms and criteria, which often align with a diagnostic manual. ADDiSS's site (http://www.addiss.co.uk/adhd.htm), for example, provides background, diagnostic criteria, and symptom lists under their ADHD "Information centre." The page refers to both the DSM-IV and ICD-10. "ADHS Deutschland e.v." (http://www.adhs-deutschland.de/desktopdefault.aspx?tabid-12/69_read-65/) in German provides a similar list under their "Diagnose" page.

These checklists, both formal and less formal, may facilitate pre and/or self-diagnosing. In a sense they are ADHD made simple, a do-it-yourself diagnosis. The origins of these checklists are in the U.S. and they often serve as a way of popularizing the DSM-IV criteria.

Advocacy Groups

Advocacy groups play an important role in spreading awareness about, and shaping policy around ADHD diagnosis and treatment. The non-profit patient organization Associacao Brasileira Do Deficit De Atencao (Brazilian Association Attention Deficit/ABDA) in Brazil, for example, provides support group services, information about diagnosis and treatment, and telephone and email support to individuals with ADHD and their families. Their webpage—which they note receives an average of 200,000 monthly visits—also provides detail about

ADHD-related policy in Brazil (http://www.tdah.org.br/br/a-abda/quem-somos.html). They describe legal protections for individuals with disabilities, and the organization's support of policy efforts to secure educational resources in school for individuals with ADHD.

This group and others like it are often funded in part by pharmaceutical companies like Novartis, Janssen-Cilag and Shire (Barbarini, forthcoming). Many such groups are also connected to the U.S.-based organization Ch.A.D.D (Children and Adults with Attention Deficit/Hyperactivity Disorder), which provides education and support about ADHD diagnosis and treatment and advocates for legal protections (e.g. at work and in school) for individuals with ADHD. The group holds conferences that bring together lay and professional groups around topics related to ADHD diagnosis and treatment and they are often listed as a resource on other groups' sites.

Such advocacy groups—online or face-to-face—are common in the U.S. and increasingly common in many other countries. Groups exist at the local (Ch.A.D.D.'s chapter in dozens of U.S. locales; ADHD Support Group Cornwall, and other cities in the UK), national (e.g. French Adult ADHD Association; Center for ADD/ADHD Advocacy, Canada (CADDAC)) and even international level (e.g. ADHD Europe, and the World Federation of ADHD), and they tend to bring together stakeholders from various backgrounds. As noted previously, AIFA collaborated with the Italian Association of Paediatricians to raise awareness about ADHD and its treatment with methylphenidate, and was influential in bringing methylphenidate back to the Italian market (Bonati et al., 2001a; Bonati, 2005; Frazzetto et al, 2007). Groups are often comprised of individuals with backgrounds in various fields, including education, psychiatry, neurology, and psychology, as well as individuals diagnosed with ADHD and their family members (ADHD Information Services [ADDISS] in the UK; HyperSupers TDAH in France; ADHS Deutschland e.V. in Germany).

Similar to online checklists, the online presence of many advocacy groups may facilitate pre and/or self-diagnosing, thus increasing the likelihood to seek or obtain a medical diagnosis and treatment. Group pages often provide information about diagnostic criteria and the online checklists. Various sites provide information about treatment as well, even providing contact information for local professionals (e.g. psychiatrists, psychologists, ADHD coaches, etc.). The U.K.-based site AADD-UK, for example, provides a "Help & Support" page with information on how to find an ADHD provider. The aforementioned ABDA site provides information about medical approaches to ADHD and includes a registry of ADHD specialists. For well-established organizations like Ch.A.D.D., an online presence provides a way to reach audiences beyond their country of origin. For newer country-based organizations it creates links to exchange information and strategies for supporting ADHD diagnoses and treatments.

POINTS OF RESISTANCE

While it seems evident that ADHD diagnosis and treatment are spreading in a wide range of countries, and that several key vehicles may facilitate that migration, this is an uneven process. In some countries the growth of ADHD diagnosis has been rapid, while in other countries we see much less use of the diagnosis. An examination of these points of "resistance" is beyond the scope of this paper but we briefly note several main points here.

In countries where the ICD remains the diagnostic touchstone, fewer people are likely to be diagnosed and treated as having ADHD. In some of these countries there is also a concern that an ADHD diagnosis is a label that carries with it a stigma an individual must manage (Mueller et al., 2012). In countries such as France, where psychoanalytic psychiatry remains strong or dominant (Misès et al., 2002), there is a resistance to adopting an ADHD diagnosis and an even greater reticence to prescribing psychoactive medications (Vallee, 2011). Forms of psychotherapy or parent engagement are much more likely responses to behavioral troubles. Psychoactive medications are often the treatment

choice of last resort (Bursztejn and Golse, 2006; Le Heuzey et al., 2006; Vallee, 2011).

In several countries including Italy and France, only specialists like child psychiatrists could historically diagnose and prescribe psychoactive medications (Debroise, 2004; Panei et al. 2010). And in many countries the number of child psychiatrists is very small. When only specialists can diagnose and treat ADHD, fewer people are likely to be diagnosed. The availability of medications can also limit treatment. In some countries few psychoactive drugs are approved for children and in many countries Ritalin and other stimulants are considered a controlled substance. As noted previously, until recently, it was illegal to prescribe Ritalin in Italy—thus restricting pharmaceutical treatment and perhaps, to a degree, diagnosis as well. Even when a diagnosis is made, psychoactive medications are also often expensive and beyond many people's reach, particularly in low-income areas or countries.

Concerns about the safety of ADHD medication may also limit treatment in certain countries. A recent safety review of methylphenidate from the European Medicines Agency, which restricts its recommendations to children >6 years of age and adolescents and does not mention use in adults, has led methylphenidate to no longer be licensed for use in countries like Norway (Kooij et al., 2010: 3). In other countries like the U.K., only some of the numerous drugs used to treat ADHD are available.

Finally, in some countries like Italy there remains a cultural skepticism toward treating behavioral problems with psychoactive drugs. This type of organized popular opposition exists in many countries (e.g. Brazil) but often appears to be limited to the Internet or to some modest protests—which are usually focused on stimulant medication rather than the diagnosis.

While these points of resistance are real and may slow the impending globalization of ADHD, they do not appear to be making a permanent impact on the increasing international spread of ADHD diagnosis and treatment.

GLOBALIZATION AND THE EXPANSION OF MEDICALIZATION

While systematic data and evidence are still often limited, signs nonetheless suggest a spread internationally of the diagnosis and treatment of ADHD. Furthermore, while each country may have its own specific history of ADHD diagnosis and treatment, we identify five vehicles that appear to facilitate the globalization of ADHD. This case can contribute to the medicalization literature (e.g. Conrad, 2007) by showing how an extant medicalized diagnostic category can migrate from one established location to multiple geographic locations globally.

The pharmaceutical industry certainly plays a significant part in this. In the past two decades, several major drug companies have heavily marketed ADHD and its pharmaceutical treatment in the U.S. (Schwarz, 2013). As the U.S. market for ADHD drugs becomes saturated and patents on drugs near expiration, pharmaceutical companies seek new markets for their products. One way to expand markets is to find new applications for existing drugs (e.g. adult ADHD). Another is to expand to more international markets. Thus there are plenty of incentives for the pharmaceutical industry to promote ADHD and its treatment in more countries around the world. This seems to be occurring first in Western Europe, but also in other countries (e.g. Brazil, Mexico, Japan) as pharmaceutical companies seek new and expanded markets for their products.

The globalization of ADHD could not occur without the influence of American-based psychiatry. While several of the countries we examined have their own "origin stories" about ADHD, the expanding influence of American psychiatry, especially biological psychiatry, is of great significance. Until the 1990s ADHD was mostly diagnosed in the U.S. and a few other countries. But since the 1990s we have seen a diffusion of the ADHD diagnosis and treatment more worldwide. This comes in part from more psychiatrists being trained in the U.S. and bringing these perspectives back to their countries of origin. It also reflects the influence biological psychiatry is having on the field; ADHD with its stimulant treatment option where available may be a harbinger of putative biological causes and treatments.

Another major vehicle for the globalization of ADHD has been the growth in the adoption of the DSM criteria for ADHD. Until the 1990s many countries used the ICD criteria for diagnosis of "hyperkinetic syndrome", which was seen as similar to ADHD. The ICD diagnostic criteria, however, are much more restrictive—with a higher threshold for diagnosis than the DSM. Beginning in the 1990s, international guidelines and psychiatrists were increasingly adopting the DSM criteria's lower threshold for ADHD diagnosis. Part of the rationale seems to be that since most of the ADHD research used the DSM criteria, other countries should adopt it as a type of standardization of diagnosis. The result appears to be a rising ADHD diagnosis and treatment worldwide.

In the past two decades ADHD has also become more well-known in the media (Horton-Salway, 2011) and information has become more accessible on the Internet. There are several ways this affects the impending globalization of ADHD. First, there is an almost endless amount of information available on various sites about ADHD, its symptoms and its treatment. This information exists from numerous sources and in many languages. Various pharmaceutical and professional websites exist, in addition to hundreds of interactive websites in dozens of countries and in numerous languages. Many of these sites are advocacy and support groups, some directly connected to U.S. support groups, spreading ideas about ADHD to anyone who seeks it. We have been particularly struck by the ADHD "checklist", simple screening devices usually based on DSM criteria, that allow Internet users to "measure" how many behaviors an individual exhibits that could lead to a possible ADHD diagnosis. These checklists are ADHD made simple, easily usable by professionals, consumers, and putative patients. Virtually all of these checklists are versions of U.S.-based checklists, and may contribute to the migration of DSM-based ADHD diagnosis.

We note that there are several points of resistance to widespread globalization of ADHD, perhaps most important being the dominance of psychoanalytic or psychodynamic psychiatry in some countries (e.g. France and Italy), the limits or restrictions on stimulant medications in some markets (e.g. France and Italy), and opposition or resistance groups skeptical of ADHD and its treatment (some on the Internet, e.g. in Italy). Our sense, however, is that while these resistance forces may slow the usage of the ADHD diagnosis and treatment in specific locales, they ultimately may only have a small impact of the impending globalization of ADHD.

It is ultimately unclear how far and wide the ADHD diagnosis will migrate and we purposely limit our claims here by using the term 'impending' in the title. Furthermore, data necessary for systematically quantifying and comparing increases in ADHD diagnosis and treatment across countries is currently limited. It is quite apparent, however, that ADHD diagnosis and treatment are on an increasingly global path. Our guess is that in a decade or less, the ADHD diagnosis will be more established and treated worldwide. In addition to making this claim, we also have attempted to show how this may happen.

This review has several important limitations. First, we selected countries using an opportunity sample of cases for which published literature on ADHD was available, and where the literature suggested there were differences over time in ADHD diagnosis and treatment. The descriptions here may thus not generalize to all contexts surrounding ADHD diagnosis and treatment. Further research is needed to explore ADHD in global context in general, and in countries that have received less attention here and elsewhere (e.g. in Asia, Eastern Europe, the Middle East, and Africa). Space constraints and a lack of systematic comparative ADHD research and data limit the scope of this paper.

The case of ADHD nonetheless raises a number of questions about the relationship between globalization and medicalization. The medicalization literature focuses on the definition of a condition and its consequences, with little attention to how the definition migrates or is manifested from one situation to another. Most of the sociological research on medicalization has focused on North America (Conrad, 2007; Clarke et al, 2010) or medicalization in specific countries. There has been some research on definitional expansion (Conrad and Potter, 2000) but considerably less on the acceptance and application of medicalized categories in different geographic locations. With an increasingly "flat" and interconnected world (Friedman, 2005) with permeable national boundaries for medical knowledge (especially in cyberspace), this may be too limited a focus for a medicalization analysis. The shifting engines of medicalization, as in Conrad's (2007) terms, may require an expanded lens. To what extent is the medicalization of human conditions a global phenomenon and how does our analytic stance change as we expand our analytic lens worldwide? Certainly, the migration and differential implementation of medical diagnoses needs to be a central part of this analysis. In this context medicalization is also likely to be a multi-directional project, rather than primarily emanating from the U.S. It might be useful to see how globalized medicalization is related to the concerns about global health and to what has come to be known as global "medical tourism" (Reisman, 2010). The medicalization of the "global mental health agenda" may divert attention from important social and structural approaches to global health (Clark, 2014). We hope the ADHD case will inspire other researchers to examine further how other medicalized conditions become global diagnoses.

ACKNOWLEDGMENTS

Our thanks to Phil Brown, Allen Horwitz and Ilina Singh for comments on an earlier version of this paper.

Note

1. The following countries were explored: Australia, Brazil, Canada, Colombia, England, Finland, Germany, Greece, Iceland, Israel, Italy, Japan, Netherlands, New Zealand, Qatar, Spain, Sweden, Taiwan, Thailand, Turkey, the United States, and Venezuela.

References

Abraham, John, 2010. The sociological concomitants of the pharmaceutical Industry and medications. In: Bird, C.E., Conrad, P., Freemont, A.M., Timmermans, S. (Eds.), The Handbook of Medical Sociology, Vanderbilt University Press, Nashville TN.

ADHS Deutschland e.v., 2011. ADHS bei Kindern und Jugendlichen (Aufmerksam-keits-Deflzit-Hyperaktivitats-Storung). http://www.ag-adhs.de (accessed September 2012).

Agence Nationale de Securite du Medicament et des Produits de Sante, 2013. Methylphenidate: donnees d'utilisation et de securite d'emploi en France. http://ansm.sante.fr/var/ansm_site/storage/original/applicafion/8d-dl277a3867155547b4dce58fc0db00.pdf.

Agency for Public Health, 2002. Document from Agenzia di Sanita' Pubblica', Lazio regarding mental health interventions, http://www.asplazio.it/asp_online/tut_soggetti_deb/files/files_sal_ment/TSMREE_2002.PDF (accessed August 2012).

Akatsu, H., Kuffner, J., 1998. Medicine and the Internet. West. J. Med. 169, 311–317.

American Medical Association, 2008. Physicians Characteristics and Distribution in the U.S., 2008 ed. American Medical Association, Chicago.

American Psychiatric Association, 1994, Diagnostic and Statistical Manual of Mental Disorders (IV). American Psychiatric Association, Washington.

Anderson, J.C., 1996. Is childhood hyperactivity a product of western culture. Lancet 348, 73–74.

Associazione Italiana Disturbi di Attenzione/Iperattivita) (AIDAI). www.aidai.org.

Associazione Italiana Famiglie (AIFA). www.aifaonlis.it.

Ayers, S.L., Kronenfeld, J.J., 2007. Chronic illness and health seeking information on the Internet. Health: Interdiscip. J. Soc. Study Health Illn. Med. 11 (3), 327–347.

Barbarini, Tatana de Andrade, July 2014. Medicalization Through ADHD: Support and Resistance Groups in Brazil. Paper prepared for the meetings of the International Sociological Association (forthcoming).

Barker, K., 2008. Electronic support groups, patient-consumers, and medicalization: the case of contested illness. J. Health Soc. Behav. 49, 20–36.

Barkley, R.A., 2002. International consensus statement on ADHD. J. Am. Acad. Child Adolesc, Psychiatry 41 (12). 1389.

Barkley, R.A., et al., 2002. International consensus statement on ADHD. Clin. Child Fam. Psychol. Rev. 5 (2). 89–111.

Basaglia, F., 1982. Conversazione: a proposito della nuova legge 180. In: Basaglia. F. (Ed.), Franco Basaglia, Scritti, dall' apertura del manicomio alla nuova legge sull' assistenza psichiatrica, vol. 2. Turin, Einaudi, pp. 1968–1980.

Behague, D.P., 2009. Psychiatry and politics in Pelotas, Brazil: equivocal quality of conduct disorder and related diagnoses. Med. Anthropol. Q. 2 (4), 455–482.

Besoli, G., Venier, D., 2003. Il disturbo di attenzione con iperattivita: indagine conoscitiva tra I pediatri di famiglia in Friuli-Venezia Giulia, vol. X. Quaderni ACP, pp. 8–9.

Bianchini, R., Postorino, V., Grasso, R., Santoro, B., Migliore, S., Burlo, C., Tata, C., Mazzone, L., 2013. Prevalence of ADHD in a sample of Italian students: a population-based study. Res. Dev. Disabil. 34 (9), 2543–2550.

Bonati, M., 2005. The Italian Saga of ADHD and its treatment. In: Lloyd, G., Cohen, D., Stead, J. (Eds.), New Critical Perspectives on ADHD. Routledge, London.

Bonati, M., Impicciatole, P., Pandolfini. C., 2001a, Reintroduction of methylphenidate in Italy needs careful monitoring. Br. Med. J. 322 (7285). 555.

Bonati, M., Impacciatole, P., Pandolfini, C., 2001b. Evidence and belief in attention deficit hyperactivity disorder: reintroduction of methylphenidate in Italy needs careful monitoring. Br. Med. J. 322, 556.

Bramble, D., 2003. Annotation: the use of psychotropic medications in children: a British view, J. Child Psychol. Psychiatry 44 (2), 169–179.

Bursztejn, C., Golse, B., 2006. L'hyperactivite avec troubles de l'attention: questions cliniques et epistemologiques. In: Neuropsychiatrie de l'enfance de l'adolescence. vol. 54, pp. 29–37.

Canino, G., Alegria, M., 2008. Psychiatric diagnosis - is it universal or relative to culture? J. Child Psychol. Psychiatry. 49 (3), 237–250.

Camerini, G.B., Coccia, M., Caffo, E., 1996. Il disturbo da deficit dell' attenzione-iperattivita': analisi della frequenza in una popolazione scolastica attraverso questionari agli insegnanti. In: Psichiatria dell' infanzia e dell' adolescenza, vol. 63, pp. 587–594.

Care Quality Commission, 2013. The Safer Management of Controlled Drugs. Annual Report (2012). http://www.cqc.org.uk/sites/default/files/media/documents/cdar_2012.pdf.

Carlat, D.J., 2010. Unhinged: The Trouble with Psychiatry – a Doctor's Revelations about a Profession in Crisis. Free Press, New York.

Chambry, J., 2006. Trouble deficit de l'attention-hyperactivite de l'enfant et l'adolescent: du diagnostic a la prise en charge. Ann. Med. Psychol. 164, 613–619.

Clark, J., 2014. Medicalization of global health 2: the medicalization of global mental health. Glob, Health Action 7, 24000.

Clarke, A.E., Shim, J.K., Maim, L., et al., 2003. Biomedicalization: technoscientific transformations of health, illness and U.S. Biomedicine. Am. Sociol. Rev. 68 (2), 161–194.

Clarke, A.E., Mamo, L., Fosket, J.R., et al. (Eds.), 2010. Biomedicalization: Technoscience, Health and Illness in the U.S., Duke University Press, Durham, NC.

Clavenna, A., Rossi. E., Derosa, M., Bonati, M., 2007. Use of psychotropic medications in Italian children and adolescents, Eur. J. Pediatr. 166, 339–347.

Cohen, R.A., Sussman, B., 2010. Health Information Technology Use Among Men and Women Aged 18–64: Early Release of Estimates Form the National Health Interview Survey, January-June 2009. http://www.cdc.gov/nchs/data/hestat/healthinfo2009/healthinfo2009.pdf (accessed January 2014).

Conrad. P., 1975. The discovery of hyperkinesis: notes on the medicalization of deviant behavior. Soc. Probl, Oct. 12–21.

Conrad, P., 1976. Identifying Hyperactive Children: the Medicalization of Deviant Behavior. DC Heath, Lexington. MA.

Conrad, P., 2005. The shifting engines of medicalization. J. Health Soc. Behav. 46 (March), 3–14.

Conrad, P., 2007. The Medicalization of Society: On the Transformation of Human Conditions into Treatable Disorders. Johns Hopkins University Press, Baltimore.

Conrad, P., 2010. The changing social reality of ADHD. Contemp. Sociol. 39, 525–527.

Conrad. P., 2013. Medicalization: changing contours, characteristics and contexts. In: Cockerham, William (Ed.). Health Sociology on the Move: New Directions in Theory. Blackwell, Oxford.

Conrad, P., Potter, D., 2000. From hyperactive children to ADHD adults: observations on the expansion of medical categories. Soc. Probl. 47, 59–82.

Conrad, P., Stults, C., 2010. The Internet and the experience of illness. In: Bird, C., et al. (Eds.), The Handbook of Medical Sociology, sixth ed. Vanderbilt University Press. Nashville TN, pp. 179–191.

Corbo, S., Maroila, F., Sarno, V., Torrioli, M.G., Vernacotola, S., 2003. Prevalenza dell'ADHD in bambini sequiti dal Pediatra di Famiglia. Med. Bambino. 1, 22–25.

De Souza, I., Mattos, P., Pina, C., Fortes, D., 2008. ADHD: the impact when it is not diagnosed, J. Braz. Psychiatry 57 (2), 139–141.

Debroise, A., 2004. Ritaline: Un Feuilleton à la Française. La Recherche 16, 34–36.

Diller, L., 1997. Running on Ritalin, Bantam Books, New York.

Dopfner, M., Frolich, J., Lehmkuhl, G., 2000. Hyperkinetische Storungen. In: Leitfaden Kinder- und Jugendpsychotherapie, Bd 1. Hogrefe, Gottingen.

Ebeling, M., 2011. "Get with the program": pharmaceutical marketing, symptom checklists and self-diagnosis. Soc. Sci. Med. 73, 825–832.

Einersdottir, J., 2008. Teaching children with ADHD; Icelandic early childhood teachers perspectives. Early Child Dev. Care 178 (4), 375–397.

Eysenbach, G., Powell, J., Englesakis, M., et al., 2004. Health related communities and electronic support groups. Br. Med. J. 328, 1166–1170.

Faraone. S.V., Seargeant, j., Gillberg, C, Biederman. J., 2003. The worldwide prevalence of ADHD: is it an American condition? World Psychiatry 2, 104–113.

Fayyad, J., De Graaf, R., Kessler. J., et al., 2007. Cross-national prevalence and correlates of adult attention-deficit hyperactivity disorder. BJP 190, 402–409.

Ferber, I., Schubert. I., Lehmkuhl, G., Spengler, A., Dopfner, M., 2001. Methylphenidat bei hyperkinetiscen Storungen: Verordnungen in den 90er-Jahren. Dtsch. Arztebl. 98 (9), A-541–A-544.

Ferber, L., Lehmkuhl, G., Koster, L, Dopfner, M., Schubert. I., Frolich, J., Ihle, P., 2003. Methylphenidatgebrauch in Deutschland: Versichertenbezogene epidemiologische Studie uber die Entwicklung von 1998 vis 2000. Dtsch. Arztebl. 100 (1–2), A-41–46.

Fox, S., 2005. Health Information Online. Pew Internet and American Life Project. http://www.pewinternet.org/~/media/Files/Reports/2005/PIP_Healthtopics_May05.pdf. http://www.pew_iternet.org/~/media/Files/Reports/2005/PIP_Healfhtopics_May05.pdf (accessed January 2014).

Fox, S., Fallows, D., 2003. Internet Health Resources. Pew Internet and American Life Project. Retrieved September 5, 2012. http://www.pewinternet.org/-/media//Files/Reports/2003/PIP_Health_ReportJuly_2003.pdf.pdf.

Frances, C., Hoizey, G., Millart, H., Trenque. T., 2004. Paediatric methylphenidate (Ritalin) restrictive conditions of prescription in France. Br. J. Clin. Pharmacol. 57 (1). 115–116.

Frazzetto, G., Keenan, S., Singh, I., 2007. 'l'Bambini e le Droghe': the Right to Ritalin vs the Right to Childhood in Italy. BioSocieties 2, 393–412.

Friedman. T., 2005. The World is Flat: A Brief History of the Twenty-first Century. Farrar, Straus and Giroux, New York.

Gallucci, F., Bird. H.R., Berardi, C., et al., 1993. Symptoms of attention-deficit hyperactivity disorder in an Italian school sample: findings of a pilot study. J. Am. Acad. Child Adolesc. Psychiatry 32, 1051–1058.

Gazzetta Ufficiale della Republica Italiana, No. 230, 3 October 2003.

Germinario, E.A.P., Arcieri, R., Bonati, M., Zuddas, A., Masi, G., Vella, S., Chiarotti, F., Panei, P., The Italian ADHD Regional Reference Centers, 2013. Attention-Deficit/Hyperactivity Disorder Drugs and Growth: An Italian Prospective Observational Study. Journal of Child and Adolescent Psychopharmacology 23 (7), 440–447.

Gogineni, R.R., Fallon, A.E., Rao, N.R., 2010. International medical graduates in child and adolescent psychiatry: adaptation, training, and contributions. Child Adolesc. Psychiatr. Clin. N. Am. 19, 833–853.

Goldman, L., Genel, M., Bezman, R., et al., 1998. Diagnosis and treatment of attention Deficit/Hyperactivity disorder in children and adolescents. Council of Scientific Affairs, American Medical Association. J. Am. Med. Assoc. 279, 1100–1107.

Golse, B., 2004. Enfant de moins de six ans: hyperactivite. Arch. Pediatr. 406–409.

Gomes, M., Palmini, A., Barbirato, F., Rohde. L.A., Mattos, P., 2007. Knowledge about attention-deficit/hyperactivity disorder in Brazil. J. Braz. Psychiatry 56 (2). 94–101.

Goodman, R.D., Neves dos Santos, D., Robatto Nunes, A.P., Periera de Miranda, D., 2005. A survey of child mental health problems in a predominantly Afro-Brazilian rural community. Soc. Psychiatry Psychiatr. Epidemiol, 40, 11–17.

Green, C., Chee, K., 1997. Understanding A.D.H.D: a Parent's Guide to Attention Deficit: Hyperactivity Disorder in Children. Vermilion, London.

Green, H., McGinnity, A., Meltzer, H., Ford, T., Goodman, R., 2005. Mental Health of Children and Young People, Great Britain. Palgrave MacMillan, London.

Guareschi-Cazzullo, A., Mazzini-Tomazzolli, C, 1971. La syndrome Ipercinetica, Contributo Casistico ala sua Validita'Nosografica, Neuropsichiatr, Infant. Ease. 118.

Hinshaw, S., 1994. Attention Deficit Disorders and Hyperactivity in Children. Sage, Thousand Oaks, CA.

Hinshaw, S.P., Scheffler, R.M., 2014. The ADHD Explosion: Myths, Medication, Money, and Today's Push for Performance. Oxford University Press, Oxford.

Hinshaw, S.P., Scheffler, R.M., Fulton, B.D., et al., 2011. International variation in treatment procedures for ADHD: social context and recent fiends, Psychiatr. Serv. 62 (5). 459–464.

Hoffmann, H., 1845. Der Sruwwelpeter. http://www.struwwelpeter.com/ (accessed January 2014).

Holowenko, H., Pashute, K., 2000. ADHD in schools: a survey of prevalence and 'Coherence' across a local UK population. Educ. Psychol. Pract. 16 (2), 181–190.

Horton-Salway, M., 2011. Repertoires of ADHD in UK newspaper media. Health: Interdiscip. J. Soc. Study Health Illn. Med. 15, 533–550.

Horwitz. A., Wakefield, J., 2007. The Loss of Sadness. Oxford University Press, New York.

Huss, M., Holling. H., Kurth, B., Schlank, R., 2008. How often are German children and adolescents diagnosed with ADHD? Prevalence based on the judgment of health care professionals; results of the German Health and Examination Survey (KiGGS). Eur. Child Adolesc. Psychiatry 17 (Suppl. 1), 52–58.

Kessler, R.C., Adler, L., Barkley, R., Biederman, J., et al., 2006. The prevalence and correlates of adult ADHD in the United States: results from the National Comorbidity Survey Replication. Am. J. Psychiatry 163, 716–723.

Knellwolf, A.L., Deligne, J., Chiarotti, F., Auley, G.R., Palmieri, S., Boisgard, C.B., Panei, P., Autret-Leca, E., 2008, Prevalence and patterns of methylphenidate use in French children and adolescents. Eur. J. Clin. Pharmacol. 64, 311–317.

Kooij, S.J.J., Bejorot. S., Blackwell, A., Caci. H., Casas-Brugue, M., Carpentier, P.J., Edvinsson, D., Fayyad, J., Foeken, K., Fitzgerald, M., Gaillac, V., Ginsberg, Y., Henry, C., Krause, J., Lensing, M.B., Manor, I., Niederhofer, H., Nunes-Filipe, C., Ohlmeier, M.D., Oswald, P., Pallanti, S., Pehlivanidis, A., Ramos-Quiroga, J.A., Rastam, M., Ryffel-Rawak, D., Stes, S., Asherson, P., 2010. European consensus statement on diagnosis and treatment of adult ADHD; the European network on adult ADHD. BMC Psychiatry 10, 67.

Kutcher. S., Aman, M., Brooks, S.J., Buitelaar, J., 2004. International consensus statement on attention-deficit/hyperactivity disorder (ADHD) and disruptive behavior disorder (DBDS): clinical implications and treatment practice suggestions, Eur. Neuropsychopharmacol. 14 (1), 11–28.

Lafortune, D., Meilleur, D., 2014. Medically defining, screening, and treating conduct disorder: a French controversy, J. Child Fam. Stud. 23. 728–737.

Le Heuzey, M.F., Vergnaud, S., Mouren, M.C., 2006. Traitements medicaux de l'enfant hyperactif: a propos des deux nouvelles formes de methylphenidate commercialisees en France. Arch. Pediatr. 13,100–103.

Lecendreux, M., Konofal, E., Faraone, S.V., 2010. Prevalence of attention deficit hyperactivity disorder and associated features among children in France. J. Atten. Disord. 15 (6). 516–524.

Lee, I.L. Schachar, R.J., Chen, S.X., Ornstein, T.J., Charach, A., Barr, C, Ickowicz, A., 2008. Predictive validity of DSM-1V and 1CD-10 criteria for ADHD and hyperkinetic disorder. J. Child Psychol. Psychiatry 49 (1), 70–77.

Lohse, M.J., Muller-Oerlinghausen, B., 2009. Psychopharmaka, in: Schwabe, U., Paffrath, D. (Eds.), Arzneiverordnungsreport 2009 Aktuelle Daten, Kosten Trends und Kommentare edn, Springer Medizin Verlag, Heidelberg, pp. 767–810.

Lohse, M., Lorenzen, A., Muller-Oerlinghausen, B., 2008. Psychopharmaka. In: Schwabe, U. Paffrath. D. (Eds.), Arzneiverordnungs-report 2008. Springer, Berlin, pp. 773–817.

Malacrida, C, 2003. Cold Comfort: Mothers. Professionals and Attention Deficit Disorder. University of Toronto Press, Toronto.

Marchini, L., Puzzo, F., Pirella. A., et al., 2000. Se non sta fermo solo in USA scatta la ricetta. Occhio Clin. Pediatr. 4, 12–14,

Marzocchi, G.M., Cornoldi, C., 2000. Una Sala di Facile uso per la Rilevazione dei Comportamenti Problematici dei Bambini con Deficit di Attenzione e lper-attivita. Psicol. Clin, dello Svilupp. 4, 43–63.

Mayes, R., Bagwell. C, Erkulwater, J., 2009. Medicating Children: ADHD and Pediatric Mental Health. Harvard University Press. Cambridge, MA.

McCarthy. S., Wilton, L, Murray, M.L. Hodgkins, P., Asherson. P., Wong, I.C.K., 2012. The epidemiology of pharmacologically treated attention deficit hyperactivity disorder (ADHD) in children, adolescents and adults in UK primary care. BMC Pediatr. 12. 78.

Mises, R., 2012. Classification française de troubles mentaux de l'enfant et de l'adolescent – R – 2012, fifth ed. Presses de l'ecole des hautes etudes en santé publique.

Misès. R., Quemada, N., Botbol, M., et al., 2002. French classification for child and adolescent: mental disorders, Psychopathology 35, 176–180.

Moffitt, T.E., Melchior, M., 2007. Why does the worldwide prevalence of childhood attention deficit disorder matter? Am. J. Psychiatry 164, 256–258.

Mueller, A.K., Fuermaier, A.B., Koerts, J., Tucha, L., 2012. Stigma in attention deficit hyperactivity disorder. Atten. Deficit Hyperact. Disord. 4 (3), 101–114.

Mugnaini. D., Masi, G., Brovedani, P., Chelazzi, C, Matas, M., Romagnoli, C, Zuddas, A., 2006. Teacher reports of ADHD symptoms in Italian children at the end of first grade, Eur, Psychiatry. 21. 419–426.

National Institute for Clinical Excellence, 2006. Methylphenidate, Atomoxetine and Dexamfetamine for the Treatment of Attention Deficit Hyperactivity Disorder in Children and Adolescents. Technology Appraisal 98. NICE, London. Available at: www.nice.org.uk/TA98.

National Institute for Clinical Excellence, 2008. Attention Deficit Hyperactivity Disorder: Diagnosis and Management of ADHD in Children, Young People and Adults. NICE Clinical Guidelines, No. 72. National Collaborating Centre for Mental Health.

National Institute for Clinical Excellence. 2009. Attention Deficit Hyperactivity Disorder: Diagnosis and Management of ADHD in Children, Young People and Adults. NICE Clinical Guidelines, No. 72. National Collaborating Centre for Mental Health (UK). British Psychological Society (UK), Leicester (UK).

Nettleton, S., Burrows. R., O'Malley. L, 2005. The mundane realities of the everyday lay use of the Internet for health and their consequences for media convergence. Sociol. Health llln. 27 (7), 972–992.

Neumarker, K., 2005. Kramer-Pullnow syndrome: a contribution on the life of Franz Kramer and Hans Pullnow. Hist. Psychiatry 16 (4), 435–451.

Orford, E., 1998. Commentary: diagnosis needs tightening. Br. Med. J. 316, 1594–1596.

Ortega, F., Barros, D., Oman. L, et al., 2010. Ritalin in Brazil: Production, Discourse and Practices. In: Interface—Comunicacao Saude Educacao, vol. 14(39), pp. 499–510.

Overmeyer, S., Ebert, D., 1999. Die hyperkinetische Störung im Jugend- und Erwachsenenalter. Dtsch. Arztebl. 96, 1275–1278.

O'Leary, K.D., Vivian, D., Cornoldi, C, 1984. Assessment and treatment of 'hyperactivity' in Italy and the United States. J. Clin. Child Psychol. 13, 56–60.

O'Leary, K.D., Vivian, D., Nisi, A., 1985. Hyperactivity in Italy. J. Abnorm. Child Psychol. 4, 485–500.

Panei, P., Addis, A., Arcieri. R., Chiarotti, F., Knellwolf, A.L., Panci, C., Rocchi, F., Vella, S., 2008, Registro nazionale dell'ADHD (Attention Deficit Hyperactivity Disorder): primo anno di attivita (2007—2008). Istituto Supeiiore di Sanita, Rome.

Panei, P., Arcieri, R., Bonati, M., Bugarini, M., Didoni, A., Germinario, F., 2010. Safety of psychotropic drug prescribed for attention-deficit/hyperactivity disorder in Italy. Adverse Drug Reaction Bulletin 260. 999–1002.

Parliamentary Office of Science and Technology, 1997. Treating Problem Behavior in Children, OST, London.

Phillips, C.B., 2006. Medicine goes to school: teachers as sickness brokers for ADHD. PLOS Med. 3 (4). 182.

Pichot, P., Guelfi, J.D., Kroll, J., 1983. French perspectives on DSM-III. In: Spitzer, R.L., Williams, J.B., Skodol, A.E. (Eds.), International Perspectives on DSM-III. American Psychiatric Press, Inc., Washington, D.C., pp, 155–173.

Polanczyk, G., de Lima, M.S., Horta, B.L., Biederman, J., Rohde, L.A., 2007. The worldwide prevalence of ADHD: a systematic review and metaregression analysis. Am. J. Psychiatry 164, 942–948.

Polanczyk, G., Laranjiera, R., Zaleski, M., Pinsky, I., 2010. ADHD in a representative sample of the Brazilian population: estimated prevalence and comparative adequacy of criteria between adolescents and adults according to item response theory. J. Methods Psychiatr. Res. 19 (3), 177–184.

Ponde, M.P., Freire, A.C.C., 2007. Prevalence of attention deficit hyperactivity disorder in school-children in the city of Salvador Bahia. Brazil. Arq. Netiro-Psi-quiarr. 65 (2). 240–244.

Prendergast, M., Taylor, E., Rapoport, J.L., Bartko. J., Donnelly. M., Zametkin, A., Ahearn. M.B., Dunn, G., Wieselberg. H.M., 1988. The diagnosis of childhood hyperactivity. A US.-U.K. Cross-National study of DSM-III and ICD-9. J. Child Psychol. Psychiatry 29, 289–300.

Reisman, D., 2010. Health Tourism: Social Welfare through International Trade. Edward Elgar Publishing, Northampton, MA.

Remschmidt. H., The Global ADHD Working Group, 2005. Global ADHD Working Group. 2005. "Global consensus on ADHD/HKD." Eur. Child Adolesc. Psychiatry 14, 127–137.

Robison, I., Sclar, D., Skaer, T., et al., 1999, National trends in the prevalence of attention-deficit/hyperactivity disorder and the prescribing of methylphenidate among school-age children 1990–1995. Clin. Pediatr. 38, 209–217.

Robison, L.M., Sclar, D.A., Skaer, T.L., Galin, R.S., 2004. Treatment modalities among US children diagnosed with attention-deficit hyperactivity disorder: 1995–99. Int. Clin. Psychopharmacol. 19, 17–22.

Rohde, L.A., 2002. ADHD in Brazil: the DSM-1V criteria in a culturally different population. J. Am. Acad. Child Adolesc. Psychiatry 41 (9), 1131–1133.

Sargeant, J., Steinhausen, H., 1992, European perspectives on hyperkinetic disorder. Eur. Child Adolesc. Psychiatry 1(1), 34–41.

Scheffler, R.M., Hinshaw, S.P., Modrek, S., Levine, P., 2007. The global market for ADHD medication. Health Aff. 26 (2), 450–457.

Schubert, I., Lehmkuhl, G., Spengler, A., Döpfner, M., Ferber, L., 2001. Methylphenidat: bei hyperkinetischen Störungen. Verordnungen in den 90er-Jahren. Dtsch. Arztebl. 98. 541–544.

Schubert, I., Koster, I., Lehmkuhl. G., 2010. The changing prevalence of attention-deficit/hyperactivity disorder and methylphenidate prescriptions. Dtsch. Arztebl. Int. 107 (36). 615–621.

Schwarz, A., December 14 2013. The Selling of Attention Deficit Disorder. New York Times, p. 1.

Schwarz, A., May 16 2014. Thousands of Toddlers are Medicated for A.D.H.D., Report Finds. Raising Worries New York Times, p. A11.

Sechter, D., 1995. Enquete sur l'utilisation des classifications internationals (DSM III-R – CIM-10) en France, en psychiatrie libérale et publique. L'Encéphale, Vol. Spéc. 35–38.

Skounti, M., Phialithis, A., Galanakis, E., 2007. Variations in prevalence of attention deficit disorder worldwide. Eur. j. Pediatr. 166, 127–133.

Smith, M., 2010. The uses and abuses of the history of hyperactivity. In: Graham, L.J. (Ed.), (De) constructing ADHD. Peter Lang. New York, pp. 21–40.

Squillante, M., 2014, Classifications in child and adolescent psychiatry. Arch. Psychiatr. Psychother. 1, 15–19.

Swanson, J.M., Sergeant, J.A., Taylor, E., et al., 1998. Attention-deficit hyperactivity disorder and hyperkinetic disorder. Lancet 351, 429–433.

Taylor, E., 1986. Overactivity, hyperactivity and hyperkinesis: problems and prevalence. In: Taylor, E. (Ed,), The Overactive Child: Clinics in Developmental Medicine. No. 97. Blackwell. Oxford.

Taylor. E., 1994. Syndromes of attention deficit and hyperactivity. In: Ruder, M., Taylor, E.,

Hersov, L. (Eds.), Child and Adolescent Psychiatry: Modern Approaches, third ed. Blackwell Scientific Publications, Oxford, pp. 285–307.

Taylor, E., Sergeant, J., Döpfner, M., Gunning, B., Overmeyer, S., Möbius, H., Eisert, H.G., 1998. Clinical guidelines for hyperkinetic disorder. Eur. Child Adolesc. Psychiatry 7, 184–200.

Thapar, A., Holmes, J., Poulton, K., Harrington, R., 1999. Genetic basis of attention deficit and hyperactivity. Br. J. Psychiatry. 174, 105–111.

Thomas, K., 2012. Drug Makers Growth is Linked to Emerging Markets. New York Times July 12.

Timimi, S., Maitra, B., 2009. ADHD and Globalization. In: Timimi, S., Leo, J. (Eds.), Rethinking ADHD: From Brain to Culture. Palgrave Macmillan, New York, pp. 198–217.

Timimi, S., et al., 2004. A critique of the international consensus statement on ADHD. Clin. Child Fam. Psychol. Rev. 7(1), 59–63.

Vallee, M., 2009. Deconstructing America's Ritalin Epidemic; Contrasting US-France Ritalin Usage (Ph.D. dissertation). University of California, Berkeley, p, 265. 3410842.

Vallee, M., 2011. Resisting American psychiatry: French opposition to DSM-III, biological reductionism, and the pharmaceutical ethos. Adv. Med. Sociol. 12. 85–110.

Watters, E., 2010. Crazy like Us; the Globalization of the American Psyche. Free Press, New York.

Winterstein, A.G., Gerhard, T., Shuster, J., Zito, J., Johnson, M., Liu, H., Saidi. A., 2008. Utilization of pharmacologic treatment in youth with attention/deficit/hyperactivity disorder in Medicaid database. Ann. Pharmacother. 42 (1), 24–31.

Wittchen, H.U., Jacobi, E, Rehm, J., Custavsson, A., Svensson, M., Jonsson, B., Olesen, J., Allgulander, C, Alonso, J., Faravelli, C, Fratiglioni, L., Jennum, P., Lieb, R., Maercker. A., van Os, J., Preisig, M., Salvador-Canilla, L, Simon, R., Steinhausen, LLC, 2011. The size and burden of mental disorders and other disorders of the brain in Europe 2010. European Neuropsychopharmacology 21. 655–679.

World Health Organization, 2005. Atlas of Psychiatric Education and Training across the World. http://www.who.int/mental_health/evidence/Atlas_tiaining_final.pdf (accessed September 2012).

Zisook, S., Balon, R., Bjorksten, K., et al., 2007. Psychiatry residency training around the world. Acad. Psychiatry 31, 309–325.

Zuddas, A., Bonati, M., 2003. Conferenza Nazionale di Consenso. Indicazioni e strategie terapeutiche per i bambini e gli adolescenti con disturbo da deficit attentivo e iperattivita'. http://www.aidaiassociazione.com/documents/ConsensusCaglRelaz.pdf (URL accessed September 2012).

INTERNATIONAL MEDICAL MIGRATION

Global Movements of Doctors and Nurses

Hannah Bradby

INTRODUCTION

While the international migration of skilled health-care professionals has a long history (Gish, 1971), its particular visibility in the early years of the 21st century and the way that it has been held responsible for health problems in resource-poor countries, is the topic of this article. Global mobility as an ongoing aspect of human existence, that is only likely to increase in scope, scale and spread, has potentially far-reaching implications for how equitable health-care provision is organized nationally and internationally. Uneven global development with associated differential markets for labour and other commodities, along with the development of new markets for medical recruitment at the end of

the 20th century, has promoted international professional migration.

The study of medicalization, whereby nonmedical problems become defined and subsequently treated as medical problems, has tended to focus on unruly bodies subject to normalization pressures such that pharmacologically treatable illnesses or disorders are defined. Despite the intention that medicalization be defined as a neutral process (Conrad et al., 2010), there is an implicit assumption in much research that medicalization must be negative (Parens, 2013). This article examines how the global migration of skilled health-care workers can be understood as part of the medicalization of global public health problems and thereby responds to Conrad's (2005) call to examine how

International Medical Migration: The Global Movements of Doctors and Nurses, Hannah Bradby in *Health, 18*(6), 580–596, 2014. Reprinted with permission from SAGE Publications, Inc.

the engines of medicalization have proliferated and are now driven by more commercial and market interests than by professional claims-makers. (p. 10)

These 'emergent engines of medicalization' need to be examined 'with political economy perspectives' to supplement social constructionist approaches (Conrad, 2005), given the contrast between the medicalization of the 1970s and 1980s (medical professional dominance and physician entrepreneurship) and the technical scientific innovations of the 1990s with associated pharmacological and medical markets (Clarke et al., 2003). The transnational capitalization of medical recruitment offers new ways for medicalization to develop at a population rather than individual level.

From the middle 20th century onwards, doctors (and subsequently nurses) from low-income countries have formed a reserve army of labour (Castles and Miller, 2009) for high-income countries, but this was not discussed as a 'crisis' until the early years of the 21st century, when the debate developed along emotive lines. In 2006, the World Health Organization (WHO, 2006) report focussed on the loss of health-care personnel from the world's poorest countries, which were also the places that were coping with the spread of HIV. In positing a causal connection between poor population health outcomes and high rates of skilled health worker emigration, the WHO report confirmed the idea of a causal connection between a higher density of health-care professionals and improved life expectancy. The insistence on trained professionals rather than socioeconomic conditions as key for ameliorating public health has been widespread and can be interpreted as medicalization. The debate about the effects of physician and nurse emigration on the countries that they were leaving, and the obligations upon those that receive them, has and continues to be emotive. Within this debate, nurses and doctors embody the importance of health as a social good such that their emigration from a place with health problems is highly charged. The presumed positive effects that skilled health-care professionals have on the health of a population is challenged by the

'task-shifting' (or task-sharing) movement, which seeks to provide health services in resource-poor settings by employing workers with reduced training.

Explanatory models and theories for international 'brain drain' and 'flow' of so-called human health-care resources do not take into account sociological theories of professional dominance and medicalization. An examination of the evidence cited in the 2006 WHO report, which promoted the idea of a causative link between health-care professional density and poor population health outcomes, considers how the link is asserted and offers a means to interrogate the policy responses to shortages of health-care professionals. In pointing to medicalization of global public health problems, the article reiterates the need to include equity in consideration of health-care staffing in rich and poor worlds alike.

METHODS

A narrative literature review followed up references using traditional scholarly methods and including articles, chapters and pamphlets to locate further references. The research sought to establish the conceptual and theoretical context in which late 20th and early-21st century migratory movements of doctors and nurses have been understood by offering a critical analysis of sources.

PROBLEMATIZING MEDICAL MIGRATION

The lack of good-quality statistical data to track the movement of physicians, midwives and nurses has been periodically lamented over the last four decades (Ahmad, 2005; The Committee on the International Migration of Talent, 1970; Van Hoek, 1970; Organisation for Economic Co-operation and Development [OECD], 2010). Despite these inadequate data, competition for the world's health workforce has been termed a global 'bidding contest' analogous to competition for other commodities in limited supply (Labonté and Schrecker,

2007). Significant skilled international migration is confined to the rich world (e.g. more than a quarter of foreign doctors in Belgium are from the Netherlands and Norwegians constitute about half of those in Denmark; Connell, 2010). Furthermore, of the skilled workers who migrate from poor to rich countries, health-care workers represent a small proportion (Stilwell et al., 2004). Thus, the migration of doctors and nurses from sub-Saharan Africa to the Global North is a subsection of wider movements, yet this aspect of migration came to dominate the global public health agenda at the start of the 21st century (Bradby, 2013). The 'embarrassing optics of rich countries exploiting the health human resources of African countries devastated by the AIDS epidemic' (Wright et al., 2008) became impossible to ignore.

The estimated 20 per cent of doctors and 10 per cent of nurses from Africa who work overseas (Clemens and Pettersson, 2008) represent a potential impediment to their source country's capacity to deliver health care and to do so equitably (Stilwell et al, 2004). The sense that the 'departure of trained professionals from low income countries to find work in high-income countries has emerged as a perverse subsidy' (Mensah et al., 2005) appeared as a strong critique that was widely taken up, including by the WHO.

Between 23 per cent and 34 per cent of practising physicians in New Zealand, the United Kingdom, the United States, Australia and Canada have been trained elsewhere, and while a small proportion of these are from sub-Saharan African, nonetheless, the damage done to poor countries losing a high proportion of medical and nursing graduates made headlines. As one of the world's poorest countries, Malawi has a low life expectancy, high infant mortality and a high prevalence of HIV/AIDS. More than 100 nurses per year have been leaving Malawi, which, in a country that produces only 50 graduates per year from its nursing schools (Record and Mohiddin, 2006), represents a significant loss. In South Africa, a regional referral centre for spinal injuries near Johannesburg had to close down when both resident anaesthetists were recruited by a new Canadian spinal injuries unit (Martineau et al.,

2004). In the Philippines, an entire cardiovascular unit in a provincial hospital was temporarily closed because of the wholesale recruitment of its nurses to overseas jobs (Alkire and Chen, 2006).

Nurses have been described as 'one of the most critical components of the workforce' (Buchan and Aiken, 2008) with the global nurse shortage adjudged 'not just an organizational challenge or a topic for economic analysis; it has a major negative impact on health care' (Buchan, 2006). Elsewhere, both doctors and nurses are referred to as the 'most precious resource' (Johnson, 2005) for sub-Saharan African countries (Coombes, 2005) and as

> crucial instruments of health, doctors and nurses should be treated differentially—indeed exceptionally well, exceptionally soon—for ethical reasons that go far beyond their own well-being. (Alkire and Chen, 2006: 116)

The loss of skilled health workers has been described in emotive and/or hyperbolic terms, as part of a confounding of the provision of doctors and nurses with the provision of health. The 'robbing', 'raiding' (Johnson, 2005) and 'poaching' of trained professionals who constitute poor countries' 'educated elite' has been lamented as 'deeply immoral' (Hooper, 2008). The 'devastating consequences for the source countries' (Larsen et al., 2005) have been indicted as criminal (Mills et al., 2008) and compared with slavery (Heath, 2007). Otherwise measured authors 'declaim the brain drain in the most strident and emotive language' (Crush et al., 2012: 927).

With the departure of trained professionals from their poor home countries for better paid jobs in the rich world making headlines, it became hard to avoid the conclusion that 'brain drain' was not only contributing to but also driving inequality in the distribution of health workers worldwide (Daniels, 2008). With significant aid being devoted to distributing antiretroviral treatment in sub-Saharan African countries, chronically depleted health services, lacking infrastructure, personnel and equipment became highly visible. Sub-Saharan

Africa's lack of health-care personnel became shame-fully apparent when the migration of doctors and nurses from South Africa, Zimbabwe and Ghana to Western countries came under scrutiny. Although research has most often focussed on particular coun-tries' loss of professionals (e.g. Chikanda, 2005a; Crush and Pendleton, 2012) and others have noted the significant differences between African countries (e.g. Niger compared to Ghana; Clemens and Pet-tersson, 2008), the emigration of skilled healthcare workers has nonetheless come to be talked about as a highly pressing *sub-Saharan African* public health problem. The delineation of 'sub-Saharan Africa' as a meaningful geographical space has been criticized as a construction of the Global North (Airhihenbuwa, 2007), but is nonetheless reproduced here as a cen-tral term of the 'brain drain' debate.

Attention to the emigration of health-care pro-fessionals from sub-Saharan African countries, coinciding with poor health outcomes in the same places, became the focus of two influential reports (Joint Learning Initiative [JLI], 2004; WHO, 2006). These two reports represent the convergence of ideas about the key role of skilled health-care pro-fessionals, not just as a correlate of population health outcomes, but as a *causative* correlation such that a higher density of professionals is seen as a major cause of improving population health. As a perpet-uation of earlier models of professional dominance, the supposition that skilled health-care profession-als 'cause' good health in resource-poor settings has influenced the global policy agenda around 'brain drain'.

JLI 2004 AND WHO 2006 REPORTS

In 2004, the 'JLI' (a funded network of over 100 'global health leaders') drew attention to the dis-mal effects of HIV spread and labour emigration coinciding with chronic underinvestment in health-care staff in African countries (JLI, 2004). Also in 2004, a High Level Forum on the Health Millen-nium Development Goals reported on '. . . a human

resources crisis in health, which must be urgently addressed'. And so in 2006, the World Health Report enumerated a shortfall in the global health workforce, suggesting there were 4.3 million too few doctors, nurses, midwives and other health-care workers worldwide, calling the situation a 'global health workforce crisis' (WHO, 2006).

These reports were key in putting health-care pro-fessional shortage on the global public health agenda, which, as a political process, relies on a compelling narrative. The story that rich countries were poach-ing doctors from poor countries is persuasive and plausible, illustrating as it does, wider international inequalities. These inequalities became encapsulated in the idea, described in the JLI's (2004) report that there were more Malawian-trained doctors in Man-chester than in Malawi. Subsequently, this idea of Malawian physicians congregating in Manchester has been queried as an urban myth http://www.bbc.co.uk/news/magazine-16545526, lacking sound numerical basis (Lizi et al., 2013).

Mythical or otherwise, the JLI report of 2004, confirmed by the World Health Report of 2006, suggested a connection between global migration flows of health professionals to indus-trialized, primarily Anglophone, countries from poorer countries, with particular attention paid to sub-Saharan African countries with impover-ished health-care provision, deteriorating health outcomes and high rates of HIV infection. Longitudinal research demonstrated a positive association between HIV prevalence rates and the departure of medical professionals from sub-Saharan Africa (Bhargava and Docquier, 2002), while poor work conditions, fear of HIV transmis-sion (Chikanda, 2005b), having family members overseas and/or employment in the private sector to accumulate money (Chikanda, 2005a) all pro-moted the departure of skilled health professionals in the case of Zimbabwe. While poor conditions, including poor health, promote emigration, the link between low health-care worker density back to health outcomes is less clear. The evidence used to assert the link between health-care worker emi-gration and poor health outcomes in these key reports is considered next.

RELATIONSHIP BETWEEN HEALTH-CARE WORKER DENSITY AND POPULATION HEALTH

The WHO (2006) report includes the following graphic, illustrating an association between the density of health-care workers per unit of population, against measures of maternal, child and infant mortality (see Figure 46.1), which was derived from a graphic that appeared in the earlier JLI report (2004; see Figure 46.2). These graphs bring to the fore some assumptions about the relationship between a population's health, the health-care provision available and the health-care professionals available.

In the JLI report, the collapse in life expectancy in, for instance, Zimbabwe and Zambia (see Figure 46.3,), is presented as evidence of the fatal effects of the combined burden of HIV, together with long-term underinvestment in health-care services. A measure of mortality is then plotted against a measure of the density of health-care professionals and titled 'More health workers–fewer deaths' (see

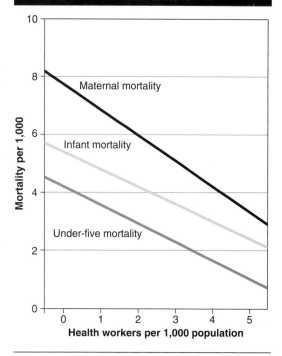

FIGURE 46.2 ■ More Health Workers— Fewer Deaths

Source: Reproduced from JLI (2004: 26).

Figure 46.2), which appropriately describes the association represented (JLI, 2004).

The 2006 World Health Report declared the global crisis in health workforce a central problem for public health and one that required both national and international governance. The graph that was first published by the JLI in 2004 was reproduced in the 2006 World Health Report, but now the title assumes a causative connection with 'Health workers save lives!' (see Figure 46.1). This title states an unambiguously causative relation between the presence of health professionals and fewer premature deaths in the population. This assertion ignores the difficulty of demonstrating an independent effect of increased health-care professional density on improved health outcomes in the face of confounding variables, which are drivers for both poor health and an attenuated healthcare workforce. For instance, studies of physicians who are absent

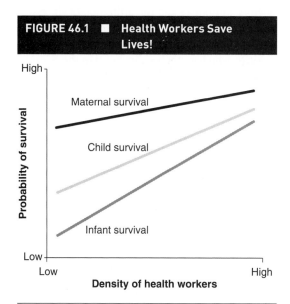

FIGURE 46.1 ■ Health Workers Save Lives!

Source: Reproduced from WHO (2006: xvi).

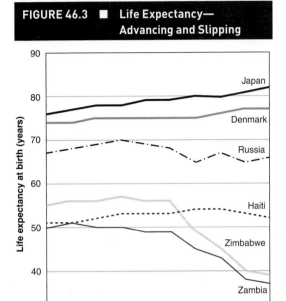

FIGURE 46.3 ■ Life Expectancy—Advancing and Slipping

Source: Reproduced from JLI (2004: 15).

from their employment because of industrial action (Cunningham et al., 2008) or due to high rates of migration (Bhargava and Docquier, 2002) show that mortality rates tend to improve or remain stable with the reduced availability of physicians, suggesting that doctors do not, in any straightforward way, save lives.

Similarly, where health-care staff shortages have led to ward closures, hospital mortality rates have remained stable rather than deteriorating (Brown, 1997). Where commentators seek to demonstrate a link between, for instance, a lack of nursing staff and poor health outcomes, the measures cited are often confined to clinical settings, for example, cross-infection rates and post-surgery adverse events, thereby capturing an aspect of professional practice rather than assessing patients' general well-being or predicted life expectancy (Buchan and Aiken, 2008).

In 1978, Alfonso Mejia noted the difficulty of measuring 'the impact of migration on the health status in donor and recipient countries' was such that any measures were rendered 'almost useless' (Mejia, 1978). More recent quantitative analyses of the association between the density of health-care professionals and mortality rates have given contradictory results. Using global data, a higher density of doctors has been shown to have a positive effect on maternal, infant and under-five mortality (Robinson and Wharrad, 2001) and a higher density of doctors, nurses and midwives was positively associated with maternal mortality rate and to a lesser extent with infant mortality rate and under-five mortality (Anand and Bärnighausen, 2004). In 'developed' countries, doctor density has been found to have a negative effect on infant and perinatal mortality and no effect on maternal mortality (Cochrane et al., 1978). Other studies using global data found no significant association between doctor density and infant mortality (Kim and Moody, 1992) and no association between doctor density and either infant or maternal mortality (Hertz et al., 1994). Three studies found no association between nurse density and maternal mortality, infant or under-five mortality, and infant mortality (Kim and Moody, 1992; Robinson and Wharrad, 2000, 2001). No association was found between the concentration of doctors and nurses and the utilization of six 'essential' health services in low- and middle-income countries, leading to speculation that other health workers, who had not been included in the research, were undertaking aspects of service provision (Kruk et al., 2009), a point to which we return.

The graphs in the JLI (2004) and the World Health Report (2006) cite one article that is notable for its demonstration of an independent effect of health-care professional density on mortality rates in a multi-country analysis (JLI, 2004; WHO, 2006). This article offers a cautious conclusion regarding the role that the density of human resources having a role to play 'in addition to other determinants' when 'accounting for the variation in rates of maternal mortality, infant mortality, and under-five mortality across countries' (Anand and Bärnighausen, 2004).

The text of the 2006 World Health report states that

... worker numbers and quality are positively associated with immunization coverage, outreach of primary care, and infant, child and maternal survival . . . The quality of doctors and the density of their distribution have been shown to correlate with positive outcomes in cardiovascular diseases. (Anand and Bärnighausen, 2004; WHO, 2006)

While immunization coverage and primary care outreach are good indicators that health services are being provided, and may be correlates of improving population health, they are not simple indicators of population health, in the way that infant, child and maternal survival undoubtedly are. Yet, the tendency to confound the provision of *health services* with the provision of *health* is routine in discussions of global 'brain drain', as is an assumption that the provision of *health services* is closely related, if not co-terminus with, providing a higher density of skilled health workers. This tendency to collapse down the careful qualification of research findings in Anand and Bärnighausen (2004) is epitomized by a commentator in the *British Medical Journal* who claims that 'there is a linear relation between health outcomes and the density of health-care workers' such that

> current policies of recruiting doctors from poor countries are a real cause of premature death and untreated disease in those countries and actively contribute to the sum of human misery. (Heath, 2007)

The oversimplified claim that 'health care professionals save lives' (WHO, 2006) suggests simple solutions to the workforce crisis, such as manipulating migration flows. A simplified model posits the emigration of trained health-care personnel as causing poor health outcomes, thereby implying simplified interventions to regulate migration 'flows' in the name of promoting health. Such 'plumbing' models render 'health-care human

resources' (HHR) a mobile commodity open to manipulation through preventing emigration, promoting return migration and introducing so-called ethical recruitment.

REGULATING THE MOVEMENT OF RESOURCES

Attempts to reduce migration out of countries with significant unmet need for healthcare betray a view of health-care workers as a mobile and transferable resource whose flow is open to regulation (Wright et al., 2008). This view potentially ignores workers' own assessment of their interests, not to mention violations of individual freedom of movement (Mackintosh et al., 2006a). Attempts to restrict international recruitment and offer incentives for skilled health-care workers to stay put have proved largely ineffective in sub-Saharan Africa (Mensah, 2005).

Even if the restriction of skilled health-care workers' emigration could be achieved, this would not necessarily increase their availability in source countries since there is no guarantee that those workers will make themselves available for public-service posts, particularly not in the rural and/or impoverished areas where the need is greatest (Clemens, 2007). Furthermore, in poor countries such as Ghana, with a small number of resident health-care workers, even if a policy of migration-reversal could be achieved, it would not bring the density of physicians up to WHO-recommended levels (Arah et al., 2008). By contrast, in richer countries such as New Zealand where physicians' numbers are much higher per head of population, it has proved easier to attract health workers to return from the OECD countries to which they had migrated (Zurn and Dumont, 2008). This suggests that on a global scale attempts to foster return migration may have widened inequalities of health-care professional density.

In parallel with emigration restriction, ethical recruitment policies, for instance through compensatory payments to sending countries that have trained a considerable proportion of a destination country's health-care staff, have sought to mitigate the damage of brain drain (Mackintosh et al., 2006a). The United Kingdom's code to restrict recruitment from 150 developing countries proved ineffective in as much as 13,000 foreign nurses and 4000 doctors arrived between 2000 and 2004 (Bevan, 2005). Restrictions on recruitment applied to public sector health-care facilities, but private health care was exempt, so the effect on overall numbers of foreign recruitment has been minimal (Daniels, 2008). In the day-to-day work of recruitment agencies, there is an over-riding concern to fill empty jobs and little consideration of ethical implications (Runnels et al., 2011). Medical recruitment agencies have been successful in mobilizing health-care personnel as a resource that responds to market demand where migration restrictions and global codes of practice without 'teeth' have been ineffective.

While skilled health-care workers are treated as a commodity by medical recruitment agencies, elsewhere they are treated as a public good. This clash of perspectives is made explicit where professionals are trained in publicly funded education systems and then recruited to work abroad. It has been suggested that the injustice of 'poaching' professionals who should be available to a local public could be addressed through financial restitution (Mackintosh et al., 2006a, 2006b). Arguably, this approach treats the emigration of skilled professionals as an issue of inequality between nation states such that the cost of creating expertise should be borne by the country that benefits from the resultant 'intellectual property' (Pang et al., 2002). Restitution and migration regulation risk reinforcing medical exceptionalism, treating health-care workers as qualitatively different compared to other essential workers. Furthermore, it promotes a view of medical workers as a resource belonging to a specific locality and, if that locality is poor, as carrying special moral obligations for their country of origin's health (Millen, 2008). Whether doctors and nurses from poor settings should carry an extra moral responsibility for their country's public health is not a question that has been much interrogated (Raghuram, 2009).

Recently, there has been a shift in the debate about the estimated 4.3 million personnel missing from global health systems (WHO, 2006) with the acknowledgment that the international migration of doctors and nurses may never have been 'the main culprit behind these shortages' (OECD, 2010). A realization that the 'global health workforce crisis' goes beyond the issue of migration (OECD, 2010) underpins alternative responses.

TASK-SHIFTING

As an alternative to manipulating migration, task-shifting interrogates whether highly trained personnel constitute the best means of providing effective and efficient health care (OECD, 2010). The gravity of the health problems facing countries such as Malawi and Zambia having created the

> necessary conditions for exploring new ways to deliver health care; ways that are possibly less expensive, more community focused, more empowering (MacLachlan and Mc Auliffe, 2005)

and possibly more effective [JH1]. Shifting tasks from highly trained professionals to less qualified, lower paid staff has been commonplace in hospitals wherever workloads are high. But so-called 'task-shifting' has taken on particular resonance as a response to chronic health-care staff shortages in low-income settings with high rates of infectious disease and/or maternal mortality (Smith and Favell, 2006). Rather than producing clinically oriented health professionals who are expensive to train and likely to migrate once qualified, health workers whose skills are appropriate to the disease burden and availability of resources in a particular setting present a better investment (WHO, 2008).

The so-called mid-level cadres (clinicians trained in specific tasks appropriate for local settings) offer clinical efficacy and economic value in the provision of emergency obstetric care (Mc Auliffe et al., 2011) and treatment for HIV (Callaghan et al., 2010;

Mdege et al., 2012). In Malawi, clinical officers and clinical assistants now constitute a significant health-care workforce and one that does not have the international mobility conferred by an internationally recognized medical degree (MacLachlan and Mc Auliffe, 2005).

Although the research evidence remains limited (Mdege et al., 2012), task-shifting initiatives have achieved success (e.g. East, Central, and Southern African Health Community (ECSA-HC), 2010; Lehmann et al., 2009; Mannan et al., 2010). With nurses successfully undertaking cataract surgery in Bangladesh and caesarean sections in Mozambique, we might ask why Western countries remain reliant upon much more expensive models of doctor-led surgery? (Crisp, 2010). Task-shifting is potentially paradoxical for the professional interests of doctors and nurses. In Western countries, redistributing menial or repetitive tasks to occupational divisions with less training and lower pay has been interpreted as one means of maintaining medical professional dominance. However, the prospect that valued medical and surgical interventions, competently undertaken by clinical officers in resource-poor settings, offers a potential threat to the justification for highly trained clinical professionals. Task-shifting as a response to the global 'crisis in HHR' has been criticized as legitimating the provision of a second-class service to resource-poor countries, accompanied by assertions of the very value of skilled professionals.

Skilled health professionals have come to represent the particular value of health as a quality that allows us to enjoy other aspects of human existence and as a common good (Daniels, 2008), and this has been an aspect of the good standing of Medical and Nursing professionals in Western countries. The market value of skilled health professionals (which is related to their symbolic value) has been realized by medical recruitment agencies, as well as private medical schools that have opened in India and, more recently, English-language programmes in Eastern Europe.

Task-shifting has been presented as a means to prevent markets from exploiting value from medical labour: health professionals who are not trained in English cannot emigrate for employment overseas (Dovlo, 2003). The tendency to take 'mid-level cadres' for granted as a stable workforce and/or to assume that they represent a short-term measure until the stock of skilled workers builds up (Mc Auliffe et al., 2011) underestimates the ability of the market for health-care workers to adapt to new circumstances. While a shortened training in a local language prevents individual health-care migration, the increased mobility of technology and patients (Labonté et al., 2013; Whittaker et al., 2010) allows value to be extracted from task-shifting in other ways. There are indications that Indian models of health care, making use both of the lower salaried professionals and of cadres with less training, offer high-quality health care at low prices, such that complex heart surgery with good outcomes can be sold to American patients in the Cayman Islands (Govindarajan and Ramamurti, 2013). New models of health-care provision exploit the gaps of uneven global development for profit.

CONCLUDING THOUGHTS

In response to the global debt crisis of the late 1970s, African countries were obliged by the World Bank and International Monetary Fund to 'de-prioritize' investment in their social sectors—including health and education—in favour of promoting export currency to enable interest payments on loans owed to foreign banks. The effects of the 'structural adjustment policies' (or 'brute neoliberalism'; Onuki, 2011) of the 1980s became apparent through the 1990s, with the suspension and mandatory early retirement of health-care professionals (Daniels, 2008), such that the public health sector shrank and the private health sector grew. This promoted the emigration of health professionals from rural settings and public-service jobs, leading to health professional shortages, which, combined with other aspects of underinvestment, exacerbated poor working conditions and therefore emigration, especially in areas where HIV was spreading (Chikanda, 2005a).

The public health problems in sub-Saharan Africa, like the emigration of skilled health-care professionals, can be seen as having common cause in the imposition of underinvestment. Analyses that emphasize the role of individual migration decisions and link this to poor population health outcomes make the 'health-care worker crisis' into a debate about doctors' and nurses' mobility, emphasizing professional rather than socioeconomic determinants of health. The arrival of the global HIV pandemic in resource-poor countries medicalized aid programmes (Ivers et al., 2010), cementing the central role of medical personnel as key to improving health outcomes. Addressing global health inequalities by focussing on health-care professional densities as achieved through their migratory movements has maintained a medicalized view of heroic doctors and nurses as improving health outcomes, thereby benefiting medical recruitment agencies' business. Task-shifting approaches offer a powerful critique to professional claims of unique expertise in specific interventions, the implications of which have been largely ignored in resource-rich settings. Conrad's (2005) call to look at the political economy of medicalization would find fertile ground if a global rather than a nationally bounded view of health-care provision could be adopted.

The amplification of migration (Castles and Miller, 2009) as part of 'the expansion and intensification of social relations and consciousness across world-time and world space' (Steger, 2009) has yet to inform research into health-care professionals' migration. The means, and crucially the motivation, to migrate between localities, nations and continents are within the grasp of an increasing proportion of humanity and the apparently irrepressible desire to migrate has proven very hard to regulate. Alongside the amplification of migration is the mobility of capital, ideas and technology that (interests in medical tourism notwithstanding) is yet to inform research into global health inequalities. In particular, the penetration of public health-care provision with the interests of private and corporate capital has received too little analytic interest in the assessment of global health inequalities. This article seeks to wrest attention away from the ideals of Hippocratically bound medical professionals operating within nationalized health systems towards the flows of capital in the provision of services that institutions and individuals will pay for. The willingness of national institutions to pay for the recruitment of medical and nursing personnel has been a crucial part of so-called 'brain drain', which task-shifting has partially circumnavigated. Anticipating the future flows of capital within and beyond the nation state is a task that perhaps ought to occupy more of our attention.

The opening up of statutorily funded health service provision to for-profit contractors underway in Western European welfare states (e.g. Davis and Tallis, 2013) means that economic exigencies, rather than social equity, will increasingly determine the commissioning of services. The effects of these changes on nationally bounded as well as global inequalities are of interest. Attending to movements of capital, as well as to human mobility in the global health-care economy might, at the very least, prevent professional migrants from being held individually accountable for public health problems with long-standing antecedents and far-reaching implications.

ACKNOWLEDGMENTS

The basis of this work was undertaken while the author was the medical diversity fellow at the Max Planck Institute for the Study of Religious and Ethnic Diversity, Gottingen, Germany, courtesy of Dr Kristine Krause. Thanks to Birgitt Sippel for preparing the figures.

References

Ahmad OB (2005) Managing medical migration from poor countries. 5M/331(7507): 43–45.

Airhihenbuwa CO (2007) *Healing Our Differences: The Crisis of Global Health and the Politics of Identity*. Lanham, MD: Rowman & Littlefield.

Alkire S and Chen L (2006) 'Medical Exceptionalism' in international migration: Should doctors and nurses be treated differently? In: Tamas K and Palme J (eds) *Globalizing Migration Regimes: New Challenges to*

Transnational Cooperation. Aldershot: Ashgate, pp. 100–117.

Anand S and Bärnighausen T (2004) Human resources and health outcomes: A cross-country econometric study. *Lancet* 364: 1603–09.

Arah OA, Ogbu UC and Okeke CE (2008) Too poor to leave, too rich to stay: Developmental and global health correlates of physician migration to the United States, Canada, Australia, and the United Kingdom. *American Journal of Public Health* 98(1): 148–154.

Bevan S (2005) Britain accused of ignoring nurse-recruitment ban. *Lancet* 366(9501): 1915–1916.

Bhargava A and Docquier F (2002) HIV pandemic, medical brain drain, and economic development in sub-Saharan Africa. *World Bank Economic Review* 22(2): 345–366.

Bradby H (2013) A review of research and policy documents on the international migration of physicians and nurses. Max Planck Institute for the Study of Religious and Ethnic Diversity Working Paper Series. Gottingen: Max Planck Institute for the Study of Religious and Ethnic Diversity. Available at: http://www.mmg.mpg.de/fileadmin/user_upload/documents/wp/WP_13-07_Bradby_A-Review-of-Research.pdf

Brown D (1997) Workforce losses and return migration to the Caribbean: A case study of Jamaican nurses. In: Pessar P (ed.) *Caribbean Circuits: New Directions in the Study of Caribbean Migration.* New York: Centre for Migration Studies, pp. 197–223.

Buchan J (2006) Evidence of nursing shortages or a shortage of evidence? *Journal of Advanced Nursing* 56: 457–158.

Buchan J and Aiken L (2008) Solving nursing shortages: A common priority. *Journal of Clinical Nursing* 17(24): 3262–3268.

Callaghan M, Ford N and Schneider H (2010) A systematic review of task-shifting for HIV treatment and care in Africa. *Human Resources for Health* 8: 8. Available at: http://www.human-resources-health.com/content/8/1/8

Castles S and Miller MJ (2009) *The Age of Migration: International Population Movements in the Modern World.* 4th ed. New York: Guilford Press.

Chikanda A (2005a) *Medical leave: The exodus of health professionals from Zimbabwe.* South African Migration Project, Migration policy series no. 34. http://www.queensu.ca/samp/sam-presources/samppublications/policy-series/policy34.htm

Chikanda A (2005b) Nurse migration from Zimbabwe: Analysis of recent trends and impact. *Nursing Inquiry* 12(3): 162–174.

Clarke AE, Shim JK, Mamo L, et al. (2003) Biomedicalization: Technoscientific transformations of health, illness, and U.S. biomedicine. *American Sociological Review* 68: 161–194.

Clemens MA (2007) *Do visas kill? Health effects of African health professional emigration.* Working paper no. 114, Washington, DC: Centre for Global Development. Available at: http://www.aspeninstitute.org//sites/default/f1les/content/images/f1le_Clemens_Do_visas_kill_3_.pdf

Clemens MA and Pettersson G (2008) New data on African health professionals abroad. *Human Resources for Health* 6:1. Available at: http://www.human-resources-health.eom/content/6/l/l

Cochrane AL, St Leger AS and Moore F (1978) Health service 'input' and mortality 'output' in developed countries. *Journal of Epidemiology Community Health* 32: 200–205.

Connell J (2010) *Migration and the Globalisation of Health Care.* Cheltenham: Edward Elgar.

Conrad P (2005) The shifting engines of medicalization. *Journal of Health and Social Behavior* 46: 3–14.

Conrad P, Mackie T and Mehrotra A (2010) Estimating the costs of medicalization. *Social Science & Medicine* 70: 1943–1947.

Coombes R (2005) Developed world is robbing African countries of health staff. *BMJ* 330(7497): 923.

Crisp N (2010) *Turning the World Upside Down: The Search for Global Health in the 21st Century.* London: CRC Press.

Crush J and Pendleton W (2012) The brain drain potential of students in the African health and nonhealth sectors. *International Journal of Population Research* 2012(274305): 10.

Crush J, Chikanda A and Pendleton W (2012) The disengagement of the South African medical diaspora in Canada. *Journal of Southern African Studies* 38(4): 927–949.

Cunningham SA, Mitchell K, Narayan KMV, et al. (2008) Doctors' strikes and mortality: A review. *Social Science & Medicine* 67(11): 1784–1788.

Daniels N (2008) *Just Health: Meeting Health Needs Fairly.* New York: Cambridge University Press.

Davis J and Tallis R (2013) *NHS SOS: How the NHS Was Betrayed – And How We Can Save It.* London: Oneworld Publications.

Dovlo D (2003) The brain drain and retention of health professionals in Africa. A case study prepared for Regional Training Conference on Improving Tertiary Education in sub-Saharan Africa: Things That Work! Available at: http://siteresources.worldbank.org/INTAFRREGTOPTEIA/Resources/dela_dovlo.pdf

East, Central, and Southern African Health Community (ECSA-HC) (2010) *Task Shifting in Uganda: Case Study.* Washington, DC: Futures Group, Health Policy Initiative, Task Order 1.

Gish O (1971) *Doctor Migration and World Health: The Impact of the International Demand for Doctors on Health Services in Developing Countries* (Occasional Papers on Social Administration), vol. 43. London: G. Bell & Sons.

Govindarajan V and Ramamurti R (2013) India's secret to low-cost health care (Blog post). In: HBR Blog Network, October 15 (Harvard Business Review, Harvard University). Available at: http://blogs.hbr.org/2013/10/indias-secret-to-low-cost-health-care/

Heath I (2007) Exploitation and apology. BMJ 334(7601): 981.

Hertz E, Hebert JR and Landon J (1994) Social and environmental factors and life expectancy, infant mortality, and maternal mortality rates: Results of a cross-national comparison. *Social Science & Medicine* 39: 105–114.

Hooper CR (2008) Adding insult to injury: The healthcare brain drain. *Journal of Medical Ethics* 34(9): 684–687.

Ivers LC, Cullen KA, Freedberg KA, et al. (2010) HIV/AIDS, undernutrition and food insecurity. *Clinical Infectious Diseases* 49(7): 1096–1102.

Johnson J (2005) Stopping Africa's medical brain drain: The rich countries of the North must stop looting doctors and nurses from developing countries. BMJ 331(7507): 2–3.

Joint Learning Initiative (JLI) (2004) *Human Resources for Health: Overcoming the Crisis.* Cambridge, MA: Harvard University Press.

Kim K and Moody PM (1992) More resources better health? A cross-national perspective. *Social Science & Medicine* 34: 837–842.

Kruk ME, Prescott MR, de Pinho H, et al. (2009) Are doctors and nurses associated with coverage of essential health services in developing countries? A cross-sectional study. *Human Resources for Health* 7(27): 1–9.

Labonté R and Schrecker T (2007) Globalization and social determinants of health: Introduction and methodological background (part 2 of 3). *Globalization and Health* 3(6): 1–17.

Labonté R, Runnels V, Packer C, et al. (eds) (2013) *Travelling Well: Essays in Medical Tourism*

(Studies in Population Health Series), vol. 4, 1st ed. Ottawa, ON, Canada: Institute of Population Health, University of Ottawa.

Larsen JA, Allan HT, Bryan K, et al. (2005) Overseas nurses' motivations for working in the UK: Globalization and life politics. *Work, Employment and Society* 19: 349–368.

Lehmann U, Van Damme W, Barten F, et al. (2009) Task shifting: The answer to the human resources crisis in Africa? *Human Resources for Health* 7(1): 49.

Lizi E, Lwanda J and Matiti H (2013) Modern medical myth: 'More Doctors in Manchester than in Malawi': A preliminary communication. *Malawi Medical Journal.* Available at: http://www.med-col.mw/mmj/? p=1374

Mc Auliffe E, Manafa O, Bowie C, et al. (2011) Managing and motivating: Pragmatic solutions to the brain drain. In: *Human Resources in Healthcare, Health Informatics and Healthcare Systems.* IGI Global, pp. 79–95. Available at: http://services.igi-global.com/resolvedoi/resolve.aspx? doi=10.4018/978-l-61520-885-2.ch005

Mackintosh M, Mensah K, Henry L, et al. (2006a) Aid, restitution and international fiscal redistribution in health care: Implications of health professionals' migration. *Journal of International Development* 18(6): 757–770.

Mackintosh M, Raghuram P and Henry L (2006b) 'A Perverse Subsidy': African-trained doctors and nurses in the National Health Service. *Soundings* 34: 103–113.

MacLachlan M and Mc Auliffe E (2005) Developed world is robbing Africa of health staff. BMJ 331(7507): 48.

Mannan H, Boostrom C, MacLachlan M, et al. (2010) A systematic review of the effectiveness of alternative cadres in community based rehabilitation. *Human Resources for Health* 10:20. DOI: 10.1186/1478-4491.10-20. Available at: www.human-resources-health.com/content/10/1/20

Martineau T, Decker K and Bundred P (2004) 'Brain Drain' of health professionals: From rhetoric to responsible action. *Health Policy* 70(1): 1–10.

Mdege ND, Chindove S and Ali S (2012) The effectiveness and cost implications of task-shifting in the delivery of antiretroviral therapy to HIV-infected patients: A systematic review. *Health Policy Planning* 28(3): 223–236.

Mejia A (1978) Migration of physicians and nurses: A world wide picture. *International Journal of Epidemiology* 7(3): 207–215 (also published in *Bulletin of the World Health Organization* 2004; 82(8): 626–630).

Mensah K (2005) International migration of health care staff: Extent and policy responses with illustrations from Ghana. In: Koivusalo M and Mackintosh M (eds) *Commercialization of Health Care: Global and Local Dynamics and Policy Responses.* Basingstoke: Palgrave Macmillan, pp. 201–215.

Mensah K, Mackintosh M and Henry L (2005) *The 'Skills Drain' of Health Professionals from the Developing World: A Framework for Policy Formulation.* London: Medact.

Millen J (2008) Health worker shortages and HIV/AIDS: Responses and linkages. *Practicing Anthropology* 30(4): 8–12.

Mills EJ, Schabas WA, Volmink J, et al. (2008) Should active recruitment of health professional from sub-Saharan Africa be viewed as a crime? *Lancet* 371(9613): 685–688.

OECD (2010) International migration of health workers. *Improving international cooperation to address the global health workforce crisis.* Available at: www.oecd.org/publications/Policybriefs

Onuki H (2011) The global migration of care labour. Filipino workers in Japan. In: Mahon R and Robinson F (eds) *Feminist Ethics and Social Policy: Towards a New Global Political Economy of Care*. Vancouver, BC, Canada; Toronto, ON, Canada: UBC Press, pp. 60–74.

Pang T, Lansang MA and Haines A (2002) Brain drain and health professionals: A global problem needs global solutions. *BMJ* 324(7336): 499–500.

Parens E (2013) On good and bad forms of medicalization. *Bioethics* 27(1): 28–35.

Raghuram P (2009) Caring about 'brain drain' migration in a postcolonial world. *Geoforum* 40(1): 25–33.

Record R and Mohiddin A (2006) An economic perspective on Malawi's medical 'Brain Drain'. *Globalization and Health* 2(1): 12.

Robinson J and Wharrad H (2000) Invisible nursing: Exploring health outcomes at a global level – Relationships between infant and under-5 mortality rates and the distribution of health professionals, GNP per capita, and female literacy. *Journal of Advanced Nursing* 32(1): 28–40.

Robinson J and Wharrad H (2001) The relationship between attendance at birth and maternal mortality rates: An exploration of United Nations' data sets including the ratios of physicians and nurses to population, GNP per capita and female literacy. *Journal of Advanced Nursing* 34(4): 445–155.

Runnels V, Labonté R and Packer C (2011) Reflections on the ethics of recruiting foreign-trained human resources for health. *Human Resources for Health* 9(2): e1–e11.

Smith MP and Favell A (2006) *The Human Face of Global Migration. International Highly Skilled Migration in Europe, North America and the Asia-Pacific. Comparative Urban and Community Research*, vol. 8. New Brunswick, NJ; London: Transaction Publishers.

Steger MB (2009) Globalisation and social imaginaries: The changing ideological landscape of the twenty-first century. *Journal of Critical Globalisation Studies* 1(1): 9–30.

Stilwell B, Diallo K, Zurn P, et al. (2004) Migration of health-care workers from developing countries: Strategic approaches to its management. *Bulletin of the World Health Organization* 82(8): 595–600.

The Committee on the International Migration of Talent (1970) *The International Migration of High-Level Manpower: Its Impact on the Development Process*. New York: Praeger Publishers.

Van Hoek FJ (1970) *The Migration of High Level Manpower from Developing to Developed Countries*. The Hague: Mouton.

Whittaker A, Manderson L and Cartwright E (2010) Patients without borders: Understanding medical travel. *Medical Anthropology* 29(4): 336–343.

World Health Organization (WHO) (2006) *Working Together for Health: The World Health Report 2006*. Geneva: WHO.

World Health Organization (WHO) (2008) *Task Shifting: Global Recommendations and Guidelines*. Geneva: WHO. Available at: http://www.who .int/workforcealliance/knowledge/resources/ taskshifting_guidelines/en/index.html

Wright D, Nathan F and Gupta M (2008) The 'Brain Drain' of physicians: Historical antecedents to an ethical debate, c. 1960–79. *Philosophy, Ethics, and Humanities in Medicine* 3: 24.

Zurn P and Dumont J-C (2008) *Health workforce and international migration: Can New Zealand compete?* OECD health working paper no. 33, 22 May. Paris: OECD.

INDEX

Ewell, Thomas, 279, 280
Experience rating, 401, 412, 413, 414, 419
External environment, 7
External risk rhetoric, 568–569
Eysenbach, Gunther, 224

Facebook, 640, 641, 644, 645–646, 649
Fagin, Claire, 341
Fair Housing Act of 1968, 53
Fanshel, David, 454, 456
Farmer, Paul, 41
Farrar, Eliza W., 335
Farrell, J. A., 299
Fashion media, body image, eating problems, and, 163
Fat-acceptance activists, body size, civil rights, and, 176 (n1)
Fatness stereotypes, 162, 163, 172
FDA. *See* Food and Drug Administration (FDA)
Federal government
   cost control measures and, 329
   financing of medical care and, 402
   medical insurance and, 277
   See also Medicaid; Medicare
Federal Poverty Line
   ACA eligibility criteria and, 417
   health insurance premiums and, 420
Fee-for-service system, 277, 294, 329
Feinberg, Joel, 335
Females. *See* Gender
Feminism
   birth perspectives, 620–621, 629, 630
   political language for nursing and, 342
Fernandez-Balsells, M., 585
Fetal heart monitoring, C-sections and, 635
Fibromyalgia syndrome (FMS)
   collectivity and electronic support groups for, 648
   embodied health movements and, 667
Fibromyalgia syndrome (FMS), electronic support group, 217, 219–234
   background and conceptual framework, 220–223
   conclusion, 232–234
   contemporary medicalization: role of patient-consumers, 220–222

contested illness and lay expertise, 222–223
data and coding, 224–225
data and methods, 223–226
discussion, 231–232
empowerment without power, 230–231
findings, 226–231
illness reification, 226–227
lay/embodied *vs.* professional/medical expertise, 229–230
nonparticipant observation, 223–224
participation at *Fibro Spot*, 225–226, 226 (exhibit)
setting, 223
skeptical dependency on medical expertise, 227–229
Financing medical care
   as big business, 401
   burden of, 419–420
   See also Health insurance; Medicaid; Medicare; Paying for health care
Finland social relationships studies, 116, 118 (figure)
First-dollar rationing, 441, 445
Fischer, Claude, 142, 152 (n5)
Fiske, Annette, 340
Flaig, D. M., 223
Flegal, Katherine, 161
Flexible resources, 505
   at contextual and individual levels, 26
   mechanism demise and death and, 32
   SES inequalities in health and, 25–27
Flexner, Abraham, 276
Flexner Report, 276, 283
Floyd, Hugh H., 229
FMS. *See* Fibromyolgia syndrome (FMS)
Food and Drug Act of 1906, 377
Food and Drug Administration (FDA), 355, 374, 377, 438
   "Blue Ribbon" Committee Report, 598
   broadcast DTCA guidelines, 375
   Center for Drug Evaluation and Research, 378
   diet supplements and, 357
   drug advertising and, 373, 376, 378

herbal medications marketing and, 349
   Viagra approved by, 375–376
Food and Drug Administration Modernization Act of 1997, 607
Food industry
   as manufacturer of illness, 41
   political economy of illness and, 99–100
Forceps
   social childbirth and, 286
   social class and doctors' use of, 289
For-profit commercial insurance companies, 401
Foucault, Michel, 532, 571, 621
France
   ADHD and points of resistance in, 726, 728
   ADHD treatment/diagnosis in, case example, 714, 716–717
   obstetric education in, 285
   percentage of children diagnosed with ADHD in, 712
   traditional midwifery in, 290
Frank, Arthur, 193
Freedom, countervailing mechanisms and, 33
Free market economy, resource allocation in, 440
Freese, Jeremy, 27, 32, 33, 505
Freidson, Eliot, 268, 298, 314, 323, 355, 595, 598, 601
Freire, Paolo, 459
French Adult ADHD Association, 725
French Classification of Child and Adolescent Mental Disorders (CFTMEA), 716, 717
Frickel, Scott, 687
Frist, Bill, 378
Fuchs, V. R., 13, 446
Fujimura, Joan H., 532
Fundamental cause theory
   contextualizing risk factors and, 34
   deployment of resources and, 25, 28
   development of, 25, 36 (n2)
   essential features in, 25
   flexible resources and, 25
   "give back effect" and, 31–32
   implications for health policy, 33–35
   limits on: countervailing mechanisms, 32–33